EXERCISE, FITNESS, AND HEALTH

A CONSENSUS OF CURRENT KNOWLEDGE

Claude Bouchard, PhD
Laval University

Roy J. Shephard, MD, PhD
University of Toronto

Thomas Stephens, PhD
Social Epidemiology and Survey Research, Ottawa, Ontario

John R. Sutton, MD
McMaster University

Barry D. McPherson, PhD
Wilfrid Laurier University

EDITORS

Human Kinetics Books
Champaign, Illinois

International Conference on Exercise, Fitness, and Health (1988 :
   Toronto, Ont.)
      Exercise, fitness, and health : a consensus of current knowledge /
   edited by Claude Bouchard . . . [et al.].
         p.   cm.
      ''Proceedings of the International Conference on Exercise, Fitness,
   and Health held May 29-June 3, 1988, in Toronto, Canada''--T.p.
   verso.
      Includes bibliographies.
      ISBN 0-87322-237-7
      1. Exercise--Health aspects--Congresses.   2. Physical fitness-
   -Congresses.   3. Health--Congresses.   I. Bouchard, Claude.
   II. Title.
   RA781.I48   1988
   613.7--dc20   89-11139
                                                          CIP

ISBN: 0-87322-237-7

The articles in this book were presented at the International Conference on Exercise, Fitness, and Health, held May 29 to June 3, 1988, in Toronto, Canada.

Developmental Editor: Marie Roy
Managing Editor: Holly Gilly
Copyeditor: Bruce Owens
Assistant Editors: Julia Anderson, Valerie Hall, Robert King, and Timothy Ryan
Proofreaders: Karin Leszczynski, Laurie McGee, and Claire Mount
Production Director: Ernie Noa
Typesetters: Brad Colson, Sandra Meier, Cindy Pritchard, and Angela Snyder
Text Layout: Jayne Clampitt, Kimberlie Henris, and Tara Welsch
Text Design: Keith Blomberg
Cover Design: Jack Davis
Cover Photo: Kirk Schlea/Berg and Associates
Illustrations: David Gregory
Printer: Edwards Brothers

Printed in the United States of America

10   9   8   7   6   5   4   3   2   1

Human Kinetics Books
A Division of Human Kinetics Publishers, Inc.
Box 5076, Champaign, IL 61825-5076
1-800-747-4HKP

Contents

Preface

In 1985, the executive committee of the Canadian Association of Sport Sciences proposed that this conference be organized in cooperation with 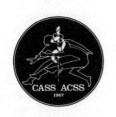 organizations in the private and public sectors that are concerned with healthy lifestyles for Canadians. For almost 3 years, the board of directors had been working to assemble a team of internationally recognized scholars to present state-of-the-art knowledge in their particular areas of expertise. All delegates were encouraged to contribute to the process, which culminated in the drafting of consensus statements concerning our current understanding of the relationships among exercise, fitness, and health.

The objectives of this conference were (a) to review the current status of our knowledge concerning the relationships among exercise, fitness, and health and (b) to develop consensus statements defining our understanding of these relationships.

The North American Life Assurance Company was the major sponsor of this conference. This company has had a long-standing commitment 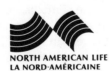 to supporting scientific research, to increasing public awareness of the benefits of exercise, and to healthier, more active lifestyles. In 1985, North American Life was also the major sponsor for the Scientific Conference held in conjunction with the World Master Games in Toronto, the proceedings of which were published in the book *Sport Medicine for the Mature Athlete.*

Representing the government of Canada, the Ministers of State for Fitness and Amateur Sport—the Honorables Otto Jelinek and Jean *Fitness Canada Condition physique Canada* Charest—and their staff at Fitness Canada have provided both financial and leadership support for the hosting of this conference. The 1986 Canadian Summit on Fitness reaffirmed the importance of regular physical activity in the lifestyle of Canadians and identified the need for both scientific research and policy analysis in the area of fitness and health. The commitment of Fitness Canada to this conference represented an important step in the development of knowledge and programs that will enhance our lifestyles and total health.

For more than a decade the government of Ontario has been actively involved in supporting and promoting fitness and healthy lifestyles Ministry of Tourism and Recreation / Ministère du Tourisme et des Loisirs / Ontario through the work of the Ontario Ministry of Tourism and Recreation, currently under the leadership of the Honorable Hugh O'Neil. Within this ministry, Fitness Ontario has been particularly supportive in many ways of both the research and the practitioner communities. This continuing support is derived from the personal commitment and creative ideas generated by the staff of this ministry.

In addition to these major sponsors, we gratefully acknowledge the contribution of the following corporations, foundations, and government agencies that committed personnel or funds to insure the quality and success of the conference:

Air Canada
Astro Dairy Products Ltd
Campbell Soup Company Ltd
Canadian Airlines International
Canadian Heart Foundation
City of Toronto
Computer Junction
Health and Welfare Canada
Heart and Stroke Foundation of Ontario
Hydrafitness Industries Ltd
Nike Canada Ltd
Ontario Ministry of Health
PARTICIPaction
Petro Canada
Xerox Canada Inc.

In addition, we gratefully recognize the contribution of Laval University, Wilfrid Laurier University, and York University. Thanks are also expressed to Lise Gosselin, Marc Landry, and Martine Marcotte for their support in the preparation of the program and proceedings of the conference and to Roy Howse, executive assistant to the board of directors of the conference. Finally, we would like to express our gratitude to the numerous volunteers, many from North American Life, who helped us to organize and conduct the conference.

The following individuals served as members of the board of directors and were responsible for the development and organization of the conference:

Barry D. McPherson, Chair
Claude Bouchard
Cora Craig
David Cunningham
Peter Gellatly
Norm Gledhill
Barbara O'Brien Jewett
Russ Kisby
Diane McPherson
Art Quinney
Art Salmon
Roy J. Shephard

Thomas Stephens
John R. Sutton

Part I of this book includes the consensus statement (chapt. 1) emanating from the conference and introductory addresses (chapts. 2 through 4). After a brief introduction by Professor P.O. Åstrand (chapt. 2) comparing issues raised during the 1966 Toronto conference with those of the 1988 conference, the papers of Professors R.S. Paffenbarger (chapt. 3) and R.J. Shephard (chapt. 4) are reproduced because of the general interest of their topics. The papers presented by the invited speakers and discussants are published in their entirety in the succeeding chapters. The consensus statement is largely based on these thematic papers. The book is divided into 6 parts:

Part I. Consensus Statement and Introductory Addresses (chapts. 1 to 4)

Part II. Assessment and Determinants of Physical Activity, Fitness, and Health (chapts. 5-17)

Part III. Human Adaptation to Physical Activity (chapts. 18-33)

Part IV. Physical Activity and Fitness in Disease (chapts. 34-54)

Part V. Physical Activity and Fitness in Growth, Reproductive Health, and Aging (chapts. 55-60)

Part VI. The Risks of Exercising (chapts. 61-62)

We now invite you to study and debate the consensus statement as well as the supporting evidence presented by the invited speakers and discussants at the 1988 International Conference on Exercise, Fitness, and Health. The success of this conference may well be measured by the debate and research that is initiated by the readers of this volume. We encourage you to be critical in your acceptance of the evidence. We hope that the state of the art by the year 2000 will render this volume obsolete and necessitate that the next generation of scientists host a similar event.

The Editors
September 1988

List of Contributors

ANDRES, Reubin, MD
Gerontology Research Center
National Institute of Aging
Francis Scott Key Medical Center
Baltimore, Maryland 21224
USA

ÅSTRAND, Per-Olof, MD
Department of Physiology III
Karolinska Institutet, GIH
S-114 33 Stockholm
Sweden

BALDINI, Fred D., MS
Exercise and Sport Research Institute
Department of Health and Physical Education
Arizona State University
Tempe, Arizona 85287
USA

BAR-OR, Oded, MD
Children's Exercise and Nutrition Centre
Department of Pediatrics and Chedoke–
    McMaster Hospitals
McMaster University
Hamilton, Ontario
L8N 3Z5
Canada

BERGER, Michael, MD
Department of Metabolic Diseases and Nutrition
Düsseldorf University
Moorenstr. 5
4000 Düsseldorf
Federal Republic of Germany

BIGLAND-RITCHIE, Brenda, PhD, DSc
John B. Pierce Foundation
Congress Avenue
New Haven, Connecticut 06519
USA

BJÖRNTORP, Per, MD
Department of Medicine I
Sahlgrenska Sjukhuset
S-143 45 Göteborg
Sweden

BLAIR, Steven N., PED
Director of Epidemiology
Institute for Aerobics Research
12330 Preston Road
Dallas, Texas 75230
USA

BLANCHET, Madeleine, MD, Présidente
Conseil des affaires sociales et de la famille
Gouvernement du Québec
1126, chemin St-Louis
Sillery, Québec
G1S 1E5
Canada

BOUCHARD, Claude, PhD
Physical Activity Sciences Laboratory
PEPS
Laval University
Ste-Foy, Québec
G1K 7P4
Canada

BRAY, George A., MD
Department of Diabetes and Clinical Nutrition
University of Southern California Medical
    Center
2025 Zonal Avenue OCD-252
Los Angeles, California 90033
USA

BRESLOW, Lester, MD, MPH
School of Public Health
University of California
Los Angeles, California 90024
USA

BRILL, Patricia A., PhD
Institute for Aerobics Research
12330 Preston Road
Dallas, Texas 75230
USA

BROWN, David R., PhD
Miami University–Ohio
Department of Physical Education, Health, and
    Sport Studies
Room 107, Phillips Hall
Oxford, Ohio 45056
USA

BUSKIRK, Elsworth R., PhD
Laboratory for Human Performance Research
119 Noll Laboratory
Pennsylvania State University
University Park, Pennsylvania 16802
USA

CALABRESE, Leonard H., DO
Section of Clinical Immunology
Departments of Rheumatic and Immunologic
  Disease
The Cleveland Clinic Foundation
9500 Euclid Avenue
Cleveland, Ohio 44106
USA

CHOW, Raphael, MD
Room 7326, Medical Sciences Building
University of Toronto
Toronto, Ontario
M5S 1A8
Canada

CHUBB, Michael, PhD
Department of Geography
315 Natural Science Building
Michigan State University
East Lansing, Michigan 48824
USA

COSCINA, Donald V., PhD
Section of Biopsychology
Clarke Institute of Psychiatry
University of Toronto
Toronto, Ontario
M5T 1R8
Canada

CUMMING, David C., MB, ChB
Departments of Obstetrics and Gynaecology
  and Medicine
1D1 Walter Mackenzie Health Sciences Centre
University of Alberta
Edmonton, Alberta
T6G 2R7
Canada

CUNNINGHAM, David A., PhD
Department of Physiology
University of Western Ontario
London, Ontario
N6A 5C1
Canada

DELA, Flemming, MD
Department of Medical Physiology B
The Panum Institute
University of Copenhagen
Blegdamsvej 3 C
2200 Copenhagen N
Denmark

DEMPSEY, Jerome A., PhD
Department of Preventive Medicine
University of Wisconsin
504 Walnut Street
Madison, Wisconsin 53705
USA

DISHMAN, Rod K., PhD
Behavioral Fitness Laboratory
Physical Education Building
University of Georgia
Athens, Georgia 30602
USA

DURNIN, John V.G.A., MA, MB, ChB, DSc
Institute of Physiology
University of Glasgow
Glasgow G12 8QO
Scotland

EDGERTON, V. Reggie, PhD
Department of Kinesiology
University of California at Los Angeles
405 Hilgard Avenue
Los Angeles, California 90024
USA

FARRELL, Peter A., PhD
Laboratory for Human Performance Research
Penn State
University Park, Pennsylvania 16802
USA

FAULKNER, John A., PhD
Department of Physiology
Medical School
University of Michigan
Ann Arbor, Michigan 48109
USA

FOLINSBEE, Lawrence J., PhD
CE-Environmental, Inc.
6320 Quadrangle Drive
Suite 100
Chapel Hill, North Carolina 27514
USA

FROELICHER, Victor F., MD
Cardiology Section
Long Beach VA Medical Center
5901 East Seventh Street
Long Beach, California 90822
USA

GALBO, Henrik, MD
Department of Medical Physiology B
The Panum Institute
University of Copenhagen
Blegdamsvej 3 C
2200 Copenhagen N
Denmark

GARDNER, Andrew W., MS
Exercise and Sport Research Institute
Department of Health and Physical Education
Arizona State University
Tempe, Arizona 85287
USA

GARFINKEL, Paul E., MD
Toronto General Hospital
University of Toronto
Toronto, Ontario
M5G 2C4
Canada

GILLIGAN, Catherine, BA
Biogerontology Laboratory
Department of Preventive Medicine
University of Wisconsin
504 Walnut Street
Madison, Wisconsin 53705
USA

GLEDHILL, Norman, PhD
Department of Physical Education, Recreation
  and Athletics
York University
Toronto, Ontario
M3J 1P3
Canada

GREEN, Howard J., PhD
Department of Kinesiology
University of Waterloo
Waterloo, Ontario
N2L 3G1
Canada

HAGBERG, James M., PhD
Center on Aging
University of Maryland
College Park, Maryland 20742
USA

HANSEN, Henrik P., MD
Department of Medical Physiology B
The Panum Institute
University of Copenhagen
Blegdamsvej 3 C
2200 Copenhagen N
Denmark

HARBER, Victoria J., PhD
Department of Obstetrics and Gynecology
McMaster University
Hamilton, Ontario
L8N 3Z5
Canada

HARRISON, Joan E., MD
Room 7326, Medical Sciences Building
University of Toronto
Toronto, Ontario
M5S 1A8
Canada

HUTTON, Robert S., PhD
Department of Psychology
NI-25
University of Washington
Seattle, Washington 98195
USA

HYDE, Robert T., MA
Department of Health Research and Policy
Division of Epidemiology
Health Research and Policy Building
Stanford University School of Medicine
Stanford, California 94305
USA

JONES, Norman L., MD
Ambrose Cardiorespiratory Unit
McMaster University Medical Centre
1200 Main Street West
Hamilton, Ontario
L8N 3Z5
Canada

KEMMER, Friedrich W., MD
Department of Metabolic Diseases and
  Nutrition
Düsseldorf University
Moorenstr. 5
4000 Düsseldorf
Federal Republic of Germany

KILLIAN, Kieran J., MD
Ambrose Cardiorespiratory Unit
McMaster University Medical Centre
1200 Main Street West
Hamilton, Ontario
L8N 3Z5
Canada

KJAER, Michael, MD
Department of Medical Physiology B
The Panum Institute
University of Copenhagen
Blegdamsvej 3 C
2200 Copenhagen N
Denmark

KOHL, Harold W., PhD
Institute for Aerobics Research
12330 Preston Road
Dallas, Texas 75230
USA

MALINA, Robert M., PhD
Department of Anthropology
University of Texas at Austin
Austin, Texas 78712
USA

MAYER, Tom G., MD
Division of Orthopedic Surgery
University of Texas
Southwestern Medical Center
5323 Harry Hines Boulevard
Dallas, Texas 75235
USA

McPHERSON, Barry D., PhD
Faculty of Graduate Studies
Wilfrid Laurier University
Waterloo, Ontario
N2L 3C5
Canada

MIKINES, Kari J., MD
Department of Medical Physiology B
The Panum Institute
University of Copenhagen
Blegdamsvej 3 C
2200 Copenhagen N
Denmark

MONTOYE, Henry J., PhD
Biodynamics Laboratory
University of Wisconsin
2000 Observatory Drive
Madison, Wisconsin 53706
USA

MOORE, Sean, MB, BCh, BAO
Department of Pathology
McGill University
3775 University Street
Montréal, Québec
H3A 2B4
Canada

NACHEMSON, Alf L., MD, PhD
Department of Orthopaedics
Sahlgren Hospital
S-413 45 Göteborg
Sweden

NEWSHOLME, Eric A., PhD
Department of Biochemistry
Merton College
University of Oxford
South Parks Road
Oxford OX1 3QU
England

OAKES, Barry W., MD
Department of Anatomy
Monash University
Wellington Road
Clayton, 3168
Australia

OLDRIDGE, Neil B., PhD
Department of Health Sciences
The University of Wisconsin
Milwaukee, Wisconsin 53201
USA

OSCAI, Lawrence B., PhD
Exercise Research Division
Department of Physical Education
University of Illinois at Chicago
Box 4348
Chicago, Illinois 60680
USA

PAFFENBARGER, Ralph S., Jr., MD, Dr PH
Department of Health Research and Policy
Division of Epidemiology
Stanford University School of Medicine
Stanford, California 94305
USA

PALMER, Warren K., PhD
Department of Physical Education
University of Illinois at Chicago
Box 4348
Chicago, Illinois 60680
USA

PARKER, Anthony W., MD
Department of Anatomy
University of Queensland
St. Lucia 4067
Brisbane
Australia

PATERSON, Donald H., PhD
Faculty of Physical Education
University of Western Ontario
London, Ontario
N6A 5C1
Canada

POWERS, Scott K., PhD
Applied Physiology Laboratory
Louisiana State University
Baton Rouge, Louisiana 70803
USA

PRIOR, Jerilynn C., MD
Endocrinology and Metabolism
University of British Columbia
Vancouver, British Columbia
V5Z 1M9
Canada

RECHNITZER, Peter A., MD
University of Western Ontario
450 Central Avenue, Suite 304
London, Ontario
N6B 2E8
Canada

SAHLIN, Kent, MD
Department of Clinical Physiology
Karolinska Institute
Huddinge University Hospital
S-141 86 Huddinge
Sweden

SALTIN, Bengt, MD
August Krogh Institute
Universitetsparken 13
DK-2100 Copenhagen Ø
Denmark

SCHULL, William J., PhD
Center for Demographic and Population
   Genetics
University of Texas Health Science Center
   at Houston
PO Box 20334
Houston, Texas 77225
USA

SECHER, Niels H., MD
Department of Medical Physiology B
The Panum Institute
University of Copenhagen
Blegdamsvej 3 C
2200 Copenhagen N
Denmark

SHEPHARD, Roy J., MD, PhD
School of Physical and Health Education
University of Toronto
320 Huron Street
Toronto, Ontario
M5S 1A1
Canada

SIME, Wesley E., PhD
Stress Physiology Laboratory
University of Nebraska
Lincoln, Nebraska 68588
USA

SIMON, Harvey B., MD
Cardiovascular Health Center and Infectious
   Disease Unit
Harvard Medical School and Massachusetts
   General Hospital
Boston, Massachusetts 02114
USA

SISCOVICK, David S., MD, MPH
Division of General Internal Medicine
University of Washington
Harborview Medical Center ZA-60
329 Ninth Avenue
Seattle, Washington 98195
USA

SKINNER, James S., PhD
Exercise and Sport Research Institute
Department of Health and Physical Education
Arizona State University
Tempe, Arizona 85287
USA

SMITH, Kristin A., BA
Biogerontology Laboratory
Department of Preventive Medicine
University of Wisconsin
504 Walnut Street
Madison, Wisconsin 53705
USA

SMITH, Everett L., PhD
Biogerontology Laboratory
Department of Preventive Medicine
University of Wisconsin
504 Walnut Street
Madison, Wisconsin 53705
USA

STALLKNECHT, Bente, MD
Department of Medical Physiology B
The Panum Institute
University of Copenhagen
Blegdamsvej 3 C
2200 Copenhagen N
Denmark

STEFANICK, Marcia L., PhD
Stanford Center for Research in Disease
   Prevention
730 Welch Road, Suite B
Stanford University School of Medicine
Stanford, California 94305
USA

STEPHENS, Thomas, PhD, Consultant
Social Epidemiology and Survey Research
Box 837
Manotick, Ontario
K0A 2N0
Canada

SUTTON, John R., MD
School of Medicine
McMaster University Medical Centre
Box 2000, Station A
Hamilton, Ontario
L8N 3Z5
Canada

TIPTON, Charles M., PhD
Department of Exercise and Sport Sciences
108 Gittings Building
University of Arizona
Tucson, Arizona 85721
USA

VAILAS, Artnur C., PhD
Department of Physical Education and Dance
University of Wisconsin
Madison, Wisconsin 53706
USA

VRANIC, Mladen, MD, DSc
Department of Physiology
Room 3358, Medical Sciences Building
University of Toronto
Toronto, Ontario
M5S 1A8
Canada

WALTER, Stephen D., PhD
Department of Clinical Epidemiology
  and Biostatistics
McMaster University
Hamilton, Ontario
L8N 3Z5
Canada

WASSERMAN, David, PhD
Department of Molecular Physiology
  and Biophysics
Vanderbilt University School of Medicine
Nashville, Tennessee 37232
USA

WHIPP, Brian J., PhD, DSc
Division of Respiratory and Critical Care,
  Physiology and Medicine
Harbor-UCLA Medical Center
1000 West Carson Street
Torrance, California 90509
USA

WHITE, Timothy P., PhD
School of Kinesiology
University of Michigan
Ann Arbor, Michigan 48109
USA

WING, Alvin L., MBA
Department of Health Research and Policy
Division of Epidemiology
Stanford University School of Medicine
Stanford, California 94305
USA

WOOD, Peter D., DSc, PhD
Stanford Center for Research in Disease
  Prevention
730 Welch Road, Suite B
Stanford University School of Medicine
Stanford, California 94305
USA

YOUNG, Archie, MD
Academic Department of Geriatric Medicine
Royal Free Hospital School of Medicine
Rowland Hill Street
Hampstead, London
NW3 2PF
England

PART I
Consensus Statement and Introductory Addresses

Chapter 1

Exercise, Fitness, and Health: The Consensus Statement

Edited by
Claude Bouchard, PhD
Roy J. Shephard, MD, PhD
Thomas Stephens, PhD
John R. Sutton, MD
Barry D. McPherson, PhD

Contents of Consensus Statement

Introduction

Attempts to reach a consensus about the status of current knowledge in the area of exercise, fitness, and health have not been numerous. At the time of the Conference on Physical Activity and Cardiovascular Health, held in Toronto in 1966, an effort was made to synthesize the existing research and clinical literature, with a particular focus on the cardiovascular system and vascular diseases (*Canadian Medical Association Journal*, Vol. 96, No. 12, 1967). More recently, four national and international meetings have reviewed the existing knowledge base on some aspects of the topic of exercise, fitness, and health. One of these conferences was held in Oslo and the proceedings were published in 1982 as a supplement (No. 29) to the *Scandinavian Journal of Social Medicine*. Another was organized by the British Sports Council in May of 1983, and a summary of the proceedings has received limited circulation as a brief report entitled "Exercise, Health and Medicine." A workshop was held by the United States Public Health Service (USPHS) Centers for Disease Control on "Epidemiologic and Public Health Aspects of Physical Activity." These proceedings have been published in an issue of *Public Health Reports* (Volume 100, No. 2, 1985). Finally, a symposium was held in 1985 in Sweden on the topic of "Physical Activity in Health and Disease" under the patronage of *Acta Medica Scandinavica*, which also published the proceedings as a supplement to the journal (Suppl. 703, Vol. 218, 1986).

The 1988 Toronto Conference on Exercise, Fitness, and Health differed from these other conferences in that a) it was designed for the sole purpose of establishing a consensus about the current status of the knowledge base, b) it was international in nature, c) it benefited from the active participation of the world's leading experts on the topics examined, and d) it covered most aspects of the field, although a few topics had to be omitted from the program because of time constraints (e.g., the gastrointestinal tract, the kidneys, the bladder, etc.).

The consensus statement emerging from the Conference is the result of an elaborate work plan that dates back to 1985 when the project was conceptualized and launched. From the beginning, the aim of the Conference organizers was to bring together scientists and clinicians who were internationally recognized authorities in each dimension of the relationships among exercise, fitness, and health. These experts were asked to prepare a comprehensive written review indicating current knowledge on their particular topic and to identify the outstanding issues from both a substantive and a methodological/technological point of view. The written reviews were circulated prior to the Conference, allowing discussants and members of the Consensus Committee to study the material and comment upon it. During the Conference, these experts and discussants heard each other out, and met each evening for further discussion and to review the draft of the Consensus statement prepared by the Conference Consensus Committee.

The final decision to include or exclude specific topics from the consensus statement was a complex issue and could not be based on a single criterion. In case of doubt, relevance to health outcomes, extent of incidence or prevalence of a health condition, and the adequacy of current evidence were used as general guidelines to assess the importance of a given topic and the quality of the data available. Knowledge was considered as firm and generally accepted if the data were from large or multiple randomized studies with clearcut results and a low statistical risk of errors. In some cases, data from small or few randomized studies were also used, particularly if trends were consistent across studies. Other types of evidence, including correlational data and studies with inconsistent results, were generally not used in developing the consensus statement, although the status of the research literature on some topics made this occasionally unavoidable.

For four and a half days during the Toronto Conference, the 33 primary speakers, the 30 invited discussants and the 5 members of the Conference Consensus Committee (See the Appendix to this chapter) discussed and debated the evidence to arrive at the Consensus Statement. In addition, they considered the written comments and verbal input from hundreds of delegates at the Conference, most of whom were active scientists. Thus, the present Consensus Statement represents the end point of an elaborate process that has enjoyed major contributions and input from literally hundreds of clinicians and scientists. However, any errors in the published text remain the responsibility of the members of the Conference Consensus Committee, who are serving as editors of the document.

The Basic Paradigm of the Conference and Key Definitions

The Paradigm

The subject matter has been approached on the assumption that there are complex relationships between the levels of habitual physical activity, physical and physiological fitness, and health. In a simplified manner, these relationships are illustrated in Figure 1.1. The model specifies that habitual physical activity can influence fitness, which in turn is correlated with the level of habitual physical activity. For instance, the fittest individuals tend to be the most active and, with increasing fitness, people tend to become more active. The model also specifies that fitness is related to health in a reciprocal manner. That is, health status influences both habitual physical activity level and fitness level.

In reality, the relationships between the level of habitual physical activity, fitness and health are more complex than suggested by Figure 1.1. Other factors are associated with individual differences in health status. Likewise, the levels of physical and physiological fitness are not determined entirely by an individual's level of habitual physical activity. Other lifestyle components, environmental conditions, personal attributes, and genetic characteristics also affect the major factors of the basic model and determine their interrelationships. A more complex model describing the relationships between habitual physical activity, fitness, and health is suggested by Figure 1.2. Both the program content of the Conference and the content of the Consensus Statement were planned in the context of the relationships specified in this figure.

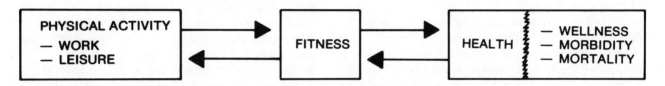

Figure 1.1. A simplified paradigm of the relationships among habitual physical activity, fitness, and health.

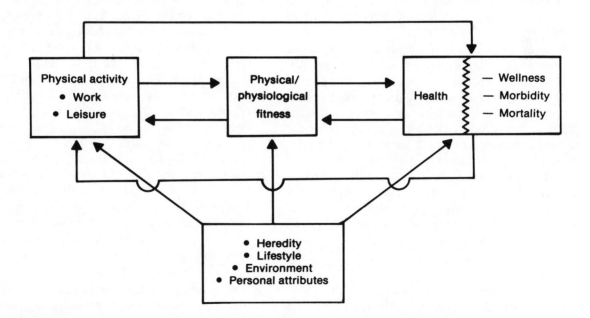

Figure 1.2. A model describing in schematic manner the complex relationships among habitual physical activity, fitness, and health.

Definitions

Several basic definitions were prepared by the Program Committee and circulated to the speakers and discussants prior to the Conference. These definitions are important to an understanding of the content of the consensus statement and they are thus reproduced here.

- **Physical Activity:** Any bodily movement produced by skeletal muscles and resulting in energy expenditure.
- **Leisure activity:** Physical activity that a person or a group chooses to undertake during their discretionary time.
- **Exercise and Training:** Exercise is leisure-time physical activity. Training is repetitive bouts of exercise, conducted over periods of weeks or months, with the intention of developing physical and/or physiological fitness.
- **Physical Activity pattern:** A comprehensive description of physical activity over a defined period of time, concerning the type, frequency, duration, and intensity of physical activity. Activity patterns can be used to calculate energy expenditure, assuming that the energy cost of the individual activities is known. The converse is not true: Physical activity patterns cannot be necessarily inferred from a knowledge of overall energy expenditure. Nevertheless, the description of physical activity patterns and the measurement of energy expenditure are the two principal approaches used to quantify physical activity.
- **Exercise intensity:** Exercise intensity can be expressed in either absolute or relative terms. Absolute intensity refers to the actual rate of energy expenditure, and is frequently used to assess physical activity in occupational and epidemiological studies. It is often expressed as a multiple of the resting metabolic rate (MET), for example, 5 METs. Relative intensity refers to the energy cost of the activity expressed as a percentage of the individual's maximal power output, and is customarily used to describe intensity in physiological studies. If allowance is made for the influence of age on maximum power output, the two approaches can be reconciled. Table 1.1 defines exercise intensity categories.
- **Energy expenditure:** The production of heat energy by the body is expressed in kilojoules. The most important components of overall energy expenditure include basal metabolic rate, physical activity, and the thermic effect of food. Basal metabolic rate accounts for the largest portion of daily

Table 1.1 Intensity of Physical Activity

	Relative intensity (%)	Absolute intensity (METs)			
		Young	Middle-aged	Old	Very old
Rest		1.0	1.0	1.0	1.0
Light	< 35	< 4.5	< 3.5	< 2.5	< 1.5
↓	> 35	< 6.5	< 5.0	< 3.5	< 2.0
	> 50	< 9.0	< 7.0	< 5.0	< 2.8
	> 70	> 9.0	> 7.0	> 5.0	> 2.8
Maximum	100	13	10	7	4

energy expenditure. Physical activity is clearly the most variable component of total daily energy expenditure.

- **Physical and Physiological Fitness:** *Fitness* is an elusive concept that cannot be defined in a universally acceptable manner in the context of exercise and health. For the purpose of this conference, a distinction is drawn between physical fitness and physiological fitness. *Physical fitness,* as defined by the World Health Organization, is "the ability to perform muscular work satisfactorily." It is generally thought that physical fitness (which comprises cardiorespiratory endurance, muscular strength and endurance, and flexibility) is determined by several variables including habitual physical activity level, diet, and heredity.

Fitness also extends to biological systems which are influenced by the level of habitual physical activity. In that sense, one may talk about physiological fitness. Variables to consider include blood pressure, glucose tolerance and insulin sensitivity, blood lipid levels and the lipoprotein profile, body composition and fat distribution, and stress tolerance. Some clinical values for these various characteristics are more desirable than others from the viewpoints of both health and performance.

In the context of fitness, adaptation refers to the processes of adjustment of the human organism to variations inthe level of habitual physical activity. Adaptation is therefore defined in terms of the responses to such activity including training and a lack of adequate physical activity.

- **Health:** Health is a human condition with physical, social, and psychological dimensions, each characterized on a continuum with positive and negative poles. Positive health is associated with a capacity to enjoy life and to withstand challenges; it is not merely the absence of disease.

Negative health is associated with morbidity and, in the extreme, with mortality.

- **Wellness:** Wellness is a holistic concept, describing a state of positive health in the individual and comprising biological and psychological well-being.

- **Morbidity and Mortality:** Morbidity is a state of ill health, generally resulting from a specific pathology. Mortality is usually defined in terms of an age and sex-specific death rate.

- **Heredity:** Inherited factors contribute to human variation in physical and physiological fitness and in health. The concept of heredity also includes the effects of genes determining the phenotypic response to lifestyle and environmental factors.

- **Lifestyle:** Lifestyle comprises the aggregate of an individual's behaviors, actions, and habits which can affect personal health (e.g., smoking, diet, habitual physical activity).

- **Environment:** The environment has physical and social characteristics (temperature, humidity, altitude, quality of air, place of residence, social network, characteristics of workplace, gross national product, etc.) which affect habitual physical activity, fitness, and health.

- **Personal attributes:** Personal attributes include such enduring sociodemographic and psychological characteristics as: age, sex, socioeconomic status, personality, and motivation.

Assessment of Physical Activity, Fitness, and Health

Assessment of Physical Activity Level and Overall Energy Expenditure

Physical activity is almost universally accepted as being relevant to health, although the pattern of activity (nature, intensity, frequency and duration of individual exercise bouts, cumulative years of participation) required to induce maximum health benefits remains uncertain. One obstacle to more definitive studies is the considerable interaction of physical activity with fitness, nutritional status, and other sociocultural variables. Isolating the specific health effects of physical activity is thus very difficult.

More conclusive investigations of the relationship between health and physical activity will de-pend upon the development of better methods of assessing both overall energy expenditure and patterns of physical activity at work and during leisure hours. Existing procedures also need more careful validation.

A prime epidemiological requirement is to increase our information about patterns of habitual physical activity in specific population groups. A diary record (preferably prospective) and/or a questionnaire are the only current methods capable of providing such information on large numbers of individuals. Careful validation of both procedures is necessary to check for systematic errors in quantifying activity patterns. Such techniques cannot be applied to children younger than ten years of age; parents can be questioned, but there remains a need to develop methods specifically applicable to young children.

The criterion to be used when validating questionnaire assessments of habitual activity remains a problem. Doubly labeled water has been used successfully to monitor energy expenditures in small animals. The development of new ratio mass spectrometers with greater precision has reduced the dose of the isotope needed and hence the cost, so that the method has potential application to human assessments made over periods of 1 to 2 weeks, provided that the number of subjects is not large.

Personal monitoring devices hold most promise for small-scale experimental validation of self-reports and for future epidemiological studies. Techniques will, in all probability, include single- or multiple-plane accelerometers, perhaps in combination with the monitoring of heart rate and/or the use of computerized activity records. The traditional approach of measuring oxygen consumption has the disadvantage of modifying the subject's movements, but a further potential approach would be a technique for accumulating information obtained from a thoracic respiration recorder.

Rapid developments in technology may soon provide suitable low-cost instrumentation for epidemiological studies. Future monitoring devices should incorporate a time base and be able to measure and store data on movement patterns or physiological responses at intervals of about one minute for a total period of 12 to 24 hours.

For the immediate future, we shall probably continue to rely very largely on diary records or questionnaires, possibly supplemented by selected measurements of movement patterns and/or heart rates, when assessing relationships between habitual physical activity and health.

Assessment of Physical and Physiological Fitness

In the assessment of physical and physiological fitness, it is important to identify whether the information relates to performance- and/or health-related fitness. Performance-related fitness refers to those components of fitness that contribute to optimal work or sport performance, whereas health-related fitness involves those components that relate to health status.

When evaluating physical fitness, the following components should be considered:

Flexibility

Flexibility is relatively easy to assess. Standard procedures are required for more reliable joint-specific measures. From a health-related perspective, additional measurements which correlate well with the risk of back disorders are needed.

Body Composition

A range of techniques is presently available, but none is completely accurate or valid and all need improvement. For most purposes, the two-component model, fat and fat-free tissue, is sufficient. For health-related fitness, the concern is not only with the amount of fat, but also with fat distribution. Since the presence of a high waist-to-hip circumference ratio and excessive trunk or abdominal fat places the individual more at risk of diabetes and cardiovascular diseases, this information should be included in the evaluation of body composition. More direct measurements are needed for an accurate description of the various body components. Simpler and more accurate indirect methods of assessing body composition and fat distribution are also needed. Imaging techniques appear promising but continued development is needed to make such methods simpler and more practical. Finally, there is a need to study the effects of such factors as age, gender, heredity, health status, level of fitness, and type of training upon the various body components.

Muscle Strength and Endurance

Strength can be assessed using isometric, isotonic, and isokinetic methods. Each has inherent limitations. While isometric tests are easy to administer, information is limited to the specific joint angles measured, and the direct applicability of data to most types of movement is questionable. Tests of isotonic strength provide more information about performance, but better standardization of measurement technique is needed. Isokinetic testing is promising, but further validation is required. Age- and gender-specific norms should be developed, describing the strength and endurance of large-muscle groups at varying speeds of contraction. Some tests of muscular strength and endurance can be dangerous, and alternative methods of measurement should be developed.

Anaerobic Abilities

There remains a need to develop standardized tests, reflecting the ability to undertake different types and durations of brief, high-intensity physical activity. Anaerobic tests are generally more relevant to performance-related fitness than to health-related fitness.

Aerobic Ability

The direct measurement of maximal aerobic power ($\dot{V}O_2$max) is the most satisfactory method for assessing aerobic ability and there are definite criteria for its measurement. Submaximal tests have often been used to predict $\dot{V}O_2$max where maximal tests are contraindicated or prevented by technical difficulties, but there are serious limitations with these methodologies. More research is needed on standardized tests of endurance capacity, the ability to sustain endurance exercise. $\dot{V}O_2$max, endurance capacity, and participation in physical activity, while usually associated with each other, cannot be used interchangeably.

During a routine medical or health examination, selected physiological and biochemical variables are of considerable importance. A normal blood pressure and concentrations of plasma lipids, insulin, and blood glucose in the low-to-normal range are signs of physiological fitness and are associated with a low body-fat content and low abdominal fat, both also characteristics of physiological fitness.

Proper interpretation of physical fitness and physiological fitness data has to take into account such characteristics of the individual as age, gender, years of education, and personal lifestyle, including inventories of tobacco use, alcohol use, diet, and leisure-time and occupational activity. In addition, any family history of hypertension, blood lipid disorders, diabetes, obesity, ischemic heart disease, or early death of relatives should be considered.

Assessment of Health

The assessment of health status has evolved considerably since the concept of positive health was first articulated. Nevertheless, traditional indices of morbidity (e.g., hospital admissions, bed-days by cause, case-fatality ratios) and of mortality (e.g., life expectancy at specified ages) continue to dominate descriptions of population health status. A major limitation in this class of indicators is their origin in administrative data. For morbidity, their application is often limited to a small and unrepresentative fraction of the total population. Mortality statistics are also of limited use in describing health status. Nevertheless, in cross-sectional studies, the prevalence of certain diseases possibly related to activity should be measured. More importantly, in prospective or longitudinal studies, the incidence rate for these diseases could serve as valuable health indices. Both short- and long-term cross-sectional and longitudinal studies are needed to better understand the relationship between habitual physical activity, fitness, and health.

In consequence, population-based measures such as two-week disability days and measures of functional status (e.g., ability to undertake the activities of daily living) have been developed. Such measures, while more comprehensive in the population covered, are fragile because of their reliance upon survey data which are not usually collected on a routine basis. Data from administrative sources, on the other hand, suffer from inconsistencies in recording, classification, or processing, and are often focused on events rather than individuals. With all such measures, it is important to distinguish between disease events (e.g., prevalence of a condition) and proxy measures based on the consequences of illness (e.g., hospital days).

The assessment of positive health has been hindered by difficulties in its conceptualization, while conceptual developments have been retarded by a paucity of data. Disability-free life expectancy and psychological well-being are two measures commonly used to describe positive dimensions of population health.

Measures of health are also needed for smaller scale intervention studies on the effects of exercise and physical activity. For such purposes, certain "surrogates" for health have proved useful. For example, the effects of exercise regimens can be related to known risk factors for the development of atherosclerotic complications (serum lipids, glucose tolerance, blood pressure), even though these variables serve only as proxies for health itself. In studies involving larger numbers of individuals and lasting for long enough periods of time, the incidence rates for specific diseases may also serve as relevant end-points (coronary artery disease, diabetes mellitus, osteoporosis). While useful, these variables are only pieces of an overall estimate of the global health of a population. Thus, scientists should, when possible, use more global measures, such as healthy life expectancy or disability-free life expectancy. These variables will allow more meaningful comparisons across cultures and nations of the impact of habitual physical activity and fitness.

Determinants of Participation in Physical Activity

Personal attributes can classify people as likely to be responsive or nonresponsive to interventions that are designed to increase their level of habitual physical activity. Available evidence from developed countries suggests many categories of individuals who are particularly inactive in their leisure time and who, to date, have been unresponsive to supervised programmes. Such target groups include blue-collar workers, low-income, less-educated individuals, ethnic minorities, housewives, middle-aged individuals, the physically disabled, smokers, and those with a Type A behavior pattern. While resistant to an increase of physical activity, such groups are of interest to public health, since they are the people most likely to benefit from an increase in their personal activity.

Those who are active tend to be self-motivated and possess self-regulatory skills: setting personal physical activity goals, planning to reach them, minimizing environmental barriers to implementation, and monitoring and reinforcing their actions. Those promoting physical activity must thus seek to develop behavioral skills and environments that will enable and reinforce participation.

There is a need to identify and rank determinants of participation in physical activity. Initiation and maintenance of physical activity must be considered separately. Interventions focused upon knowledge, attitudes, intentions, health beliefs, self-efficacy, and expectancies about activity outcomes, while helpful in the planning and adoption of physical activity, have only a weak influence upon the maintenance of such behaviour unless individuals are taught the self-regulation of behaviour, are prepared for relapses, and receive tangible reinforcement of physical activity that is undertaken. Traditional techniques of health promotion and education, medical and fitness screening and health-risk appraisal can stimulate initiation of an activity programme. However, they cannot, alone, sustain participation because they focus on abstract concepts of health rather than specific incentives to an active lifestyle.

Community and personal social support of physical activity is important in removing barriers and reinforcing behavioural change. It will encourage maintenance of physical activity, but is unlikely to be fully effective in the absence of concrete rewards such as enjoyment and personal satisfaction.

Moderate rather than strenuous physical activity seems likely to favour the adoption of an unsupervised exercise programme, particularly among those who are initially unfit. However, in supervised programs where the intensity of exercise is appropriate to fitness level, adherence is apparently unrelated to the intensity or duration of activity bouts, except where injury has occurred.

Little progress has yet been made in determining how perceived exertion, exercise sensations, and perceived barriers to exercise influence habitual physical activity patterns. Precise methods of measuring these variables are needed for population studies.

We need to identify and rank both personal attributes and environmental factors (both sociocultural and physicochemical) that influence patterns of habitual physical activity. This would not only advance theoretical understanding, but would allow a selection of more effective methods of intervention in various segments of the population and in different environmental settings.

We need to discover how determinants of physical activity vary with age, race, gender, ethnicity, socioeconomic status, fitness, and health. There is a need to explore how perceptions of and preferences for various types and intensities of physical activity are formed, and to decide whether such factors influence participation.

Much more information is needed on how the determinants of physical activity change with age, with particular reference to factors influencing the participation of children and of middle-age and elderly people.

Human Adaptation to Physical Activity

Nervous System and Sensory Adaptation

It is generally recognized that motor units within a motor pool are recruited in a relatively fixed order, associated with the size of the unit, the smaller motoneurons being recruited first. This is not to say that the size principle is one of complete functional rigidity, nor that it has to be assumed to be based exclusively on the size of the motoneuron. This principle is important in understanding neural strategies for the control of movement and related phenomena, such as the metabolic response of muscle to exercise. The size principle serves as a basis for the rationale of functional order among hundreds of enzyme and substrate properties within and across muscle units. Furthermore, the sensory response to movement is an integral part of the size-principle schema, as the spindles and tendon organs are organized around muscle fibers that are innervated by the smaller and more excitable motoneurons. Finally, the size principle goes far in explaining the quality and quantity of adaptation that occurs in specific types of motor units.

Given the current technology and the present views of the neural control of movement and homeostasis, a number of important issues should be pursued. For example, the physiological and anatomical features of the nervous system that determine the order of motor unit recruitment remain to be fully defined. Other questions include: To what degree is there order in recruitment across motor pools? How are the sensory endings within the muscle, tendon, joints, skin, etc. and their central projections integrated into the alpha and gamma motoneuron pools? Furthermore, the metabolic properties and the energy demands of central neural function in neuronal and glial tissue in brain, brain stem and cord are important to define.

It is of interest also to identify the mechanism(s) through which the nervous system exerts its influence on specific protein expression in muscle fibers. This information will help clarify qualitative and quantitative differences among motor units. Other issues related to motoneuron-muscle fiber interrelationship include the following: What determines the number of muscle fibers that a motoneuron can innervate and sustain functionally? What regulates the eventual selection between a muscle fiber and axon terminal? And how plastic is the motoneuron-muscle fiber interdependence? Additionally, how adaptable are the neural networks that control the motor unit?

Further issues of plasticity of the neuromuscular system are related to optimizing neuromuscular function with respect to human growth and development, aging, arthritis, and neuromuscular impairments. An understanding of the mechanisms and etiology of neuromuscular impairments are essential in the development of useful diagnostic, preventive, and rehabilitative procedures.

Hormonal Responses

The hormonal response to exercise is a complex, highly integrated system that involves activation of the sympathetic nervous system and the hypothalamic pituitary axis. In response to these hormonal changes, several physiological responses occur to increase delivery of oxygen and metabolic fuels to working muscles for energy production and to maintain other body homeostatic mechanisms including regulation of body temperature, circulating blood volume, and electrolyte balance. There is release or suppression of a large number of hormones that regulate the mobilization and/or metabolism of glucose, free fatty acids, and amino acids or alter fluid and electrolyte balance. The magnitude and pattern of the hormonal adaptation to physical activity depends on multiple factors which include but are not limited to the intensity and duration of the exercise performed and the level of training. Conditions influencing metabolic fuel availability and hormonal adaptation include the amount and composition of the antecedent diet and the influence of feeding prior to or during exercise. The hormonal adaptation to exercise may be modified by age and sex, although it is difficult to differentiate these effectsfrom other factors. Physical training will reduce all the hormonal responses to exercise at a given absolute intensity.

Physical activity is associated with activation of the sympathetic nervous system and a rise in plasma norepinephrine and epinephrine concentrations. The increase in plasma norepinephrine represents a spillover from sympathetic nerve terminals and gives only a rough approximation of sympathetic nerve stimulation. Plasma norepinephrine increases with increasing work intensity and duration in relation to the muscle mass involved. Several other factors also increase the norepinephrine response to exercise. These include hypoxemia, hypovolemia, exposure to hot or cold environments; and assuming and performing work in an upright position. Epinephrine responses are less than the increases in norepinephrine and are seen primarily with exercise of high-intensity or in response to a falling blood glucose concentration.

The major physiological effects of sympathetic nervous system activation during exercise include effects on the cardiovascular system, stimulating perspiration, stimulating the renin-angiotensin system, and the regulation of metabolic fuel mobilization and utilization. Lipolysis and glycogenolysis in both liver and muscle tissue are stimulated while insulin secretion is suppressed. In addition, increased blood flow to working muscles results in increased insulin delivery to these tissues. The falling insulin concentrations in plasma have major effects on glucose, lipid, and amino acid metabolism, thereby making these fuels more readily available. Insulin inhibits hepatic glucose production and affects glucose utilization.

Glucagon responses are minimal during mild to moderate intensity exercise. However, with prolonged exercise, glucagon concentrations increase. The hepatic effect of glucagon is augmented as insulin concentration decreases. Elevation of growth hormone and cortisol concentration with increasing work loads may contribute to the control of energy substrates during prolonged exercise.

There appears to be considerable redundancy in the adaptive responses so that a deficiency of one hormonal system may be compensated by overactivity of another. A number of hormonal systems interact in fuel metabolism, so that, with an acute deficiency in one, some compensation is possible.

Prolonged endurance training is associated with increased plasma epinephrine responses to various stimuli, including insulin-induced hypoglycemia, hypoxia, hypercapnia, glucagon, and caffeine. Taking into account the various effects of epinephrine it is clear that a high capacity to secrete epinephrine represents an advantage in competitive sports.

Training also increases insulin sensitivity. Thus less insulin is needed to handle a given carbohydrate load and glucose homeostasis is maintained or improved. Hence, the decreased insulin secretory capacity of the pancreatic beta cells appears to be an adaptive response to increased peripheral insulin sensitivity rather than a state of insulin deficiency.

Bone and Connective Tissue Adaptation

There is only limited knowledge about the effects of physical activity on the structure and functions of bones, joints, ligaments, and tendons. It has been known for centuries that these structures respond to altered levels of mechanical stimulation. What is lacking is the quantification of the responsible mechanism(s).

A gap remains between the scientific understanding of these tissues and applications of this knowledge to clinical medicine and public health. However, we do know that immobilization has detrimental effects on the structure and function of these tissues. This has led to a change of clinical management; immobilization is now minimized and early passive mobilization is encouraged.

Bone mineral content can now be measured accurately, using quantitative single- or dual-photon absorptiometry, neutron activation or quantitative computerized tomography scanning to localize changes. Ultrasound has also been used to monitor changes in bone with loading, but the interpretation of such data requires clarification. A combination of the above information with biochemical data such as urine and serum hydroxyproline concentrations may be useful in predicting individuals who will develop problems when subjecting themselves to severe musculoskeletal stress.

The relative contributions of the genome—the mechanical and hormonal environments of bone remodeling and maintenance of bone mass—are still not well understood. Recent work supports the concept of an optimal strain, genetically programmed but specific to a given region of bone and its functional loading. The approximate type and magnitude of strain required to maintain bone mass and to induce fatigue fractures is now known. However, current knowledge has not allowed total prevention of bone loss after prolonged recumbency or weightlessness (spaceflight). Further studies are required to predict which patients and which bones are particularly vulnerable to stress fractures. The minimization of bone loss in experimental animal models by application of pulsed electromagnetic fields is encouraging. It remains important to undertake longitudinal studies to determine the influence of various intensities of activity upon bone growth in children.

Much has been learned about cartilage and especially the details of proteoglycan structure and metabolism. Loading increases the concentration of proteoglycans within articular cartilage. In vitro tissue culture systems have been well established and characterized. However, little of this knowledge and technology has been applied to human cartilage either in vivo or in vitro.

Our understanding of the repair processes in articular cartilage is still very rudimentary. The normal adult has a complex three-dimensional array of collagen fibres embedded in a rich proteoglycan matrix; this is difficult to repair and/or replace. Loading and joint motion appear to be important determinants of chondrogenic stem-cell differentiation toward a chondrocyte which will synthesize a neoarticular cartilage matrix. The nature of the molecular signals determining these events needs to be established.

There has been overwhelming animal evidence that the insertions of knee ligaments are weakened by inactivity. The loss in bone-ligament junction strength due to inactivity occurs within weeks and takes much longer to return to normal. It also exceeds the potential gain from increased activity, suggesting that the normal junction strength is close to maximum and that the demands of daily physical activity are sufficient to maintain the integrity of the bone-ligament junction. However, demands must include physical activities (stair or hill climbing) that place an appropriate stress at the insertion sites. The meniscal cartilages are essential to normal knee-joint function, and their surgical removal leads to premature osteoarthritis. Although previously there was a propensity to treat individuals with meniscal knee problems by surgical removal, this has largely been replaced by other procedures. Preliminary studies indicate that, far from being metabolically and physiologically inert tissues, these cartilages are responsive to mechanical stimuli and can undergo healing.

Isolated ligaments and tendons follow the pattern observed with junctions. Namely, they exhibit more changes with decreased physical activity than with increased physical activity. Not only do they become smaller and weaker, but the biomechanical properties indicate molecular changes in the collagen. When immobilized, there are marked reductions in the aerobic enzyme activity of ligaments and tendons. This suggests that the cellular environment has become more anaerobic and possibly more acidotic. Unlike skeletal tissue, normal ligaments and tendons show little increase in their aerobic enzyme activity with chronic physical activity. This finding complements the ligament-bone junction strength results, indicating that limited functional improvement will occur with regular physical activity.

The weakness and healing of repaired tissue is protracted if the affected tissues are immobilized.

Since immobilization is essential during the early stages of repair, the clinical use of continuous passive motion has provided a link between the time of surgery and the moment when it is appropriate to begin the prescription of light physical activity. Return of normal function is facilitated by regular physical activity, but the optimum intensity, frequency, duration, mode, and specificity of exercise remains obscure. If major advances are to be made in our understanding of the mechanisms by which physical activity alters bones and connective tissues, the techniques of molecular biology must be incorporated into this research.

Skeletal Muscle Adaptation

The forces developed during muscular activation provide a stimulus for adaptive responses in skeletal muscle fibers. The adaptations are characterized by modifications of morphological, biochemical and molecular variables. These in turn alter functional attributes of the fibers, and are readily reversible when the stimulus is altered. The changes in functional attributes range from a diminished capacity to generate and maintain power in response to reduced physical activity, to an enhanced capacity to sustain power for long periods of time following endurance training, or to an enhanced capacity to develop high power following strengthtraining. Adaptations are observed primarily at the level of single motor units. The adaptations appear to be induced primarily by changes in the pattern of recruitment of motor units interacting with the force and velocity (i.e., power) of the contractions. Additional variables include the duration of a single session of physical activity, the frequency of the sessions, and the duration of the overall training program. Although a relationship exists between the training stimulus and the adaptive response, the relationship is complex and not stoichiometric. Variations in the adaptive response to training stimuli may exist for subjects of different genotype, gender, age, and nutritional status, but the data are equivocal.

Immobilization of limbs and suspension of the hind limbs provide useful models of reduced physical activity. Atrophic responses result from the decrease in recruitment and/or load, and include a loss of muscle mass, fiber cross-sectional area and capacity for maximum force development. The relative amount of fast myosin increases, which leads to an increased velocity of shortening.

Endurance training involving repetitive contractions for prolonged periods with relatively low forces increases the capacity for oxidative metabolism and delays the onset of metabolic acidosis. In the muscles trained for endurance exercise, world-class endurance athletes have high percentages of fibers which are low in myosin ATPase activity and are presumed to be slow fibers. In spite of this observation and the fact that experimental paradigms can change fiber types, the ability of voluntary endurance activities to modify myosin characteristics of individual fibers has not been demonstrated definitively, and the issue remains controversial.

Strength training involving few contractions for short periods of time with relatively high forces may produce an increase in muscle mass due primarily to hypertrophy of individual fibers. Following training, the increased capacity to develop maximum force and especially power exceeds the increase in total fiber cross-sectional area. The excess is explained in part by an optimization of motor unit recruitment. Adaptations to skeletal muscle fibers have a direct influence on the physical fitness level of the individual. Increases or decreases in the ability of skeletal muscle to develop and sustain power can have a corresponding positive or negative impact upon the quality of a person's life.

Substantive issues regarding the adaptation of skeletal muscle fibers that remain unresolved include: clarification of the mechanistic linkages between specific training stimuli and the resultant adaptive responses; the relationship between measures of intensity and duration of training and the muscle adaptations produced in individuals of differing initial characteristics; and clarification of the role, if any, of contraction-induced injury in the adaptive response to training.

Adipose Tissue Adaptation

Lipid mobilization during exercise is determined by the stimulatory and inhibitory mechanisms of the adipose tissue hormone-sensitive triglyceride lipase. This enzyme hydrolyses triglycerides to free fatty acids and glycerol. In humans, the sympathetic nervous system is the main factor stimulating this system, while insulin is the main inhibitor.

The trained state is characterized by a greater reliance on free fatty acid oxidation during submaximal exercise and a sparing of carbohydrate. In the trained individual, serum free fatty acid and blood glycerol concentrations are unchanged or slightly lower than control levels when exercise is performed at a standardized work rate. This pattern of response occurs even though endurance training reduces the catecholamine response to submaximal exercise.

It has recently been confirmed in humans that exercise training results in an increased capacity to release free fatty acids from adipocytes. The sensitivity of adipose tissue to the lipolytic action of catecholamines is enhanced. However, if endurance training is stopped, after a short period of inactivity, the plasmafree fatty acid and glycerol responses to epinephrine infusion are decreased, while that of lactate is increased.

Exercise training thus produces enhanced lipolysis in adipose tissue, resulting in a smaller fat cell. It appears that training adapts fat cells for an increased mobilization followed by a rapid replenishment of energy stores. The replenishment phase is facilitated by an increase of insulin sensitivity. There is a need for more research about sex differences and regional fat depot variation in the lipolytic and replenishment processes.

Carbohydrate, Lipid, and Amino Acid Metabolism

Intense exercise of short duration requires a high amount of energy. This is obtained from the breakdown of skeletal muscle endogenous phosphocreatine and glycogen. With increasing duration of exercise, the contribution of the oxidative pathways to the muscle ATP needs becomes more important. During prolonged exercise of moderate intensity, the contribution of anaerobic replenishment of ATP is negligible. Instead, blood glucose, glucose from liver glycogen, glucose from muscle glycogen, and fatty acids from adipose tissue lipolysis are providing most of the energy for ATP needs. Both glucose and fatty acids are oxidized simultaneously during prolonged exercise. It is unlikely that muscle triacylglycerol, ketone bodies, and amino acid oxidation make a major contribution to the energy demands of exercise.

Anaerobic and power training only slightly increase the capacity of the skeletal muscle to store and break down the endogenous substrates of anaerobic metabolism. On the other hand, endurance training greatly increases the oxidative capacity of skeletal muscle. Both at a given absolute power output and at the same relative intensity, training results in 1) an increased fat oxidation, and 2) a decreased formation of lactic acid, with less fatigue. At the same absolute work intensity, there is also a decreased formation of ammonia. Aerobic training increases the sensitivity of liver, adipose tissue, and skeletal muscle to insulin.

Prolonged exercise increases the rate of energy expenditure for a period after exercise has finished. There is likely to be an effect of both intensity and of duration of exercise on this phenomenon. This might be caused, in part, by an increase in the rates of substrate and other metabolic cycles.

Pulmonary Adaptation

Breath pattern and timing and alveolar gas exchange have been described exhaustively for every type, intensity, and duration of exercise, at various altitudes and in most healthy populations. The acute effects of exercise on arterial blood gases, alveolar-to-arterial gas exchange, and ventilation-to-perfusion distribution are adequately documented. There is a consensus that the alveolar-to-arterial O_2 difference increases about threefold in heavy exercise in normal untrained subjects. This is due, in part, to a more nonuniform distribution of ventilation to perfusion. Arterial PO_2 is adequately defended until the oxygen consumption exceeds about 60 to 65 ml per kg body weight per minute. Beyond this level, some subjects develop arterial hypoxemia due to a combination of an inadequate hyperventilatory response and an excessively wide $A\text{-}aDO_2$. A diffusion limitation to alveolar-capillary equilibration probably occurs in maximum exercise. This diffusion limitation is established for O_2 transport; limitations to CO_2 equilibration probably also occur but have not as yet been quantified. The turnover of extravascular lung water increases during even mild exercise. We do not know if this fluid accumulates or where it might accumulate during exercise.

Inspiratory intercostal muscles and the expiratory muscles of the rib cage and abdomen are recruited even during mild exercise. This recruitment increases with increasing work rate, so that the end-expiratory lung volume is progressively reduced. As a consequence, the length of the inspiratory muscles prior to inspiration is optimized, permitting improved tension generation. During maximum exercise, the major inspiratory muscles are heavily recruited. Intrathoracic pressure and local blood flow reach very high levels, but it is unlikely that the respiratory muscles become fatigued. In humans, the proportion of total body cardiac output and oxygen consumption diverted to the respiratory muscles during exercise has not yet been quantified accurately. Maximum dilation of both the extrathoracic and intrathoracic airways occurs during exercise, so that the pulmonary airflow resistance remains unchanged in the face of up to 10- to 20-fold increases in inspiratory and expiratory flow rates.

The primary mechanism for exercise hyperpnea remains unclear. Acting in concert with descending feed-forward neurogenic stimuli originating in the higher CNS and increasing in proportion to locomotion, there is an ascending neurogenic stimulus. The latter originates in contracting skeletal muscle in response to as yet unspecified neurochemical stimuli. Chemoreceptor feedback—especially from peripheral chemoreceptors—is crucial for the fine tuning of this ventilatory response. Fine tuning is especially important in transitions from rest to work and from one work load to the next. In addition, a relatively small but significant portion of the total stimulus to exercise hyperpnea arises from a compensatory response to the normal mechanical impedance presented by the lungs and airways during exercise.

During very heavy exercise, a variable hyperventilation occurs, due only in part to peripheral chemoreceptor stimulation via the accompanying metabolic acidosis. The receptor sites and neural pathways necessary for mediation of any mechanical feedback from the lungs or chest wall during exercise remain largely unexplored. The contribution of vagal feedback to the regulation of breathing pattern and expiratory muscle recruitment in exercising humans also remains untested. Finally, we do not know how the complex array of feed-forward and feedback mechanisms interact during exercise to assure recruitment of upper airway and chest wall muscles (acting as respiratory, postural, and locomotor muscles).

Few attempts have been made to document morphologic and functional aspects of chest wall adaptation in various types of chronic exercise. Current dogma suggests that chronic physical training has no significant effect on lung structure or function, and that it has relatively little effect on the structure or metabolic capacity of respiratory muscles. The capacity of the more trainable organ systems (cardiovascular and locomotor muscle) may then surpass in some circumstances that of the untrainable pulmonary system. Arterial hypoxemia, then, reflects the absence of a hyperventilatory response appropriate to the extreme maximal metabolic requirements of highly trained athletes.

The effects of aging upon lung and chest wall function have received only cursory examination. What effects do age-related changes in the compliances of the lung and chest wall have on respiratory muscle coordination, endurance, and strength? What are the implications of these mechanical changes for the distribution of ventilation and the adequacy of gas exchange during heavy exercise?

Cardiovascular Adaptation

The key issues are: the factors limit oxygen transport capacity and utilization during exercise, the adaptations to habitual physical activity of the various components involved in the oxygen transport system, the functional significance of the adaptations to exercise, and the stimuli required for the regulation of the observed adaptations.

There is seldom less than 95% oxygen saturation of the hemoglobin in arterial blood in healthy young sedentary, trained, and well trained individuals during intense exercise at sea level. Arterial hypoxemia has been reported in endurance runners but the prevalence is debated. When the level of habitual physical activity is increased, so is the blood volume. The latter changes over a rather short period (weeks and months), without any significant alterations in the blood hemoglobin content. The largest blood volumes are found in those well trained for endurance. They also tend to have low normal hemoglobin concentrations. It remains unclear whether the low hemoglobin is a physiological adaptation, or is a sign of maladaptation.

The dimensions of the heart increase with habitual physical activity, as does the stroke volume. Over a broad spectrum ranging from healthy but inactive individuals to endurance trained athletes, there is a very close relationship between the amount of oxygen offered to the tissues during brief exhaustive exercise and maximal oxygen uptake. The factors which determine the maximal oxygen transport capacity are arterial oxygen content, maximal heart rate, and stroke volume. Of these three variables, only the last changes significantly with training. This observation has led many to conclude that cardiac dimensions and cardiac filling limit maximal oxygen uptake in humans.

Some evidence is accumulating to support the notion that the large blood vessels of heart and skeletal muscles are all positively affected by training. The magnitude of the microcirculatory bed also adjusts to the needs of the working muscles. Adaptations seem to allow a larger muscle blood flow without a reduction of mean transit time. Indeed, with training, the capillary density (capillary blood volume) may increase more than the muscle blood flow, thereby increasing the mean transit time through the exercising muscles.

In heavy exercise involving a large fraction of the muscle mass (as in running or bicycling), some 10% of the oxygen delivered to the working tissues is not extracted. However, after training, as little as 4 to 5% of the blood oxygen content is returned from the exercising limbs. It is still debated whether the oxygen remaining in the venous blood that leaves trained contracting muscle reflects a peripheral limitation of oxygen diffusion or an admixture of blood with a high residual oxygen content from inactive muscle and other tissues.

The conductance of skeletal muscle is larger than the pump capacity of the heart in both sedentary and trained conditions. To maintain blood pressure during intense exercise that involves a large muscle mass, the sympathetic nervous system adjusts the peripheral resistance to match the output of the heart. Such a vasoconstriction affects not only the viscera and inactive muscles, but also, to a lesser extent, the vessels of the exercising limbs.

The lungs can transfer and the skeletal muscle can utilize oxygen at rates which are greater than what the heart can deliver. In trained individuals, the heart has a greater oxygen transport capacity than in the sedentary, coming close to the upper limit of the lungs, but still lagging behind that of the skeletal muscles.

Behavioral Adaptation

In addition to affecting biochemical, physiological, and morphological parameters, exercise may affect other health-related behaviors such as smoking, alcohol use, and dietary habits. Understanding such behavioral consequences of exercise is relevant to both health promotion and epidemiology. For both purposes, data on changes in behavior are more informative than associations. Within the severe limitations of the available data, which mostly pertains to leisure activities, the following conclusions can be drawn.

Persons who exercise in their leisure time are less likely to be smokers, but the relationship between the two behaviors is weak, and available evidence is largely correlational. Smoking rates differ little between sedentary and moderately active groups, but highly active individuals are much less likely to smoke than their sedentary peers. There is very little evidence from controlled trials that exercise programs enhance smoking cessation, although exercise may be useful in controlling the immediate weight gain which sometimes follows cessation. Exercise appears to be beneficial in treating

alcohol and drug abuse, but the evidence is scanty and the bases for its therapeutic use are not clear.

In the general population, exercise is positively associated with energy intake. Epidemiologic studies and clinical trials alike show a higher energy intake in more active individuals. There is also limited longitudinal evidence that an increase of exercise may be associated with a shift to a more healthful diet.

Cross-sectional data from population surveys and a variety of narrowly defined groups reveal weak positive correlations between exercise and other health practices. The common characteristic of these practices is a requirement for some deliberate effort, e.g., regular medical or dental checks, updated immunizations, or the use of seat belts. Positive associations are found in both sexes, all age groups, and across social classes. However, they are weak and the data are correlational. It is unlikely that these practices represent a behavioral adaptation to exercise. A more likely explanation is that some common characteristic, such as concern for health, predisposes people to exercise and to adopt other healthy practices. Finally, there is some evidence that exercise is associated with social factors such as maintenance of good interpersonal relationships, job performance, and other aspects of social functioning.

The way in which exercise, physical activity, and changes in physical activity fit into the total lifestyle needs much more exploration. Additional studies are needed to determine if converting from a sedentary to an active status is accompanied by changes in dietary habits, whether in terms of improved diet or the development of eating disorders. Physical activity programs for children and adolescents need to be studied to determine whether such activity helps to develop and maintain a lifelong active lifestyle. The role of regular physical activity in prevention of smoking adoption should be examined, as well as the potential contribution of exercise to smoking cessation and treatment of alcohol abuse.

Physical Activity, Fitness, and Reproductive Health

Reproductive Function

There is little doubt that strenuous physical activity influences the hypothalamic-pituitary-gonadal axis in men and women. Although acute exercise results in an increased serum concentration of sex hormones in females and males, prolonged strenuous activity may have a suppressive effect. Subclinical changes include decreased pulsatile release of luteinizing hormone, reduced gonadotropin response to gonadotropin-releasing hormone, and reduced gonadal steroid levels. Chronically depressed levels of gonadal steroids may result in reduced trabecular bone mass. Serum estradiol and progesterone are reduced at appropriate phases of the menstrual cycle. In men, serum androgens are reduced with potential impairment of spermatogenesis. The long-term significance of these changes is not known.

Cross-sectional studies suggest that delayed puberty, amenorrhea, and oligomenorrhea may occur with regular strenuous exercise. The prevalence of secondary amenorrhea is only slightly higher than that seen in the general population.

For women who have been ovulating regularly (usually by 12 years after menarche), the most prevalent change with training is a decrease in molimina (normal premenstrual symptoms) followed by luteal phase shortening. Molimina includes breast tenderness or enlargement, symptoms of fluid retention, and sometimes an increase in appetite or mood changes which predict ovulation. With more intense exercise, anovulation may occur. The young woman (within 12 years of menarche) or the woman who has not established ovulatory cycles may develop oligomenorrhea (cycle interval >36 days). She may even become amenorrheic (cycle interval >180 days) if there is an associated weight loss or situational stress. The reproductive changes occurring with training are reversible. Those that persist are often compounded by such additional factors as weight loss, illness, or psychological stress.

The suppression of reproductive functions appears to originate in the hypothalamus, but the mechanisms are unknown. Management of individuals with significant reproductive symptoms depends on the nature of the symptoms and reproductive requirements. Treatment involves encouragement to restore physiological norms of dietary intake and body composition, as well as reexamination of the exercise load.

Pregnancy

In general, the well-being of the mother and fetus is not harmed by moderate physical activity, provided that exercise is in keeping with the mother's prior level of conditioning. Research is required to establish what types and intensities of exercise are safe for the mother and fetus. Research is also needed on 1) the acute effects of exercise on the fetus, 2) the role of fitness on labor, delivery, and the health of the mother in the postpartum period, and 3) the effects on fetal outcome.

Physical Activity, Fitness, and Growth

Physical activity is only one of many factors which influence the developing individual. The growing and maturing individual does not necessarily respond to environmental stimuli in a similar manner to that of an adult.

Changes in physical, motor, and physiological fitness are influenced by the processes of growth and maturation, and it is often difficult to distinguish the effects of regular physical activity upon fitness from the changes associated with growth and maturation. There tends to be intraindividual stability of many morphological and physiological characteristics. The degree of this stability throughout growth varies among characteristics. Knowledge of such tracking is important when assessing intervention programs.

The normal response to training is clearly established at the time of puberty. Prepubescents respond to training with improvement in their maximal aerobic power, muscle strength, and muscle power, but some evidence suggests that trainability is perhaps lower than that of more mature groups.

Information on the effects of regular childhood physical activity on risk factors for cardiovascular disease is equivocal. While cross-sectional studies suggest that active children have a favorable lipid and lipoprotein profile, there are no controlled longitudinal studies to suggest a causal relationship. Lasting benefits to health (e.g., in obesity) may be achieved only if physical activity is augmented as part of a multidimensional intervention. Schools can provide the environment for large-scale programs which should include physical exercise, nutritional education, and general lifestyle education.

There is a need for both appropriate instrumentation and quantitative assessment of amounts and patterns of physical activity during childhood and adolescence. There is a paucity of longitudinal data describing the transitional years from adolescence into adulthood. Cross-sectional data from North America and Europe suggest a pronounced decline in physical activity which generally coincides with the end of high school.

The following issues merit more detailed study: Can regular physical activity alter age- and maturity-associated variation in such risk factors as HDL-cholesterol or insulin sensitivity? Which is more important: a satisfactory level of fitness or a lifestyle with a pattern of regular physical activity? Should more time and effort be devoted to the assessment and encouragement of physical activity in children and youth than to fitness per se?

Physical Activity, Fitness, and Aging

Among older people, and particularly with the onset of senescence, there is a trend to ever-decreasing physical activity. In spite of the apparent increase in physical activity among older adults in North America, there is little hard evidence to support this perception. For the active older adult, there is a reduction in the levels of certain traditional coronary risk factors.

Many functional abilities are reduced with aging, such as static and dynamic strength, muscular speed and power, and maximal aerobic power. Hypotrophy of muscle begins earlier in life but is accelerated after the age of 60 years. This hypotrophy is caused by a general loss of fibres, without predominant effect on any one fibre type. Muscle fibre size is also reduced, and this reduction is most evident in Type II fibres. Muscle fibre loss appears due to a reduction in the number of functioning motor units. The trainability of skeletal muscle at various ages has not been clearly defined.

The decrease in absolute $\dot{V}O_2$max is about 10 percent per decade from age 20 to 60 years. Exercise training in the fifth and sixth decades of life may alleviate this decline, but more importantly will induce a functional gain, equivalent to as much as 10 to 15 years of aging in many individuals.

Physical Activity, Fitness, and Mental Health

The mental health benefits of physical activity include reductions in anxiety, tension, depression, and reactivity to stressors. These and other factors may contribute to a sense of ''well-being'' in the active person, but this concept is difficult to define and assess. Reduced arousal prior to, during, and after exposure to stressors, quicker autonomic recovery following exposure to a stressor, and attenuated emotional reactions to some stressors are all associated with self-reported habitual activity and/or physical fitness. It is unknown whether these responses are linked to changes in aerobic power.

High levels of muscle tension may produce pain. Rest as well as relaxation training are effective in reducing both state anxiety and muscle tension. However, aerobic exercise of moderate to high intensity is also followed by reduced muscle tension, as well as reductions in state anxiety and blood pressure which last from 2 to 5 hours after a bout of activity. Acute exercise of low intensity and short duration reduces muscle tension, but is not associated with any reduction in state anxiety.

Chronic exercise may be associated with lower-than-average levels of anxiety, and/or muscle tension. It is also associated with reductions of depression in individuals who are mildly or moderately depressed. Nevertheless, patients who are taking psychotropic medication should be closely monitored during exercise bouts.

The quality and quantity of sleep is influenced positively by chronic exercise and negatively by exercise deprivation. Exercise deprivation can also lead to irritability and increases of anxiety and depression in some individuals. The intense and prolonged chronic exercise of endurance competition, if pursued to excess, may lead to a performance decrement, with increased fatigue, anxiety, and depression in some individuals.

While it is clear that exercise can benefit many areas of mental health, details of a programme that will optimize mental health have yet to be determined.

Physical Activity and Fitness in Disease Prevention and Treatment

Atherosclerosis

Evidence relating exercise or fitness level directly to the progression of atherosclerosis in humans is scarce. Nevertheless, findings characterized as appropriately sequenced, biologically graded, plausible, and coherent with existing knowledge strongly support the idea that physical activity is inversely and causally related to the incidence of ischemic heart disease, the most important clinical manifestation of atherosclerosis. The relationships of regular physical activity to the progression of atherosclerosis and incidence of stroke and peripheral vascular disease require further study.

Several potential mechanisms contribute to the plausibility of the exercise-ischemic heart disease relationship. The evidence for the influence of exercise on the thrombosis and fibrinolytic processes, which might reduce the risk of coronary events, is conflicting. As well, the relationships among platelet activation, coagulation, and exercise need much more study. Resting blood pressure tends to be reduced by regular exercise, possibly through a reduction in catecholamine levels. Active people exhibit high plasma concentrations of high-density lipoprotein (HDL) cholesterol, the ratio of HDL to low-density-lipoprotein (LDL) cholesterol, and especially of the apparently atherosclerosis-inhibiting HDL_2 subfraction. Recent studies on the biology of the arterial wall in both dietarily induced atherosclerosis, and that resulting from arterial wall injury, indicate that the HDL to LDL ratio is important because low density lipoprotein and very low density lipoproteins bind to altered proteoglycans in lesions. In contrast, HDL shows very little activity. Apolipoprotein A-I is also frequently elevated in active individuals, again predicting a low risk of ischemic heart disease. The activities of lipoprotein lipase (directly) and of hepatic lipase (inversely) are correlated with a favorable lipid profile. Adiposity is closely related to habitual exercise, plasma lipoprotein pattern, and lipase activities. Consequently, from a practical perspective, exercise and a loss of excess body fat may be regarded as a single health prescription.

Major risk-reducing effects are associated with regular aerobic exercise. Much remains to be learned about the type of activity and the optimal duration, intensity, and frequency of exercise, particularly in a context of long-term health. It seems that an improvement in measures such as HDL-cholesterol concentration occurs across the total spectrum of physical activity. In several training studies, $\dot{V}O_2$max increased, but significant improvement in plasma lipoproteins could not be detected. The increased energy expenditure coincident with long-term exercise is typically accompanied by an increased energy intake. This association should not be overlooked in seeking to understand causal relationships between physical activity and cardiovascular risks; and it may confer health benefits in relation to an adequate intake of nutrients and fiber.

Ischemic Heart Disease

Exercise-trained animals show an increased coronary artery luminal cross-sectional area, greater myocardial capillary density, and reduced amount of infarcted myocardial tissue. Whether myocardial collateralization is increased remains controversial, but exercise most likely improves perfusion when ischemia is already present. Myocardial function is also improved secondary to exercise training, with increased intrinsic contractility, faster relaxation, enzymatic alterations, greater calcium availability, and enhanced autonomic and hormonal control of function.

Morphologic and metabolic adaptations to training enhance the ability of the cardiovascular system to withstand a wide variety of stressors. An exercise-diet study using monkeys showed a reduction of exercise-induced ischemia, by increasing coronary artery luminal cross-sectional area, but only a nonatherogenic diet stopped progression of coronary atherosclerosis. Exercise should thus be adjunctive to modification of other risk factors with a well demonstrated influence on atherosclerosis. Miniature-swine studies show that myocardial ischemia is a necessary stimulus for the development of collateral vessels, but exercise appears to enhance their development. Atherosclerotic lesions are present in coronary arteries enlarged by exercise, but are less of a threat to the myocardium.

In young humans, cross-sectional and longitudinal training studies commonly show increased ventricular mass, wall thickness, volume, and function. However, increases in left-ventricular mass may not occur in younger subjects unless high levels of exercise are used and may not occur at all in older subjects. In cardiac patients, most exercise studies have not altered the double product (i.e., heart rate times systolic blood pressure) at which ischemia occurs, although thallium scintigraphy has revealed improvement in angina patients after training.

An association between the level of physical activity and degree of atherosclerosis has not been demonstrated. Prospective studies assessing physical activity and fitness support the hypothesis that regular exercise can decrease the risk of cardiac events and help reduce other risk factors.

In patients with established ischemic heart disease, an exercise program can result in the hemodynamic changes of training. However, whether cardiac changes can occur is controversial. Though more dramatic beneficial changes have been associated with training at 85% of maximal oxygen uptake, this prescription is also associated with a higher rate of cardiac complications.

Imaging techniques, such as positron emission tomography, magnetic resonance imaging, and computer angiographic tomography offer promise for documenting cardiac adaptations to exercise training. The most significant changes in myocardial function will likely occur during exercise. Consequently, imaging techniques that can be applied during exercise hold the greatest promise for increasing our knowledge about exercise adaptations.

Hypertension

Individuals with essential hypertension can decrease their resting systolic and diastolic blood pressures by approximately 10 mmHg through regular endurance exercise. Thus, endurance training should be recommended as an important component in the nonpharmacological management of moderate essential hypertension (pressures 140/90 to 160/105 mmHg). Individuals with more marked elevations in blood pressure (>160/105 mmHg) should add exercise to their treatment regimen only after initiating pharmacologic therapy to lower their pressures. In such patients, exercise training may well reduce their blood pressure further, allowing a decrease of antihypertensive medication.

Moderate-intensity exercise training (40% to 60% of VO_2max) may be as efficacious in correcting borderline hypertension as is higher-intensity training. Moderate exercise may be particularly applicable to the elderly and those with orthopedic conditions. Individuals with low body mass, those with high diastolic blood pressures, and women may show greater decreases in both systolic and diastolic blood pressures with exercise training. However, regular endurance exercise induces some reduction of resting blood pressures in individuals of all ages. The systemic hemodynamic changes, and any neurohumoral mechanisms underlying such reductions in blood pressure, remain unclear.

The acute blood pressure lowering effects of single bouts of submaximal endurance exercise needs further study. Other nonpharmacological interventions, such as weight loss, behavioral modification, diet, and drug therapy, must also be investigated to assess potential synergistic, additive, or inhibitory interactions with exercise.

Diabetes Mellitus

Exercise should be recommended for the diabetic as for the nondiabetic, despite problems of glucose regulation. In the presence of insulin deficiency, exercise may result in hyperglycemia and ketosis, whereas in the presence of insulin excess, hypoglycemia may arise. Ketosis and hyperglycemia are indications to postpone exercise until effective treatment has been instituted.

In contrast to Type I diabetes, glucose regulation during exercise is not normally a problem in Type II diabetes, except for patients who are being treated with sulphanylurea medications.

Exercise has not been shown to improve long-term glycemic control in Type I diabetes mellitus. However, all Type I diabetic patients should be encouraged to participate in physical activity for the same reasons as the general population. A number of particular exercise-associated risks must be minimized for Type I diabetic patients. Long-term complications of diabetes mellitus include preproliferative retinopathy, autonomic neuropathy, hypertension, peripheral polyneuropathy and central and peripheral cardiovascular disease. These may all be relative or absolute contraindications to exercise.

Comprehensive educational programmes are needed for the diabetic patient. These should teach systematic blood glucose self-monitoring and autonomous self-therapy, including alterations of insulin dosage and carbohydrate intake appropriate for exercise. Only patients who have learned responsible self-management will be able to avoid exercise-induced hypoglycemia (or ketosis) and to perform at optimal levels in competitive sports and games.

Exercise is expected to improve insulin sensitivity and thus forms a major component of rational therapy in Type II diabetes mellitus. Along with hypocaloric diets, exercise should improve glycemic control in Type II patients. While such benefits may be anticipated in young and middle-aged hyperinsulinemic Type II diabetic patients, there is a need to weigh the particular efficacy of exercise against its risks at all ages. Physical exertion presents particular risks in elderly patients with a high prevalence of cardiovascular disease and orthopedic degenerative problems. Such risks must be minimized in relation to potential benefits.

Newly applied methodologies include Nuclear Magnetic Resonance Spectroscopy, modeling of C-peptide data to measure the rates of insulin secretion and the modification of tracer techniques to monitor changes in metabolic fluxes at the onset of exercise. Outstanding issues include the explanation of discrepancies between in vitro and in vivo observations on the role of insulin in regulating glucose uptake, the localization of acute and chronic effects of insulin to receptor and postreceptor sites, and the determination of the possible regulatory role of a variety of neuropeptides. More epidemiological studies are also necessary, examining the role of exercise as an adjunct to other forms of treatment and as a possible method of alleviating diabetic complications.

Obesity

Energy expenditure includes such components as basal metabolism, the thermic effects of food, the energy cost of exercise, and the level of habitual physical activity. The obese are generally less physically active than nonobese individuals. Basal metabolic rate is related to body mass, particularly the fat-free mass. Since body mass and probably fat-free mass are greater in the obese, the obese expend more energy at rest than the nonobese. With improved methods of measuring energy expenditure in free-living individuals, further research on the relationship between energy expenditure and obesity is required.

Skeletal muscle tissue from obese and lean individuals shows similar adaptations during physical training. An increase in habitual physical activity is usually associated with a decrease of body fat in moderately obese individuals. An acute bout of physical activity in an obese individual lowers insulin levels and improves glucose tolerance for a few days.

Chronic physical activity leading to a decrease of body mass in obese individuals is associated with increased insulin sensitivity and improved glucose tolerance. High-density-lipoprotein cholesterol is lower in obese individuals. Although exercise training increases HDL cholesterol in nonobese individuals, the effect of exercise is less clear in the obese.

Further research is needed to explore differences in the response of hypertrophic and hyperplastic obese individuals to regular exercise and to explain the differences observed in fat loss; to determine mechanisms for differences in the thermic effect of food and its interaction with exercise in the obese; to understand why exercise in obese individuals may not increase blood HDL cholesterol; to explain mechanisms which limit the decrease

in fat-cell size with training; and to increase our understanding of the ways in which exercise can be used effectively as a part of treatment for obesity.

Pulmonary Diseases

Exercise limitation in chronic airflow obstruction is mainly due to dyspnea, but in some patients leg-muscle fatigue or a cardiac impairment may be important. A number of factors contribute to dyspnea: increased ventilatory demands, airflow limitation, and reduced respiratory muscle strength.

Mechanisms contributing to exercise limitation are best assessed by physiological measurements and quantifying dyspnea *during* exercise.

Exercise rehabilitation programmes in pulmonary patients need to be designed in concert with optimal management of airflow obstruction, and in relation to the activities of daily living. Supplemental O_2 may play a useful role in some hypoxemic patients. Exercise rehabilitation programmes can reduce disability and handicap.

Assessment may thus be considered in terms of impairment, disability, and handicap where: a) impairment refers to reductions in pulmonary function expressed in relation to normal standards; b) disability is defined in terms of reductions in functional exercise capacity, again expressed in terms of normal standards; and c) handicap describes the impact of impairment and disability on the subject's quality of life (expectations versus capabilities).

Asthma is a common condition which can impair exercise performance. Asthmatics have hyperreactive airways which constrict in response to various stimuli, including exercise. This occurs especially when the air is cold and/or dry. Most patients with exercise-induced asthma will respond to specific treatment used prophylactically, thereby allowing them to take part in recreational and competitive activities.

Aerobic training induces an increase in exercise performance of asthmatics. However, data are conflicting regarding its effect on reducing the incidence and severity of exercise-induced asthma.

Osteoarthritis

Careful review indicates that the perceived association between athletic training and subsequent osteoarthritis is due to either thematic injury or joint malalignment. To avoid inducing osteoarthritis, exercise programs should therefore stress safety. The person with established osteoarthritis should avoid large or abrupt forces on the affected joints because these could further damage subchondral bone and cause pain. Nevertheless, immobilization and overuse are both detrimental, while moderate non-weight-bearing activity may be beneficial for the patient with osteoarthritis. Further research, both clinical and population based, is needed to quantify an appropriate amount of exercise. In addition, participants in exercise programs should avoid extreme fatigue, as such a state may lead to joint injury and subsequent development of clinical osteoarthritis to the disease process.

Osteoporosis

The mechanical function of the skeleton is to provide protection for vital organs and a framework for mobility. Mechanical force, through gravity and muscle pull, is a major factor in maintaining or increasing bone mass and bone strength. The calcium-regulating hormones may cause bone resorption in their function of maintaining calcium homeostasis.

The skeleton is a living tissue, constantly undergoing repair and restructuring through the action of bone cells. In general, maximum bone mass is achieved during the third or fourth decade of life, and a gradual loss of bone mass occurs in subsequent decades. The maximum level of bone mass and the subsequent rate of bone loss depend, at least in part, on the level of habitual physical activity. Physically active individuals generally have greater bone mass than more sedentary individuals. Conversely, immobilization and bed rest result in profound bone loss. In experimental animals, bone loss caused by immobilization can be prevented by the daily application of intermittent compression forces. The mass of bone thus produced is proportional to the magnitude of the force that is applied regularly. In humans, maintenance of a high physical activity level may be an effective means of attenuating age-related bone loss.

Profound loss of bone mass and bone strength, or osteoporosis, is a common problem of elderly people. This can cause recurrent fractures with application of little or no abnormal force. Many diseases and some drugs can cause osteoporosis, but in most cases, no underlying cause can be identified. In addition to genetic predisposition, osteoporosis has been attributed to such factors as age, a decrease in female sex hormones at menopause,

suboptimal nutrition, and a sedentary lifestyle.

Physical activity is important both for the prevention of osteoporosis and for the rehabilitation of the osteoporotic patient. However, more research is required to establish optimal exercise programs that are attractive as well as beneficial, programs that avoid the possible deleterious effects of fatigue, starvation diets, or altered sex hormone activity. Prevention of osteoporosis also requires attention to overall good health.

Back Pain

Major human suffering and economic costs accompany back pain. Costs are concentrated in the relatively small group of individuals who suffer chronic back pain. The greatest impact on the problem can thus be made by preventing chronic back pain.

The detrimental effect of immobilization is clear for all the structures of the back. Both experimental and clinical evidence suggest the beneficial effect of graded physical activity. The therapeutic response is facilitated by associated behavioral approaches. Perceived disability may be lessened by changing monotonous and taxing work, while paying more attention to the overall psychological well-being of workers.

When a pathologic problem is proven and has been treated surgically or medically, physical activity rather than rest and deconditioning should be incorporated into the rehabilitation process. Supervised physical rehabilitation, based on a simple quantification of function, should become a standard approach. However, conclusive studies supporting the preventive value of physical activity or fitness have yet to be reported.

Immune Function and Infection

Biologic roles of the immune system include the protection of the host from infectious and neoplastic disorders. The role of exercise and training in influencing the adaptation of this response has yet to be clearly defined. Acute exercise seems an influential variable that modulates the immune response, with changes in: the trafficking of immunocompetent cells, immunologic functions of lymphocytes, and release of lymphokines. These immunologic adaptations are modest in degree and brief in duration.

Training induces immunologic adaptations that persist even in the resting state. These adaptations are heterogeneous, but also modest in degree and of unclear clinical significance. There is no clinical evidence that the immunologic adaptation to either exercise or training modifies host defences against infectious diseases.

In vitro assays demonstrate that exercise affects host defence mechanisms, including granulocyte count, lymphocyte count and function, cytotoxicity, cytokine production, and secretory immunoglobulin concentrations. However, changes are small in magnitude, last only a few hours, and their biologic significance is uncertain. Observations have generally not been controlled for confounding variables such as psychologic stress, nutrition, and energy expenditure. Little is known about the influence of exercise, training, or "overtraining" on susceptibility to infection. There is a need for carefully designed clinical trials investigating the effects of exercise and training on the host response to infectious disease. This should include in vitro and in vivo testing of immunologic responsiveness, as well as a careful clinical assessment.

Although bed rest has been prescribed more often than necessary in people with hepatitis and mononucleosis, extreme exertion and contact sports should be avoided until recovery from these conditions. Patients with mild upper-respiratory infections, on the other hand, need not restrict their exercise schedules. Patients with lower-respiratory infections and those with fevers and myalgias suggesting a systemic infection should avoid strenuous exertion until recovery.

Cancer

Epidemiologic studies suggest a lower risk of colon cancer in physically active individuals. The mechanisms of this potential protective effect are unknown, although decreased intestinal transit time and/or lifestyle alterations such as differences in dietary fiber may be involved.

Epidemiologic evidence also suggests a lower risk of cancers of the breast and reproductive tract in physically active women, and hormonal mechanisms for the finding have been proposed. Further studies are needed to confirm this observation. Exercise is unlikely to induce remissions in patients with established cancer, but it may improve their quality of life.

Recovery from Surgery, Disease, or Trauma

The limb muscles lose strength after abdominal surgery. The loss of function appears to be greater than can be explained by bed rest alone.

The functional capacity of many elderly patients is so low that it is highly desirable to prevent any further reduction of fitness. In younger patients, endurance training before surgery prevents the postoperative functional capacity from dropping below the initial pretraining level. This points to a need for studies of preoperative training for elderly surgical patients.

Vascular surgery may be performed to improve exercise tolerance. Under such circumstances, postoperative endurance training improves functional capacity.

Risks of Engaging in Physical Activities

Exercise is associated with risks as well as benefits. Two important exercise-related risks are sudden cardiac events and musculoskeletal injuries. Sudden exercise-related cardiac death is a very rare event. Exercise-related musculoskeletal injuries often requiring medical attention are common. They result, on occasion, in severe disability.

Sudden Death

Epidemiologic studies on men have demonstrated that the risk of sudden cardiac death is transiently increased during vigorous exercise. The increase in risk during a given bout of exercise is less for men who exercise regularly than for men who are less active. Men with prior clinical ischemic heart disease are at increased risk for exercise-related sudden cardiac death. The net effect of habitual vigorous exercise by symptom-free men is to reduce the overall risk of sudden cardiac death. The incidence of sudden cardiac death is much lower for women than for men. Although data are lacking, the same benefits of endurance training reported for men seem likely to apply to women.

Additional research is needed to identify potential predictors of exercise-related sudden cardiac death and to determine if other factors alter the transient increase in risk of sudden cardiac death during exercise.

Musculoskeletal and Other Injuries

Individuals who participate in either exercise or sport have a high likelihood of being injured. In North America and elsewhere, millions of people experience sports-related injuries each year. The vast majority of these injuries are mild and occur in young men.

The most severe sports-related injuries occur in contact-type sports. Many of these injuries can be prevented with adequate equipment and training. The most common sports injuries arise from overuse, related to very frequent and intense training and competition.

Growing bones are particularly vulnerable to injury. Of special concern are the apparently causal relationships between children performing selected movements and an increased incidence of musculoskeletal injuries. For example, repeated hyperextension of the back and excessive impact on the long bones and growth plates are potentially injurious. The lack of adequate data underscores the need for definitive longitudinal studies and prudent public policy.

A few epidemiologic studies have estimated the risks of exercise-related musculoskeletal injuries. Running-related musculoskeletal injuries are directly related to the distance run per week and occur with equal frequency in both sexes at all ages. Among participants in aerobic dance, prior orthopedic injuries or a lack of participation in other sports are associated with an increased risk of exercise-related musculoskeletal injuries. For most commonly performed types of aerobic exercise, estimates of the incidence of musculoskeletal injuries are still required.

Factors that alter the risk of exercise-related musculoskeletal injuries also need further examination. A priority area of research should be the immediate risks of changing exercise levels.

Heredity, Lifestyle, and Environment

Heredity, Fitness, and Health

Health is the culmination of many interacting factors, including our genetic constitution. Humans are quite diverse in their response to life events, but pay a price for this diversity. As a result of their genetic endowments, some individuals are unable to survive or thrive in particular environments as well as others. Given these circumstances, health must be relative. It cannot imply an equal state of physical and mental well-being for all, but it can imply achievement of the highest level of well-being consonant with a given individual's genetic potential.

Many genetic influences on health do not operate independently; they interact, i.e., they amplify or diminish the effects of one another. We are not all equally prone to become obese or diabetic, whatever our nutritional or exercise habits. Intervention to achieve better health must therefore take cognizance of these complexities. If a disease has a strong genetic component and is common, the best preventive strategy may be to change the general environment which is unmasking the genetic predisposition.

In the particular case of exercise and fitness, only a small fraction of the individual differences in the habitual level of physical activity is associated with genetic variation. In the case of physical and physiological fitness, the situation is more complex as many components are involved. A small-to-moderate genetic effect is generally reported for body fat and fat distribution, cardiorespiratory adaptation to submaximal exercise, submaximal power output, $\dot{V}O_2max$, glucose tolerance, and insulin sensitivity. Larger genetic effects are found for muscular strength, anaerobic capacities, blood pressures, and blood lipids and lipoproteins.

The most significant finding is undoubtedly that the genotype is responsible for much of the observed variation in response to regular exercise. For instance, the training response to aerobic training ranges from near-zero improvement to about a 1-fold increase in the initial $\dot{V}O_2max$. As much as 75% of individual differences in the response to training are associated with the genotype. The genotype also determines the adaptive response to regular exercise of other indicators of physical and physiological fitness. This situation makes it difficult to predict the exact benefits that a given individual may derive from regular exercise. These benefits are easier to identify for a group or population.

Lifestyle Components, Fitness, and Health

Lifestyle factors play an important role in the major disease problems of our time in the industrialized world: cardiovascular disease, cancer, chronic respiratory disease, motor vehicle crashes, chronic liver disease, and others. Thus, attention must be paid to lifestyle changes as a means of improving health. It is currently the most important way of extending longevity and of maintaining health through the years.

Exercise constitutes an important element of lifestyle that pertains to health, but is only one of several which are relevant. Others include eating behavior, sexual activity, use of alcohol, tobacco, and other drugs, motor vehicle driving. In fact, all behaviors, actions, and habits, as well as social relations, must be considered. Lifestyle is shaped and can be altered by changes in living circumstances, social influences on personal choices, and by individuals themselves.

We have to recognize the broad context in which exercise should be seen in relation to health. Efforts to improve fitness and health must include adequate and proper exercise as one healthful change of lifestyle. Exercise may also play an indirect role in smoking cessation, improved nutrition, addiction therapy, and other lifestyle improvements, although the evidence for this is still weak.

Environment, Fitness, and Health

Our ability to exercise is influenced to a marked degree by environmental conditions. The effects of temperature, ambient pressures, humidity, radiation, environmental contaminants, and gravity alter physiological responses to exercise and, in some instances, may produce specific health hazards.

Patterns of leisure-time physical activity are related to seasons. In societies in the northern hemisphere with wide annual temperature fluctuations, there is a pronounced increase in activity in May through August and a sharp drop in December through March. Activity is positively related to both mean daily temperature and hours of daylight. Participation in activity is also affected by geographic variations in climate, being highest on the temperate west coast of both Canada and the United States.

The ability to exercise in the face of acute environmental changes requires both behavioral and physiological adaptations. Physiological adjustments to cold and heat aim to maintain the internal milieu as close to normal as possible. In cold environments, homeostasis is accomplished by reducing the outer-core blood flow to maintain internal heat and also by generating more heat through shivering. In warm environments, the initial responses require increased skin blood flow to transfer heat from the core to the periphery and also to stimulate sweating, the most efficient heat-loss mechanism. Acclimatization occurs with continued exposure to a changed climate. Under extremely hot or cold conditions, exercise performance is reduced in spite of acclimatization.

Although performance levels are impaired, exercise can be performed at high altitudes as long as adequate acclimatization has occurred. Physiological adaptations optimize and improve the internal oxygen milieu, including increases of ventilation, increased erythrocyte production, and oxygen extraction.

Frostbite and hypothermia resulting from cold exposure and heat stroke, heat syncope, and hyperthermia resulting from heat stress are potentially fatal problems coincident with thermal stress. These problems are preventable through an understanding of basic physiological principles, an awareness of situations in which difficulties can occur, and preventive measures such as the use of appropriate clothing and maintenance of adequate hydration. Organizers and medical personnel of mass-participation events must be equipped and educated to respond to environmental medical emergencies on-site.

As more people engage in physical activity at unaccustomed elevations, altitude-related problems have become of more than theoretical interest. Acute mountain sickness, high-altitude pulmonary and cerebral edema are serious and potentially fatal conditions. Appropriate acclimatization can significantly reduce such risks.

Pollution of the environment with sulfur oxides, nitrogen oxides, particulate matter, ozone, and carbon monoxide can create specific health hazards, and may also impair exercise performance. Individuals, with increased airway reactivity or cardiopulmonary impairment are particularly susceptible to pollutants. Comprehension of situations in which air pollutants may constitute a health hazard and guidelines concerning unwise conditions for exercise or competition are currently required.

Health Status of the Participant Versus the Nonparticipant and the Fit Versus the Unfit

Physical activity can develop physical and physiological fitness. Lack of fitness can limit activity. Disease can reduce or destroy fitness and decrease or prevent activity. Activity leading to fitness can avoid or delay disease and disability, improve the quality of life, or even extend it.

Epidemiology began as a study of infectious diseases. Its application to chronic diseases such as coronary heart disease, and their relationships to physical activity, fitness, and survival, are quite a different matter. The problems are more complex, and most of the available evidence must be labeled as "circumstantial". The data concern frequencies and distributions of lifestyle elements versus morbidity and mortality patterns, all to be rated by probabilities and interpreted by logic and common sense. Nevertheless, the circumstantial evidence we have today about physical activity, physical fitness, and health is quite strong and has been gaining acceptance in the scientific and medical communities. It is also increasingly supported by more direct experimental behavioral, biological, and medical research.

The modern story of physical activity, fitness, and health began 35 years ago when the coronary heart disease risks of sedentary drivers and physically active conductors on London double-decked buses were contrasted. The conductors had significantly less coronary heart disease, what disease they had was less severe,and they were more likely to withstand an attack than the drivers. After checking and discarding many other explanations, it was concluded that the best explanation for the findings was a difference in energy expenditure on the job. In the United States, similar findings were obtained from a study of 6,000 San Francisco long-shoremen who had been followed for 22 years. Those who were cargo handlers did very heavy work. When tasks were translated into energy expenditure demands, the men in jobs requiring 35 MJ or more per week had much lower risks of fatal coronary heart disease than men who held physically less demanding jobs. Sudden-death heart attacks were less common among the cargo handlers, either because they had fewer heart attacks, or because they were better able to withstand one.

Although physical activity patterns seemed to be at somewhat lower levels, similar contrasts in risks were found among still larger study populations of middle-aged men who worked at sedentary jobs and obtained most of their physical exercise during their leisure time. Although many studies agree as to the inverse relationship between physical activity and health, investigators have disagreed concerning the influence of quantity versus intensity of the exercise required for optimum benefit. However, findings arenot necessarily contradictory. Discrepancies may be due to differences in definitions, classification and diagnostic criteria, and in the personal characteristics among study populations. Future studies should thus be designed to reconcile these observations. Nevertheless, the important point is that all large-scale investigations concur that adequate physical activity is essential to soundness of cardiovascular health. This view is being confirmed and extended by many other types of studies.

Studies of physical fitness also point in the same direction as the physical activity findings. However, studies of physical fitness should be broadened to cover other body systems as well as the cardiovascular system.

Controlling for the influence of physical activity is complicated because it may have a positive or beneficial influence upon other lifestyle components (e.g., cigarette smoking) whose influence is adverse. We need to determine the mechanisms by which physical activity promotes good health and longevity, whether by cardiovascular modifications, metabolic processes, or various other physiological and lifestyle considerations.

The rationale for a focus on physical activity and fitness stems from at least the following considerations: a) Physical activity is a natural requirement of the body. b) Physical fitnessis a continuum that describes the physiological state of the body, and determines its vitality or capacity to be active. c) History suggests that present sedentariness is a recent development, which may be at least partly responsible for such adverse health trends as the 20th-century "epidemic" of coronary heart disease. d) In "developed" countries, nearly two thirds of the population are habitually sedentary. e) Physical activity is a positive influence that tends to further positive health, and that counters an adverse lifestyle. f) A concomitant of sound health maintenance is likely to be an optimization of longevity, together with an enhancement of the quality of life. The concepts of activity and fitness are key determinants of whole-body, or total, health (i.e., physical, psychological, social, cultural, and spiritual well-being), helping to meet the life goals of both the individual and the community.

Costs and Benefits of Activity Versus Inactivity

Good health and the prevention of disease are basic human needs. Since substantial public resources are currently invested with the intention of satisfying these needs, cost-effectiveness analyses should be used to distinguish the merits of various health promotion tactics from traditional medical approaches. The prevention of disease is generally better than its cure in terms of reducing both social and economic costs.

Evidence suggests that regular physical activity may reduce the incidence and severity of chronic disease and perhaps extend the life span by a few years. Techniques for quality adjustment of the observed life span are in the early stages of development. However, gains in quality-adjusted life expectancy are likely to exceed any extension of absolute life span. Regular physical activity also contributes positively to mental health and to self-assessed health. The latter has been taken as a general indicator of health status.

Although it is difficult to obtain rigorous epidemiological evidence, it is likely that the industrial benefits from appropriate types of fitness programming include an enhancement of corporate image, an increase of worker satisfaction and productivity, a decrease of absenteeism and personnel turnover, and in some situations, a decrease of industrial injuries. In addition to an improvement of overall lifestyle, potential societal benefits of greater personal physical fitness may include a reduction in demands for acute and chronic medical services, lower indirect costs of illness, and less costly physical dependence during the retirement years.

There remain many gaps in our current understanding of costs and benefits of physical activity. Economic analyses have been complicated by a lack of consensus as to which exercise programmes are most effective in improving health. Issues include the marginal societal costs of implementing greater physical activity in target populations, the impact of exercise on the quality of life, long-term rates of participation in exercise programmes, and the impact of social changes upon these various statistics. Further information should be obtained from prospective controlled trials. However, current analyses suggest that exercise produces fiscal benefits which can outweigh immediate programme costs.

Appendix: Participants Involved in Developing the Consensus Document

Speakers:

P.O. Åstrand, Stockholm, Sweden
P. Björntorp, Göteborg, Sweden
M. Blanchet, Québec City, Québec
S.N. Blair, Dallas, Texas
G.A. Bray, Los Angeles, California
L. Breslow, Los Angeles, California
D.R. Brown, Oxford, Ohio
E.S. Buskirk, State College, Pennsylvania
L.H. Calabrese, Cleveland, Ohio
R.K. Dishman, Athens, Georgia
J.V.G.A. Durnin, Glasgow, Scotland

R. Edgerton, Los Angeles, California
J. Faulkner, Ann Arbor, Michigan
V.F. Froelicher, Long Beach, California
J. Hagberg, Gainesville, Florida
E.S. Horton, Burlington, Vermont
N.L. Jones, Hamilton, Ontario
R.M. Malina, Austin, Texas
A. Nachemson, Göteborg, Sweden
E.A. Newsholme, Oxford, England
R.S. Paffenbarger, Palo Alto, California
J.C. Prior, Vancouver, British Columbia
B. Saltin, Copenhagen, Denmark
J. Schull, Houston, Texas
R.J. Shephard, Toronto, Ontario
D.S. Siscovick, Seattle, Washington
J. Skinner, Tempe, Arizona
E.L. Smith, Madison, Wisconsin
J.R. Sutton, Hamilton, Ontario
C.M. Tipton, Tucson, Arizona
M. Vranic, Toronto, Ontario
P. Wood, Palo Alto, California
A. Young, London, England

Discussants and Other Invited Guests:

R. Andres, Baltimore, Maryland
O. Bar-Or, Hamilton, Ontario
B. Bigland-Ritchie, New Haven, Connecticut
M. Berger, Düsseldorf, Federal Republic of Germany
C. Bouchard, Ste-Foy, Québec
M. Chubb, East Lansing, Michigan
D. Cummings, Edmonton, Alberta
D. Cunningham, London, Ontario
J. Dempsey, Madison, Wisconsin
B. Drinkwater, Vashon, Washington
L. Folinsbee, Triangle Park, North Carolina
H. Galbo, Copenhagen, Denmark
P.E. Garfinkel, Toronto, Ontario
N. Gledhill, North York, Ontario
H. Green, Waterloo, Ontario
J. Harrison, Toronto, Ontario
F.W. Kemmer, Düsseldorf, Federal Republic of Germany
T. Mayer, Dallas, Texas
H.J. Montoye, Madison, Wisconsin
S. Moore, Montréal, Québec
B. Oakes, Melbourne, Australia
N. Oldridge, Milwaukee, Wisconsin
L. Oscai, Chicago, Illinois
A. Quinney, Edmonton, Alberta
P. Rechnitzer, London, Ontario
K. Sahlin, Stockholm, Sweden
W. Sime, Lincoln, Nebraska

H.B. Simon, Boston, Massachusetts
T. Stephens, Ottawa, Ontario
S. Walter, Hamilton, Ontario
B. Whipp, Torrance, California
T. White, Ann Arbor, Michigan

R.J. Shephard, Toronto, Ontario
T. Stephens, Ottawa, Ontario
J.R. Sutton, Hamilton, Ontario

Consensus Committee:

C. Bouchard, Ste-Foy, Québec
B.D. McPherson, Waterloo, Ontario

Chapter 2

Issues in 1966 Versus Issues in 1988

Per-Olof Åstrand

I was honored by the invitation to present the concluding remarks at the 1966 International Symposium on Physical Activity and Cardiovascular Health held in Toronto. This was a pleasure. It was a stimulating meeting from both a scientific and a social point of view. It was the first time I met the conditions of the deal that, unless you bring manuscripts, you do not get reimbursed for travel expenses. A staff of editors took the manuscripts and raised questions, and 4 months later the proceedings were in print (7)!

Now I have the privilege to speak at the opening session of this conference, and for a few minutes I am supposed to look into the rearview mirror.

Since 1966 there has been an impressive development of high-technology apparatus and methods. Thus, many publications related to exercise, fitness, and health are based on data made possible by the use of echocardiography, radionuclide cardiography, Doppler echocardiography, nuclear magnetic resonance imaging, computed tomography scanning, optoelectronic systems (e.g., the Selspot system) to study movements, and more sophisticated computer programs to analyze data (e.g., EMG and ECG), promoted by computers being more advanced but less expensive. Telemetric systems to relay signals without disturbing the subjects have been improved, and small, easy-to-carry recording systems have been developed.

In 1966 the human skeletal muscle biopsy had just been introduced. The classical study by Bergström and Hultman (2) in the proceedings (7, p. 719), in which each leg was exercised on a cycle ergometer, was presented in a figure illustrating a carbohydrate-loading procedure. The more elaborate studies related to diet and physical performance that followed this first step were reported as "to be published," and surely they were (1).

In 1966 there were, for evident reasons, no discussions of fiber types in human skeletal muscle or of the effects of training and deconditioning on its enzyme systems, capillary density, and myoglobin concentration. The biopsy technique initiated numerous investigations (9).

Apparatuses for the exact control of speed of movement when measuring maximal dynamic strength came later (e.g., Cybex). Cavagna's studies (3) of the storage of energy in the elastic components of the muscles were first published in the 1970s.

In 1966 there were no papers dealing with the relationships among exercise, fitness, and reproductive health (which now is an exciting issue) or with osteoporosis. Very little attention was devoted to exercise and the endocrine system. The terms *anabolic steroids* and *strength training* were not combined. The first report of the effect of so-called blood doping appeared in 1972. Actually, the original studies were conducted in our department (4). We have been told that such experiments should not be done! Our defense is that we were not paid by the Swedish Olympic Committee. We call it basic research.

Wasserman discussed the *anaerobic threshold*, a concept that has initiated many studies. There were questions raised about which factor or factors could limit maximal aerobic power. Today I think that we have the answer; that is, when large-muscle groups are involved it is the central circulation.

Refined techniques have been developed to diagnose and treat sports-related injuries, coronary artery diseases, and hypertension, to give three examples. Kannel presented data from the Framingham Study, and several papers were devoted to coronary heart disease (CHD). In my concluding remarks at the 1966 symposium I stated that I was personally convinced that habitual physical activity could reduce the risk of a coronary heart attack and that the chances of surviving a heart attack were statistically better in those who are active than in those who are sedentary. Studies on the relationship between physical activity and cardiovascular health are very difficult. However, I think I was too pessimistic when I thought that it might take 100 years for this final proof (see chapt. 3).

It should be emphasized that the epidemiological studies of blood cholesterol concentration as a risk factor for CHD in a way had to start all over again by the development of methods that make it possible to fractionate cholesterol compounds into subfractions, notably high-density lipoprotein (HDL), low-density lipoprotein (LDL), and very low density lipoprotein (VLDL). Endurance training can increase the capillary density in the skeletal muscles. The enzyme lipoprotein lipase is located in the capillary walls and has the potential to transfer triglycerides to HDL (and free fatty acids) and to release it into the plasma compartment, thereby increasing its HDL concentration.

With the development of more sophisticated equipment and methods, longitudinal studies have certainly become more complicated. How do we compare data sampled in 1966 with data obtained in 1988? One wants to apply the most modern apparatus available, as the methods in 1966 and 1988 may differ markedly.

In 1966 there was no mention of a topic that I find quite fascinating, namely, that oxygen, being a requisite for our survival, also has toxicological potentials. In aerobic metabolism there is a production of molecules that are intermediates in electrical charge between O_2 and H_2O. These intermediates, also named free oxygen radicals, include superoxide ion, hydroxyl radical, and derivates of these radicals such as H_2O_2 and singlet oxygen. They can elicit lipid peroxidation, enzyme inactivation, denaturation of proteins, and structural changes in nucleic acids. A particular problem is that the oxidizing free radicals apparently can damage membranes by lipid peroxidation mediated by some sort of chain reactions. During evolution, living organisms had to develop adequate antioxidant defenses to combat the destructive capability of these oxygen radicals. Thus aerobic cells, such as muscle fibers, have been equipped with enzymes and nonenzymatic scavenger systems against these radicals (there are antioxidants like peroxidases, catalases, and superoxide dismutases; the other line of defense is to bring oxygen to carriers such as hemoglobin, myoglobin, and cytochrome P-450).

There are speculations that physically very active individuals would also be more exposed to the destructive tendency of oxygen. Cytochrome oxidase, which is responsible for most of the biological oxygen consumption, produces water without the release of intermediates. In other words, there is not a proportional increase in the production of free oxygen radicals with an increase in the body's oxygen uptake. There are also reports about an adaptive increase in the biosynthesis of the scavenger superoxide dismutases with an increasing metabolic rate and therefore production of free radicals (5, p. 263). Salminen and Vihko (8) report that endurance training of a mouse increased the resistance of skeletal muscles to injuries caused by lipid peroxidation. It may also be a question of an efficient replacement of damaged molecules by resynthesis.

From a nutritional viewpoint it should be pointed out that selenium is a cofactor for glutathione peroxidase (which is an effective scavenger of singlet oxygen and which protects lipids) and that vitamin C can be an antioxidant.

"Oxygen possesses a good Dr. Jekyll-evil Mr. Hyde personality" (5, p. 386). The overall picture we get is the Dr. Jekyll aspect that an increased whole-body metabolism (and thereby oxygen consumption) by regular physical activity is essential for optimal body function. Now I am curious whether there will be any discussion of free oxygen radicals during this conference.

For a physiologist it is a pleasure to quote Starling: "The physiology of today is the medicine of tomorrow." Physiologists constitute one scientific group that should use the most advanced technology to understand normal function of living systems and mechanisms of diseases. Studying the normal human individual provides an important baseline for the study of disease. There is a definite trend toward the new scientific frontiers (e.g., molecular biology, genetics, immunology, developmental biology, and the neurosciences) dominating both research and teaching much more now than 22 years ago. It is, however, the responsibility of physiologists to put together the lifeless pieces of molecular and cellular biology into living systems. Morgan, a past president of the American Physiological Society, emphasizes that

the research approach that is taken should not impact on the ability of the physiologist to teach a broad-based course in human physiology to medical students. Those physiologists who work at the systems level must be fully aware of advances at the cellular and molecular level, whereas those who work on molecular mechanisms must be able to integrate their data into a model of systemic function (6, p. 325).

In my opinion exercise physiology from these viewpoints is particularly important because an exercise situation in various environments gives the unique possibility of studying how different functions are regulated and integrated. In fact, most functions and structures are in some way affected by acute and chronic (i.e., in a training program) exercises. Therefore, exercise physiology is to a high degree an integrated science whose goal is to reveal the mechanisms of overall bodily function and its regulation. Therefore, meetings like that held in 1966 and the one today, which includes almost all aspects of exercise, are very important.

It is regrettable that so few pages in standard textbooks in physiology are devoted to discussions of the effects of exercise on different functions and structures, and the past 22 years have hardly improved the situation. That may explain why most physicians do not recommend regular physical activity!

I list here some journals related to sports medicine that appeared after 1966: *Canadian Journal of Applied Sports Science, International Journal of Sports Medicine, Medicine and Science in Sports Medicine and Exercise, Physical Fitness/Sports Medicine, Scandinavian Journal of Sports Medicine,* and *Sports Medicine.* I hope we will find the time also to read classical periodicals such as *Science, Nature, Journal of Physiology, American Journal of Physiology,* and *Journal of Applied Physiology* as well as basic journals in various specialties.

Scientifically well supported arguments were presented at the 1966 conference for a lifestyle that included habitual physical activity. I am convinced that this conference will strengthen the arguments and elucidate a more holistic view of an optimal lifestyle. Considering the dramatic increase in the population of older individuals, key issues are the extent to which impairment, morbidity, and mortality are inevitable consequences of an individual's genetic composition (i.e., to intrinsic factors) and the extent to which environment and the individual's lifestyle pattern (i.e., extrinsic factors) can modify these processes. I am sure that some thought and discussion will be devoted to this question at this conference.

We are all looking forward to tonight's lecture and to an exciting week.

References

1. Bergström, J., L. Hermansen, E. Hultman, and B. Saltin. Diet, muscle glycogen and physical performance. *Acta Physiol. Scand.* 71: 140-150, 1967.

2. Bergström, J., and E. Hultman. Muscle glycogen synthesis after exercise: An enhancing factor localized to the muscle cell in man. *Nature* 210: 309-310, 1966.

3. Cavagna, G.A., L. Komarek, and S. Mazzoleni. The mechanics of sprint running. *J. Physiol.* 217: 709-722, 1971.

4. Ekblom, B., A.N. Goldberg, and B. Gullbring. Response to exercise after blood loss and reinfusion. *J. Appl. Physiol.* 33: 175-180, 1972.

5. Gilbert, D.L., ed. *Oxygen and living processes: An interdisciplinary approach.* New York: Springer-Verlag, 1981.

6. Morgan, H.E. The American Physiological Society in its centenary year. *Physiol. Rev.* 67: 325-328, 1987.

7. Proceedings of the International Symposium of Physical Activity and Cardiovascular Health. *Can. Med. Assoc. J.* 96(12): 693-915, 1967.

8. Salminen, A., and V. Vihko. Endurance training reduces the susceptibility of mouse skeletal muscle to lipid peroxidation in vitro. *Acta Physiol. Scand.* 117: 109-114, 1983.

9. Saltin, B., and P.D. Gollnick. Skeletal muscle adaptability: Significance for metabolism and performance. In: Peachey, L.D., R.H. Adrian, and S.R. Geiger, eds. *Handbook of physiology: Skeletal muscle.* Baltimore: Williams & Wilkins, 1983, pp. 555-631.

Chapter 3

Physical Activity and Physical Fitness as Determinants of Health and Longevity

Ralph S. Paffenbarger, Jr.
Robert T. Hyde
Alvin L. Wing

The importance of leisure-time physical activity in sedentary populations has become well recognized, and many lifestyles are being modified by fashion or by professional advice to include frequent sessions of exercise. This social trend has led to a surge of interest in developing more specific knowledge about the various influences of physical activity or exercise on fitness and health. The interrelationships among exercise, fitness, and health and their opposites can be represented by a series of ratios:

$$\frac{\text{Active}}{\text{Sedentary}} : \frac{\text{Fit}}{\text{Unfit}} : \frac{\text{Healthy}}{\text{Diseased}} : \frac{\text{Long-lived}}{\text{Short-lived}}$$

Both above and below the line, the progression of these characterizations is a cause-and-effect sequence leading to either desired or unfavorable results. Surely the desired results are improved quality of life and longevity in terms of both individual and community health, but the requirements for promoting these are not yet well understood. Even the basic definitions of exercise, fitness, and health are still subject to discussion and debate, revealing that their interrelationships are indeed complex.

Some approaches have defined *physical activity* or *exercise* as bodily movement accomplished by muscle power and the expenditure of energy. Fitness is then taken to be a set of attributes that represent the capacity to perform the physical activity. Health is not merely the presence or absence of disease; rather, it is a continuum that represents all levels of bodily vitality from the highest end point to the lowest end point, which is death. But levels of physical activity and fitness, as well as life and longevity (the postponement, not avoidance, of death), also extend over a considerable range, and this seems to parallel in many respects the concept of health as a continuum.

Furthermore, when we look at this pattern of ratios more closely, we see other paths of influence besides the cause-and-effect mainline from beginning to end. Activity can develop fitness. Lack of fitness can limit activity. Disease can reduce or destroy fitness and alter or deny activity. Activity leading to fitness can avoid or delay disease and disability and improve the quality of life or even extend it. These patterns reveal the complexity of the total picture, which often requires epidemiological methods for its assessment and interpretation.

Epidemiological Evidence

Epidemiology began as a search for the causes and means of the spread of infectious diseases. Its applications to chronic diseases such as coronary heart disease (CHD) and their relationships to physical activity and fitness and survival are quite a different matter. From some points of view most of the best evidence we have has been labeled circumstantial. Nevertheless, the circumstantial evidence we have today about physical activity, fitness, and health is quite strong and has gained respect. The data concern frequencies and distributions of lifestyle elements versus morbidity and mortality patterns, all of which are rated by probabilities and interpreted by logic and common sense. There is something to be said for this approach. If the scientific method is "trial and error," the legal method would be "error and trial" and the epidemiological method "playing the odds" or "considering the numbers." All three methods must rely on one basic concept—that of *probable cause*—and this term is used in all of them.

In this chapter, we consider three groups of studies that deal with physical activity, physical fitness, and longevity. They relate mostly to CHD because more work has been done in that area and because CHD in the Western world is the foremost cause of premature death. We examine the fortunes and misfortunes of exercisers and nonexercisers and of the fit and the unfit, that is, their status in health and disease and their longevity or premature death.

Occupational Physical Activity and CHD

The modern story of exercise and CHD begins with Professor Jeremy N. Morris of London, who, in 1953 with his colleagues, contrasted the CHD risks of thousands of sedentary drivers and physically active conductors on the double-deck buses in that city (12, 16, 17). The conductors had significantly less CHD, what disease they had was less severe, and they were more likely to withstand an attack than were the drivers. Morris et al. checked and discarded many other explanations before concluding that this was due to differences in energy expenditure on the job. Today we would conclude also that the conductors were physically more fit than were the drivers.

In the United States we obtained similar findings from a study of 6,351 San Francisco longshoremen, whom we followed for 22 yr, from 1951 through 1972 (1a, 19, 24). Those who were cargo handlers did very heavy work loading and unloading shipments in the holds of big oceangoing vessels—pulling, pushing, shoving, lifting, heaving, and shoveling, mostly by might and main. When these tasks were translated into their energy expenditure demands, the men in jobs requiring 8,500 kcal or more per week were found to have much lower risks of fatal CHD than were men who held less demanding jobs, such as tally clerks, hoist operators, and foremen. Sudden-death heart attacks were less common among the cargo handlers either because they had fewer heart attacks or because they were better able to withstand them.

Because all longshoremen had to begin as cargo handlers and serve at least 5 yr doing that heavy work (the average was 13 yr), even those who became clerks must have been fit already. Individual job tasks were assessed by ergometer tests, and blood pressures and other physiological parameters of fitness were obtained by a multiphase screening at the start of the study in 1951. Some aspects of their total fitness presumably were modified by their socioeconomic status, cigarette smoking, and other lifestyle elements, but their highly vigorous physical activities on the job were undoubtedly responsible for their lower risks of fatal CHD. These patterns held at all ages and with or without other characteristics known to influence CHD risk.

Leisure-Time Physical Activity and CHD

Similar contrasts in CHD risk were found among still larger study populations of middle-aged men who worked at sedentary jobs and obtained most of their physical exercise during their leisure time, although their physical activity patterns represented somewhat lower levels of energy output. Morris et al. (13, 14) studied the lifestyles and health records of 17,944 British civil servants whose deskwork assignments deprived them of virtually any vigorous physical activity on the job. Most may have been rather less fit than were the San Francisco longshoremen. But some of these Britishers were habitually brisk about their household duties, gardening, and recreational sports play after work and on holidays. Those who enjoyed vigorous yard work, hiking, running, and sturdy games had a CHD incidence half as high as that of their fellow workers who were less active in their leisure time.

Morris and his colleagues became interested in a number of epidemiological issues relating to the assessment of physical activity and fitness and their influences on CHD risk. In this study population the strongest evidence of a protective effect pointed to intensity of exercise rather than totals of all physical activity whether light or strenuous. The top deck of Table 3.1 shows that relative risks of CHD dropped significantly as levels of vigorous sports play increased among the British civil servants. Men reporting eight or more sports-play episodes in 4 wk (or at least twice a week) had only 36% the CHD risk of men who played no sports at all.

Morris et al. concluded (10, 11) that the aerobic or cardiovascular benefits of vigorous endurance-type sports play, likely to require 7.5 kcal $\cdot$ min^{-1} or more were responsible for the lower risk of CHD. These findings persisted when they tested

Table 3.1 Relative Risks of Coronary Heart Disease (CHD) by Gradients of Physical Activity

	Episodes of vigorous sports play in past 4 wk	CHD rate per 100 men[a]			Relative risk of CHD		
		Fatal	Nonfatal	Total	Fatal	Nonfatal	Total
British civil servants;	0	2.6	3.7	6.3	1.00	1.00	1.00
7,820 men aged 45-59 at	1-3	1.4	3.7	5.1	0.54	1.00	0.81
entry; 9 or more yr of	4-7	1.0	2.5	3.6	0.38	0.68	0.57
follow-up, 1976-1985	8+	0.7	1.3	2.0	0.27	0.35	0.32

	Tertiles of leisure-time physical activity in kcal/d	No. CHD cases	CHD rate per 1,000 men[b]	Relative risk of CHD
Multiple Risk Factor Intervention	Low	286	71.8	1.00
Trial; 12,138 men aged 35-57 at	Moderate	260	63.5	0.88
entry; 8 yr of follow-up (7 yr	High	235	58.0	0.81
average), 1973-1981				

	Study subjects[c]	No. subjects	Relative risk of CHD by regular exercise in years of play				
			None	< 5	5-10	11+	Any
Residents of Auckland, New Zealand; Caucasian	**Men**						
men and women aged 35-64; case-control study	Controls	653					
of nonfatal myocardial infarction and sudden	MI	363	1.0	1.2	0.5	0.2	0.4
death (within 24 hr) from CHD, 1981-1982	Sudden death	130	1.0	1.9	0.5	0.1	0.4
	Women						
	Controls	390					
	MI	100	1.0	0.9	0.7	0.2	0.1
	Sudden death	32	1.0	—	—	0.2	0.1

	Physical activity index in kcal/wk	Worker-years of observation (worker-years)	No. CHD cases	CHD rate per 1,000 worker-years[d]	Relative risk of CHD
Harvard alumni; 16,936	< 2,000	56,459	307	5.8	1.00
men aged 35-74 at entry;	2,000+	38,027	122	3.5	0.61
10-yr follow-up for					
nonfatal and fatal CHD,					
1962-1972					

[a]Adjusted for age differences; $p = 0.03$.

[b]Adjusted for age differences; $p < 0.01$.

[c]Age matched.

[d]Adjusted for differences in age, cigarette habit, and blood pressure status; $p < 0.01$.

several different methods of assessing total physical activity and intensity of energy output. Style or kind of exercise seemed important in that vigorous sports play, especially endurance-type, large-muscle exercise, was more beneficial than was heavy work (such as gardening) per se. Fitness assessments such as skinfold tests and electrocardio-grams were of some indicative value but were less impressive than was the inverse relationship of vigorous habitual exercise to CHD risk.

Corroborative trends were also noted in energy and weight studies of a subgroup of these British men, as the most active men consumed more calories yet weighed less than did their counter-parts who were less active. Also, a gradient effect was seen across the three activity-level subsets in the study. These observations were interpreted to signify that the differences in physical activity representing types and amounts of vigorous sports play were important enough to influence risks of CHD apparently because of their presumed effects on cardiovascular fitness, body composition or weight, and perhaps muscularity and other aspects of total fitness. Metabolic fitness tests, such as those for serum cholesterol, failed to predict CHD risk in this British study. It is unknown whether differences in diet, smoking, or other lifestyle ele-ments may have masked or confounded any in-fluences of serum cholesterol level.

The second deck in Table 3.1 shows incidence rates of CHD among 12,138 middle-aged men dur-ing a 7-yr follow-up in the Multiple Risk Factor In-tervention Trial (MRFIT) reported by Leon et al. (8). When classified into tertiles by their levels of leisure-time physical activity in kilocalories per day, the middle group was more than twice as ac-tive as was the low group, and the high group was more than twice as active as was the middle group. A consistent gradient of benefit against CHD is seen across the three physical activity tertiles of the MRFIT population. Their range of activity in kilocalories per week was similar to that of the Har-vard University alumni summarized in the bottom deck of Table 3.1. As is discussed later, a number of fitness observations were also reported for the MRFIT men.

In a case control study, summarized in the third deck of Table 3.1, Scragg et al. (30) found that risks of myocardial infarction and sudden death were progressively reduced in New Zealand men and women aged 35-64 who habitually had engaged in vigorous sports play or exercise (such as running) for at least 5 yr, after which their relative risk dropped to half that of nonexercisers as the 10-yr mark was passed. After additional years the risks were 0.20 or less for both men and women. The longer intervals seem to imply that the exercise had become a well-established habit and had been sufficient to maintain cardiovascular fitness at a protective level.

In the United States we studied large cohorts of Harvard University alumni, some of whom had been varsity athletes in college, some players of intramural sports, and some physically inactive during their student days (23, 25). The investiga-tions showed that the physical activity habits of the alumni, not their athletic histories as students, influenced their middle-age patterns of CHD risk. Here again was an inverse relationship between middle-age physical activity level and CHD. The consistent parallelisms of the findings as to physi-cal activity and CHD in all the diverse study popu-lations described here have been corroborated further by prior and subsequent studies in other populations (2, 4, 6, 7, 28, 29). Although this evi-dence of cause and effect must be considered cir-cumstantial, it is quite strong, and by now most of it has been accepted as valid and important.

The 16,936 Harvard alumni aged 35-74 at entry were followed for 10 or 16 yr for CHD and other morbidity and mortality. Their exercise status was expressed by a physical activity index in kilo-calories per week compiled from their habitual walking, stair climbing, and leisure-time sports play and similar activities. About 40% had an in-dex of 2,000 kcal per week or more, and their rela-tive risk of developing CHD during the 10-yr follow-up interval (Table 3.1, bottom deck) was 39% lower than the CHD risk for less active men (i.e., those with an index of less than 2,000 kcal per week).

Although many studies (4) agree as to the in-verse relationship of physical activity and CHD, the findings have varied concerning the influence of quantity versus intensity of the exercise required for optimum benefit. In contrast to the experience of the Harvard alumni, the MRFIT study showed little or no added benefit for exercising beyond a moderate level. However, the MRFIT study popu-lation was selected as middle-aged men at pre-sumed high risk of CHD, and their participation in vigorous physical activity or sports play was much less prevalent than it was among the Har-vard alumni. Both of these studies contrast with the experience of the British civil servants, whose CHD risk was lowered only if their physical activity included vigorous sports play. However, the respective findings from these three studies are not necessarily contradictory. To a considerable ex-tent their departures are likely to be accounted for by confounding due to differences both in defini-tions, classification, and diagnostic criteria and in personal characteristics among study populations. The important point here is that all these substantial, large-scale investigations concur that adequate physical activity is essential to soundness of cardiovascular health, and this view is being confirmed and extended by many other studies.

Although the advantage of continuing adequate exercise to cardiovascular health was consistent over a broad range of ages and life experiences among the Harvard alumni, this advantage was enhanced by including vigorous activity in regular exercise programs (Figure 3.1A). Of the alumni who expended 2,000 or more kcal per week, 89% participated in active sports play of some kind and 67% in vigorous sports play. Corresponding figures for men who expended less than 2,000 kcal per week were 30% and 20%. Men participating in vigorous sports play who expended 1,000 kcal or more per week in walking, stair climbing, and other light activities had less than half (relative risk = 0.42) the CHD incidence of their nonvigorous, mostly sedentary classmates, who expended less than 500 kcal per week in such activities. A gradient response of declining disease incidence was evident with increasing energy expenditure.

The saving effect of current exercise of low-level intensity is increased by vigorous sports play (Figure 3.1B). In a multiple logistic regression analysis that adjusted for differences in age and the alternate type of activity, each curve showed

a significant reduction in CHD incidence as energy output increased. At any point along the scale of physical activity in kilocalories per week, the extra benefit attached to playing vigorous sports was gained even though total energy expenditure was not increased. The advantage for vigorous over more moderate activities was appreciable (p = 0.019) and might have shown a parallel in fitness assessments if they had been available for study.

Table 3.2 shows the relative influence of selected types of physical activity on *cardiovascular disease mortality* among Harvard alumni during the 16-yr follow-up period (1962-1978). It lists the age-adjusted death rates and relative risks of death from cardiovascular disease associated with specified levels and combinations of three types of physical activity assessed per week: walking 6 mi or more, stair climbing up and down 36 or more floors (or stories), and actively playing sports of any type or amount.

Among men denying participation in all three activities (16% of the worker-years), there were 41 deaths per 10,000 worker-years. When this rate was used as a standard for comparison, relative risks less than 1.00 were observed in the presence of any activity or combination of activities and were 0.80 for any single activity, 0.62 for any two, and 0.53 for all three.

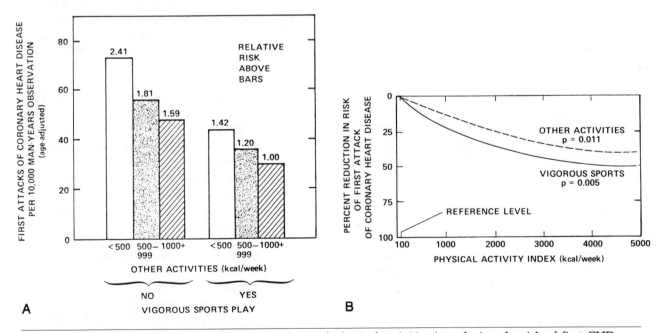

Figure 3.1. Relative importance of vigorous and casual physical activities in reducing the risk of first CHD attack among 16,936 Harvard alumni, 1962-1972: A, age-adjusted incidence rates and relative risks of CHD by combinations of vigorous sports play and other activities; B, percent reduction in incidence rates of CHD by vigorous sports play and other activities. Curves adjusted for differences in age and the alternate type of activity.

Table 3.2   Rates and Relative Risks of Death From Cardiovascular Diseases (CVD) Among 16,936 Harvard Alumni by Types of Weekly Physical Activity, 1962-1978

Weekly physical activity					
Walk 6+ mi	Climb 36+ floors	Sports play	Prevalence in worker-years (%)	CVD death rate per 10,000 worker-years[a]	Relative risk of CVD death
−	−	−	16	41	1.00
−	−	+	17	28 }	.69 }
−	+	−	7	30 } 33	.72 } .80
+	−	−	14	38 }	.93 }
−	+	+	8	27 }	.66 }
+	−	+	16	19 } 26	.48 } .62
+	+	−	10	34 }	.82 }
+	+	+	12	22	.53

[a]Adjusted for age differences.

In the 16-yr follow-up interval, sports play was the most influential in leading to decreased mortality and was followed closely by walking and stair climbing being about equally important. Although intensity and persistence of these activities were not measured and are not considered in this analysis, it is likely that sports play generally was more vigorous and sustained than were walking and stair climbing.

Physical Fitness and Health

Studies not only of physical activity but also of physical fitness have revealed important relationships to health. Surely this is not an either/or situation. These questions are often asked: Can there be fitness without physical activity? Can there be health without fitness? Can there be health without physical activity? The answer is probably not. The fitness studies point in the same direction as the physical activity findings we have just reviewed.

These issues are bridged rather effectively by Leon et al. (8) in the MRFIT report mentioned previously. Physical fitness data obtained from the baseline exercise treadmill tests were compared by tertile of leisure-time physical activity. Both treadmill time and the percentage of subjects achieving the target heart rate were significantly higher with increasing level of leisure-time physical activity, whereas resting and intermediate exercise heart rates were lower. The upper third of subjects by leisure-time physical activity had normal or average estimated mean functional capacity, whereas the least active group was below average in fitness.

We have already seen that the relative risks of CHD in the MRFIT men corresponded to their levels of leisure-time physical activity and fitness.

The study by Peters et al. (27) of physical fitness and risk of myocardial infarction among 2,779 Los Angeles fire and police personnel touches on a number of relationships between fitness and cardiovascular health (Table 3.3, top deck). Continued employment in these stressful jobs was contingent on maintenance of fitness and avoidance of debilitating disease. Physical fitness testing included spirometry, bicycle ergometry, resting and exercise electrocardiograms, and assessments of flexibility and strength. Physical fitness reflected physical activity level rather more strongly than did influences of blood pressure, serum cholesterol level, and cigarette smoking. Below-median physical fitness doubled the risk of myocardial infarction during the 8-yr (average of 4.8 yr) follow-up over the risk for men with above-median fitness. Incidence was tripled among 196 men who were unable to complete their exercise tests.

Low physical fitness scores did not predict higher risk of myocardial infarction unless the men also had above-median levels of systolic blood pressure or serum cholesterol or were smokers. Men with low fitness plus two or three of these other adverse characteristics were at 6 or 7 times the risk of experiencing a myocardial infarction within the next few years of follow-up. Conversely, men with any of those other characteristics were deemed to be protected against myocardial infarction if they maintained above-average fitness. This appears to parallel the Harvard alumni findings, which showed that a physical activity index of 2,000 kcal or more per week tended to counter the influences

Table 3.3 Relative Risks of Coronary Heart Disease (CHD) by Gradients of Physical Fitness

	Men with selected characteristic[a]	Physical work capacity	No. MI cases	Relative risk of MI (95% CL)
Los Angeles public safety officers; 2,779 men aged 35-54 at entry; 8-yr follow-up (4.8 yr average) for symptomatic myocardial infarction (MI), 1971-1978	Systolic BP above-median level	Low	19	5.1 (1.7-21.7)
		High	3	1.0
	Serum cholesterol above-median level	Low	22	4.4 (1.7-14.9)
		High	4	1.0
	Cigarette smoker	Low	22	3.4 (1.4-10.1)
		High	5	1.0
	Any two or all three of above	Low		6.6 (2.3-27.8)
		High		1.0

	Quartiles of fitness by submaximal bicycle ergometry	No. CHD deaths	CHD death rate[b] (%)	Relative risk of CHD death
Norwegian industry and government workers; 2,014 healthy men aged 40-59 at entry; 7-yr follow-up for CHD mortality, 1972-1982	1 (lowest)	29	5.7	1.00
	2	12	2.4	0.42
	3	11	2.2	0.39
	4 (highest)	6	1.1	0.19

	Exercise test heart rate	No. of men	Death rate per 100 men[c]			Relative risk of death*		
			All causes	CVD	CHD	All causes	CVD	CHD
U.S. railroad workers; 2,431 men aged 22-79 at entry; 20-yr follow-up for CHD, cardio-vascular disease (CVD), and all-cause mortality, 1957-1977	128+	526	31.4	18.7	13.2	1.00	1.00	1.00
	116-127	692	27.8	15.7	11.6	0.89	0.84	0.88
	106-115	665	22.3	12.6	8.7	0.71	0.67	0.66
	<106	548	22.8	12.4	9.1	0.73	0.66	0.69

	Quartiles of fitness by stage 2 heart rates on submaximal treadmill test	CHD death rate (%)	CVD death rate (%)	Ratio of death rates 1:4 (95% CL)	
				CHD	CVD
North American (Lipid Research Clinics) men; 4,276 aged 30-69 at entry; 8.5-year average follow-up for CHD and cardiovascular (CVD) mortality, 1972-1984	1 (lowest)	1.69	2.21	6.5	8.5
	2	0.91	1.56	(1.5-28.7)	(2.0-36.7)
	3	0.91	1.30		
	4 (highest)	0.26	0.26		

	Quintiles of fitness by maximal treadmill test	No. of all-cause deaths	Death rate per 10,000 worker-years[c]	Relative risk of death (95% CL)
Cooper Clinic men; 10,244 middle-aged; 8 year average follow-up for all-cause mortality	1 (lowest)	75	64.0	3.4 (2.0-5.8)
	2	40	25.5	1.4 (0.8-2.5)
	3	47	27.1	1.5 (0.8-2.6)

(Cont.)

Table 3.3 (Continued)

Quintiles of fitness by maximal treadmill test	No. of all-cause deaths	Death rate per 10,000 worker-years[c]	Relative risk of death (95% CL)
4	43	21.7	1.2 (0.6-2.2)
5 (highest)	35	18.6	1.0

[a]Age matched.

[b]Adjusted for age differences; $p < 0.001$.

[c]Adjusted for age differences.

*$p < 0.01$ for each cause of death.

of smoking, hypertension, and parental disease on the risk of developing CHD (25).

Lie et al. (9) studied fitness in relation to characteristics associated with CHD and incidence of CHD among 2,014 men from Oslo, Norway, during a 7-yr follow-up (Table 3.3, second deck). In the analysis, subjects in four age-groups were cross-tabulated into quartiles by estimated levels of fitness derived from submaximal ergometer tests rated by cumulative work and body weight, or km • min^{-1} • kg^{-1}. Although fitness declined with age, the most fit men in each age group had lower blood pressures, lower heart rates, lower serum lipids, higher maximal heart rates and maximal blood pressures during exercise, and higher spirographic results. Also, they smoked less than did the men in lower fitness quartiles. Gradient patterns were generally consistent but not always significant. Interview-assessed physical activity data were considered too fragmentary to establish relationships to physical fitness, but leisure-time levels of physical activity and sports play tended to parallel levels of physical fitness by quartiles. The data are presented as rates and relative risks of CHD by fitness quartiles. Although unable to ascertain whether physical fitness mediated influences of physical activity on risks of CHD, the investigators concluded that physical fitness as assessed in this study was a very strong inverse predictor of risk of fatal CHD. Because the upper fitness quartile had a CHD risk as low as that of a comparison group of highly fit expert cross-country skiers (not tabulated here), the possibility of a threshold, or optimum, level of fitness benefit was suggested. Physical activity sufficient to achieve a training effect was advocated for asymptomatic middle-aged men in the belief that it might help maintain a high enough level of fitness to protect against CHD.

Slattery and Jacobs (32) reported a 20-yr follow-up for CHD mortality, cardiovascular disease mortality, and all-cause mortality among 2,431 U.S. railroad workers aged 22-79 at entry. They had undergone treadmill fitness tests in 1957-1960 and 1,914 were retested in 1962-1964 (Table 3.3, third deck). Exercise heart rate was the strongest predictor of cardiovascular disease risk and mortality but was most closely related to exercise systolic blood pressure. The investigators decided that the greater cardiovascular disease risk associated with high exercise heart rate was due largely to the higher blood pressure levels. Like the other recent studies of physical fitness mentioned previously, this one concluded that long-range investigations of the relationships among physical activity, physical fitness, and health are needed to determine whether physical activity reduces risks of CHD and premature mortality by enhancing physical fitness or by some other mechanisms such as metabolic changes. The parallelisms of the findings as to physical fitness and CHD described here are corroborated by studies in other populations (3, 5, 33, 34). We begin to see that studies of physical fitness should be broadened to *whole-body fitness*, which involves metabolic and other body systems as well as the cardiovascular system. Many questions about whether and how physical activity influences fitness and health thus might be answered more readily and the mechanisms of each better understood.

Ekelund et al. (2a) reported an 8.5 year follow-up for CHD and cardiovascular disease mortality among 4,276 Lipid Research Clinic study men, aged 30 to 69 at entry, who had undergone treadmill exercise testing and assessment of potential predictors of CHD at baseline. The heart rate at stage 2 of a submaximal exercise test and time-on-treadmill were used as fitness measures. The fourth deck of Table 3.3 shows that the unadjusted cumulative mortality was substantially higher in the quartile of subjects with the lowest level of fitness than in the most fit quartile—6.5 times higher for coronary heart disease mortality and 8.5 times higher for all cardiovascular disease mortality. Adjustment for age differences did not alter these ratios. In multivariate analyses, adjustment for other covariables (e.g., cigarette smoking, blood pressure level, and lipoprotein-cholesterol profile) did not change the relative risks meaningfully, indicating that the relations between physical fitness and death for coronary heart and cardiovascular disease mortality were independent of those other variables.

In a follow-up of 10,244 middle-aged men for relationship between physical fitness as measured by maximal time-on-treadmill and all-cause mortality, Blair et al. (1) found that mortality rates declined across physical fitness quintiles by 70 percent from the least to the most fit men (Table 3.3, bottom deck). Trends remained after accounting for differences among quintiles in age; cigarette smoking habit; blood cholesterol, blood pressure, and blood glucose levels; and parental history of CHD. The higher levels of physical fitness led to a delay in all-cause mortality, primarily cardiovascular disease and cancer mortality.

Lifestyles and Longevity

We turn now to the topics of all-cause mortality and longevity as influenced by exercise, fitness, and other considerations of lifestyle. Pekkanen et al. (26) studied the influence of high physical activity on the incidence of premature death from any cause among 636 healthy Finnish men aged 45-64 at entry who were followed for 20 yr (1964-1984). There were 287 deaths, 106 due to CHD; but the men who had been most active lived 2.1 yr longer (Table 3.4, top deck) than did the men who had been less active, mainly because of their differences in CHD risk. Thus the saving was in avoidance of premature death, and the survival curves of high actives and low actives converged in the last 5 yr of follow-up. Those who died differed more in fitness elements such as body mass index than did those who survived, but the differences seemed too small to account for the survival advantage associated with the more active men. In fact, low body mass index was an adverse characteristic relative to all-cause mortality even though obesity tends to promote CHD risk. The converging survival curves of the high- and low-activity groups might reflect converging levels of activity, altered influences of activity with aging, or both. However, the results show that the longevity benefits ascribed to high activity or vigorous

Table 3.4   Age Effects, Rates, and Relative Risks of Death From All Causes by Gradients of Physical Activity

	Physical activity at baseline	No. men at baseline	Mean age at baseline	Mean age at death (yr)			
				First 10% dead***	First 20% dead*	First 30% dead*	All men dead**
Finnish men; 636 aged 45-64	Low	386	54.9	60.3	62.6	64.5	67.4
at entry; 20-yr follow-up,	High	250	55.2	62.5	64.6	66.8	69.1
1964-1984							
Added years of life from high activity[a]				1.4	2.0	2.4	2.1

	Physical activity index (kcal/wk)	Prevalence in worker-years (%)	No. of deaths	Deaths per 10,000 worker-years[b]		Relative risk of death	
Harvard alumni; 16,936 men	< 500	15.4	308	93.7	⎫	1.00	⎫
aged 35-74 at entry; 16-yr	500- 999	20.9	322	73.5	⎬ 75.2	0.78	⎬ 1.00
follow-up, 1962-1978	1,000-1,499	15.2	202	68.2	⎭	0.73	⎭
	1,500-1,999	10.4	121	59.3		0.63	
	2,000-2,499	8.1	89	57.7	⎫	0.62	⎫
	2,500-2,999	6.9	62	48.5	⎬ 54.4	0.52	⎬ 0.72
	3,000-3,499	5.0	42	42.7		0.46	
	3,500+	18.1	203	58.4	⎭	0.62	⎭

[a]Adjusted for differences in age, blood pressure, serum cholesterol, and cigarette smoking.

[b]Adjusted for age differences; $p < 0.0001$.

*$p < 0.001$.

**$p = 0.002$.

***$p = 0.006$.

exercise were appreciable regardless of whether their relationships to characteristics of fitness remain to be clarified. The investigators interpreted the survival patterns as showing that physical activity tends to promote longevity by preventing premature death but is unlikely to extend the natural life span of humans.

The Finnish longevity study invites a number of comparisons to reports on physical activity and longevity among Harvard alumni (21, 23). The Finnish men constituted a smaller study population that was followed over a longer interval and that represented a higher percentage of deaths, so the analyses did not need to rely on actuarial projections and estimates of survival as did the Harvard alumni study. Therefore, the more literal Finnish observations substantiate the Harvard findings. Despite what would seem to be obvious differences in lifestyles, the results of the two studies are remarkably in agreement in most respects.

Before discussing the longevity patterns of the alumni, we may consider their rates and relative risks of all-cause mortality by gradients of physical activity assessed by their physical activity index (Table 3.4, bottom deck). As in other analyses, the breaking point between the low and the high physical activity index is taken at 2,000 kcal per week, and death rates are expressed per 10,000 worker-years. The more active of the 16,936 alumni had 28% lower risk of death from any cause during the 16 yr of follow-up (1962-1978) than did the less active men. The gradient shows a steady

decline as activity levels increase from less than 500 to an optimum of 3,500 kcal per week, and the trend is highly significant ($p < 0.0001$).

From the all-cause mortality data in the Harvard alumni study it is possible to estimate an individual's added years of life to be gained by having the benefits of favorable lifestyle elements, including the habit of adequate contemporary physical activity with an index of 2,000 kcal or more per week (Table 3.5). The bottom line of the table shows that the greatest gain would be achieved by avoiding hypertension, the second greatest by not smoking cigarettes, and the third greatest by exercising enough to have a high index (i.e., for men with these specific adverse characteristics). Because the influence of physical activity is partly independent of the others, whose contributions are also partly cumulative, a lifestyle that combines several of these virtues might be expected to gain perhaps more years of added life than it would from any single item alone. We have already seen that exercise promotes longevity mainly by preventing premature death from CHD. Appropriate exercise seems to have a similar influence in staving off hypertension, which is highly predictive of increased CHD risk and shortened survival (22).

Cigarette smoking is associated with death from lung cancer and other afflictions as well as with promoting CHD; therefore, avoidance of cigarette smoking might be expected to postpone mortality in several ways, and this may account for its larger benefit. Nonsmokers might be reducing their

Table 3.5 Added Years of Life From Favorable Lifestyle Patterns in Men Up to Age 80 as Estimated From Harvard Alumni Mortality Experiences, 1962-1978

Age at entry	Physical activity index 2,000+ vs. < 2,000 (kcal/wk)	Cigarette nonsmoking vs. smoking	Normotensive vs. hypertensive	Net weight gain of 7+ vs. < 7 (kg)	Parental longevity 65+ vs. < 65 (yr)
35-39	1.50	2.68	3.48	1.22	1.15
40-44	1.39	2.62	3.31	1.16	0.98
45-49	1.10	2.38	2.60	1.05	0.76
50-54	1.20	2.23	2.20	1.03	0.76
55-59	1.13	2.00	1.84	1.14	0.45
60-64	0.93	1.64	1.51	1.01	0.22
65-69	0.67	0.98	1.20	0.59	0.09
70-74	0.44	0.51	0.37	0.34	0.06
75-79	0.30	0.03	0.18	−0.04	0.04
35-79[a]	1.25	2.26	2.72	1.09	0.81

Note. Each lifestyle pattern is adjusted for differences in all the other patterns listed.

[a]Weighted average adjusted for differences in age and all the other patterns listed.

risk of premature death from CHD, lung cancer, and so on, whether or not they are vigorous exercisers; if they are exercisers, so much the better their chances for extended longevity.

Net weight gain since college may have somewhat conflicting implications, as high weight gain tends to predict CHD and low weight gain other fatal diseases, such as cancer, the ravages of alcoholism, and so on. Table 3.5 shows that it is better to gain 7 kg or more than it is less, which appears to be a low-end cut point hinting at the latter causes of death. If we also had an upper cut point relating to CHD, the table would offer a midrange or scope within which weight gain would be most likely to enhance longevity. Then the years gained by optimum weight control might be somewhat increased over the present numbers in that column. The differing implications for CHD and all-cause mortality may help explain why obesity is often found to be weak or ambivalent as an element of health risk. Individuals who weigh the same may be quite different in their body compositions, for example, one fat and the other muscular (and it is likely that they will differ also in their habits of physical activity, which also influence body composition). Therefore, some combined assessment of physical activity and weight gain might reveal even more pertinent implications for longevity than do the separate columns tabulated here.

Controlling for the influence of physical activity versus other elements of lifestyle or physiology is complicated by the fact that physical activity is usually a positive, or beneficial, influence that modifies the impact of others, such as obesity or cigarette smoking, whose influences are adverse. It is often suggested that much of the benefit of vigorous exercise or physical activity may consist of countering adverse influences of unwise habits (smoking or alcohol) or unfortunate characteristics (hypertension or heredity). We need to sort out the mechanisms by which physical activity promotes both short- and long-term health and longevity, whether these be cardiovascular modifications, metabolic processes, or other physiological considerations. By exploring the elements of fitness we ought to arrive at a clearer picture of the most important aspects of influences of physical activity on the various systems of the body and the processes by which these influences determine health status and longevity. Have there been any studies designed to reveal the influences of physical fitness on longevity? Where does fitness fit in? Some might approach that topic by looking at the lifestyles and health patterns of athletes. But ath-

leticism may not be a satisfactory synonym for physical fitness because one might be considered fit without being an athlete. What observations can we make about fitness and longevity from the studies described earlier of the British civil servants, the San Francisco longshoremen, the Harvard alumni, the Los Angeles safety workers, the Norwegians, and the Finns? Although the epidemiological patterns of fitness can be expected to parallel those of physical activity, it is obvious that we need much more epidemiological study of fitness to apply and extend the information so far obtained from clinical studies.

One point often made about physical activity and fitness is that the kind or intensity of physical activity influences fitness. For example, aerobic endurance exercise or some vigorous sports play is needed to develop cardiovascular fitness and functional capacity. It can even reduce resting heart rate by increasing stroke volume. Another point offered is that habitual physical activity will help maintain fitness if it is frequent enough and constant enough (18, 31). Table 3.6 shows the rewards in longevity for devoting 3 or 4 hr a week to incidental and deliberate exercise such as

Table 3.6 Added Life From 3 or 4 Hours of Weekly Exercise to Age 80 as Estimated From Harvard Alumni Mortality Experiences, 1962-1978

Age at entry	Days active	Days of life gained	Hours gained per hour active
3 hr exercise/wk			
40	260	507	1.95
50	195	438	2.25
60	130	339	2.61
70	65	161	2.47
4 hr exercise/wk			
40	347	507	1.46
50	260	438	1.68
60	173	339	1.96
70	87	161	1.86

Note. Data are for recreational activities, including sports play, and stair climbing and walking. Results are for the expenditure of energy at 2,000 kcal/wk or more vs. expending less than 2,000 kcal/wk. Days and hours of life gained are adjusted for differences in cigarette smoking, blood pressure status, net gain in body mass index since college, and parents' ages at death.

recreational activities (including sports play), as estimated from the experience of the alumni and their mortality during the interval 1962-1978. The table suggests that the same amount of longevity is gained (say 507 d by a 40-yr-old man) if he exercises for 260 d at 3 hr per week or for 347 d at 4 hr per week. One assumption seems to be that he did the same amount of exercise in each case but that he did it faster (i.e., in less time) in one schedule than in the other. However, the faster (3 hr per week) exercise may have been 25% more vigorous than was the slower (4 hr per week) exercise and so may have had a somewhat different influence on physical fitness and on CHD risk (Figure 3.1A, B). Furthermore, the table says nothing about what the vigorous (3-hr) alumnus did with the 87 d (347 − 260) he had free after fulfilling his quota of exercise. These differences, in turn, might have been enough to alter the implications for longevity, a point that seems not to have been built into the calculations in these tables. If so, the hours gained per hour of exercise may also be imprecise, as the 3-hr subtraction and division has not allowed for any such adjustment. This is a small illustration of why important considerations of fitness need to be included in the assessment of physical activity levels and the planning of exercise programs.

Even in this highly hypothetical situation, we need to hypothesize further that the faster man not only might have 87 d of extra time for his leisure and for additional exercise over that of his slower comrade but also that he might be expected to live somewhat longer as a result of his greater intensity of effort in expending 2,000 kcal per week or more (Figure 3.1B). Therefore, if the slower man has gained 507 d of added life, the faster man has the likelihood of gaining appreciably more for three reasons: (a) He has the opportunity to exercise 87 d more than the slower man. (b) The exercise he did in the 260 d should give him extra longevity benefit because it was vigorous. (c) The exercise he does in the 87 d (after overtaking the slow man) also is likely to be vigorous.

Ultimately, the study of exercise, fitness, and lifestyle is likely to involve some assessments of their potential impact on the well-being of the individuals and communities we have been talking about. Part of the answer may be seen in longevity estimates such as have been mentioned. A further approach is to consider the implications of attributable risk estimates.

Relative and attributable risks of death, derived from a multivariate analysis and contrasting the presence and absence of five adverse personal characteristics, with adjustment for age and for each of the other four characteristics, are given in Table 3.7. Note that in this analysis we begin with a condition of sedentariness and then show what effect conversion to a level of adequate physical activity might be expected to have on the health status of individuals and communities. The levels of the other characteristics, such as cigarette smok-

Table 3.7 Relative and Attributable Risks of Death From All Causes Among 16,936 Harvard Alumni (1962-1978) by Selected Adverse Characteristics

Adverse characteristic	Prevalence in worker-years (%)	Relative risk of death	Clinical attributable risk (%)	Community attributable risk (%)
Sedentary lifestyle[a]	62.0	1.31	23.6	16.1
Cigarette smoking[b]	38.2	1.73	43.2	22.5
Hypertension[c]	9.4	1.76	42.1	6.4
Low net weight gain[d]	35.1	1.33	24.6	10.3
Early parental death[e]	33.3	1.15	13.1	4.8
One or more of the above[f]	90.5	1.94	47.7	45.3

Note. Risks are adjusted for differences in age and all the other characteristics listed.

[a]Energy expenditure of less than 2,000 kcal/wk in walking, climbing stairs, and playing sports.

[b]Any amount.

[c]Physician diagnosed.

[d]Net gain in body mass index of less than 3 English units since college (i.e., not more than 7 kg or 15 lb).

[e]One or both parents dead before the age of 65.

[f]Adjusted for differences in age only.

ing, are likewise shifted from adverse to favorable health implications. First, the relative risk estimates are used to describe the respective levels, in this case referring to a 16-yr follow-up in the Harvard alumni study.

Men with sedentary lifestyles (i.e., those expending fewer than 2,000 kcal per week) were at 31% higher risk of death during the follow-up interval than were more active men; cigarette smokers had a 73% higher risk than did nonsmokers; hypertensive men were at a 76% higher risk than were normotensive men; men with a net weight gain of less than 7 kg after college were at 33% greater risk than were men who had gained more; and men who had lost one or both parents before the age of 65 were at 15% greater risk than were men whose parents survived to age 65 or beyond. Alumni with one or more of these adverse characteristics were at 94% greater risk of death from any cause than were classmates with none of the characteristics.

Clinical attributable risks shown in the table give estimates of potential percentage reductions in the risk of death for persons who might exchange an adverse characteristic for its more healthful counterpart. Sedentary men who become more active might reduce their risk of death by 24%. Reformed cigarette smokers might have 43% lower mortality experience; and hypertensive men who achieved normal blood pressures might have 42% lower mortality. Men with low net weight gains since college might have 25% lower risk of death if they had gained more; and men with histories of early parental mortality might have experienced a 13% reduced death risk if both parents had been more long-lived. If an alumnus with one or more of these adverse characteristics could have avoided all of them, his risk of death from any cause during the follow-up interval might have been reduced by 48% over the experience of classmates who had one or more of the adverse characteristics.

Community attributable risks estimate the potential reductions in death rates in a population or group of people whose unfavorable characteristics were converted to more healthful features. These estimates take the prevalence of the characteristics into account. As seen in Table 3.7, the risk of death might have been reduced among the Harvard alumni by 16% if every man had expended 2,000 kcal per week or more in walking, stair climbing, and recreational activities. Total abstinence from cigarettes might have cut the community death rate by 22%, abolition of hypertension by 6% (relatively small because of its low prevalence), a

greater weight gain by 10%, and survival of both parents to age 65 or older by 5%. If all five adverse characteristics had been eliminated completely from the Harvard community, the death rate from all causes might have been reduced by nearly one half (45%).

Conclusion

We have reviewed a series of recent studies of physical activity and fitness as they relate to health and longevity and have described some likely cause-and-effect associations in a series of ratios. Their complexities can be expressed by a Venn diagram (Figure 3.2). We know that the circles overlap, but we need to find out where, how much, why, and how they do so. The areas they have in common should represent the chief interests and objectives of our next round of research in this field.

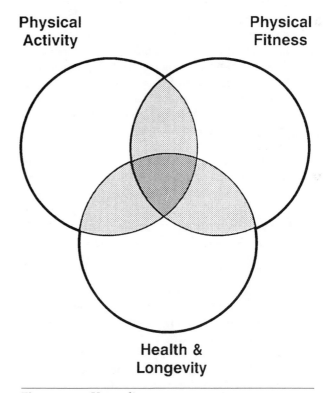

Figure 3.2. Venn diagram.

To translate these circles into specific terms as proposals for further study, we need to consider suggestions such as the following:

- *Taxonomy, definitions, and criteria.* There is need for simple, meaningful terminology. Its definitions should be established on a sequential basis that recognizes that insofar as physical activity influences physical fitness both are alterable determinants of health. Fitness also may be modified by other influences, such as diet, disease, and heredity. It will be expedient to consider and accept a priority of influences on health, perhaps in this order: activity, fitness, diet, other lifestyle habits, and heredity.

- *Physical activity.* For purposes of prescription and evaluation, the following questions need to be answered to characterize physical activity: (a) What type (endurance, resistance, sports play, do-it-yourself)? (b) How much (frequency and duration)? (c) How intense (level of energy demand)? and (d) For whom (age, gender, clinical status, personal goal)? There is pressing need to establish standards for individual prescriptions and for community interventions.
- *Physical fitness.* There is need to accept that physical fitness means a functional integration of *all* body systems influenced by physical activity, particularly the following: (a) cardiovascular-respiratory, (b) musculoskeletal, (c) metabolic-endocrine, (d) neuropsychological, (e) hematological, and (f) gastrointestinal. Studies need to establish the kinds and amounts of acute and chronic (short- and long-term) changes (and the consequences of those changes) induced in each body system by physical activity (20).
- *Health.* Our present interest centers on aspects of health and physical fitness that result from muscular and bodily activities. The aim is not only to avoid or delay disease but also to achieve and maintain optimum levels of physical fitness, total health, and longevity insofar as these states are influenced by appropriate choices and patterns of physical activity.
- *Research in exercise science.* The rationale for our focus on physical activity stems from at least the following considerations: (a) Engagement in activity is a natural procedure and requirement of the body. (b) Physical fitness (like health) is a continuum that describes the physiological state of the body systems and determines its vitality or capacity to be active. (c) Records of history reveal that sedentariness is a recent development and was not previously a characteristic of humanity. Technological progress has engineered this change, which is at least partly responsible for adverse health trends such as the so-called 20th-century epidemic of CHD. (d) In developed countries,

nearly two thirds of the population are habitually sedentary and thus at risk of developing health problems that should be mitigated by adopting wiser habits of adequate physical activity. Because cardiovascular disease, the first cause of premature death, tends to be reduced or delayed by adequate activity, substitution of more activeness for sedentariness is a major priority in programs for promotion of good health. (e) Physical activity is a positive influence that tends to further positive health, and it counters adverse lifestyle elements that tend to promote negative health and the development of CHD and other chronic diseases such as hypertension, osteoporosis, Type II diabetes mellitus, and syndromes of anxiety and depression. More information is needed on the effect of physical activity on respiratory disease, arthritis, and cancer. (f) A concomitant of sound health maintenance is likely to be an extension of longevity to its optimum, together with enhancement of the quality of life. These outcomes represent goals for the foreseeable future.

In summary, activity and fitness are key determinants of whole-body, or total, health (i.e., physical, psychological, social, cultural, and spiritual well-being) and help both the individual and the community achieve life goals.

Acknowledgments

This work was supported by U.S. Public Health Service research grants HL 34174 from the National Heart, Lung and Blood Institute and CA 44854 from the National Cancer Institute. This is report No. XXXVI in a series on chronic disease in former college students.

References

1. Blair, S.N., H.W. Kohl III, R.S. Paffenbarger, Jr., D.G. Clark, K.H. Cooper, and L.W. Gibbons. Physical fitness and all-cause mortality: A prospective study of healthy men and women. *JAMA*. In press.
1a. Brand, R.J., R.S. Paffenbarger, Jr., R.I. Scholtz, and J.B. Kampert. Work activity and fatal heart attacks studied by multiple logistic risk analysis. *Am. J. Epidemiol.* 110: 52-62, 1979.

2. Donahue, R.P., R.D. Abbott, D.M. Reed, and K. Yano. Physical activity and coronary heart disease in middle-aged and elderly men: The Honolulu Heart Program. *Am. J. Public Health* 78: 683-685, 1988.

2a. Ekelund, L.-G., W.L. Haskell, J.L. Johnson, F.S. Whaley, M.H. Criqui, and D.S. Sheps. Physical fitness as a predictor of cardiovascular mortality in asymptomatic North American men. The Lipid Research Clinics mortality follow-up study. *N. Engl. J. Med.* 319:1379-1384, 1988.

3. Erikssen, J. Physical fitness and coronary heart disease morbidity and mortality. *Acta Med. Scand.* Suppl. 711: 189-192, 1986.

4. Fentem, P., and N. Turnbull. Benefits of exercise for heart health: A report on the scientific basis. In: *Exercise-heart-health.* London: The Coronary Prevention Group, 1987, p. 110-125.

5. Gyntelberg, F., L. Lauridsen, and K. Schubell. Physical fitness and risk of myocardial infarction in Copenhagen males aged 40-59. *Scand. J. Work Environ. Health* 6: 170-178, 1980.

6. Hinkle, L.E., Jr., H.T. Thaler, D.P. Merke, D. Renier-Berg, and N.E. Morton. The risk factors for arrhythmic death in a sample of men followed for 20 years. *Am. J. Epidemiol.* 127: 500-515, 1988.

7. Kannel, W.B., A. Belanger, R. D'Agostino, and I. Israel. Physical activity and physical demand on the job and risk of cardiovascular disease and death: The Framingham Study. *Am. Heart J.* 112: 820-825, 1986.

8. Leon, A.S., J. Connett, D.R. Jacobs, Jr., and R. Rauramaa. Leisure-time physical activity levels and risk of coronary heart disease and death: The Multiple Risk Factor Intervention Trial. *JAMA* 258: 2388-2395, 1987.

9. Lie, H., R. Mundal, and J. Erikssen. Coronary risk factors and incidence of coronary death in relation to physical fitness: Seven-year follow-up study of middle-aged and elderly men. *Eur. Heart J.* 6: 147-157, 1985.

10. Morris, J.N. Exercise and the incidence of coronary heart disease. In: *Exercise-heart-health.* London: The Coronary Prevention Group, 1987, p. 21-34.

11. Morris, J.N. Physical activity in the prevention of cardiovascular disease. In: *Inspanning en voeding,* edited by A.M.J. van Erp-Baart, M.B. Katan, H.C.G. Kemper, J.A.M. van der Laan, J.N. Morris, E. de Nobel, W.H.M. Saris, and H.W.H. Weeds. Alphen aan den Rijn/Brussels: Samson/Stafleu, 1985, p. 54-63.

12. Morris, J.N. *Uses of epidemiology* (3rd ed.). Edinburgh: Churchill Livingstone, 1975, p. 159-186.

13. Morris, J.N., S.P.W. Chave, C. Adam, C. Sirey, L. Epstein, and D.J. Sheehan. Vigorous exercise in leisure-time and the incidence of coronary heart-disease. *Lancet* i: 333-339, 1973.

14. Morris, J.N., M.G. Everitt, R. Pollard, S.P.W. Chave, and A.M. Semmence. Vigorous exercise in leisure-time: Protection against coronary heart-disease. *Lancet* ii: 1207-1210, 1980.

15. Morris, J.N., M.G. Everitt, and A.M. Semmence. Exercise and coronary heart disease. In: Macleod, D., R. Maughan, M. Nimmo, T. Reilly, and C. Williams, eds. *Exercise: Benefits, limits and adaptations.* London: E. & F.N. Spon, 1987, p. 4-19.

16. Morris, J.N., J.A. Heady, P.A.B. Raffle, C.G. Roberts, and J.W. Parks. Coronary heart disease and physical activity of work. *Lancet* ii: 1053-1057, 1111-1120, 1953.

17. Morris, J.N., A. Kagan, D.C. Pattison, M. Gardner, and P.A.B. Raffle. Incidence and prediction of ischaemic heart disease in London busmen. *Lancet* ii: 552-559, 1966.

18. Noakes, T. *Lore of running.* Cape Town, South Africa: Oxford University Press, 1985.

19. Paffenbarger, R.S., Jr., and W.E. Hale. Work activity and coronary heart mortality. *N. Engl. J. Med.* 292: 545-550, 1975.

20. Paffenbarger, R.S., Jr., and R.T. Hyde. Exercise as protection against heart attack [Editorial]. *N. Engl. J. Med.* 302: 1026-1027, 1980.

21. Paffenbarger, R.S., Jr., R.T. Hyde, A.L. Wing, and C.-c. Hsieh. Physical activity, all-cause mortality, and longevity of college alumni. *N. Engl. J. Med.* 314: 605-613; 315: 399-401, 1986.

22. Paffenbarger, R.S., Jr., A.L. Wing, R.T. Hyde, and D.L. Jung. Physical activity and incidence of hypertension in college alumni. *Am. J. Epidemiol.* 117: 245-257, 1983.

23. Paffenbarger, R.S., Jr., R.T. Hyde, A.L. Wing, and C.H. Steinmetz. A natural history of athleticism and cardiovascular health. *JAMA* 252: 491-495, 1984.

24. Paffenbarger, R.S., Jr., M.E. Laughlin, A.S. Gima, and R.A. Black. Work activity of longshoremen as related to death from coronary heart disease and stroke. *N. Engl. J. Med.* 282: 1109-1114, 1970.

25. Paffenbarger, R.S., Jr., A.L. Wing, and R.T. Hyde. Physical activity as an index of heart

attack risk in college alumni. *Am. J. Epidemiol.* 108: 161-175, 1978.

26. Pekkanen, J., B. Marti, A. Nissinen, and J. Tuomilehto. Reduction of premature mortality by high physical activity: A 20-year follow-up of middle-aged Finnish men. *Lancet* i: 1473-1477, 1987.

27. Peters, R.K., L.D. Cady, Jr., D.P. Bischoff, L. Bernstein, and M.C. Pike. Physical fitness and subsequent myocardial infarction in healthy workers. *JAMA* 249: 3052-3056, 1983.

28. Powell, K.E., P.D. Thompson, C.J. Caspersen, and J.S. Kendrick. Physical activity and the incidence of coronary heart disease. *Annu. Rev. Public Health* 8: 253-287, 1987.

29. Salonen, J.T., J.S. Slater, J. Tuomilehto, and R. Rauramaa. Leisure time and occupational physical activity: Risk of death from ischemic heart disease. *Am. J. Epidemiol.* 127: 87-94, 1988.

30. Scragg, R., A. Stewart, R. Jackson, and R. Beaglehole. Alcohol and exercise in myocardial infarction and sudden coronary death in men and women. *Am. J. Epidemiol.* 126: 77-85, 1987.

31. Simon, H.B., and S.R. Levisohn. *The athlete within: A personal guide to total fitness.* Boston: Little, Brown, 1987.

32. Slattery, M.L., and D.R. Jacobs. Physical fitness and cardiovascular disease mortality: The U.S. Railroad Study. *Am. J. Epidemiol.* 127: 571-580, 1988.

33. Sobolski, J., M. Kornitzer, G. de Backer, M. Dramaix, M. Abramowicz, S. Degre, and H. Denolin. Protection against ischemic heart disease in the Belgian physical fitness study: Physical fitness rather than physical activity? *Am. J. Epidemiol.* 125: 601-610, 1987.

34. Wilhelmsen, L., J. Bjure, B. Ekström-Jodal, M. Aurell, G. Grimby, K. Svärdsudd, G. Tibblin, and H. Wedel. Nine years' follow-up of a maximal exercise test in a random population sample of middle-aged men. *Cardiology* 68(Suppl. 2): 1-8, 1981.

Chapter 4

Costs and Benefits of an Exercising Versus a Nonexercising Society

Roy J. Shephard

Both governments and corporations are increasingly applying the techniques of cost-benefit and cost-effectiveness analyses to the evaluation of health programs (25, 26, 27, 28, 31, 32, 33), including initiatives that fall within the scope of this conference.

As professionals concerned with positive health, we should welcome and encourage this trend, given that expenditures on the prevention of disease still account for no more than 4%-6% of medical spending (32) and that exercise will likely prove to be a cost-effective health measure. Indeed, perhaps the best method of assuring a more appropriate distribution of funding between health promotion and acute medical care is to counter the mistaken notion that few preventive measures are cost-effective (27, 28).

The intent of cost-benefit and cost-effectiveness analyses is to express the costs of a program (both financial and social) in dollar equivalents, weighing these charges against the anticipated benefits (e.g., reduced demands for medical care, increased industrial productivity, and decreased absenteeism). In a cost-benefit analysis, such gains are also expressed in dollar terms.

Methodological Problems

Cost-Benefit Versus Cost-Effectiveness Analysis

The investigator must immediately decide on the relative merits of cost-benefit and cost-effectiveness analyses. In a cost-effectiveness analysis, the community is asked to establish some criterion of effectiveness (e.g., a decrease of medical costs or a reduction in absenteeism); program options are then compared in terms of their costs per unit change in the chosen measure of effectiveness. Sometimes the cost-benefit and cost-effectiveness approaches may overlap. For example, effectiveness might be measured in terms of the average number of years of normal quality life (1) added by a fitness program; the community might then decide that a cost of $20,000 per year of quality-adjusted life span was a worthwhile investment of public funds but that if the cost exceeded $100,000 per year the program would be too expensive to justify further consideration (7).

Some people are uncomfortable with both cost-benefit and cost-effectiveness analyses because they set a finite value on human life and health. However, ethical decisions are inevitably involved when making medical expenditures. If money is spent on a single individual for a heart, lung, or liver transplant, this money is no longer available for preventive initiatives such as fitness programs. Accordingly, it is more ethical to weigh policy alternatives in quantitative fiscal terms than it is to respond to emotional appeals from special interest groups such as surgeons or hospital administrators.

The main advantage of cost-effectiveness over cost-benefit analysis is that the former can make an appropriate allowance for life beyond retirement. In contrast, most cost-benefit analyses view the worth of continuing life simply in terms of labor, adding either the entire income of the individual or that portion that remains after personal needs have been satisfied (typically, 25% of income). From a harsh economic point of view, it could be argued that the best type of fitness program keeps a person productive until retirement but allows death shortly afterward. As one becomes older, this argument becomes increasingly unpalatable, for one recognizes that the life to be saved is one's own! We would be rash to suggest either that senior citizens make no contribution to society or that they have no continuing claims on society based on their previous labor. A further problem of a rigid cost-benefit analysis is that it becomes more profitable to provide services to a high-level executive than to a minimum wage earner. Again, this concept might be appropriate in Nazi philosophy, but it does not appeal to a Canadian humanitarian.

Currently, cost-benefit analysis is thus offered as a tool for ethical decision making rather than as a rigid balance sheet to be followed slavishly.

Inflation

In Canada, as in most other countries, the real value of a unit of currency is constantly diminishing. Accounts must thus be expressed relative to an arbitrary reference point, for example, the value of the Canadian dollar in June 1983 or May 1988. The usual method of converting data collected at other times is to apply the consumer price index (CPI), which expresses the current cost of a fixed basket of goods and services relative to their prices on the specified date. When using the CPI, we should note that economists have occasionally altered the contents of the basket to reflect cultural changes. Complications have also arisen from modifications in the base equipment attached to, for example, a motorcycle, a car, or a refrigerator. Moreover, the method of estimating the cost of shelter has differed between the United States and Canada. The U.S. figures have assumed the purchase of a house rather than the rental of an apartment, so that the American CPI has risen relative to the Canadian CPI when interest rates have been high. A further source of difficulty is differential inflation. For example, between 1972 and 1982 the CPI increased by 150%, but the costs of the average bicycle increased by only 83%; on the other hand, the costs of medical services substantially outpaced the general rate of inflation.

Discount Rate

Some of the benefits of enhanced physical activity, such as protection against a future heart attack, may not be recouped for many years. Economists thus tend to discount the benefits of physical activity (26, 27, 28, 42). In essence, discounting ex-

presses the willingness of a typical individual (or of society) to invest now for future benefit (13). This is an important issue because the discount rate greatly reduces the apparent fiscal benefit from exercise. Suggestions of an appropriate figure range from the real (inflation-corrected) rate at which governments can borrow money (2.5%-3.0%) to the opportunity forgone in the private sector (which, even after allowance for taxation, might rise as high as 10%). On occasion, high discount rates have been proposed not because they were thought to be correct but rather as a means of tempering the enthusiasm of experts in preventive medicine (27, 28)!

There have been occasional attempts to check the evidence of interest rates against the willingness of the public to pay for safety devices (e.g., smoke detectors and car seat belts) or to accept work in hazardous occupations at premium pay (3, 8). However, the findings remain somewhat equivocal; in the first case, it is necessary to assume that the prime motivation for purchase of the protective device is personal safety rather than the protection of property, and in the second case one must assume that (a) the labor market is fully competitive, (b) all workers are aware of the true risks of a given employment and respond in a rational manner, and (c) wage differentials reflect the danger rather than the discomfort associated with hazardous work. Moreover, any discount rate deduced from such responses applies only to a given population living in a given era.

That sector of the population most in need of prevention unfortunately seems the least willing to sacrifice immediate gratification for future good. Moreover, the present generation as a whole seems less willing to invest in the future than were earlier generations. A further imponderable is the real growth in productivity (currently 1%-2% per year). From the viewpoint of society, the value of a year of productive life may be much less now than it would be 20 yr hence. On the other hand, in a longer-term perspective, automation may reduce the need for labor to the point that an increased working span has little commercial value.

There are several practical difficulties in applying any of the proposed discount rates to the specific tactic of exercise promotion. In particular, there is an uncertain lag period between the individual's commencement of an exercise program and the onset of any resultant health benefit. Also, because of poor compliance with the proposed regimen and interindividual variations in response to any exercise that is undertaken, the extent and timing of the resultant health benefit vary from one person to another. More fundamentally, although there is a lag period when an exercise program is first starting up, once it has been operating for several years one cohort of subjects is realizing a health benefit at the same time that funds are being invested to promote exercise in a subsequent cohort. Thus, it seems inappropriate to discount the health benefits of exercise except during the start-up phase (27).

Participation Rates

In determining the health benefits derived from acute medical care, statistics are available only for that portion of the population that accepts treatment, and a patient who insisted on premature discharge from a hospital would likely be excluded from calculations of prognosis. However, with a preventive tactic such as regular exercise, the numerator becomes the entire population of a region, cooperative and uncooperative alike. Everyone is offered treatment irrespective of susceptibility to heart disease or some other condition that may be prevented by vigorous exercise, and the resultant attenuation of cost-effectiveness is further exacerbated because not everyone adheres to the proposed exercise prescription.

The long-term participation rate is indeed a major source of uncertainty in our calculations. Some authors have advanced very pessimistic figures, suggesting that the 6-mo participation rate is unlikely to exceed 20% of the target community (30, 39). Clearly, more information is needed. However, there is increasing evidence that many of the people who are stimulated to greater physical activity by a formal employee fitness program continue to exercise in an informal manner even if they drop out of structured classes at the work site (18).

A further imponderable is the importance of social climate to the shaping of exercise behavior (11). If there were a massive investment in the molding of public attitudes, it is possible that the rate of recruitment might be increased and the rate of recidivism much lower.

Marginal Costs

Most of the available information on program costs refers to the current steady state. However, the real issue on the cost side of the ledger is not the expense of operating current programs but rather the added investment in facilities and advertising that would be needed to increase participation by a

specified amount (12). Likewise, in unfortunate situations in which there is a clamor to cut programs, information is needed on the compensating variation (the willingness of the consumer to make good any shortfall in funding), the equivalent variation (the substantial alternative incentives that would be needed to secure reelection of a government or the satisfaction of employees), or both (21).

Opportunity Costs

Some analyses have only partially examined the consumer costs incurred by participation in physical activity programs. Given that one must pursue physical activity several hours per week for the rest of one's life to obtain many of the proposed benefits, note should be taken of the time invested by the participant. Skeptics have suggested that one's life can be lengthened by some 2 yr by jogging long distances, but almost all this time must be spent on the track! Certainly, the opportunity cost depends greatly on the pleasure the individual derives from exercising.

The estimation of opportunity cost thus becomes important when comparing possible program alternatives. In large cities, long hours can be spent traveling to and from exercise facilities (38), and, at least in theory, a saving of travel time is one important advantage of an employee fitness program over many rival types of exercise prescription. In practice, the quality of the recreational experience must be weighed against this opportunity cost, and many people seem prepared to travel long distances to a lake or a ski resort rather than obtaining a similar amount of physical activity by taking the stairs to an office basement.

Multiplier Effects

Many analyses of program benefits have focused simply on changes in the health and productivity of the individual participant. However, a complete analysis must include the impact of recreational investment on other sectors of the economy. In general, expenditures on exercise programs will stimulate the regional economy, but some specific sectors (e.g., passive entertainment, brewing, and the manufacture of cigarettes) may be depressed if a given population becomes more active and health conscious (32).

One analysis conducted in Ontario estimated that each dollar that the provincial government invested in fitness programming generated some

$4.60 of investment from the private sector (9). Other analyses have suggested a relatively small multiplier effect for consumer recreational expenditures because those employed in recreational facilities often receive relatively low salaries (2). A further important variable is the area of the country in which the economic multiplication occurs; in a region of chronically high unemployment, even a small stimulation of consumer expenditures may be very helpful to economic growth.

In addition to its general multiplier effect, the construction of an attractive park or conservation area may add substantially to personal property values for individuals whose homes border the new recreational facility (14).

Societal Change

Social change is another important variable in terms of both costs and benefits. Over the past 20 or 30 yr, Canadian society has seen a progressive migration from rural areas and small towns to large metropolises and a corresponding change in both the needs and the opportunities for physical activity. The proportion of school-age dependents has steadily diminished, but at the same time the proportion of senior citizens, particularly the very old, has progressively increased (34). Immigration has also changed the fabric of Canadian society from that of a well-established white, Anglo-Saxon, and Protestant stronghold to a multicultural and multiracial community.

All these social changes have influenced both the demand for fitness services and the ability of society to respond to this demand.

Types of Benefits

Beneficial effects of physical activity programming may be noted at the levels of the individual, the corporation, and the government. This raises the question as to how the economic benefits from a program should be distributed. Cost-benefit and cost-effectiveness analyses usually ignore any transfer of payments between one sector of the economy and another, although it is possible to draw up a narrower balance sheet and look, for example, at the costs and benefits to a corporation that has invested in an employee fitness program.

Individual Benefits

Individual benefits, or *opportunity dividends*, should be set against the opportunity costs of time that is allocated to exercise and tangible exercise-related expenditures on clothing, equipment, and travel. Many people will declare that the main reason they exercise is to feel better. Arousal, elevation of mood, increase in the range of experiences, enhancement of personal appearance and self-image, improved current health, avoidance of chronic disease, and the anticipation of a 1- to 2-yr extension of life span are all possible personal benefits of an active lifestyle (34).

The concept of the quality of life is plainly a major variable in any cost-benefit or cost-effectiveness analysis of life span, but techniques of measuring life quality are still in their infancy (1, 7, 33, 42). The quality of life differs substantially between a person who has just enough energy to meet the minimum demands of daily living and a peer who is in abundant health. Some allowance can be made for prolonged disability if convalescent months are discounted at 0.5 or 0.6 of their calendar values, but major personal and social costs of prolonged disability remain that are not adequately described in this manner. For example, charges may be incurred for additional transportation and home modifications, and other family members may lose income because they are assisting the disabled individual (22).

The total burden of health costs also extends to an employer, who must deal not only with time lost due to the illness itself, but also with poor productivity before an acute deterioration of health, postdisability loss of productivity, costs of retraining and replacing workers with permanent disability, and increased pension costs for those who must take premature retirement (33).

Industrial Benefits

Possible benefits from company-sponsored fitness programming, in addition to changes of health status, include an upgraded corporate image, increased worker satisfaction and productivity, decreased absenteeism and employee turnover, and a decreased industrial injury rate.

The impact of an employee fitness program on corporate image depends on the product being marketed. Food manufacturers and insurance companies seem particularly interested in developing an image of concern for good health. Within the company hierarchy, a fitness program may also improve managerial image and thus increase worker satisfaction (5, 6). In the company we studied, the initial level of worker satisfaction was quite high, and although gains of satisfaction were statistically significant, the practical impact of participation in the fitness program was marginal (Shephard and Cox, in press, 1988). A much larger effect might be anticipated in a company in which labor relations were initially poor, although in such a situation it would also be difficult to carry out a successful investigation of the magnitude of response.

Much of the research to date has concentrated on white-collar occupations, in which it is difficult to measure productivity precisely (Table 4.1). In the year following the introduction of an employee fitness program, Cox et al. (5) found a 7% rise of productivity at the Canada Life Assurance Company. However, a part of this gain was apparently a Hawthorne-type effect because there was also a 4.3% jump in productivity at a matched control company. The net effect of 2.7% nevertheless represented a substantial payroll saving to the experimental company.

The analysis of absenteeism is also quite difficult because much of the total absenteeism is attributable to a small proportion of staff, and about half of absences are brief and unrelated to health. A number of recent studies have suggested some impact of employee fitness programming on absenteeism (31, 32), although most of these investigations have been short-term and uncontrolled (Table 4.2). At the Canada Life Assurance Company, Cox et al. (5) did not see any significant benefit in the company as a whole in the year following introduction of an employee fitness program. Nevertheless, when data were broken down post hoc in terms of program participation, those who adhered highly to the exercise program developed a 22% decrease of absenteeism relative to other members of the company. Moreover, this change was significantly correlated with changes in both maximum oxygen intake and employee satisfaction. In many companies, the total loss of work from absenteeism averages as many as 10 out of 220 d per year, and because replacement labor is used about 75% less efficiently, absenteeism increases payroll costs by almost 8% (32). If there were 20% adherents to an employee fitness program, and their absenteeism decreased by 22%, this would diminish payroll costs by about 0.35%.

Turnover is a major cost for many companies. In the Canada Life project, management set the average cost of training a new employee at about $7,000 (5). Before the fitness program was started, the annual turnover rate was about 18%. However, in those adhering highly to the fitness program, turnover during the following year dropped to 1.8%. This could not be attributed to the participation of a specially conscientious group

Table 4.1 Impact of Fitness and Lifestyle Programs on Productivity

Author	Benefit
Rohmert (1973)	Less fatigue; faster recovery
LaPorte (1966)	Greater strength and hand steadiness; less eye fatigue
Pravosudov (1978)	Output standard +2%-5% to +10%-15%
Reville (1970)	31% decrease of errors
Geissler (1960)	Reduced fatigue
Manguroff et al. (1960)	Reduced fatigue
Galevskaya (1970)	Reduced fatigue
Pravosudov (1978)	Greater creativity; less fatigue
Heinzelman (1975)	Greater self-reported productivity
Howard and Mikalachki (1979)	No benefit in middle managers
Finney (1978, 1979)	No benefit from recreational programs
Stallings et al. (1975)	No effect on teaching or research output
Blair et al. (1980)	No effect on supervisor assessments, merit pay, or promotions
Health & Welfare Canada (1974)	4% gain of productivity
Mealey (1979)	39% increase of police-officer commendations
Briggs (1975)	Improved memory, muscle control, work performance
Shephard et al. (1981)	2.7% gain of productivity
Andrevsky (1982)	76% of participants at Hospital Corporation of America more productive
Danielson and Danielson (1982)	Doubling of productivity of forest-fire fighters under arduous conditions
Groves and de Carlo (1981)	15%-25% gain of productivity with programs, 25%-35% loss if withdrawn

Note. Classes of work and details of fitness programs differ among studies. For detailed discussion of each, see Shephard (32).

of long-term employees because their initial length of service was rather comparable with that of other workers. If we assume that the reduction of turnover is program related, the benefit would amount to about 2.2% of payroll costs.

Table 4.2 Impact of Fitness and Lifestyle Programs on Industrial Absenteeism: A Summary of Published Reports

Impact of absenteeism
11 times that of strikes 5.9 d/yr nonunion, 9.6 d/yr union

Impact of exercise

Author	Benefit
Lindén (1969)	Correlation of low absenteeism; high $\dot{V}O_2$max
Condon (1978) Erwin (1978)	23% decrease of absenteeism
Barhad (1979)	Decrease of absenteeism
Pafnote et al. (1979)	Decrease of absenteeism
Keelor (1970)	50% decrease of absenteeism
Pravosudov (1978)	Decrease of 4.0 d per worker-year
Mealey (1979)	Decrease of 34% (1.4 d per worker-year)
Wilbur (1982)	Decrease of 22%
Bjurstrom and Alexiou (1978)	Decrease of .59 d per worker-year
Blair et al. (1980) (1986)	No effect Reduced absenteeism
Richardson (1974)	Decrease of .82 d per worker-year
Garson (1977)	Decrease of 47% (2.8 d per worker-year)
Cox et al. (1981)	Decrease of 23% (1.3 d per worker-year)
Andrevsky (1982)	Marked drop in absenteeism (Boeing Corp.)
Wilson (1982)	Decrease of .62 d per year in adherents (13% change)
Baun et al. (1986)	Reduced absenteeism

Mean of percentage changes *30*
Mean decrease of absences *1.6 d per worker-year*
Replacement cost = *1.6 (1.75) d per worker-year*

Note. For detailed discussion of individual studies, see Shephard (32).

Little impact on physical injuries would be expected in a white-collar industry. However, among groups such as police the institution of a regular fitness program has reduced the number of claims presented for disabling back injuries (20) (Table 4.3).

Table 4.3 Impact of Fitness and Lifestyle Programs on Industrial Injuries

Impact of injuries in Canada
11.5 d production loss per worker-year
1,400 hospital beds per day occupied by injured
11% of workers injured
1 in 6,000 workers killed

Impact of exercise
Pravosudov (1978)—industrial trauma 2-10 times less frequent

Mealey (1979)—reduced low-back problems, pulled muscles, and strained ankles and wrists

Jacobson and Webber (1987)—compensable injury rate reduced to zero

Note. For detailed discussion of individual studies, see Shephard (32).

National Benefits

The anticipated national benefits of greater personal fitness include reductions in both the direct and the indirect costs of illness, an improvement of overall lifestyle, and a reduction of charges for geriatric care.

The direct costs of real or perceived illness include expenditures for personal services and supplies (e.g., hospital care, services of physicians and nurses, and drugs) together with nonpersonal items (e.g., medical research, training, public health services, capital construction, and insurance schemes). The indirect costs include losses of production from illness, premature death, and grief (15, 16).

Medical Services

Several authors have suggested that those engaged in fitness programs make fewer visits to physicians and require less medical attention (Table 4.4). In the Canada Life study, Shephard et al. (36) were able to obtain grouped Ontario Hospital Insurance Plan (OHIP) data on the charges for hospital usage and medical consultations, including costs *caused* by exercise involvement (26, 27). Over the first year after initiation of the program, the experimental company showed a small benefit relative to the matched control company; the advantage of the experimental group averaged some 0.5 d less of hospital bed usage per worker-year, plus the equivalent of three less physician consultations per year (36). However, the benefit was shown by both participants and nonparticipants in the exercise program and may thus have reflected a general increase of worker satisfaction or health awareness at the experimental company.

Table 4.4 Impact of Fitness and Lifestyle Programs on Demand for Medical Services

Author	Benefit
Pravosudov (1978)	Fourfold reduction in medical consultations 22.5% vs. 55% granted sick leave 4-d shorter duration of illness
Quasar (1976)	Average fitness would reduce OHIP claims 5.5% and would save $13 million per year in ischemic heart disease.
Corrigan (1980)	Fitness participants had lower dollar claims on university health insurance than did program dropouts.
Shephard et al. (1983)	Reduced hospital bed usage and OHIP charges relative to employees at control company
Jacobson and Webber (1987)	Compensable injury rate reduced to zero
Dedmon (1987)	Reduced medical claims
Barker (1987)	Reduced medical claims

Note. For detailed discussion of individual studies, see Shephard (32).

Because our study was short-term, it did not examine possible changes in bed usage resulting from a decrease of ischemic heart disease (IHD). The gains that we saw were essentially in short-term perceived health. It remains a matter of debate whether chronic conditions such as IHD would show a long-term decrease in an exercised population and, if so, by how much. Klarman (15) estimated that in 1962 the direct cost to the U.S. economy from all forms of cardiovascular disease was $3.1 billion; participants in a vigorous activity program could possibly reduce their portions of this charge by at least 50% (23, 24). To the $3.1 billion direct cost of cardiac disease must be added the loss of output from premature death. On the assumption that total earnings were lost, Klarman set output item at $19.4 billion; however, some authors have suggested that one should al-

low only the value added to the national economy by the worker, perhaps 25% of earnings. Survivors of a heart attack usually lose 3-6 mo of gainful employment; Klarman put the cost of the resultant loss of production at a further $3 billion. Finally, there is the very difficult item of disturbances created by grief, widowhood, and orphanhood. One possible method of estimating this last entry in our ledger is to consider court awards for the pain and distress suffered by relatives. However, most economists, in what seems a measure of despair, simply take a fixed percentage of other costs; Klarman suggested that $5 billion was an appropriate charge to the U.S. economy of 1962.

Several major assumptions are inherent in these calculations of the economic losses from illness. One is the figure accepted for the employment rate. Prolonged illness has less economic impact in a society that already has much unemployment. A related variable is the labor participation rate, or that proportion of people of working age who choose to enter the labor force. Finally, due allowance must be made for the unpaid services contributed by a spouse in activities such as child rearing. Often this is set at the worth of a full-time domestic servant, but this may be an underestimate (16).

Lifestyle

Physical activity often brings about an improvement of lifestyle, including such specific health benefits as a decreased usage of tobacco and alcohol. The health hazard appraisal schema was applied at the beginning and at the end of the Canada Life trial. The results suggested that improvements of lifestyle among men who adhered highly to the program had been sufficient to reduce their effective "appraised age" by an average of more than 2 yr (35) (Table 4.5).

A decrease of smoking also has more general benefits for society. Workers allocate less time to the ritual of the cigarette. Damage to furnishings is reduced, other workers are not annoyed by the smoke, money is saved on heating and ventilation, and reductions in fire insurance premiums can be negotiated (17).

Geriatric Services

A third potential social benefit from regular exercise is a reduced demand for geriatric services. The causes of institutionalization vary among senior citizens, but one major consideration is

Table 4.5 Impact of Fitness and Lifestyle Program on Appraised Age of Subjects

Nature of program participation	Change of appraised age (yr)		
	Men	Women	All
Control subjects	−0.92	0.87	−0.03
Nonparticipants	−0.25	1.37	0.56
Dropouts	−0.74	−0.77	−0.75
Low adherents	−0.94	0.03	−0.46
High adherents	−2.41	−0.11	−1.26

Note. Data expressed as change relative to calendar age.

undoubtedly a decrease of aerobic power, muscular strength, and flexibility, to a point where the normal minimum activities of daily living can no longer be carried out unaided (34). Regular training can restore maximum oxygen intake, deferring this situation for 10 yr or more. If the active person then experiences a period of dependency similar to that of the sedentary senior, there would be no fiscal advantage in the extended life span. However, if we make the more reasonable assumption that life span is not materially extended by exercise, then two thirds of the active group will die of intercurrent disorders before expensive, long-term institutional care is required (34).

Program and Social Costs

The techniques of increasing personal physical activity at various ages are so many and so varied that it is almost impossible to specify either the direct program or the social costs of increasing fitness. However, a few simple examples follow.

Walking

Fast walking is often considered a zero-cost means of improving the fitness of an older person. Nevertheless, at the personal level the active person faces some additional costs. Time will be invested, perhaps two pairs of comfortable shoes will be worn out every year, and (unless walking is intended to reduce body mass) additional food must be purchased to match the extra energy that is expended. From a societal point of view, there may also be some expense in providing paved sidewalks and in ensuring that these are plowed and sanded in the winter months. On the other hand,

if walking is built into the daily round, there may be a net saving to the community due to, for example, a lesser demand for public parking and for feeder bus routes to subway stations.

Employee Fitness Programs

Costs vary greatly with the nature of the facility, and varying modes of payment are also adopted (4, 41). Some companies provide only showers or subsidize membership at an external exercise facility. If a gymnasium is provided on-site, the recommended floor area ranges from 0.25 to 1.50 m² per employee, and additional space is allowed for fitness testing and personal exercise outside of scheduled class times. The annual cost of an on-site facility is typically $500-$750 per participant. About a third of the companies meet the entire expense of exercise programs, whereas others require full payment by participating employees. The most common arrangement is a sharing of cost; payroll deductions of $5.00-$6.00 per month do not seem to influence participation adversely (37), and indeed some authors have argued that a financial commitment of this order stimulates attendance at exercise classes.

A more critical issue may be the purchase of special clothing. Employees perform with peers and supervisors, and thus may be reluctant to exercise in other than the latest-fashion gym shoes and sweat suits. The cost of such items may have an appreciable negative impact on program recruitment.

Community Exercise Resources

The cost of various forms of community recreation can be assessed from the maximum potential occupancy of a facility relative to the costs of land plus construction (29, 32). If we assume 20% participation by members of the community, the likely costs range from $35 per resident per year for a mass pursuit such as public ice or roller skating to $200 per resident per year for a team game such as ice hockey (where the number of participants in any one arena is quite limited).

Outdoor pursuits such as swimming in a park or cross-country skiing are very rewarding aesthetically, but costs are relatively high in terms of improving cardiovascular health, because the operating season for the facility is short.

The cost of land, including access routes and parking, is a major expense when developing public recreational facilities. The cost-benefit ratio for community sports would thus be substantially improved if controls on land speculation were more effective.

Some Outstanding Issues

Tentative Balance Sheet

A tentative balance sheet is presented in Table 4.6. The main area for which cost estimates can be provided is the private sector. Even here, many of the items listed are gross approximations at best. There is considerable scope for putting costs on unknown items and refining estimates for the remainder.

One unresolved factor that has a major bearing on calculations for the government sector is whether a charge should be levied for an additional medical expenses that may be incurred if exercise allows a person to live longer (3, 28, 40). This may be an appropriate tactic when assessing a preventive measure such as vaccination (which has little effect on general health), but it does not seem correct for an active population, for which the annual medical expenses are likely to fall substantially below the population average even during old age (32, 35, 36). Moreover, the person who lives longer generally makes an increased contribution to society. Although the extra productive years are acknowledged in a cost-benefit analysis, they are ignored by a cost-effectiveness analysis. Incidental medical charges consume only a small part of the added productive capacity, and it is no more reasonable to include such charges in the imputed cost of treatment than it is to levy a charge for food, clothing, and housing (which the patient will merit through a longer productive life).

Despite arguments of this sort that need to be resolved, the currently available cost-benefit figures are encouraging in suggesting that benefits outweigh immediate program costs by a substantial margin. It is worth emphasizing that a substantial part of the anticipated benefits of exercise lie in the industrial sector (the impact on productivity, absenteeism, and turnover). The reason is that almost everyone works and is thus susceptible to an increase of output or a decrease of turnover. On the other hand, the costs of medical treatment are concentrated on relatively few individuals with real or perceived sickness, and however hard the rest of the population exercise, they are unable to change the health of the sick group by other than the force of their example.

Table 4.6 Costs and Benefits of Enhanced Physical Activity

Costs	Benefits
Personal	
Food: $20/yr	Better intake of nutrients and vitamins
Clothing	Reduced expenditure on alcohol, tobacco, and drugs; other forms of recreation; dress clothing
Equipment	
Admission fees	
Travel and lodging	New experiences
Time: $250-$500/yr	Meaning for age of leisure/ employment
Injury	
Death	Reduced industrial and domestic injury
	Improvements of perceived health; reduction of acute and chronic disease; enhanced quality of geriatric life
	Control of alcohol, tobacco, and drug dependency; less passive smoking and fires
	Improved personal appearance
	Enhanced property values
	Fewer problems from social deviancy
Private sector	
Exercise facilities: $100-$150/yr	Worker satisfaction large, but enhanced productivity $116/yr
Medical supervision and exercise personnel	Reduced turnover and absenteeism $260/yr reduced industrial injuries $40/yr reduced health insurance premiums
Time	
Sports injuries	
	Enhanced company image
	Enhanced employment and economic growth
	Entrepreneurial opportunities
	Enhanced property values
Government	
Fitness promotion	Reduced hospital and health care costs $233/yr
Exercise facilities: $35-$200/yr	Reduced social deviancy (vandalism, law enforcement, detention)
Recreational workers	
Land acquisition	Reduced geriatric dependency $35/yr
Infrastructure (roads, mass transit, etc.)	Enhanced employment
	Economic stimulation and increased tax base; enhanced environment

(Cont.)

Table 4.6 (Continued)

Costs	Benefits
	Improved balance of payments
	Benefits as for private sector in government-controlled enterprises
	Military fitness

Note. Costs and benefits calculated on the basis of 20% participation in the fitness and lifestyle program and expressed in 1982 U.S. dollars. For detailed discussion of individual studies, see Shephard (32).

Value Judgments

Cost-benefit and cost-effectiveness analyses allow decisions between program alternatives to be taken logically. To evaluate alternative demands on scarce health resources, it is necessary to understand both the economic and non-economic costs and benefits (8). However, once the necessary information has been assembled, the analyst must make a series of value judgments.

For example, how far does the social value of an active lifestyle merits its costs? How much money should be allocated to either the prevention or the treatment of disease relative to the treatment of acute disease and other social priorities? How, indeed, can one compare the social acceptability of prevention versus acute care (19)? It might seem obvious that most consumers would choose preventing rather than treating disease, even if the former were more costly. However, in practice, decisions are not always made in terms of an optimized combination of economic and noneconomic factors. Sometimes publicity for so-called miracle medicine, such as heart and liver transplants, has an irrational impact on the decisions taken by both the patient and medical planners.

Purpose of Society

Issues regarding the costs of exercise and health promotion touch on the fundamental purpose of Canadian society. We have suggested that employee fitness programs are likely to be a good corporate investment. However, let us suppose that after careful fiscal analysis a company finds that the economic benefits of its fitness program fall short of the anticipated fiscal dividends. How far,

then, is the employer justified in spending money to increase worker satisfaction or health? What is the purpose underlying our economy: to maximize the gross national product, or to ensure the happiness of Canadian citizens? Can we agree with Pope John Paul II on the principle of the priority of labor over capital, the latter serving merely as an instrument of the laborers?

Authority for Decisions

Finally, we must ask who has the authority to choose when major budgetary decisions are required? Is there an elite who supposedly know what is best for society? Or should we allow some Canadians to adopt a poor lifestyle at the expense of their more disciplined fellow citizens (10)? Is the individual responsible for poor personal health, or should we blame a society that provides too many incentives to drink, smoke, and overeat and too few incentives to exercise?

Decisions about fitness and health are often made by professionals who have relevant expertise but who also have a strong vested interest in specific solutions. Alternatively, solutions may be left to the general public, who are often poorly informed and at the mercy of the powerful forces of consumer advertising. Recourse is sometimes made to parliamentarians, but they unfortunately are strongly influenced by pressure groups in marginal constituencies. The ideal would be an appeal to an absolute scale of values, such as the Judeo-Christian ethic, the Kantian moral imperative, or the Golden Rule. However, society has yet to reach the stage of maturity where all cost-benefit and cost-effectiveness decisions are made on this basis.

Suggested Research Priorities

The unresolved issues mentioned previously suggest a number of research priorities. To these questions may be added more explicit tasks.

Definition of the Beneficial Type of Exercise

Most analyses to date have considered merely the benefits of exercise. However, exercise is not a single entity but varies both in intensity and in quality. If a cardiac health benefit is sought, a threshold of intensity, amount, or both must be surpassed; if increases in life satisfaction, perceived health, and willingness to work are the goals, then the quality of the recreational experience may be much more important than is the intensity or the amount of activity that is undertaken.

Determination of Long-Term Participation Rates

Long-term participation rates are needed for various forms of exercise and active recreation. It is also desirable to determine how far these rates can be increased by favorable changes in the social climate.

Program Costs

Although the cost of current programs is known fairly accurately, more information is needed on the marginal costs that would be required to interest that segment of the population that is presently inactive.

Cost Uncertainties

Various items in the cost-benefit ledger that need clarification have been noted previously. In particular, more work is needed on the indirect costs of ill health and the value that the average person would place on so-called abundant health, which is implicit in the concept of fitness.

Acknowledgment

The research of this laboratory on the economics of fitness was supported in part by a grant from the Directorate of Fitness and Amateur Sport.

References

1. Berg, R.L. Establishing the values of various conditions in life for a health status index. In: Berg, R.L., ed. *Health status indexes*. Hospital Research and Educational Trust, 1973, p. 120-127.
2. Berger, E. *Recreation—A changing society's economic giant*. Toronto: Ministry of Tourism and Recreation, 1983.
3. Blomquist, G. Value of life-saving. *J. Pol. Econ.* 87: 540-558, 1979.
4. Collis, M. *Employee fitness*. Ottawa, ON: Queen's Printer, 1977.
5. Cox, M., R.J. Shephard, and P. Corey. Influence of an employee fitness programme upon fitness, productivity and absenteeism. *Ergonomics* 24: 795-806, 1981.
6. Cox, M., R.J. Shephard, and P. Corey. Physical activity and alienation in the workplace. *Proceedings of the North American Society of Sport Sociology*, Toronto, 1982.
7. Criqui, M., and R.M. Kaplan. *Behavioral epidemiology and disease prevention*. New York: Plenum Press, 1985.
8. Dardis, R. The value of life: New evidence from the market place. *Am. Econ. Rev.* 70: 1077-1082, 1980.
9. Ellis, J.B. *Economic impacts of sport, recreation and fitness activities in Ontario: A preliminary review*. Toronto: Ontario Ministry of Tourism and Recreation, 1982.
10. Godin, G., and R.J. Shephard. Physical fitness: Individual or societal responsibility? *Can. J. Public Health* 75: 200-203, 1982.
11. Godin, G., and R.J. Shephard. Psychosocial predictors of exercise intentions among spouses. *Can. J. Appl. Sport Sci.* 10: 36-43, 1985; 8: 104-113, 1983.
12. Haggerty, R.J. Changing lifestyles to improve health. *Prev. Med.* 6: 276-289, 1977.
13. Hodgson, T.A. The state of the art of cost of illness estimates. *Adv. Health Econ. Health Services Res.* 4: 129-164, 1982.
14. Jensen, C.R. *Leisure and recreation: Introduction and overview*. Philadelphia: Lea & Febiger, 1977.
15. Klarman, H.E. Socio-economic impact of heart disease. In: Andrus, E.C., ed. *The heart and circulation*. Second National Conference on Cardiovascular Diseases. Washington, DC: U.S. Public Health Service, 1964, vol. 2.
16. Klarman, H.E. Economics of health. In: Clark, D.W., and B. MacMahon, eds. *Preventive and community medicine* (2nd ed.). Boston: Little, Brown, 1981, p. 603-615.
17. Kristein, M.M. The economics of health promotion at the work site. *Health Educ. Q.* 9(Suppl.): 27-36, 1982.
18. Leatt, P., H. Hattin, C. West, and R.J. Shephard. Seven-year follow-up of employee fitness program. *Can. J. Public Health* 79: 20-25, 1988.
19. McPherson, P.K. The political argument on health costs. *Br. Med. J.* 290: 1679-1680, 1985.
20. Mealey, M. New fitness for police and firefighters. *Phys. Sports Med.* 7: 96-100, 1979.
21. Morey, R.C. Cost-effectiveness of an employer-sponsored recreational programme: A case study. *Omega* 14: 67-74, 1983.

22. Mushkin, S.J., and S. Landfeld. *Non-health sector costs of illness* (Report No. A-7). Washington, DC: Georgetown University, Public Services Laboratory, 1978.

23. Paffenbarger, R. Physical activity and fatal heart attack: Protection or selection? In: Amsterdam, E.A., J.H. Wilmore, and A.N. deMaria, eds. *Exercise in cardiovascular health and disease.* New York: Yorke Books, 1977.

24. Paffenbarger, R.S., R.T. Hyde, A.L. Wing, and C.-c. Hsieh. Physical activity, all-cause mortality and longevity of college alumni. *N. Engl. J. Med.* 314: 605-613, 1986.

25. Russell, D. *The cost of doing nothing: An assessment of initiatives in fitness and health for the Hillary Commission.* Dunedin, New Zealand: University of Otago, 1987.

26. Russell, L.B. The economics of prevention. *Health Policy* 4: 85-100, 1984.

27. Russell, L.B. Issues in the design of future preventive medicine studies. In: Whelan, D., and J. Evered, eds. *The value of preventive medicine.* Bath, ME: Pitman Press, 1985, p. 203-217 (CIBA Foundation Symposium 110).

28. Russell, L.B. *Is prevention better than cure?* Washington, DC: Brookings Institution, 1986.

29. Shephard, R.J. *Endurance fitness* (2nd ed.). Toronto: University of Toronto Press, 1977.

30. Shephard, R.J. Factors influencing the exercise behaviour of patients. *Sports Med.* 2: 348-366, 1985.

31. Shephard, R.J. The impact of exercise upon medical costs. *Sports Med.* 2: 133-143, 1985.

32. Shephard, R.J. *The economics of enhanced endurance fitness.* Champaign, IL: Human Kinetics, 1986.

33. Shephard, R.J. The economics of prevention: A critique. *Health Policy* 7: 49-56, 1987.

34. Shephard, R.J. *Physical activity and aging* (2nd ed.). London: Croom Helm, 1987.

35. Shephard, R.J., P. Corey, and M. Cox. Health hazard appraisal—The influence of an employee fitness programme. *Can. J. Public Health* 73: 183-187, 1982.

36. Shephard, R.J., P. Corey, P. Renzland, and M. Cox. The impact of changes in fitness and lifestyle upon health care utilization. *Can. J. Public Health* 74: 51-54, 1983.

37. Shephard, R.J., P. Morgan, R. Finucane, and L. Schimmelfing. Factors influencing recruitment to an occupational fitness program. *J. Occup. Med.* 22: 389-398, 1980.

38. Smith, S.L.J. *Recreation geography.* Harlow, Essex, England: Longman, 1983.

39. Song, T.K., R.J. Shephard, and M. Cox. Absenteeism, employee turnover and sustained exercise participation. *J. Sports Med. Fitness* 22: 392-399, 1982.

40. U.S. Congress Office of Technology Assessment. *Cost-effectiveness of influenza vaccination.* Washington, DC: U.S. Government Printing Office, 1981.

41. Wanzel, R.S. Rationale for employee fitness program. In: Wanzel, R.S., ed. *Employee fitness: The how to.* Toronto: Ministry of Culture and Recreation, 1979, p. 1-16.

42. Weinstein, M.C. Cost-effective priorities for cancer prevention. *Science* 221: 17-23, 1983.

PART II

Assessment and Determinants of Physical Activity, Fitness, and Health

Chapter 5

Assessment of Physical Activity During Leisure and Work

John V.G.A. Durnin

This is a conference on exercise, fitness, and health. With your permission, I will devote my attention to the relevance of physical activity to health in the general population without special reference to extremely fit people or to athletes. I should also like to think that we are considering health in a positive fashion and not just as an absence of disease.

I know that many people in this audience are athletes of some kind, perhaps not competitive but still sufficiently interested in physical exercise to undertake it relatively frequently at a fairly high level. Although I hope this chapter will have some secondhand relevance to them, they do not constitute the group on whom I want to concentrate. Indeed, I am not at all sure how beneficial exercise that is frequent, habitual, and *strenuous* is from the point of view of the health of the community. Proper statistical information on this is scanty and somewhat controversial. Something that frequently worries me about the supposed health benefits of strenuous exercise is that such exercise appears almost never part of the normal life of people living a traditional rural existence. In the populations we have studied in parts of New Guinea and Burma, no one, if they could possibly avoid it, did anything really energetic. They would have thought it quite mad to choose voluntarily to exert themselves to near-maximal levels. Indeed, I have not infrequently had similar thoughts myself.

My concern is with the large mass of ordinary people who, in the sort of society that characterizes industrialized countries, are rather inactive most of the time. They are also relatively unfit, and moderate obesity is usually relatively common (my statements are all qualified!). These variables—inactivity, lack of physical fitness, and obesity, as well as eating patterns that may also be less than desirable—might all interact in relation to health

or lack of health in the community, and isolating the one variable of physical activity is often difficult and confusing. The fact is also that hard, wide-ranging evidence is remarkably scarce.

I should interject at this stage that I am making an assumption that work plays almost no part in the lives of a very large proportion of the population as far as physical activity is concerned. Industrialized society has very successfully eliminated most forms of even moderate activity from one's occupations. Therefore, almost all my analysis of this topic is concerned with physical activity as something undertaken voluntarily in leisure time.

Assessment in Relation to Population Group

When we consider the assessment of physical activity at varying levels of strenuousness in different groups of the population, assessment needs to be examined in ways appropriate for the particular population group. The first and (to me) obvious differentiation concerns the possibly distinctive attitudes of, and differing benefits to, males and females. Excluding that major subdivision, groups who may have their own special characteristics to bear in mind are infants and young children, older children and adolescents, middle-aged people, and, very importantly, the elderly. The assessment of physical activity in the elderly may well help to elucidate its importance in making some older people more physically active and agile, feel better, have more social contacts, and eat more and thus be less likely to suffer from nutritional deficiencies.

The baseline group against which it might be useful to contrast activity in other groups consists of young adult males. I am not suggesting that they set a standard that other groups should try to emulate but simply that they probably have the highest level of physical activity and therefore are a useful prototype for comparison. In a fashion similar to one that I have used in the past to set a standard of desirable fatness, I will use the young adult male as a sort of frame of reference that serves as a starting point for this discussion, as long as it is quite clear that this does not imply that exercise levels appropriate for young-adult males are also desirable for women, children, and other groups.

In relation to *fatness*, the basic criteria I employed to theorize about the possible desirable level for young adult males starts off with the same premise that can be used for physical activity, namely, that much of the present anatomy and physiology of the human body has developed because of the necessities of humans during the long process of evolution, during which they were hunter-gatherers most of the time. "Gathering" did not require any special physical attributes. The hunter, of course, did have specific needs, for example, a fair amount of muscular strength to lift and carry heavy objects and the ability to move very fast for brief periods of time. (Incidentally, on that basis I suggested that the ideal amount of fat in the male body was the *minimal* amount [8].) It is at least plausible that these requirements of muscular strength and speed of movement did not demand extraordinary cardiovascular fitness nor the facility of long endurance. If agility, speed, and moderate strength were what was needed for survival, then they were likely to be the faculties receiving preferential genetic treatment. The body of the young adult male might then be constructed anatomically and physiologically to have these characteristics, and maintaining them at a reasonable level would not necessarily require frequent and prolonged periods of heavy physical exercise. If indeed young males were the most active groups, the basic norm of desirable physical activity could therefore be a level that involved frequent periods of physical activity but not necessarily activity of more than a moderate degree.

The requirement for and benefits from activity for groups other than young-adult males might, theoretically at least, be expected to differ significantly from theirs. It seems to me that the clearest division must be between males and females, if not of any age certainly for young and middle-aged adults. Although a superficial impression gained from seeing the considerable numbers of red-faced, sweating women jogging in many North American towns and cities might easily be that women were as intent as were men on exercising at high levels, thus increasing their $\dot{V}O_2$max and becoming slim and muscular, this impression would undoubtedly entail an error of judgment. These women represent a female aberration. They constitute .0001% of the world's population of women and are typical only of a small section of middle-class American and European females. Physical activity in women has, I suspect, relatively little in common with its male counterpart, at least until fairly old age, when there might well be considerable overlap.

The evolutionary aspect of the female anatomy and physiology might also suggest that only very moderate physical activity was necessary in any significant way to maintain their different physical attributes. None of the hard labor that is the normal role of rural women (e.g., carrying babies, carrying water, carrying vegetables and fruit, working in the fields, and doing much walking) involves high levels of energy expenditure, to judge from data collected in the Gambia (15), India (9), New Guinea (21), and other countries; and both the activity required in daily life and the activity levels needed to maintain health and fitness seem to be satisfied by quite moderate exercise.

It seems to me that a basic consideration of the role of physical activity in the welfare of the individual might be influenced by the way in which we try to assess physical activity. We might have preconceived ideas of which types of activity are important, and the results we obtain might, at least in part, reflect these preconceptions.

I like to believe that we are examining physical activity and health in a broad way, encompassing many varying positive aspects of health and not restricting ourselves in any way simply to a consideration of the role of physical activity in attaining fitness or in preventing disease.

Various Forms of Influence of Physical Activity

Although the importance of physical activity certainly varies with gender and age, a few generalities might have some relevance to all groups. One of these might be some degree of *physical fitness*, not because of any particular intrinsic usefulness of being fit, but simply because, in all age groups, it reflects the ability to move—to walk, run, work, play games, or do any number of active pursuits—with minimal physical distress to the individual.

Another factor is the *mobility* and *suppleness* of limbs that is maintained by physical activity and that, frequently I should imagine, is not a conscious component of physical activity but an automatic concomitant of being active.

Yet another aspect is the feeling of *well-being* generated by physical activity. This could easily be the most generally recognized benefit resulting from physical activity and the most appreciated short-term health gain. Although well-being is important at all ages, it is especially advantageous to those elderly people who are habitually active (11). The level, duration, and type of activity necessary to produce this feeling of well-being surely differ very much between genders, groups, and individuals within groups. Children of both genders, young and middle-aged women, and older people might obtain this from levels of activity that would not necessarily be very strenuous nor have a long duration. Many young adult or middle-age men (and especially perhaps the type we find at a conference such as this) would obtain the sensation of well-being only by exercise done several times weekly and at perhaps 60% or more of their $\dot{V}O_2$max. I am sure there is a strong cultural component here. Although I recognize the real pleasure to be obtained from severe exertion, and although I accept also the pandemic nature of this modern phenomenon, I feel there is something of the Protestant ethic here that has even contaminated other cultures. The idea of "no gain without pain" has infiltrated our subconscious so that activity, to be really satisfactory, must be strenuous. We must guard against the judgments of people who hold such views, in the overall assessment of the relationships of physical activity to health.

Another aspect of this relationship is connected with *body image*, perhaps not very closely a component of health but something that clearly contributes to personal satisfaction. There is probably some element of the body image incentive in almost anyone, at any age, who is deliberately physically active.

Finally, the aspect of physical activity that motivates a large percentage of middle-aged men who exercise actively and possibly a rather small percentage of women relates to *disease prevention*, particularly the degenerative diseases of the cardiovascular system. The level and duration of exercise required to decrease the likelihood of premature cardiovascular disease is still, I regret to say, a subject of much speculation and remarkably little hard evidence. This is an unfortunate but understandable gap in our knowledge because to obtain good factual evidence we need highly controlled studies on large populations over many years—almost a practical impossibility, although a few admirable investigations have attempted this.

There are many references to an apparent negative relationship between physical activity and the incidence of cardiovascular disease (4, 12, 13, 19, 22, 23, 26, 27, 31). However, only in the cases of the Framingham (13), British civil servant (6, 18), and Harvard alumni activity (23) studies (and perhaps one or two more) was there a determined attempt to obtain not only general information on physical activity but also some sort of assessment of *duration* and *intensity*. The attempts, praiseworthy though they were, were not scientifically convincing.

To form any moderately correct impression of whether, and by how much, activity is related to health, we need valid information about exercise habits. Also, if we are attempting to persuade large sections of the population to increase their levels of activity, we need some baseline data as reference levels.

To obtain the baseline data (or any really useful information about physical activity), we need to categorize it with regard to its intensity, duration, and frequency. The methods available for this are limited and unfortunately rather imprecise and open to considerable error.

Methods of Acquiring Information on Physical Activity

Methods of acquiring information may involve (a) questioning or self-recording, (b) some form of measurement of movement, (c) heart rate recording, or (d) measuring energy expenditure. Several useful general reviews of these methods have been published recently, particularly those by Montoye et al. (17, 29). The most common technique of assessment is to measure physical activity by *questionnaire* or by a *diary record*. Some questionnaires require a skilled interviewer and can take up to 1-1/2 hr, whereas others can be self-administered and completed in 10-15 min. Testing the validity of the different types of questionnaires is difficult (5), and there is still great uncertainty in this field. One is often left with a final impression of a mixture of rather rough and vague information (24) and quite unjustified precision in which statements are made such as "The mean leisure time physical activity index . . . was 677 [sic] kcal/week" (3).

The decision on which form the investigation of physical activity will take depends on what the information is intended for. If reasonably high precision is required on limited numbers of individuals, then a diary record that is based on a recall interview might be adequate. This might be done as a recall in detail of physical activity over the previous 24 hr and might include an element of history; that is, the 24-hr recall would be put into the context of its relationship to activity patterns during the previous week, whether this was reasonably representative of a long-term pattern, whether there were marked seasonal influences, and whether at some time in the past a significant alteration in physical activity pattern had occurred. A diary method can also be employed prospectively, with the individual recording his or her activity during periods of 2 or 3 d or longer. However, without very close and time-consuming supervision it is difficult to know how accurately the prospective record has been kept, and in the end it may be possible to subdivide a population into only a relatively few categories on the basis of duration of physical activity, frequency, and an indication of whether any activity of high intensity took place. Heikkinen et al. (10) used this approach to subdivide a population into only a few categories, and the Baecke questionnaire (2) is another fairly straightforward way of doing this. In general, some form of questionnaire or diary record usually assumes top priority as an assessment of usable information on physical activity.

If methods of direct measurement of activity are to be employed, the whole investigation undergoes a considerable alteration in scope. First, the number of individuals becomes reduced on a logarithmic scale. Information by some form of questionnaire can be obtained on hundreds or even thousands of individuals. Data from direct recording will be restricted to tens of individuals. However, such data might be extremely useful as an adjunct to questionnaires, particularly in acquiring validatory information; statistically chosen subsamples analyzed by direct recording can give information on the validity or reliability of the general results from the questionnaires.

If we undertake direct measurement of the activity of the individual, several techniques are available. The *recording of movement* can be done by various kinds of instruments, from the old-fashioned and rather unsatisfactory pedometers to accelerometers, actometers, and electrical devices for counting steps. Cinephotography, which can be used for assessing certain types of complex activities, is obviously not appropriate in the present context. *Pedometers* are in common use (they can be purchased easily in sporting goods stores), but, although they have a much improved design over older instruments, they are still open to considerable error in both over- and under-recording. They are also not suitable for measuring swimming, cycling, or activities done in a more or less static position. Not many scientific articles have described their use critically, and one relies more on hearsay, which is seldom very positive in their favor. Saris and Binkhorst (25) found them to be inaccurate when used for children, and we have not found them (even in laboratory studies) to be acceptably reliable and accurate, notwithstanding our willingness to accept very rough data. For general scientific use in the assessment of physical activity they are unsuitable.

Other instruments of relevance are *accelerometers*, which measure horizontal, lateral, or vertical movement and can be of considerable benefit in intensive laboratory-based studies. However, because the output is in the form of electrical signals that need retrieval and sometimes complex analysis, the use of this instrument is not really convenient for large-scale fieldwork. Perhaps I am being unduly restrictive in my interpretation of the theme of this conference, but it seems to me that we will obtain statistically satisfactory information only by studies on relatively large numbers of individuals, and this is not practicable using accelerometers.

An instrument with greater potential in our present context is an *actometer*, which seems to be a generic term for any type of instrument that records activity. The practical use of such meters was described some years ago by Saris and Binkhorst (25) and La Porte et al. (14), all of whom seemed to find them satisfactory for discriminating between groups of individuals with differing activity patterns. The more recent form of actometer is a modified wristwatch that is capable of recording not only movement but also acceleration or intensity of movement. Recent papers by Tryon (28) and Avons et al. (1) provided extra information about their usefulness when worn by subjects during several days.

The study by Avons et al. (1) is perhaps worth quoting in some detail. Counts from the actometers were related to actual measurements of energy expenditure during a 17.5-hr period inside a whole-body indirect calorimeter. Twelve men were studied while performing activities such as sitting, cycling, stepping, and walking. The actometers were then worn for 7 d of normal living. There were very high correlations, varying from 0.80 to 0.97, between energy expenditure and actometer counts. Unfortunately, however, the data as presented fall into an elementary statistical trap, and the correlations are virtually meaningless.

Apart from this criticism, the conclusion of Avons et al. (1) is that "when actometers are used to monitor energy expenditure in the community, their performance was disappointing." Calibration was needed for individual subjects, for types of activity, and for the instruments. It seems difficult to envisage that this technique can become, in the immediate future, something that can be employed on large-scale community studies. Its likely use may still be important but seems to be in the controlled laboratory investigation.

Instruments for recording electrically each time the foot touches the ground are also available. These devices may have a place in the general context of recording activity, but they (like pedometers) do not necessarily record all forms of physical activity (e.g., activity of the trunk and arms, cycling, and swimming), and their information is therefore limited although again may be helpful in roughly subdividing groups of individuals.

Heart rate recording will obviously, at least theoretically, give us information about physical activity. I will not comment on the instrumental aspect of recording heart rate; many relatively inexpensive instruments on the market are capable of recording the duration of activities of differing severity, for example, a heart rate of 130 beats/min or more, 110 beats/min or more, or whatever levels are particularly desired. These recorders can also be worn easily and continuously for at least 24 hr and often for much longer. They are capable of providing complex information on reasonably sized population groups, and I am convinced that they have an important place in monitoring physical activity.

Nevertheless, it is tedious and sometimes difficult to analyze and interpret the data accumulated, and there still seem to have been relatively few large-scale studies of a kind to interest us here using this technique. There are, of course, also many problems about relating heart rate to the intensity of activity, especially at the level of or below moderately strenuous activity. Many factors other than the activity may affect heart rate, and the bulk and site of the muscle groups involved may also influence the heart rate. In the study by Avons et al. (1), the relationship between heart rate and energy expenditure (measured inside the whole-body calorimeter) varied to the extent that again calibration was needed for individuals and for types of activity.

Measurements of *oxygen consumption* or of *energy expenditure* do not seem to be very relevant to our present needs other than as indicators of the intensity of activity monitored by other means, for example, by questionnaires or by instruments.

A reasonable conclusion from this discussion might be that we still need to rely very largely on questionnaires or diary recording (recall or prospective). Possibly, actometers or heart rate recording might be utilized on a subsample, but this complicates the study considerably and may not, depending on the objective, help us much in our basic conclusions.

Methods Relative to Age of Population

I now revert briefly to my earlier discussion about the relevant level and duration of physical activity for the different population groups in whom we might be interested. I deal with these mostly in relation to age.

With infants and young children, questionnaires completed by the mother might not always provide adequate data, and it might be necessary to gather functional information by heart rate recording. We have been doing this recently on 2- to 3-yr-olds in a study relating activity to growth. However, there are problems in using this method in very young children both from the point of view of interpretation of the data and from the simple practical problems (e.g., children often tamper with the electrodes or the connecting wires).

In the case of older children and adults of any age, a questionnaire or a diary (retrospective or prospective) is still probably the method of choice for large groups, and perhaps one of the alternative techniques can be employed on a subsample. Validating the diary records is difficult, and many errors, some of them biased, are likely to occur. For example, many (even most) people tend to exaggerate both the duration and the intensity of their physical activities. As long as this exaggeration is more or less equally biased within or between groups, it will not have too much influence on a comparative study. However, the bias may not be even, and it is also a problem to determine the minimum level of activity in any population group with much confidence.

Intensity of Physical Activity

As far as the intensity of activity is concerned, I tend to be sympathetic to the idea that for all groups, excluding young adults and perhaps young-middle-aged men, the level of interest is activity of moderate intensity, with heart rates no higher than 120-130 beats/min (or the equivalent for older people). All the really important beneficial effects of exercise can almost certainly be acquired as a result of activity at that level.

For young and young-middle-aged men, the hard evidence in favor of a much higher level of exercise seems to me very scanty. Morris et al. (18, 20) suggested that only habitual exercise at a level of at least 7.5 kcal $\cdot$ min^{-1} (which in fact probably corresponds to a heart rate of 120-130 beats/min), lasting at least 30 min and occurring no less infrequently than every second day, was needed to reduce the incidence of coronary heart disease. However, the data on which these recommendations are based are very rough and imprecise, and I suspect that a very large part of the justification for the supposition that activity (if it is to be effective as a means of preventing or delaying cardiovascular disease) must be of moderately high intensity depends on an extrapolation of physiological findings on what level of exercise is needed to improve cardiovascular capabilities. Whether this extrapolation is entirely relevant to disease prevention is open to some dispute.

Conclusion

I will conclude by restating my view that the critical assessment of habitual physical activity has widespread importance from the points of view of health and of the prevention of disease. However, the information needs to be gathered with care and interpreted with appropriate circumspection. We should not allow ourselves to be seduced into facile and unjustified conclusions because of our own proper predilections. The fact that physical activity is certainly beneficial should not dissuade us from attempting a careful appraisal of which kind of physical activity is most beneficial for which result on which particular population group. There is no doubt that the type of exercise and its intensity and duration may have a marked effect on muscle tone, muscular function, the feeling of well-being, general bodily function, body composition, nutritional intake, and other aspects of body function and be-

havior; however, we need much more valid information on these topics.

More than 20 yr ago I gave a paper here in Toronto (at a similarly distinguished gathering of people interested in physical activity) on *activity patterns in the community* (7). At that time I tried to relate activity to anthropometric and social data, defining activity in terms of actual energy expenditure. We had detailed data then of daily energy expenditure on several hundred individuals, and we have collected similar data since then on several hundred more. However, the number of individuals in the separate cells or subgroups—when allowance is made for gender, age, socioeconomic status, occupations, diet, fatness, and so on—becomes far too small for any really useful statistical analyses to be done. We were driven to use different and simpler methods to obtain the necessary volume of data.

In relation to the specific topic I am dealing with, we have not advanced all that much further in the past 20 yr. The two useful monographs "Habitual Physical Activity and Health" (30) and "Physical Activity in Disease Prevention and Treatment" (16) still leave us with many unanswered questions on our topic today. Perhaps I am only stating the obvious when I say that, within my suggestion that it is the duration and frequency and type of *moderate* physical activity that are important, we need information on several very large population groups. Although some small-scale validation (e.g., by heart rate recording or by actometer) may be helpful, the basic requirement can be accomplished only by some form of questionnaire; and that in itself may be quite complicated, laborious, expensive, and time consuming.

We will never get answers that will convince the scientific unbeliever in exercise on such a complex problem as exercise, fitness, and health (with all the confounding variables) by small-scale studies, no matter how well the studies are executed.

References

1. Avons, P., P. Garthwaite, H.L. Davies, P.R. Murgatroyd, and W.P.T. James. Approaches to estimating physical activity in the community: Calorimetric validation of actometers and heart rate recording. *Europ. J. Clin. Nutr.* 42: 185-196, 1988.
2. Baecke, J.A.H., J. Burema, and J.E.R. Fritters. A short questionnaire for the measurement of physical activity in epidemiological studies. *Am. J. Clin. Nutr.* 48: 1-6, 1982.

3. Brooks, C.M. Leisure time physical activity assessment of American adults through an analysis of time diaries collected in 1981. *Am. J. Public Health* 77: 455-460, 1987.

4. Brunner, D., S. Altman, K. Loebl, S. Schwartz, and S. Levin. Serum cholesterol and triglycerides in patients suffering from ischemic heart disease and in healthy subjects. *J. Atheroscl. Res.* 28: 197, 1977.

5. Buskirk, E.R., D. Harris, J. Mendez, and J. Skinner. Comparison of two assessments of physical activity and a survey method for caloric intake. *Am. J. Clin. Nutr.* 24: 1119-1125, 1971.

6. Chave, S.P.W., J.N. Morris, and S. Moss. Vigorous exercise in leisure time and the death rate: A study of male civil servants. *J. Epidemiol. Community Health* 32: 239-243, 1978.

7. Durnin, J.V.G.A. Activity patterns in the community. *Can. Med. Assoc. J.* 96: 882-886, 1967.

8. Durnin, J.V.G.A. Possible interaction between physical activity, body composition and obesity in man. In: Bray, G.A., ed. *Recent advances in obesity research.* London: Newman, 1978, vol. 2, p. 237-241.

9. Durnin, J.V.G.A., and S. Drummond. Adaptations to seasonal fluctuations in food availability in a group of Indian rural women. *Europ. J. Clin. Nutr.* (in press).

10. Heikkinen, E., W.E. Waters, and Z.J. Brzezinski. The elderly in eleven countries. In: *Public health in Europe.* Copenhagen: World Health Organization, 1983.

11. Jagger, C., M. Clarke, and R.A. Davies. The elderly at home: Indices of disability. *J. Epidemiol. Community Health* 40: 139-142, 1986.

12. Kahn, H. The relationship of reported coronary heart disease mortality to physical activity of work. *Am. J. Public Health* 53: 1058, 1963.

13. Kannel, W.B., T.R. Daeber, G.D. Friedann, W.E. Glennon, and P.M. McNamara. Risk factors in coronary heart disease. The Framingham Study. *Ann. Int. Med.* 61: 888-899, 1964.

14. La Porte, R.E., L.H. Kuller, D.J. Kupfer, R.J. McPartland, G. Matthews, and C. Caspersen. An objective measure of physical activity for epidemiologic research. *Am. J. Epidemiol.* 109: 158-168, 1979.

15. Lawrence, M., and R.G. Whitehead. Physical activity and total energy expenditure of child-bearing Gambian village women. *Europ. J. Clin. Nutr.* 42: 145-160, 1988.

16. Masironi, R., and H. Denolin. *Physical activity in disease prevention and treatment.* London: Butterworth, 1985.

17. Montoye, H.J., and H.L. Taylor. Measurement of physical activity in population studies. *Hum. Biol.* 56: 195-216, 1984.

18. Morris, J.N., C. Adam, S.P.W. Chave, C. Sirey, and L. Epstein. Vigorous exercise in leisure-time and the incidence of coronary heart disease. *Lancet* i: 333-339, 1973.

19. Morris, J.N., J.A. Heady, P.A.R. Raffle, C.G. Roberts, and J.W. Parks. Coronary heart disease and physical activity of work. *Lancet* ii: 1053, 1953.

20. Morris, J.N., R. Pollard, M.G. Everitt, and S.P.W. Chave. Vigorous exercise in leisure time: Protection against coronary heart disease. *Lancet* ii: 1207-1210, 1980.

21. Norgan, N.G., A. Ferro-Luzzi, and J.V.G.A. Durnin. The energy and nutrient intake and the energy expenditure of 204 New Guinean adults. *Philos. Trans. R. Soc. London [Biol.]* 268: 309-348, 1974.

22. Paffenbarger, R.S., and W.E. Hale. Work activity and coronary heart mortality. *N. Engl. J. Med.* 292: 545-550, 1975.

23. Paffenbarger, R.S., A.L. Wing, and R.T. Hyde. Physical activity as an index of heart attack risk in college alumni. *Am. J. Epidemiol.* 108: 161-175, 1978.

24. Sallis, J.F., W.L. Haskell, P.D. Wood, S.P. Fortmann, T. Rogers, S.N. Blair, and R.S. Paffenbarger. Physical activity assessed methodology in the 5-city project. *Am. J. Epidemiol.* 121: 91-106, 1985.

25. Saris, W.H.M., and R.A. Binkhorst. The use of pedometer and actometer in studying daily physical activity in man. Part I: Reliability of pedometer and actometer. *Eur. J. Appl. Physiol.* 37: 219-228, 1977.

26. Shapiro, S., E. Weinblatt, C.W. Frank, and R.V. Sager. Incidence of coronary heart disease in a population insured for medical care (HIP). *Am. Public Health Assoc. Yearbook* (59): 1969.

27. Taylor, H.L., E. Klepetar, A. Keys, W. Parlin, H. Blackburn, and T. Puchner. Death rates among physically active and sedentary employees of the railroad industry. *Am. J. Public Health* 52: 1697, 1962.

28. Tryon, W.W. Activity as a function of body weight. *Am. J. Clin. Nutr.* 46: 451-455, 1987.

29. Washburn, R.A., and H.J. Montoye. The assessment of physical activity by questionnaire. *Am. J. Epidemiol.* 123: 563-576, 1986.

30. World Health Organization. *Habitual physical activity and health* (WHO Regional Publications European Series No. 6). Copenhagen: World Health Organization, 1978.

31. Zukel, W., R.H. Lewis, P.E. Ehterline, R.C. Painter, L.S. Ralston, R.M. Fawcett, A.P. Meredith, and B. Paterson. A short-term community study of the epidemiology of coronary heart disease. *Am. J. Public Health* 49: 1630, 1959.

Chapter 6

Discussion: Assessment of Physical Activity During Leisure and Work

Henry J. Montoye

I was pleased to read and hear Dr. Durnin's thoughtful presentation. His work on the energy cost of activities is known and respected in the United States and Canada as well as in Europe, and his data are used in the scoring of many activity questionnaires and interviews. The interpretations and conclusions of someone who has worked for so long in this area are certainly valued.

There is convincing evidence that a sedentary lifestyle in some people contributes to obesity, coronary heart disease, osteoporosis, and perhaps other medical problems. I agree with Dr. Durnin that the importance of intensity, duration, frequency, and circumstances surrounding the physical activity in these relationships with health is not clear. Much of the evidence that exercise is associated with the maintenance of health comes from studies in which the significant source of exercise is occupational activity of a relatively low intensity. The classical studies of Morris (9, 10) are early examples. In the Tecumseh study (8), in which men from an entire community were classified on the basis of habitual physical activity, occupational work was more decisive than was leisure-time exercise.

Modern technology reduced greatly the occupational physical work in highly developed countries (even among farmers), but some workers still expend significant amounts of energy on their jobs. For many of us it is true that the only source of exercise is our leisure time, including going to and from our jobs. Frequently, it is hoped that high-intensity exercise for relatively brief periods of time three or four times a week will provide the equivalent protection from chronic disease that low-intensity occupational work of longer duration seems to provide. Dr. Paffenbarger presented some data in chapter 3 indicating that this might

be so, but I must agree with Dr. Durnin that the evidence for this is far from conclusive.

I also agree with our speaker that the possible association of exercise to health should not be our only concern. For example, allowing one's physical fitness and activity to reach a low level may prevent participation in enjoyable leisure-time activities. The shrinking of our world of activities may eliminate some of the sources of joy in our lives.

Because we do not know which characteristics of physical activity are related to health, we must keep all our options open in developing ways of assessing physical activity. Perhaps the greatest contribution exercise can make to health is in the control of obesity and the many medical problems associated with being overweight. This would suggest that energy expenditure is most important. On the other hand, the effects of high-intensity exercise may have significance in the maintenance of health of the cardiovascular system, in which case the estimation of total energy expenditure is insufficient and we should measure the rate of energy expenditure as well.

I am not in agreement with Dr. Durnin that "physical activity in women has relatively little in common with its male counterpart." In recent years the world has changed in this regard, at least in the United States. Opportunities and encouragement for exercise for girls and women have increased by leaps and bounds. Their skill and participation rates are approaching those of males. Income and television exposure for female professional athletes are increasing rapidly. Almost as many women as men work outside the home and in many of the same kinds of jobs, including mail delivery, fire protection, factory work, and so on. Women are patronizing health clubs to about the same extent as are men. Although Dr. Durnin's statement would have been true a few years ago, it is becoming increasingly less true now.

In his concluding paragraph our speaker indicated that we have not come very far in the past 20 yr in methods of assessing physical activity. With regard to questionnaires and interviews this is true. There is still a great need for validated methods of estimating habitual physical activity for use in epidemiological studies and in particular in children and older adults. However, on some fronts considerable progress has been made. I devote the rest of my remarks to a discussion of these advancements.

Questionnaires and interviews at the moment still appear to be the methods for assessing exercise habits in epidemiological studies, but other possibilities are on the horizon. New questionnaires and interviews have appeared, but none have been validated, mainly because of a lack of an acceptable criterion. Energy expenditure is only one aspect of physical activity, but until recently there has been no adequate criterion for even this assessment in free-living subjects. The use of portable instruments such as the Oxylog (P.K. Morgan, Ltd., 4 Bloors Lane, Rainham, Gillingham, Kent, England ME8 7ED) are sufficiently uncomfortable and restricting as to distort normal activity. However, an adequate criterion—doubly labeled water—appears to be feasible for validation studies of energy expenditure.

The rationale for using doubly labeled water stems from the fact that a subject can ingest a known amount of $^2H^{18}O$ water and that after a suitable period (overnight) the urine sample provides an estimate of total body water and a baseline value of the concentration of ^2H and ^{18}O in body fluids. After a week or two, another urine sample reflects the decrease in ^{18}O, part of which was lost in H_2O, urine, perspiration, and respiratory water and part in the CO_2 produced. The ^2H is lost in water. The CO_2 output can then be calculated by subtraction (6). If an average respiratory quotient of .85 is assumed, the O_2 consumption during the period can be estimated. The respiratory exchange ratio exceeds 0.85 during strenuous exercise. However, this kind of exercise likely represents only a small percentage of a 24-hr day, even among more active subjects, so the error in this assumption would not be great.

Schoeller and van Santen (14) first used the method in a controlled study with humans and reported an average difference of 2% compared to dietary intakes. Later, Schoeller et al. (13) studied 9 males housed in a metabolic chamber for 4 d. The

men exercised vigorously for about 1 hr 15 min twice per day. Near-continuous respiratory gas exchange data were compared with the doubly labeled water estimate of energy expenditure, and agreement was good. The doubly labeled method overestimated CO_2 production by 1% with a standard deviation of 7%.

Mechanical and electronic devices that record movement, physiological parameters, or both appear to hold the promise for the future in assessing habitual physical activity, and much recent work has been accomplished in this area. Dr. Durnin mentioned pedometers and their limitations. I agree that they are inaccurate (4, 16). This device has been around for a long time. According to the *World Almanac of Presidential Facts*, Thomas Jefferson, the third U.S. president, invented the pedometer, but this is incorrect. Figure 6.1 probably represents the first pedometer designed, and by Leonardo da Vinci about 500 years ago (5). A pedometer is constructed to count steps in walking and possibly running and should not be expected to measure other kinds of activities or total energy expenditure. The tension in the spring of each instrument may vary so the instruments of even the same brand are not uniform (4). The same pedometer will give different results when worn by different individuals. Other devices have been employed for counting steps (7) but more sophisticated devices hold greater promise. The rapid developments in micro-electronics make this an exciting field.

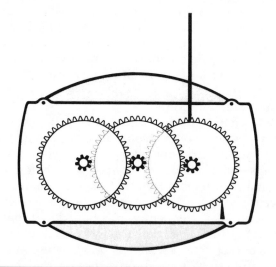

Figure 6.1. Pedometer designed by Leonardo da Vinci. *Note.* From *The Inventions of Leonardo da Vinci* (p. 84) by C. Gibbs-Smith, 1978, London: Phaidon Press. Reprinted by permission of Phaidon Press and Biblioteca Ambrosiana, Milan.

The characteristic of physical activity which is most troublesome to estimate is the intensity (strenuousness) of the exercise. For this reason, portable accelerometers and physiologic recorders will likely be incorporated in the instruments of the future. The actometer (11, 12) was mentioned by our speaker. This is a mechanical accelerometer and therefore it is difficult to standardize. For this reason, when developing a portable vertical accelerometer, we used a piezoelectric bending element as the transducer (15). This instrument, available under the trade name Caltrac, appears to be reasonably accurate for estimating energy expenditure, although it too has not been adequately validated. The price (about $75) makes it affordable for epidemiological studies. There are several problems with a single-plane accelerometer of this kind. It underestimates energy expenditure when movements have significant lateral and forward-backward elements. It also underestimates or fails to record energy expenditures in isometric muscular contraction, weightlifting, and activities in which the trunk is fairly stationary (e.g., rowing). Finally, the inexpensive portable accelerometers that are available do not have the capacity to store accelerations (energy expenditure estimates) over a time base. Thus, variations in intensity cannot be retrieved but only averaged over the entire period.

I have been assured that three-dimensional portable accelerometers can be constructed of the same size (78 g; 9 cm × 7 cm × 1.5 cm) and that they would cost as much as the Caltrac (Hemokinetics, Inc., 1923 Osmundsen Road, Madison, Wisconsin, 53706, USA). Thus, lateral and forward-backward movements may be recorded. Also, storage capacity may be added at little additional cost or weight so that intensities over many brief periods of time may be stored and retrieved. There remains the problem of underrecording activities that involve isometric contractions or limb movements while the trunk is stationary.

Because of the difficulties encountered in measuring $\dot{V}O_2$ in the field, there is interest in the simpler but less direct method of recording physiological data associated with energy expenditure. Advancements in telemetry and other aspects of bioengineering have made such techniques more attractive.

Almost from their beginning, humans must have observed that pulse rate and ventilation increase during strenuous activity. In 1907, Benedict (1) reported that heart rate and heat production were related. Systolic blood pressure, ventilation, and body temperature are also roughly proportional to the intensity of exercise. All these variables can be telemetered or entered on portable recorders, but heart rate is most easily recorded.

Remarkable progress has been made in the development of heart rate recorders. They are now reliable and relatively inexpensive. In themselves they do not provide good estimates of energy expenditure in the field (2, 3) because, as pointed out by Dr. Durnin, factors other than exercise influence heart rate. Dancing raises the heart rate as a result of increased energy expenditure, but how high it goes may be as much a matter of who our dancing partner is. Also, individual $\dot{V}O_2$-heart rate calibration curves are required to translate heart rates into energy expenditure.

As the previous discussion indicates, there are limitations and problems with all devices proposed to estimate physical activity or energy expenditure in freely moving subjects. As a result, a number of instruments have been developed that attempt to combine movement sensors and physiological data (7). Most of these utilize heart rate recording and a movement counter or counters. At present, such combination instruments are expensive, but as costs come down they probably will be the method to use in epidemiological studies and smaller experimental investigations. Questionnaire and interview methods likely will continue to be used in national surveys. Doubly labeled water needs to be investigated further, but with the greater precision of new ratio mass spectrometers (and consequently the need for less ^{18}O) we are beginning to see more studies utilizing this technique.

In closing let me say that I am pleased to be participating in this important conference and to share the podium with Dr. Durnin, whom I have known for a long time.

References

1. Benedict, F.G. *The influence of inanition on metabolism* (Publication No. 77). Washington, DC: Carnegie Institute, 1907, p. 542.
2. Campbell, I.T. The use of heart rate to measure habitual energy expenditure. *Am. J. Clin. Nutr.* 39: 494-496, 1984.
3. Christensen, C.C., H.M.M. Frey, E. Foenstelien, E. Aadland, and H. Refsum. A critical evaluation of energy expenditure estimates based on individual O_2 consumption/heart rate curves and average daily heart rate. *Am. J. Clin. Nutr.* 37: 468-472, 1983.

4. Gayle, R., H.J. Montoye, and J. Philpot. Accuracy of pedometers for measuring distance walked. *Res. Q.* 48: 632-636, 1977.

5. Gibbs-Smith, C. *The inventions of Leonardo da Vinci.* London: Phaidon Press, 1978, p. 31-43.

6. Lifson, N., and R. McClintock. Theory of use of the turnover rates of body water for measuring energy and material balance. *J. Theoret. Biol.* 12: 46-74, 1966.

7. Montoye, H.J. Activity instrumentation. In: *Encyclopedia of medical devices and instrumentation,* edited by J.G. Webster. New York: John Wiley & Sons, 1988, vol. 1, p. 1-15.

8. Montoye, H.J., H.L. Metzner, J.B. Keller, B.C. Johnson, and F.H. Epstein. Habitual physical activity and blood pressure. *Med. Sci. Sports* 4: 175-181, 1972.

9. Morris, J.N., and M.D. Crawford. Coronary heart disease and physical activity of work. *Br. Med. J.* 2: 1485-1496, 1958.

10. Morris, J.N., J.A. Heady, P.A.B. Raffle, C.G. Roberts, and J.W. Parks. Coronary heart disease and physical activity of work. *Lancet* ii: 1053-1057, 1111-1120, 1953.

11. Saris, W.H.M., and R.A. Binkhorst. The use of pedometer and actometer in studying daily physical activity in man. Part I. Reliability of pedometer and actometer. *Eur. J. Appl. Physiol.* 37: 219-228, 1977.

12. Saris, W.H.M., and R.A. Binkhorst. The use of pedometer and actometer in studying daily physical activity in man. Part II. Validity of pedometer and actometer measuring the daily physical activity. *Eur. J. Appl. Physiol.* 37: 229-235, 1977.

13. Schoeller, D.A., E. Ravussin, Y. Schutz, K.J. Acheson, P. Baertschi, and E. Jequier. Energy expenditure of doubly labeled water: Validation in humans and proposed calculations. *Am. J. Physiol.* 250: R823-R830, 1986.

14. Schoeller, D.A., and E. van Santen. Measurement of energy expenditure in humans by doubly labeled water method. *J. Appl. Physiol.* 53: 955-959, 1982.

15. Servais, S.B., J.G. Webster, and H.J. Montoye. Estimating human energy expenditure using an accelerometer device. *J. Clin. Eng.* 9: 159-171, 1984.

16. Washburn, R., M.K. Chin, and H.J. Montoye. Accuracy of pedometer in walking and running. *Res. Q. Exerc. Sport* 51: 695-702, 1980.

Chapter 7

Determinants of Participation in Physical Activity

Rod K. Dishman

The midcourse review (29) of the 1990 physical fitness and exercise objectives for the United States (30) recommended that the determinants of physical activity and exercise be known by the year 2000. Specifically recommended were that the following be known: (a) the relationship between participation in various types of physical activities during childhood and adolescence and the physical activity practices of adults, (b) the relationship between the accessibility of facilities and the physical activity practices of adults, and (c) the behavioral skills associated with a high probability of adopting and maintaining a regular exercise program. These areas were not presented to represent all the important potential determinants of physical activity but were intended to reflect those for which public health interventions might be effectively implemented with great benefit for the population. Because behavioral objectives for the determinants of physical activity and exercise were not included in the original 1990 objectives (30), consideration of their possible inclusion in the revised objectives for the year 2000 is noteworthy.

It is now acknowledged that the impending failure to meet the 1990 participation rate objectives for vigorous and frequent activity (118) is in part due to the lack of understanding of the predisposing, enabling, impeding, and reinforcing determinants that influence free-living physical activity and adherence to supervised exercise programs (40). Population estimates (141) indicate that current participation rates in the United States fall far below the 1990 objectives (20, 118) (Figure 7.1) and below the guidelines indicated by epidemiological evidence (111, 119) and consensus among sports medicine experts (2). The prevalence of vigorous and frequent activity in the United States is estimated at 10% of all adults (14, 15, 19). This rate is comparable to estimates from Australia (105), whereas about 25% of Canadians are be-

lieved to be highly active (142). Evidence does suggest that free-living activity has increased among North Americans during the past 15 yr (144) (Figure 7.2), and this is encouraging for future promotions designed to increase contemporary activity. The magnitude of the increase is not clear, however, because the available technology for assessing physical activity in a population has not permitted precise quantification of activity intensity, time spent in activity, or periodicity of activity (89, 102, 135, 156). Less encouraging are estimates (Figure 7.3) that the prevalence of sedentary leisure time during the past 15 yr has remained at 30%-60% (19, 20, 142) in Canada and the United States while the typical dropout rate (Figure 7.4) from supervised exercise programs has remained at roughly 50% (36). A review of what is known about the determinants of physical activity, as well as suggestions for future study, is thus timely.

My purpose in this chapter is fivefold. I will (a) describe what is currently known about the personal attributes, environments, and physical activity characteristics associated with participation in supervised and free-living physical activity; (b) discuss the demonstrated effectiveness of behavior change interventions designed to increase physical activity; (c) suggest ways that existing theoretical models may clarify the behaviors, population segments, and methods that appear most likely to enhance the effectiveness of interventions to increase physical activity; (d) review the limitations in methods and research design that have hindered our knowledge; and (e) propose, in appropriate places throughout the text, questions and approaches that may add to our knowledge or facilitate effective interventions.

In some areas, new information will alter or expand accepted conclusions about the determinants. In others, little will be changed from earlier

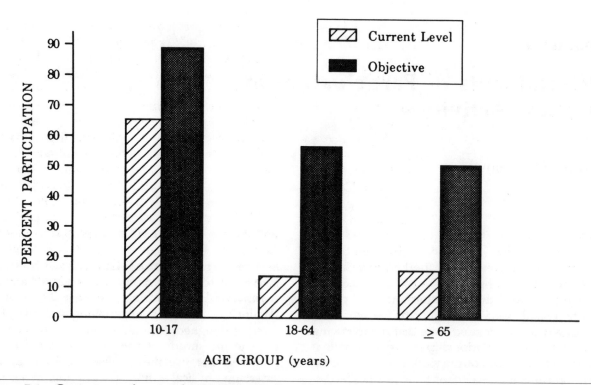

Figure 7.1. Current prevalence and 1990 objectives for appropriate physical activity by age-group. From "The Status of the 1990 Objectives for Physical Fitness and Exercise" by K.E. Powell, K.G. Spain, G.M. Christenson, and M.P. Mollenkamp, 1986, *Public Health Reports, 101,* p. 17. Reprinted by permission.

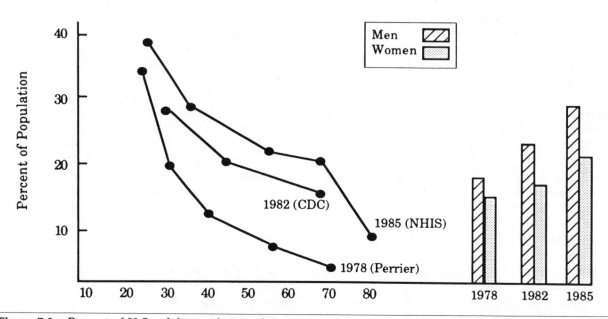

Figure 7.2. Percent of U.S. adult population who are vigorously active, 1978-1985 (3 kcal/kg/d or more of leisure-time activity). From "Secular Trends in Adult Physical Activity: Exercise Boom or Bust?" by T. Stephens, 1987, *Research Quarterly for Exercise and Sport, 58,* p. 96. Reprinted by permission.

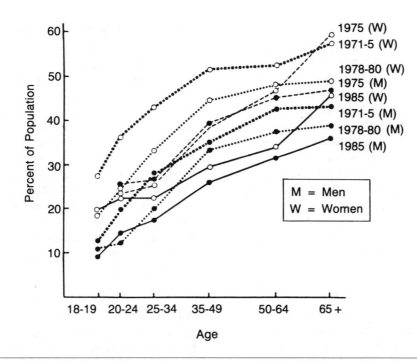

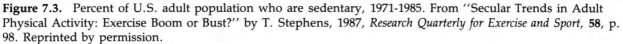

Figure 7.3. Percent of U.S. adult population who are sedentary, 1971-1985. From "Secular Trends in Adult Physical Activity: Exercise Boom or Bust?" by T. Stephens, 1987, *Research Quarterly for Exercise and Sport*, **58**, p. 98. Reprinted by permission.

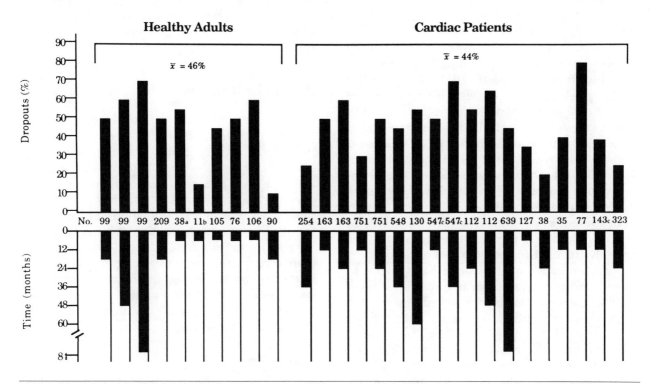

Figure 7.4. Relationship between the dropout rate (%) and the duration of exercise training (months) in studies of healthy adults and cardiac patients. The number (no.) of participants in each study is designated thus: a = assigned to individual exercise program, b = assigned to YMCA group exercise program, c = men only. From "Program Factors That Influence Exercise Adherence: Practical Adherence Skills for the Clinical Staff" by B.A. Franklin, 1988, in R.K. Dishman (Ed.), *Exercise Adherence: Its Impact on Public Heath* (p. 238). Champaign, IL: Human Kinetics. Reprinted by permission.

reviews (35, 40, 95, 107). The studies come from computerized searches (e.g., MEDLINE and Psychological Abstracts) and a personal retrieval system. For some determinants only one or a few studies have been reported in the literature, and thus original sources are referenced. For other determinants, the individual studies reported are so numerous that it is necessary to reference review articles rather than all the specific studies available. Small-sample reports using measures of unknown reliability and validity were excluded when low internal and external validities rendered findings uninterpretable. However, population surveys are considered, even when their internal validities are unknown, because of their potential for generalizability.

Known Determinants

The known determinants of physical activity can be categorized as past and present personal attributes, past and present environments, and physical activity itself (35, 40). This categorization effectively organizes the empirical literature that is available, provides a descriptive framework for evaluating the potential of behavioral and psychological theories as explanations for physical activity patterns, and offers guidance for interventions designed to increase physical activity while clarifying their relative effectiveness. Admittedly, the distinctions drawn about the origins of determinants are at times vague because the assessment of determinants is often based on correlational studies of self-reported beliefs and perceptions of the participant. Thus, the true origin or causal impact of many determinants remains to be shown by objective experiments.

For these reasons, the term *determinant* will be used to denote a reproducible association or predictive relationship other than cause and effect. Because few experimental studies have been conducted, the confidence that can be placed in most findings depends on their repeated observation across different settings, methods, and subjects. Some determinants appear to differ truly, however, when physical activity occurs in a supervised setting where time, place, activity, and type of participant may be restricted in range relative to spontaneous or free-living activity in a population base and when distinctions are drawn between planning for participation, initial adoption of physical activity, continued participation or maintenance, and periodicity of participation. These differences

are noted when data are available to allow comparisons of determinants across people or settings.

The absence of uniform standards for defining and assessing physical activity and its determinants and the diversity of the variables, population segments, time periods, and settings sampled in published studies make it difficult to interpret and compare results. Often only a few studies have been done in a particular area. Most studies come from supervised settings, and relatively few population studies of determinants have been reported. Available population surveys have used questions with unknown reliability and validity, and generalizability to the population of the more controlled small-sample results is unknown in many instances.

Too few studies are available on, for example, children (38), the elderly (113, 132, 145), the disabled (59, 88), and ethnic, cultural, and minority groups (16, 129, 151) to permit conclusions about how determinants in these cases may differ from general observations. There are also few comparative animal studies (65). This lack of uniformity prevents a relative weighting or ordering of the importance of determinants and their interactions. Although the determinants of physical activity are conceptually multivariate in action, the current empirical literature limits our view to one that is univariate.

Personal Attributes

Personal attributes are defined as demographic variables, biomedical status, past and present behaviors, activity history, and psychological traits and states associated with physical activity. Determinants that reside or originate in the individual are important because they can identify personal variables or population segments that may be targets for interventions to increase physical activity or, conversely, can describe impediments or people resistive to physical activity interventions. It is important to know what might be changed for whom and the personal determinants or types of people that may make change difficult or impractical.

Demographic Variables

When physical activity is defined by observation, those who do not adopt or adhere to supervised rehabilitative and work-site exercise programs typically have high coronary heart disease risk profiles. Smokers and blue-collar workers are likely dropouts from rehabilitative exercise programs for post-myocardial infarction patients (107) and are unlikely to utilize work-site exercise facilities (25, 50, 131). The robustness of these determinants for other supervised settings and the population is less clear. Although blue-collar workers are less likely to be active when total leisure activity is considered (18, 22, 141, 142), neither smoking nor occupational status appear related to participation in leisure sport (100, 114). In the population it appears that smoking is unrelated to total physical activity (106), but those who engage in high-intensity, high-frequency fitness regimens may be less likely to be smokers (12). Sedentary smokers are likely to complain of exertional fatigue regardless of fitness level (73), and this might deter their participation.

Participants in a supervised preventive medicine exercise program have been shown to have more formal education than have nonparticipants (107), and education level is associated with free-living activity in the population (22, 141, 142). Because concomitant associations seen in the population for low activity with age, fewer years of education, and low income occur in cross-sectional comparisons, the degree to which they signal causal circumstances or a selection-bias effect remains unclear. Prospective comparisons of age effects on activity between birth cohorts and cross-sectional age-groups in Harvard alumni (117) and users of the Cooper Aerobic Center in Dallas, Texas (11), indicate that age is a selection bias, not a cause of inactivity. Age is unrelated to adherence to supervised exercise (40, 107). However, the generalizability of these results for age in other population groups and settings and for other demographics such as smoking, education, and socioeconomic status has apparently not been tested. This must be done if demographics associated with activity are to be interpreted as targets for interventions to increase physical activity.

The degree to which geographic differences in activity patterns across the United States and Canada either reflect differences in climate, access, and the culture inherent in the regions or reflect population distributions on age, education, and socioeconomic status is unknown (22). For example, in the population women are less active than are men when total activity and fitness regimens are considered. However, gender may interact with the type of activity to influence participation. Community study reveals that women are more likely than are men (127) to adopt and maintain moderate activity routines such as walking, and, although accurate estimates are not available, there is no doubt that participation rates in commercial dance-exercise classes are highest among women.

Biomedical Status

The overweight are less likely to stay with a fitness program (34, 43, 64, 97, 101, 131, 159), and the obese may better respond to alternative routines of moderate activity such as walking than they will to fitness regimens (43, 64). Even so, excess weight is still a barrier to activity, and the obese remain less responsive to public health interventions that include walking and climbing than are normal-weight inactives (16). Even in gentle walking programs, 60%-70% of the obese will stop within 6-12 mo (43, 64), and this dropout rate exceeds that typically seen in supervised programs for normal-weight individuals (36, 107).

Circulatory disability or low metabolic tolerance ($\dot{V}O_2$peak) for physical activity (like body weight variables) are not reliable predictors of adherence to clinical exercise programs (17, 40, 95, 107). However, in one study of apparently healthy men, initial fitness predicted a higher volume of participation in a yearlong running program (70). Men in cardiac rehabilitation exercise programs are more likely to adhere if they have documented heart disease or angina or have had one myocardial infarction (34, 107). These factors could affect reinforcing or aversive exercise sensations and disease symptoms or provide concrete signs of health vulnerability that could interact with beliefs about the health benefits of exercise to facilitate participation (35). However, knowledge of disability or health-risk factors alone seems insufficient to prompt exercise behavior. Men at risk for coronary heart disease are less likely to enter fitness (131) or wellness (25) exercise programs or to adhere after entry (107, 132). Moreover, neither fitness testing nor knowledge of fitness status or health-risk appraisal influences activity levels or intentions to be active physically (61, 62).

In supervised settings, predictive approaches using biomedical and demographic entry profiles suggest that select groups who are prone to comply with or drop out of certain types of programs can be identified fairly accurately, but not with predictive accuracy adequate for practical use with individuals (34, 39, 108, 155). Moreover, pragmatic constraints have generally limited the variables examined to those routinely revealed in medical screening and history taking, exercise tolerance testing, and self-reporting of sociodemographics. This approach has its roots in the design of research on supervised exercise (107) because if there are few differences in lifestyle, health risks, morbidity, and mortality between dropouts and the active, there will be little loss of generalizability of results on these outcomes from exercise trials if dropouts are excluded from outcome analyses. But biomedical and sociodemographic factors have low sensitivity for predicting behavior (53). Also, participant scores on medical, fitness, and sociodemographic measures vary from program to program. Several factors that are useful for predicting dropout in some patient groups (e.g., smoking, blue-collar work status, obesity, and angina) are not prevalent in other groups and therefore are not helpful for predicting dropout in those groups.

Smoking and occupation and body weight (including body mass index and skinfold estimates of fatness), exercise tolerance, and cardiovascular health status have been considered to be demographic and biomedical variables, respectively, and usually have been assessed by indirect methods on a cross-sectional basis. Thus, as they have been measured, their reliability and validity as true behavioral determinants have been undemonstrated, and there is no empirical evidence that they provide effective targets in interventions for increasing physical activity. It is more likely that they can provide ways to segment large populations into relatively homogeneous categories. Although such categories will be imprecise predictors and unlikely causes of behavior, they may serve as sentinel variables hinting at other factors more directly linked with the determinants of physical activity.

Past and Present Behaviors

Smoking, occupation, socioeconomic status, and being overweight could collectively indicate other habits or behaviors that reinforce sedentary living or create barriers to adopting or maintaining physical activity. Many blue-collar occupations may carry with them the perception of on-job activity adequate for health and fitness despite low actual exertion, and the normative behaviors within low socioeconomic groups may reinforce inactivity. Smoking and being overweight could exert direct barriers for high-intensity activities or signal a generalized pattern of low-frequency health behaviors. Although cross-sectional, correlational studies show little association between physical activity and other health-related behaviors (12, 106, 129, 143), many theories of human behavior assume that increasing the occurrence of other behaviors that share common precursors, environments, or outcomes with physical activity will facilitate increases in physical activity.

The degree to which habitual exercise contributes to other changes in risk behavior and the degree to which it is dependent on them has not

been directly studied (12). However, data from a successful stress management trial involving business executives who manifested the Type A behavior pattern (125) suggested an increase in leisure-time physical activity at a 6-mo follow-up even though subjects were instructed to maintain preexperiment activity levels. Reported diets did not change, but subjects lost weight and had lower serum cholesterol; each change is consistent with increased exercise. Moreover, a recent survey of a 9-mo community fitness campaign in Ontario (52) found that a generalized perception of lifestyle change was the best estimate of self-reported activity levels, which were also related to reported changes in the specific health behaviors of smoking, drinking, and weight control. A U.S. population survey also showed a link between perceived increases in physical activity and other changes in health habits (54), but the more controlled Canada Health Survey of health practices showed that physical activity was related only to polio immunization (143). In a large population-based trial in the United States, several health-risk behaviors were favorably influenced by an educational media campaign, whereas self-reported physical activity remained unchanged across 1 yr (99).

A new or altered behavior is more likely to persist when several behaviors facilitate or are compatible with one another and are cued by a range of common environmental stimuli and reinforcers. A role for other health behaviors as determinants of physical activity thus remains tenable but untested by experimental methods.

Activity History

If demographic or biomedical factors and other behaviors are found to represent selection biases rather than causes of physical activity, the importance of past activity history assumes great significance for interpreting both past and present determinants, designing and evaluating plausible interventions, and predicting future activity.

Supervised and free-living activity. In supervised programs in which activity can be directly observed, past participation in the program is the most reliable correlate of current participation (40). This prediction holds for adult men and women in supervised fitness programs and is consistent with observations in treatment programs for patients with coronary heart disease and obesity. As shown in Figure 7.5, the rate of participation typically drops within the initial 3-6 mo and then plateaus and continues a gradually decreasing but

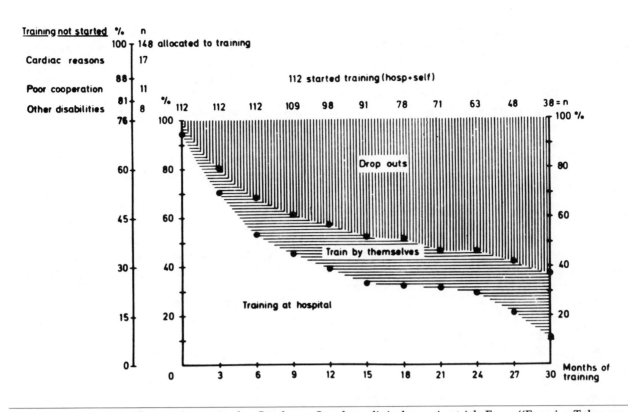

Figure 7.5. Exercise adherence rates in the Göteborg, Sweden, clinical exercise trial. From "Exercise Tolerance and Physical Training of Non-Selected Patients After Myocardial Infarction" by H.M. Sanne, D. Elmfeldt, G. Grimby, C. Rydin, and L. Wilhelmsen, 1973, *Acta Medica Scandinavica*, **551**(Suppl.), p. 60. Copyright 1973 by *Acta Medica Scandinavica* and H.M. Sanne, D. Elmfeldt, G. Grimby, C. Rydin, and L. Wilhelmsen. Reprinted by permission.

linear pattern across the next 12-30 mo. Individuals who are still active after 6 mo are likely to remain active 1 yr later (34, 107). Recent findings for free-living activity are similar (42, 58, 127).

The impact of past free-living activity on supervised physical activity is less clear. Studies have shown that inactive leisure time at entry correlates with dropping out from supervised rehabilitative exercise programs (36, 107). This has been seen among homogeneous groups of either healthy or post-myocardial infarction males. No correlation between program adherence and self-reported intensity, duration, or frequency of preenrollment exercise has been seen across a broad spectrum of cardiovascular health (34). A recent study of a walking program for postmenopausal women found differences in preprogram self-reports of daily stair climbing, number of city blocks walked per day, and daily caloric expenditure between adherents and dropouts (87). Thus, discrepancies about past free-living activity as a determinant of supervised exercise may be specific to the population or activity studied.

Youth Sport. Organized-sport experience might contribute knowledge, skills, and predispositions useful for activity in later years and is amenable to large-scale public intervention. Thus, a causal relationship between sport participation and adult activity would have strong implications for public health.

No prospective study has shown a relationship for adherence to cardiac rehabilitation exercise programs or for free-living physical activity with participation in interscholastic or intercollegiate athletics. This illustrates the need for cautious interpretation of the cross-sectional, retrospective studies that link youth sport history with contemporary adult physical activity. Indeed, one early study has shown that former college athletes become less active than do former nonathletes by middle age (103). Yet it remains unclear whether physical activity determinants for the individual who begins habitual activity at middle age are the same as those of the person who has been active since childhood, and prospective studies of childhood sport or physical education as a determinant of contemporary adult activity have not been reported. A search of the scientific literature reveals a single abstracted report (70) of a direct predictive relationship (in a self-selected group of 48 men) between voluntary jogging mileage and a retrospective measure of a perceived positive elementary school experience in physical education.

In their recent review, Powell and Dysinger (116) reported six research articles on youth participation in sport and physical education as antecedents to adult activity patterns. They concluded that available data are equivocal and that future studies should standardize definitions and measures as well as control confounding variables, recall bias, selection bias, and the content and quality of sport and physical education programs. A recent report (37) on Caucasian males was able to control confounding effects by age, fitness, fatness, and cardiovascular health and employed standardized activity measures. No association was seen between a self-report of past participation in school sports and either a cross-sectional sample of free-living physical activity or a prospective sample of supervised exercise. Future studies should quantify activity intensity, use objective measures of both school and community sport participation and subjective and objective measures of the sport experience, and sample women and other races and ethnic or cultural groups.

Although childhood sport experience can be an agent in socializing adult roles, it can also be overridden by other personal and environmental influences that exert a more immediate effect in adulthood. Furthermore, it will be difficult to separate behavioral influence learned from sport involvement (e.g., activity skills and interests) from the influence of other personal traits that may mediate both youth sport involvement and adult exercise patterns. Personality, body build and composition, and cardiovascular fitness have been related to both sport success and adult activity patterns (35, 40), yet each has a substantially heritable origin.

There is a growing literature on participation motivation and determinants of dropout in organized youth sport (49) that parallels public health concerns about childhood activity patterns. However, interpretation of this literature is also difficult because studies have typically involved cross-sectional and correlational comparisons of static groups, and the validity of the self-reports used to assess determinants has not been confirmed. Because the available data are descriptive rather than predictive or experimental, guidelines for interventions to increase youth sport participation are not available. Moreover, the influences of participation motivation or dropping out of youth sport on adult physical activity have not been studied either prospectively or retrospectively.

The findings on activity history as a determinant of adult physical activity collectively challenge education and public health agencies to make a positive impact on physical activity, exercise, and health-related physical fitness in children (75). More important, they signal a challenge to fields of study concerned with public health problems to advance knowledge about the determinants of physical activity patterns among children and youth (31, 32) and about how these determinants and activity patterns might relate to the determinants and activity patterns of adults (38).

Psychological Traits and States

It is important to know whether either stable or transient psychological constructs are causal determinants of physical activity. Psychological constructs can account for variability in behavior within population segments that are demographically homogeneous and across settings that differ in place and time. Because these constructs can reflect past behavior history but exist in the present, they offer promise for more precise predictions of physical activity than do the determinants considered up to this point. Whether heritable or learned, some psychological constructs (e.g., personality factors like temperament) are viewed as traits that are relatively resistant to environmental influence, whereas others (e.g., attitudes, beliefs, values, expectancies, and intentions) are behavioral dispositions that appear more amenable to change. Both are better predictors of a specific behavior when psychological responses to a given situation (i.e., states) are also measured.

Studies of psychological traits and states as determinants of physical activity have been scarce and have yielded mixed results. This seems largely the case because most of the studies have been atheoretical, have not permitted a complete test of the theory used, or have not adequately accounted for how the setting in which the study took place or how the subjects studied might have affected the variance observed on both determinants and physical activity. These concerns are addressed later in this chapter in sections on theory and methodology. To understand how advancements in psychological theory and methodology may clarify the determinants of physical activity, it is instructive first to examine the results from empirical studies.

Personality. Cross-sectional comparisons have shown habitually active adult males to be more extroverted than are those who are sedentary (93, 158), but prospective studies have found extroverts to be both likely adherents (13) and dropouts (97) in supervised exercise programs. In a like manner, ego strength has been found to be positively related to program adherence among post-myocardial infarction patients (13) but unrelated to exercise training in college women (39). Self-perceived mood disturbance is related to early dropout from adult fitness (155) and cardiac rehabilitation programs (13), whereas a depressive personality (93) and somatization (24) have also been associated with free-living inactivity.

A trait measure of self-motivation (39) has been a more consistent correlate of physical activity (85, 138). Evidence (68) suggests that self-motivation may reflect willpower or self-regulatory skills such as effective goal setting, self-monitoring of progress, and self-reinforcement, all believed to be important for maintaining physical activity (35) and intentions to change behavior (4). Successful endurance athletes have consistently scored high on self-motivation, and self-motivation has discriminated between adherents and dropouts across a wide variety of settings, including athletic conditioning, adult fitness, preventive medicine, cardiac rehabilitation, commercial spas, corporate fitness (85, 138), and free-living activity in college students (42). The settings studied have varied in length from 5 wk to 2 yr and have included men and women of various fitness levels. Other studies have shown no differences between adherents and dropouts on self-motivation in adult fitness, dance exercise, and interscholastic sports (85, 138). Our initial classification model (39) was most accurate when self-motivation scores were combined with body weight and composition. This seems to support the usefulness of interactions between psychological and biological traits in accounting for exercise behavior; recent work has confirmed this prediction model for adherents to supervised exercise but not for dropouts (155). The lack of specificity for self-motivation in predicting dropouts (53) supports the idea that psychological traits probably interact with aspects of the physical activity setting to determine behavior. Programs with strong social support or reinforcement in settings requiring low-frequency, low-intensity activity may negate differences in self-motivation (154). The self-motivated individual may also be likely to leave a supervised program but to continue a personal program of free-living activity (42).

A role for motivational traits as determinants of physical activity is consistent with a reported relationship between supervised exercise adherence and the Jenkins Activity Survey (JAS) of Type A behavior (122). There is a significant overlap between self-motivation and the JAS, suggesting a common achievement motivation dimension. Although male post-myocardial patients assessed as Type A have been early dropouts from exercise rehabilitation (107) and infrequent users of work-site facilities (133), they are more likely to exercise at high intensity in supervised settings and show larger increases in fitness than are Type Bs (122). Self-reports and interview assessments of Type A behavior are each associated positively with free-living physical activity in population-based studies (71, 83, 90). Because Type A behavior is not consistently related to cardiovascular morbidity and mortality in these population studies (130), whereas low fitness and physical inactivity are (90, 136), evidence suggests that associations of Type A behavior with fitness gains and physical activity are not confounded by health status but reflect a motivated behavioral predisposition.

Although psychological traits do change, they are resistive to change over the narrow ranges of time, exposure, and settings characteristic of medical and public health interventions. The findings described here may best indicate the types of individuals prone to be active or inactive, not the determinants that are targets for behavior change. Factors related to knowledge, attitudes, values, and beliefs have proven more responsive to population-based education and persuasion campaigns designed to alter health behaviors. They have also been studied as determinants of physical activity.

Knowledge, attitudes, and beliefs. Knowledge and belief in the health benefits of physical activity may motivate initial involvement and return to activity following relapse, but feelings of enjoyment and well-being seem to be stronger motives for continued participation in work-site (131) and gerontologic (145) exercise programs. Similarly, in the population the inactive are as likely as are the active to view physical activity as a positive health behavior (55, 114). Knowledge of health and exercise was associated with regular activity of moderate intensity (e.g., routine walking) for both men and women in a population-based study but did not predict participation in vigorous exercise (127). Inactive members of minority and low-socioeconomic groups are relatively uninformed about the health benefits of exercise and its appropriate forms or amounts (18, 19, 114, 151), but in the U.S. population only about 5% of those currently inactive and those active believe that more information on fitness benefits would likely increase their participation (114). Paradoxically, however, only 5% of the U.S. population can accurately identify the optimal intensity, duration, and frequency of physical activity for cardiopulmonary fitness (19). Estimates from several countries indicate that more than half of the public is aware of fitness promotion programs, but less than 20% of the active respondents in one survey felt that they were influenced by such programs (98). Thus, although the active may be more knowledgeable about exercise, it is unclear whether such knowledge is an antecedent or a consequence of activity.

Education campaigns may more effectively increase physical activity if they dispel misinformation that might impede activity for some groups and if knowledge about effective goal setting and behavioral skills is reinforced by successful experience or peer models who demonstrate the skills, successful strategies for overcoming barriers, and desirable outcomes.

Those who perceive their health as poor are unlikely to enter or adhere to an exercise program (92, 104) and, if they do, are likely to participate at a low intensity and frequency (134). Those who do not expect or value health outcomes from physical activity, and who also believe that health outcomes are out of their personal control, have been found to exercise less frequently and to drop out sooner in fitness-related programs than have peers holding opposite views (39, 41). However, because most entrants into supervised programs share similarly positive attitudes and beliefs about expected outcomes from exercise, their self-perceptions of exercise ability, feelings of health responsibility, and attitudes toward exercise do not reliably predict who will adhere to the program (3, 35, 39). Health beliefs, positive attitudes toward activity, subjective norms, and beliefs in the outcome-expectancy value of physical activity can influence the intention to be active, but intentions have also failed to predict subsequent participation (58, 60).

It is likely that a lack of knowledge about appropriate physical activity and negative or neutral attitudes and beliefs about physical activity outcomes may impede physical activity for some people, but positive knowledge, attitudes, and beliefs about general health outcomes to physical activity alone appear inadequate to ensure participation in physical activity.

Efficacy and Outcome Expectancies. There are also mixed findings from both supervised and free-living settings about the roles of efficacy and outcome expectancies as determinants of physical activity. Specific efficacy beliefs about the ability to exercise have predicted compliance with an exercise prescription in both heart (46, 47) and lung (77) patients and with free-living activity in a population base (127). In young, healthy adults, however, a belief in personal control over health outcomes predicts free-living activity, but beliefs and values held specifically for exercise outcomes and personal ability to control them appear unrelated to both free-living and supervised physical activities (41). In one study, low exercise self-efficacy predicted intentions to adopt a worksite exercise program (28).

The mixed findings on attitudes, values, and beliefs regarding exercise outcomes and self-efficacy highlight the need to distinguish physical activity as a health-corrective behavior in patients, when disease symptoms make health outcomes from exercise salient, from physical activity as a health-protective behavior (157) in healthy individuals, when health risks are abstract, not tangible (35). Other expectancy-value beliefs about physical activity outcomes and perceived barriers to participation have been understudied, apparently because of lack of a measurement technology. Valid self-report measures of reinforcing expected outcomes of participation and perceived barriers are developing (140).

Environmental Factors

At present, many of the potentially enabling, reinforcing, and impeding determinants of physical activity are regarded as environmental. Yet they have been usually assessed by self-reported perceptions by participants and nonparticipants. Because the objectivity, reliability, and validity of the self-reports have seldom been verified, the degree to which the true origin of the determinants resides in the person or the environment remains to be determined. This must be done before interventions for decreasing or removing impediments and for facilitating, enabling, and reinforcing conditions can be effectively directed toward people or places.

Facility Convenience

Access to facilities is a necessary, but not sufficient, facilitator of community sport and exercise participation (114). It is perceived in the population as an important participation influence (18), particularly among the elderly (132). Also, both perceived convenience of the exercise setting (3, 56) and actual proximity to home or place of employment (56, 66, 146) are consistent discriminators between those who choose to enter or forgo involvement and between those who adhere or dropout in supervised exercise programs. Yet in one supervised exercise program those most likely to drop out actually lived closer to the chosen activity setting, although they perceived inconvenience as a factor leading to their return to inactivity (56). In the population, the already active paradoxically are twice as likely as are the inactive (22% vs. 10%) to feel that greater availability of facilities would increase their participation (114).

Depositing a fee that is returnable on completing a program successfully is a common and effectively short-term intervention for facilitating supervised exercise adherence (44, 85), but commercial exercise programs experience dropout rates similar to other programmatic exercise settings (152), faring only as well as do work-site and community programs that provide free access to exercise and activity facilities (36, 50, 131).

Time

A similar incongruity between perceived and actual barriers is seen for time. A lack of time is the principle and most prevalent reason given for dropping out of supervised clinical and community exercise programs (35, 40, 95, 107) and for inactive lifestyles (40, 54, 55, 114). For many, however, this may reflect a lack of interest or commitment to physical activity, as population surveys indicate that regular exercisers are as likely as are the sedentary to view time as an activity barrier (18, 54, 55, 114). Also, in one survey of the U.S. population (114), the already active were twice as likely as were the inactive (22% vs. 10%-11%) to believe that a 4-d work week or more flexibility in the daily work schedule would lead to an increased likelihood of sport involvement and fitness. Moreover, among family members working women have been more likely than have nonworking women to be regular exercisers; half of the single

parents in this survey were regularly active, and a third of parents in other parental groups were regularly active (55).

It is not yet clear whether time and facility convenience truly represent environmental determinants, perceived determinants, or poor behavioral skills such as time management or whether they simply are rationalizations of a lack of motivation to be active. Effective interventions cannot be guided by current knowledge about these factors until this uncertainty is resolved.

Climate or Region

Surveys of habitual runners (126) reveal that only among the most committed do weather conditions have no impact on activity patterns. Most runners commonly interrupt their routines if the environment is inclement, but it is not known how many seek substitute settings. The type of leisure-sport participation is influenced by seasonal availability, but most who are active remain involved in activities year-round (18, 100); schoolchildren are most active in spring and summer (31, 32). In a like manner, climate clearly influences choices of outdoor leisure activities (100), but it is unknown whether overall participation rates differ by region. Highly active American adults are more likely to live in the West and the Midwest, whereas inactive adults live in the East and the South (114, 141). Similarly, the most active Canadians reside in the West (British Columbia), whereas the least active are in the Atlantic provinces and Quebec (141, 142). However, these geographic distributions are as likely to reflect age and socioeconomic factors as they are to reflect differences in climate (22). Although in one U.S. survey one fourth of the public stated that nicer weather would likely increase their sport involvement, nearly twice as many active as inactive people stated this (114).

Physical Activity Characteristics

Of the possible determinants of physical activity participation, characteristics of physical activity have received the least study. They are fundamentally critical, however, for establishing desirable participation goals. In addition to establishing fitness and epidemiological criteria for setting national participation objectives, it is important to determine whether activity characteristics predispose or impede participation in the population or in specific population segments and settings.

Self-reported discomfort has been associated with dropping out of an endurance training program in college women (74), but most studies of supervised exercise programs in adults do not show an association between dropout rates and exercise intensity or perceived exertion (115). Intensity in these studies is relativized according to an individual's metabolic tolerance for exercise, and this minimizes variation in physical strain and its role as a determinant. For example, no difference in cumulative dropout rate has been seen between male post-myocardial infarction patients randomly assigned to either high-volume activity (60%-85% $\dot{V}O_2$peak, 4 d/wk) or to low-volume activity (50% $\dot{V}O_2$peak, 1 d/wk) in a 4-yr clinical exercise trial (108). Injuries from high-intensity running can directly lead to dropout, but this should not become a problem in the typical case until durations of 45 min, frequencies of 5 d per week, or both are performed by the previously untrained (115).

In free-living settings in which the energy cost of standard activities may require varying percentages of metabolic capacity, exertional perceptions and preferences may be a more important influence on participation. Walking has been a successful adherence strategy in supervised exercise (7), and the estimated metabolic intensity of activity was also a determinant of free-living activity participation in a large community sample (127). In the latter study, although more men (11%) than women (5%) adopted vigorous exercise such as running during a year's time, a comparatively higher proportion of women (33%) than men (26%) took up such moderate activities as routine walking, stair climbing, and gardening. Both genders were much more likely to adopt moderate activity than they were a fitness regimen. Moderate activities showed a dropout rate (25%-35%) roughly one half of that seen for vigorous exercise (50%) (127).

It is well established that the unfit and untrained perceive a standard activity intensity as more effortful than do the fit and trained. At rest the sedentary and unfit complain of chronic fatigue (21, 86), and sedentary smokers report excessive fatigue during treadmill exercise (73). However, it is not now known whether chronic fatigue creates a barrier to participation or whether alleviation of chronic fatigue with increased fitness is an incentive for participation.

The relationships among fitness, physical activity, perceived exertion, and preferred levels of exertion have not been systematically studied as determinants of participation. It is noteworthy, however, that behavior change interventions have shown increased overall energy expenditure or frequency of activity but not increased intensity of physical activity. The influence on participation of type of activity is equally unclear, although one community-based study has shown that a perceived choice of activity type increased attendance in a supervised program (147).

Behavior Change Interventions

Although some recent reports suggest that community (16, 26) and work-site (10) health promotions can increase physical activity, the collective evidence indicates no predictable impact of health education promotions on the fitness or activity of adults (50, 57, 61, 99, 121); physician or medical office interventions and school and community promotions with children may hold more promise but have received little study (75). Behavioral effectiveness seems increased when promotions include social support and individualized goal setting, planning, and monitoring rather than focusing only on health education and provision of facilities. When public health-based promotions of physical activity are effective, the impact is likely to be short-lived if skills related to self-motivation of behavior are not imparted (36).

For many, self-motivated physical activity appears to stem from rational goal setting, self-monitoring of behavior, and self-reinforcement of a valued behavior (39, 68). It is believed that many who have the intention to be active but remain sedentary lack these self-regulatory skills; studies have shown that interventions incorporating appropriate goal orientations and planning, together with conscientious self-monitoring and self-reward, can support participation among activity-intentioned but undermotivated individuals (85, 96). The usefulness of these goal-setting and reinforcement skills for maintaining involvement has been demonstrated for short periods (4-10 wk) among those already motivated to adopt activity. This could, however, have an indirect impact over the longer term, as self-report evidence suggests that intrinsically concrete rewarding states (e.g., feeling better or enjoyment from goal attainment) can augment initial abstract incentives (e.g., anticipation of health benefits or desire for weight loss) (35).

Relatively few experimental studies of changes in physical activity have been attempted. Those conducted have applied general principles and techniques of behavior modification to alter exercise behavior rather than to manipulate determinants of exercise behavior. This has been partly a pragmatic decision because several known exercise determinants (e.g., smoking, occupation or socioeconomic status, and being overweight) are themselves difficult or impractical to change. However, when determinants of physical activity are not controlled in behavior change studies, they may confound the outcomes.

Behavior Modification

The techniques and principles of behavior modification can be viewed either as reinforcement control or stimulus control strategies that are based on behavioral or cognitive-behavioral principles (85). Behavioral approaches, including written agreements (109), behavior contracts and lotteries (44, 150, 158), stimulus control (78, 79, 110), and contingency incentives (1, 78, 113), have been used successfully in case control studies. Cognitive-behavioral approaches, including self-monitoring (96, 109, 110), sensory distraction (96), goal setting (96, 110, 113), feedback (96, 110, 113), and decision making (72, 152), have appeared equally effective when used alone or when combined in intervention packages. Behavior modification tech-

niques are collectively associated with an increase of 10%-25% in frequency of physical activity, but their impact on changes in intensity and duration of activity is less clear.

With few exceptions (43), studies have not focused on health outcomes as the dependent variable for determining intervention effectiveness. Likewise, most interventions have lasted only 3-10 wk, and only a few show maintenance of activity in follow-up assessments. Follow-up studies typically show that increases in physical activity associated with behavior modification are short-lived after the intervention is removed (Figure 7.6). Also, placebo control comparisons have been infrequent. Therefore, generalizations are not possible about specific components of the interventions that are effective for specific populations. Strategies that effect a change have in common a dimension of social reinforcement or support (139), and they appear more successful when carried out in groups rather than outside supervised settings.

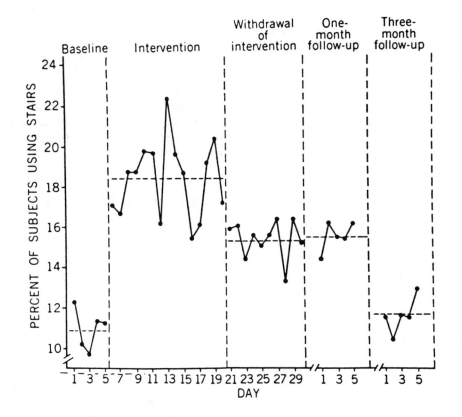

Figure 7.6. Percent of subjects using stairs before, during, and after behavior change intervention. From ''Evaluation and Modification of Exercise Patterns in the Natural Environment'' by K.D. Brownell, A.J. Stunkard, and J.M. Albaum, *American Journal of Psychiatry*, **137**, p. 1542. Copyright 1980, The American Psychiatric Association. Reprinted by permission.

Relapse Prevention

Even among the habitually active, unexpected disruptions in activity routines or settings can interrupt or end a previously continuous exercise program (35, 95, 107). Relocation, medical events, and travel can impede the continuity of activity reinforcement and create new activity barriers. It is believed, however, that interruptions and life events have less impact as the activity habit becomes more established (35); their impact may also be diminished if the individual anticipates and plans their occurrence, recognizes them as only temporary impediments, and develops self-regulatory skills for preventing relapses to inactivity (9, 84, 94, 96).

Setting management appears to be a particularly important behavioral skill for individuals who intend to increase activity levels but have a history of inactivity or relapse. A consistent daily routine in a convenient place and time that is flexible enough to accommodate existing activity preferences and daily fluxes in motivation but that is planned to achieve tangible long-term activity objectives within a reasonable time (e.g., 6-10 wk) should facilitate the reinforcing potential of participation while minimizing major impediments (85, 94, 95). Understanding that relapses are normal and reversible seems important to ensuring that attempts to be active are persistent (85, 94, 95).

For many adults personalized social support from program staff or an activity partner sharing similar interests and ability are potent exercise and activity reinforcers (96, 152). Social support can provide an important behavioral boost for those who intend to be active but who do not possess self-regulatory skills or self-motivation.

Psychological Models of Determinants

Although the behavior change interventions and health promotions that have been applied to physical activity have systematic methods and traditions with conceptual and empirical bases, they are essentially technologies. Psychological theories can guide the effective implementation of intervention technologies. Several theories are prominent and may have implications for public health promotions of physical activity. Figure 7.7 depicts my conception of the likely roles of these theories in understanding the determinants of physical activity. It is important to examine how their predictions for interactions of personal attributes, environments, and physical activity characteristics are borne out by empirical study of free-living and supervised physical activity in various population segments. Several goals are apparent.

First, the estimated 20%-60% of sedentary individuals who have no intention to exercise (18, 54, 55, 60, 100, 114) ought to be motivated to do so. Although most people view exercise as beneficial, they may have little personal incentive to act on that belief and may expect the cost of exercise to outweigh any gains. Second, the estimated 40%-60% who now exercise only mildly or irregularly (19, 20, 141, 142) will need to increase their commitment. Reinforcement for participation must overcome barriers and lack of skills if good intentions are to be implemented as sustained action. But little is known about what reinforces high exertion by some and inactivity among others.

Thus, the psychological models described in Table 7.1 can be directed at various stages of planning, adopting, and maintaining physical activity. These models encompass attitudes, beliefs, or expectations about physical activity and health outcomes, personal ability (or efficacy), control, social norms, and behavioral skills for reducing barriers to activity and reinforcing participation.

Although each of the models describes aspects of physical activity participation, it is unknown whether any model or combination thereof can explain the determinants of physical activity adequately for public health purposes of increasing physical activity. It seems unlikely that psychological models that exclude or minimize considerations about biological and environmental aspects of physical activity will be sufficient to explain and predict physical activity.

Limitations in Methods and Research Design

Population surveys can be generalized to a large population. However, surveys rely on subjective, possibly inaccurate, estimates of activity and a narrow set of possible determinants with unknown reliability and validity. Surveys often use cross-sectional or retrospective designs and have not permitted a weighting of relative influence among variables.

Studies of supervised exercise programs and community-based physical activity have permitted more precise measures of activity and determinants, and they frequently examine variable interactions. However, their ability to be generalized to other populations, settings, and activities usually has not been tested and is therefore restricted. Although

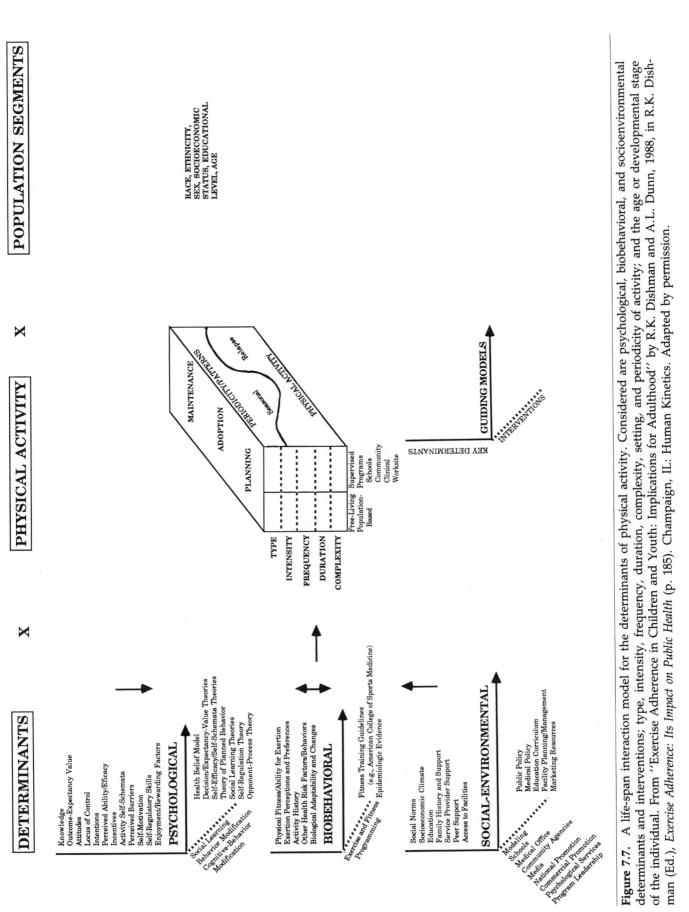

Figure 7.7. A life-span interaction model for the determinants of physical activity. Considered are psychological, biobehavioral, and socioenvironmental determinants and interventions; type, intensity, frequency, duration, complexity, setting, and periodicity of activity; and the age or developmental stage of the individual. From "Exercise Adherence in Children and Youth: Implications for Adulthood" by R.K. Dishman and A.L. Dunn, 1988, in R.K. Dishman (Ed.), *Exercise Adherence: Its Impact on Public Health* (p. 185). Champaign, IL: Human Kinetics. Adapted by permission.

Table 7.1 Summary of Psychological Models of Physical Activity Determinants

Psychological model and summary statement	Results of studies	General conclusions

A. Models that have generated research

1. **Health belief model**
Compliance with any health behavior depends on perceived vulnerability to a disorder, belief that health risk is increased by noncompliance, and belief that the health effectiveness of the behavior outweighs barriers (124).

a. Not valid for all health behaviors (e.g., health-related vs. health-directed) (76).
b. Validity for exercise has been mixed (138), but most studies have not tested the total model (92, 104). Valid and reliable measures for perceived exertion benefits and barriers have been available only recently (140). Physical activity is perceived as requiring more time and effort than are other health behaviors (149), and free-living activity is unreliably associated with other health behaviors in the population (12, 106, 143). Thus, physical activity appears unique among health-related actions.

a. Failure to predict may be due to the positive view of health behaviors held by the general public or the wide range in behavioral demands or complexity of physical activity.
b. Active individuals often perceive their health as good and not vulnerable to disease. Time, convenience, and exertion are viewed as barriers but equally so by the already active. The model was designed for risk-avoidance behavior, not health-promotive behavior. Thus, its effectiveness may be less for those who view physical activity as a health-promotive or wellness behavior more than for those who see it as an illness-reducing behavior.

2. **Locus of control theory**
Belief in personal control over reinforcement outcomes from behavior influences motivation, particularly in novel circumstances in which little information is available for decision making (123).

a. Studies with adults have yielded mixed results. Cross-sectional comparisons show exercisers to have a more internal locus, whereas prospective studies show inconsistent relationships with supervised adherence (39, 41). The validity and reliability of exercise-specific measures have not been demonstrated (41).

a. Because locus of control encompasses, but does not clearly distinguish the importance of, beliefs about outcomes of behavior and personal control, it lacks precision for predicting specific behaviors in specific contexts (e.g., supervised exercise).
b. Health locus of control shows promise for predicting free-living physical activity in young adults (41) and as a moderating variable for other models, such as self-efficacy (8) and planned behavior (51).

3. **Theory of reasoned action**
Attitudes about a specific exercise prescription (i.e., time, place, and type of exercise) can predict behavior through its interaction with social norms. Both influence exercise intention (5).

a. No studies show that social desirability of activity can predict supervised exercise (39), and studies of free-living physical activity show mixed results (58, 59, 60). Spouse impact is reliable, but personal attitudes are not (45, 69).
b. Available data from supervised and community settings suggest that only 25%-50% of intentions to begin and maintain an exercise program translate to sustained action. The model predicts about one third of exercise intentions (58, 59, 60, 61, 62, 112, 138).

a. Intentions seem largely necessary but not sufficient to predict physical activity. The extent to which the active plan their exercise routines and the impact of interventions on intentions and subsequent exercise remains unknown.

Psychological model and summary statement	Results of studies	General conclusions
4. Self-efficacy To attempt and persist at a behavior change, one must perceive a personal ability to carry out the behavior when the outcome is known. Self-efficacy develops by (a) actual mastery, (b) modeling, (c) verbal persuasion, and (d) emotional signs of coping ablity (8).	a. Among post-MI patients, beliefs about ability to exercise can increase following fitness testing or training (47, 128). b. Self-efficacy beliefs distinguish patients who exceed or do not attain their exercise intensity prescriptions (46); are better predictors of exercise compliance than are health control beliefs for chronic obstructive-lung patients (77); and relate to adoption of vigorous activity in men and adoption and maintenance of moderate activity for men and women in free-living settings (33, 127). c. Dropouts and adherents in a preventive medicine program were equally likely to perceive increased ability for safe exertion as a benefit of exercise (128). Low exercise self-efficacy predicted intention to adopt a work-site exercise program (28).	a. Feelings of self-efficacy most accurately predict when they are specific to a narrow range of behaviors and times. b. Self-efficacy is influenced by actual experience and subjective signs of inability. Therefore, past experience and perceived exertional strain must be considered; self-efficacy does not predict persistence of behavior change when incentives are not present. c. General feelings of physical ability might be a better predictor of overall physical activity patterns across time, settings, and activities than are specific self-efficacy beliefs, but this has not been tested.

B. Models understudied in physical activity settings

5. Theory of planned behavior Expands theory of reasoned action by considering perceived and actual control over behavior. Recognizes that intentions are often not implemented because of inability, situational barriers, or transience of intentions (4).	a. No physical activity studies are reported.	a. May help explain failure of reasoned-action theory to predict physical activity by integrating self-control and self-efficacy variables.
6. Physical activity model Attraction to physical activity is reinforced by increased self-esteem and is mediated by perceived increases in physical ability and fitness due to increased activity (138).	a. Studies of adult fitness programs show a weak relationship with sustained participation but suggest an influence on initial adoption (39, 138).	a. Lacks specificity for activity, place, and time, but this may not be a problem for predicting total activity patterns. b. Attractive model because it provides a link between past activity history, fitness self-perceptions, and attitude. c. Permits an empirical contrast with more complex models of attitude (4, 5), perceived ability (8), and self-schemata (80). Similarity with models of perceived competence could integrate the literature on youth sport participation with determinants of physical activity (49).

(Cont.)

Table 7.1 (Continued)

Psychological model and summary statement	Results of studies	General conclusions
7. Expectancy-value decision theories Behavior is a function of self-expectations of the outcomes from a behavior and the evaluation of these outcomes in contrast to outcomes of alternative actions (8).	a. May predict intention or interest in adopting free-living physical activity (81) but has not predicted participation in either free-living or supervised activity (33, 39, 41, 81).	a. Useful global framework for understanding the unique aspects of the preceding six models; each has emanated from the broader decision-theory base. b. Integration of self-efficacy (8) and planned behavior (4) within an expectancy-value umbrella may offer a parsimonious model for explaining adoption of physical activity.
8. Self-regulatory theory Behavior is controlled much like a servomechanism, in which goal setting, self-monitoring of behavior, and self-reinforcement are necessary skills to implement behavioral intentions and overcome personal and situational barriers to motivation (82, 91).	a. Some evidence supports the effectiveness of interventions that include goal setting, self-monitoring, and self-reinforcement (85, 95, 96). Cross-sectional study suggests that these skills combine with self-motivation to explain variance in free-living activity (68). Most effective in multiple-component packages, particularly using principles of relapse prevention (85, 94).	a. Apears particularly important for explaining maintenance and periodicity of physical activity in free-living physical activity. Can be an important adjunct to prevent or reduce the incidence of dropout in supervised settings.
9. Opponent-process theory A two-phase process underlies motivated behavior. The primary phase to a stimulus is excitatory, and it initiates a secondary, inhibitory (or opponent) phase that returns arousal to a hedonic neutrality acceptable to the individual. The opponent process grows faster and stronger with stimulus exposure, whereas the initial phase grows weaker and decays more rapidly. Thus, an initially pleasurable or aversive response requires increasing stimulus exposure, whereas its absence produces a growing opponent response (137).	a. No physical activity studies reported.	a. May help explain maintenance or adherence to habitual physical activity. The theory's biobehavioral nature can account for tangible sensations that may reinforce continued participation. The exclusive reliance of the previous models on cognition has been inadequate for conceptualizing tangible or concrete reinforcing mechanisms for participation among the active (35).

Note. From ''Exercise and Adherence in Children and Youth'' by R.K. Dishman and A.L. Dunn, 1988, in R.K. Dishman (Ed.), *Exercise Adherence: Its Impact on Public Health* (pp. 170-175). Champaign, IL: Human Kinetics. Adapted by permission.

prospective studies have been used commonly in supervised exercise programs, there are relatively few controlled experiments of determinants. Thus, there is some imbalance in methods and knowledge across populations, settings, and activity (Table 7.2).

The studies reviewed each have specific limitations because of inadequacies in measurement of determinants or activity patterns, sample size, or representativeness or because of inadequate control or quantification of possible confounding variables. All these factors limit the ability of the

Table 7.2 Summary of Variables That May Determine the Probability of Physical Activity

Determinant	Changes in probability	
	Supervised program	Free-living activity
Personal attributes		
Past program participation	++	+(≠)
Past free-living activity	+	+
Contemporary program activity		0
School sports	0	0
Health behaviors	00	+(≠)
Blue-collar occupation	−−	−
Smoking	−−	0
Overweight (fatness or body mass index)	−	−
High risk for coronary heart disease[a]	−	−
Type A behavior pattern	−	+
Health and exercise knowledge	0	0
Health locus of control	+	+
Attitudes	0	0
Enjoyment of activity	+	+(≠)
Perceived health or fitness	++	−(≠)
Mood disturbance	−	−
Education (yr)[a]	+	++
Age[a]	00	−
Expect personal health benefit	0	+(≠)
Value exercise outcomes	0	0
Self-efficacy for exercise	+	+
Intention to be active	0	+
Active self-schemata		+
Self-motivation	+	++
Behavioral skills (goal setting, self-monitoring, self-reinforcement, relapse planning)		+
Environmental factors and interventions		
Spouse support	++	+
Perceived lack of time	−−	−(≠)
Facilities access or convenience	++	0
Disruptions in routine	−	
Social reinforcement or support (staff, exercise partner)	+	
Past family influences		+(≠)
Peer influence (past or present)		+(≠)
Physician influence		+
School programs	+	+(≠)
Cost	0	0
Medical screening or fitness testing	0	0
Climate (or geographical region)[a]	−	−
Contracts, agreements, contingencies	++	+(≠)
Stimulus control and reinforcement control	++	
Benefit and cost decision analysis	++	
Relapse prevention training	++	+(≠)
Physical activity characteristics		
Activity intensity	−	−
Choice of activity type (perceived)	+	
Perceived effort	−−(≠)	−(≠)

Note. ++ = repeatedly documented increased probability; + = weak or mixed documentation of increased probability; 00 = repeatedly documented that there is no change in probability; 0 = weak or mixed documentation of no change in probability; − = weak or mixed documentation of decreased probability; −− = repeatedly documented decreased probability; (≠) indicates unknown validity of measures employed. Blank spaces indicate no data. From "The Determinants of Physical Activity and Exercise" by R.K. Dishman, J.F. Sallis, and D. Orenstein, 1985, *Public Health Reports*, **100**(2), p. 162. Adapted by permission.

[a]Likely a selection bias, not a causal determinant.

studies to be generalized to other population groups. Differences in sample size, reliability of measures, and the range of scores on determinants and physical activity also influence the variability of results from studies of the same population group or type of setting. Thus, both the internal validity and the robustness of many determinants remain unclear. Also, most studies have been descriptive, relying on correlational rather than experimental data.

There exists a need to standardize exercise programs and the methods used for assessing physical activity and its correlates if reproducible and generalizable results are to be obtained. The reported range in supervised program adherence rates of 10%-90% (36, 40, 95, 107) attests to the magnitude of program diversity. The absence of standardized psychometric and behavioral methods in studies examining psychological variables was previously described.

In supervised exercise studies, widely varying definitions of adherent behaviors are used. For example, in two studies that observed cardiac rehabilitation patients, one defined *dropout* as absence from supervised sessions for more than 8 consecutive wk (108), whereas another (34) defined it as absence for 2 wk. Although the most reliable influence on program adherence appears to be length of the program period studied, attempts have been made to compare studies in which the period of interest may range from less than 1 mo to 36 mo. The impact of this on results is best illustrated by the observation that some factors related to adherence early in a program can no longer be related later (101, 155).

There are also very different types and volumes of activity employed as the exercise stimulus for very different types of subjects. These have ranged from a study of male prison inmates who ran for 20 wk at an intensity of 85%-90% of maximum heart rate for a duration of 30 min 5 d per week (115) to a group of urban females in a community-based exercise dance class that met for 1-1/4 hr once per week for 10 wk (154). This diversity represents varying behavioral demands on participants and provides differing social support, both of which can likely interact with personal attributes of individuals to influence physical activity participation.

A need also exists to standardize the measures of physical activity. Measurement approaches have included job classification; retrospective self-report; daily self-recording; mechanical, electronic, and physiological surveillance; and observation. There are problems in standardizing results for studies of determinants that cannot use direct observation of physical activity. Although questionnaires validated against biological estimates of activity (e.g., metabolic tolerance and heart rate monitors, or motion sensors) are useful in dichotomizing between highly active and sedentary individuals, they are less accurate in distinguishing between levels of activity intensity (42). Also, behavior does not ensure that predicted biological change will occur. Importantly, the psychometric properties of self-reported physical activity (i.e., reliability and construct validity) are also largely unknown. The usefulness of activity questionnaires validated from epidemiological studies for detecting behaviorally significant amounts of activity variance remains unknown for small samples.

Recall assessment of physical activity is a pragmatic approach for large populations for which direct observation or objective monitoring cannot be implemented. Validation of recall methods has been limited by the absence of a consensus standard or criterion for comparison (89). The assessment of physical activity is discussed in detail elsewhere in chapters 5 and 6. The lack of uniform assessment methods for physical activity is important for studies of determinants because it makes it difficult to evaluate whether determinants of physical activity truly differ across people, settings, and time; whether certain determinants, interventions, or theoretical models are associated with unique aspects of the physical activity; or whether the various measures each are simply poor estimates of true physical activity. Therefore, for practical and research purposes it currently seems desirable to evaluate both subjective and objective evidence of exercise behavior when direct observation is not feasible.

There is also a need to determine a reliable baseline expectancy for adherence to supervised exercise programs. Clinical trials with post-myocardial infarction patients indicate that a substantial number of dropouts are due to medical contraindications. These have represented 15%-40% of dropouts from 2-, 3-, and 4-yr programs (107). Similarly, uncontrollable inactivity can result from injury (115). True conflicts in schedule and relocation also occur that are beyond the personal control to influence participation (107), but they will not be well explained by most psychological theories.

Conclusion

The midcourse review of the U.S. Public Health Service's 1990 objectives has recommended that the determinants of physical activity and exercise be known by the year 2000. Study of the determinants of physical activity has a 20-yr history in North America and Scandinavia, yet the typical dropout rate from supervised exercise programs has remained at 40%-50% during this time. In the population, estimates indicate that 30%-60% of Americans and Canadians engage in no leisure-time physical activity, whereas only 10% of Americans and 25% of Canadians are regularly and vigorously active. Research on determinants has largely relied on predictive models based on personal attributes of participants or on generalized intervention models for behavior change and promotion campaigns. The success of these approaches for facilitating physical activity patterns has been limited because physical activity appears to be a complex set of behaviors, requiring much time and effort, that may not be responsive to the same prompts and reinforcers as are most other health habits.

In this chapter I have discussed personal attributes, environments, and physical activity characteristics that predispose, enable, impede, and reinforce the planning, adoption, and maintenance of physical activity in supervised and free-living settings. Perceived values or abilities and expected or real outcomes combine with age, education level, socioeconomic and biomedical status, personality, lifestyle habits, and perceived or real environments and barriers to shape a person's disposition to plan, adopt, maintain, increase, or return to a physical activity pattern. This disposition may also be shaped by activity history; by social norms, modeling, and reinforcement by family, peers, educators, and medical or health care providers; by prompts to action from the environment; by accessibility of facilities; and by the type, frequency, duration, intensity, and complexity of physical activity.

The effectiveness of behavior change interventions, promotions, and self-regulatory skills for increasing physical activity was also discussed, and prominent psychological models that can be evaluated as guides for physical activity interventions were presented. It will continue to be important to identify psychological models that explain the various stages of participation in physical activity, and it is likely that different models may best explain different stages, such as planning, adopting, maintaining, and returning to an activity pattern in supervised and free-living settings.

Methodological problems encountered in measuring determinants and assessing physical activity patterns were also addressed because they influence the reproducibility and behavioral interpretations of the physical activity determinants that have been investigated. There has been little uniformity of method, theory, subjects, setting, and measurement in past studies of the determinants of physical activity. The number of studies conducted on relatively small numbers of demographically homogeneous subjects in supervised settings and for purposes of adult fitness and preventive medicine has far outnumbered population surveys and community-based studies. More balance is needed for the future. Population studies are important to describe the generalizability of causal determinants to populations and their segments. However, small-sample studies, particularly prospective experiments, must continue. They are needed to unravel the causal mechanisms underlying the determinants of physical activity and to evaluate practical applications for optimizing participation in specific settings.

All the potentially important determinants are not known, and it is not precisely known in what ways established determinants interact to influence participation. Participation in supervised exercise training and in free-living physical activity may be influenced in somewhat different ways by different determinants, which may differ for specific population segments and settings. Too few studies have directly compared homogeneous groups (e.g., children, the elderly, race and ethnic or cultural groups, socioeconomic levels) across heterogeneous settings (e.g., medical, work site, community and commercial programs, and spontaneous leisure) or heterogeneous groups across homogeneous settings to know how to increase physical activity in a population or its segments economically and predictably. However, enough is known to increase the likelihood of physical activity for individuals and small groups under supervision.

References

1. Allen, L.D., and B.A. Iwata. Reinforcing exercise maintenance using high-rate activities. *Behav. Mod.* 4: 337-354, 1980.

2. American College of Sports Medicine. Position statement on the recommended quantity and quality of exercise for developing and maintaining fitness in healthy adults. *Med. Sci. Sports Exerc.* 10: vii-x, 1978.

3. Andrew, G.M., N.B. Oldridge, J.O. Parker, D.A. Cunningham, P.A. Rechnitzer, N.L. Jones, C. Buck, T. Kavanagh, R.J. Shephard, J.R. Sutton, and W. McDonald. Reasons for dropout from exercise programs in post coronary patients. *Med. Sci. Sports Exerc.* 13: 164-168, 1981.

4. Ajzen, I. From intentions to actions: A theory of planned behavior. In: Kuhl, J., and J. Beckman, eds. *Action-Control: From cognition to behavior*, Heidelberg, FRG: Springer, 1985: 11-39.

5. Ajzen, I., and M. Fishbein. Attitude-behavior relations: A theoretical analysis and review of empirical research. *Psychol. Bull.* 84: 888-918, 1977.

6. Atkins, C.J., T.L. Patterson, B.E. Roppe, R.M. Kaplan, J.F. Sallis, and P.R. Nadar. Recruitment issues, health habits, and the decision to participate in a health promotion program. *Am. J. Prev. Med.* 3: 87-94, 1987.

7. Ballantyne, D., A. Clark, G.S. Dyker, C.R. Gillis, V.M. Hawthorne, D.A. Henry, D.S. Hole, R.M. Murdoch, T. Semple, and G.M. Stewart. Prescribing exercise for the healthy: Assessment of compliance and effects of plasma lipids and lipoproteins. *Health Bull.* 36: 169-176, 1978.

8. Bandura, A. Self-efficacy: Toward a unifying theory of behavioral change. *Psychol. Rev.* 1984: 191-215, 1977.

9. Belisle, M., E. Roskies, and J.M. Levesque. Improving adherence to physical activity. *Health Psychol.* 6: 159-172, 1987.

10. Blair, S.N., P.V. Piserchia, C.S. Wilbur, and J.H. Crowder. A public health intervention model for worksite health promotion: Impact on exercise and physical fitness in a health promotion plan after 24 months. *JAMA* 255: 921-926, 1986.

11. Blair, S.N., R.T. Mulder, and H.W. Kohl. Reaction to "secular trends in adult physical activity: Exercise boom or bust?" *Res. Q. Exerc. Sport* 58: 106-110, 1987.

12. Blair, S.N., D.R. Jacobs, Jr., and K.E. Powell. Relationships between exercise or physical activity and other health behaviors. *Public Health Rep.* 100: 172-180, 1985.

13. Blumenthal, J.A., R.S. Williams, A.G. Wallace, R.B. Williams, and T.L. Needles. Physiological and psychological variables predict compliance to prescribed exercise therapy in patients recovering from myocardial infarction. *Psychosom. Med.* 6: 519-527, 1982.

14. Brooks, C.M. Leisure time physical activity assessment of American adults through an analysis of time diaries collected in 1981. *Am. J. Public Health,* 77: 455-460, 1987.

15. Brooks, C.M. Adult participation in physical activities requiring moderate to high levels of energy expenditure. *Phys. Sportsmed.* 15: 119-132, 1987.

16. Brownell, K.D., A.J. Stunkard, and J.M. Albaum. Evaluation and modification of exercise patterns in the natural environment. *Am. J. Psychiatry* 137: 1540-1545, 1980.

17. Bruce, E.H., R. Frederick, R.A. Bruce, and L.D. Fisher. Comparison of active participants and dropouts in CAPRI cardiopulmonary rehabilitation programs. *Am. J. Cardiol.* 37: 53-60, 1976.

18. *Canada Fitness Survey. Fitness and lifestyle in Canada.* Ottawa, ON: Fitness Canada, 1983.

19. Caspersen, C.J., G.M. Christenson, and R.A. Pollard. Status of the 1990 physical fitness and exercise objectives—Evidence from NHIS 1985. *Public Health Rep.* 101: 587-592.

20. Centers for Disease Control. Sex-, age-, and region-specific prevalence for sedentary lifestyle in selected states in 1985—the Behavioral Risk Factor Surveillance System. *Morbid. Mortal. Week. Rep.* 36: 195-198, 203-204, 1987.

21. Chen, M.K. The epidemiology of self-perceived fatigue among adults. *Prev. Med.* 15: 74-81, 1986.

22. Chubb, M., and H.R. Chubb. *One third of our time? An Introduction to Recreation Behavior and Services.* New York: John Wiley & Sons, 1981.

23. Clarke, H.H., ed. National adult physical fitness survey [Special edition]. *President's Council on Physical Fitness and Sports newsletter.* Washington, DC: President's Council on Physical Fitness and Sports, May 1973.

24. Collingwood, T.R., I.H. Bernstein, and D. Hubbard. Canonical correlation analysis of clinical and psychological data in 4,351 men and women. *J. Cardiac Rehabil.* 3: 706-711, 1983.

25. Conrad, P. Who comes to work-site wellness programs? A preliminary review. *J. Occup. Med.* 29: 317-320, 1987.

26. Crow, R., H. Blackburn, and D. Jacobs. Population strategies to enhance physical activity. *Acta Med. Scand. Suppl.* 711: 93-112, 1986.

27. Cunningham, D.A., P.A. Recheitzer, J.H. Howard, and A.P. Donner. Exercise training of men at retirement: A clinical trial. *J. Gerontology* 42: 17-23, 1987.

28. Davis, K.E., K.L. Jackson, J.J. Kronenfeld, and S.N. Blair. Intent to participation in worksite health promotion activities: A model of risk factors and psychosocial variables. *Health Educ. Q.* 11: 361-377, 1984.

29. Department of Health and Human Services. *Midcourse review: 1990 physical fitness and exercise objectives.* Washington, DC: U.S. Government Printing Of   ., 1986.

30. Department of Heal   nd Human Services. *Promoting health/preventing disease: Objectives for the nation.* Washington, DC: U.S. Government Printing Office, Fall 1980.

31. Department of Health and Human Services. The National Children and Youth Fitness Study. *JOPERD* 56(1): 44-90, 1985.

32. Department of Health and Human Services. The National Children and Youth Fitness Study, II. *JOPERD* 58(9): 50-96, 1987.

33. Desharnais, R., J. Bouillon, and G. Godin. Self-efficacy and outcome expectations as determinants of exercise adherence. *Psych. Rep.* 59: 1155-1159, 1986.

34. Dishman, R.K. Biologic influences on exercise adherence. *Res. Q. Exerc. Sport* 52: 143-15 , 1981.

35. Dishman, R.K. Compliance/adherence in health-related exercise. *Health Psychol.* 1: 237-267, 1982.

36. Dishman,   ., ed. *Exercise adherence: Its impact on pu   ealth.* Champaign, IL: Human Kinetics, 1988.

37. Dishman, R.K. Supervised and free-living physical activity: No differences in former athletes and nonathletes. *Am. J. Prev. Med.* 4: 153-160, 1988.

38. Dishman, R.K., and A.L. Dunn. Exercise adherence in children and youth: Implications for adulthood. In: Dishman, R.K., ed. *Exercise adherence: Its impact on public health.* Champaign, IL: Human Kinetics, 1988: 145-189.

39. Dishman, R.K., and W. Ickes. Self-motivation and adherence to therapeutic exercise. *J. Behav. Med.* 4: 421-438, 1981.

40. Dishman, R.K., J.F. Sallis, and D. Orenstein. The determinants of physical activity and exercise. *Public Health Rep.* 100: 158-171, 1985.

41. Dishman, R.K., and M.A. Steinhardt. Internal health locus of control predicts free-living, but not supervised, physical activity: A test of exercise-specific control and outcome expectancy hypotheses. *Res. Q. Exerc. Sport.* In press.

42. Dishman, R.K., and M. Steinhardt. Reliability and concurrent validity for a seven-day recall of physical activity in college students. *Med. Sci. Sports Exerc.* 20: 14-25, 1988.

43. Epstein, L.H., R. Koeske, and R.R. Wing. Adherence to exercise in obese children. *J. Cardiac Rehabil.* 4: 185-195, 1984.

44. Epstein, L.H., R. Wing, J.K. Thompson, and R. Griffin. Attendance and fitness in aerobics exercise: The effects of contract and lottery procedures. *Behav. Mod.* 4: 465-479, 1980.

45. Erling, J., and N.B. Oldridge. Effect of a spousal-support program on compliance with cardiac rehabilitation. *Med. Sci. Sports Exerc.* 17: 284, 1985.

46. Ewart, C.K., K.J. Stewart, and R.E. Gillilan. Usefulness of self-efficacy in predicting overexertion during programmed exercise in coronary artery disease. *Am. J. Cardiol.* 57: 557-561, 1986.

47. Ewart, C.K., C.B. Taylor, C.B. Reese, and R.F. DeBusk. Effects of early postmyocardial infarction exercise testing on self-perception and subsequent physical activity. *Am. J. Cardiol.* 51: 1076-1080, 1983.

48. Feather, N.T. *Expectations and actions: Expectancy value models in psychology.* Hillsdale, NJ: Lawrence Erlbaum Associates, 1982.

49. Feltz, D.L., and M.E. Ewing. Psychological characteristics of elite young athletes. *Med. Sci. Sports Exerc.* 19: S98-S105, 1987.

50. Fielding, J.E. Effectiveness of employee health improvement programs. *J. Occup. Med.* 24: 907-916, 1982.

51. Fielding, J.E. Health promotion and disease prevention at the worksite. *Annu. Rev. Public Health* 5: 237-265, 1984.

52. Fitness Ontario. *The relationship between physical activity and other health-related lifestyle behaviors: A research report from the Ministry of Culture and Recreation.* Toronto: Government of Ontario, Sports and Fitness Branch, 1982.

53. Gale, J.B., W.T. Eckhoff, S.F. Mogel, and J.E. Rodnick. Factors related to adherence to an exercise program for healthy adults. *Med. Sci. Sports Exerc.* 16: 544-549, 1984.

54. Gallup Organization. *American health: Public attitudes and behavior related to exercise.* Princeton, NJ: Author, 1985.

55. *The General Mills American family report, 1978-1979: Family health in an era of stress.* New York: Yankelovich, Skelly and White, 1979.

56. Gettman, L.R., M.L. Pollock, and A. Ward. Adherence to unsupervised exercise. *Phys. Sportsmed.* 11: 56-66, 1983.

57. Godin, G., and R.J. Shephard. Physical fitness promotion programmes: Effectiveness in modifying exercise behavior. *Can. J. Appl. Sport Sci.* 8: 104-113, 1983.

58. Godin, G., P. Valois, R.J. Shephard, and R. Desharnais. Prediction of leisure-time exercise behavior: A path analysis (LISREL V) model. *J. Behav. Med.* 10: 145-158, 1987.

59. Godin, G., A. Colantonio, G.M. Davis, R.J. Shephard, and C. Simand. Prediction of leisure time exercise behavior among a group of lower-limb disabled adults. *J. Clin. Psychol.* 42: 272-279, 1986.

60. Godin, G., R.J. Shephard, and A. Colantonio. The cognitive profile of those who intend to exercise but do not. *Public Health Rep.* 101: 521-526, 1986.

61. Godin, G., R. Desharnais, J. Jobin, and J. Cook. The impact of physical fitness and health-age appraisal upon exercise intentions and behavior. *J. Behav. Med.* 10: 241-250, 1987.

62. Godin, G., M. Cox, and R.J. Shephard. The impact of physical fitness education on behavioral intentions towards regular exercise. *Can. J. Appl. Sports Sci.* 8: 240-245, 1983.

63. Green, L.W. Modifying and developing health behavior. *Annu. Rev. Public Health* 5: 215-236, 1984.

64. Gwinup, G. Effect of exercise alone on the weight of obese women. *Arch. Intern. Med.* 135: 676-680, 1975.

65. Hanson, D.L., W. Van Huss, and G. Strautneik. Effects of forced exercise upon the amount and intensity of the spontaneous

activity of young rats. *Res. Q. Exerc. Sport* 37: 221-230, 1967.

66. Hanson, M.G. Coronary heart disease, exercise and motivation in middle-aged males. (Doctoral dissertation, University of Wisconsin–Madison, 1976). *Dissertation Abstracts International*, 37, 2755B, 1977.

67. Haskell, W.L., H.J. Montoye, and D. Orenstein. Physical activity and exercise to achieve health-related physical fitness components. *Public Health Rep.* 100: 202-212, 1985.

68. Heiby, E.M., V.A. Onorato, and R.A. Sato. Cross-validation of the self-motivation inventory. *J. Sport Psychol.* 9: 394-399, 1987.

69. Heinzelmann, F., and R.W. Bagley. Response to physical activity programs and their effects on health behavior. *Public Health Rep.* 86: 905-911, 1970.

70. Ho, P., L. Graham, S. Blair, P. Wood, W. Haskell, P. Williams, R. Terry, and J. Farquhar. Adherence prediction and psychological/behavioral changes following one-year randomized exercise programs [Abstract]. Proceedings of Pan American Congress and International Course on Sports Medicine and Exercise Science, Miami, May 1981: 9.

71. Howard, J.H., P.A. Rechnitzer, D.A. Cunningham, and A.P. Donner. Change in Type A behavior a year after retirement. *Gerontology* 26: 643-649, 1986.

72. Hoyt, M.F., and I.L. Janis. Increasing adherence to a stressful decision via a motivational balance-sheet procedure: A field experiment. *J. Pers. Soc. Psychol.* 31: 833-839, 1975.

73. Hughes, J.R., R.S. Crow, D.R. Jacobs, M.B. Mittlemark, and A.S. Leon. Physical activity, smoking, and exercise-induced fatigue. *J. Behav. Med.* 7: 217-230, 1984.

74. Ingjer, F., and H.A. Dahl. Dropouts from an endurance training program. *Scand. J. Sports Sci.* 1: 20-22, 1979.

75. Iverson, D.C., J.E. Fielding, R.S. Crow, and G.M. Christenson. The promotion of physical activity in the U.S. population: The status of programs in medical, worksite, community, and school settings. *Public Health Rep.* 100: 212-224, 1985.

76. Janz, N.K., and M.H. Becker. The health belief model: A decade later. *Health Educ. Q.* 11: 1-47, 1984.

77. Kaplan, R.M., C.J. Atkins, and S. Reinsch. Specific efficacy expectations mediate exercise compliance in patients with COPD. *Health Psychol.* 3: 223-242, 1984.

78. Kau, M.L., and J. Fisher. Self-modification of exercise behavior. *J. Behav. Ther. Exp. Psychiatry* 5: 213-214, 1974.

79. Keefe, F.J., and J.A. Blumenthal. The life fitness program: A behavioral approach to making exercise a habit. *J. Behav. Ther. Exp. Psychiatry* 11: 31-34, 1980.

80. Kendzierski, D. Self-schemata and exercise. *Basic Appl. Soc. Psychol.* (in press).

81. Kendzierski, D., and V.D. LaMastro. Reconsidering the role of attitudes in exercise behavior: A decision theoretic approach. *J. Appl. Soc. Psychol.* 18: 737-759, 1988.

82. Kirschenbaum, D.S., and A.J. Tomarken. On facing the generalization problem: The study of self-regulatory failure. In: Kendall, P.C., ed. *Advances in cognitive-behavioral research and therapy.* New York: Academic Press, 1982: vol. 1, 221-300.

83. Kittel, F., M. Kornitzer, G. DeBacker, M. Dramaix, J. Sobolski, S. Degre, and H. Denolin. Type A in relation to job stress, social and bioclinical variable: The Belgian physical fitness study. *J. Hum. Stress* 9: 37-45, 1983.

84. King, A.L., and L.W. Frederiksen. Low-cost strategies for increasing exercise behavior: Relapse preparation training and support. *Behav. Mod.* 3: 3-21, 1984.

85. Knapp, D.N. Behavioral management techniques and exercise promotion. In: Dishman, R.K., ed. *Exercise adherence: Its impact on public health.* Champaign, IL: Human Kinetics, 1988: 203-236.

86. Kohl, H., D.L. Moorefield, and S. Blair. Is cardiorespiratory fitness associated with general chronic fatigue in apparently healthy men and women? [Abstract]. *Med. Sci. Sports Exerc.* 19(Suppl.): S6, 1987.

87. Kriska, A.M., C. Bayles, J.A. Cauley, R.E. LaPorte, R.B. Sandler, and G. Pambianco. A randomized exercise trial in older women: Increased activity over two years and the factors associated with compliance. *Med. Sci. Sports Exerc.* 8: 557-562, 1986.

88. LaPorte, R.E., L.A. Adams, D.D. Savage, G. Brenes, S. Dearwater, and T. Cook. The spectrum of physical activity, cardiovascular disease and health: An epidemiologic perspective. *Am. J. Epidemiol.* 120: 507-517, 1984.

89. LaPorte, R.E., H.J. Montoye, and C.J. Caspersen. Assessment of physical activity in epidemiologic research: Problems and prospects. *Public Health Rep.* 100: 131-146, 1985.

90. Leon, A.S., J. Connett, D.R. Jacobs, and R. Rauramaa. Leisure-time physical activity levels and risk of coronary heart disease and death: The multiple risk factor intervention trial. *JAMA* 258: 2388-2395, 1987.

91. Leventhal, H., R. Zimmerman, and M. Gutmann. Compliance: A self-regulatory perspective. In: Gentry, D., ed. *Handbook of behavioral medicine.* New York: Guilford Press, 1984: 369-436.

92. Lindsay-Reid, E., and R.W. Osborn. Readiness for exercise adoption. *Soc. Sci. Med.* 14: 139-146, 1980.

93. Lobstein, D.D., B.J. Mosbacher, and A.H. Ismail. Depression as a powerful discriminator between physically active and sedentary middle-aged men. *J. Psychosom. Res.* 27: 69-76, 1983.

94. Marlatt, G.A., and J.R. Gordon, eds. *Relapse prevention: Maintenance strategies in the treatment of addictive behaviors.* New York: Guilford Press, 1985.

95. Martin, J.E., and P.M. Dubbert. Adherence to exercise. *Exerc. Sport Sci. Rev.* 13: 137-167, 1985.

96. Martin, J.E., P.M. Dubbert, A.D. Katell, J.K. Thompson, J.R. Raczynski, M. Lake, P.O. Smith, J.S. Webster, T. Sikova, and R.E. Cohen. The behavioral control of exercise in sedentary adults: Studies 1 through 6. *J. Consult. Clin. Psychol.* 52: 795-811, 1984.

97. Massie, J.F., and R.J. Shephard. Physiological and psychological effects of training—A comparison of individual and gymnasium programs with a characterization of the exercise "dropout." *Med. Sci. Sports* 3: 110-117, 1971.

98. McIntosh, P. *"Sport for All" programs throughout the world* (Contract No. 207604). New York: UNESCO, 1980.

99. Meyer, A., J. Nash, A. McAlister, N. Maccoby, and J.W. Farquhar. Skills training in a cardiovascular health education campaign. *J. Consult. Clin. Psychol.* 48: 129-142, 1980.

100. *The Miller Lite report on American attitudes toward sports.* New York: Research and Forecasts, Inc., 1983.

101. Mirotznik, J., E. Speedling, R. Stein, and C. Bronz. Cardiovascular fitness program: Factors associated with participation and adherence. *Public Health Rep.* 100: 13-18, 1985.

102. Montoye, H.J., and H.L. Taylor. Measurement of physical activity in population studies: A review. *Hum. Biol.* 56: 195-216, 1984.

103. Montoye, H.J., W.P. Van Huss, H. Olson, W.R. Pierson, and A. Hudec. *Longevity and morbidity of college athletes.* Indianapolis: Phi Epsilon Kappa, 1957.

104. Morgan, P.P., R.J. Shephard, and R. Finucane. Health beliefs and exercise habits in an employee fitness programme. *Can. J. Appl. Sport Sci.* 9: 87-93, 1984.

105. National Heart Foundation of Australia. *Risk factor prevalence study* (No. 2-1983). Canberra, Australia: Author, 1985.

106. Norman, R.M.G. *The nature and correlates of health behavior* (Health Promotion Studies Series No. 2). Ottawa, ON: Health and Welfare, 1986.

107. Oldridge, N.B. Compliance and exercise in primary and secondary prevention of coronary heart disease: A review. *Prev. Med.* 11: 56-70, 1982.

108. Oldridge, N.B., A. Donner, C.W. Buck, N.L. Jones, G.A. Anderson, J.O. Parker, D.A. Cunningham, T. Kavanagh, P.A. Rechnitzer, and J.R. Sutton. Predictive indices for dropout: The Ontario Exercise Heart Collaborative Study Experience. *Am. J. Cardiol.* 51: 70-74, 1983.

109. Oldridge, N.B., and N.L. Jones. Improving patient compliance in cardiac rehabilitation: Effects of written agreement and self-monitoring. *J. Cardiac Rehabil.* 3: 257-262, 1983.

110. Owen, N., C. Lee, L. Naccarella, and K. Haag. Exercise by mail: A mediated behavior-change program for aerobic exercise. *J. Sport Psychol.* 9: 346-357, 1987.

111. Paffenbarger, R.S., Jr., and R.T. Hyde. Exercise adherence, coronary heart disease, and longevity. In: Dishman, R.K., ed. *Exercise adherence: Its impact on public health.* Champaign, IL: Human Kinetics, 1988: 41-73.

112. Pender, N.J., and A.R. Pender. Attitudes, subjective norms and intentions to engage in health behaviors. *Nurs. Res.* 35: 15-18, 1986.

113. Perkins, K.A., S.R. Rapp, C.R. Carlson, and C.E. Wallace. A behavioral intervention to increase exercise among nursing home residents. *Gerontology* 26: 479-481, 1986.

114. *The Perrier study: Fitness in America.* New York: Perrier–Great Waters of France, Inc., 1979.

115. Pollock, M.L. Prescribing exercise for fitness and adherence. In: Dishman, R.K., ed. *Exercise adherence: Its impact on public health.* Champaign, IL: Human Kinetics, 1988, p. 259-277.

116. Powell, K.E., and W. Dysinger. Childhood participation in organized school sports as

precursors of adult physical activity. *Am. J. Prev. Med.* 3: 276-281, 1987.

117. Powell, K.E., and R.S. Paffenbarger, Jr. Workshop on epidemiologic and public health aspects of physical activity and exercise: A summary. *Public Health Rep.* 100: 118-126, 1985.

118. Powell, K.E., K.G. Spain, G.M. Christenson, and M.P. Mollenkamp. The status of the 1990 objectives for physical fitness and exercise. *Public Health Rep.* 101: 15-21, 1986.

119. Powell, K.E., P.D. Thompson, C.J. Casperson, and J.S. Kendrick. Physical activity and the incidence of coronary heart disease. *Annu. Rev. Pub. Health* 8: 253-287, 1987.

120. Ramlow, J., A. Kriska, and R.A. LaPorte. Physical activity in the population: The epidemiologic spectrum. *Res. Q. Exerc. Sport* 58: 111-114, 1987.

121. Reid, E.L., and R.W. Morgan. Exercise prescription: A clinical trial. *Am. J. Pub. Health* 69: 591-595, 1979.

122. Rejeski, W.J., D. Morley, and H.S. Miller. The Jenkins Activity Survey: Exploring its relatinship with compliance to exercise prescription and MET gain within a cardiac rehabilitation setting. *J. Cardiac Rehabil.* 4: 90-94, 1984.

123. Rodin, J. Aging and health: Effects of the sense of control. *Science* 233: 1271-1276, 1986.

124. Rosenstock, I.M. Historical origins of the health belief model. *Health Educ. Monogr.* 2: 1-9, 1974.

125. Roskies, E., H. Kearney, M. Spevak, A. Surkis, C. Cohen, and G. Gilman. Generalizability and durability of treatment effects in an intervention program for coronary-prone (Type A) managers. *J. Behav. Med.* 2: 195-207, 1979.

126. Sacks, M.H., and M.L. Sachs, eds. *Psychology of running.* Champaign, IL: Human Kinetics, 1981.

127. Sallis, J.F., W.L. Haskell, S.P. Fortmann, K.M. Vranizan, C.B. Taylor, and D.S. Solomon. Predictors of adoption and maintenance of physical activity in a community sample. *Prev. Med.* 15: 331-341, 1986.

128. Sanne, H.M., D. Elmfeldt, G. Grimby, C. Rydin, and L. Wilhelmsen. Exercise tolerance and physical training of non-selected patients after myocardial infarction. *Acta Med. Scand. Suppl.* 551: 1-124, 1973.

129. Schoenborn, C.A. Health habits of U.S. adults, 1985: The "Alameda 7" revisited. *Public Health Rep.* 101: 571-580, 1986.

130. Shekelle, R.B., S.B. Hulley, J.D. Neaton, J.H. Billings, N.O. Borhani, T.A. Gerace, D.R. Jacobs, N.L. Lasser, M.B. Mittlemark, and J. Stamler. The MRFIT behavior pattern II. Type A behavior and incidence of coronary heart disease. *Am. J. Epidemiol.* 122: 559-570, 1985.

131. Shephard, R.J. Exercise adherence in corporate settings: Personal traits and program barriers. In: Dishman, R.K., ed. *Exercise adherence: Its impact on public health.* Champaign, IL: Human Kinetics, 1988: 305-320.

132. Shephard, R.J. *Physical activity and aging* (2nd ed.). London: Croom Helm, 1987.

133. Shephard, R.J., and M. Cox. Some characteristics of participants in an industrial fitness programme. *Can. J. Appl. Sport Sci.* 5: 69-76, 1980.

134. Sidney, K.H., and R.J. Shephard. Attitude toward health and physical activity in the elderly: Effects of a physical training program. *Med. Sci. Sports* 8: 246-252, 1976.

135. Slater, C.H., L.W. Green, S.W. Vernor, and V.M. Keith. Problems in estimating the prevalence of physical activity from national surveys. *Prev. Med.* 16: 107-118, 1987.

136. Sobolski, J., M. Kornitzer, G. DeBacker, M. Dramaix, M. Abramawicz, S. Degre, and H. Denolin. Protection against ischemic heart disease in the Belgian Physical Fitness Study: Physical fitness rather than physical activity? *Am. J. Epidemiol.* 125: 601-610, 1987.

137. Solomon, R.L. The opponent process theory of acquired motivation. *Am. Psychol.* 35: 691-712, 1980.

138. Sonstroem, R.J. Psychological models. In: Dishman, R.K., ed. *Exercise adherence: Its impact on public health.* Champaign, IL: Human Kinetics, :~8: 125-154.

139. Stalonas, P.M., W.G. Johnson, and M. Christ. Behavior modification for obesity: The evaluation of exercise, contingency management, and program adherence. *J. Consult. Clin. Psychol.* 46: 463-469, 1978.

140. Steinhardt, M.A., and R.K. Dishman. The reliability and validity of expected outcomes and barriers for habitual physical activity. *J. Occupational Med.* 31: 536-546, 1989.

141. Stephens, T., D.R. Jacobs, Jr., and C.C. White. A descriptive epidemiology of leisure-time physical activity. *Public Health Rep.* 100: 147-158, 1985.

142. Stephens, T., C.L. Craig, and B.F. Ferris. Adult physical activity in Canada: Findings from the Canada Fitness Survey I. *Can. J. Public Health* 77: 285-290, 1986.

143. Stephens, T. Health practices and health status: Evidence from the Canada Health Survey. *Am. J. Prev. Med.* 2: 209-215, 1986.

144. Stephens, T. Secular trends in adult physical activity: Exercise boom or bust? *Res. Q. Exerc. Sport* 58: 94-105, 1987.

145. Stones, M.J., A. Kozma, and L. Stones. Fitness and health evaluations by older exercisers. *Can. J. Public Health* 78: 18-20, 1987.

146. Teraslinna P., T. Partanen, A. Koskela, K. Partanen, and P. Oja. Characteristics affecting willingness of executives to participate in an activity program aimed at coronary heart disease prevention. *J. Sports Med. Phys. Fitness* 9: 224-229, 1969.

147. Thompson, C.E., and L.M. Wankel. The effects of perceived choice upon frequency of exercise behavior. *J. Appl. Soc. Psychol.* 10: 436-443, 1980.

148. Tsai, S.P., W.B. Baun, and E.J. Bernacki. Relationship of employee turnover to exercise adherence in a corporate fitness program. *J. Occup. Med.* 29: 572-575, 1987.

149. Turk, D.C., T.E. Rudy, and P. Salovey. Health protection: Attitudes and behaviors of LPNs, teachers, and college students. *Health Psychol.* 3: 189-210, 1984.

150. Vance, B. Using contracts to control weight and to improve cardiovascular physical fitness. In: Krumboltz, J.D., and C.E. Thoresen, eds. *Counseling methods.* New York: Holt, Rinehart and Winston, 1976.

151. Vega, W.A., J.F. Sallis, T. Patterson, J. Rupp, C. Atkins, and P.R. Nader. Assessing knowledge of cardiovascular health-related diet and exercise behaviors in Anglo- and Mexican-Americans. *Prev. Med.* 16: 696-709, 1987.

152. Wankel, L.M. Decision-making and social support strategies for increasing exercise involvement. *J. Cardiac Rehabil.* 4: 124-135, 1984.

153. Wankel, L.M., and C.E. Thompson. Motivating people to be physically active: Self-persuasion vs. balanced decision-making. *J. Appl. Soc. Psychol.* 7: 332-340.

154. Wankel, L.M., J.K. Yardley, and J. Graham. The effects of motivational interventions upon the exercise adherence of high and low self-motivated adults. *Can. J. Appl. Sport Sci.* 10: 147-155, 1985.

155. Ward, A., and W.P. Morgan. Adherence patterns of healthy men and women enrolled in an adult exercise program. *J. Cardiac Rehabil.* 4: 143-152, 1984.

156. Washburn, R.A., and H.J. Montoye. The assessment of physical activity by questionnaire. *Am. J. Epidemiol.* 123: 563-576, 1986.

157. Wurtele, S.M., and J.E. Maddox. Relative contributions of protection motivation theory: Components in predicting exercise intentions and behavior. *Health Psychol.* 6: 453-466, 1987.

158. Wysocki, T., G. Hall, B. Iwatce, and M. Riordan. Behavioral management of exercise: Contracting for aerobic points. *J. Appl. Behav. Anal.* 12: 55-64, 1979.

159. Young, R.J., and A.H. Ismail. Comparison of selected physiological and personality variables in regular and nonregular adult male exercisers. *Res. Q. Exerc. Sport* 48: 617-622, 1977.

Chapter 8

Discussion: Determinants of Participation in Physical Activity

Michael Chubb

Dr. Dishman's review is impressive and most useful, being based on more than a dozen exercise determinant articles he authored or coauthored and on a recently published book entitled *Exercise Adherence* (5), which he compiled with a distinguished group of exercise researchers. With more than 380 citations from 159 sources (including some 50 scientific journals), it seems almost presumptuous to raise any questions about its methodologies, conclusions, or recommendations. However, in examining a scientific review, a number of questions need to be explored if the importance and implications of its contribution are to be understood fully:

- Is the methodology appropriate?
- How complete is the information?
- How useful are the data in implementing change?
- What, given the answers to these questions, should be the direction of future research?
- How can this goal be best achieved?

These questions are addressed in that order in the following paragraphs.

Is the Methodology Appropriate?

The Epidemiological Approach

Dr. Dishman used normal epidemiological methods by searching the medical and fitness literature diligently and grouping his findings by type of determinant. Successful use of this traditional compilation approach appears to depend on five circumstances that play a major role in controlling key variables.

First, most of the compiled studies must focus directly on the specific problem being investigat-

ed. Second, these studies should describe research that

- employs clinical or laboratory procedures where research subjects are carefully selected, properly documented, and closely observed using standardized techniques;
- tests hypotheses that primarily involve biotic relationships and investigates interventions consisting of treatments administered by health care or exercise professionals who ensure that correct techniques are used; and
- concerns subjects who generally accept the expertise and authority of these professionals and who are motivated to follow prescribed treatments because they sought professional help to remedy a specific troublesome condition.

Clinical or laboratory studies of supervised exercise usually come close to meeting all these conditions except for the predominance of social and psychological variables rather than biotic variables. However, the clinical or laboratory environments often make it possible to use testing methods or experimental procedures that quantify or control such variables. The epidemiological approach is therefore appropriate for most clinical or laboratory-based physical activity studies and provides much useful information concerning determinants and the efficacy of various interventions.

The situation is significantly different in the case of most other types of studies cited in this and other explorations of physical activity determinants and impacts. Often the physical activity component is only a minor part of the investigation rather than the main research problem. Usually, little is known about the subjects other than information gathered concerning the specific problem under investigation, so it is difficult to carry out more sophisticated types of stratification and sampling. The emphasis is on the measurement and analysis of behaviors controlled primarily by psychological and social variables, and little or no uniformity in methodology exists among studies. Interventions aimed at fitness improvement are usually self-initiated and self-administered and seldom follow any type of standardized procedure. When professionals are involved, they are mostly exercise or recreation practitioners rather than trained researchers. Clearly, the conditions under which these types of studies are carried out lack the relative uniformity of research methods and conditions that are characteristic of clinical or laboratory studies.

Thus, it is not surprising that compiling findings from predominantly nonclinical studies does not produce the same type of reliable conclusions generated by typical epidemiological work. A similar situation existed in recreation research during the 1960s and early 1970s. Increasing affluence, more cars, better recreation equipment, and interstate highways made it easier to reach beaches, parks, forests, cottages, and resorts. Lineups, overcrowding, and environmental damage resulted. Governments scrambled to investigate this so-called crisis in outdoor recreation, to predict its magnitude, and to alleviate its problems.

Hundreds of site- or activity-oriented studies of recreation behavior were conducted by federal, state, and regional agencies or university researchers (3). Scores of statewide and regional recreation plans resulted, many of which attempted to analyze and predict recreation demand by compiling the findings of numerous dissimilar studies. But it soon became apparent that this was not empirically sound. There were huge gaps in the representation of activities, populations, and sites. Most of the data concerned recreation at extraurban public sites, so little or nothing was known about the determinants or magnitude of recreation at private, commercial, or urban locations. Plans for the recreation needs of the entire population were being based on data gathered from atypical samples of the citizenry (4).

In addition, studies began to show considerable differences in recreation behavior patterns between some groups that appeared to have similar basic socioeconomic characteristics. Recreation-demand prediction equations using such variables were much less reliable than were similar equations used previously for other types of human activity (1). Researchers concluded that recreation participation determinants are more complex and vary more between relatively similar individuals than

was hypothesized. Psychological and social variables, together with opportunity supply factors, were found to be more powerful determinants and harder to identify and quantify than was expected.

As a result, recreation researchers and planners modified their methods. The compilation of recreation participation data from a number of dissimilar studies to quantify participation and predict future demand was dropped in favor of population wide telephone or interview surveys that obtained information concerning key recreation attitude and behavior data. Participation-determinant investigations changed from attempts to quantify and test elaborate multivariable predictive equations to in-depth studies of the role and variability of one or a few factors (8).

Research on unsupervised physical activity determinants may be following a similar path. The shortcomings of compiling results from a number of scattered, dissimilar, and localized studies of unsupervised exercise are becoming apparent. Such compilations do not contribute substantially to determining which possible exercise interventions will produce worthwhile increases in general population exercise participation. Similarly, although general population studies of health or fitness have provided useful data on broad physical activity behavioral patterns, they shed little light on the determinant problem as Dr. Dishman points out. As in the case of recreation behavior, the complex psychological aspects of physical activity adoption and adherence are being acknowledged. Exercise research may follow a course similar to recreation research as investigators turn away from attempting to compile empirically based paradigms that explain exercise participation and focus instead on exploring the workings of a few key determinants.

Composition of Dishman's Supporting Sources

One quarter of the sources used and one fifth of the individual citations in Dr. Dishman's review are from articles describing studies of supervised exercise (Table 8.1). In addition, about 5% of the paper's sources and citations from multiple-study review articles and 3% from the studies involving both types of exercise are likely to be of this type if the proportions are similar. Therefore, an estimated one third of the sources and one quarter of the citations concern supervised exercise research (Figure 8.1). If the premise that such investigations provide the most trustworthy determinant information is correct, then it can be concluded that between 25% and 35% of the cited findings are likely to be highly reliable, at least in the context of supervised exercise.

Table 8.1 Partial Analysis of Dishman's Citations by Exercise and Subject Type

Exercise and subject type	Sources used No.	%	Times cited No.	%	No. of subjects
Supervised exercise					
Public and quasi agencies	2	2	4	1	287
Commercial fitness	2	2	1	—	136
College students and staff	9	9	25	9	790
Employees, police, etc.	2	2	4	1	2,088
Patient treatment	14	14	27	9	3,813
Total	29	28	61	21	7,114
Unsupervised exercise					
General population	16	15	57	20	302,437
Employees, police, etc.	4	4	9	3	574
Patient treatment	4	4	7	2	396
Total	24	23	73	25	303,407
Supervised or unsupervised					
College students and staff	2	2	5	2	449
Employees, police, etc.	6	6	11	4	839
Total	8	8	16	6	1,288
Total (discrete studies)	61	59	150	52	311,809
Multistudy reviews	19	18	87	30	—
General materials	24	23	52	18	—
Total (reviews, etc.)	43	41	139	48	—
Grand total	104	100	289	100	311,809

Note. Based on analysis of 104 of the 159 sources listed in chapter 7 and 289 of the 380 citations used. Excludes in-press articles and other sources not readily available.

However, the organizations supplying exercise opportunities in the studies of supervised exercise are not representative of the actual distribution of providers of such programs. More than two thirds of the sources and 90% of the citations concerning supervised exercise are estimated to be from clinical or laboratory studies of patients undergo-

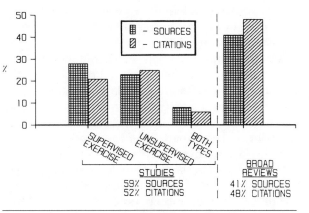
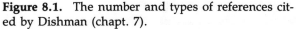

Figure 8.1. The number and types of references cited by Dishman (chapt. 7).

ing medical treatment or of college students and staff. Substantial numbers of subjects were involved, especially in the case of the patients (Table 8.1). In contrast, few sources and citations involve commercial, public, or quasi-public supervised exercise programs, and these data concern only about 400 subjects in a very limited number of settings (Figure 8.2). This is unfortunate because organized exercise programs provided by public agencies (such as municipal park and recreation departments), quasi-public organizations (YMCA, YWCA, etc.), and commercial fitness enterprises are major sources of supervised physical activity opportunities. Special emphasis should be given to undertaking studies of the determinants and efficacies of these types of programs to provide more data regarding their contribution and potential. Similarly, supervised exercise programs for employees are disproportionately few, and such studies usually concern atypical situations (e.g.,

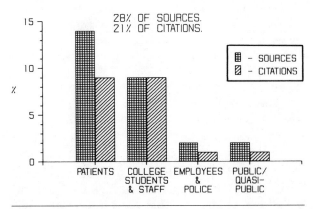

Figure 8.2. Dishman's supervised exercise sources, citations, and subjects.

large companies rather than small firms) and therefore may not be indicative of average workplace exercise program determinants.

The remaining sources in Dishman's chapter generally pertain to unsupervised physical activity monitored by methods that do not involve clinical or laboratory settings. These sources constitute an estimated two thirds of the literature cited and contribute three quarters of the citations used.

A major subdivision in this group consists of reports on specific studies involving unsupervised physical activity; these produced almost one quarter of the sources and citations (Table 8.1). Most came from general population surveys, that is, interview or self-administered questionnaire surveys of samples of the entire population within a specific area. Fifteen percent of the sources and 20% of the citations tabulated are of this type, and over 302,000 people were included in the cited surveys (Table 8.1 and Figure 8.3). Determinant information from general population surveys is highly desirable because all types of people are represented if sampling and data gathering are performed correctly. Using good general population data avoids the problem of particular determinant patterns being associated with atypical subgroups. For example, police department employees and patients in medical treatment programs are clearly responding to determinants in environments that are very different from those affecting average members of the public.

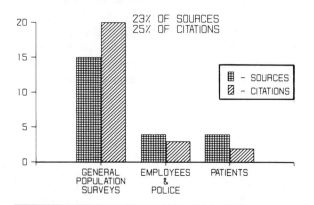

Figure 8.3. Dishman's unsupervised exercise sources, citations, and subjects.

It is unfortunate that only about one fifth of the supporting data comes from general population sample surveys. In addition to these data being applicable to the population as a whole, such surveys are the only way that good information will be obtained about the people we should be most concerned about: the individuals who are not involved in any exercise activity at a school, workplace, health care institution, community center, church, or fitness enterprise. These people constitute most of the population, and yet we have little reliable information about their physical activity attitudes and behaviors.

How Complete Is the Information?

Current knowledge of the identity and functioning of physical activity determinants is fragmentary and largely inconclusive, as Dr. Dishman indicates. Even such fundamental questions as the role of people's attitudes are still being debated (6). As indicated in the previous section, empirical data on determinants tend to be most complete for supervised exercise programs provided for college populations or patients undergoing treatment. Data are limited or absent for many large segments of the population, including minorities, the elderly, and the economically disadvantaged.

Much of the information is also incomplete in the sense that only a few selected aspects of people's perceptions and motivations concerning exercise adoption are recorded. For example, three of the general population surveys, the General Mills, Miller Lite, and Perrier studies, which were cited a total of 19 times, included only one or two questions concerning exercise beliefs. On the other hand, the Canada Fitness Survey (5 citations) had five questions that focused on reasons for exercising or not exercising. Three of these were fixed-alternative questions for which respondents were asked to check the appropriate response. The other two were open-ended questions that produced largely unprompted responses regarding activity inhibitors. This type of question, especially when asked orally by skilled interviewers, is much more likely to obtain full and accurate responses to difficult questions regarding determinants.

Completeness in reviews in which many sources are compiled is therefore a function of the representativeness of the sources, the number and nature of the questions asked, and the way in which the surveys have been administered. Investigators should properly evaluate all sources used and clearly indicate their relative applicability and reliability by appropriate qualitative and quantitative analyses. Tabulation of salient features of cited studies is a helpful method of evaluating and reviewing literature (2). This is both time and space consuming, so it should be done in technical reports or articles concerning a few determinants that can then be cited in complex compilations.

Obviously, the average reader of a large compilation depends completely on the perceptiveness, thoroughness, and integrity of the author when thousands of fragments of information are presented and referenced primarily by hundreds of numbers.

How Useful Are the Data in Implementing Change?

Much of the data can help identify appropriate interventions in the case of clinical treatment or laboratory experimentation. Even in such cases, however, the psychological factors are often poorly documented because of a lack of in-depth free-response interviews with a good cross section of subjects. In the case of the general population, little is known that helps prescribe interventions that will substantially increase both the proportion of people exercising and the amount and quality of that physical activity. The paucity of this kind of determinant information should be our major concern if we truly believe that prevention is better than cure. We need to be able to help municipal, quasi-public, and commercial fitness directors initiate programs that will move a significant proportion of the general population away from their television sets and into home, neighborhood, school, community center, or health club physical activities. Providing more of the traditional supervised programs does not appear to be the answer, although there is some unmet demand because of local deficiencies or municipal agency budget cuts. A constant flow of new ideas concerning ways to exercise while having fun and enjoying social interaction is needed (7, 9). For example, volleyball, walking, bicycling, and social dancing should be vigorously stimulated and new activities of this type developed. Compilations of existing data provide useful guidelines (often negative ones) but are unlikely to produce any speedy solutions to the problems of inactivity.

What Should Be the Direction of Future Research?

Epidemiological compilations of this type will continue to be helpful when assessing trends and efficacies. Because of the nonclinical methodologies often employed and the dissimilar nature of the behaviors involved, a more structured systematic analysis would be helpful in which findings are initially grouped by types of subjects and physical activity rather than only by determinant.

Clinical and laboratory studies of physical activity behaviors must be continued and expanded if possible. Therapeutic uses of exercise are growing and will likely increase even faster as the range of applications expands and the efficacies of such treatments are better documented. However, these studies are not likely to provide the types of data needed to produce large-scale increases in the physical activity of the general population.

The slow pace at which the general public is changing its exercise behavior patterns demands a vigorous, large-scale experimental program. Its goal should be finding and testing ways of substantially increasing participation throughout the population, not just documenting how or why people do or do not participate. Canada's federal government, provincial governments, and municipalities have led the way with the Canada Fitness Survey, a great variety of exercise-stimulating programs, and funding for a limited amount of related research. The problem is unlikely to be solved by anything less than large, well-funded national programs of applied research.

Such programs should focus on the typical sedentary or largely sedentary individuals in the general public and should include a good cross section of socioeconomic and geographic situations. Interview surveys should document past, present, and desired exercise patterns and concentrate on inhibitors. Open-ended questions should probe attitudes toward physical activity, especially home and neighborhood types of exercise that are or could be readily available to most people. Paired communities should be selected and a wide range of promotional, incentive, and programming interventions tested in the experimental community of each pair. Emphasis should be on testing interventions that involve existing resources (homes, yards, streets, neighborhood parks, schools, churches, rooftops, parking areas) but that utilize as wide a range of traditional and new techniques as possible. Perhaps an international institute for exercise stimulation could be established.

Who Should Provide the Leadership?

An applied research program of the scope and magnitude necessary to make a substantial impact on the problem will not evolve by itself but will require large amounts of well-directed leadership.

Currently, no professional group appears likely to provide such leadership. The public health organizations are preoccupied with AIDS and other immediate problems. The park and recreation professional associations endorse fitness and promote exercise programs, but only some of their constituent groups are actively involved in fitness, and current financial limitations generally preclude any substantial expansion of these efforts.

From a review of the literature and an examination of this conference's program, it appears likely that most professionals involved in exercise research investigate physical activity in clinical and laboratory settings and are not vitally interested in the participation problem of the general population. However, only the mix of professionals represented by this conference has the necessary understanding of the benefits and the technical skills needed to lead a major frontal assault on physical inactivity in developed societies. I suggest that this meeting initiate the formation of an international institute for exercise stimulation to focus attention on the problem and to coordinate programs.

References

1. Bammel G., and L.L. Burrus-Bammel. *Leisure and human behavior.* Dubuque, IA: Wm. C. Brown, 1982.

2. Benfari, R.C., E. Eaker, and J.G. Stoll. Behavioral interventions and compliance to treatment regimes. *Annu. Rev. Public Health* 2: 431-471, 1981.

3. Chubb, M. Recreation behavior studies: Empirical indicators of change. In: *Indicators of change in the recreation environment—A national research symposium* (Penn State HPER Series No. 6). University Park, PA: Penn State University, 1975, 129-174.

4. Chubb, M. Recreation use surveys and the ignored majority. In: *Proceedings of the State Outdoor Recreation Planning Workshop.* Ann Arbor, MI: U.S. Department of the Interior, Bureau of Outdoor Recreation, 1971, 47-75.

5. Dishman, R.K., ed. *Exercise adherence: Its impact on public health.* Champaign, IL: Human Kinetics, 1988.

6. Godin, G., and R.J. Shepard. Importance of type of attitude to the study of exercise-behavior. *Psychol. Rep.* 58: 991-1000, 1986.

7. Rea, P.S. Using recreation to promote fitness. *Parks Recn.* 22(7): 32-36, 59, 1987.

8. Stynes, D.J. Recreation forecasting methods. In: *A literature review: The President's Commission on American Outdoors.* Washington, DC: The Commission, 1986, Demand 33-49.

9. Summerfield, L.M., and L. Priest. Using play as motivation for exercise. *JOPERD* 58(8): 56-58, 1987.

Chapter 9

Assessment of Fitness

James S. Skinner
Fred D. Baldini
Andrew W. Gardner

Physical fitness, as defined for this conference, is characterized by the ability to perform work satisfactorily. This chapter discusses (a) the assessment of the various components of physical fitness (flexibility, body composition, muscular strength and endurance, anaerobic abilities, and cardiovascular-respiratory abilities); (b) methodological and technical problems associated with that assessment; (c) the effect of such factors as age and gender; and (d) current research and future needs.

Flexibility

Flexibility is an integral and separate aspect of fitness (29, 36). Its value to performance and prevention of injury is apparent in various sports and in health- and fitness-related fields (5, 12, 27). De Vries (29) defined *flexibility* as the possible range of movement (ROM) in a joint or a series of joints. *Static* flexibility refers to the ROM without considering speed of movement (26), and *dynamic* flexibility refers to the quick use of the full ROM (36).

The assessment of flexibility has been reviewed in detail by Corbin (26), Fleischman (36), Holland (48), and Mee (76). In general, it is easy to measure and requires a minimal amount of equipment (e.g., goniometers, fleximeters, anthropometers, tape measures, measuring sticks, and calipers). Electrogoniometers, photogoniometers, and radiogoniometers have also been used. For mass screening and a rough index of flexibility, the most widely used is the sit-and-reach test.

Structural factors influencing flexibility include skin, muscle, connective tissue, tendon, bone, and joint capsule (26, 29); muscles and ligaments seem to be the most important factor (26). In general,

active individuals tend to be more flexible (74), as are females, especially at younger ages (84). Flexibility increases until young adulthood and then decreases (22, 84). Flexibility is not necessarily reduced with weight training. If flexibility training is used at the same time, the result is equal to or better than that seen in nonathletes (29). Other factors that might influence flexibility are length of the body part involved, temperature, and ischemia (110).

Two major factors to consider when assessing flexibility are measurement variation (48) and joint specificity. When standardized procedures are used, reliability improves significantly (78). Additionally, ROM may differ markedly from one joint to another in the same person. Therefore, standard procedures for more reliable measurements and joint-specific measures for more valid profiles are needed.

Body Composition

The assessment of body composition has been studied extensively. Early work was described at a national conference (18) and in a recent symposium (67). Behnke and Wilmore (13) put forth a theoretical model for "reference man and woman" on the basis of the study of physical dimensions and relative proportions of muscle, fat, and bone in many subjects.

Body Density

Hydrostatic weighing is considered the "gold standard" of indirect body fat estimates (20, 105). Body density is a function of the densities of the various body components and the proportion each represents relative to the entire body mass. Studies using cadavers have reported the densities of these components (39, 72, 77, 103), which are used to estimate body density and body composition using various equations (19, 95).

Hydrostatic weighing uses a two-component model of fat and fat-free tissue. This model assumes that (a) the density of each component is known; (b) densities are constant among individuals; (c) the density of individual lean tissue components are constant within and among individuals, with a constant proportional contribution to the density of fat-free mass; and (d) individuals being assessed differ only in the amount of fat when compared to reference man (19, 101, 105). With repeated weighings, the range does not exceed 0.005 g • ml^{-1} (3). Garrow et al. (41) found that the standard deviation on subjects with considerable variation in fat was less than 0.3 kg fat. Lohman (66) and Bakker and Struikenkamp (8) reported standard errors of estimate as high as 2.7% fat.

The major concern with using body density to estimate body fat is that young and old populations tend to be overestimated, although some athletic populations are underestimated (1, 106, 107). Better, alternative methods have been developed (3, 35, 41, 42, 44, 95, 104), including residual volume measurement and the use of water- and air-displacement systems.

A more serious source of error may lie with the assumptions; that is, although the density of fat is fairly constant with age, gender, and location, muscle and bone densities vary greatly (11, 72, 105, 106, 107). As an example, bone density increases up to age 20 and decreases after age 50 (66). In addition, men and women differ in the amount of fat they store (32, 66). Martin et al. (72) have also shown that both density and the proportion of components vary greatly.

With improved techniques, hydrostatic weighing is relatively easy to perform, economical, and highly repeatable (41, 57, 66). The disadvantages include the problems with the previous assumptions, the need for complex equipment, and the ability to measure or estimate residual volume and gastrointestinal gas. Hydrostatic weighing is still important, however, for comparing fatness among people from a homogeneous population and for measuring changes within a person over time (8).

Wilmore (105) states that the standard equations used today are not appropriate for all populations.

Direct measurements are thus needed for accurate description of the body components.

Anthropometry

Skinfolds can be used to assess body composition. Although the assumption is that 50% of the body fat is subcutaneous (57, 60), it may be more or less (23, 31). Correlation coefficients of -0.71 to -0.84 have been reported between skinfolds and hydrostatic weighing in different populations. Predictions based on skinfolds are usually within 3%-5% of values estimated from hydrostatic weighing data (73).

Due to the variation in body density related to gender and age, many population-specific equations have been developed (32, 51, 85, 109, 111), but debate continues whether to use these or more general equations (86). Some of this debate centers on the use of a linear regression model to fit curvilinear data. Using quadratic regression analysis, Jackson and colleagues (50, 52) developed generalized equations independent of age and body composition. Although the sum of skinfolds is a good index of fatness to use with persons who modify their lifestyles (73), the choice of population-specific and general equations needs further study.

The skinfold method is inexpensive, and measures are easily obtained (40), but there are methodological problems. Caliper pressure should not vary more than 2 g • mm^{-2} over a range of 2-40 mm and should be 9-20 g • mm^{-2} (33). Pollock and Jackson (86) suggest using the same calipers used to develop a given regression equation. Other problems include interobserver error, difficulty obtaining accurate measures on obese people (40), and the considerable expertise needed to obtain accurate measurements (57). Universal standards and guidelines for skinfold measurement are needed.

Various techniques have been used to image the thickness of subcutaneous fat at various sites, including roentgenography (56), ultrasound (57), and nuclear magnetic resonance imagery (68). They are similar to skinfold methods in that selected sites are measured and total fat is estimated using mathematical equations. Muscle and bone can also be imaged and perhaps directly measured. These techniques show promise as advances in hardware and software make their use more practical.

Body stature, circumferences, and girths also have been used to profile various populations and to estimate relative fatness (57, 73, 87). They are relatively easy to measure and give estimates of body structure and composition.

Total Body Water

The use of isotopic tracers to estimate total body water (TBW) is based on the dilution principle; that is, the concentration of a compound in a solvent depends on the amount of compound and solvent. It is estimated that fat-free mass (FFM) contains a large, stable amount of water (73.2%), whereas fat is relatively water free. Thus, FFM can be estimated if TBW is known. Tracers include antipyrine, ethanol, tritiated water, and deuterated water. An ideal tracer should distribute evenly in the body and only in water and be nonmetabolizable and nontoxic. Possible sources of error include a 2% exchange of the isotope with H^+, the state of hydration, and variation in FFM water from 73.2%.

Dilution techniques are easy to use and are safe. When combined with hydrostatic weighing, a multiple-component system can estimate fat, water, and FFM. The disadvantages include the need for specialized equipment, as well as time, cost, and assumptions involved.

Because of the high conductive properties of water, bioelectrical impedance may also be used to estimate TBW and FFM. Studies comparing this with other indirect methods (4, 63, 69, 91) reported mixed results because it tends systematically to underpredict young, lean, and active populations and to overpredict old, obese, and nonactive populations. Although this method is rapid, safe, and easy to use, impedance at the electrode-tissue interface may change (47), FFM may not be 73.2% water, fat may not be water free, and normal hydration is needed.

Muscle Mass Estimation

The total body potassium (K+) method assumes that fat contains little or no K+, whereas FFM has a relatively constant proportion, with approximately 98% being intracellular. Of the naturally occurring K+ isotopes, K^{40} contributes 0.12% (37). Once the amount of K+ in the body has been determined, mathematical equations derive lean body mass (38). In general, the K^{40} method yields higher body fat percentages than does hydrostatic weighing (62, 79). Men tend to have more K+, which tends to drop with age due to a lower FFM (10, 38, 79, 80).

This method is safe and easy to use. The disadvantages include the availability and expense of equipment, difficulty in calibrating whole-body counters for different body builds, underestimation of K+ in large and obese subjects, the assumption that all cells have the same amount of K+, and the possibility that athletes have different distributions of K+ (21, 40).

Although K^{40} gives an indication of muscle cell mass, total body nitrogen (TBN) gives an indication of muscle cell protein. Cohn et al. (25) suggest that muscle tissue and nonmuscle lean tissue contain known amounts of K+ and N. After measuring K^{40} and TBN, one can estimate muscle mass from the assumption that fat tissue contains neither. Disadvantages include the complicated techniques involved, the cost, radiation, and the time needed.

Another method to estimate muscle mass is to measure creatinine excretion (CE). Creatinine is produced in the muscle, from which it diffuses into the blood and eventually into the urine. Animal studies show that CE is directly proportional to total body creatinine. If we make the following assumptions, CE can be used to predict muscle mass.

- Creatinine is almost totally in muscle.
- After a creatine-free diet, muscle creatine concentration remains constant.
- Conversion of creatine to creatinine is irreversible and occurs at a constant rate.
- Creatinine excretion is constant.

One caution concerning this method: Although CE is linearly related to muscle mass during growth (24), 24-hr CE in adults may vary considerably because of strenuous exercise, emotional stress, diet, disease, infection, or trauma.

Another way to estimate muscle mass is by means of 3-methylhistidine (3-MH). It is released during the breakdown of actin and myosin and is eventually excreted in the urine. The largest portion of 3-MH is in skeletal muscle (about 75%), varying little with different muscles. The assumption is that protein synthesis equals protein breakdown during steady state. If so, then 3-MH excretion should be proportional to muscle mass (21). The effects of gender, age, menstruation, nutrition, hormone status, fitness, exercise, injury, and training are unknown. Also, the ratio of myofibrillar protein to sarcoplasmic and stromal protein may be different among and within trained subjects (21).

Future Needs

Roche (87) concluded that none of the current methods are completely accurate or valid and that all need improvement. More direct chemical data, simpler and more accurate indirect methods, and further study of such factors as age, gender, disease, and population differences are needed.

Muscle Strength and Endurance

The strength or force-generating ability of muscle is important in rehabilitation and sports and can be determined by using various types of muscular contractions. Isometric (ISOM) strength is primarily assessed by a cable tensiometer for isolated muscle groups across a single joint or by a dynamometer for large-muscle groups (e.g., legs, hip, and back). Valid inter- and intraindividual comparisons require using identical joint angles. Back and leg dynamometers were developed in 1925 (14), whereas such isokinetic (ISOK) and ISOM dynamometers as the Cybex, Orthotron, and Kincom were developed more recently.

Maximal voluntary contraction (MVC) strength is often assessed isometrically because ISOM forces are easy to measure, even though their relationship with the dynamic contractions characteristic of most physical activities is questionable. Correlation coefficients between ISOM and isotonic (ISOT) strength range between 0.62 and 0.80 (29).

Isotonic strength is assessed by the maximal weight lifted once by a muscle group (i.e., the 1-repetition maximum, or 1 RM). Because progressively heavier loads are lifted until this maximum is reached, the subjectivity in guessing the number of trials needed may vary greatly such that fatigue influences the outcome. Tests not requiring lifting weights include chinning, dipping, push-ups, sit-ups, and rope climbing. Although these tests are easy to administer, variability may be high during maximal effort, and the number of repetitions at a given resistance (endurance) is related to a subject's strength.

Although 1-RM ISOT contractions are limited by the lowest maximal force obtained at any joint angle throughout the ROM, ISOK devices allow the maximal force to be exerted and measured throughout the ROM under conditions of relatively constant velocity (81). Kannus et al. (55) feel that these machines are safe and reliable, but Winter et al. (108) are less certain about their reliability and validity. Although ISOK machines are quite popular, it is not clear how well strength measured at one speed reflects strength at a faster or slower speed (81). Also, the force generated during the high accelerations characteristic of most athletic events cannot be measured.

Regardless of how strength is assessed, several factors are important. Both ISOM and ISOT strength increase from 10 to 14 yr to 20 to 29 yr, remain unchanged until 40 to 49 yr, and then decline (64). Lower strength in children is explained more by a smaller muscle mass than by a reduced force-generating capacity of muscle fibers (29). Reduced strength in old age is due to muscle atrophy (especially fast-twitch, or FT, fibers), reduced number of muscle fibers, and decreased ability to recruit FT fibers (64). Although strength training in older men has increased their fiber size similar to that of younger men, strength was still less, suggesting that some loss with age is neurological (65).

Few gender differences occur in children, whereas differences after puberty are due mainly to a smaller muscle mass in women. When expressed relative to FFM or muscle cross-sectional area, gender strength differences are eliminated or reduced (102), suggesting that the force-producing capability of individual muscle fibers is similar.

Muscular endurance may be expressed in absolute (lifting the same load) and relative (lifting the same percent MVC) terms. Absolute values correlate closely with strength, but relative values do not (29). The assessment of relative endurance can be made with ISOM, ISOK, and ISOT contractions.

The ability to hold an ISOM contraction depends on the percent MVC applied (2). Over time, the maximal ISOM tension drops, and a characteristic fatigue curve is found (88). With ISOM contractions above 60% MVC, there is complete occlusion of blood vessels to the muscle (88), and the fatigue curves are steeper.

Muscular fatigue may be determined by electromyography at a constant ISOM tension from the increase in muscle electrical activity during the contraction (28). One can also measure both the recovery of force production at given percentages of maximum following fatiguing ISOM exercise or the drop in ISOM holding time after a given recovery period.

Several measures of ISOT endurance include lifting light weights more than 20-25 times or counting the number of sit-ups and push-ups. Asmussen (6) used an ergograph to measure the reduction in ROM during successive contractions. Finally, ISOK devices may provide reliable and valid measures of endurance by determining the reduction in force with repeated contractions.

Age and gender may influence muscular endurance. Strength and absolute endurance (ISOM and ISOT) decline at the same rate with age, whereas relative endurance is unchanged or increases slightly (64); this may be explained by a decreased proportion of FT fibers. Absolute endurance in men is greater because of strength differences, whereas relative endurance is similar (29). In fact, women may have better relative endurance because of a higher percent MVC before muscle blood flow is occluded (46).

Age- and gender-specific norms for strength and endurance are needed for specific populations, especially at varying speeds of contraction. Although further validation is needed, ISOK testing is promising.

Anaerobic Abilities

Tests of anaerobic (AN) ability involve very high intensity exercise lasting less than 1 s up to several minutes (97). Bar-Or (9) criticized many AN tests for being nonspecific, invalidated, and too dependent on skill and motivation. It is generally agreed that most AN tests are reliable in motivated subjects and that they correlate highly with one another, but there is less agreement about what they measure. There is also no so-called gold standard with which to compare test results and, unlike the steady-state $\dot{V}O_2$ in submaximal tests or the plateau in $\dot{V}O_2$ seen in maximal aerobic tests, there are no accepted criteria for what should be measured or how.

Part of this lack of agreement is caused by terminology. For example, the terms *AN power* and *AN capacity* have been used to describe the highest 5-s and average 30-s power outputs, respectively, on the Wingate AN test (WANT). Other AN tests lasting from 1 to 10 s (71) also use the term *AN power*. Bar-Or (9) now prefers to define AN power as peak power (PP) and AN capacity as mean power (MP). Reducing the use of labels should permit more discussion of the measures themselves and what they might mean.

Methodological Problems

It is difficult to determine the amount of aerobic and AN (alactic and lactic) involvement in tests lasting more than a few seconds. Estimates of relative contributions are questionable because of the difficulty in assessing mechanical efficiency (100) and thus the total energy required. Given the large individual differences in mechanical efficiency (45),

$\dot{V}O_2$max, and the kinetics of the rise in $\dot{V}O_2$ at the onset of exercise, estimates of aerobic energy production and its relative contribution can vary greatly.

Along with the lack of accepted criteria of what constitutes the various types of AN ability, there are large differences in the sophistication of devices used for their measurement. As a result, differences in measurement accuracy and the frequency with which they are taken often make it difficult to compare results on the same AN test obtained from different laboratories.

Even within the same test, there is not always agreement on methodology. A good example involves the optimal resistance for the WANT. The original test used 75 g • kg^{-1} body weight (7). Using various resistances, Dotan and Bar-Or (30) later found that the highest 30-s MP was obtained at 87 g • kg^{-1}; there was no plateau in the 5-s PP values, however. As other studies have found even higher optimal resistances for the 30-s test, Bar-Or (9) now recommends 90 and 100 g • kg^{-1} with adult nonathletes and athletes, respectively. Although these recommendations recognize that athletes respond differently, the suggested resistances do not necessarily yield the highest 5-s PP. Optimal resistance may therefore vary with the test duration as well as with the age, gender, and type and level of training of the subjects.

Effects of Age, Gender, and Training Status

The effect of these factors has been studied with the WANT. The resistance of 75 g • kg^{-1} has been suggested for children (7) compared to 87 g • kg^{-1} for adults (30). Vandewalle et al. (100) reported that peak power on a cycle ergometer occurred at a velocity of 95 rpm in young boys and 125 rpm in male power athletes. Because power athletes tend to have more FT muscle fibers, it is not surprising that Sargeant et al. (89) also found that men with more than 50% FT fibers reached their maximal power at 119 rpm compared to 104 rpm in those with less than 50% FT fibers. Although the reason for any gender differences is not clear, Dotan and Bar-Or (30) found that the optimal resistance was slightly lower and that the optimal pedaling velocity was about 20% slower in women; this may be associated with their smaller active muscle mass or their larger potential for oxidative metabolism (43). Evans and Quinney (34) proposed an equation to predict optimal resistance from leg volume and body weight, but Dotan and Bar-Or (30) and Patton et al. (82) did not find this extra information useful.

Present Research and Future Needs

A standardized, generally accepted system for classifying AN ability is needed. Skinner and Morgan (97) proposed such a modified system based on characteristics and limitations of the body's energy systems. There were two aerobic, two AN, and one mixed (aerobic and AN) activity classes in this system. The two types of AN activity can be differentiated by relative intensity and duration. Maximal intensity AN activity requiring 275%-400% $\dot{V}O_2$max can be done for 1-10 s and is associated with the phosphagen (ATP and CP) levels and their rates of degradation. Very high intensity AN activity, on the other hand, requires 200%-250% $\dot{V}O_2$max, can be done for 20-45 s, and is associated with the rate of anaerobic glycolysis.

Because longer tests become more aerobic and less strenuous, Vandewalle et al. (100) suggested that tests longer than 1 min are not necessary, especially because Katch et al. (59) found a correlation coefficient of 0.95 between total work output in a 40-s test and a 120-s test. Regardless of the resistance applied, Raveneau (unpublished thesis cited in Vandewalle et al., 100) found that the correlation coefficient between total work done at 20 s and 30 s of an all-out test was very high ($r = 0.99$). Thus Vandewalle et al. (100) suggest that AN tests need be only 15-20 s because they are easier to perform than are 30- to 40-s tests.

Using the WANT, Skinner and O'Connor (98) did a cross-sectional study on athletes who performed the five types of activities in the proposed classification system previously mentioned (power lifters, gymnasts, wrestlers, 10-km runners and ultramarathoners in the continuum from high AN to high aerobic ability). Although the 5-s PP differentiated the AN power lifters (12.7 W · kg⁻¹) from the aerobic runners (11.3-11.4 W · kg⁻¹), there were no differences (8.8-9.3 W · kg⁻¹) in the 30-s MP of the different athletes. Thus, it appears that a 5-s test measures AN abilities that are different from those measured by a 30-s test. Given that these tests were done at a resistance of 75 g · kg⁻¹ and that this is probably not the optimal resistance for all types of athletes (especially the power athletes) and for both 5-s and 30-s AN tests, any discussion of the optimal duration for an AN test should also consider the optimal resistance and the AN ability that one wishes to measure.

It is obvious that there are different types of AN ability and many kinds of AN tests. As stated by Vandewalle et al. (100), there is no AN test that measures the different components of AN metabolism equally well. Thus, more research on the biochemical and neural events associated with each is warranted so that we can better understand AN metabolism. As we gain a better understanding of general AN ability, more sport-specific tests can be developed in the laboratory and then modified and applied to the athlete.

Aerobic Abilities

Aerobic ability may be assessed by several methods, including maximal aerobic power ($\dot{V}O_2$max) and endurance capacity (EC, or the ability to sustain a high percentage of $\dot{V}O_2$max for a prolonged time). Although $\dot{V}O_2$max is considered a major factor in EC, these variables are not closely related (16, 83), suggesting that each involves different aspects of aerobic ability.

Many types of ergometers can be used to determine $\dot{V}O_2$max, and each has its advantages and disadvantages (93). There is an intraindividual, day-to-day variability of 4%-6% (58) due to such factors as errors in gas analysis and calibration, equipment calibration, change in environmental conditions, prior eating and sleeping patterns, preliminary familiarization with the task, and time of day (93). Reproducibility on the bicycle ergometer and treadmill are similar, but bicycle $\dot{V}O_2$max values are 7%-8% below the treadmill values (15). The high power output during cycling restricts quadriceps muscle blood flow, resulting in more peripheral than central limitation. Regardless of modality, maximal effort is judged by a plateau in $\dot{V}O_2$ and the attainment of maximal values for heart rate (HR), respiratory exchange ratio, and blood lactate (LA) concentration.

When $\dot{V}O_2$max is not measured, estimations can be made from submaximal exercise tests. This estimation is based on the linear relationship between HR and $\dot{V}O_2$ (assuming a constant mechanical efficiency) and on extrapolation from several submaximal HRs to a predicted or known maximal HR (93). Although a 10% prediction error exists (92), submaximal tests estimate fitness with less risk and are particularly useful for testing large samples in a short time. The predicted group mean values of $\dot{V}O_2$max are similar to the measured values, but individual estimates are less precise.

Few standardized tests have been developed to assess aerobic ability using EC. One such test by Boulay et al. (17) determines maximal aerobic capacity (MAC) by measuring the total work done in 90 min on a cycle ergometer at the ventilatory threshold (VT). Three major methodological concerns with this test are (a) the subjectivity of determining VT, (b) the certainty that this represents the highest steady-state exercise that a person can do for 90 min, and (c) the required test duration. Péronnet et al. (83) developed an endurance index (EI) derived from $\dot{V}O_2$max, the relationship between running speed and $\dot{V}O_2$, and a representative performance at a distance equal to or greater than 10 km. They found a correlation coefficient of 0.85 between EI and the percent $\dot{V}O_2$max at VT but one of only 0.11 between $\dot{V}O_2$max and EI.

Measures of blood LA are related to EC and are sensitive to training adaptations (53). The LA concentration at a given submaximal intensity is as powerful a predictor of EC as are more exhaustive tests (54). Additionally, an inverse relationship exists between EC and exercise intensity expressed relative to the anaerobic threshold (75). Thus, the time to fatigue at an intensity eliciting the highest steady-state LA concentration may also characterize EC.

Effects of Age and Gender

Accurate assessment of aerobic ability in children is a challenge because they may not be motivated to exercise to exhaustion, as indicated by a less frequent plateau in $\dot{V}O_2$ with maximal exercise (61). Mode of exercise may also be a concern; for example, the cycle ergometer may not be as desirable when proper cadence is required for the appropriate power output (61). Schmücker and Hollmann (90) found that familiarization with bicycle exercise increased peak $\dot{V}O_2$, suggesting that practice trials be given before testing. Thus treadmills may be preferred because they are machine paced and yield higher $\dot{V}O_2$max values (15, 49, 70). The relationship between $\dot{V}O_2$max and EC is not as high as it is in adults (61) because of other factors (e.g., economy). Sjödin (96) found a higher relation in children between running speed at the onset of blood LA accumulation (V_{OBLA}) and EC than for V_{OBLA} and $\dot{V}O_2$max, suggesting that this LA threshold is a more sensitive indicator of EC.

There are also problems in the assessment of aerobic ability in the elderly. As the main concern is safety, a physician should be in visual contact or in close proximity during testing. Thomas et al. (99) found test-retest reliability coefficients of 0.67, 0.87, and 0.90 on three different treadmill protocols in 224 men aged 55-68; test repetition yielded higher $\dot{V}O_2$max values. Only one third of the men had a plateau in $\dot{V}O_2$, suggesting that such peripheral factors as reduced leg strength are more limiting than are central factors. A more obscure problem relates to sample bias, as not all older individuals can perform maximal exercise because of health problems. For example, medical screening eliminated 21% of elderly volunteers for a physical training problem involving $\dot{V}O_2$max tests (94). Therefore, a more pragmatic approach may be to report data at absolute and relative submaximal power outputs so that more elderly people can be assessed with less risk.

Similar criteria for determining $\dot{V}O_2$max apply to men and women. Although women have lower values—primarily because of lower cardiac output, hemoglobin concentration, and lean body mass (102)—gender differences do not appear until about age 12 (61). The $\dot{V}O_2$max (ml $\cdot$ kg^{-1} $\cdot$ min^{-1}) of boys remains unchanged as they physically mature, whereas that of girls drops (61). Although social influences and the greater accumulation of subcutaneous fat may explain such findings, women are able to reach a plateau in $\dot{V}O_2$ as well as are men (94). Boulay et al. (17) found that women had lower $\dot{V}O_2$max and VT values but also were able to exercise 90 min at VT without problems and had similar values during retests.

Promising Avenues of Current Research and Future Needs

The ability of LA thresholds to estimate EC and their sensitivity to changes in aerobic ability are noteworthy. This has implications for assessing fitness because submaximal LA values may be more accurate and reliable than is $\dot{V}O_2$max in adults and because there is considerably less risk when testing older adults. Because too little is known about EC, more research on tests of prolonged exercise (e.g., MAC and the EI) is needed. The time to fatigue at varying intensities expressed relative to the LA threshold may be one way to better characterize this aspect of aerobic ability.

Conclusion

It is obvious that there are many ways to assess the different aspects of fitness. Although some aspects (e.g., maximal aerobic power) and the techniques and criteria for measuring them are generally accepted (e.g., a plateau in $\dot{V}O_2$ with increasing exercise), many other methods and criteria are not. These other aspects need more research to develop valid and reliable tests (e.g., tests of anaerobic ability and body composition).

When assessing fitness, one should also consider the reason for doing each test. For example, tests to evaluate the fitness of an elite athlete should relate to performance, tests of normal children and adults should relate more to health, and tests of the elderly and people with such chronic diseases as coronary heart disease, diabetes, and emphysema should be related more to those factors that are important for health, well-being, and independence. Thus, fitness assessment should be specific to the particular aspect being measured, to the population being studied, and to the reasons why they are tested.

References

1. Adams, J., M. Mottola, K. Bagnalland, and K. McFadden. Total body fat content in a group of professional football players. *Can. J. Appl. Sport Sci.* 7: 36-40, 1982.

2. Ahlborg, B., L. Ekelund, G. Guarnieri, R. Harris, E. Hultman, and L. Nordesjö. Muscle metabolism during isometric exercise performed at constant force. *J. Appl. Physiol.* 33: 224-228, 1972.

3. Akers, R., and E. Buskirk. An underwater weighing system utilizing "force cube" transducers. *J. Appl. Physiol.* 26: 649-652, 1969.

4. Albright, A. *Validation of bioelectrical impedance in obese, lean, adolescent, and aging populations.* Unpublished master's thesis, California State University, Sacramento, 1987.

5. Anderson, B. *Stretching.* Bolinos, CA: Shelter Publications, 1980.

6. Asmussen, E. Muscle fatigue. *Med. Sci. Sports* 11: 313-321, 1979.

7. Ayalon, A., O. Inbar, and O. Bar-Or. Relationships among measurements of explosive strength and anaerobic power. In: Nelson, R., and C. Morehouse, eds. *Biomechanics IV.* Baltimore: University Park Press, 527-532, 1974.

8. Bakker, H., and R. Struikenkamp. Biological variability and lean body mass estimates. *Hum. Biol.* 49: 187-202, 1977.

9. Bar-Or, O. The Wingate anaerobic test—an update on methodology, reliability and validity. *Sports Med.* 4: 381-397, 1987.

10. Barter, J., and G. Forbes. Correlation of potassium-40 data with anthropometric measurements. *Ann. N.Y. Acad. Sci.* 110: 264-270, 1963.

11. Baumgartner, J., and A. Jackson. *Measurement and evaluation in physical education.* 2nd ed. Dubuque, IA: Wm. C. Brown, 1982.

12. Beaulieu, J. *Stretching for all sports.* Pasadena, CA: Athletic Press, 1980.

13. Behnke, A., and J. Wilmore. *Evaluation and regulation of body build and composition.* Englewood Cliffs, NJ: Prentice Hall, 1974.

14. Berger, R. *Applied exercise physiology.* Philadelphia: Lea & Febiger, 1982.

15. Boileau, R., A. Bonen, V. Heyward, and B. Massey. Maximal aerobic capacity on the treadmill and the bicycle ergometer of boys 11-14 years of age. *J. Sports Med. Phys. Fit.* 17: 153-162, 1977.

16. Bouchard, C., and G. Lortie. Heredity and endurance performance. *Sports Med.* 1: 38-64, 1984.

17. Boulay, M., P. Hamel, J. Simoneau, G. Lortie, D. Prud'homme, and C. Bouchard. A test of aerobic capacity: Description and reliability. *Can. J. Appl. Sport Sci.* 9: 122-126, 1984.

18. Brožek, J. Body composition: Parts I and II. *Ann. N.Y. Acad. Sci.* 110: 1-1018, 1963.

19. Brožek, J., F. Grande, J. Anderson, and A. Keys. Densitometric analysis of body composition: Revision of some quantitative assumptions. *Ann. N.Y. Acad. Sci.* 110: 113-140, 1963.

20. Brožek, J., and A. Keys. The evaluation of leanness-fatness in man: Norms and interrelationships. *Br. J. Nutr.* 5: 194-206, 1951.

21. Buskirk, E., and J. Mendez. Sports science and body composition analysis: Emphasis on cell and muscle mass. *Med. Sci. Sports Exerc.* 16: 584-593, 1984.

22. Buxton, D. Extension of the Kraus-Weber test. *Res. Q.* 28: 210-217, 1957.

23. Caldwell, F. Cadaver study challenges body fat computations. *Phys. Sportsmed.* 9: 21-22, 1981.

24. Cheek, D. *Human growth, body composition, cell growth, energy and intelligence.* Philadelphia: Lea & Febiger, 1978.

25. Cohn, S., D. Vartsky, S. Yasumura, A. Sawitsky, I. Zanzi, A. Vaswani, and K. Ellis. Compartmental body composition based on total body nitrogen, potassium and calcium. *Am. J. Physiol.* 239: E524-E530, 1980.

26. Corbin, C. Flexibility. *Clin. Sports Med.* 3: 101-117, 1984.

27. Corbin, C., and M. Noble. Flexibility: A major component of physical fitness. *J. Phys. Educ. Rec.* 51: 23-24, 57-60, 1980.

28. deVries, H. Method for evaluation of muscle fatigue and endurance from electromyographic fatigue curves. *Am. J. Phys. Med.* 47: 125-135, 1968.

29. deVries, H. *Physiology of exercise*. 3rd ed. Dubuque, IA: Wm. C. Brown, 1980.

30. Dotan, R., and O. Bar-Or. Load optimization for the Wingate anaerobic test. *Eur. J. Appl. Physiol.* 51: 409-417, 1983.

31. Durnin, J., and J. Womersley. Body fat assessed from total density and its estimation from skinfold thickness: Measurements on 481 men and women aged from 61 to 72 years. *Br. J. Nutr.* 32: 77-97, 1974.

32. Edwards, D. Differences in the distribution of subcutaneous fat with sex and maturity. *Clin. Sci.* 10: 305-315, 1951.

33. Edwards, D., W. Hammond, M. Healy, J. Tanner, and R. Whitehouse. Design and accuracy of calipers for measuring subcutaneous tissue thickness. *Br. J. Nutr.* 9: 133-143, 1955.

34. Evans, J., and A. Quinney. Determination of resistance settings for anaerobic power testing. *Can. J. Appl. Sport Sci.* 6: 53-56, 1981.

35. Falkner, F. An air displacement method of measuring body volume in babies: A preliminary communication. *Ann. N.Y. Acad. Sci.* 110: 75-79, 1963.

36. Fleischman, E. *The structure and measurement of physical fitness*. Englewood Cliffs, NJ: Prentice Hall, 1964.

37. Forbes, G. Methods for determining the composition of the human body. *Pediatrics* 29: 477-491, 1962.

38. Forbes, G., and J. Hursh. Ages and sex trends in lean body mass calculated from K^{40} measurements, with a note on the theoretical basis for the procedure. *Ann. N.Y. Acad. Sci.* 110: 225-263, 1963.

39. Forbes, R., A. Cooper, and H. Mitchell. The composition of the adult human body as determined by chemical analysis. *J. Biol. Chem.* 203: 359-366, 1953.

40. Garrow, J. New approaches to body composition. *Am. J. Clin. Nutr.* 35: 1152-1158, 1982.

41. Garrow, J., S. Stalley, R. Diethelm, P. Piltet, R. Hesp, and R. Halliday. A new method for measuring body density of obese adults. *Br. J. Nutr.* 42: 173-183, 1979.

42. Gnaedinger, R., E. Reineke, A. Pearson, W. Van Huss, J. Wessel, and H. Montoye. Determination of body density by air displacement, helium dilution and underwater weighing. *Ann. N.Y. Acad. Sci.* 110: 96-108, 1963.

43. Green, H., I. Fraser, and D. Ranney. Male and female differences in enzyme activities of energy metabolism in vastus lateralis muscle. *J. Neurol. Sci.* 65: 323-331, 1984.

44. Gundlach, B., H. Nijkrake, and J. Hautuast. A rapid and simplified plethysmographic method for measuring body volume. *Hum. Biol.* 52: 23-33, 1980.

45. Hermansen, L., and J. Medbo. The relative significance of aerobic and anaerobic processes during maximal exercise of short duration. In: Marconnet, P., J. Poortmans, and L. Hermansen, eds. *Physiological chemistry of training and detraining*. Basel, Switzerland: Karger, 1984, p. 56-57, vol. 17.

46. Heyward, V., and L. McCreary. Comparison of the relative endurance and critical occluding tension levels of men and women. *Res. Q.* 49: 301-307, 1978.

47. Hill, R., J. Jansen, and J. Fling. Electrical impedance plethysmography: A critical analysis. *J. Appl. Physiol.* 22: 161-168, 1967.

48. Holland, G. The physiology of flexibility: A review of the literature. *Kinesiol. Rev.* 1: 49-62, 1968.

49. Ikai, M., and K. Kitagawa. Maximal oxygen uptake in Japanese related to sex and age. *Med. Sci. Sports* 4: 127-131, 1972.

50. Jackson, A., and M. Pollock. Generalized equations for predicting body density of men. *Br. J. Nutr.* 40: 497-504, 1978.

51. Jackson, A., and M. Pollock. Steps toward the development of generalized equations for predicting body composition in adults. *Can. J. Appl. Sports Sci.* 7: 189-196, 1982.

52. Jackson, A., M. Pollock, and A. Ward. Generalized equations for predicting body density of women. *Med. Sci. Sports Exerc.* 12: 175-182, 1980.

53. Jacobs, I. Blood lactate: Implications for training and sports performance. *Sports Med.* 3: 10-25, 1986.

54. Jacobs, I., R. Schele, and B. Sjödin. Blood lactate vs. exhaustive exercise to evaluate aerobic fitness. *Eur. J. Appl. Physiol.* 54: 151-155, 1985.

55. Kannus, P., M. Järvinen, and K. Latvala. Knee strength evaluation. *Scand. J. Sports Sci.* 9: 9-13, 1987.

56. Katch, F., and A. Behnke. Arm x-ray assessment of percent fat in men and women. *Med. Sci. Sports Exerc.* 16: 596-603, 1984.

57. Katch, F., and V. Katch. The body composition profile: Techniques of measurement and applications. *Clin. Sports Med.* 3: 31-63, 1984.

58. Katch, V., S. Sady, and P. Freedson. Biological variability in maximum aerobic power. *Med. Sci. Sports Exerc.* 14: 21-25, 1982.

59. Katch, V., A. Weltman, R. Martin, and L. Gray. Optimal test characteristics for maximal anaerobic work on the bicycle ergometer. *Res. Q.* 48: 319-327, 1977.

60. Keys, A., F. Fidanza, M. Karvonen, N. Kimura, and H. Taylor. Indices of relative weight and obesity. *J. Chron. Dis.* 25: 329-343, 1971.

61. Krahenbuhl, G., J. Skinner, and W. Kohrt. Developmental aspects of maximal aerobic power in children. In: Terjung, R., ed. *Exercise and Sport Sciences Reviews.* New York: Macmillan, 1985, p. 503-538, vol. 13.

62. Krzywicki, H., G. Ward, D. Rahman, R. Nelson, and C. Consolazio. A comparison of methods for estimating human body composition. *Am. J. Clin. Nutr.* 27: 1380-1385, 1974.

63. Kushner, R., D. Schoeller, and B. Bowman. Comparison of total body water determination by bioelectrical impedance analysis, anthropometry, and H_2O dilution. *Am. J. Clin. Nutr.* 39: 658, 1984.

64. Larsson, L. Morphological and functional characteristics of the aging skeletal muscle in man. *Acta Physiol. Scand. Suppl.* 457, 1978.

65. Larsson, L. Physical training effects on muscle morphology in sedentary males at different ages. *Med. Sci. Sports Exerc.* 14: 203-206, 1982.

66. Lohman, T. Skinfolds and body density and their relation to body fatness: A review. *Hum. Biol.* 53: 181-225, 1981.

67. Lohman, T. Preface to body composition assessment: A reevaluation of our past and a look toward the future. *Med. Sci. Sports Exerc.* 16: 578, 1984.

68. Lohman, T. Research progress in validation of laboratory methods of assessing body composition. *Med. Sci. Sports Exerc.* 16: 596-603, 1984.

69. Lukaski, H., W. Bolonchuk, P. Johnson, G. Lykken, and H. Sandstead. Assessment of fat-free mass using bioelectrical impedance measurements of the human body. *Am. J. Clin. Nutr.* 39: 657, 1984.

70. Mǎcek, M., J. Vavra, and J. Novasadova. Prolonged exercise in prepubertal boys. *Eur. J. Appl. Physiol.* 35: 291-298, 1976.

71. Margaria, R., P. Aghemo, and E. Rovelli. Measurement of muscular power (anaerobic) in man. *J. Appl. Physiol.* 21: 1662-1664, 1966.

72. Martin, A., D. Drinkwater, J. Clarys, and W. Ross. Estimation of body fat: A new look at some old assumptions. *Phys. Sportsmed.* 9: 21-22, 1981.

73. McArdle, W., F. Katch, and V. Katch. *Exercise physiology: Energy, nutrition, and human performance.* Philadelphia: Lea & Febiger, 1981.

74. McCue, B. Flexibility of college women. *Res. Q.* 24: 316-324, 1953.

75. McLellan, T., and J. Skinner. Submaximal endurance performance related to the ventilation thresholds. *Can. J. Appl. Sport Sci.* 10: 81-87, 1985.

76. Mee, C. *Staying flexible: Full range of motion.* Alexandria, VA: Time-Life Books, 1987.

77. Mitchell, H., T. Hamilton, F. Steggerda, and H. Bean. The chemical composition of the adult human body and its bearing on the biochemistry of growth. *J. Biol. Chem.* 158: 625-637, 1945.

78. Moore, M. The measurement of joint motion. *Phys. Ther. Review* 29: 256-264, 1949.

79. Myhre, L., and W. Kessler. Body density and potassium 40 measurements of body composition as related to age. *J. Appl. Physiol.* 21: 1251-1255, 1966.

80. Novak, L. Aging, total body potassium, fat-free mass, and cell mass in males and females between ages 18 and 85 years. *J. Gerontol.* 27: 483-543, 1972.

81. Osternig, L. Isokinetic dynamometry: Implications for muscle testing and rehabilitation. In: Pandolf, K., ed. *Exercise and sport sciences reviews.* New York: Macmillan, 1986, p. 45-80, vol. 14.

82. Patton, J., M. Murphy, and F. Frederick. Maximal power outputs during the Wingate anaerobic test. *Int. J. Sports Med.* 6: 82-85, 1985.

83. Péronnet, F., G. Thibault, E. Rhodes, and D. McKenzie. Correlation between ventilatory threshold and endurance capability in marathon runners. *Med. Sci. Sports Exerc.* 19: 610-615, 1987.

84. Phillips, M. Analysis of results from Kraus-Weber test of minimum muscular fitness in children. *Res. Q.* 26: 314-323, 1955.

85. Pollock, M., T. Hickman, Z. Kendrick, A. Jackson, A. Linnerud, and G. Dawson. Prediction of body density in young and middle-aged men. *J. Appl. Physiol.* 40: 300-304, 1976.

86. Pollock, M., and A. Jackson. Research progress in validation of clinical methods of

assessing body composition. *Med. Sci. Sports Exerc.* 16: 606-613, 1984.

87. Roche, A. *Body-composition assessments in youth and adults.* Columbus, OH: Ross Laboratories, 1985.

88. Royce, J. Isometric fatigue curves in human muscle with normal and occluded circulation. *Res. Q.* 29: 204-212, 1958.

89. Sargeant, A., P. Dolan, and A. Young. Velocity for maximal short-term (anaerobic) power output in cycling. *Int. J. Sports Med.* 5: 124-125, 1984.

90. Schmücker, B., and W. Hollmann. The aerobic capacity of trained athletes from 6 to 7 years of age on. *Acta Paediatr. Belg. Suppl.* 28: 92-101, 1974.

91. Segal, K., B. Gutin, E. Presta, and T. Van Itallie. Comparison with densitometry of a localized current injection method and a uniform current induction method for estimating human body composition. *Am. J. Clin. Nutr.* 39: 658, 1984.

92. Shephard, R. A nomogram to calculate the oxygen cost of running at slow speeds. *J. Sports Med. Phys. Fit.* 9: 10-16, 1968.

93. Shephard, R. Tests of maximum oxygen intake: A critical review. *Sports Med.* 1: 99-124, 1984.

94. Sidney, K., and R. Shephard. Maximum and submaximum exercise tests in men and women in the seventh, eighth, and ninth decades of life. *J. Appl. Physiol.* 43: 280-287, 1977.

95. Siri, W. Apparatus for measuring human body volume. *Rev. Sci. Instruments* 27: 729-738, 1956.

96. Sjödin, B. The relationships among running economy, aerobic power, muscle power, and onset of blood lactate accumulation in young boys (11-15 years). In: Komi, P., ed. *Exercise and sport biology.* Champaign, IL: Human Kinetics, 1982, 57-60.

97. Skinner, J., and D. Morgan. Aspects of anaerobic performance. In: Clarke, D., and H. Eckert, eds. *Limits of human performance.* Champaign, IL: Human Kinetics, 1985, p. 31-44.

98. Skinner, J., and J. O'Connor. Wingate test—Cross-sectional and longitudinal analysis. *Med. Sci. Sports Exerc.* 19: S73, 1987.

99. Thomas, S., D. Cunningham, P. Rechnitzer, A. Donner, and J. Howard. Protocols and reliability of maximal oxygen uptake in the elderly. *Can. J. Sport Sci.* 12: 144-151, 1987.

100. Vandewalle, H., G. Peres, and H. Monod. Standard anaerobic exercise tests. *Sports Med.* 4: 268-289, 1987.

101. Wedgewood, R. Inconsistency of lean body mass. *Ann. N.Y. Acad. Sci.* 110: 141-152, 1963.

102. Wells, C. *Women, sport and performance.* Champaign, IL: Human Kinetics, 1985.

103. Widdowson, E., R. McCance, and C. Spray. The chemical composition of the human body. *Clin. Sci.* 10: 113-125, 1951.

104. Wilmore, J. A simplified method for determination of residual lung volumes. *J. Appl. Physiol.* 27: 96-100, 1969.

105. Wilmore, J. Body composition in sports and exercise: Directions for future research. *Med. Sci. Sports Exerc.* 15: 21-31, 1983.

106. Wilmore, J., and J. McNamara. Prevalence of coronary disease risk factors in boys, 8 to 12 years of age. *J. Pediatr.* 84: 527-533, 1974.

107. Wilmore, J., H. Miller, and M. Pollock. Body composition and physiological characteristics of active endurance athletes in their eighth decade of life. *Med. Sci. Sports* 2: 113-117, 1974.

108. Winter, D., R. Wells, and G. Orr. Errors in the use of isokinetic dynamometers. *Eur. J. Appl. Physiol.* 46: 397-408, 1981.

109. Womersley, J., J. Durnin, K. Boddy, and M. Mahaffy. Influence of muscular development, obesity and age on the fat-free mass of adults. *J. Appl. Physiol.* 41: 223-229, 1976.

110. Wright, V., and R. Johns. Physical factors concerned with the stiffness of normal and diseased joints. *Bull. Johns Hopkins Hosp.* 106: 215-231, 1960.

111. Young, C., J. Blondon, R. Tensuan, and J. Fryer. Body composition studies of "older" women thirty to seventy years of age. *Ann. N.Y. Acad. Sci.* 110: 589-607, 1963.

Chapter 10

Discussion: Assessment of Fitness

Norman Gledhill

In the previous chapter, Skinner and his colleagues provided a comprehensive summary of the components of physical fitness and their assessment. The present overview is intended to complement their summary and to focus the topic of fitness assessment more specifically on health status implications. It is informative at the outset to distinguish between performance-related fitness and health-related fitness (perhaps the latter should be wellness-related fitness). Performance-related fitness refers to those components of fitness that enable optimal work or sport performance, and each sport has very specific fitness requirements (e.g., anaerobic endurance, leg power, and upper-body muscular endurance). Health-related fitness refers to those components of fitness that exhibit a relationship with health status (e.g., muscle or joint disorders and cardiovascular risk factors). Further, for the purpose of this conference, and as it pertains to exercise and health, a distinction is made between physical fitness and physiological fitness. Physical fitness is the ability to perform muscular work satisfactorily. It is determined by the level of several attributes (e.g., cardiovascular-respiratory endurance, muscular strength, muscular endurance, flexibility, and body composition) that are influenced by activity. Physiological fitness encompasses both physical fitness and those biological systems (e.g., blood pressure, glucose tolerance, and the blood lipid profile) that exhibit a relationship with health status and that are influenced by the level of physical activity.

Screening Candidates for Fitness Assessments

Candidates for performance-related fitness assessments are generally both symptom free and chronically active, and it is not necessary to screen them

medically before an exercise test. However, when assessing apparently healthy, sedentary individuals, caution should always be taken. These individuals should be cleared for exercise testing either by a physician or through a valid medical screening device such as the Physical Activity Readiness Questionnaire (PAR-Q) (6). The PAR-Q is employed to identify those individuals for whom physical activity might be inappropriate or who require medical advice concerning the type of activities that would be most suitable or that should be avoided. The PAR-X is a follow-up questionnaire to this screening, designed for use by physicians from whom advice is sought by individuals who are not symptom free and hence not cleared for exercise testing by the PAR-Q. This topic has been reviewed in detail recently by Shephard (21).

Waiver forms are sometimes utilized by fitness appraisers to absolve themselves of responsibility if participants are injured. However, if the appraiser is negligent, such waivers are generally invalid and serve only to dissuade falsely the injured parties from pursuing their legal rights. In this light the use of a waiver form is unethical. Instead, participants should provide their informed consent to take part in the fitness assessment. The basis of informed consent is that the participant is fully aware of the procedures plus any attendant risks and is free to discontinue at any time. If an injury should occur while someone is participating with informed consent, and negligence is not involved, the fitness appraiser generally is not liable.

Standardization of Testing Procedures

Careful control of both the environmental conditions and the state of the participant is imperative if the results of the assessment are to be valid and reliable. For example, repeat testing should be conducted at the same time of day; the temperature of the testing area should be maintained in the 18-22 °C range; dietary guidelines should be adhered to; the use of stimulants such as coffee, tea, nicotine, and alcohol should be avoided; and subjects must not participate while under the influence of drug interventions. In addition, blood samples for the evaluation of such conditions as cholesterolemia and glucose intolerance must be collected under strictly controlled standard conditions.

Physical Fitness

Body Composition

Excess body weight and obesity are very common and very serious health problems that are linked with hypercholesterolemia, hypertension, diabetes, and coronary heart disease (CHD). The assessment of body composition has been reviewed in detail recently (4, 5). When the information derived from assessing body composition has a performance-related fitness application, the two-component model of fat and fat-free tissue is sufficient, as knowledge of total fat (percent fat) is the primary concern. In most sports a recommended percent fat for optimal performance has been identified. For such applications the body composition techniques summarized by Skinner et al. are all appropriate (e.g., hydrostatic weighing, skinfolds, total body water, and muscle mass estimation). However, for health-related fitness the concern is not only with the amount of fat but also with the pattern of fat distribution. The relationship between excess total body fat and the risk of cardiovascular disease has long been known (4, 5). In recent years it has also been demonstrated convincingly that an excessive amount of fat in the trunk region is associated with a higher mortality rate and an increased morbidity: glucose intolerance (14), blood lipid disorders (13), and hyperinsulinemia (9).

The body mass index (wt/ht²), combined with selected skinfold fat measurements (to distinguish between muscularity and adiposity), provides a functional index of the total amount of fat on the body. Also, the ratio of waist girth to hip girth, combined with skinfold fat measurements from the hip and back, provides a useful index of fat distribution (1). This information has recently been incorporated into the assessment of body composition in the Canadian Standardized Test of Fitness (11). First, the body mass index (BMI) is calculated

as an index of proportional weight. If the BMI falls within an age- and a gender-related risk zone, the sum of five skinfolds (triceps, biceps, subscapula, iliac crest, and medial calf) is examined to determine whether the high BMI is due to excessive muscularity or to excessive adiposity. Next, the distribution of fat is examined using the waist-to-hip ratio (WHR) and the sum of two skinfolds (SOTS) (iliac crest and subscapula). Determining whether the WHR and SOTS fall into age- and gender-related risk zones then permits the fitness appraiser to evaluate whether the pattern of fat distribution places the participant at risk for CHD (2).

Skinner et al. referred to other techniques for determining the amount of body fat: ultrasound, computed tomography, and nuclear magnetic resonance. The use of radioactivity in assessing body composition is ethically questionable, and generally it is not economically feasible to utilize these techniques on a practical basis (although a portable ultrasound system has been developed). However, they are useful as research tools and can provide valuable information not attainable with other techniques. For example, it has been illustrated through computed tomography that skinfold assessments of subcutaneous fat are reasonably accurate except at the abdomen, where skinfold measurements considerably underestimate intra-abdominal fat (3).

Flexibility

Performance in selected sports depends on very specific flexibility characteristics. Hence, for performance-related fitness the assessment of flexibility at a number of articulations is of considerable importance. Skinner et al. point out that as a rough index of flexibility for general screening, the most widely used test is the sit-and-reach test. They caution the reader to pay attention to joint specificity in assessing flexibility; the degree of flexibility among articulations in the same body varies markedly, and no single articulation can be taken as an overall index of flexibility. In fact, the sit-and-reach assessment of lower-back flexibility is popular because of its relevance to health-related fitness. Poor flexibility in the lower back is an indication of susceptibility to lower-back disorders (19), and it is well documented that, in addition to the related suffering, back problems have a significant economic impact (22). Additional measurements of flexibility and other components of physical fitness that correlate with back disorders are required.

Other examples of health-related applications of the flexibility assessment techniques described by

Skinner et al. include evaluating the degree of impairment caused by arthritis, determining the effectiveness of rehabilitation programs, and evaluating sedentary older adults who are susceptible to flexibility-related injuries.

Muscle Strength and Endurance

Strength and endurance are very important considerations in performance-related fitness because in virtually all sports improvements in these components generally lead to improvements in performance. Strength and muscular endurance are likewise important in health-related fitness because they are required in many everyday activities as well as for occasional emergencies. Minimum levels of strength and muscular endurance are essential for all individuals but in particular for older adults, for whom the quality of life often depends substantially on their capacity for self-help. Decisions concerning the need for institutional care, home assistance care, or complete independence for seniors are commonly based on the performance of functions requiring strength, muscular endurance, or both. Hence, in fitness programs for older adults it is important to maintain muscular strength and endurance. To monitor the development of these capacities, the various techniques described by Skinner et al. are applicable, although future attention should be directed to providing appropriate standards.

The evaluation of muscular endurance in both performance-related and health-related fitness assessments is most often accomplished by means of push-ups and sit-ups. However, because health-related fitness assessments are normally conducted on sedentary individuals, the inclusion of tests that require maximal effort can be dangerous and are generally contraindicated. Further, the performance of common sit-up protocols can result in injuries. A recently proposed safer alternative to the classic bent-knee sit-up is the partial curl-up conducted in time with a metronome (25 curl-ups per min to a maximum of 75) with the knees bent 90°, the arms stretched forward alongside the legs, and during the curl-up the palms of the hands sliding 8 cm along the floor (11).

Anaerobic Abilities

The assessment of anaerobic endurance is essentially restricted to performance-related fitness applications.

Aerobic Ability

The relationship between a high level of cardiovascular-respiratory fitness and a reduced risk for CHD is well established. In addition, aerobic power is the best single index of work capacity. The most widely employed index of cardiovascular-respiratory fitness is the maximal oxygen uptake ($\dot{V}O_2$max). Although the results from direct assessments of $\dot{V}O_2$max are considerably more accurate than are the predicted results, apparently healthy, sedentary individuals should not normally be exercised to maximum, especially if they are age 40 or over. For this reason the direct measurement of $\dot{V}O_2$max is generally reserved for performance-related fitness assessments. In spite of the 10% to 15% error associated with the results of predictive tests, these protocols are recommended for the assessment of cardiovascular-respiratory fitness in apparently healthy, sedentary individuals. On the other hand, if a high degree of accuracy is desired when determining the $\dot{V}O_2$max of such individuals (especially those 40 or over), it is advisable to consider the participants as high-risk individuals and to test them in the presence of medical personnel while constantly monitoring ECG and blood pressure.

Leisure-Time and Occupational Activity

Recent evidence has demonstrated convincingly that when the influences of all other risk factors in the cause of death are removed, there is a significant inverse relationship between activity level and mortality rate. Paffenbarger et al. (17) reported that death rates due to cardiovascular or respiratory causes declined steadily as the energy expended on such self-selected activities as walking, stair climbing, and sports increased from less than 500 to 3,500 kcal per week. Increasing the energy expenditure beyond 3,500 kcal per week produced less substantive improvements. Their findings indicate that an energy expenditure of 2,000 kcal per week is associated with a 30% lower death rate than is that of normal, sedentary individuals. Similarly, Leon et al. (16) concluded that a higher level of leisure-time physical activity is related to a lower incidence of CHD and overall mortality in middle-aged high-risk males. These were both retrospective studies, but in a recent prospective study Salonen et al. (18) observed that when adjustments were made for the influence of all other risk factors, participants in both leisure-time physical activity and occupational physical activity significantly lowered their risks of CHD.

The assessment of leisure-time physical activity and occupational physical activity can be accomplished by using self-reported inventories of the nature and quantity of physical activity. For example, information on leisure-time and occupational physical activity (including the intensity, frequency, and duration) and the physical activity associated with traveling to and from work can be converted to caloric expenditure and compared with a positive physical activity profile.

In this regard it is possible that those individuals who are genetically endowed with a high $\dot{V}O_2$max derive the associated high stroke volume and cardiac output from large ventricular volumes and not from enhanced myocardial contractility. On the other hand, those individuals who exercise vigorously on a regular basis yet who have a low $\dot{V}O_2$max may be genetically endowed with small ventricular volumes in spite of an enhanced myocardial contractility. Which individual has the lower risk for CHD? I speculate that the latter individual is at a lower risk due to a stronger heart and a variety of other exercise-related benefits (e.g., lower total cholesterol, elevated high-density lipoproteins, lower blood pressure, and decreased body weight). If this hypothesis is correct, then in health-related fitness evaluations $\dot{V}O_2$max results should be interpreted in conjunction with the individual's physical activity profile. Further, the risk factor calculated for cardiorespiratory fitness status should incorporate a significant activity component independent of the $\dot{V}O_2$max value.

Special Populations

Rheumatoid arthritis is characterized by pain, stiffness, weakness, and restricted mobility. Its etiology is unknown, and it occurs most commonly between 25 and 65 years of age with a female preponderance of 3:1. Although the cardiorespiratory and locomotor fitness levels of persons with rheumatoid arthritis limit their physical performance, the common cycle ergometer and strength and flexibility testing protocols are applicable (7).

The ability of disabled persons to use manually operated wheelchairs is dependent on their muscular strength, muscular endurance, and cardiorespiratory fitness. This topic has been reviewed in detail recently (20). Although wheelchair ergometers have been developed (12), the fitness testing of wheelchair-dependent individuals is commonly performed using modified cycle ergometers or arm ergometers. The upper-limb strength and muscular endurance of disabled persons is generally assessed through standard laboratory techniques as described by Skinner et al.

Physiological Fitness

Physiological fitness encompasses both physical fitness (as examined previously) and those biological systems that exhibit a relationship with health status and that are influenced by the level of physical activity. The values that are measured to characterize biological systems typically include a transitional zone from normal to abnormal. Hence, some clinically acceptable normal values are more desirable than are others, and it is therefore possible to assess the "fitness" of certain biological systems. This information, combined with information pertaining to physical fitness, is collectively termed *physiological fitness*.

Blood Pressure

Hypertension is not a disease but rather a symptom of a variety of possible disorders in the cardiovascular system. Information on cardiovascular fitness as it relates to the risk for CHD can be gained by measuring the systolic and diastolic blood pressures by the auscultatory technique on the left arm in the sitting position and following 15 min of rest. In adults, diastolic pressure should be less than 95 mmHg and systolic pressure less than 160 mmHg (24). However, blood pressures between 140/90 and 160/95 mmHg are associated with an increased incidence of cardiovascular disorders. Exercise testing is useful for identifying inappropriate blood pressure responses and for evaluating the effectiveness of drug interventions in normalizing the blood pressure response.

Blood Lipids and Lipoproteins

Abnormalities in blood lipids (notably, cholesterol and triglycerides) and the lipid carriers (lipoproteins) are assessed by means of a blood sample collected with the subject in a fasting condition. These variables are of great significance to physiological fitness. The triglyceride-rich very low-density lipoproteins (VLDLs) and the cholesterol-rich low-density lipoproteins (LDLs) transport (and perhaps deposit) lipids throughout the body. The high-density lipoproteins (HDLs) are thought to remove lipids from the body. The assessment of triglycerides, total cholesterol (cholesterol content per 100 ml of plasma of all lipoproteins combined), and LDL or the associated apolipoprotein B can be compared with expected values, and high levels are associated with an increased risk for CHD. Conversely, an elevated HDL, or the associated apolipoprotein A-I, is associated with a reduced risk of CHD. Further, a low HDL-LDL ratio is associated with a high risk of CHD. Hence, optimal physiological fitness is associated with relatively high plasma levels of HDL and relatively low plasma levels of triglycerides, total cholesterol, and LDL (8).

Glucose Intolerance

Diabetes is a leading cause of premature death and, in addition to its independent risk, also leads to cardiovascular disorders (15). The assessment of urinary sugar (glucosuria) using commercial test paper or a 2-hr postprandial (postmeal) blood glucose level provides simple screening procedures for glucose intolerance and the potential presence of diabetes. For a more definitive evaluation, an oral glucose tolerance test can be performed employing a glucose load of 40 g $\cdot$ m^{-2} body surface area (or 100 g) following a 3-d carbohydrate diet and an overnight fast. Blood samples taken pre-ingestion and at 30, 60, 90, and 120 min post-ingestion are analyzed for glucose, with the glucose response calculated as the integral area under the 2-hr curve. In addition, by using radioimmunoassay determinations of the plasma insulin levels before and after the glucose challenge, glucose intolerance due to either insulin deficiency or insulin resistance can be distinguished.

Personal Lifestyle Inventory and Family History

Proper interpretation of physical fitness and physiological fitness data must take into account age, gender, and years of education. Additional assessment areas worthy of examination are inventories of personal lifestyle data (e.g., tobacco use, alcohol use, and diet) and family histories of hypertension, blood lipid disorders, diabetes, obesity, CHD, and longevity. This information can be ascertained by using self-reported questionnaires (possibly supplemented by an interview to probe questionable responses) and assigned a risk factor on the basis of existing epidemiological data.

Conclusion

Given the extent and complexity of health-related fitness information that can be assessed, efforts should be concentrated on devising an optimal approach to integrating and providing this information to participants. One possible approach is a computer-processed "composite" physiological fitness score customized to the age, gender, and aspirations of the participant, with weighed contributions for the various fitness components of importance in the profile of each participant (e.g., 25% $\dot{V}O_2$max; 25% weekly caloric expenditure; 20% body composition; 10% strength, muscular endurance, and flexibility; 10% blood pressure; and 10% tobacco and alcohol use). Blood lipid and glucose-tolerance information could also be incorporated, perhaps triggered by information in the personal lifestyle inventory or family history.

Because it is strongly recommended that information concerning weekly activity profiles be incorporated into future fitness assessments, it is necessary to develop functional standardized techniques for quantifying physical activity profiles as well as standards of "desirable" physical activity profiles for various populations, together with realistic and achievable goals for monitoring the participants' progress. Some direction in this regard has already been provided (10).

Given that insufficient physical activity (hypokinetic disease) is associated with a risk for CHD and premature death that is similar to that of any other major risk factor (18), and given that the portion of the general population manifesting hypokinetic disease is approximately 3-5 times that of any other risk factor (23), the primary target in preventive medicine should be the reversal of hypokinetic disease. Hence, the assessment and reversal of hypokinetic disease and its correlates should be established as the highest-priority health initiative.

References

1. Ashwell, M., T.J. Cole, and A.K. Dixon. Obesity: New insight into the anthropometric classification of fat distribution shown by computed tomography. *Br. Med. J.* 290: 1692-1694, 1985.

2. Björntorp, P. Hazards in subgroups of human obesity. *Eur. J. Clin. Invest.* 14: 239-241, 1984.

3. Borkan, G.A., D.E. Hults, S.G. Gerzof, B.A. Burrows, and A.H. Robbins. Relationship between computed tomography tissue areas, thickness and total body composition. *Ann. Human Biol.* 10: 537-546, 1983.

4. Brodie, D.A. Techniques for measurement of body composition, Part I. *Sports Med.* 5(1): 11-40, 1988.

5. Brodie, D.A. Techniques of measurement of body composition, Part II. *Sports Med.* 5(2): 74-98, 1988.

6. Chisholm, D.M., M.L. Collis, L.L. Kulak, W. Davenport, and N. Gruber. Physical activity readiness. *Br. Columbia Med. J.* 17: 375-378, 1975.

7. Ekblom, B., and R. Nordemar. Rheumatoid arthritis. In: Skinner, J.S., ed. *Exercise testing and exercise prescription for special cases: Theoretical basis and clinical applications.* Philadelphia: Lea & Febiger, 1987, Chapt. 7, p. 101-114.

8. Ernst, N.D., and J. Cleeman. Reducing high blood cholesterol levels: Recommendations from the national cholesterol education program. *J. Nutr. Educ.* 20(1): 23-29, 1988.

9. Evans, D.J., R.G. Hoffman, R.K. Kalkhoff, and A.H. Kissebah. Relationships of body fat topography to insulin sensitivity and metabolic profiles in premenopausal women. *Metabolism* 33(1): 68-75, 1984.

10. Ferris, B., F. Landry, and C.L. Craig. Toward a Canadian standard for physical activity and fitness. *Sport Sci. Rev.* (January): 32-39, 1987.

11. Fitness and Amateur Sport Canada. *Canadian Standardized Test of Fitness operations manual.* 4th ed. Ottawa, ON: Author, 1988.

12. Glaser, R.M., M.N. Sawka, M.F. Brune, and S.W. Wilde. Physiological responses to maximal effort wheelchair and arm crank ergometry. *J. Appl. Physiol.: Respir. Environ. Exerc. Physiol.* 48(6): 1060-1064, 1980.

13. Kalkhoff, R.K., A. Hartz, D. Rupley, A.H. Kissebah, and S. Kelber. Relationship of body fat distribution to blood pressure, carbohydrate tolerance and plasma lipids in healthy obese women. *J. Lab. Clin. Med.* 102: 621-627, 1983.

14. Kissebah, A.H., N. Vydelingum, N. Murray, D.J. Evans, A. Hartz, R.K. Kalkhoff, and P.W. Adams. Relation of body fat distribution to metabolic complications of obesity. *J. Clin. Endocrinol. Metab.* 54: 254-260, 1982.

15. Leon, A.S. Diabetes. In: Skinner, J.S., ed. *Exercise testing and exercise prescription for special cases: Theoretical basis and clinical applications.* Philadelphia: Lea & Febiger, 1987, Chapt. 8, p. 115-133.

16. Leon, A.S., J. Connett, D.R. Jacobs, and R. Rauramaa. Leisure time physical activity levels and risk of coronary heart disease and death: The multiple risk intervention trial. *JAMA* 258(17): 2388-2395, 1987.

17. Paffenbarger, R.S., R.T. Hyde, A.I. Wing, and C.-c. Hsieh. Physical activity, all cause mortality, and longevity of college alumni. *N. Engl. J. Med.* 314(10): 605-613, 1986.

18. Salonen, J.T., J.S. Slater, J. Tuomilehto, and R. Rauramaa. Leisure time and occupational physical activity: Risk of death from ischemic heart disease. *Am. J. Epidemiol.* 127(1): 87-94, 1988.

19. Sharkey, B.J. *Physiology of fitness.* Champaign, IL: Human Kinetics, 1979.

20. Shephard, R.J. Sports medicine and the wheelchair athlete. *Sports Med.* 4: 226-247, 1988.

21. Shephard, R.J. PAR-Q, Canada Home Fitness Test and exercise screening alternatives. *Sports Med.* 5: 185-195, 1988.

22. Shephard, R.J. *Economic benefits of enhanced fitness.* Champaign, IL: Human Kinetics, 1986.

23. Stephens, T., C.L. Craig, and B.F. Ferris. Adult physical activity in Canada: Findings for the Canada Fitness Survey. *Can. J. Public Health* 77(4): 285-295, 1986.

24. World Health Organization. *Report of the WHO Expert Committee: Arterial hypertension* (WHO Technical Report No. 628). Geneva: WHO, 1978.

Chapter 11

Assessment of Health Status

Madeleine Blanchet

Traditionally, assessment of health status tended to concentrate on measures of mortality, morbidity, and other manifestations of ill health, measuring progress by the reduction in negative factors and outcomes. Even today in most countries, annual reports on health, such as the well-known *Surgeon's General Report on Health* in the United States, use decreases in death rates over time to represent gains in health.

Other traditional measures have been positively expressed such as life expectancy at various ages and potential years of life lost, which is currently in use in Canada and gives additional weight to deaths occurring at younger ages, such as those due to motor vehicle accidents. However, mortality is not the only criterion of ill health, as it fails to take into account other problems that are equally important but that do not involve a life-threatening prognosis, for example, physical and mental disabilities, rheumatic complaints, sensory impairments, sequel of accidents, and mental disorders.

Data reporting contacts with health services can provide a tool for epidemiological inquiry as well as a measure to monitor whether any improvement is taking place. This approach has been applied mostly to the surveillance of infectious diseases such as influenza epidemics and, more recently, to the monitoring of AIDS and other sexually transmitted diseases. Attempts have been made to adapt this method to other chronic and acute diseases. The "sentinel" health events being outlined rely on routine recording of mortality and morbidity as a method of identifying avoidable events.

Changes in health status cannot usually be inferred from contacts that relate to treatment or hospitalization. These existing systems rarely provide information on individuals that may be used for epidemiological analysis, although systems that link the episodes for an individual may be able to identify first admissions. Disease registers overcome some of these problems by creating a record for an individual and may include patients seen at the primary care level as well as in hospitals. However, theses registers are restricted to give information only about specific causes of ill health. Trend data from these registers may be used to identify changes in the incidence of specific diseases, although the completeness of registration always has to be considered in interpreting these data.

Deriving measures of health status from routinely collected statistics is further limited by the fact that only a few developed countries collect information on patient contacts at the primary care level on a routine basis, except where primary care practitioners are paid on a fee-for-service basis. Even in this case, the most valid and reliable information relates to the various medical and surgical procedures rather than to the diagnoses of patients' conditions. However, the utilization of diagnosed morbidity has been attempted by the Quebec Ministry of Health and Social Services to obtain data on the prevalence of chronic diseases such as cancer; nevertheless, assessment of health through such a system is limited because the same diagnosis (e.g., diabetes) can cover a whole range of functional states (from coma to stabilized, mild diabetes). A traditional measure that is expressed positively such as life expectancy free from disability or healthy life expectancy, represents a step toward the development of more significant health indicators.

For the limited and well-defined purposes of geographical planning of services and overall evaluation of health policies, it is of interest to adopt an aggregate indicator of health status that combines both mortality and functional disability. Life expectancy expresses the health status of a population in the form of the average number of years of life without disability. There are several advantages in using an index of this kind:

- From the methodological point of view, life expectancy free from disability is calculated using simple demographic methods because it is merely an extension of the concept of life expectancy.
- Both health professionals and lay users can easily understand this concept. To the extent that life expectancy is widely used, healthy life expectancy can also be used.
- It may be said to have its own frame of reference because, by comparing healthy life expectancy and life expectancy, an immediate picture is obtained of the extent of disability within a population.
- An increase in this aggregate index reflects rising aspirations concerning the quality of life and therefore is a positive factor in the health field.

An example of this aggregate index as applied to the Quebec population is shown in Figure 11.1. Life expectancy free from disability was calculated by Dillard (2) by breaking down life expectancy at a given age into the following categories:

- Life expectancy in institutional care
- Life expectancy with temporary limitation of activity
- Life expectancy with permanent limitation of activity

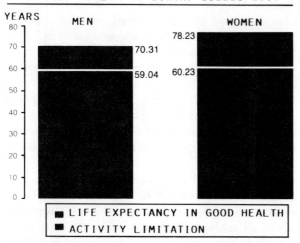

Figure 11.1. An aggregate index of health status, combining mortality and functional disability.

In Quebec in 1980, total life expectancy was 70.31 yr for men and 78.23 yr for women, whereas life expectancy free from disability was only 59 yr for men and 60 yr for women. The institutionalization rate was higher for women than it was for men. Moreover, women reported more limitations of various degrees, but men experienced more severe permanent limitations.

Wilkins and Adams (9) have studied life expectancy free from disability trends for Canada, comparing results of the 1979-1980 survey to a previous survey carried out in 1950-1951. They found little improvement in health status over the last 30 yr when various forms of disability rather than simple life expectancy were taken into account. Using data from surveys conducted in the United States, Colvez and Blanchet (1) arrived at the same conclusions.

Dillard (2) made it possible to rank the main disease categories in terms of their repercussions on life expectancy free from disability. Cardiovascular diseases as a top priority for healthy life expectancy is strengthened by the fact that these diseases are not only the first cause of death but also major causes of disability. However, musculoskeletal disorders and impairments rank second among women and fourth among men. Accidents and injuries rank second among men, and tumors rank third.

A new perspective of priorities for health programs can be derived from this method of assessing health. This technocratical view of priorization may nevertheless have little relevance for most health services consumers.

Physiological and Biological Measures

Measures of health status that refer to a total population require information from those not using services and from those who do and normally imply a need for some kind of population survey. Charts on the distribution of height and weight by age are required to evaluate the development and nutritional status of children as well as of adults. Such charts have been developed by research groups in universities and by insurance companies. They are used in underdeveloped and industrialized countries. Evaluation of dental status and detection of hearing and vision problems exist where the population is subject to routine screening procedures. Moreover, information on biological and physiological measures need to be gathered in health examination surveys. Surveys such as those conducted in the United States are much less common than are health interview surveys because of their greater cost and complexity. Nevertheless, small-scale health examination surveys are being conducted within the framework of routine examination provided by local primary care practitioners (physicians and nurses). Most of these surveys provide information on blood pressure, serum cholesterol, and smoking. They report the beneficial effects of interventions by practitioners. The two Canadian reports on periodic health examinations provide a set of standard examinations that have proved to be effective in the field of preventive care and that are applicable within the context of primary care practice. Recent and well-known surveys on fitness among Canadians provide data for the planning and evaluation of physical activity policies and programs.

It is very likely that future health examination surveys in Canada would be more cost-effective if they drew a sample from the offices of family practitioners rather than launching a separate survey. This could then be done better at the provincial level.

In Quebec, the Rochon Commission released its report in February 1988 (4). Two issues were dealt with by this controversial report: the measurement of the impact of health services and the fact that determinants of health status may have little to do with the present modes of delivery of health and social services. The commission felt that an urgent priority for the coming years will be the development of the measures of impact of health and social services. Another priority will be the development of health objectives and methods of measuring the impact of programs on the attainment of the proposed objectives.

Assessment of Health: The Canadian Government's Position

In 1984 there was a major evaluation of the health status program component by the Health Division of Statistics Canada. This evaluation is known as the Owen Report (5). One of the central recommendations of the report was that governmental offices should pay more attention to health outcomes, not to the resource consumption of the health sector. Although outcomes are more diffi-

cult to measure than are inputs, they do represent the bottom line of health programs and policies. There is increasing recognition that information on resources is of limited value and use if such information cannot be linked to impacts on the health of the population.

In Canada recent publications by Dillard (2), Wilkins and Adams (9), and Peron and Strohmenger (6) have explored old and new measures of health outcomes. Some of these have been based on generalizations of the concept of longevity observed from life tables, particularly Evans's (3) terminology of *healthful equivalent life expectancy* or *quality adjusted life years*. The concept of healthful equivalent life expectancy seems promising as a summary measure of health outcomes.

Therefore, one major focus should be on the people and their healthfulness. Health outcomes should have primary emphasis. There should be an overall indicator for the average or median healthfulness of the population. This could be a statistic (like the healthy life expectancy measure) and could be called the "GNP statistic." This type of measurement would give a reasonable indication of the nation's health status.

This is recognized as a risky procedure, given the problems in measuring health status. Any single-valued indicator for an individual will need to be an index defined over a vector of health status attributes. In turn, each attribute will raise substantial measurement issues, and any aggregate index will embody important matters of judgment. Nevertheless, conceptual problems of similar depth have not prevented the government from producing sets of poverty lines or a consumer price index.

Disability-free life expectancy (DILE) is an index of the average length of a healthy life. It aims at measuring the evolution in health status of the population. The first calculations of this index were made at the end of the 1960s (8). Ten calculations have been made since then, mostly in the United States, Canada (and the province of Quebec), Japan, and France. Its major qualities are its usefulness for setting health targets and determining the present and future needs. Is DILE's future a conjunctional index of health status? The circumstances are undoubtedly favorable. Nevertheless, for DILE to be used routinely as is the current life expectancy concept, two conditions that do not fulfill the current approach must be satisfied; that is, disability measurements for comparisons over time must be reliable, and the recording of the reversible or irreversible character of disability must be available. Further research is undoubtedly needed to clarify these points and to add more precision and reliability to this aggregate index of health.

Assessment of Health: France's Viewpoint

The main objective of the health and social services system is not only to extend life but also to maintain the quality of life, in terms of autonomy and social functioning, for as long as possible and for as long as desired by the people.

So that we can notice changes in health status over a period of time and be able to compare populations to subgroups, the right indicator must depend on the functions or roles that are common to every individual. This research has led the World Health Organization to the identification of six so-called survival functions (10) to measure health consequences. We should emphasize only a small number of fundamental dimensions of the human body that are relatively independent of social contexts to evaluate the development of population health status.

Among these six survival functions, the simplest and most universal ones are concerned with the abilities to satisfy independently the immediate physical needs of the body and to move effectively in its environment. Further research on the elderly has led to the need for a better classification of elderly people who are in need of services from the institutions. As a result, researchers from France (7) have proposed a set of measures that could accurately answer the questions pertaining to the degree of autonomy of the elderly.

Assessment of Health: Quebec's Viewpoint

The commission's inquiry (4) on health and social services throws light on the importance of assessing the population's health as a basic tool for planning and evaluation. According to the commission, it is essential to focus the health system and its resources on the health and social needs of the population. Professional and institutional interventions should also be oriented toward results, one of which is the impact on the health of the population.

The diagnosis made by the commission points out that our existing health system is focused on resources and processes. In the future it should be oriented toward health objectives and should be able to measure the impact of programs on the health status of the population.

If the system is result oriented, it means that the individual, the family, and the community are placed in a system whose mission is to respond to the needs of the person. This implies that the population participates in the debates on priorities, objectives, allocation of resources, results, methods, and evaluation processes. It means that the responsibilities are in the hands of the population and its representatives, including deputies, ministers, and mayors. The population itself, not only the professionals or administrators, should judge the priorities and the successes obtained.

Such a reform implies well-educated and well-informed citizens. It also implies a political willingness to transfer the power from the central government to the regional and local governments. We are far from this vision, but in my opinion we will be forced into it in the coming decades. This situation will occur because of the growing pressures on public financing of health and social services. People will ask for results not only at the individual level but also at the community level.

A major recommendation of the commission is to regionalize the process of resource allocation to come closer to the needs of the population as perceived by the population itself rather than by professionals and technocrats.

Perspectives on the Development of Health Status Measurement

The commission indicates that the present information system contains mostly data on resources (inputs) and processes, little information on services (outputs) and even less on results (impact on health and social status of the population) (4). The commission foresees an important development in the field of health and social indices that will have many implications. For the scientific community it means that research should focus on methodology to develop a set of relevant and valid indicators of impact. For the political forces it means that party programs would include some indications of priorities in terms of health status. For the public administrators it means that programs and resource allocation will need to be revamped to take into account health objectives and the impact of the programs as well as objectives of efficiency and managerial performance.

Aside from the existing obstacles to the development of indicators, conceptual and methodological problems remain important. Global and classical indicators are easy to collect and to follow up, but their limitations are well known. The present definitions of health are based on the concepts of functional autonomy, social accomplishments, and quality of life. These definitions are undoubtedly more positive and closer to the values of our society. But admittedly, it becomes more difficult to build indicators that measure the level of attainment of these health objectives. Whenever we move from a biomedical concept of health and disease to a more relevant and consensual definition of health, the subjectivity appears striking. Nevertheless, we should not stop reflecting on this important aspect.

The problem of defining and validating health and welfare indicators has become an international preoccupation. New cultural and multisectorial research is needed, and this will undoubtedly bring some kind of improvement.

Conclusion

This overview of the various methods of assessment of health status and of the synthesis of recent reports from Canada, the United States, and France leads to the conclusion that, in spite of the ongoing research, an integrating model has yet to be developed. The very nature of health in all its components (objective, subjective, social, mental, and physical) remains mysterious. There is a need for transcultural research on the methods of assessing health and, more basically, on the concept of health itself. Besides health care, the new paradigm of health involves many components, such as genetic, cultural, economic, and social factors (Figure 11.2).

References

1. Colvez, A., and M. Blanchet. Potential gains in life expectancy free of disability: A tool for health planning. *Int. J. Epidemiol.* 12: 86-91, 1983.
2. Dillard, S. *Durée ou qualité de la vie. Conseil des affaires sociales et de la famille.* Quebec: Les Publications du Québec, 1983.

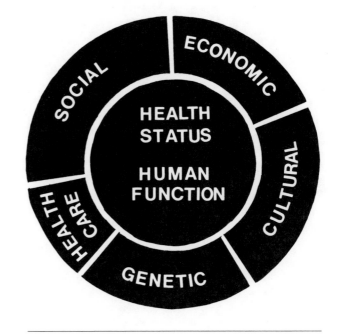

Figure 11.2. The many components of the new paradigm of health.

3. Evans, R.G. *Strained mercy: The economics of Canadian health care.* Toronto: Butterworth, 1984.
4. Gouvernement du Québec. *Rapport de la Commission d'enquête sur les services de santé et les services sociaux.* Quebec: Les Publications du Québec, 1988. (English version available)
5. Owen Consulting Group Ltd. *Health status statistics program evaluation.* Ottawa, ON: Statistics Canada, 1985.
6. Peron, Y., and C. Strohmenger. *Demographic and health indicators, presentation and interpretation.* (Catalog No. 82-5438). Ottawa, ON: Statistics Canada, 1985.
7. Robine, J.M. *Les indicateurs de type Espérance de vie sans incapacité (EVSI).* Quebec: Conseil des affaires sociales et de la famille, 1986.
8. Sullivan, D.F. A single index of mortality and morbidity. *HSMHA Health Rep.* 86: 347-354, 1971.
9. Wilkins, R., and O. Adams. *Healthfulness of life.* Montreal: Institute of Research in Public Policy, 1983.
10. World Health Organization. *Development of indicators for monitoring progress towards health for all by the year 2000.* Washington, DC: WHO, 1981.

Chapter 12

Discussion: Assessment of Health Status

Reubin Andres

The story goes that Poinsot, the French philosopher-mathematician, was once asked to define time. His response (I am paraphrasing it) was "Do you know whereof we speak when we discuss time? If so, let us talk about it. If you do not know what we mean by 'time,' let's change the subject." I feel a bit that way about health. We all have a general concept of what we are talking about. We certainly will not be permitted to change the subject, as Dr. Blanchet so clearly demonstrated to us in chapter 11. It is difficult to devise a simple global concept of health. There is no generally accepted measure of that, so we tend to use surrogates for health. It hardly needs pointing out that even in the titles of the individual sessions of this conference the word *health* occurs repeatedly. In some sessions health is stated overtly in the title; if not, health lurks behind the name of a disease or a morbid condition. So in Dr. Paffenberger's review (chapt. 3) of the health status of his subjects, he was actually reporting the presence or absence of coronary heart disease. The chapters that follow discuss lifestyle and health, environment and health, heredity and health, mental health, and so forth. The fact that the speakers were able to prepare their texts before they heard Dr. Blanchet tell them how difficult it was to define health illustrates the fact that there seem to be, in fact, some reasonably acceptable surrogates for the concept of total health.

I thus see the role of this session as one that will increase the participants' appreciation for the complexity of the concept of health. It is not a simple matter to assess the impact of physical activity or fitness on health. It is necessary for each of us to think about a broader measure of health than the one we are perhaps accustomed to measuring. These surrogates for health tend to fall into several categories. The first of these substitutes is longev-ity, or mortality, or years of life remaining at certain fixed ages. Death, if I may say so, is a very attractive variable. Mortality is not a graded or distributed variable. There are no shades of gray. There is no borderline category. The techniques for determining it are quite the same in developed and in developing nations, and indeed there is a clear relationship between mortality and health status. Unhealthy individuals are more likely to die. But there is more to life than being alive, and so we need measures for the quality of life. Quality is a difficult variable to measure. It is multidimensional, and the weight of each of the dimensions in this equation to compute quality will vary with each person as he or she is asked to assess the quality of his or her life. Or it may vary with scientists, who may need to measure many variables and then to weight each of these variables to create an equation applicable to the entire population.

In an effort to create a measure that is more specific than is quality of life (more specific and therefore more quantifiable), Dr. Blanchet summarized other mortality-derived variables in her very interesting review. She pointed out that there is not only life expectancy—total life expectancy—but also life expectancy that is free from disability, a very important concept. Or, we might consider quality-adjusted life years (a term that Dr. Blanchet used in her review) or healthful equivalent life expectancy. All these are difficult to measure, and we may not hear those terms again during this conference. It may be that when we reassemble for a follow-up conference in the year 2000, we will hear more about them. All these measures are aimed at providing a global index of the health of individuals and collectively of a society. Improvement can be expected in all those measures if physical activity or fitness does have a significant impact on health as we understand health.

But it is conceivable that total life span might not be increased perceptibly even though the quality of life or the disabilityfree life expectancy is increased. Indeed that concept is currently creating some controversy, that is, Fries's concept of *compression of morbidity*. There is no time to describe that concept in detail except to say that Fries and others have pointed out that the survivorship curves for developed societies are becoming more square, that is, the number of people who remain alive at increasing ages tends to stay quite constant until late in life, when, at some fixed age near the end of the life span, everybody dies on close to the same day, perhaps at age 85 if that is the life expectancy. That is the direction that the survivorship curve has been moving since cave-dweller times. The controversial extension of this concept is that the period of disability will actually shorten as the curve becomes more square. That is a very optimistic view but unfortunately is probably wrong. The weight of the evidence is that as longevity increases and as the drop in the curve gets sharper or more square, the period of disability is actually getting longer.

Let me point out that this conference is full of other surrogates for this elusive concept of health. As you listen to the presentations on the impact of exercise and fitness on physiological and anatomical or structural systems (e.g., cardiovascular, pulmonary, nervous, endocrine, immune, etc.) and on specific disease states (e.g., coronary disease and hypertension, COPD, diabetes, etc.), you are in each case listening to an analysis of a piece of the health picture. When the effect of fitness (e.g., on HDL_2) is measured, it is again understood that a surrogate for health is being assessed. It reminds one of the parable of the blind men and the elephant. (Several men each grasped a different part of the elephant and mistook the creature for something else.) Verily, physical activity is like unto a diabetes preventer. But the organizers of this conference and the participants have not been blind. The very structure of the conference demonstrates the understanding of the awesome complexity of these topics. My point is that the lack of adequate global measures of health really has not very much hindered the accumulation of a vast amount of valid and persuasive evidence concerning the roles of exercise and fitness in health.

Let me close these remarks with a brief sense of discomfort over one of the themes that Dr. Blanchet emphasized strongly, namely, that of an increased role for the general public and for regional authorities to set priorities and to determine programs. It seems that the terms *administrators, politicians,* and *technocrats* were used in a somewhat pejorative sense. As my beard has turned gray and I have taken up some of the characteristics of an administrator and a technocrat, it bothers me just a bit. It seems to me that the goals of getting individual people and regions involved can be accomplished through the democratic process of the election of representatives of the people who, whether in Parliament or in Congress, can set the broader goals and the objectives. And then, quite correctly, one can turn to experts—to scientists, technocrats, and administrators—to carry out the extraordinarily complex details. Those experts, I might say, are also required in the planning phase of legislation, and I imagine that is going to be one of the results of a conference such as this one. Smallpox was wiped off the face of the earth not by a regional or a national effort but by a global effort that was obviously aided in an essential way be regional processes. So I believe that the deliberation of this conference not only will have a profound effect on Canada and its regions but also will create waves that will be global.

Now let me give you an illustration of another complexity in assessing health. Figure 12.1 illustrates the effect of age on the relationship of body mass index (BMI) to overall mortality (1). The data have been derived by us from the most recent large U.S.-Canadian insurance study (2). I would like to have shown data on physical activity or fitness, but such data are not available, and BMI will illustrate the point. The figure shows what is now well recognized as a U- or J-shaped relationship between BMI and mortality. The curves drawn to fit these data were derived by regressing mortality to Age and on Age² (i.e., the data are fit to a quadratic regression). Age is seen to be a highly significant influence on the relationship of BMI to mortality.

Figure 12.2 breaks down the data for specific causes of death for men aged 40 to 69. It would be of great interest to have such data for physical activity and fitness, but studies far beyond those now available are needed. In any case, what you see in the figure are very different sorts of curves among the individual causes of death. Consider coronary heart disease. Only the right-hand side of the U-shaped curve is seen. For this cause of death it is best to be very lean. The same is true of diabetes, as we know. Lowest mortality occurs in the men of lowest BMIs. In deaths from pneumonia and influenza, only the left-hand side of the U-shaped curve is seen; it appears to be best to be on the distinctly overweight side. The same is true for deaths from suicides. Other causes of death

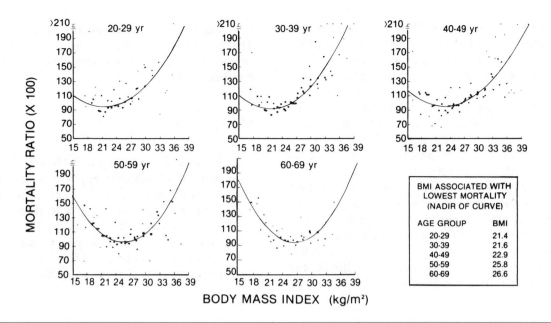

Figure 12.1. Effect of body mass index (BMI) on total mortality. Data for men in 5 decades of life. Curves were constructed from the following regression equation: mortality ratio = a + b Age + c Age². Sizes of symbols in the figure are related to the number of deaths in each BMI group.

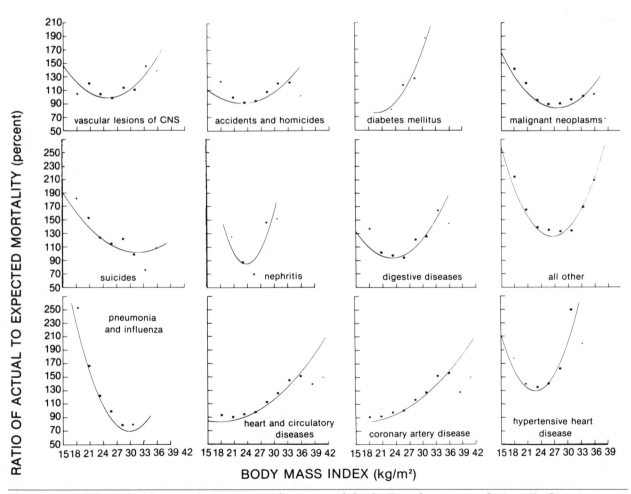

Figure 12.2. Effect of body mass index on specific causes of death. Data for men aged 40 to 69. Curves were constructed as indicated in the legend of Figure 12.1.

have other sorts of curves. Thus, one can influence one's mode of death. We can give advice on that. To lower mortality from heart and circulatory diseases and from diabetes (surrogates of health), you try to stay on the very lean side. On the other hand, if your goal in life is not to die of pneumonia or not to commit suicide, it seems best to stay on the fat side. The point again is that in each case we are looking at surrogates of health, and we need to look at a variety of them.

I ask all of us then to stay alert when we hear talks about specific variables or specific diseases. Ultimately, we also must keep in mind the larger concept of health as Dr. Blanchet pointed out. In essence, then, I think we have brought you bad news and good news in this session of the conference. The bad news is that we really do not yet have simple, reliable measures of global health. The good news is that it has not mattered too much. Despite the gaps in knowledge, a great deal has been learned.

References

1. Andres, R. Mortality and obesity: The rationale for age-specific height-weight tables. In: *Principles of Geriatric Medicine*, edited by R. Andres, E. Bierman, and W.R. Hazzard. New York: McGraw-Hill, 1985, p. 311-318.
2. *Build Study 1979*. Chicago: Society of Actuaries and Association of Life Insurance Medical Directors of America, 1980.

Chapter 13

Heredity, Fitness, and Health

William J. Schull

We are what we were. As human beings we are the culmination of a long evolutionary history, and our genetic past conditions our individual and collective responses to the stresses of the present. To understand these responses, we need more than mere phenomenological description; we must delineate the role of genetic factors for at least two reasons. First, heuristically, one would like to be able to define a process (biochemical or physiological) completely in all its complexities and ramifications, and in this context it is important to bear in mind that the same gene can behave advantageously in one environment and disadvantageously in another. For example, individuals heterozygous for the gene that in a homozygous state produces sickle-cell anemia do not normally have hematologic crises under conditions of normal oxygen pressure but can if that pressure is significantly reduced. Second, examining the role of genetic factors is a means to identify individuals at high risk of some aberrant, possibly pathological outcome in their responses to stress. Informed intervention in these instances ultimately depends on the capacity to anticipate events. It is difficult to see how this can occur without an appreciation of the molecular and cellular processes that are involved.

Does this mean, for example, that one should search for or even expect a gene for maximal oxygen uptake ($\dot{V}O_2max$)? Certainly not. Contrarily, does this imply that one's $\dot{V}O_2max$ is an epigenetic phenomenon, free of genetic modulation? Again no, as $\dot{V}O_2max$ varies with conditioning and doubtlessly with other factors as well. It can be high in some who lead a sedentary life and low in some who are strenuously active. Proper oxygenation is more than a simple respiratory function; it involves transport, in which the structural form of hemoglobin is important; diffusion in tissues; and cellular utilization. Genetic factors can be important at all these levels. However, this variation must be seen in the context of the process and the variables that one can or does measure. But how is this to be done?

The Unmeasured Genotype

Studies to identify the role of genetic factors in the origin of continuously varying traits (e.g., health and fitness, in which our genetic constitutions and our environments interact) have traditionally been one of two broad types: the unmeasured genotype and the measured genotype. The unmeasured genotype attempts to dissociate genetic from nongenetic factors using the general principles and models, some quite elegant, of quantitative genetics. It seeks to assign components of variation in the trait in question to genetic factors on the one hand and to environmental forces on the other and to determine the presence and possibly the chromosomal location of a major gene, that is, one that makes a disproportionate contribution to the total observed variation. It does so through the examination of the correspondence between a response and the known segregation of genes. Commonly, it culminates in statements about the collective importance of genetic variation (often expressed in terms of heritability) and cultural transmission.

Although studies of this nature are often necessary and are frequently all that can be done at a particular time, they should be seen merely as first steps, not as ends in themselves. They are essentially phenomenological. Their limitations are numerous, but two in particular loom large. First, because they begin with some statistical preconception of the mode of gene action or, in the case of path analysis, impose on the data a hierarchical cause-and-effect structure, the results are no more realistic than the model is appropriate, and different models frequently lead to quite different results. Second, they provide no insight into the molecular or cellular bases of the processes that subtend the phenotype itself, although they may be useful in predicting or even assessing the probable impact of broad strategies of intervention, that is, interventions aimed at populations rather than at specific individuals.

The Measured Genotype

The other approach, the measured genotype, employs some of the same statistical tools as does the unmeasured genotype but develops somewhat differently. It attempts to decompose variation into components attributable to specific genetic loci rather than to the totality of genes involved. For example, it might seek to measure the component of variation in serum cholesterol assignable to allelic variation at the locus responsible for the apo-E lipoprotein (13). Its principal shortcoming is that its application presupposes the existence of genetic loci at which different genotypes can be identified electrophoretically, immunophoretically, or by some other technique. As a consequence, because the number of such genetic loci remains small (possibly no more than 1% or 2% of the entire genome), the situations in which it has been applied have been limited. However, as the number of restriction fragment length polymorphisms grows and the number of genes actually cloned increases, this approach—coupled with other recent developments in molecular biology that make possible the amplification of specific segments of DNA, such as the polymerase chain reaction—will in time undoubtedly become the method of choice. Its merits are that it can provide evidence of the effects of specific genes and thereby a means of recognizing individuals at high risk. It promises directed intervention through the molecular or cellular processes associated with a particular genetic locus.

Obesity: A Paradigm

To provide a more specific discussion of these general remarks, I will consider obesity, one of the most important risk factors associated with a wide variety of states of ill health and commonly the focus of many fitness programs. It is abundantly clear that obesity is significantly associated with the onset of non-insulin-dependent diabetes mellitus (54), premature myocardial infarctions and hypertension (41), cholecystitis and cholelithiasis

(1), cancer of the corpus of the uterus (56), gout (57), and possibly fatal cancer of the prostate (47). Adiposity is second only to age as a risk factor for non-insulin-dependent diabetes, and it is similarly important in hypertension, although here there are apparently gender-related differences in the association of the distribution of subcutaneous fat with cardiovascular risk factors (27). Obesity threatens health in other ways as well; for example, obese hypertensives, particularly males, are more resistant to antihypertensive medications (37). Hyperinsulinemia and insulin resistance are more common among the obese, particularly those with a centralized distribution of body fat (31, 34). It is interesting to note too that response to dietary cholesterol is inversely correlated with body mass index; hyperresponders are invariably leaner (30). Similarly, obese individuals commonly have lower caloric intakes than do nonobese individuals. Moreover, body weight and fatness have been shown to be potential confounders in the assessment of the risk of physical activity (3).

Many of the clinical conditions we have enumerated appear to be familial in nature and thus possibly genetic in origin; however, the chain or chains of events that lead to their association with obesity have been obscure. Some of the difficulties are the length of time that generally intervenes between the onset of obesity and the occurrence of disease and the definition of obesity, which varies. Obesity is often defined merely as some percentage excess over an ideal body weight, as the percentile standing of the individual, or as his or her body mass index (taken to be the weight in kilograms divided by the height in meters squared). It has been a widespread practice also to treat obese individuals as if their obesity had the same causal basis even though experimental evidence has shown that there are at least two separable components in the deposition of excess body fat: hyperphagia and increased metabolic efficiency. Each of these may in turn have heterogeneous origins, but this is conjectural because there has not existed the biochemical or physiological means to characterize such heterogeneity rigorously. The remarks that follow focus on what might be termed *idiopathic* obesity, but not the type associated with simply inherited genetic disorders, such as the Prader-Willi or the Laurence-Moon-Biedl-Bardet syndrome, in which obesity is merely a part of the constellation of effects associated with the syndrome. These latter disorders, interesting in their own right, can provide insights into the underlying biological processes; however, their impact on public health is undoubtedly small.

A variety of conventional strategies have been employed to determine the role of genetic variation in the origin of obesity. Each has its strengths and limitations. The approaches include the correspondences in weight between monozygous twins on the one hand and dizygous twins on the other, the correlation in weight between foster children and their adoptive and biological parents (4, 5, 50), and traditional family investigations (for a review of these various studies, see refs. 8, 39). These studies have focused on weight at different ages from birth to adulthood but rarely on the process of weight gain itself, and the results frequently have been contradictory. Techniques of measurement have not been well standardized if at all. Some studies are based on direct but single observations of weight and some on weight as self-reported, and others have employed silhouettes. Some have used skinfold thickness as measures of corpulence (23); others have not. Few have examined the pattern of fat distribution or the tracking of weight over time, and concomitant sources of variation, such as activity or temporal trends, have been poorly controlled or ignored.

This unsatisfactory situation seems likely to persist until more pertinent measurements are used (35). These include variation in lean body mass, fat distribution, and biochemical or physiological measures associated with specific genes. Until recently, this has not been practicable; however, a corner of this curtain of uncertainty may have been lifted at last. Several lines of evidence, many still tentative, suggest this to be so. Some of these are briefly reviewed here. The intention is to urge a strategy that has been used successfully in other contexts and not to defend the importance or long-term pertinence of any of these specific developments.

Ionic Pathways

First, there is the apparent role of the ionic pathways associated with the red blood cell membrane. Four pathways are presently recognized (more may exist): (a) the so-called Na-K pump, an active pathway that is inhibited by ouabain, a glycoside obtained from the wood or seeds of several plants; (b) the sodium cotransport system, a passive pathway inhibitable by furosemide, a complex anthranilic acid often used as a diuretic; (c) the sodium-lithium countertransport system, another passive pathway inhibited by phloretin, a glucoside derived from the bark of many of the *Rosaceae*; and (d) the so-called leak, a minor pathway that seems to reflect a random loss of the ion in ques-

tion. Each of these major pathways of ionic transport has been the object of considerable research and has been shown to be associated with some form of ill health. For example, elevated red blood cell sodium-lithium countertransport is more common among individuals with essential hypertension than it is among normotensive persons (51), and Boerwinkle et al. (7) have shown that about 50% of the normal variability between individuals in sodium-lithium countertransport is attributable to the segregation of genetic factors (52).

York et al. (58) have demonstrated that an enzymatic defect exists in the obese mouse, a common animal model for obesity in humans. There is a loss of thyroid-induced sodium- and potassium-dependent ATP; the homozygous, obese mouse has reduced levels of sodium-potassium ATPase. This observation prompted De Luise et al. (16) (see also refs. 15, 17) to look for evidence of reduced energy use in the cells of obese persons, as ATP is the principal energy currency of the body. They found that the number of sodium-potassium pump units in the erythrocytes from obese subjects was reduced about 22% when compared with nonobese controls and that the number of pump units was significantly and negatively correlated with the percentage of ideal body weight. Normally, the sodium pump is responsible for 20%-50% of total cellular thermogenesis (some estimates are as high as 70%). The weights of the obese individuals in this study ranged from 147%-277% above their ideal body weights. They clearly satisfy most operational definitions of obesity, but the selection criteria used may inadvertently compromise the inferences that can be drawn because the causal mechanisms that give rise to extreme measurements in a continuous distribution are often more limited in number than are those seen more centrally in the distribution. For example, it has been argued that some of the effect they observe is attributable to ethnic differences in obesity and that the ethnic origins of the patient and the comparison person were not controlled in De Luise's studies (6). This caveat notwithstanding, their observations suggest that within these obese individuals there exists some subset in which the pump may be defective, cellular utilization of ATP is diminished, and the calories that would normally find their way to glycolysis are stored.

Given the quantitative nature of the findings of De Luise et al., one might assume that the Na^+-K^+ pump is genetically controlled but then suspect a multifactorial basis for the inheritance of differences. However, most enzymatic variation appears continuously distributed if measured in terms of activity levels, even when the underlying structural differences in the enzyme are known to be inherited simply and discretely (see, e.g., the situation with respect to the red cell enzyme acid phosphatase). The seemingly continuous nature of the variation in the pump may merely reflect the metric used to assess differences and not the nature of the genetic variability. Although it is patently too early to know whether these findings will be supported with time, there are observations that suggest they may be. For example, there is evidence that some obese humans have an impaired thermogenetic response to a stimulus such as a rise in circulating catecholamines (29). Or that weight gain is a commonly observed phenomenon among manic depressives on lithium therapy where it has been thought that this was due to the known effects of lithium on water balance; polydipsia and polyuria are frequently seen in manics on lithium therapy. Although this seems undoubtedly to be one of the mechanisms contributing to weight gain, there is also a gain in weight not attributable to retained water (18). Lithium impinges on the sodium-potassium pump and can seemingly do so at lithium concentrations in the range of 1 mg/L water (11). Thus, weight gain with lithium therapy and possibly at still lesser levels of lithium absorption suggests a change in the sodium-potassium pump that is either inherited or directly due to the competitive effects of this metal. Weight is known to be significantly associated with sodium-lithium countertransport (7), but whether obesity per se has a disproportionate effect is not presently clear. These observations aside, a defect in the pump, when it occurs, makes the widespread effects of obesity more easily understood.

Sex-Hormone-Binding Globulin (SHBG)

Second, there is evidence that sex-hormone-binding globulin (SHBG), a genetically controlled protein, is instrumental in weight gain and fat patterning. Although the precise functions of this protein are not fully defined, DeMoor and Joosens (19) found a significant inverse correlation between SHBG and body weight using an estradiol-binding index constructed from the binding capacity and affinity association constant. This correlation was independent of nine other factors, including blood pressure, cholesterol, age, and height. Other studies have reported similar effects. Low serum testosterone and SHBG have been found in massively obese men. Kopelman et al. (33) have reported increased plasma testosterone and decreased SHBG levels in obese woman when compared to lean controls.

Two studies on humans have looked specifically at the relationship between fat deposition and levels of SHBG. Purifoy et al. (43) compared levels of serum androgens and SHBG in obese female Pima Indians and normal-weight Caucasians. Although the Pimas, who have a strong propensity for android obesity, had decreased SHBG compared to controls, a strong age effect confounded the association. Nevertheless, one can speculate that the female predisposition for upper-trunk adiposity in this ethic group may involve the action of androgens during development and later life. Evans et al. (21), in a study of the relationship of androgenic activity to body fat topography, fat-cell morphology, and metabolic aberration in premenopausal women, found a decrease in SHBG and an increase in the percentage of free testosterone to be accompanied by (a) increasing hip-to-waist girth ratios; (b) increasing size of abdominal, but not femoral, adipocytes; (c) increasing plasma glucose and insulin levels; and (d) dimished in vivo insulin sensitivity. They concluded tentatively that in premenopausal women increased tissue exposure to unbound androgens may be partially responsible for fat localization in the upper body and the associated upset of glucose-insulin homeostasis. However, none of these studies have examined the role of genetic factors in a rigorous or quantitative manner, presumably reflecting the absence of good methods for visualizing the protein in sera. This situation seems to be changing, and methods soon may be at hand to examine these issues in the context of known genotypes (see, e.g., ref. 36).

Other Genetic Factors

Finally, there is other evidence of the role of genetic factors in human obesity. Some is of a biochemical nature, such as the apparent functioning of the enzyme lipoprotein lipase as the gatekeeper for the entry of lipids into the cell, and some is not. Mueller (39) has reviewed this latter evidence and concludes that there is low to moderate heritability of adult static obesity (see also refs. 8, 9, 45). He asserts that one third or so of the variation between individuals in fatness appears ascribable to genetic causes, and further notes that changes in fatness in the course of life and the anatomical positioning of fat are important modifiers of the health effects of obesity. Notable in this regard is the apparent centripetal distribution of fat seen in diabetes (see, e.g., ref. 28). Obesity and, for that matter, leanness appear inherited. For example, Moll et al. (38) have recently examined this issue in children who were part of the Muscatine Study. They selected four groups of children and their families for investigation: a random sample, a group of children in the lowest quintile of weight on three successive examinations, a group of students that gained at least two quintiles over the survey, and a group of students who were in the fifth quintile of all three examinations. Evidence of heritability was seen in all four groups.

Over the past decade or so, the role of the so-called satiety hormones or brain-gut peptides has grown larger and genetically more intriguing. Cholecystokinin and bombesin, for example, are peptides found in the gut and in the central and peripheral nervous system, and both are known to inhibit food intake after peripheral and central administration. Unfortunately, the literature on the function of these hormones and their interrelationships is extensive and often contradictory and places a burden on the reader's perseverance as well as perspicacity. Recently, attention has focused heavily on cholecystokinin, bombesin, somatostatin, and glucagon. It warrants note that, as yet, many of these peptides are identified through radioimmunological techniques, and the reproducibility of such tests often leaves much to be desired. Little study apparently has been done in assessing the role of genetic factors in the determination and variability of these hormones, although the genes responsible for cholecystokinin (20), glucagon (55), and somatostatin (22) have been cloned and sequenced. Many of these hormones (neurotransitters) influence the action of the gallbladder and thus fat absorption.

Cholecystokinin has been one of the more extensively investigated of the various satiety hormones. It clearly plays a major role in integrating the intestinal phase of digestion, and its effects on satiation are specific, although the mechanism of the effect is not fully known. However, it is clear that gastric vagal fibers are necessary for the effect to occur. Because cholecystokinin circulates in the blood in very low concentrations (a few pmol), it is unlikely that blood-borne cholecystokinin is a satiety signal. It has been conjectured therefore that the satiety effect is due to the activation of vagal afferent fibers that inhibit the central control of feeding and that cholecystokinin acts either directly on its numerous vagal receptors that have been recently described or indirectly through a gastric smooth-muscle effect to which vagal receptors

are sensitive (44, 46). It has been suggested that its role may be to titrate the passage of calories, that is, to serve as a gating mechanism that controls the flow of food through the pylorus.

Patently, the origins of obesity and fat patterning are complex, and there are numerous opportunities for genetic variation to impinge on the process or processes involved. Few if any studies have examined more than one of the numerous interacting factors. It seems unlikely that our knowledge will be materially furthered until a more holistic approach becomes practicable; as these brief remarks have attempted to convey, such an approach grows progressively more feasible and essential. Collectively, the number of measurable genotypes with apparent effects on obesity has increased at a pace that warrants consideration of an analysis based on measured genotypes. In this regard, although obesity appears to be a characteristic of all human populations under appropriate circumstances, those populations with unusually high frequencies of obese individuals may be particularly informative.

Among such populations are the indigenous inhabitants of the New World, the islands of the Pacific (e.g., the Nauruans, the Samoans, and so on), the blacks of the Americas, and many admixed groups, such as the Mexican Americans of the United States. Prevalence patterns in the latter populations commonly parallel the degree of Amerindian admixture, suggesting a genetic mechanism. Among Mexican Americans, a group of particular interest for its size and accessibility, Mueller et al. (40) used a body mass index of 30 or greater, which corresponds roughly to the 90th percentile of the HANES distribution (2, 24), and found that in those over age 20 the percentage of Mexican Americans residing in Starr County, Texas, with a body mass index equaling or exceeding 30 ranged from 22% to 53% in women and from 27% to 40% in men. This population is known to have age-specific prevalences of non-insulin-dependent diabetes that are 3-5 times greater than those seen in non–Mexican Americans in Texas (25), and this situation seems to prevail generally among Mexican Americans (see, e.g., refs. 48, 49). Age-specific prevalences of gallbladder disease, as revealed by cholecystectomy and ultrasonography, are equally elevated in this group of individuals, and cases of cholecystitis and cholelithiasis are known to cluster within families (26). Moreover, there is evidence that in females under the age of 45 a significant association between gallbladder disease and diabetes exists that is not explicable by increased body mass alone. Most if not all of the stones are cholesteric, and the precocity of their appearance is startling. Cases of acute cholecystitis with dozens of stones have been seen in females as young as 12. Invariably, in such cases other close female relatives have exhibited early, if not always equally precocious, onset of gallbladder disease. Qualitatively, the diets of these individuals appear to have changed little in the recent past, although the quantities of the limited number of foodstuffs eaten have increased.

The molecular and cellular events that underlie these observations are unclear, but current studies of lipid metabolism, including extensive apolipoprotein genotyping and the use of specific restriction endonucleases, may clarify the situation. A search for variation at the loci responsible for those satiety hormones that have been cloned and sequenced might also be profitable. However, it must be borne in mind first that the study of the insulin gene, where a similar opportunity exists, has not as yet been especially rewarding and second that the molecular structure of, for example, cholecystokinin appears to have been highly conserved for at least 500 million yr and may therefore be a poor candidate for much interindividual variability (53).

Conclusion

In closing, as one examines the nature-nurture or gene-environment interaction, it is important to bear in mind that genetic constitution programs not only the limits of response to environmental challenges but also the rate at which that response occurs. Too commonly, conditioning is seen as an epigenetic phenomenon, one devoid of any genetic control (see, e.g., ref. 14), but no end of conditioning will make a world-class runner of all of us, although we would undoubtedly be somewhat faster after conditioning than before. A more profitable avenue of inquiry into mechanisms thus is one that focuses on variability in response to a standardized regimen, particularly among those individuals who can be construed as falling outside the customary range of variation. Rates of change and velocities are often more informative than is the end ultimately attained because the latter can be achieved in a variety of ways. For example, Poehlman et al. (42) (see also ref. 9) have shown that changes in body fat following short-term (22 d) overfeeding (1,000 cal per day) of monozygous twins appears to be genetically con-

trolled. The intrapair correlation in gains of adiposity and fat-free mass were impressive when viewed in the context of the heterogeneity between the sets of twins. Much of the effect was mediated through alterations in the energy expenditure components assessed in the study. Similar studies that treat weight gain as a dynamic rather than a static process are desperately needed and ideally should examine dizygous and monozygous twins with the measured-genotype approach.

As we have seen, a growing causal role is being recognized for seemingly simply inherited variation in such phenomena as sodium-potassium cotransport and sodium-lithium countertransport and can be shown also in apolipoprotein variability. All these are directly or indirectly associated with the production and utilization of ATP, the energy currency of the body. Ultimately, events that affect the cellular dynamics involved in the formation of adenosine mono-, di-, and triphosphates must impinge on physical fitness and health, as these are the sources of energy that fuel physical achievement. It can be anticipated that similar variability will be seen to be instrumental in the proneness to obesity. Whether this variability will prove to be advantageous in terms of health, and the circumstances under which it is, has yet to be established.

References

1. Abbruzzese, A., and P.J. Snodgrass. Diseases of the gallbladder and bile ducts. In: Wintrobe, M.M., G.W. Thorn, R.D. Adams, I.L. Bennett, Jr., E. Braunwald, K.J. Isselbacher, and R.G. Petersdorf, eds. *Harrison's principles of internal medicine.* 6th ed. New York: McGraw-Hill, 1970.

2. Abraham, S., C.L. Johnston, and M.F. Najjar. Weight and height of adults 18-74 years of age, United States, 1971-1974. *Vital and health statistics* (Series 11, No. 211). Washington, DC: Department of Health, Education and Welfare, 1981.

3. Albanes, D. Potential for confounding of physical activity risk assessment by body weight and fatness. *Am. J. Epidemiol.* 125: 745-746, 1987.

4. Annest, J.L., C.F. Sing, P. Biron, and J-G. Mongeau. Familial aggregation of blood pressure and weight in adoptive families. I. Comparisons of blood pressure and weight

statistics among families with adopted, natural, or both natural and adopted children. *Am. J. Epidemiol.* 110: 479-491, 1979.

5. Annest, J.L., C.F. Sing, P. Biron, and J-G. Mongeau. Familial aggregation of blood pressure and weight in adoptive families. II. Estimation of the relative contributions of genetic and common environmental factors to BP correlations between family members. *Am. J. Epidemiol.* 110: 492-503, 1979.

6. Beutler, E., W. Kuhl, and P. Sacks. Sodium-potassium-ATPase is influenced by ethnic origin and not by obesity. *N. Engl. J. Med.* 309: 756-760, 1983.

7. Boerwinkle, E., S.T. Turner, R. Weinshilboum, M. Johnson, E. Richelson, and C.F. Sing. Analysis of the distribution of erythrocyte sodium lithium countertransport in a sample representative of the general population. *Genet. Epidemiol.* 3: 365-378, 1986.

8. Bouchard, C., and L. Pérusse. Heredity and body fat. *Annu. Rev. Nutri.* 8: 259-277, 1988.

9. Bouchard, C., L. Pérusse, C. Leblanc, A. Tremblay, and G. Thériault. Inheritance of the amount and distribution of human body fat. *Int. J. Obes.* 12: 31-41, 1988.

10. Bouchard, C., A. Tremblay, J-P. Després, E.T. Poehlman, G. Thériault, A. Nadeau, P. Lupien, S. Moorjani, and J. Dussault. Sensitivity to overfeeding: The Quebec experiment with identical twins. *Prog. Food Nutri. Sci.* (in press).

11. Clench, J., R.E. Ferrell, W.J. Schull, and S.A. Barton. Hematocrit and hemoglobin, ATP and DPG concentrations in Andean man. In: Brewer, G.F., ed. *Proceedings of the Fifth International Conference on Red Cell Metabolism.* New York: Alan R. Liss, 1981.

12. Dahl, L.K. Possible role of chronic excess salt consumption on the pathogenesis of essential hypertension. *Am. J. Cardiol.* 8: 571-575, 1961.

13. Davignon, J., R.E. Gregg, and C.F. Sing. Apolipoprotein E polymorphism and atherosclerosis. *Arteriosclerosis* 8: 1-21, 1988.

14. Dejours, P. Extreme environments: An overview. In: Sutton, J.R., C.S. Houston, and G. Coates, eds. *Hypoxia and cold.* New York: Praeger, 1987, p. 3-11.

15. De Luise, M., and J.S. Flier. Functionally abnormal Na$^+$-K$^+$ pump in erythrocytes of a morbidly obese patient. *J. Clin. Invest.* 69: 38-44, 1982.

16. De Luise, M., G.L. Blackburn, and J.S. Flier. Reduced activity of the red-cell sodium-potassium pump in human obesity. *N. Engl. J. Med.* 303: 1017-1022, 1980.

17. De Luise, M., E. Rappaport, and J.S. Flier. Altered erythrocyte Na$^+$-K$^+$ pump in adolescent obesity. *Metabolism* 31: 1153-1158, 1982.

18. Dempsey, G.M., D.L. Dunner, R.R. Fieve, T. Farras, and J. Wong. Treatment of excessive weight gain in patients taking lithium. *Am. J. Psychiatry* 133: 1082-1084, 1976.

19. DeMoor, P., and J.V. Joosens. An inverse relation between body weight and the activity of the steroid binding B-globulin in human plasma. *Steroidologia* 1: 129-136, 1970.

20. Deschenes, R.J., L.J. Lorenz, R.S. Haun, B.A. Roos, K.J. Collier, and J.E. Dixon. Cloning and sequence analysis of cDNA encoding rat preprocholecystokinin. *Proc. Natl. Acad. Sci. USA* 81: 726-730, 1984.

21. Evans, D.J., R.G. Hoffman, R.K. Kalkhoff, and A.H. Kissebah. Relationship of androgenic activity to body fat topography, fat cell morphology, and metabolic aberrations in premenopausal women. *J. Clin. Endocrinol. Metab.* 57: 304-310, 1983.

22. Goodman, R.H., J.W. Jacobs, W.W. Chin, P.K. Lund, P.C. Dee, and J.F. Haebner. Nucleotide sequence of a cloned structural gene coding for a precursor of pancreatic somatostatin. *Proc. Natl. Acad. Sci. USA* 77: 5869-5873, 1980.

23. Haines, A.P., J.D. Imeson, and T.W. Meade. Skinfold thickness and cardiovascular risk factors. *Am. J. Epidemiol.* 126: 86-94, 1987.

24. Hamill, P.V.V., T.A. Drizd, C.L. Johnson, R.B. Reed, and A.F. Roche. NCHS growth curves for children birth to 18 years United States. *Vital and health statistics* (Series 11, No. 165). Washington, DC: Department of Health, Education and Welfare, 1977.

25. Hanis, C.L., R.E. Ferrell, S.A. Barton, L. Aguilar, A. Garza-Ibarra, B.R. Tulloch, C.A. Garcia, and W.J. Schull. Diabetes among Mexican-Americans in Texas. *Am. J. Epidemiol.* 118: 659-672, 1983.

26. Hanis, C.L., R.E. Ferrell, B.R. Tulloch, and W.J. Schull. Gallbladder disease epidemiology in Mexican Americans in Starr County, Texas. *Am. J. Epidemiol.* 122: 820-829, 1985.

27. Harlan, L.C., W.R. Harlan, J.R. Landis, and N.G. Goldstein. Factors associated with glucose tolerance in adults in the United States. *Am. J. Epidemiol.* 126: 674-684, 1987.

28. Joos, S.K., W.H. Mueller, C.L. Hanis, and W.J. Schull. Diabetes Alert Study: Weight history and upper body obesity in diabetic and non-diabetic Mexican American adults. *Ann. Hum. Biol.* 11: 167-172, 1984.

29. Jung, R.T., P.S. Shetty, W.P.T. James, M.A. Barrand, and B.A. Callingham. Reduced thermogenesis in obesity. *Nature* 279: 322-323, 1979.

30. Katan, M.B., and A.C. Beynan. Characteristics of human hypo- and hyperresponders to dietary cholesterol. *Am. J. Epidemiol.* 125: 387-399, 1987.

31. Kissebah, A.H., N. Vydelingum, R. Murray, D.J. Evans, A.J. Hartz, R.K. Kalkhoff, and P.W. Adams. Relationship of body fat distribution to metabolic complications of obesity. *J. Clin. Endocrinol. Metab.* 54: 254-260, 1982.

32. Klimes, I., M. Nagulesparan, R.H. Unger, S.L. Aronoff, and D. M. Mott. Reduced Na$^+$, K$^+$-ATPase activity in intact red cells and isolated membranes from obese man. *J. Clin. Endocrinol. Metab.* 54: 721-724, 1982.

33. Kopelman, P.G., T.R.E. Pilkington, N. White, and S.L. Jeffcoate. Abnormal sex steroid secretion and binding in massively obese women. *Clin. Endocrinol.* 12: 363-369, 1980.

34. Krotiewski, M., P. Björntorp, and C. Sjoström. Impact of obesity on metabolism in men and women: Importance of regional adipose distribution. *J. Clin. Invest.* 72: 1150-1162, 1983.

35. Laporte, R.E., L.L. Adams, D.D. Savage, G. Brenes, S. Dearwater, and T. Cook. The spectrum of physical activity, cardiovascular disease and health: An epidemiologic perspective. *Am. J. Epidemiol.* 120: 507-517, 1984.

36. Meikle, A.W., W.M. Stanish, N. Taylor, C.Q. Edwards, and C.T. Bishop. Familial effects on plasma sex-steroid content in man: Testosterone, estradiol and sex-hormone-binding globulin. *Metabolism* 31: 6-9, 1982.

37. Modan, M., H. Halkin, A. Lusky, Z. Fuchs, A. Shitrit, and B. Modan. Resistance of obese hypertensives to antihypertensive medications. *Am. J. Epidemiol.* 124: 507-508, 1986.

38. Moll, P., T. Burns, and R. Lauer. Obesity and leanness in children is heritable: The Muscatine Study. *Am. J. Epidemiol.* 124: 517-518, 1986.

39. Mueller, W.H. The genetics of human fatness. *Yearbook Phys. Anthropol.* 26: 215-230, 1983.

40. Mueller, W.H., S.K. Joos, C.L. Hanis, A.N. Zavaleta, J. Eichner, and W.J. Schull. The Diabetes Alert Study: Growth, fatness, and fat patterning, adolescence through adulthood in Mexican Americans. *Am. J. Phys. Anthropol.* 64: 389-399, 1984.

41. Pickering, G. *High blood pressure.* New York: Grune & Stratton, 1968.

42. Poehlman, E.T., A. Tremblay, J.-P. Després, E. Fontaine, L. Pérusse, G. Thériault, and C. Bouchard. Genotype-controlled changes in body composition and fat morphology following overfeeding in twins. *Am. J. Clin. Nutri.* 43: 723-731, 1986.

43. Purifoy, F.E., L.H. Koopmans, R.W. Tatum, and D.M. Mayes. Serum androgens and sex hormone binding globulin in obese Pima Indian females. *Am. J. Phys. Anthropol.* 55: 491-496, 1986.

44. Rehfeld, J.F. Cholecystokinin as satiety signal. *Int. J. Obes.* 5: 465-469, 1980.

45. Savard, R., C. Bouchard, C. Leblanc, and A. Tremblay. Familial resemblance in fatness indicators. *Ann. Hum. Biol.* 10: 111-118, 1983.

46. Smith, G.P., J. Gibbs, C. Jerome, F.X. Pi-Sunyer, H.R. Kissileff, and J. Thornton. The satiety effect of cholecystokinin: A progress report. *Peptides* 2: 57-59, 1981.

47. Snowdon, D.A., R.L. Phillips, and W. Choi. Diet, obesity and risk of fatal prostate cancer. *Am. J. Epidemiol.* 120: 244-250, 1984.

48. Stern, M.P., S.P. Gaskill, C.R. Allen, Jr., V. Garza, J.L. Gonzales, and R.H. Waldrop. Cardiovascular risk factors in Mexican Americans in Laredo, Texas. I. Prevalence of overweight and diabetes and distributions of serum lipids. *Am. J. Epidemiol.* 113: 546-555, 1981.

49. Stern, M.P. Diabetes in Hispanic Americans. In: Harris, M.I., and R. Hamman, eds. *Diabetes data in America: Diabetes data compiled in 1984.* (NIH Publication No. 85-1468). Washington, DC: U.S. Government Printing Office, 1985.

50. Stunkard, A.J., T.I.A. Sorenson, C.L. Hanis, T.W. Teasdale, R. Chakraborty, W.J. Schull, and F. Schulsinger. An adoption study of human obesity. *N. Engl. J. Med.* 314: 193-198, 1986.

51. Turner, S.T., E. Boerwinkle, M. Johnson, E. Richelson, and C.F. Sing. Sodium-lithium countertransport in ambulatory hypertensive and normotensive patients. *Hypertension* 9: 24-34, 1987.

52. Turner, S.T., M. Johson, E. Boerwinkle, E. Richelson, H.F. Taswell, and C.F. Sing. Sodium-lithium countertransport and blood pressure in healthy blood donors. *Hypertension* 7: 955-962, 1985.

53. Vigna, S.R., M.C. Thorndyke, and J.A. Williams. Evidence for a common evolutionary origin of brain and pancreas cholecystokinin receptors. *Proc. Natl. Acad. Sci.* USA 83: 4355-4359, 1986.

54. West, K.M. *Epidemiology of diabetes and its vascular lesions.* New York: Elsevier, 1978.

55. White, J.W., and G. Saunders. Structure of the human glucagon gene. *Nucleic Acids Res.* 14: 4719-4730, 1986.

56. Wynder, E.L., G. Escher, and N. Mantel. An epidemiological investigation of cancer of the endometrium. *Cancer* 19: 489-520, 1966.

57. Wyngaarden, J.B. Gout and other disorders of uric acid metabolism. In: Wintrobe, M.M., G.W. Thorn, R.D. Adams, I.L. Bennett, Jr., E. Braunwald, K.J. Isselbacher, and R.G. Petersdorf, eds. *Harrison's principles of internal medicine.* 6th ed. New York: McGraw-Hill, 1970.

58. York, D.A., G.A. Bray, and Y. Yukimura. An enzymatic defect in the obese (ob/ob) mouse: Loss of thyroid-induced sodium- and potassium-dependent adenosine triphosphate. *Proc. Natl. Acad. Sci.* USA 75: 477-481, 1978.

Chapter 14

Discussion: Heredity, Fitness, and Health

Claude Bouchard

The notions that humans are genetically similar but different from one another and that health and disease are the results of a large number of interacting genetic and nongenetic (environment and lifestyle) influences were described in an elegant manner by Dr. Schull. I center my discussion of these issues directly on the paradigm of exercise, fitness, and health.

An important concept, one that is ubiquitous in human genetics, is that of the biochemical individuality of each person (with the exception of identical twins) (13). We are not all alike within the species, and genetic heterogeneity is considerable (8). One consequence of this observation is that the average person, the average phenotype, or the average response to exercise are only constructs of the observers. In reality, we find diversity both in phenotype and in response to various stresses. Human genetics is a powerful science that can greatly increase our understanding of human biology in health and disease (12). However, the complexity of the genetic effect increases the farther removed the phenotype of interest is from the genes (e.g., physical fitness). Networks of interacting genes, themselves in constant interactions with environmentally and lifestyle-generated stresses or pressures, are operating to maintain biological and behavioral homeostasis or to improve acclimatization. In this sense, physiological genetics and behavioral genetics have become important for health scientists and exercise scientists who are interested in the complexities of the paradigm of exercise, fitness, and health.

The Basic Paradigm

We are part of this conference because we feel that there are reasons to believe that regular physical activity (mainly leisure-time physical activity or exercise) can increase physical and physiological fitness in most individuals. In addition, we also feel that the levels of both habitual physical activity and fitness exert influences on mortality, morbidity, and the sense of well-being. However, there remains many controversial issues in this basic paradigm. Further progress in our understanding of the conditions affecting the relationships among exercise, fitness, and health in humans requires the recognition of the critical importance of genetic variation among individuals. Figure 14.1 illustrates how the paradigm should be viewed to take into account human genetic diversity.

The figure emphasizes the fact that genotype should be considered as an important determinant not only because of its potential contributions to the phenotypes of the model (i.e., level of habitual physical activity, physical and physiological fitness, and health status) but also because it is an affector of the adaptive responses (from the level of habitual physical activity to fitness and from both to health status).

In this chapter, I illustrate these various effects of the genotype. The results of recent studies from our laboratory will be used to demonstrate that all five effects of the genotype shown in Figure 14.1 are important to consider in our study of the paradigm of exercise, fitness, and health. These data will also suggest clearly that overall the genotype is a major determinant of the paradigm, or one that accounts for a strikingly large fraction of human variation.

Level of Habitual Physical Activity

In a recent report we have shown that biological inheritance was involved in determining some of

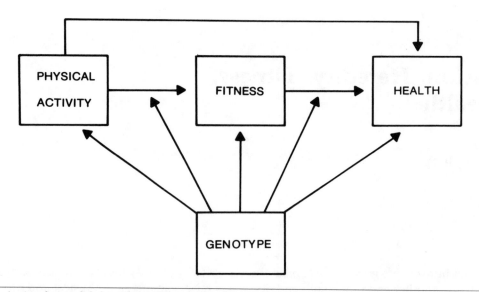

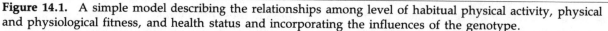

Figure 14.1. A simple model describing the relationships among level of habitual physical activity, physical and physiological fitness, and health status and incorporating the influences of the genotype.

the individual differences in the level of habitual physical activity (10). On the basis of a 3-d diary obtained from 1,610 subjects from 375 families, which included nine different types of relatives, we showed that the genetic effect for the level of habitual physical activity reached about 20% of the variance adjusted for age and gender variation. In contrast, participation in sports did not seem to be determined by any genetic mechanism (Table 14.1)

Table 14.1   Genetic Variance and Other Variance Components for the Level of Habitual Physical Activity

Variables	Level of physical activity (work and leisure)	Participation in sports
Total transmissible variance	.27	.12
Genetic transmission	.20	.00
Cultural transmission	.06	.12
Nontransmissible variance	.73	.88

Note. Data are from a 3-d activity record in 1,610 subjects from 375 families. The estimates were derived from the path analysis BETA model using the full-model solution. From "Genetic and Environmental Influences on Level of Habitual Physical Activity and Exercise Participation" by L. Pérusse, A. Tremblay, C. Leblanc, and C. Bouchard, 1989, *American Journal of Epidemiology*, **129**(5), p. 1019. Copyright 1989 by American Journal of Epidemiology. Adapted by permission.

Thus, it seems from these results that the general level of activity of the individual is a phenotype exhibiting some dependence on the genotype. However, nongenetic influences are largely responsible for most of the individual differences observed in habitual physical activity, including participation in sports and other forms of voluntary exercise.

Physical and Physiological Fitness

The contribution of the genotype to fitness was shown by the results of two reports dealing with $\dot{V}O_2max$ (2) and body fat (4). In the case of $\dot{V}O_2max$, data were obtained in regular brothers, dizygotic twins, and identical twins under the same standardized laboratory conditions. After controlling statistically for the unwarranted effects of age, gender, and body mass, we found that the genetic effect for maximal aerobic power reached less than 40% when expressed per kilogram body weight but only about 10% of the variance relative to fat-free mass. Parent-child data are quite compatible with these low estimates (6).

As for variation in human body fat, the data available are more abundant (3), and more sophisticated analytical strategies could be applied to large data sets. Using the sum of six skinfolds as a surrogate for the amount of subcutaneous fat and using body density derived from underwater weighing to compute fat mass in kilograms, we were able to assess the genetic effect on the basis

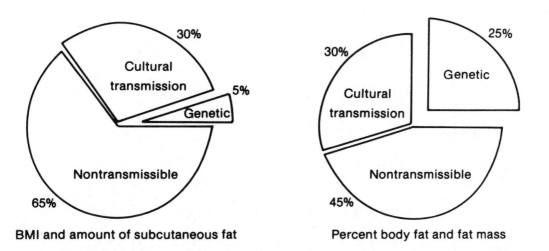

Figure 14.2. Total transmissible variance and its genetic component for subcutaneous fat and fat mass. Adapted from Bouchard et al. © Macmillan Press. (4).

of data obtained from nine different kinds of relatives (4). Using a complex path analysis procedure, we concluded that the genetic effect in the body mass index and subcutaneous fat reached only about 5% of the variance but 25% for fat mass and percent body fat (Figure 14.2). Fat distribution among various regions of the body is also characterized by a genetic effect of the order of 25%-30%.

Health Status

Inherited biological characteristics are related to mortality causes, life duration, and morbidity in the populations of industrialized societies. The abundant literature on genetics and diseases and on genetics and risk factors (e.g., blood pressure, obesity, blood lipids, and lipoproteins) testifies to that effect. One illustration from a recent study completed in our laboratory may serve as an illustration of this phenomenon.

Blood cholesterol, LDL cholesterol, and HDL cholesterol were obtained in a large sample of 375 families. Using a path analysis technique developed to solve problems in genetic epidemiology, we concluded that more than half of the variance in LDL cholesterol, HDL cholesterol, and the ratio of HDL cholesterol to total cholesterol was determined by the genotype even after we allowed for the contribution of factors such as age, gender, body fat, regional fat distribution, level of fitness, level of habitual physical activity, energy intake, fat intake, smoking, and alcohol consumption (9) (Figure 14.3).

Response to Exercise Training

The main questions are (a) whether the response to exercise training is heterogeneous in the population, (b) whether the heterogeneity in trainability is related to the genotype, (c) whether the alterations in health status as a result of regular exercise and the concomitant changes in fitness are heterogeneous, and (d) whether the heterogeneity in the changes of health status induced by regular exercise and increased fitness is dependent on or independent of the genotype.

Several experiments have been performed in our laboratory to establish the importance of the individual differences among sedentary subjects in the response to a precise training stimulus. In one study that was designed to estimate the effects of endurance training on $\dot{V}O_2$max and endurance performance, 13 women and 11 men were subjected to a 20-wk cycle ergometer training program (7). Subjects trained initially four times per week and then increased to five times per week. Each session lasted 40 and then 45 min, starting at 60% intensity early in the program and increasing progressively to 85% of the maximal heart rate reserve. Each training session was fully standardized and monitored for each subject. These sedentary males and females improved their $\dot{V}O_2$max from 2.3 to 2.9 L • min⁻¹, a group gain of 0.6 L • min⁻¹, or about 26%. But when each individual's improvement was computed, a mean training change of 30% with a standard deviation of 15% was registered. Of interest was the observation that training response in $\dot{V}O_2$max ranged

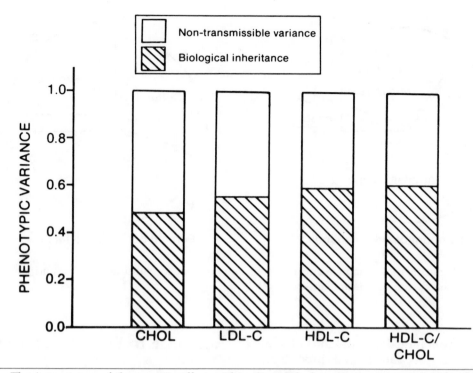

Figure 14.3. The importance of the genetic effect within the total phenotypic variance for blood cholesterol and lipoproteins after adjustment for a variety of covariates. Adapted from Pérusse et al. (9).

from 7% to 87%. The maximal aerobic power data reported per kilogram of body weight revealed the same variation in response.

Age and gender of subjects, as well as their prior training experience, do not seem to contribute much to human variation in trainability. The major causes of human variation in the response to training are the current phenotype level (i.e., the pretraining status of the trait considered) and a genetically determined capacity to adapt to exercise training that is probably unique for each biological characteristic or family of characteristics. The latter represents the so-called role of heredity in trainability or, more rigorously, the genotype-training interaction. Evidence from our laboratory for a role of the genotype in the response to training has been discussed elsewhere (1).

One study will be sufficient to illustrate the phenomenon. Ten pairs of monozygotic twins were subjected to a 20-wk endurance training program as described previously. Under this program, $\dot{V}O_2$max improved by 16%. However, there were considerable interindividual differences in training gains as illustrated by a range of 0%-41% for $\dot{V}O_2$max per kilogram of body weight. However, differences in the response to training were not distributed randomly among the twin pairs. Thus, intraclass correlations computed with the amount

of training gain in $\dot{V}O_2$max (L • min⁻¹) was 0.77, indicating that members of the same twin pair yielded a fairly similar response to training; that is, 77% of the variance in the training response seemed to be genotype dependent (11). These results suggest that the sensitivity of maximal aerobic power to endurance training is largely genotype dependent. Figure 14.4 illustrates the similarities in the twin response to training for training gains in ml • kg⁻¹ • min⁻¹ (intraclass = 0.74; $p < 0.01$) and in percent changes (intraclass = 0.82; $p < 0.01$).

Much more research is needed on the role of the genotype in the changes of health status brought about by an increase in both habitual physical activity and fitness. It is quite clear, however, that the phenomenon of a heterogeneous adaptive response extends also to indicators of health status, particularly risk factors. Again, we use the case of blood lipids to illustrate the case of heterogeneity in response and the role of the genotype in adaptation.

Six pairs of male monozygotic twins were subjected to a cycle ergometer exercise program that induced a 92.4 mJ energy deficit over 22 consecutive days (5). Plasma triglycerides and the insulin response to an oral glucose load decreased significantly with the short-term training program, and there was an important energy deficit. A significant increase in the ratio of HDL cholesterol to total cholesterol was also seen with the program. However, the heterogeneity in the response to the treatment was quite remarkable, particularly for

the insulin response to the glucose challenge, plasma triglycerides, plasma LDL and HDL cholesterol, and the ratio of HDL cholesterol to total cholesterol. These variations in response were not random (Table 14.2).

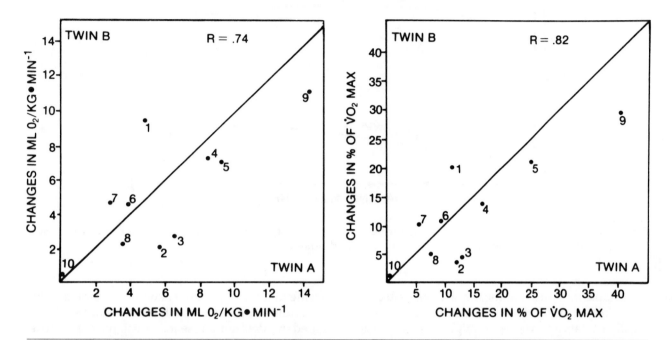

Figure 14.4. Intrapair resemblance (intraclass coefficient) in 10 pairs of identical twins for training changes in maximal aerobic power following 20 wk of endurance training. Adapted from D. Prud'homme, C. Bouchard, C. Leblanc, F. Landry, and E. Fontaine, "Sensitivity of maximal aerobic power to training is genotype-dependent," *Medicine and Science in Sports and Exercise,* **16**(5), pp. 489-493, 1984, © by American College of Sports Medicine.

Table 14.2   Twin Resemblance in Blood Lipids and Lipoproteins as a Result of Training Causing an Energy Deficit

Variables	Effect of treatment (*F* ratio)	Genotype-training interaction (*F* ratio)	Intrapair resemblance in response (intraclass)
Plasma cholesterol	3.0	23.8***	.92***
Plasma LDL cholesterol	3.7	18.3**	.90**
Plasma HDL cholesterol[a]	1.7	5.1*	.67*
HDL/total cholesterol[a]	6.3*	10.9**	.83**

Note. Six pairs of male monozygotic twins were submitted to a 2-hr daily exercise program for 22 consecutive days. Although energy intake was kept constant, the training program caused an energy deficit of 4.2 mJ/d. From "Heredity and Changes in Plasma Lipids and Lipoproteins and Short-Term Exercise Training in Men" by J.P. Després, S. Moorjani, A. Tremblay, E.T. Poehlman, P.J. Lupien, A. Nadeau, and C. Bouchard, 1988, *Arteriosclerosis,* **8**, p. 405. Copyright 1988 by American Heart Association. Adapted by permission.

[a]Twin resemblance in response to training remained significant for these variables after control over relative trunk fat (0.72 and 0.59 for HDL cholesterol and the ratio of HDL to total cholesterol, respectively).

*p < .05. **p < .01. ***p < .001.

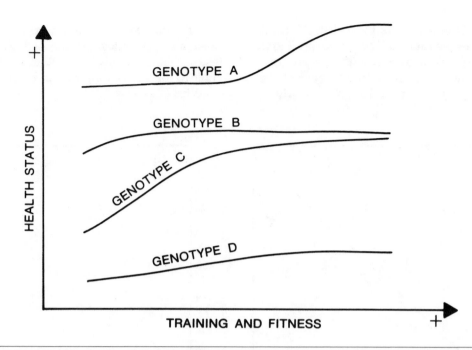

Figure 14.5. Schematic illustration of the contribution of the genotype in mediating the changes in health status as a result of an increase in physical activity level and fitness.

The table indicates that the intrapair resemblance in the response of blood cholesterol variables to the 22-d treatment was quite high. A role for the genotype in determining the alterations was particularly evident for HDL cholesterol and the ratio of HDL cholesterol to total cholesterol. This is an important issue that deserves more extensive investigations.

Conclusion

Because of inherited factors whose exact nature is presently undetermined, there are considerable individual differences in the components of the paradigm of exercise, fitness, and health. In addition, one finds that the genotype is also strongly involved in determining the response to regular exercise and to an increase in fitness. The situation is illustrated in Figure 14.5, which indicates that the genotype is clearly a major determinant of the changes in health status observed with increasing activity level and fitness.

These observations suggest that some individuals will profit much from a higher level of habitual physical activity, whereas others may be little affected by such a change in lifestyle. In other words, there are low responders, who may not achieve a better health status as a result of regular exercise. We need to recognize this situation when trying to understand how habitual physical activity and fitness influence health status. More sophisticated models and research designs than those commonly used in sport science and sports medicine are needed to allow for the pervasive influences of the genetically determined biological and behavioral individuality.

References

1. Bouchard, C., M.R. Boulay, J.A. Simoneau, G. Lortie, and L. Pérusse. Heredity and trainability of aerobic and anaerobic performances: An update. *Sports Med.* 5: 69-73, 1988.
2. Bouchard, C., R. Lesage, G. Lortie, J.A. Simoneau, P. Hamel, M.R. Boulay, L. Pérusse, G. Thériault, and C. Leblanc. Aerobic performance in brothers, dizygotic and monozygotic twins. *Med. Sci. Sports Exerc.* 18: 639-646, 1986.
3. Bouchard, C., and L. Pérusse. Heredity and body fat. *Annu. Rev. Nutr.* 8: 259-277, 1988.
4. Bouchard, C., L. Pérusse, C. Leblanc, A. Tremblay, and G. Thériault. Heredity, human body fat and fat distribution. *Int. J. Obes.* 12: 205-215, 1988.
5. Després, J.P., S. Moorjani, A. Tremblay, E.T. Poehlman, P.J. Lupien, A. Nadeau, and C.

Bouchard. Heredity and changes in plasma lipids and lipoproteins and short-term exercise training in men. *Arteriosclerosis* 8: 402-409, 1988.

6. Lesage, R., J.A. Simoneau, J. Jobin, J. Leblanc, and C. Bouchard. Familial resemblance in maximal heart rate, blood lactate and aerobic power. *Hum. Hered.* 35: 182-189, 1985.

7. Lortie, G., J.A. Simoneau, P. Hamel, M.R. Boulay, F. Landry, and C. Bouchard. Responses of maximal aerobic power and capacity to aerobic training. *Int. J. Sports Med.* 5: 232-236, 1984.

8. Neel, J.V. A revised estimate of the amount of genetic variation in human proteins: Implications for the distribution of DNA polymorphisms. *Am. J. Hum. Genet.* 36: 1135-1148, 1984.

9. Pérusse, L., J.P. Després, A. Tremblay, C. Leblanc, J. Talbot, C. Allard, and C. Bouchard. Genetic and environmental deter-

minants of serum lipids and lipoproteins in French Canadian families. *Arteriosclerosis* 9: 308-318, 1989.

10. Pérusse, L., A. Tremblay, C. Leblanc, and C. Bouchard. Genetic and familial environmental influences on level of habitual physical activity. *Am. J. Epidemiol.* 129: 1012-1022, 1989.

11. Prud'homme, D., C. Bouchard, C. Leblanc, F. Landry, and E. Fontaine. Sensitivity of maximal aerobic power to training is genotype dependent. *Med. Sci. Sports Exerc.* 16: 489-493, 1984.

12. Scriver, C.R. Presidential address: Physiological genetics—Who needs it? *Am. J. Hum. Genet.* 40: 199-211, 1987.

13. Williams, R.J. *Biochemical individuality: The basis for the genetotrophic concept.* New York: John Wiley & Sons, 1956.

Chapter 15

Lifestyle, Fitness, and Health

Lester Breslow

Although physical activity as a factor in fitness and health is the main concern of this conference and its proceedings, the organizers have asked for some consideration of other aspects of lifestyle that relate to fitness and health. To be discussed here are eating behavior; sexual activity; use of alcohol, tobacco, and other drugs; motor vehicle driving; and social network. Lifestyle consists of behavior regarding all such options in living, including exercise or leisure-time physical activity. In a more complete sense it also embraces work; but space limitation precludes attention to that important aspect of lifestyle here.

This chapter focuses on lifestyle, apart from exercise, as it affects physiological fitness and health. According to this conference's definition, physiological fitness includes physical fitness but extends to all bodily systems that underlie health status. How well these systems are functioning may be determined by such measures as blood pressure, glucose tolerance, visual acuity, and lipoprotein profile. Both physiological fitness and the aspects of lifestyle discussed here are related to exercise as indicated in the conference model.

Until fairly recently, and still in many circles concerned with health, the paradigm for health improvement has been biomedical. Advances in understanding microorganisms and how to control them as agents of disease (along with progress in biomedical science generally) has led to widespread adoption of that approach to health. However, a growing body of evidence indicates that the noncommunicable diseases such as cancer and heart disease, which have become the major causes of morbidity and mortality, are mainly caused by lifestyle factors. The presumption and increasing evidence that these diseases can also be controlled largely by attention to lifestyle is rapidly expanding the scope of health endeavor. The fact that longevity in Canada, the United States, and several other countries has already reached 75 yr (and

prospects for good health during those years have increased) has stimulated examination of ways to achieve the full potential of life. That examination is becoming more directed to lifestyle, including physical activity, as a key factor in health.

Nature and Determinants of Lifestyle

The patterns of living that constitute an individual's lifestyle are made up of behaviors that a person adopts from among those available in the context of that person's life circumstances. Increasing recognition of how greatly these behaviors influence health has prompted inquiry into their nature and determinants.

Some observers emphasize the voluntary aspect of lifestyle and focus on what can be done to encourage selection of healthful options by individuals. Others contrast the difficulty of changing personal behavior as a means of improving health with what they see as the relative ease of implementing environmental measures that do not require individual action. Still others are concerned with the ethical dimensions of the problem, especially the idea of blaming the victim. These varying points of view all relate to what supposedly can be done to correct lifestyle as a factor in health.

It may be useful here to examine the origins of lifestyle as a basis for considering what can be done to improve health. Three sets of factors largely determine lifestyle: (a) biological, such as hunger and susceptibility to addiction; (b) circumstantial, for example, the availability of food and persons of the opposite gender; and (c) social influences on choice from the general community milieu and special groups of peers.

It is true that man does not live by bread alone, but food does come first in sustaining life and health. Hunger extends its influence on human behavior from seeking food when it is practically unobtainable to excessive indulgence when that becomes possible. Also, people try using various substances other than food to minimize hunger, for example, coca leaves, opiates, and nicotine-containing tobacco. They may find these substances pleasurable but then often become hooked on them because withdrawal evokes several kinds of discomfort and pain. The biological nature of humans thus forms the basis of behavior.

However, the expression of biological propensities is limited by the conditions of life. In North American cities those with income sufficient to eat in restaurants can obtain food from almost any part of the world, prepared according to recipes from scores of nationalities and ethnic groups. Along the Sepik River in Papua New Guinea, on the other hand, people have been so isolated and impoverished that they derive a very substantial portion of their calories from the carbohydrate obtained by running water through the chopped-up interior of sego palm trees (personal observation, 1985). Turning to another kind of appetite, heterosexuality cannot be expressed when no persons of the opposite sex are available. Thus, a human's innate urges can be satisfied only when the circumstances of life permit.

Within the limits established by biology and living situations, and with the latter expanding throughout the world, social influences largely determine lifestyle choices. As greater affluence extends the availability of options, both the larger social milieu and the closer social networks surrounding individuals overwhelmingly guide a person's lifestyle. For example, although national patterns of alcohol consumption are changing, the French are still known for wine, Germans for beer, and Scots for whiskey; North American drink all three. However, among people in some religious groups in North America, as well as in some Moslem countries, alcohol consumption is so deeply frowned on that very few drink at all. Tobacco use in many parts of the world is often strongly encouraged both by peers and by the social milieu, and establishing the habit before the age of 20 frequently leads to addiction.

Another evidence of social influence on lifestyle may be seen in the patterns of people who migrate from one country or region to another and begin to adopt the lifestyle of those who already live there. For example, Asians and people from Mexico and other parts of Latin America who move to the United States bring much of their social heritage and corresponding behavior with them; but they also begin to mix that lifestyle with the mores that they find in their new living circumstances.

The Relationship of Lifestyle to Physiological Fitness and Health

Lifestyle affects health through its impact on biological systems, principally the physiological, chemical, immunologic, and anatomical systems. For example, overeating results in obesity, a structural impairment that can adversely affect the cardiovascular system; overeating may also engender the disturbance of carbohydrate metabolism known as Type II, or non-insulin-dependent, diabetes. Tobacco smoke can alter the bronchial epithelium to the point of bronchogenic carcinoma besides affecting the cardiovascular system.

Through such observations the concept of risk factors is appearing more often in consideration of lifestyle, physiological fitness, and health (3). As usually employed, the term risk factors includes two categories: unhealthy elements of lifestyle and indicators of physiological or other biological disturbance. Either or both of these mean greater-than-normal risk of various diseases and premature death. Thus, elevated blood cholesterol (especially LDL cholesterol), high blood pressure, glucose intolerance, chewing snuff, drinking alcohol to excess, and a low level of physical activity are all risk factors. A new approach to health maintenance and health improvement has grown up around the notion of health risk appraisal (10). People are offered a series of physical measurements and questions about lifestyle designed to ascertain their prospects for health; sometimes the latter is formulated in terms of a so-called health age, which is based on population norms and can then be contrasted with one's chronological age.

Although the health-risk appraisal does convey significant information about health prospects, it is important also to differentiate behavior (lifestyle) clearly from bodily characteristics (physiological and other biological indicators) and particularly to examine their interrelationships. Within biological limits, behavior (lifestyle) largely determines one's bodily characteristics, that is, how far toward the healthful or the unhealthful end of the spectrum one's physical parameters will go. In turn these physiological and other biological characteristics underlie physical health status. This formulation gets us away from the notion of pure chance as the all-important factor in health (unfortunately still held by many people) and toward the concept of probability, which can be measured. Although the measurements in health risk appraisals are still relatively crude, progress is being made toward their improvement, and enough is already known for them to serve as a guide to health improvement. The extent to which this may be possible is illustrated in the discussion of lifestyle items that follows.

Selected Aspects of Lifestyle and Their Influence on Physiological Fitness and Health

Eating Behavior

One's place on the poverty-affluence scale in the community where one lives profoundly influences what one eats. People within a country (even residents of a whole country) who live at a low socioeconomic level tend to subsist largely on carbohydrates. These are mainly grains, roots, and other foods taken directly from the ground. Access to hunting and fishing permits a more varied diet.

As people attain greater means, they begin to use more meat and meat products from domesticated animals (along with other foods). As the economy moves increasingly toward feeding grain to animals, protein and the proportion of calories in the diet from fat increase.

People who are emerging from poverty into relative affluence encounter considerable risk of obesity from excessive consumption of calories, often largely in the form of fat. For example, an epidemic of Type II diabetes from excessive eating is now affecting people from the rural areas of Papua New Guinea who have recently entered commercial life in Port Moresby, enabling them for the first time to eat as much as they want (personal observation, 1985). A similar phenomenon can be seen among certain socially and economically disadvantaged minority groups in the United States as they come out of extreme poverty (6). With even greater affluence, people begin to eat fewer calories and especially less fat, perhaps responding to the notion that in so doing they may become less obese and thereby more attractive and healthy.

The two greatest problems in the eating behavior of Americans that have a substantial impact on physiological fitness and health are that many people do not eat enough of either total food or specific nutrients, and many people consume food, especially calories and fats, far beyond their bio-

logical needs and are actually overfilling their bodies.

Thus, being underweight or critically deficient in certain nutrients such as vitamins A and C is one nutritional affliction, and excessive bodily fat is the other. Each of these imposes well-known hazards onto health status: susceptibility to infection and other debilitating consequences on the one hand and increased likelihood of cardiovascular disease and possibly certain cancers on the other.

Within this general framework, other common and specific features of nutrition pertinent to health should be noted, including excessive consumption of salt, which appears to increase the risk of hypertension for some people; saturated fat, which contributes to elevated blood cholesterol and the consequent atherosclerosis; and sugar, which accelerates dental caries.

It should be emphasized that the biological taste for salt, fat, and sugar is quickly established. The influence of poverty on eating behavior, especially hunger, commonly gives way to overindulgence in unhealthful foods as soon as poverty is even partially overcome. That is why people living on relatively low incomes but not in extreme poverty manifest the greatest amount of obesity.

Sexuality

Next to hunger, sexual activity seems to be the most powerful biological urge. It takes many forms. Ideally, of course, sexual activity contributes tremendously both to direct satisfaction in life and to stability in the most profound human social relationship and support system, which itself enhances health and life. Unfortunately, biological urges and strong social influences converge on many individuals to provoke sexual behavior that carries the danger of seriously harmful consequences to health. Paramount risky behaviors are sexual promiscuity and beginning to engage in sexual intercourse at too young an age. Adding to the risks are failure to guard against the specific dangers themselves, for example, unwanted pregnancies and sexually transmitted diseases.

The age at which sexual activity starts varies with time and place. For example, in North America, under the influence of many factors during the 1980s, sexual intercourse typically begins in the teens (4).

Each year during the early 1980s, 8% of 18- to 19-yr-old girls in the United States were having babies; other rates were 5% of 17-yr-olds, 3% of 16-yr-olds, and 1.5% of 15-yr-olds. Among all girls in the age-group 15 to 17, 3.2% annually gave birth during 1978-1983 (13). Some high schools in urban areas with very high rates of pregnancy have had to establish day-care centers for infants so that the mothers can attend school. Not only does sexual activity start early in the United States, but it is evidently largely unprotected against sexually transmitted diseases as well as pregnancy.

In modern China on the other hand, at least until recently, sexual intercourse has apparently been uncommon before the age of 20. This difference in the sexual behavior of the Chinese severely limits teenage pregnancy and thus the extent of low-birth-weight infants and further consequences, both biological and social.

Unwanted pregnancies among teenage girls lead to huge numbers of low-birth-weight infants in the United States and is a substantial factor in that country's continuing relatively high infant mortality rate compared with other industrialized countries (14). Not only are an unnecessarily high number of babies thus lost but the mother's health and other prospects in life are often damaged by constriction of education and the opportunity to work. Many of the surviving daughters, raised without benefit of both parents, go on to repeat the cycle.

Promiscuity is not as well documented as is the early start of sexual intercourse, but it is obviously widespread in the United States, as evidenced by the high frequency of sexually transmitted diseases (13). The AIDS outbreak of the 1980s in North America and Western Europe that was originally due largely to homosexual promiscuity appears to be dampening that sexual practice. How much the AIDS epidemic will influence sexual behavior patterns remains to be determined.

Although sexual promiscuity often begins in the teens, at any age it is largely responsible for the spread of sexually transmitted diseases. The classical venereal diseases, syphilis and gonorrhea, continue to affect, respectively, tens of thousands and hundreds of thousands of Americans annually. Although reasonably effective therapy is generally available, the occurrence of cases and associated harm fundamentally reflect the lifestyle of those involved. In recent years two other sexually transmitted diseases have been attracting attention: chlamydial infections (previously often called nongonoccocal urethritis) and herpes. Not only are more than a million Americans affected with one or both of these infections annually, but chlamydial pneumonia strikes an estimated 720 per 100,000 children under 1 yr of age annually, and

neonatal disseminated herpes affected 17 per 100,000 neonates in 1979 (16).

Use of Alcohol

From antiquity, humans learned the pleasure of drinking fermented and, later, distilled liquors made principally from grain and fruit. Alcoholic beverages became a part of much ceremonial life, including religious and other festivities. They have been extensively incorporated into eating behavior and also are used simply for enhancing social occasions.

People of different cultures follow various patterns of alcohol consumption. For example, the Jews and the Irish have been known historically for contrasting drinking customs; on the other hand, observant Seventh Day Adventists and Mormons avoid alcohol completely. Poor people tend not to drink, apparently because they find it necessary to spend money on other things; but some slum dwellers who are in that situation because of alcohol problems spend a large portion of their incomes on the substance.

In the United States as of 1985, 35% of adults did not drink alcohol (13). Thirty-five percent were light drinkers (up to 1/5 oz of alcohol per day on average); 22% were moderate drinkers (1/5 to 1 oz), and 8% were heavy drinkers (1 oz or more per day). Almost one fourth of all adults sometimes consume five or more drinks in 1 day. The extent of alcohol consumption increases with level of income and is substantially greater among males than among females. About 5% of American adults are diagnosable as alcohol abusers or alcohol dependent. Excessive alcohol indulgence, as well as dependence (in the sense of increased tolerance and withdrawal symptoms), occurs especially among people with greater-than-usual vulnerability. There is a substantial familial (including genetic) component to that state.

As a toxic agent, alcohol affects the gastrointestinal system, especially the liver, causing cirrhosis. It also provokes digestive metabolic abnormalities resulting in nutritional deficiencies. In the nervous system, excessive alcohol can result in brain damage, sometimes with delirium tremens or depression; in the cardiovascular system, it can cause cardiomyopathy and arrhythmias. It also is a substantial factor in cancer of the oral cavity, larynx, and esophagus as well as in motor vehicle accidents and other types of trauma. Its involvement in the fetal-alcohol syndrome has only recently come into view. Finally, adverse effects, including physical trauma, of excessive alcohol on family and other social life are tremendous.

Alcohol-induced disease accounts for 20,000 deaths a year in the United States in addition to the 24,000 motor vehicle deaths involving alcohol and 30,000 deaths in other alcohol-related situations.

Because excessive alcohol causes so much distress to the individuals affected and to those around them, social efforts are periodically undertaken to reduce or even to eliminate consumption. For example, the temperance movement in the United States reached a climax in the early part of the 20th century with the enactment of a national prohibition. Experience with that policy, however, led to its abandonment after a few years. Other countries have taken advantage of the price elasticity in alcohol purchasing to lower consumption through taxation and to raise revenues. Many jurisdictions now seek control by limiting the time and places of purchase.

Although experience with alcohol by individuals apparently brings biological factors into play, trends in its use among groups of people and over time strongly reflect social influences.

Tobacco

American Indians were smoking tobacco when Europeans started colonization during the 16th century. Use of tobacco in various forms (smokeless, pipe, etc.) subsequently spread to many parts of the world. Its pleasant effects, compounded by the distress of unsatisfied craving for tobacco following habituation, leads to continuing dependence on the psychoactive component, nicotine. Withdrawal symptoms can be quite severe and make nicotine a difficult addiction to overcome; also, relapse is common. Although the use of tobacco was not uncommon before the 19th century, only when the cigarette appeared on the market did smoking become a daily activity among masses of people. Special impetus came from free distribution of the product to American soldiers who carried the cigarette home during and after World War I.

Although thoracic surgeons noted the connection between cigarettes and lung cancer in the 1930s, cigarette consumption kept expanding among men. The habit spread to women somewhat during the 1920s and did so on a mass scale about the time of World War II with the rise of feminism. It reached a peak about 1964, when the U.S. Surgeon General's report on smoking and health turned the tide (12). Since that time, smoking cigarettes has declined among men in the United States from more than 50% to about 30%. Women's smoking never reached the height of men's addiction and has also fallen to less than 30% (8).

North American and British tobacco companies, confronted by dwindling cigarette sales, have adopted a multifaceted strategy that includes an aggressive marketing approach to blacks, sports followers, and women through cultivating their special interests and linking smoking to those interests. The industry also has been making a bold effort to addict young people to snuff; at least until recently, that effort has achieved considerable sales among adolescents, with increasing oral cancer as a consequence. Finally, U.S. and British tobacco interests have been establishing markets in developing countries, often in collaboration with local companies.

Thus, tobacco use has become an element of lifestyle among hundreds of millions of people worldwide. Meanwhile, its economic roots in both centrally planned and market economies make it a huge societal problem for those concerned with health. In developing as well as in developed countries, cynical national leaders have been all too willing to trade short-term personal, corporate-economic, and political gains for long-term societal health consequences that are disastrous.

Although most of the knowledge concerning the health impact of tobacco has come directly from epidemiological studies, a fair amount is known about its physiological effects. Outstanding among these is nicotine's psychoactive properties. Habituated tobacco users suffer substantial withdrawal symptoms, including irritability, anxiety, and loss of the ability to concentrate. These symptoms may continue for weeks unless relieved by nicotine; this is why it is difficult to quit tobacco. Smoking cigarettes also leads to aortic and possibly coronary atherosclerosis, peripheral vascular disease, reduced cerebral blood flow, increased blood pressure, heart rate and myocardial contractility, and loss of the blood's oxygen-carrying capacity through formation of carboxy-hemoglobin (15). Furthermore, tobacco is carcinogenic to several tissues of the body, particularly the oral cavity, esophagus, larynx, lung, and bladder.

These profound effects on the body are responsible for the huge health toll: approximately 350,000 premature deaths annually in the United States alone, or almost 1,000 deaths per day. About one third of this excess mortality is due to lung cancer, even more to cardiovascular disease, and the remainder to other forms of cancer, chronic lung disease, and other conditions. In addition to this mortality, tobacco of course imposes a tremendous disability burden on the population. The economic cost of smoking in the United States is estimated at $50 billion, with about $15 billion in direct health care costs and $35 billion due mainly to lost productivity (5). Tobacco is the plague of our time.

Use of Other Drugs

Alcohol and tobacco consumptions are now so widespread that one tends to overlook the fact that these substances essentially are drugs and are sought largely for their psychoactive effects.

The human tendency to take advantage of substances with such properties may be seen further in the way people approach other groups of drugs. Poor people in the Andes Mountains long ago found relief from the pain of their lives by chewing coca leaves. That experience fountained the use of cocaine in various forms and social groups. Recently, many middle-class Americans have adopted the cocaine habit, and it now appears on the upswing in the United States (7). The popularity of LSD and similar psychedelic substances reached a peak in the 1960s and has since declined.

The cannabinoids, including marijuana, depend for their psychoactive effects on delta-9-textrahydrocannabinol. Marijuana in the United States is smoked primarily in social situations for inducing relaxation or making one intoxicated. Marijuana is tried by a high proportion of American teenagers, and a recent report indicates regular use by American high school seniors in about the same proportion as alcohol, or 6% (7). About 7% of adult Americans in 1982 reported marijuana use at least monthly, about 1% cocaine, 57% alcohol, and 32% cigarettes. The use of these substances, however, is substantially higher among young people, especially men aged 20-30, than among older adults.

Because of the magnitude of their effects on individuals, as well as the illegality and criminality associated with them, opiates and cocaine attract the most attention as drug problems. From the standpoint of lifestyle, however, few people take those drugs without earlier having used cigarettes, marijuana, or excessive amounts of alcohol.

Cocaine stimulates the cardiovascular system in a manner similar to that of nicotine, but cocaine more strongly induces euphoria. Addiction occurs, and withdrawal can become extremely uncomfortable. The combination of cocaine, alcohol, and sedatives to maintain a desired mental state often leads to profound disturbances and sometimes death.

Heroin, morphine, and other opiates, especially when taken intravenously, induce pleasurable mood changes as well as analgesia, peripheral vasodilatation, intestinal atony, and respiratory depression. After addiction, withdrawal results in agonizing gastrointestinal symptoms and other distress. Opiates may be the hardest of the so-called abused drugs because the effects are profound, addiction proceeds rapidly, and withdrawal symptoms are severe. Historically, traffic in illegal opiates has generated a considerable amount of crime, and the drug has even brought international conflict, as in the British-Chinese opium war. Criminal activity associated with the distribution of opiates and, increasingly, cocaine usually is countered by police efforts to deal with the problem. Violence often enters the lives of both those involved and some of those not involved in the use or the distribution of those substances.

Drug dependence and its consequences are extremely complex phenomena. Both individuals and society suffer substantial damage. Health effects of the drugs described here include death from overdose or violence in connection with obtaining a drug; personality deterioration and the increasing centrality of drug use in one's life; alienation from much social life; and the distress of actual or threatened withdrawal. Society also incurs tremendous harm from use of the drugs, including the loss of productivity and other social contributions by the individuals affected, expenditures for medical care and rehabilitation, and the cost of the struggle to contend with the deviant behavior as well as the extensive criminality associated with it.

Social efforts to deal with the drug problem are confounded because the problem has its roots in the biological propensity to explore various experiences and then, unfortunately in the case of many drugs, to become addicted. Furthermore, there is lack of clarity and social consensus on how far to proceed (or even whether to proceed) toward restricting the use of the various drugs.

Motor Vehicles

Motor vehicles have become the common mode of transportation in the industrialized parts of the world. Most adults travel in them from home to work, to go shopping, and to enjoy many leisure activities; and children are often carried in them.

The almost universal use of automobiles in many countries, coupled with the hazards involved in their operation, makes them important to health.

Injury from automobile use causes an estimated 250,000 deaths annually worldwide (17). The United States accounts for almost one fifth of these fatalities along with more than 1.5 million impairments, of which about one tenth are permanent. One fifth of the fatal crashes affect pedestrians, but this proportion is higher in urban areas; two fifths involve a single vehicle, and another two fifths involve two vehicles. Although the death rate from motor vehicle crashes has declined from about 40 per 100,000 registered vehicles in 1910 to 10 per 100,000 in 1920 and further to 2.8 in 1982, such deaths have continued to result in a very high rate of years of potential life lost.

Although a major factor in this toll is the youthfulness of those involved, the condition of the vehicle, the environmental circumstances, and the condition of the driver all contribute substantially to motor vehicle crashes.

From the standpoint of lifestyle, alcohol use is the paramount factor in fatal crashes. It is involved in about half of all killed drivers and in about one third of all adult pedestrians killed, overwhelmingly in amounts equal to or exceeding a blood alcohol concentration (BAC) of 0.10% by weight (17). Most killed passengers have BACs similar to those of their fatally injured drivers. The combination of young drivers and alcohol is especially hazardous. Lesser experience of young people with both alcohol and driving appears to increase their vulnerability to crashes. Irrespective of age or experience with alcohol, however, driving is impaired with BACs of 0.10 or above. Alcohol consumption shortly before or even while driving motor vehicles considerably increases the risk associated with them. Some countries, notably those in Scandinavia, enforce severe penalties for operating automobiles while under the influence of alcohol. Other countries, such as the United States, are quite lax in that regard.

Over the years many features of automobiles have improved safety. However, their potential for speed and the increased risk of crashes from the large numbers of them on streets and highways have tended to increase their hazard.

Although seat belts have become standard equipment for safety in automobiles, at least in North America, they are by no means always fastened for either adults or children. Pressure for more complete use of seat belts is gradually mounting, as reflected in legislation by the end of 1985 mandating seat-belt use in 16 states and the District of Columbia. Such legislation is being considered elsewhere. The prospect of air bags that inflate automatically at the time of a crash should also be noted. Corresponding to those who do not fasten seat belts in automobiles, motorcycle (and bicycle) riders who fail to wear helmets increase their risk of injury and death considerably.

Regarding automobile crashes as accidents complicates the problem. It conveys the notion that the events are acts of God or random occurrences that cannot be avoided. In fact, the evidence strongly supports the existence of a causative network that, if understood and dealt with, offers considerable promise of prevention.

Social Network

Besides all the features of lifestyle that have negative connotations for health, it is useful to consider the other side of the coin, for example, the positive effect of eating a healthy diet, wholesome sexual behavior, and driving automobiles safely. Prominent among the positive influences on one's health is the social network, or the connection between an individual and his or her social surrounding: family; close friends and relatives; and groups to which one belongs, such as churches, clubs, unions, and other socially organized institutions and agencies (2).

The social milieu (e.g., food, motor vehicles and drugs in the physical environment) exists independently of one's behavior toward it. The support for one's health, however, derives from a special kind of relationship in the case of social surroundings. Individuals enter into their social milieu and become part of it. The latter in turn influences behavior and in important ways affects health.

Families probably constitute the strongest social network. The absence of such ties (e.g., in divorced couples) is associated with elevated mortality (9). Recognition of that fact is increasing concern about social network as a lifestyle factor in health.

Industrialized society and the associated urban life has weakened family ties. For example, in the United States a substantial proportion of all marriages end in divorce; each year about half as many divorces occur as do marriages. Also, many couples now live together for lengthy periods (usually childless) without legal or religious ceremony or even much personal commitment. Sometimes, especially among older persons, that arrangement merely reflects financial (e.g., tax and social benefit) considerations; in many other situations, however, the tendency apparently signifies a more profound break with the traditional family.

Further evidence of family attenuation may be seen in the United States, particularly in the substantial proportion of single-parent families with young children. Fathers who abandon pregnant teenagers contribute significantly to the proportion of one-parent families, which sometimes extend through generations when young daughters follow the pattern of their mothers.

People living alone, especially those with no family members or other relatives or close friends living nearby, constitute another important group in American society whose health is adversely affected by an inadequate social network. The failure to provide appropriate community support for the deinstitutionalized mentally ill has aggravated their problems.

The support for health that is derived from a person's social network (often called *social support*) is increasingly recognized as very substantial. For many years investigators have noted that single, divorced, and widowed people experience poorer health and higher mortality than do married people. Now evidence indicates that one's entire social network, not just family ties, is involved in this phenomenon (2). That larger network extends beyond family to include close friends and relatives as well as church and other groups. Weakness in one element may be compensated by strength in another. The strength of the entire social network is strongly and positively associated with subsequent health and longevity.

The physiological or other mechanisms by which health support comes from the social network remain to be unraveled. Although plausible explanations have been advanced to explain the phenomenon (which is an epidemiological finding), research has made little progress in confirming or rejecting any of the hypotheses.

Lifestyle Patterns

Single elements of lifestyle, or individualized bits of behaviors reflecting biological nature and social circumstances, occur mainly in combination. An extreme and well-recognized constellation of lifestyle elements occurs among, for example, young, urban-ghetto residents in the United States who exhibit poor eating habits; use of tobacco, excessive alcohol, and other drugs; dangerous driving habits; early and promiscuous sexual ac-

tivity; and an inadequate social network. At the other end of the spectrum, middle-aged and older persons in more favored sections of the same cities tend to follow a lifestyle that has elements opposite to those of the ghetto residents. Of course, lifestyles adverse to health include inadequate physical exercise in addition to the elements noted here. The extent to which such lifestyle affects health in North America and other industrialized nations, though not fully documented, is obviously considerable.

One's standard of living underlies and profoundly affects one's lifestyle. In fact, one's basic social conditions (e.g., level of income and education, place of dwelling, and job opportunities) constitute an overwhelming determinant of lifestyle. It is within that pervasive situation, called the standard of living, that the detailed elements of lifestyle described in this section are subject to social influences at their interface with biology.

One effort to delineate lifestyle pattern for the purpose of evaluating its health impact focused on seven so-called health practices: eating moderately, exercising at least moderately, eating breakfast, eating regularly (not just snacking), not smoking cigarettes, drinking moderately or not at all, and sleeping 7-8 hr each night (1). The number of these items one followed yielded one's health practice score. At all ages from 20 to 70, those with a health practice score of 7 had better health status than did those with 6; 6 was better than 5, 5 was better than 4, 4 was better than 3, and 3 was better than 2 or fewer. The health practice score was also strongly and positively associated with subsequent longevity. A beginning effort to track the seven practices over time revealed a decline in smoking from 1977 to 1983, but results for the other practices showed no improvement and some losses or were equivocal (11).

From a consideration of individual components of lifestyle such as those described here and from an examination of lifestyle as a pattern, it is evident that lifestyle is profoundly related to health.

Although it is useful to focus on individual items (e.g., physical activity), this should be done with an understanding of that piece as an element of a larger pattern of behavior that affects health.

References

1. Belloc, N.B., and L. Breslow. Relationship of physical health status and health practices. *Prev. Med.* 13: 409-421, 1972.

2. Berkman, L.F., and S.L. Syme. Social networks, host resistance and mortality. *Am. J. Epidemiol.* 109: 186-204, 1979.

3. Breslow, L. Risk factor intervention for health maintenance. *Science* 200: 908-912, 1978.

4. Eubank, D. Population and public health. In: Last, J.M., ed. *Public health and preventive medicine.* Norwalk, CT: Appleton-Century-Crofts, 1986, Chapt. 3, p. 75-99.

5. Fielding, J.F. Smoking: Health effects and control. In: Last, J.M., ed. *Public health and preventive medicine.* Norwalk, CT: Appleton-Century-Crofts, 1986, Chapt. 26, p. 999-1038.

6. Heckler, M.M. *Report of the Secretary's Task Force on Black and Minority Health* (DHHS Publication No. 0-487-637 [QL3]). Washington, DC: U.S. Government Printing Office, 1985.

7. Johnson, C.A. Prevention and control of drug abuse. In: Last, J.M., ed. *Public health and preventive medicine.* Norwalk, CT: Appleton-Century-Crofts, 1986, Chapt. 28, p. 1075-1087.

8. Massachusetts Medical Society. Cigarette smoking in the United States. *Morbid. Mortal. Week. Rep.* 36: 581-585, 1987.

9. Ortmeyer, C.F. Variations in mortality, morbidity, and health care by marital status. In: Erhardt, L.L., and J.E. Berlin, eds. *Mortality and morbidity in the United States.* Cambridge, MA: Harvard University Press, 1974, p. 159-188.

10. Robbins, L.C., and J.W. Hall. *How to practice prospective medicine.* Indianapolis: Slaymaker Enterprises, 1970.

11. Schoenborn, C.A., and B.H. Cohen. Trends in smoking, alcohol consumption, and other health practices among U.S. adults, 1977 and 1983. *Advance Data from Vital and Health Statistics, No. 118* (DHHS Publication No. [PHS] 86-1250). Hyattsville, MD: Public Health Service, June 1986.

12. U.S. Department of Health, Education and Welfare. Public Health Service. The Surgeon General's Advisory Committee on Smoking and Health. *Smoking and health* (PHS Publication No. 1103). Washington, DC: U.S. Government Printing Office, 1964.

13. U.S. Department of Health and Human Services. *Health United States* (DHHS Publication No. [PHS] 88-1232). Washington, DC: U.S. Government Printing Office, 1988.

14. U.S. Department of Health and Human Services. Public Health Service. National Center for Health Statistics. *Proceedings of the International Collaborative Effort on Perinatal and Infant Mortality* (DHHS Publication No. [PHS] 85-1252). Washington, DC: U.S. Government Printing Office, 1985, vol. 1.

15. U.S. Department of Health and Human Services. Public Health Service. Office of Smoking and Health. *The health consequences of smoking, cardiovascular disease* (DHHS Publication No. [PHS] 84-50204). Washington, DC: U.S. Government Printing Office, 1983.

16. U.S. Department of Health and Human Services. *Promoting health/preventing disease—Objectives for the nation.* Washington, DC: U.S. Government Printing Office, 1980.

17. Waller, J.A. Prevention of premature death and disability due to injury. In: Last, J.M., ed. *Public health and preventive medicine.* Norwalk, CT: Appleton-Century-Crofts, 1986, Chapt. 50, p. 1543-1576.

Chapter 16

Exercise and the Environment

John R. Sutton

Among the most enjoyable experiences available to us are walking in the mountains, cross-country skiing on a cold winter's day, or jogging in the spring or on a summer's evening. Yet our physiological responses to exercise will be very different under each of these environmentally different circumstances. Each response is intended to maintain internal thermal or oxygen homeostasis. Furthermore, if the exposure is gradual and prolonged, adaptations occur that will promote the success of exercise in these surroundings. Our level of cardiorespiratory fitness is also important in our ability to exercise in these environments, but an important distinction must be made between the ability to perform exercise and the predisposition to the specific health hazards associated with exercise in the heat or the cold or at various altitudes. In this chapter, I briefly review the physiological responses but emphasize the interaction of humans in these environments as well as the potential health hazards and their prevention and treatment. For more details about the basic physiology, see the *Handbook of Physiology* (6) and other basic texts (13, 15, 21, 24, 26, 27, 42, 48, 51, 55, 61, 64, 65, 71, 76, 79, 98, 99, 102, 116, 118, 121).

Thermal Effects

Exercise in the Heat and Cold

For maximum efficiency, we must maintain our internal body temperatures. This feature is unique to birds and mammals only during the past 70 million yr but has conferred an important evolutionary advantage, making them independent of the environment (32). Thus, at the expense of a high metabolic rate, we can maintain our core temperatures within narrow limits in spite of a wide range

of environmental temperatures. In fact, at 37 °C we are close to the ceiling of thermal viability compared with the lower end of the temperature scale. So we have evolved much more elaborate temperature regulatory mechanisms to prevent overheating rather than overcooling. Figure 16.1 illustrates how we are able to preserve deep body temperature throughout a wide range of environmental temperatures and the mechanisms that operate to achieve this.

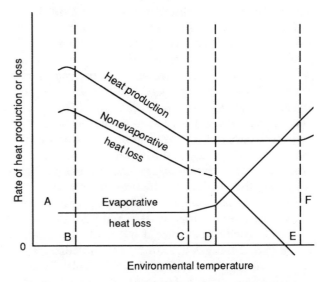

Figure 16.1. Relationship between heat production, evaporative and nonevaporative heat loss, and deep body temperature in a homeothermic animal. A = zone of hypothermia; B = temperature of summit metabolism and incipient hypothermia; C = critical temperature; D = temperature of marked increase in evaporative loss; E = temperature of incipient hyperthermial rise; F = zone of hyperthermia; CD = zone of least thermoregulatory effort; CE = zone of minimum metabolism; and BE = thermoregulatory range. These zones were defined by Mount (74).

165

Thermal Exchange

There are three bidirectional avenues of thermal exchange between the body and the environment: conduction, convection, and radiation. There is one unidirectional change: evaporation of heat lost from the body to the atmosphere. This is expressed in the heat storage equation of Winslow (125):

$$S = M \pm R \pm Cv \pm Cd - E$$

where S is heat storage, M is metabolic heat production, R is heat gained or lost through radiation, Cv is heat gained or lost by convection, Cd is heat gained or lost by conduction, and E is heat loss from evaporation. Although one can respond physiologically to a hot or a cold environment, it is important to emphasize that the most important factors enabling us to exercise under conditions of environmental extremes are behavioral, not physiological. That is, we really depend on protecting ourselves with insulated clothing and seeking shelter from immoderate heat or cold; these measures have allowed us to survive and exercise in such situations.

In the cold, the two primary physiological responses are the abilities to regulate blood flow within the body and to increase skin blood flow when there is a need to dissipate heat from the core to the surface or restrict skin blood flow when it is necessary to reduce skin heat loss and maintain the body's core temperature. Additionally, we can increase heat production several fold. Thus, we have a thermoregulatory system that appears to operate around a thermal set-point, sensing information from the core and the skin so that, whenever the core temperature varies from that set-point, the appropriate heatproducing or heat-losing mechanisms are stimulated during exercise or by a primary change in skin temperature at a constant core temperature if the heat load is external (54). Changes in skin blood flow also alter the central circulation in both heat and cold. Training improves our adaptation to cold (1); Raven et al. (91) demonstrated that shivering caused an increase in cardiac output, predominantly by increasing stroke volume. Rowell et al. (103) and Hales (40) have demonstrated that any increase in skin blood flow will be accompanied by decreases in renal and splanchnic blood flow. Exercising in the heat will also result in an increase in skin blood volume, a factor that will be clinically important in the production of syncope when people stop exercising at the end of a race but remain upright, develop venous pooling in the legs, and become syncopal.

The combination of heat acclimatization and increased physical fitness has been well demonstrated to enhance performance in the heat. Wyndham (126), Piwonka and Robinson (83), and Gisolfi and Robinson (33) showed that trained individuals had a greater heat dissipating capacity than did the untrained. Part of this is due to the increased sensitivity of sweating mechanisms with training and a lowering of the sweating threshold (75). Another important factor in the increased heat tolerance of the fit individual is the increased blood volume induced by training. This was recently demonstrated by Senay et al. (104), Convertino et al. (18), Fortney et al. (28), and Green et al. (34). This topic was well reviewed by Harrison (45).

Women have been considered to be at a disadvantage compared with men when exercising in the heat because of their substantially lower sweat rate (30, 49, 127). A further gender-related difference is the greater ratio of surface area to weight (A_D/wt) of women. However, this issue is considerably more complex. When skin temperature is above ambient temperature, an increased A_D/wt would be an advantage to women because of the relatively larger surface area available for heat loss in comparison to the mass available for heat production. Per unit of volume of sweat produced, women reach a lower body core temperature than do men and therefore have been considered more efficient temperature regulators (23). Differences in cardiorespiratory fitness between men and women may also be responsible for differences in thermal response (22, 23, 80, 123). The importance of cardiorespiratory fitness in determining the differences in temperature regulation between men and women was recently addressed by Avellini et al. (7), who selected men and women with identical cardiorespiratory fitness, equal surface areas, and equal ratios of surface area to mass. Although the numbers were small (4 in each group), in an acute heat stress study the women in the follicular phase had lower sweat rates, rectal temperatures, and heart rates than did the men. Following 10 d of acclimatization, the differences between the genders were eliminated. The rectal temperatures and heart rates were similar. The sweat rate increased during exercise in both groups, but more so in the men, suggesting that sweating was more effective in the women.

Thermal Maladaptations to Exercise in the Cold

Hypothermia results when the rate of heat loss exceeds that of heat production. The symptoms at progressively decreasing body core temperatures are shown in Table 16.1. Although we tend to think of hypothermia as occurring in wilderness areas associated with outdoor activities such as hiking, skiing, or climbing, the recreational athlete is also vulnerable. I was first made aware of hypothermia in joggers in an article called "Jogging in Tasmania," in which the author mistakenly referred to athletes dying of heatstroke (100). The author had confused September weather in the Southern Hemisphere with that in North America and compared the deaths in Tasmania with a jogger's similar death by heat stroke in a hot, polluted summer environment in Boston. The unfortunate victims in Hobart had actually become hypothermic and froze to death (110)! As most joggers and fun runners are very lightly clad, it is a common occurrence that more poorly trained, inexperienced runners may start off running at a pace at which their heat production outstrips heat loss; however, in the later stages of the race, this situation is reversed so that they become hypothermic, as Maughan et al. have established (67).

Table 16.1   Clinical Symptoms of Hypothermia

Core temperature (°C)	Symptoms and signs
37	Feeling of cold; skin cooling; decreased social interaction
36	Goose pimples
35	Shivering; muscle tension; fatigue
34.5	Deep cold Numbness Loss of coordination Stumbling Dysarthria Muscle rigidity
32	Disorientation Decreased visual acuity
31-30	Semicoma—coma
28	Ventricular fibrillation and cardiovascular death

Note. From L.E. Hart and J.R. Sutton, 1987, *Clinical Cardiology*, **5**, p. 246.

The various factors associated with hypothermia in the mountains were well illustrated in Pugh's article about four Boy Scouts who died during the Four Inns Walking Competition in 1964 (85). First,

under cold, wet, and windy conditions, Pugh demonstrated that the walkers were less efficient, requiring a greater $\dot{V}O_2$ for the constant external work up to an oxygen uptake of nearly 2-2.5 L when compared with exercise in dry, warm conditions. Achieving the same speed necessitated working at a higher percentage of $\dot{V}O_2max$, with the result that they tired more readily. Second, at low work levels, rectal temperature was lower. Finally, when exercise stopped, heat generation decreased and rectal temperature plummeted, increasing the likelihood of death from hypothermia (85). In all circumstances, the physiological factors were less important than were the behavioral ones, that is, knowing how to prepare and dress and judging when to seek rest and shelter (87).

Immersion Hypothermia

In all the instances mentioned previously, the decrease in body temperature is relatively slow in contrast to the situation that occurs with immersion hypothermia, when the rate of cooling may be 20 to 30 times faster, and death may ensue very rapidly. This is an ever-present risk for canoeists, rafters, Windsurfers, and sailors in northern regions, especially in the early spring or autumn. Although body habitus plays a role, with the more obese being better protected (90), exercise will result in an increased temperature in more of the body surface area, thus promoting more heat loss (47). Most advantages are derived from the use of flotation devices such as U-Vic Thermofloat and wet suits (47). Best of all are survival rafts such as Sea-Seat, which enables a subject to sit out of the water, thus removing high heat-loss areas from the water and minimizing heat loss.

Prevention and Treatment of Hypothermia

An appreciation that hypothermia is a constant danger when exercising in the outdoors is essential to survival. It is important to appreciate the early subtle symptoms of mild disorientation, shivering, and personality changes. In the wilderness, seeking a campsite early, erecting shelter, and warming an individual with food and fluids before his or her state deteriorates or becomes life threatening is of fundamental importance.

Once hypothermia has developed, the most appropriate actions to be taken in the field are to prevent further heat loss. These have been reviewed recently by Bangs (8), Moss (72), and Mills et al. (70). The management of hypothermia in the field and in the hospital is beyond the scope of this presentation, but the reader is referred to recent works of Mills et al. (70) and Bohn (10). The old adage of no one being dead until he or she is "warm dead" is still a worthwhile approach; a recent report from Switzerland in which three supposedly dead skiers were treated aggressively and recovered completely emphasizes this point (4). The most severely affected of those three who were caught in an avalanche was a 42-yr-old male with a rectal temperature of 19 °C. He had a cardiorespiratory arrest and was transferred to a hospital by helicopter where he was given CPR, was actively rewarmed by partial femorofemoral bypass, and then made a complete recovery. It should be remembered that in our society hypothermia most commonly occurs in association with drugs, especially alcohol (81).

Frostbite

Like hypothermia, localized freezing of tissues is preventable. The most vulnerable sites usually are the digits of the hands and feet, the nose, the ears, the chin, and any other exposed skin. Any numbness of the fingers or toes, as well as patches of white skin in these exposed areas, requires immediate warming (for more detail on this subject, see refs. 69, 82).

Hyperthermia

Hyperthermia is a normal concomitant of exercise and has been documented in marathons (89) and fun runs (114). The problems related to an excessive body core temperature may occur when the environmental circumstances do not appear to be particularly extreme or even when the day is cold (114). With exercise, there is a normal shift in the circulating fluid volume. Adolph (3) demonstrated that water was disproportionately lost from plasma compared with other body tissues. Moreover, if significant dehydration occurs, the heat-dissipating mechanisms will be compromised further. In the competition between the skin and muscle for blood flow (a competition accentuated by exercise), for a comparable external heat stress skin blood flow will be lower compared with the resting state (103). Studies by Hales et al. (43) have demonstrated that during severe heat stress skin blood flow begins to fall. The same situation pertains when central venous pressure is reduced by lower body negative pressure (74, 128). When these data are taken in concert, Rowell (101) concluded that the hierarchy of homeostatic mechanisms favors the maintenance of arterial pressure and circulation to the vital organs at the expense

of skin vasodilatation and thermoregulation. In the most recent publication concerning circulatory changes in collapsed fun runners, Hales et al. (43) have demonstrated a marked reduction in skin blood flow when compared to control runners. They postulated that the reduction in skin blood flow occurred when right-heart filling pressures were reduced. To date, no human data are available to support this hypothesis, although supportive animal data do exist (41).

Heat Exhaustion and Heatstroke

The organs affected in exertional heat injury are tabulated in Table 16.2. Although most of the early reports emphasized the importance of dehydration and described patients arriving with dry, parched skin, various clinical manifestations are relevant to marches in the desert but not to collapsed fun runners. More than 80% of these patients have been reported to have moist, cold skin, yet their rectal temperatures may well be 42-43 °C (96, 97, 114; for a detailed description of the pathophysiological changes seen in heatstroke, see refs. 17, 19, 44, 46, 58, 59, 60, 63, 77, 106, 108, 111). Heat syncope is common when runners stop running and develop gravitational venous pooling in association with the decreased effect of the muscle pump to stimulate venous return.

Prevention and Management of Heatstroke, Heat Exhaustion, and Heat Syncope

Exertional heatstroke and other thermal illnesses are preventable, but the athlete and the organizers and medical directors of fun runs need to be aware that such possibilities exist. Furthermore, a simple understanding of the pathophysiological mechanisms involved in the genesis of heatstroke will prevent tragedies such as army recruits running in wet suits and succumbing to heatstroke (11). The interaction of the susceptible runner with a given set of environmental circumstances sets the stage for heat illness and heatstroke. It is important to appreciate that high humidity with high solar radiation on a windless day reduces the body's ability to lose heat by the most effective means, evaporation. Evidence suggests that the most susceptible individuals include the young, the old, and those who are dehydrated, ill, obese, unfit, and lack heat acclimatization (112). Also, many fun runs are held in the spring, when runners are still unacclimatized. They often train in the cool of the

Table 16.2 Clinical Manifestations of Exertional Heat Injury

System	Comment
Cardiovascular	
Sinus tachycardia	Invariable finding
Transient hypertension	Rare
Hypotension and shock	Rare
Acute left-heart failure	Rare; higher incidence in older population
Pulmonary	
Hyperventilation	Common finding
Pulmonary edema	Rare: present as final complication before death
Pulmonary infarction	Rare
Neurologic	
Delirium, hallucinations, status epilepticus, oculogyric crises, opisthotonus	Occur fairly commonly; manifestations of hyperirritability that often occur in association with nervous system depression
Coma	A feature of moderate to severe heat stroke
Cerebellar syndromes	Rare
Hemiplegic episodes	Rare
Renal	
Acute nephropathy	Occurs in 50% of patients who develop heat stroke
Chronic interstitial nephritis	Uncommon
Hematologic	
Purpura; conjunctival hemorrhage; manifestation of bleeding into lungs, kidneys, myocardium, liver, or central nervous system	Occurs with bleeding diathesis. Rare, but when it occurs, prognosis is very poor.
Gastrointestinal	
Diarrhea and vomiting	Common, especially during first 24 hr
Hematemesis and melena	Rare; occur in association with bleeding diathesis
Endocrine	
Clinical signs of hypoglycemia (blood sugar levels of < 25 mg/dl)	Uncommon
Musculoskeletal	
Muscles rigid and contracted	Common finding; associated with elevation in serum enzymes and myoglobinuria

Note. From L.E. Hart and J.R. Sutton, 1987, *Clinical Cardiology,* **5,** p. 250.

morning or evening but compete when the environmental conditions are hottest. Also, at this time of year an unseasonably hot day following weeks of cold weather is not uncommon. Hughson et al. (53) have shown that many of the runners who collapse with heatstroke are trying to outdo themselves with their best-ever times and fail to heed the early warning signals of impending disaster.

Management of Heat Illness

Heat exhaustion and heat stroke are part of a continuum, the principle difference between them being the alteration of consciousness in heat stroke. Hyperthermia usually above 39.5 °C and sometimes as high as 43 °C is seen in both (95). The most important point to emphasize is that treatment must begin on-site. This highlights organizational strategies and the need to be able to diagnose accurately with measurement of core temperature and to institute cooling therapy, including that with intravenous fluids at the race site. Delay can be fatal. Many race organizers identify the nearest hospital emergency room facilities to be used for collapsed runners or casualties; however, this will postpone the onset of treatment and may jeopardize the patient unnecessarily. In the experience of several hundred thousands of runners, no serious sequelae have resulted when resuscitation and cooling have been instituted at the race site. However, the converse has not been the case (46, 93, 94, 96). We are aware of more than a dozen fatalities that have occurred when resuscitation facilities were not available immediately on-site. Furthermore, when the runner reaches the emergency room, the realization of a potentially life-threatening illness may not always be apparent to the attending staff; there may be a delay in establishing the correct diagnosis by measuring core temperature and a further lag in instituting treatment.

With the diagnosis established, the essential features of treatment include intravenous therapy to reestablish the circulation and cooling. Cooling with a fan and a fine warm spray (122) was a method introduced to treat Mecca pilgrims, an approach that Keilblock (57) has shown to be the most effective means to reduce the elevated temperature when compared with several alternatives.

It is important to appreciate that both hypothermia and hyperthermia can occur in the same race. The 30-km Billy Sherring Round the Bay race held in Hamilton, Ontario, is the oldest distance race in North America; it was established in 1894 and has been held annually at the end of March, when weather conditions are usually cool. Although the front runners will finish with elevated temperatures, the winds off the lake invariably cool the slower runners to the extent that some become hypothermic. At this time of year, unseasonably hot days may also occur before any runner has had a chance to become acclimatized to heat. The medical directors of runs held in the spring and autumn must prepare to treat some casualties who are too hot as well as others who may be too cold. Accurate measurement of rectal (core) temperature with an "IVAC" or low-reading thermometer is essential to establish the diagnosis and follow with the corresponding treatment.

In an attempt to educate organizers of fun runs to the potential hazards, the American College of Sports Medicine (5) has issued a position stand, "Prevention of Thermal Injuries During Distance Running," a revision of which will be available in 1989. This document also has been translated into language suitable for the lay public and is available from the college.

Altitude

On ascent to altitude, the primary stress is that of the low oxygen pressure paralleling the decreased barometric pressure. This decreases in an exponential manner until, at the equivalent of the summit of Mount Everest, barometric pressure is approximately 250 torr, giving an inspired oxygen pressure of 43 torr (84, 124). In addition, many of the stresses we have considered under the topic of hypothermia are also present in the mountain environment. The combination of cold and hypoxia appears to be additive; these interactions have been addressed recently at the International Hypoxia Symposium (115).

The physiological responses to increasing altitude attempt to restore oxygen homeostasis, and adaptations occur in most of the links in the oxygen transport chain from air to tissue as well as structural and biochemical changes within various tissues. Nevertheless, the actual response that occurs will depend on the duration of exposure to hypoxia and will be very different in the case of acute hypoxia, such as an aviator who loses an oxygen mask compared to a climber who has spent weeks to months in a mountain environment. This is again quite different from the high-altitude native who has lived in central Asia or the Andes for many years.

Responses to Moderate Altitude

The selection of Mexico City (elevation 2,270 m above sea level) as the venue for the 1968 Olympic Games demonstrated the effects of even moderate altitude on physical performance. A decrease in wind resistance allowed sprinters to perform better at higher elevations than they could at sea level, but most middle- and long-distance runners were severely affected. It appeared that athletes who came from sea level were at a definite disadvantage; this was graphically demonstrated in the final of the 10,000-m track event when Ron Clarke, then the holder of the world record for that distance, finished in sixth place in a state of collapse. All those finishing ahead of him were either native to high altitude or had lived there for prolonged periods (48). The winning time, which was almost 2 min slower than that of the world record, reflected the general trend seen in most of the distance events (48, 88).

Several studies examining the effects of moderate altitude on athletic performance were stimulated by the Mexico City Olympics (14, 25, 48, 88, 107). Pugh (88) and Sime et al. (107) found a reduction in the performances of athletes at moderate altitude, concluding that submaximal exercise at sea level is nearly maximal at even moderate altitudes and that relatively little can be done to improve performance. Pugh examined the effect of acclimatization on his distance runners. In 3-mi time trials conducted 4 d after arrival in Mexico City, the athletes took an average of 8.5% longer to complete their runs than they did at sea level. On the 29th day following arrival, performances were 5.7% slower. This gain of 2.8% translated into a 20-s gain over 3 mi following acclimatization. The slowing effect of altitude on the longer events is even more pronounced, amounting to 17%-22% over the marathon distance (48).

Thus, an athlete's chance of success during competition at altitudes comparable to that of Mexico City depends on his or her response to hypoxia, the time allowed for acclimatization, and the competitor's usual resident altitude. The changes recorded in Pugh's subjects following 1 mo of acclimatization seem minimal; nonetheless, there was some measure of improvement. Perhaps adaptation periods of months rather than weeks are necessary for more significant changes.

The effect of altitude training on athletic performance at sea level is also of great interest (48, 105). Findings so far have been inconclusive, and the benefits seem little more than marginal (2).

Physiological Responses to Prolonged Hypoxia

Increased ventilation is one of the most important responses to prolonged hypoxia. Set at the beginning of the oxygen transport chain, this has a profound effect on adaptations downstream. The immediate response is a decrease in PCO_2, which will result in increased alveolar oxygen and therefore arterial oxygen. This has been most recently studied in the project Operation Everest II (52). The arterial blood gases found at the equivalent of the summit of Mount Everest were 11 torr PCO_2 and 30 torr PO_2 (120). The major adaptations in oxygen transport are illustrated in Figure 16.2. Hematologic responses are also important; at the equivalent of the Everest base camp, there is approximately a one-third increase in hemoglobin and hematocrit. Although this was one of the first adaptations described in the literature, Cerretelli (16) has questioned what an optimal hemoglobin might be. A detailed discussion of this is found in the articles by Buick et al. (12) and Winslow (125).

An increase in cardiac output is seen in response to exercise, and the relationship is accentuated with acute hypoxia. Following prolonged exposure, however, this relationship is similar to findings at sea level (37, 86). Groves et al. (37) have also shown a significant pulmonary hypertension

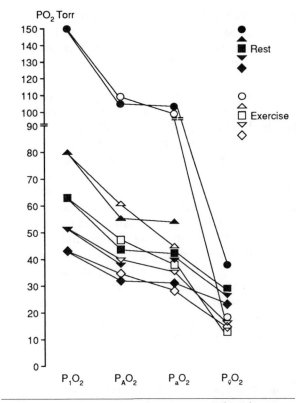

Figure 16.2. Oxygen tension at rest and with exercise at crucial steps in the oxygen transport cascade from inspired air to mixed venous blood. Closed circles = sea level P_IO_2 of 149 torr; closed deltas = P_IO_2 of 80 torr; closed squares = P_IO_2 of 63 torr; closed inverted deltas = P_IO_2 of 49 torr; and closed diamonds = P_IO_2 of 43 torr.

that is not completely reversed following administration of 100% oxygen, suggesting that chronic structural changes may occur. At the tissue level, maximal oxygen extraction appears to occur, but at altitudes beyond 6,100 m, evidence from Operation Everest II suggests that the mixed venous oxygen at 10 torr cannot be lowered (120). Studies in human muscle showed that mountaineers have reduced muscle fiber size; this results in an increased muscle capillary density, which may be an additional advantage in oxygen diffusion to the cell (66, 78). These workers also found an increased mitochondrial density. Metabolic pathways also are altered at altitude, and although glycolysis appears to be enhanced, maximum glycolytic flux is reduced with reductions in maximum muscle and plasma lactate (35).

Altitude Maladaptations

Provided that the ascent to altitude has been sufficiently gradual, the physiological responses previously mentioned will occur, and the individual will make appropriate adjustments; however, one will never be able to perform exercise at extreme altitude as well as one can at sea level. On the other hand, if the rate of ascent and the altitude reached have been too great for the individual, certain problems may arise, some of which may be life threatening. All altitude illnesses, with the exception of acute hypoxia, take some time to develop, usually hours after the initial hypoxic insult (Table 16.3); therefore, it is not the hypoxia per se that is responsible for the pathophysiological changes. Marked changes in the cerebral and pulmonary circulation occur. Sutton and Lassen (119) have hypothesized that the changes in both these circulations may be primarily responsible for the development of the cerebral and pulmonary manifestations of altitude illness. The best description of acute mountain sickness (AMS) was given by Dr. T.H. Ravenhill, a physician for a small mining company in the Andes:

It is a curious fact that the symptoms of puna [AMS] do not usually evince themselves at once. The majority of newcomers have expressed themselves at being quite well on first arrival. As a rule, towards evening, the patient begins to feel rather slack and disinclined to exertion. He goes to bed but has a restless and troubled night and wakes up the next morning with a severe frontal headache. There may be vomiting; frequently there is a sense of oppression in the chest, but there is rarely any respiratory distress or alteration in the normal rate of breathing so long as the patient is at rest. The patient may feel slightly giddy on rising from the bed, and any attempt at exertion increases the headache, which is nearly always confined to the frontal region. . . . The headache increases towards evening, so also does the pulse rate; all appetite is lost and the patient wishes to be alone—to sleep if possible. Generally, during the second night he is able

Table 16.3   Features of the Different Forms of Altitude Illness

Illness	Description
Acute mountain sickness (AMS)	Symptoms include headache, insomnia, nausea, vomiting, ataxia, and disturbed consciousness Affects anyone who goes high enough, quickly enough Symptoms are accentuated by physical exercise Unpleasant but not serious Descent brings dramatic relief
Chronic mountain sickness (CMS)	Also known as Monge's disease Only seen in long-term altitude dwellers Pulmonary hypertension, polycythemia, mental deterioration Descent to sea level ensures recovery
High-altitude pulmonary edema (HAPE)	Develops as dyspnea and dry cough but later progresses to cough with pink frothy sputum, indicative of severe hypoxemia; cyanosis Serious; rapid descent mandatory or death ensues Oxygen administration may be useful Some investigators recommend diuretic therapy (Furosemide, 40 mg intravenously)
High-altitude cerebral edema (HACE)	Severe headache, mental confusion, hallucinations, ataxia, weakness, and coma Rare but very serious Descent to lower altitude mandatory Intravenous steroids (betamethasone, 4 mg every 4 hr) recommended

Miscellaneous conditions	High altitude retinal hemorrhage (HARH)
	  Common above 5,000 m; usually asymptomatic; resolves without treatment
	Edema of face and periphery
	Circulation problems such as thrombophlebitis and embolism
	  Unusual but serious when they do occur
	Sickle-cell crises
	  Persons with sickle-cell trait may develop crises at even moderate altitudes

Note. From J.R. Sutton, 1983, *Seminars in Respiratory Medicine*, **5**, pp. 129-130.

to do so and, as a rule, wakes the next morning feeling much better. . . . By the fourth day, he is probably much better and at the end of a week is fit again. (92)

Although epidemiological studies have been difficult, Hackett et al. (38) described a 50% incidence of acute mountain sickness in trekkers on the route to Everest. These workers also noted that the incidence was considerably higher in those who flew to altitude than in those who gradually acclimated by walking.

High-Altitude Pulmonary Edema (HAPE)

High-altitude pulmonary edema was also recognized by Ravenhill, although the first clear description in English was given by Charles Houston (50). We now recognize this to be a life-threatening illness whose principle symptoms are extreme breathlessness and a dry cough that later produces frothy and sometimes bloody sputum. Clinical examination reveals marked respiratory distress, cyanosis, tachycardia, and crepitations.

High-Altitude Cerebral Edema (HACE)

High-altitude cerebral edema was also recognized by Ravenhill (92), although the clear evidence that HACE occurs alone is by no means certain (20). The principle symptoms are those of acute mountain sickness but with extreme fatigue, dizziness, hallucinations, double vision, nightmares, bizarre and irrational behavior, emotional lability, ataxia, and incoordination. These symptoms may worsen rapidly as the patient becomes unconscious and begins to die.

High-Altitude Retinal Hemorrhage (HARH)

High-altitude retinal hemorrhage is another common finding at altitude but is usually asymptomatic. It was first described on Mount Logan by Frayser et al. (31). More detailed studies from that environment showed a 56% incidence in people above 5,300 m with an increased incidence following severe exercise (68).

Other high-altitude syndromes such as thromboses, chronic mountain sickness, and high-altitude deterioration are beyond the scope of this chapter; nor have I considered various maladies such as sickle-cell disease and heart and lung disorders, which may be aggravated on exposure to altitude (for further details on these topics, see ref. 39).

As with most environmental problems, altitude disorders are preventable. By the same token, they can also be life threatening and must be taken very seriously. There is considerable individual variation, and although attempts have been made to predict those who are most at risk of developing mountain sickness (they appear to be the underventilators; see ref. 62), such studies are unlikely to be performed before exposure to altitude (113). Of all the time-honored preventative measures, that of slow acclimatization remains the simplest and the safest. The following schedule is recommended for the average person but in no way guarantees prevention of symptoms. If an individual experiences using this rate of ascent, it has been too fast. There is no evidence that increased cardiorespiratory fitness makes a person less susceptible to these altitude maladies. In fact, the young, fit, and energetic who almost attack the mountains may be most at risk, probably because of the rate of ascent or exercise intensity.

1. Begin below 2,500-3,000 m whether arriving by automobile or aircraft.
2. Exert oneself little for the first 24 hr.
3. Avoid or minimize alcohol consumption for the first 48 hr.
4. Keep the daily rate of ascent below 300 m.
5. If you climb higher than that during the day, sleep lower.
6. Keep well hydrated and avoid sedatives.

Of all the medications available, that of the carbonic anhydrase inhibitor acetazolamide has proven to be the most successful (29, 117). The mechanisms are rather complex, but one possibly important one is that of the reduction of sleep hypoxemia (117). These studies have been confirmed by important double-blind crossover studies in the mountain environment (9, 36). As carbonic anhydrase is a rather ubiquitous enzyme, it is not entirely clear by which mechanism acetazolamide minimizes the symptoms of AMS. More recently, studies by Johnson et al. (56) have demonstrated that prior treatment with dexamethasone will tend to prevent AMS.

The treatment of HAPE and HACE constitutes a medical emergency. Oxygen, furosemide, acetazolamide, and (in the case of cerebral edema) dexamethasone should be given and the patient evacuated by immediate descent. One cannot emphasize too strongly the importance of removing the patient to a lower altitude (for more detailed information, see ref. 39).

High-Pressure (Diving) and Polluted Environments

Specific effects of high-pressure environments (diving) recently have been reviewed by Strauss (109) and are beyond the scope of this chapter. In urban environments, air pollution is a serious health concern; numerous pollutants may affect the oxygen transport ability by combining with hemoglobin (as with carbon monoxide) or by causing respiratory difficulties (as with ozone and sulphur dioxide), especially in those subjects with increased airway reactivity. Again, this topic is beyond the scope of this chapter, and the reader is referred to the next chapter.

Conclusion

Maximum enjoyment of exercise often occurs in exotic environments, be they cold, hot, or high. The body is capable of making many adjustments, but the behavioral factors are more important than is physiology in such adaptations. Failure to adapt can be fatal, and all the illnesses associated with exercise in these environments are preventable. It seems paradoxical that we advocate exercise as an essential ingredient to the enrichment of our lives and the improvement of our health because it may be a double-edged sword. Injudicious exercise in the susceptible individual carries with it a high risk. However cautious we are, we will never completely eliminate such dangers.

References

1. Adams, T., and E.J. Haberling. Effects of training on response to cold. *J. Appl. Physiol.* 13: 226-230, 1958.
2. Adams, W.C., E.M. Bernauer, D.B. Dill, and J.B. Bomar, Jr. Effects of equivalent sea level and altitude training on $\dot{V}O_2$max and running performance. *J. Appl. Physiol.* 39: 262-266, 1975.
3. Adolph, E.F. Blood changes in dehydration. In: Adolph, E.F., ed. *Physiology of man in the desert.* New York: Interscience, 1947, p. 160-171.
4. Althaus, U., P. Aeberhard, P. Schupbach, B.H. Nachbur, and W. Mishlemann. Management of profound accidental hypothermia with cardiorespiratory arrest. *Am. Surg.* 195: 492-495, 1982.
5. American College of Sports Medicine. Position stand: Prevention of thermal injuries during distance running. *Med. Sci. Sports Exerc.* 16(5): ix-xiv, 1984.
6. American Physiological Society. *Handbook of physiology: Environmental physiology.* Bethesda, MD: Author, 1986.
7. Avellini, B.A., E. Kamon, and J.T. Krajewski. Physiological responses of physically fit men and women to acclimation to humid heat. *J. Appl. Physiol.* 49: 254-261, 1980.
8. Bangs, C. Cold injuries. In: Strauss, R.H., ed. *Sports medicine.* Philadelphia: W.B. Saunders, 1984, p. 323-343.
9. Birmingham Medical Research Expeditionary Society Mountain Sickness Group. Acetazolamide in control of acute mountain sickness. *Lancet* i: 180-183, 1981.
10. Bohn, D.I. Treatment of hypothermia: In the hospital. In: Sutton, J.R., C.S. Houston, and G. Coates, eds. *Hypoxia and Cold.* New York: Praeger, 1987, p. 286-305.
11. Brahams, D. Death of a soldier: Accident or neglect? *Lancet* i: 485, 1988.
12. Buick, F.J., N. Gledhill, A.B. Froese, and L.L. Spriet. Red cell mass and aerobic performance at sea level. In: Sutton, J.R., N.L. Jones, and C.S. Houston, eds. *Hypoxia: Man at altitude.* New York: Thieme-Stratton, 1982, p. 43-50.
13. Burton, A.C, and O.G. Edholm. *Man in a cold environment.* New York: Hafner, 1969.
14. Buskirk, E.R., J. Kollias, R.F. Akers, E.K. Prokop, and E.P. Reategui. Maximal performance at altitude and on return from altitude in conditioned runners. *J. Appl. Physiol.* 23: 259-266, 1967.
15. Cena, K., and J.A. Clark. *Bioengineering, thermal physiology and comfort.* Amsterdam: Elsevier, 1981.
16. Cerretelli, P. Limiting factors to oxygen transport on Mount Everest. *J. Appl. Physiol.* 40: 658-667, 1976.
17. Clowes, G.H.A., and T.F. O'Donnell. Heat stroke. *N. Engl. J. Med.* 291: 564-567, 1974.
18. Convertino, V.A., J.E. Greenleaf, and E.M. Bernauer. Role of thermal and exercise factors in the mechanism of hypervolemia. *J. Appl. Physiol.* 48: 657-664, 1980.
19. Costrini, A.M., H.A. Pitt, A.B. Gustafson, and D.E. Uddin. Cardiovascular and metabolic manifestations of heat stroke and severe heat exhaustion. *Am. J. Med.* 66: 296-302, 1979.

20. Dickinson, J.G. High altitude cerebral edema: Cerebral acute mountain sickness. *Semin. Respir. Med.* 5: 151-158, 1983.

21. Dill, D.B. *Life, heat and altitude.* Cambridge, MA: Harvard University Press, 1938.

22. Dill, D.B., L.F. Soholt, D.C. McLean, T.F. Drost, Jr., and M.T. Loughran. Capacity of young males and females for running in desert heat. *Med. Sci. Sports* 9: 137-142, 1977.

23. Drinkwater, B.L., J.E. Denton, I.C. Kupprat, T.S. Talag, and S.M. Horvath. Aerobic power as a factor in women's response to work in hot environments. *J. Appl. Physiol.* 41: 815-821, 1976.

24. Edholm, O.G., and A.L. Bacharach. *The physiology of human survival.* London: Academic Press, 1965.

25. Faulkner, J.A., J. Kollias, C.B. Favour, E.R. Buskirk, and B. Balke. Maximum aerobic capacity and running performance at altitude. *J. Appl. Physiol.* 24: 685-691, 1968.

26. Folk, G.E. *Textbook of environmental physiology.* Philadelphia: Lea & Febiger, 1974.

27. Folinsbee, L.J., J.A. Wagner, J.F. Borgia, B.L. Drinkwater, J.A. Gliner, and J.F. Bedi. *Environmental stress.* New York: Academic Press, 1978.

28. Fortney, S.M., C.B. Wenger, J.R. Bove, and E.R. Nadel. Effect of blood volume on forearm venous and cardiac stroke volume during exercise. *J. Appl. Physiol.* 55: 884-890, 1983.

29. Forwand, S.A., M. Landowne, J.N. Follansbee, and J.E. Hansen. Effect of acetazolamide on acute mountain sickness. *N. Engl. J. Med.* 279: 839-845, 1968.

30. Fox, R.H., B.E. Lofstedt, P.M. Woodward, E. Erikkson, and B. Werkstrom. Comparison of thermoregulatory function in men and women. *J. Appl. Physiol.* 26: 444-453, 1969.

31. Frayser, R., C.S. Houston, A.C. Bryan, I.D. Rennie, and G. Gray. Retinal hemorrhage at high altitude. *N. Engl. J. Med.* 282: 1183-1184, 1970.

32. Frim, J. Fundamentals of thermoregulation. In: Sutton, J.R., C.S. Houston, and G. Coates, eds. *Hypoxia and cold.* New York: Praeger, 1987, p. 19-32.

33. Gisolfi, C., and S. Robinson. Relations between physical training, acclimatization and heat tolerance. *J. Appl. Physiol.* 26: 530-534, 1969.

34. Green, H.J., R.L. Hughson, J.A. Thomson, and M.T. Sharratt. Supramaximal exercise after training-induced hypervolemia. I. Gas exchange and acid-base balance. *J. Appl. Physiol.* 62: 1944-1953, 1987.

35. Green, H.J., J.R. Sutton, P. Young, A. Cymerman, and C.S. Houston. Operation Everest II: Muscle energetics during maximal exhaustive exercise. *J. Appl. Physiol.* 66: 142-150, 1989.

36. Greene, M.K., A.M. Kerr, I.B. McIntosh, and R.J. Prescott. Acetazolamide in prevention of acute mountain sickness: A double-blind controlled cross-over study. *Br. Med. J.* 283: 811-813, 1981.

37. Groves, B.M., J.T. Reeves, J.R. Sutton, P.D. Wagner, A. Cymerman, M.K. Malconian, P.B. Rock, P.M. Young, and C.S. Houston. Operation Everest II: Elevated high-altitude pulmonary resistance unresponsive to oxygen. *J. Appl. Physiol.* 63: 521-530, 1987.

38. Hackett, P.H., D. Rennie, and H.D. Levine. The incidence, importance, and prophylaxis of acute mountain sickness. *Lancet* ii: 1149-1155, 1976.

39. Hackett, P.H., R. Roach, and J.R. Sutton. High altitude illness. In: Auerbach, P., and E. Geehr, eds. *Management of wilderness and environmental emergencies.* St. Louis: C.V. Mosby, 1989, p. 1-34.

40. Hales, J.R.S. Effects of exposure to hot environments on the regional distribution of blood flow and on cardiorespiratory function in sheep. *Pflugers Arch.* 344: 133-148, 1973.

41. Hales, J.R.S. A case supporting the proposal that cardiac filling pressure is the limiting factor in adjusting to heat stress. *Yale J. Biol. Med.* 59: 237-245, 1986.

42. Hales, J.R.S., and D. Richards. *Heat stress.* Amsterdam: Excerpta Medica, 1987.

43. Hales, J.R.S., F.R.N. Stephens, A.A. Fawcett, R.A. Westerman, J.D. Vaughan, D.A.B. Richards, and C.R.B. Richards. Lowered skin blood flow and erythrocyte sphering in collapsed fun-runners. *Lancet* i: 1494-1495, 1986.

44. Hanson, P.G., and S.W. Zimmerman. Exertional heatstroke in novice runners. *JAMA* 242: 154-257, 1979.

45. Harrison, M.H. Effect of thermal stress and exercise on blood volume in humans. *Physiol. Rev.* 65: 149-209, 1985.

46. Hart, L.E., B.P. Egier, S.G. Shimizu, P.J. Tandan, and J.R. Sutton. Exertional heatstroke: The runner's nemesis. *Can. Med. Assoc. J.* 122: 1144-1150, 1980.

47. Hayward, J.S., J.D. Eckerson, and M.L. Collis. Effect of behavioral variables on cooling

rate of man in cold water. *J. Appl. Physiol.* 38: 1073-1077, 1975.

48. Heath, D., and D.R. Williams. *Man at high altitude.* Edinburgh, Scotland: Churchill Livingstone, 1981.

49. Hertig, B.A., and F. Sargent II. Acclimatization of women during work in hot environments. *Fed. Proc.* 22: 810-813, 1963.

50. Houston, C.S. Acute pulmonary edema of high altitude. *N. Engl. J. Med.* 263: 478-480, 1960.

51. Houston, C.S. *Going higher.* Boston: Little, Brown, 1987.

52. Houston, C.S., J.R. Sutton, A. Cymerman, and J.T. Reeves. Operation Everest II: Man at extreme altitude. *J. Appl. Physiol.* 63: 877-882, 1987.

53. Hughson, R.L., H.J. Green, M.E. Houston, J.A. Thomson, D.R. MacLean, and J.R. Sutton. Heat injuries in Canadian mass participation runs. *Can. Med. Assoc. J.* 122: 1141-1144, 1980.

54. Jessens, C. Thermoregulatory mechanisms in severe heat stress with exercise. In: Hales, J.R.S., and D. Richards, eds. *Heat stress.* Amsterdam: Excerpta Medica, 1987, p. 1-18.

55. Jokl, E., and P. Jokl. *Exercise and altitude.* Basel, Switzerland: Karger, 1968.

56. Johnson, T.S., C.S. Fulco, L.A. Trad, R.S. Spark, and J.T. Maher. Prevention of acute mountain sickness by dexamethazone. *N. Engl. J. Med.* 310: 683-686, 1984.

57. Keilblock, A.J. Strategies for the prevention of heat disorders with particular reference to the efficacy of body cooling procedures. In: Hales, J.R.S., and D. Richards, eds. *Heat stress.* Amsterdam: Excerpta Medica, 1987, p. 489-497.

58. Kew, M.C., I. Bersohn, H.C. Seftel, and G. Kent. Liver damage in heatstroke. *Am. J. Med.* 49: 192-202, 1970.

59. Kew, M.C., O.T. Minick, R.M. Bahu, R.J. Stein, and G. Kent. Ultrastructural changes in the liver in heatstroke. *Am. J. Pathol.* 90: 609-618, 1978.

60. Kew, M.C., R.B.K. Tucker, I. Bersohn, and H.C. Seftel. The heart in heatstroke. *Am. Heart J.* 77: 324-335, 1969.

61. Khogali, M., and J.R.S. Hales. *Heat stroke and temperature regulation.* Sydney, Australia: Academic Press, 1983.

62. King, A.B., and S.M. Robinson. Ventilatory response to hypoxia and acute mountain sickness. *Aviat. Space Environ. Med.* 43: 419-421, 1972.

63. Knochel, J.P. Dog days and siriasis: How to kill a football player. *JAMA* 233: 513-515, 1975.

64. Lloyd, E.L. *Hypothermia and cold stress.* Rockville, MD: Aspen, 1986.

65. Loeppky, J.A., and M.L. Riedesel. *Oxygen transport to human tissues.* New York: Elsevier, 1982.

66. MacDougall, J.D. Structural changes in muscle with chronic hypoxia. In: Sutton, J.R., C.S. Houston, and G. Coates, eds. *Hypoxia: The tolerable limits.* Indianapolis: Benchmark Press, 1988, p. 93-100.

67. Maughan, R.J., I.M. Light, P.H. Whiting, and J.D.B. Miller. Hypothermia, hyperkalaemia and marathon running. *Lancet* ii: 1336, 1982.

68. McFadden, M., C.S. Houston, J.R. Sutton, G.W., and A.C.P. Powles. High altitude retinopathy. *JAMA* 245: 581-586, 1980.

69. Mills, W.J., R. Gower, P.H. Hackett, R.B. Schoene, R. Roach, and B. Okonek. Cold injury, dehydration, multiple system trauma on Mt. McKinley, Alaska. In: Sutton, J.R., C.S. Houston, and G. Coates, eds. *Hypoxia and cold.* New York: Praeger, 1987, p. 340-362.

70. Mills, W.J., P.H. Hackett, R.B. Schoene, R. Roach, and W. Mills III. Treatment of hypothermia: In the field. In: Sutton, J.R., C.S. Houston, and G. Coates, eds. *Hypoxia and cold.* New York: Praeger, 1987, p. 271-285.

71. Monteith, J.C., and L.E. Mount. *Heat loss from animals and man.* London: Butterworth, 1974.

72. Moss, J. Accidental severe hypothermia. *Surg. Gynecol. Obstet.* 162: 501-513, 1986.

73. Mount, L.E. The concept of thermal neutrality. In: Monteith, J.L., and L.E. Mount, eds. *Heat loss from animals and man.* London: Butterworth, 1974.

74. Nadel, E.R., G.W. Mack, H. Nose, and A. Tripathi. Tolerance to severe heat and exercise. Peripheral vascular responses to body fluid changes. In: Hales, J.R.S., and D. Richards, eds. *Heat stress.* Amsterdam: Excerpta Medica, 1987, p. 117-131.

75. Nadel, E.R., K.B. Pandolf, M.F. Roberts, and J.A.J. Stolwijk. Mechanisms of thermal acclimatization to exercise and heat. *J. Appl. Physiol.* 37: 515-520, 1974.

76. Newburgh, L.H. *Physiology of heat regulation and the science of clothing.* New York: Hafner, 1968.

77. O'Donnell, T.F., and G.H. Clowes. The circulatory abnormalities of heat stroke. *N. Engl. J. Med.* 287: 734-737, 1972.

78. Oelz, O., H. Howald, R. Jenni, H. Hoppeler, H. Claassen, J-C. Bruckner, P.E. di Prampero, and P. Cerretelli. Cardiorespiratory and muscle physiology of elite extreme altitude climbers. In: Sutton, J.R., C.S. Houston, and G. Coates, eds. *Hypoxia and cold*. New York: Praeger, 1987, p. 464-470.

79. Paolone, A.M., C.L. Wells, and G.T. Kelly. Sexual variations in thermoregulation during heat stress. *Aviat. Space Environ. Med.* 49: 715-719, 1978.

80. Pandolf, K.B., M.N. Sawka, and R.R. Gonzalez. *Human performance physiology and environmental medicine at terrestrial extremes*. Indianapolis: Benchmark Press, 1988.

81. Paton, B. Accidental hypothermia in an alcoholic. In: Sutton, J.R., C.S. Houston, and G. Coates, eds. *Hypoxia and cold*. New York: Praeger, 1987, p. 264-270.

82. Paton, B. Pathophysiology of frostbite. In: Sutton, J.R., C.S. Houston, and G. Coates, eds. *Hypoxia and cold*. New York: Praeger, 1987, p. 329-339.

83. Piwonka, R.W., and S. Robinson. Acclimatization of highly trained men to work in severe heat. *J. Appl. Physiol.* 22: 9-12, 1967.

84. Pugh, L.G.C.E. Resting ventilation and alveolar air on Mount Everest: With remarks on the relation of barometric pressure to altitude in mountains. *J. Physiol. (Lond.)* 135: 590-610, 1957.

85. Pugh, L.G.C.E. Deaths from exposure on Four Inns walking competition, March 14-15, 1964. *Lancet* i: 1210-1212, 1964.

86. Pugh, L.G.C.E. Cardiac output in muscular exercise at 5,800 m (19,000 ft). *J. Appl. Physiol.* 19: 441-447, 1964.

87. Pugh, L.G.C.E. Clothing insulation and accidental hypothermia in youth. *Nature* 209: 1281-1286, 1966.

88. Pugh, L.G.C.E. Athletes at altitude. *J. Physiol. (Lond.)* 192: 619-646, 1967.

89. Pugh, L.G.C.E., J.L. Corbett, and R.H. Johnson. Rectal temperatures, weight losses, and sweat rates in marathon running. *J. Appl. Physiol.* 23: 347-352, 1967.

90. Pugh, L.G.C.E., O.G. Edholm, R.H. Fox, H.S. Wolff, G.R. Hervey, W.H. Hammond, J.M. Tanner, and R.H. Whitehouse. A physical study of channel swimming. *Clin. Sci.* 19: 257-273, 1960.

91. Raven, P.B., I. Niki, T.E. Dahms, and S.M. Horvath. Compensatory cardiovascular responses during an environmental cold stress, 5 °C. *J. Appl. Physiol.* 29: 417-421, 1970.

92. Ravenhill, T.H. Some experiences of acute mountain sickness in the Andes. *J. Trop. Med. Hyg.* 20: 313-320, 1913.

93. Richards, C.R.B., and D. Richards. Prevention of exercise-induced heat stroke. In: Sutton, J.R., and R.M. Brock, eds. *Sports medicine for the mature athlete*. Indianapolis: Benchmark Press, 1986, p. 151-166.

94. Richards, R., and D. Richards. Medical management of fun runs. In: Hales, J.R.S., and D. Richards, eds. *Heat stress*. Amsterdam: Excerpta Medica, 1987, p. 513-525.

95. Richards, R., D. Richards, P. Schofield, V. Ross, and J.R. Sutton. Reducing the hazards in Sydney's *The Sun* "City-to-Surf" runs, 1971-1979. *Med. J. Aust.* 2: 453-457, 1979.

96. Richards, R., D. Richards, P. Schofield, V. Ross, and J.R. Sutton. Management of heat exhaustion in Sydney's *The Sun* "City-to-Surf" fun runners, 1971-1979. *Med. J. Aust.* 2: 457-461, 1979.

97. Richards, R., D. Richards, P. Schofield, V. Ross, and J.R. Sutton. Organization of *The Sun* "City-to-Surf" fun run, Sydney. *Med. J. Aust.* 2: 470-474, 1979.

98. Rivolier, J., P. Cerretelli, J. Foray, and P. Segantini. *High altitude deterioration*. Basel, Switzerland: Karger, 1985.

99. Robertshaw, D. *Environmental physiology*. London: Butterworth, 1974.

100. Robinson, C.R. Jogging in Tasmania. *N. Engl. J. Med.* 285: 1267, 1971.

101. Rowell, L.B. Human cardiovascular adjustments to exercise and thermal stress. *Physiol. Rev.* 54: 74-159, 1974.

102. Rowell, L.B. *Human circulation: Regulation during physical stress*. London: Oxford University Press, 1986.

103. Rowell, L.B., J.M.R. Detry, G.R. Profant, and C. Wyss. Splanchnic vasoconstriction in hyperthermic man: Role of falling blood pressure. *J. Appl. Physiol.* 31: 864-869, 1971.

104. Senay, L.C., Jr., D. Mitchell, and C.H. Wyndham. Acclimatization in a hot, humid environment: Body fluid adjustments. *J. Appl. Physiol.* 40: 786-796, 1976.

105. Shephard, R.J. The athlete at high altitude. *Can. Med. Assoc. J.* 109: 207-209, 1973.

106. Shibolet, S., M.C. Lancaster, and Y. Danon. Heat stroke: A review. *Aviat. Space Environ. Med.* 47: 280-301, 1976.

107. Sime, F., D. Penaloza, L. Ruiz, N. Gonzales, E. Covarrubias, and R. Postigo. Hypoxemia, pulmonary hypertension, and low cardiac

output in newcomers at low altitude. *J. Appl. Physiol.* 36: 561-565, 1974.

108. Sohal, R.S., S.C. Sun, H.L. Colcolough, and G.E. Burch. Heatstroke: An electron microscopic study of endothelial cell damage and disseminated intravascular coagulation. *Arch. Intern. Med.* 122: 43-47, 1968.

109. Strauss, R.H. Medical aspects of scuba and breath-hold diving. In: Strauss, R., ed. *Sports medicine*. Philadelphia: W.B. Saunders, 1984, p. 361-377.

110. Sutton, J.R. Community jogging vs. arduous running. *N. Engl. J. Med.* 286: 951, 1972.

111. Sutton, J.R. Heat illness. In: Strauss, R.H., ed. *Sports medicine*. Philadelphia: W.B. Saunders, 1984, p. 307-322.

112. Sutton, J.R., and O. Bar-Or. Thermal illness in fun running. *Am. Heart J.* 100: 778-781, 1980.

113. Sutton, J.R., A.C. Bryan, G.W. Gray, E.S. Horton, A.S. Rebuck, W. Woodley, I.D. Rennie, and C.S. Houston. Pulmonary gas exchange in acute mountain sickness. *Aviat. Space Environ. Med.* 47: 1032-1037, 1976.

114. Sutton, J.R., M.J. Coleman, A.P. Millar, L. Lazarus, and P. Russo. The medical problems of mass participation in athletic competition. The ''City-to-Surf'' Race. *Med. J. Aust.* 2: 127-133, 1972.

115. Sutton, J.R., C.S. Houston, and G. Coates, eds. *Hypoxia and cold*. New York: Praeger, 1987.

116. Sutton, J.R., C.S. Houston, and G. Coates. *Hypoxia: The tolerable limits*. Indianapolis: Benchmark Press, 1988.

117. Sutton, J.R., C.S. Houston, A.L. Mansell, M. McFadden, P. Hackett, and A.C.P. Powles. Effect of acetazolamide on hypoxemia during sleep at high altitudes. *N. Engl. J. Med.* 301: 1329-1331, 1979.

118. Sutton, J.R., N.L. Jones, and C.S. Houston. *Hypoxia: Man at altitude*. New York: Thieme-Stratton, 1982.

119. Sutton, J.R., and N. Lassen. Pathophysiology of acute mountain sickness and high altitude pulmonary oedema. *Bull. Eur. Physiopath. Respir.* 15: 1045-1052, 1979.

120. Sutton, J.R., J.T. Reeves, P.D. Wagner, B.M. Groves, A. Cymerman, M.K. Malconian, P.B. Rock, P.M. Young, S.D. Walter, and C.S. Houston. Operation Everest II: Oxygen transport during exercise at extreme simulated altitude. *J. Appl. Physiol.* 64: 1309-1321, 1988.

121. Ward, M. *Mountain medicine*. London: Crosby, Lockwood & Staples, 1975.

122. Weiner, J.S., and M. Khogali. Physiological body cooling unit for treatment of heat stroke. *Lancet* i: 507-509, 1980.

123. Weinman, K.P., Z. Slabochova, E.M. Bernauer, T. Morimoto, and F. Sargent II. Reactions of men and women to repeated exposure to humid heat. *J. Appl. Physiol.* 22: 533-538, 1967.

124. West, J.B., S.J. Boyer, D.J. Graber, P.H. Hackett, K.H. Maret, J.S. Milledge, R.M. Peters, Jr., C.J. Pizzo, M. Samaja, F.S. Sarnquist, R.B. Schoene, and R.M. Winslow. Maximal exercise at extreme altitudes on Mount Everest. *J. Appl. Physiol.* 55: 688-698, 1983.

125. Winslow, R.M. Hypoxia and polycythemia: The optimal hematocrit. In: Sutton, J.R., N.L. Jones, and C.S. Houston, eds. *Hypoxia: Man at altitude*. New York: Thieme-Stratton, 1982, p. 40-42.

126. Wyndham, C.H. The physiology of exercise under heat stress. *Annu. Rev. Physiol.* 35: 193-220, 1973.

127. Wyndham, C.H., J.F. Morrison, and C.G. Williams. Heat reactions of male and female Caucasians. *J. Appl. Physiol.* 20: 357-364, 1965.

128. Zoller, R.P., A.L. Mark, F.M. Abboud, P.G. Schmid, and D.D. Heistad. The role of low pressure baroreceptors in reflex vasoconstrictor responses in man. *J. Clin. Immunol.* 51: 2967-2972, 1972.

Chapter 17

Discussion: Exercise and the Environment

Lawrence J. Folinsbee

This chapter elaborates on two areas briefly discussed by Dr. Sutton: the effect of our air environment on fitness and human health, specifically the effects on the lungs; and the thermal effects of water immersion.

Outdoor pursuits may be conducted in the near-pristine environments of the Rocky Mountains or, more frequently, in the contaminated air environments of North American cities. The principle air pollutants of concern in such cities and their environs include ozone, sulfur dioxide, carbon monoxide, lead, and particulates or aerosols (including the politically important acid aerosol precursors of acid rain). Although we generally consider the outdoor environment in the context of air pollution, there is also a considerable body of evidence describing the health effects of indoor-air contaminants, of which those of major concern for human health include secondary tobacco smoke, carbon monoxide, nitrogen dioxide, wood smoke, formaldehyde, radon, and volatile organic compounds.

Indoor Air

The importance of indoor-air contaminants for long-term health is obvious. We spend much of our waking hours and most of our sleeping hours in the indoor environment, and with the increase in the number of energy-efficient (usually poorly ventilated) homes, the potential risk from indoor-air contamination is increased. For example, the presence of radon is known to increase the risk of lung cancer. Environmental tobacco smoke (ETS) significantly increases the risk of respiratory illness in children exposed by their smoking parents. Furthermore, lung growth and development may be influenced by exposure to ETS. The extent of in-

volvement of ETS with lung cancer risk is uncertain, although the evidence tends to suggest some increase in risk associated with so-called passive smoking. In addition to ETS and radon, volatile organic compounds and wood smoke present the potential for increased levels of carcinogenic compounds in the home. Although wood smoke (and smoke from other types of fires) is less of a risk in the modern North American home, the level of wood smoke contamination in the domiciles of less advanced cultures may be substantial and associated with chronic lung diseases, including cancer (20). Formaldehyde, in addition to its possible role as a carcinogen, causes symptoms of headache, eye irritation, and irritation of mucus membranes; and in some individuals hypersensitivity may lead to more severe neuropsychological and behavioral effects. The issues of indoor-air contamination and health effects have recently been reviewed comprehensively by Samet et al. (27, 28).

Dosimetry

Exposure to air pollutants is consistent with the general rule that the influence of an external factor on the physiological response of an organism is related to the amount, or dose, received. Just as the influence of hypoxia on acute mountain sickness depends at least in part on the altitude to which one is exposed, the effects of various pollutant contaminants in the environment depend on the quantity that acts on various target organs. With respect to air pollution, the major factors in determination of the dose are the concentration of the pollutant, the duration of exposure, and the volume of air inhaled (i.e., minute ventilation). Because ventilation increases proportionately with the severity of exercise, any interpretation of the effects of an air pollutant must be considered in the context of the activity level of the persons being exposed. Consequently, pulmonary health effects of air pollutants that have been shown at low levels are usually observed only when the exposed individuals are working or playing.

Ozone

The photochemical oxidant ozone is an air pollutant whose effects are of considerable public health concern. Ozone exists in the stratosphere, where it is essential for filtering ultraviolet light; this is the so-called good ozone, as depletion of this ozone layer may lead to increased incidence of skin cancer. Ozone in the troposphere (which is the air that most of us breathe) is formed by a complex reaction of ultraviolet light and the emissions from internal combustion engines that include nitrogen oxides and hydrocarbons. The levels that exist in certain urban areas depend on the interaction of meteorological factors (including pollution transport), traffic density, and industrial output.

Early studies of the effects of ozone on human health and performance indicated that effects occurred only at the relatively high levels achieved in cities such as Los Angeles or Tokyo. The earliest study (12) of the effects of ozone on exercise performance indicated a reduction in peak oxygen consumption following a 2-hr exercising exposure to 0.75 ppm ozone, a level that is never reached in the United States and Canada under present-day conditions. This reduction in performance was accompanied by pronounced respiratory symptoms of cough and pain on deep inspiration, alteration of the respiratory pattern during exercise, and marked decrements in spirometric measurements of lung function. Gong et al. (14) have recently demonstrated that exercise performance was impaired after a 1-hr exposure of heavily exercising, well-trained cyclists to an ozone concentration of 0.20 ppm. This level is reached in the Los Angeles basin over a hundred times per year and with considerably lower frequency in some other cities. The effects of ozone on exercise performance have been recently reviewed by Adams (1).

Significant effects on lung function have been observed following 1- to 2-hr exposures to ozone levels as low as 0.12 ppm, the current ambient air quality standard in the United States. The ozone literature is replete with studies using a 2-hr intermittent exercise exposure protocol, originally used by Bates et al. (2) at McGill University, that was intended to simulate light exercise during peak levels of ozone exposure such as might occur in the Los Angeles basin. However, it is now recognized that other metropolitan areas experience substantial elevation of ozone levels for much longer periods than 2 hr; levels as high as 0.12 ppm may persist for 6-8 hr (26). A recent study of subjects exposed to 0.12 ppm of ozone for approximately 6-1/2 hr while they performed nearly continuous moderate exercise produced pronounced decrements in lung function (e.g., a 12% decrease in $FEV_{1.0}$), increased respiratory symptoms, and increased airway reactivity to methacholine (11). These effects have now been observed at concentrations as low as 0.08 ppm (the current ambient air quality standard in Canada).

The effects of ozone on lung function may persist for up to 24 hr, although they are generally resolved in a few hours. However, an inflammatory response and cellular damage in the lung may persist for longer periods. Indeed, following an initial ozone-induced injury to the lung, the response to subsequent exposures is markedly enhanced for up to 48 hr (10). Repeated exposure results in a diminished response that has been called *adaptation* (9). Frequent ambient exposure to ozone in areas such as Los Angeles results in seasonal changes in response. Anecdotal reports (to the author) from runners indicate that ozone responses are greatest in the spring at the beginning of the smog season and subsequently tend to be minimal during the remainder of the summer and fall. Responsiveness typically returns the following spring after a winter of low ozone levels. These anecdotes recently have been substantiated by experimental ozone exposure studies indicating a similar seasonal variation in response (15).

It remains unclear what effect continued exposure to ozone may have on aging of the lungs. A recent epidemiological study (8) from Los Angeles suggests that the decline in lung function with age may be more rapid in areas with high levels of air pollution. This provocative finding requires confirmation. This study suggests that it would be prudent for long-term lung health to avoid heavy exercise during the time of day when ozone or other pollutant levels are elevated.

Sulfur Dioxide

Sulfur dioxide is emitted from smelters, refineries, and other stationary sources. In addition to its direct effects, SO_2 is the precursor for the formation of acid aerosols and subsequently acid rain. However, neither SO_2 nor acid sulfates have important effects on lung function in normal healthy individuals at concentrations that currently exist in the ambient air. Nevertheless, sulfur dioxide is a potent bronchoconstrictor in asthmatics. Brief exposures of only 2-3 min (17) to SO_2 levels as low as 0.40 ppm cause increased airway resistance and symptoms of wheezing and chest tightness. The responses of asthmatics to SO_2 are modified appreciably by changes in temperature and humidity of the inspired air. The response to SO_2 is exacerbated by cold, dry air (31), a combination that can occur during the winter months. Of course, low temperature and humidity of inspired air are well-known as being important in the exacerbation of exercise-induced asthma (7). Because considerable "scrubbing" of SO_2 occurs in the nasal airways, breathing through the mouth tends to produce a more pronounced response.

In modeling the responses to SO_2, considerable attention has been directed to the mechanisms of switching between oral and oronasal breathing. Niinimaa et al. (21) indicate that the average ventilation for the transition from oral to oronasal breathing during exercise is approximately 35 L• min^{-1}. However, this transition point is highly variable, and the mechanisms governing this transition are not well understood. Asthmatics, who commonly suffer from allergic rhinitis, may be forced to breath more through the mouth, thus worsening their response to SO_2. Recovery from SO_2-induced bronchoconstriction is relatively rapid (15-30 min), and the response may be partially blocked by cromolyn sodium or beta-2-sympathomimetics, which are frequently prescribed medications for asthma.

Carbon Monoxide

Carbon monoxide is a commonly occurring air pollutant that can have substantial effect on human performance, specifically by causing a reduction in maximum oxygen uptake (23). The well-known mechanism by which carbon monoxide exerts some of its effects is to occupy sites on the hemoglobin molecule that could otherwise be used for oxygen transport. A 10% increase in carboxyhemoglobin (i.e., hemoglobin bound with carbon monoxide or HbCO) results in an approximate 10% decrease in maximum oxygen uptake in nonsmokers at sea level (18). The effect appears to be due entirely to the reduction in the oxygen-carrying ca-

pacity of the blood, as the maximal cardiac output is not altered significantly. Despite the effects on maximal oxygen uptake, performance of moderate submaximal exercise in healthy individuals does not appear to be affected by accumulation of CO up to about 15% carboxyhemoglobin, a level requiring substantial exposure (i.e., in excess of 100 ppm CO for several hours) (13). Cardiac patients with angina may be at increased risk from CO exposure because elevation of their HbCO levels to about 5% or higher may accelerate the onset of chest pain during exercise. Because of the relatively slow clearance of CO from the blood (the clearance half-time is on the order of 2-4 hr), exposures that occur some time before an event (e.g., on crowded freeways or in smoke-contaminated rooms) could still influence later performance.

The potential for an interaction between carbon monoxide exposure and altitude in the limitation of performance has been known for some time. The use of gas stoves within the confines of a tent or other poorly ventilated enclosure, particularly for the purpose of melting snow, can give rise to a substantial increase in the CO level (> 100 ppm) within the tent, especially tents made of coated fabrics, which reduce air exchange. Pugh (22) reported on the effects of carbon monoxide exposure in Antarctic explorers. In volunteers who melted ice in a tent for approximately 2 hr, the HbCO increased to about 10%, a level that would cause a significant reduction in maximum oxygen uptake. A 10% increase in HbCO is equivalent to an increase in altitude of about 1,000 m and could potentially cause substantial exacerbation of the symptoms of acute mountain sickness.

Immersion Hypothermia

As mentioned by Dr. Sutton, the rate of loss of body heat is much greater in water than it is in air. In addition to the involuntary immersion in cold water experienced by boaters, kayakers, windsurfers, and river rafters, there are a large number of people who voluntarily immerse themselves in water that is cool enough to cause hypothermia. In fact, the thermoneutral temperature in water for an average resting man (4) is in excess of 33 °C (91 °F), much warmer than that of most swimming pools. Thus, seemingly warm ocean or lake temperatures present the potential risk of immersion hypothermia.

The capability to exercise in cold water without becoming hypothermic is greatly dependant on subcutaneous fat thickness. It is no accident that successful long-distance cold-water swimmers have substantial quantities of subcutaneous fat. Rennie (24) indicates that in water colder than 25 °C (77 °F) and with energy expenditures up to 500 W/m² (approximately 2.9 L • min⁻¹ oxygen uptake), a subject with increased subcutaneous fat is at a considerable advantage in preventing a decline in core temperature. For individuals involuntarily immersed in very cold water, the survival time is brief; with a water temperature of 6 °C (43 °F) the average survival is about 20 min, and few survive beyond 75 min (19). However, there is a case in which a fully-clothed fat fisherman (mean subcutaneous fat thickness of 14 mm; fat thickness averaged 25-26 mm over the trunk) survived in 5-6 °C water for some 5-6 hr while swimming to shore after his fishing boat capsized (19). The range of water temperatures in which individuals with minimal subcutaneous fat can swim and still maintain core temperature is much narrower. Furthermore, the rate of fall of core temperature is considerably more rapid in young children, who have a large surface-to-volume ratio. Sloan and Keatinge (30) reported a decline of core temperature of approximately 3 °C during a half-hour swim in 20 °C water by three lean, young swimmers. The mean ocean temperature for Canadian and western U.S. waters during the summer months is typically less than 20 °C.

At the moderate energy outputs sustained by long-distance swimmers, thick subcutaneous fat is essential to thermal homeostasis. The swimmer must also be able to sustain an energy output above a certain critical level so that heat production exceeds heat loss and core temperature can be preserved. Another factor that contributes to successful thermoregulation in cold water is the ability to reduce heat loss by peripheral vasoconstriction, a physiological characteristic that may be modified by repeated cold immersion (29).

One of the potential problems for individuals engaged in recreational swimming in cold water is that there may be no warning of impending hypothermia. Because of the relatively high skin temperature, the swimmer may not feel uncomfortably cold despite a substantial drop in core temperature (16). Persons repeatedly exposed to cold water tend to shiver at a lower core temperature and to shiver less than do those who are unaccustomed to cold (3, 25, 29). Once an individual becomes hypothermic, maximum aerobic power (6) as well as muscular strength (5) and coordination are markedly reduced while the oxygen cost of submaximal exercise increased (6).

Conversely, thick layers of subcutaneous fat are not advantageous for competitive swimmers. Water temperatures for competitive swimming are normally restricted to a narrow range of from 25-26.5 °C. The increased insulation provided by subcutaneous fat becomes a liability for individuals exercising heavily in warmer water. Cutaneous blood flow must be increased to promote heat loss, and this may compromise perfusion of exercising muscle. Indeed, the optimal subcutaneous fat thickness for competitive swimming is on the order of 2-5 mm (rather lean). Because of the short duration of the standard swimming events (< 17 min), neither hypo- nor hyperthermia is likely to be problematic.

References

1. Adams, W.C. Effects of ozone exposure at ambient air pollution episode levels on exercise performance. *Sports Med.* 4: 395-424, 1987.
2. Bates, D.V., G. Bell, C. Burnham, M. Hazucha, J. Mantha, L.D. Pengelly, and F. Silverman. Short term effects of ozone on the lung. *J. Appl. Physiol.* 32: 176-181, 1976.
3. Bittel, J.H.M. Heat debt as an index for cold adaptation in man. *J. Appl. Physiol.* 62: 1627-1634, 1987.
4. Craig, A.B., and M. Dvorak. Thermal regulation during water immersion. *J. Appl. Physiol.* 21: 1577-1585, 1966.
5. Coppin, E.G., S.D. Livingstone, and L.A. Kuehn. Effects on handgrip strength due to immersion in a 10 °C water bath. *Aviat. Space Environ. Med.* 49: 1322-1326, 1978.
6. Davies, M., B. Ekblom, U. Bergh, and I. Kanstrup-Jensen. The effects of hypothermia on submaximal and maximal work performance. *Acta Physiol. Scand.* 95: 201-202, 1979.
7. Deal, E.C., E.R. McFadden, R.H. Ingram, R.H. Strauss, and J.J. Jaeger. Role of respiratory heat exchange in production of exercise-induced asthma. *J. Appl. Physiol.* 46: 467-475, 1979.
8. Detels, R., D.P. Tashkin, J.W. Sayre, S.N. Rokaw, A.H. Coulson, F.J. Massey, and D.H. Wegman. The UCLA population studies of chronic obstructive respiratory disease. 9. Lung function changes associated with chronic exposure to photochemical oxidants—a cohort study among never smokers. *Chest* 92: 594-603, 1987.

9. Folinsbee, L.J., J.F. Bedi, J.A. Gliner, and S.M. Horvath. Concentration dependence of pulmonary function adaptation to ozone. In: Lee, S.D., M.G. Mustafa, and M.A. Mehlman, eds. *The biomedical effects of ozone and related photochemical oxidants.* Princeton Junction, NJ: Princeton Scientific, 1983, Chapt. 13, p. 175-187.

10. Folinsbee, L.J., and S.M. Horvath. Persistence of the acute effects of ozone exposure. *Aviat. Space Environ. Med.* 57: 1136-1143, 1986.

11. Folinsbee, L.J., W.F. McDonnell, and D.H. Horstman. Pulmonary function and symptom responses after 6.6 hour exposure to 0.12 ppm ozone with moderate exercise. *JAPCA* 38: 28-35, 1988.

12. Folinsbee, L.J., F. Silverman, and R.J. Shephard. Decrease of maximum work performance following ozone exposure. *J. Appl. Physiol.* 42: 531-536, 1977.

13. Gliner, J.A., P.B. Raven, S.M. Horvath, B.L. Drinkwater, and J.C. Sutton. Man's physiologic response to long term work during thermal and pollutant stress. *J. Appl. Physiol.* 39: 628-632, 1975.

14. Gong, H., P.W. Bradley, M.S. Simmons, and D.P. Tashkin. Impaired exercise performance and pulmonary function in elite cyclists during low-level ozone exposure in a hot environment. *Am. Rev. Respir. Dis.* 134: 726-733, 1986.

15. Hackney, J.D., and W.S. Linn. *Evaluating relationships among personal risk factors, ambient oxidant exposure, and chronic respiratory illness.* Paper presented at the Symposium on Susceptibility to Inhaled Pollutants, Williamsburg, VA, September 29-October 1, 1987.

16. Hayward, M.G., and W.R. Keatinge. Progressive symptomless hypothermia in water: Possible cause of diving accidents. *Br. Med. J.* 1: 1182, 1979.

17. Horstman, D.H., E. Seal, L.J. Folinsbee, P. Ives, and L.J. Roger. The relationship between exposure duration and sulfur dioxide-induced bronchoconstriction in asthmatic subjects. *Am. Ind. Hyg. Assoc. J.* 49: 38-47, 1988.

18. Horvath, S.M. Impact of air quality in exercise performance. *Exer. Sport Sci. Rev.* 9: 265-296, 1981.

19. Keatinge, W.R., S.R.K. Coleshaw, C.E. Millard, and J. Axelsson. Exceptional case of survival in cold water. *Br. Med. J.* 292: 171-172, 1986.

20. Mumford, J.L., X.Z. He, R.S. Chapman, S.R. Cao, D.B. Harris, X.M. Li, Y.L. Xian, W.Z. Jiang, C.W. Xu, J.C. Chuang, W.E. Wilson, and M. Cooke. Lung cancer and indoor air in Xuan Wei, China. *Science* 235: 217-220, 1987.

21. Niinimaa, V., P. Cole, S. Mintz, and R.J. Shephard. Oronasal distribution of respiratory airflow. *Respir. Physiol.* 43: 69-75, 1981.

22. Pugh, L.G.C.E. Carbon monoxide hazard in Antarctica. *Br. Med. J.* 1: 192-196, 1959.

23. Raven, P.B., B.L. Drinkwater, R.O. Ruhling, N. Bolduan, S. Taguchi, J. Gliner, and S.M. Horvath. Effect of carbon monoxide and peroxyacetyl nitrate on man's maximal aerobic capacity. *J. Appl. Physiol.* 36: 288-293, 1974.

24. Rennie, D.W. Tissue heat transfer during exercise in water. In: Shiraki, K., and M. Yousef, eds. *Man in stressful environments.* Springfield, IL: Charles C. Thomas, 1987, p. 211-223.

25. Rochelle, R.D., and S.M. Horvath. Thermoregulation in surfers and nonsurfers immersed in cold water. *Undersea Biomed. Res.* 5: 377-390, 1978.

26. Rombout, P.J.A., P.J. Lioy, and B.D. Goldstein. Rationale for an eight-hour ozone standard. *JAPCA* 36: 913-917, 1986.

27. Samet, J.C., M.C. Marbury, and J.D. Spengler. Health effects and sources of indoor air pollution. Part I. *Am. Rev. Respir. Dis.* 136: 1486-1508, 1987.

28. Samet, J.C., M.C. Marbury, and J.D. Spengler. Health effects and sources of indoor air pollution. Part II. *Am. Rev. Respir. Dis.* 137: 221-242, 1988.

29. Skreslet, S., and F. Aarefjord. Acclimatization to cold in man induced by frequent scuba diving in cold water. *J. Appl. Physiol.* 24: 177-181, 1968.

30. Sloan, R.E.G., and W.R. Keatinge. Cooling rates of young people swimming in cold water. *J. Appl. Physiol.* 371-375, 1973.

31. U.S. Environmental Protection Agency. *Controlled human exposure studies of sulfur dioxide health effects. Second addendum to air quality criteria for particulate matter and sulfur oxides (1982)* (EPA/600/8-86/020F). Washington, DC: U.S.E.P.A., 1986, p. 4-1 to 4-46.

PART III
Human Adaptation to Physical Activity

Chapter 18

Cardiovascular and Pulmonary Adaptation to Physical Activity

Bengt Saltin

Since the days of Harvey in the 17th century, experimental studies have become more common in establishing first the dimensions of the cardiovascular system and later its detailed function and regulation (11, 22). Early studies are also available on the role of the circulatory system for endurance performance (31).

In the 20th century the literature on this topic is overwhelming in many areas, including how acute and chronic exercise affects the circulation (50). In this brief review, certain aspects of the broad field that the title covers are highlighted. First, I focus on the magnitude of aerobic work capacity and the effects of training and age. Then a more detailed discussion follows on what limits maximal oxygen uptake. The final part deals with the regulation of the cardiovascular system in the light of uneven functional capacities of various links in oxygen transport.

Maximal Aerobic Power in Humans

One of the major functions of the cardiovascular system is to supply tissues and organs continuously with oxygen. Thus, it may be appropriate initially to give an account of its magnitude and how it is affected by the degree of habitual physical activity and age.

Sedentariness

The first major study of maximal oxygen uptake in humans was performed by Robinson (47), who studied male schoolchildren and employees at Harvard University. During growth the aerobic capacity increased until it peaked among old teenagers. Thereafter, it declined at a steady rate with increasing age (Figure 18.1). A small elevation in maximal oxygen uptake (normalized for body weight) is seen during adolescence. At the ages of 15-20, mean value is around or just above $50 \text{ ml} \cdot \text{kg}^{-1} \cdot \text{min}^{-1}$. Included in the figure are data from the 1980s collected in Denmark (1, 57). The similarity in results is worth noting. Except for the oldest age group, the present generations appear to be as good as the pre-World War II generations, maybe slightly better. This statement is based on the fact that the recent investigation was performed on a random sample of the population, whereas the subjects in Robinson's Boston study constituted a positive selection. In the latter study no women were included. The Danish data reveal considerably lower values for the women, except for the older age groups, in which women and men are more alike.

Role of Physical Activity

It is common to attribute variations in aerobic capacity mainly to genetic factors (5) (see also chapt. 14). Regular training has been proposed to affect an individual's maximal oxygen uptake only by some 20%. In contrast are the findings from bed-rest and training studies (59), which reveal that inactivity for some weeks may cause maximal oxygen uptake to become reduced to $25 \text{ ml} \cdot \text{kg}^{-1} \cdot \text{min}^{-1}$, or to two thirds of its control level. Train-

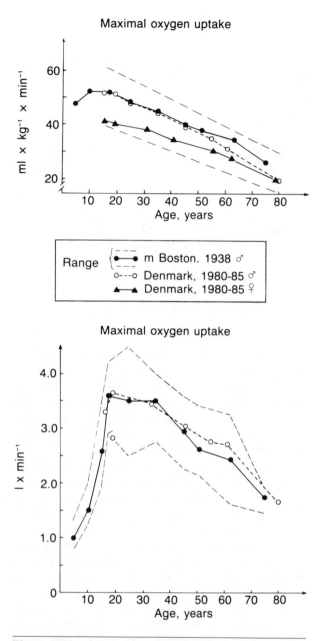

Maximal oxygen uptake

The role of genetic factors is decisive in achieving a high or very high maximal aerobic power. However, the impact of genetic endowment is of less importance for an average person's aerobic capacity. The critical upper level in maximal oxygen uptake that is impossible to surpass for most individuals may be 55 (women) to 60 (men) ml · kg⁻¹ · min⁻¹. Regardless of will and training regimens, most healthy people cannot reach such a high value; even fewer can reach 70 or 80 ml · kg⁻¹ · min⁻¹. A more proper statement than to attribute 80% to genetic and 20% to environmental

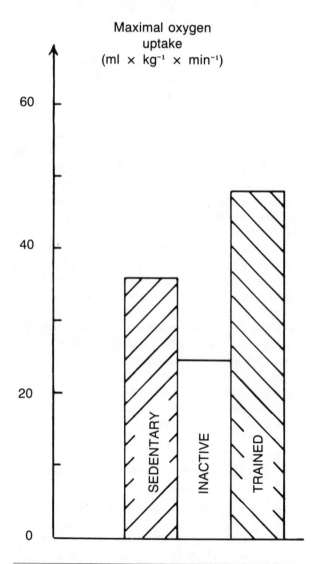

Figure 18.1. Maximal oxygen uptake in Robinson's study (47) and in recent population studies on men and women (see refs. 1, 57).

ing for some months did result in an elevation beyond control values, finally reaching close to 50 ml · kg⁻¹ · min⁻¹ (Figure 18.2). Thus, comparing the trained with the inactive stage shows a difference of almost 100%; that is, a healthy individual can double aerobic capacity in 3-4 mo through variations in leisure-time physical activity. Although these studies were performed on only a few subjects, there are reasons to believe that they would apply to a healthy population (Figure 18.3).

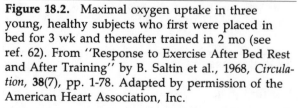

Figure 18.2. Maximal oxygen uptake in three young, healthy subjects who first were placed in bed for 3 wk and thereafter trained in 2 mo (see ref. 62). From ''Response to Exercise After Bed Rest and After Training'' by B. Saltin et al., 1968, *Circulation, 38*(7), pp. 1-78. Adapted by permission of the American Heart Association, Inc.

PHYSICAL ACTIVITY

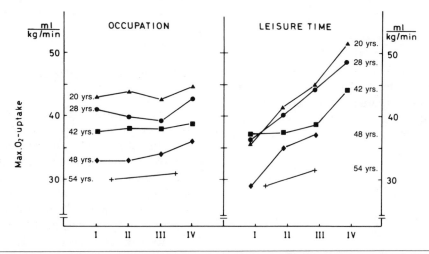

Figure 18.3. The relation between physical activity on the job and during leisure time classed from I to IV and the maximal oxygen uptake (see ref. 54). From "Physiological Effects of Physical Conditioning" by B. Saltin, 1977, in A. Tybjaerg-Hansen, P. Schnor, and G. Rose (Eds.), *Ischaemic Heart Disease. The Strategy of Postponement* (pp. 104-115). Copenhagen: FADL's. Reprinted by permission.

(training) factors would be to say that only 20% of the population have a genetic endowment to achieve 50-55 ml · kg⁻¹ · min⁻¹ or above in maximal oxygen uptake if properly trained.

Support for this notion is obtained from studies of conscripts in Sweden, where military service is compulsory. During the first 2-3 mo of military training, regular physical exercise two or three times a week is also performed. From a mean maximal oxygen uptake of 44-48 ml · kg⁻¹ · min⁻¹, an improvement of 15%-20% is achieved. Thus, an aerobic work capacity above 50 ml · kg⁻¹ · min⁻¹ is observed in most of these men of about 20 yr of age (40, 45, 60, 61). These studies also confirmed earlier findings that showed that the lower the initial maximal oxygen uptake, the larger the improvement with training (53).

A problem that has attracted special attention is whether training during adolescence is necessary for achieving a very high aerobic work capacity. Ekblom (18) was the first to propose this and to supply support for early training being advantageous. His view was later challenged by Eriksson (20), who made the point that when growth-related increases of the cardiac dimensions to training were taken into account, the observed improvements were not unique. Indeed, studies are available that indicate less aerobic adaptability during periods of accelerated growth (6, 12). Some recent Finnish studies are of special interest in this respect. Evovainio and Sundberg (21) followed a

group of male teenagers who trained up to 40-60 km per week and had a maximal oxygen uptake of 71.6 ml · kg⁻¹ · min⁻¹ at ages 12-13. Five years later the aerobic work capacity was barely improved, and none had reached an extremely high value for maximal oxygen uptake. The heart volume both in absolute number and normalized for body size had increased significantly, suggesting that cardiac dimensions do not adapt easily in the very young.

Endurance Athletes

Robinson et al. (48) was also the first to report on peak values for aerobic power. In a middle-distance runner, 80 ml · kg⁻¹ · min⁻¹ was achieved. A slightly higher value was found in a runner in 1955 by Åstrand (4). Since then, numerous reports have been published, with values reaching 90 ml · kg⁻¹ · min⁻¹ in cross-country skiers (8). In this group of athletes and in rowers the highest absolute maximal oxygen uptake values (7-7.5 L · min⁻¹) are observed (8, 68). The issue, which has been discussed at length, is why top performance in endurance events over the last 50 yr has improved much more than has maximal aerobic power. Part of the explanation is that endurance performance is not synonymous with maximal oxygen uptake (23) (see also the following discussion). Another factor is that technical developments improving efficiency and thus reducing energy turnover for a given exercise intensity also have contributed to improved performance.

Elderly Endurance Athletes

With age a decline occurs in maximal oxygen uptake even in athletes who continue with extreme training and who participate continuously in endurance competitions (Figure 18.4). Of note is that the reduction in maximal oxygen uptake with age

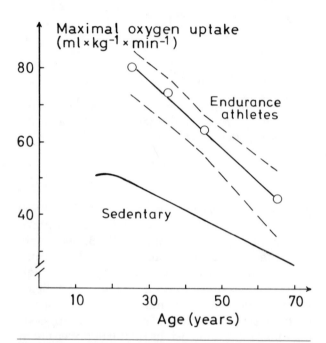

Figure 18.4. Maximal oxygen uptake in young and elderly, top-trained and still-active endurance athletes (Grimby and Saltin, in press). For comparison the mean values for men (Fig. 18.1) are also included.

and in endurance athletes is at least as large as the one observed in sedentary men (about 0.5-0.8 ml • kg^{-1} • min^{-1} per year of age). Several longitudinal training studies of previously sedentary middle-aged men have revealed that the age-related decline in aerobic capacity can be inhibited and even reversed (27, 30, 37, 65, 70). This may last for several years or perhaps for a full decade. This is of no surprise, as aerobic capacity can markedly be elevated with training also in the elderly (7, 28, 29). Thus, it appears that the training-induced improvement in maximal oxygen uptake of sedentary men can counteract an age-related decline. It is noteworthy, however, that there is a limit to the effect of the training in the elderly. The limit is given in Figure 18.4 by the values for the well-

trained endurance athlete. If this upper level is reached, maximal aerobic capacity will decline with age regardless of how well the training is performed.

Pulmonary Function

The only question to be addressed on the subject is whether during heavy exercise the blood returning to the lungs in the pulmonary artery becomes properly oxygenated when passing through the lungs. During intense exhaustive exercise, young sedentary men have a 94% saturation of their arterial blood, and moderate training does not alter the degree of oxygenation (18, 59) (Table 18.1). In endurance athletes with a maximal oxygen uptake of 74 ml • kg^{-1} • min^{-1}, a mean value of 93% was measured during peak exercise. In a few athletes a slightly more pronounced desaturation was noted but was not severe (19). In later studies in our laboratory some individual endurance athletes have been found to desaturate somewhat (72), but none to the extent reported by Dempsey et al. (16) (see also chapt. 19). Therefore, the conclusion is that, in general, the function of the lungs is adequate to maintain an optimal saturation. However, in some rare cases of young endurance athletes, the cardiovascular capacity has surpassed the capacity of the lungs to transfer oxygen. These individuals have very high aerobic capacities but not the highest.

Also, the oxygen saturation of the arterial blood is well maintained during intense exercises in the elderly (Table 18.1). Among the very well trained, a saturation below 95% was not observed. In the older age-groups of men 80 yr old, the oxygen saturation was above 92% in all subjects at a work load that demanded above 95% of their maximal oxygen uptake.

Cardiovascular System

Heart Dimension and Function

The close coupling between the arterially delivered oxygen during exhaustive exercise and the observed maximal oxygen uptake of healthy individuals over a range from 2-7 L • min^{-1} point at the heart function as being crucial for the training response (18, 19, 59) (Figure 18.5). Maximal heart rate is basically unaltered with training, as is arterial oxygen content (Table 18.1). Thus, the

Table 18.1 Mean Value and Range for Oxygen Saturation (SO$_2$), Hemoglobin (Hb), and Arterial Oxygen Content (C$_a$O$_2$) During Exhaustive Work in Studies of Young and Older Men With Different Degrees of Physical Training

	SO$_2$ (%)	Hb (g · L^{-1})	C$_a$O$_2$ (ml · L^{-1})
A. Young men[a]			
Young, sedentary ($n = 18$)	94	158	200
(38 ml · kg^{-1} · min^{-1} = $\dot{V}O_2$max)	92-96	149-169	188-218
Young, trained ($n = 18$)	94.5	159	201
(52 ml · kg^{-1} · min^{-1} = $\dot{V}O_2$max)	92-96	151-163	191-208
Endurance athletes ($n = 8$)	93	151	188
(74 ml · kg^{-1} · min^{-1} = $\dot{V}O_2$max)	89-95	147-162	179-204
B. Older men[b]			
Middle-aged, sedentary ($n = 15$)	97[c]	152	197
(mean age = 47 yr; 35 ml · kg^{-1} · min^{-1} = $\dot{V}O_2$max)	95-99	137-159	178-208
Middle-aged, sedentary ($n = 15$)	96.2[c]	149	189
(mean age = 47.5 yr; 40 ml · kg^{-1} · min^{-1} = $\dot{V}O_2$max)	93-98	141-156	177-204
Middle-aged, top-trained ($n = 7$)	96.7	154	200
(mean age = 55 yr; 43 ml · kg^{-1} · min^{-1})[d]	95-99	138-161	189-209
Old, sedentary ($n = 12$)	96.4	156	202
(mean age = 70 yr; 24 ml · kg^{-1} · min^{-1})[d]	92-99	147-164	193-210

Note. Oxygen uptake observed during exercise is given.

[a]Data are from Ekblom (18), Ekblom and Hermansen (19), and Saltin et al. (62).

[b]Data are from Granath and Strandell (24), Hartley et al. (29), and Wahren et al. (75).

[c]The mean arterial oxygen tension was 93 and 89 mmHg before and after training, respectively.

[d]The top-trained middle-aged men had a maximal oxygen uptake of 48 ml · kg^{-1} · min^{-1} and the older sedentary men approximately 26 ml · kg^{-1} · min^{-1}.

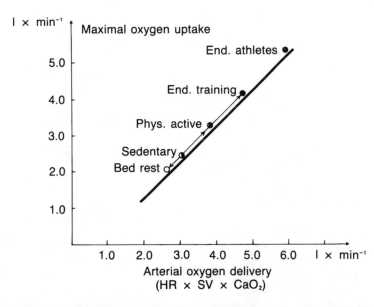

Figure 18.5. Schematic illustration of the close relation found between arterially delivered oxygen during exhaustive work and maximal oxygen uptake (see refs. 18, 19, 62).

conclusion was reached that the stroke volume of the heart was the factor that determined the maximal oxygen delivery and oxygen uptake and the variable that had to become affected by the physical training for an improvement to occur.

The size of the heart is closely related to the aerobic work capacity and to the stroke volume (9) (Figure 18.6). However, the stroke volume of the

heart is also determined by factors other than its anatomical size. One is the blood volume (35), and experimentally induced hypervolemia results in an elevation in stroke volume and maximal cardiac output (36). The notion that the ventricles of the heart eject what they contain is further substantiated by the studies on pericardectomized dogs performing maximal exercise (71). These dogs had elevated stroke volumes of some 15 ml ($\approx$ 20%-25%), which caused maximal cardiac output to increase by 3.5 L • min^{-1} ($\approx$ 20%), and maximal oxygen uptake became significantly elevated.

The notion is that the large stroke volumes observed in trained humans are associated with high filling pressures. It is also true that sedentary subjects reach slightly lower filling pressures than do trained subjects (9) (Figure 18.7), but that is only

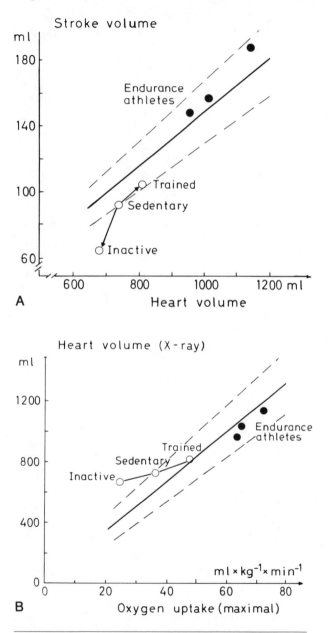

A

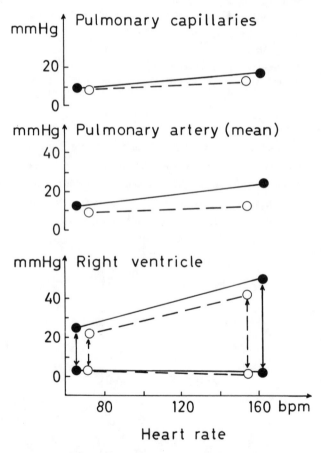

Figure 18.6. A, the relationship between aerobic work capacity and heart volume. The mean values with ± 1 *SD* are from a study of healthy men (slightly modified) (see ref. 33) and the mean values for specific groups (see refs. 9, 18, 19, 62); B, the same material as in Figure 18.6A, but the relationship between heart volume determined from biplane X ray and stroke volume is depicted.

Figure 18.7. Blood pressure in right ventricle, pulmonary artery, and pulmonary capillaries (wedge pressure) in healthy controls and trained bicyclists (see ref. 9). From "Circulatory Studies in Well Trained Athletes at Rest and During Heavy Exercise, With Special Reference to Stroke Volume and the Influence of Body Position" by S. Bevegard, A. Holmgren, and B. Jonsson, 1963, *Acta Physiologica Scandinavica,* **57**, pp. 26-50. Adapted by permission.

part of the explanation. In training studies engaging only one limb, a lower heart rate and a larger stroke volume were encountered when the same submaximal work load was performed with trained as compared with untrained muscles (Table 18.2). Further preliminary observations indicate that the filling pressures of the right ventricle

Table 18.2 Stroke Volume, Cardiac Output, and Heart Rate in Healthy Controls Exercising Submaximally With Inactive and Control Legs

Leg	$\dot{V}O_2$ (L · min⁻¹)	$\dot{Q}$ (L · min⁻¹)	HR (beats/min)
Inactive	1.3	12.4	148
Control	1.2	12.0	122

were the same in the two situations (Kanstrup-Hansen, personal communication). However, end-diastolic volume was larger when the trained muscles were engaged in the exercise. This finding is of interest in view of the results depicted in Figures 18.6 and 18.8. Endurance-trained athletes have slightly larger stroke volumes than was anticipated from the size of their hearts (Figure 18.6). Further, the end-diastolic diameter is also larger than that found in age- and weight-matched controls (38) (Figure 18.8). This points to the possibility

that the compliance of the myocardium is affected by the training and perhaps by the training status of the muscles performing the exercise. Any major alteration in ejection fraction does not occur with training. The small elevation that may be obtained can be related to a reduced after-load (10).

In conclusion, physical activity affects the dimension and function of the heart as well as the blood volume, contributing to the observed alterations in exercise stroke volumes and resulting in a lowered heart rate at submaximal exercise and an elevated maximal cardiac output in exhaustive exercise with improved training status. Elevation of the stroke volume is brought about not only by changes in size of the heart but also by an altered feedback reflex related to the training status of the muscles recruited to perform the exercise. The heart in a well-trained subject produces a larger stroke volume than is expected for the size of the heart.

Cardiovascular Function in the Elderly

It is apparent from the summary in Table 18.3 that the reduction in maximal oxygen uptake in the elderly is due to a lower capacity both to elevate the cardiac output and to widen the (a-v)O_2 difference, where the latter variable has only a small functional significance. This relates to sedentary as well as to trained subjects. The decline in maximal heart rate with age is the key to lower maximal cardiac output, but especially in the older-age

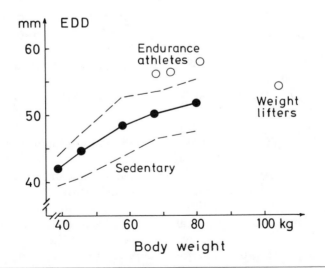

Figure 18.8. End-diastolic diameter in relation to body weight in a control material and in graphs of trained subjects (see ref. 38). From "Effect of Static and Dynamic Exercise on Heart Volume, Contractility, and Left Ventricular Dimensions" by J. Keul, H.-H. Dickhuth, G. Simon, and M. Lehmann, 1981, *Circulation Research*, **48**(6), pp. I162-I170. Adapted by permission of the American Heart Association, Inc.

Table 18.3 Summary of Data From Studies of Cardiovascular Responses to Maximal Exercise in Men of Different Ages and Degrees of Training

Variable	Young[a]			Middle-aged[b]			Elderly[c]
	Sedentary	Trained	Athletes	Sedentary	Trained	Athletes	Sedentary
Oxygen uptake							
$L \cdot min^{-1}$	3.10	3.60	5.51	2.68	3.09	3.56	1.98
$ml \cdot kg^{-1} \cdot min^{-1}$	43	50	74	34	40	52	26
Cardiac output ($L \cdot min^{-1}$)	20.6	23	32.4	18.7	21.1	26.6	13.6
Heart rate (beats/min)	194	190	183	180	176	171	153
Stroke volume (ml)	106	128	177	103	120	156	89
Arteriovenous O_2 difference ($ml \cdot L^{-1}$)	150	156	170	142	145	134	145
Mean arterial blood pressure (mmHg)	112	111	109	143	146	132	143

[a]$N = 17$. The young, trained men were 20-26 yr old and were studied by Rowell (49), Saltin et al. (62), and Ekblom et al. (18). The young athletes were studied by Ekblom and Hermansen (19) and Hermansen and Saltin (32).

[b]$N = 15$. The middle-aged, trained men were 38-55 yr old and were studied by Hartley et al. (29).

[c]The athletically trained, elderly men ($n = 9$) were 49-55 yr old and were studied by Grimby et al. (26). The sedentary, elderly men ($n = 12$) were studied by Granath and Strandell (24) during intense, but not always exhaustive, exercise.

group the reduction in stroke volume is also apparent. In this respect these data are in sharp contrast to the finding of Gerstenblith, Weisfeldt, and Lakatta reported in Lakatta (42) that in aging, healthy, sedentary men an enlarged stroke volume compensates for the lower maximal heat rate, resulting in a maintained peak cardiac output. The various age-related effects are more fully described by Buskirk (see chapt. 59). A more specific analysis on cardiovascular adaptation of the elderly is found elsewhere (27, 56, 66).

Distribution of the Cardiac Output

Very early in a training regimen, a widening of the maximal systemic (a-v)O_2 difference can be demonstrated. The explanation is that a smaller fraction of the cardiac output is perfusing noncontracting tissues, leaving only brain and skin blood flow unaltered. This results in more oxygen being extracted. More detailed studies have revealed that both splanchnic and kidney blood flow are reduced in relation to the relative work load (25, 51). These regulations should make a larger blood flow available to the contracting muscles.

When investigators sought to prove the hypothesis that there would be a larger peak blood flow in trained than in untrained muscles, no (or only very small) differences were found. In fact, only 0.5-0.7 $L \cdot kg^{-1} \cdot min^{-1}$ in maximal muscle

blood flow could be demonstrated (13). This led Mellander and Johansson (43) to conclude that all muscles of the body had to be exercising maximally to tax the pump capacity of the heart. In accordance with this view, for the maximal oxygen uptake to become elevated, not only the central hemodynamics but also peripheral factors (e.g., the muscle capillary bed and mitochondria) had to be improved. Experimental data supporting such a proposal became available from studies of training only one leg. The trained leg revealed an expansion of the capillary network and the mitochondrial volume that was accompanied by a larger peak oxygen uptake (62). The muscles of the untrained limb showed no local adaptations and only a small increase in peak oxygen uptake. In 1976 and 1977, Clausen (14, 15) reviewed the field and pointed at the close match between links in oxygen transport. He drew special attention to the fact that the highest maximal oxygen uptake was found among those who could elevate their vascular conductances the most. He proposed that the critical factor in the cardiovascular adaptation to physical training was to be able to reduce the peripheral resistance.

This was the setting when Secher et al. (67) published their study in 1977. They had subjects exercise with their legs on a bicycle, then, while continuing the leg exercise at the same load, the arms were also made to exercise. Cardiac output increased slightly, reaching the ceiling of the pump capacity of the heart. In addition, and most important, the leg blood flow was reduced. This occurred with an unaltered blood pressure. The question was then: Why did a reduction in limb blood flow occur? Although the answer at the time was not apparent, the results gave rise to concerns about the true perfusion capacity of skeletal muscles. Could it be that the plethysmographic and [33]Xe-clearance measurements underestimate the skeletal muscle blood flow?

Muscle Blood Flow

With the introduction in the 1980s of the microsphere technique to determine regional blood flows in various species came the finding that the skeletal muscle blood flow of a rat while running was markedly higher than those flows observed earlier in electrically stimulated, vascularly isolated muscles (3). Other methods had to be developed for humans. In addition, if the heart constituted a limitation, it was important that only a small fraction of the muscle mass was engaged in the exercise. Thus, the exercise chosen was either dynamic or intermittent static knee-extension contraction of the quadriceps femoris muscle of one leg (2, 52, 73, 76). Peak perfusion was estimated using the Doppler technique to determine velocity of the flow in the femoral artery and was well above 1 L $\cdot$ kg^{-1} $\cdot$ min^{-1}. This occurred without any increase in perfusion pressure. In dynamic exercise, blood flows were achieved that were equally high or higher (Figure 18.9). In light of this new information, the results of Secher et al. (67) could be explained. The vasoconstriction of the lower-limb vessels when the arms are added to ongoing intense leg exercise is a necessity to maintain blood pressure because the total peripheral conductance of skeletal muscle surpasses the pump capacity of the heart. The question raised by Clausen (15) about which factor will reduce vascular resistance with training can now also be answered: The improved capacity of the heart to provide a blood flow allows for a higher peripheral conductance.

The muscle blood flow can be estimated fairly accurately. The total perfusion of noncontracting tissues during exercise amounts to 3-4 L $\cdot$ min^{-1} in an average-size man. Thus, if maximal cardiac output can reach 15 L $\cdot$ min^{-1}, some 11-12 L $\cdot$ min^{-1} of blood perfuses the exercising muscles. If the exercise is performed by legs, up to 15 kg of muscle may be engaged in the exercise. The perfusion is then less than 1 L $\cdot$ kg^{-1} $\cdot$ min^{-1}. After a period of physical training, maximal cardiac output may

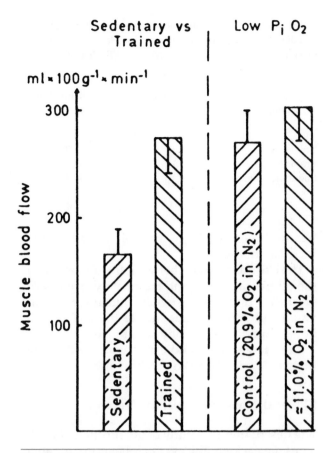

Figure 18.9. Mean values for limb (muscle) blood flow in healthy controls during exhaustive one-legged known-extensor exercise (see refs. 2, 52). From "Capacity of Blood Flow Delivery of Exercising Muscle in Humans" by B. Saltin, 1988, *American Journal of Cardiology*, **62**, pp. 30E-35E. Adapted by permission.

be increased to 20 L $\cdot$ min^{-1}. Now 16-17 L $\cdot$ min^{-1} of blood flow is available to the same muscle mass, and the perfusion of the muscles is above 1 L $\cdot$ min^{-1} $\cdot$ kg^{-1}. Endurance-trained athletes may reach 30 L $\cdot$ min^{-1} in cardiac output, which allows them a muscular blood flow of close to 2 L $\cdot$ kg^{-1} $\cdot$ min^{-1}. From these calculations it is apparent that if the intense exercise is swimming or rowing, almost the whole muscle mass ($\approx$ 25-30 kg) is involved in the exercise, and the muscle blood flow is then lowered accordingly.

The critical factor is (as discussed in detail previously) the pump performance of the heart coupled with its size. This is exemplified in Table 18.4, where heart volume is related to its peak ejected volume normalized for body weight. The untrained heart with values up to 10 ml $\cdot$ kg^{-1} of body weight can produce a cardiac output of 0.25 L $\cdot$ min^{-1} $\cdot$ kg^{-1} of body weight, whereas a top-trained

Table 18.4   Heart Volume and Observed Maximal Cardiac Output Both Normalized for Body Weight in Groups With Different Degrees of Physical Training

Training status	Heart volume (ml · kg⁻¹)	Cardiac output (L · min⁻¹ · kg⁻¹)
Sedentary	10	0.26
Trained	12	0.33
Endurance athletes	16	0.50

heart can produce twice that volume with a 50% increase in size.

The close association between the dimension of the central circulation and maximal oxygen uptake is further documented when humans are compared with other species such as the dog and the horse. In relation to body weight, the horse has 3 times larger heart and cardiac output than the human. Maximal oxygen uptake is also tripled (58).

Skeletal Muscle Capillary Network

The description and study of the function of capillaries have a long history, but reliable quantitative data have been available for only about a decade (63). In humans, 300-350 capillaries per square millimeter are found in most muscles that are not specifically trained. These capillaries are rather equally distributed among the various muscle fiber types with two to four capillaries found around each fiber. As the sharing factor is close to 3, the average number of capillaries per fiber is 0.8-1.2 in muscles of sedentary individuals. One reason for the similar capillary supply of the various fiber types in the muscle of humans as compared with other species could be that the fiber types are mixed; that is, fast-twitch fibers of the b type (FTb) are surrounded by FTa, or slow-twitch (ST), fibers. Because the two types share capillaries, there will be equal numbers of each. In this perspective it is noteworthy that the number of capillaries around enclosed FTb fibers is close to that of enclosed FTa and ST fibers (69). This pattern of capillary supply observed in human muscle is in harmony with a smaller difference in the metabolic profile of its muscle fiber types than that of other species.

Oxygen Delivery and Extraction

The question now is: How large a perfusion does the capillary network receive? As discussed previ-

ously, the upper limit is above 1.5 and could be 2.0-2.5 L · kg⁻¹ · min⁻¹, which is three- to fourfold higher than that reported in ordinary two-legged exercise (see Figure 18.9). Peak oxygen delivered to the muscle is then in the order of 0.4 L · kg⁻¹ · min⁻¹, of which 20%-25%, or 0.08-0.10 L · kg⁻¹ · min⁻¹, returns to the main circulation, as it is not extracted. This lack of complete extraction of the oxygen can have many explanations. One possibility would be a-v shunting, which is very unlikely to occur in human skeletal muscle. A mismatch between the distribution of the blood flow in the muscle and energy turnover of individual fibers of the muscle could well exist, but whether it is present has not been investigated in humans. What has been examined is the role of the time needed for the passage of blood through the capillaries, or mean transit time (MTT). The number of capillaries in the muscle is known (Table 18.5), as are their diameters (6-6.1 µm) and average length (1 mm) (34). These data give estimates of volume of the capillary net of 1%-1.5% in the skeletal muscle of sedentary humans.

A pertinent question is whether all capillaries have a flow. There are two lines of evidence that they all have a flow during intense dynamic exercise. Krogh (41) described the alternating recruitment of capillaries and the opening of more capillaries when blood flow increased. Studies supporting this concept showed that approximately 20% of the capillaries in skeletal muscle have a blood flow at rest; and with a recruitment factor of 4-5 when going to intense contractions, all (or nearly all) capillaries have indeed opened (46). Results from studies using vital microscopy described the pattern slightly differently. These investigations demonstrated that all capillaries have a flow at rest, but the velocity and hematocrit of blood in capillaries varies markedly, with blood flow velocity in some capillaries being close to zero (17). With increased blood flow the velocity of the flow increases and becomes more even. Despite this discrepancy, it appears valid to conclude that the whole capillary network is utilized in intense exercise.

In a resting muscle, MTT has been estimated to be 6 s or longer (55). During intense dynamic contraction performed with a small-muscle group like the knee extensors of one leg, MTT drops to 0.5 s or less, whereas it is close to 1 s during two-legged exercise. Inversely related to the MTT is the arterio-venous oxygen difference over the exercising limb (Figure 18.10). This relationship appears to be hyperbolic, suggesting that a further fall in MTT below a certain critical value will result in a

Table 18.5 Data on Skeletal Muscle Capillaries of the Lateral Head of the Medial Gastrocnemius in Groups With Different Degrees of Physical Training

| | | Oxidative capacity | |
Training status	Capillaries (per mm²)	Mitochondrial volume (vol %)	Citrate synthase (V_{max}) (mmol · kg⁻¹ · min⁻¹)
Young, inactive	280	2.4	4.6
Young, sedentary	310	3.7	6.8
Trained	380	4.8	12.4
Endurance athlete	780	11.4	27.4

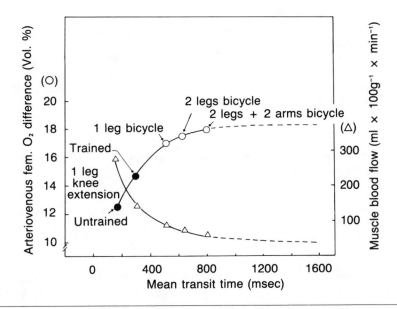

Figure 18.10. Observed $(a-\bar{v}_{fem})O_2$ differences during maximal work and estimated mean transit times in relation to muscle blood flow (see ref. 55). From "Central Cardiovascular Factors as Limits to Endurance; With a Note on the Distinction Between Maximal Oxygen Uptake and Endurance Fitness" by G. Savard, B. Kiens, and B. Saltin, 1987, in Macleod, Maughan, Nimmo, Reilly, and Williams (Eds.), *Exercise: Benefits and Limits and Adaptations* (p. 169). London: E. & F.N. Spon Ltd. Reprinted by permission.

pronounced drop in oxygen extraction. The precision and quantity of data on this topic do not allow an exact identification of the MTT when a reduced extraction occurs. However, it is easily understood why it does (Figure 18.11). As muscle perfusion increases in relation to elevation in exercise intensity, a larger fraction of the capillary network is utilized until the entire capacity is reached. At this point a sharp drop in MTT occurs, resulting in less oxygen being extracted. In intense one-legged knee-extensor exercise, this point has been surpassed, whereas in two-legged maximal exercise it has not.

Thus, the functional significance of a capillary proliferation in muscle with training should be viewed in this way. A larger capillary bed and

blood volume are needed to maintain or possibly elongate the MTT at intense exercise when peak muscle blood flow is enlarged. An illustration of this is found in men with different exercise capacities of their knee extensors (Table 18.6). In spite of the fact that men with the best work performances had the largest blood flows, they had the lowest femoral vein oxygen contents and the largest oxygen differences over the exercising limbs because of more capillaries (55).

The finding that during maximal exercise in humans there is some oxygen left in the vein blood that drains contracting muscles has been used as an argument for a peripheral limitation to maximal oxygen uptake (74; see also ref. 58). Actual PO_2 values are in the range of 8- to 12 mmHg and

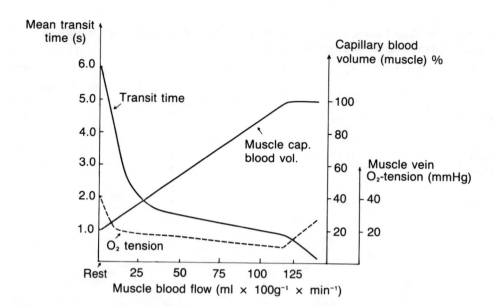

Figure 18.11. A theoretical account for the relationship between muscle blood flow, mean transit time, and oxygen tension in a vein draining a muscle.

Table 18.6   Mean Values for Certain Variables for Subjects Grouped as Low or High Performers and for 6 Subjects Who Have Trained One Leg

	Flow $(ml \cdot kg^{-1} \cdot min^{-1})$	$(a-v_{fem})O_2$ $(ml \cdot L^{-1})$	Capillary density (mm^2)	Capillary blood volume (vol %)	Mean transit time (ms)
Low[a]	2,100	123	280	0.8	380
Nontrained leg	2,350	131	320	0.9	395
High[b]	2,750	149	440	1.4	425
Trained leg	2,600	138	380	1.1	510

[a]$n = 5$.

[b]$n = 3$.

oxygen contents in the range of 10-18 ml · L⁻¹ (Table 18.7). In humans, most of the blood in the femoral vein distal to the saphenous vein drains contracting muscle, but it is unlikely that all blood is from active muscle. The blood flow in the femoral vein of the leg during two-legged maximal exercise of sedentary humans is in the order of 7-9 L · min⁻¹. If only half a liter comes from skin and other tissues and if it contains 50 ml O₂, it can almost account for the oxygen found in the femoral vein blood, suggesting that only very little oxygen remains in blood after passing through intensely contracting skeletal muscle capillaries. However, it is unlikely that some O₂ is left. A complete extraction of O₂ would be unlikely, as there has to be a driving force for the O₂ to diffuse out of the capillary. At least two conditions are to be considered at this point. The unloading of O₂ from the red cells in the capillaries follows an exponential curve; that is, after an initial fast lowering of the PO₂ of the blood, it slowly approaches zero. At these very low oxygen tensions the affinity of the hemoglobin for oxygen also counteracts a complete O₂ extraction. In many respects the situation in the skeletal muscle capillary is the reverse of that observed in the lungs, where the blood becomes saturated with O₂ but never fully. In addition, if there is some countercurrent exchange of O₂ between arteries and veins, it could account for some of the observed amount of O₂ present in the venous-blood-draining muscle. Thus, there is not much need either for a mismatch between flow dis-

Table 18.7   Oxygen Tension and Content in Femoral Vein Blood During Exhaustive Running in Men With Different Degrees of Physical Training

Training status	PO₂ (mmHg)	O₂ content (ml · L⁻¹)
Inactive	12	11
Sedentary	18	22
Physical training		
Some months	10	18
Years	8	10

tribution and muscle fiber activation or for a diffusing limitation at the level of the capillary endothelial and sarcolemmal interface to explain that some oxygen is left in the veins that drain contracting skeletal muscle.

The conclusion then is that although a small volume of oxygen is left in the vein blood returning from an exercising limb, it is not an indication of a limitation by the muscles to extract or utilize the oxygen that is offered. Rather, it is the result of some admixture of blood from noncontracting tissues and the need for a driving force for oxygen to accomplish a flux of oxygen along the whole length of the muscle capillary.

Matching Central and Regional Circulation

In the scheme presented by Mellander and Johansson (43), the central circulation provided the blood flow that the skeletal muscles demanded during exercise. Local factors controlling vasodilatation induce an increase in the peripheral conductance of skeletal muscle. The cardiac output is concomitantly increased to maintain pressure. The elevation of the cardiac output response is brought about by a combined central drive and a peripheral input from the contracting muscles (50). This pattern is valid in both small- and large-muscle-group exercise. When both legs perform the exercise, additional regulations come into play. This is most apparent with more intense exercise. What is needed is not only strict control of vasomotor tonus in vessels feeding noncontracting tissues or organs but also an adjustment of the degree of vasodilatation of the arterial tree in the exercising legs to match the output of the heart. The sympathetic nervous system serves this function. Its

activity in contracting muscles is gradually enhanced the higher is the work intensity and the larger is the fraction of muscle mass involved in the exercise (64). There appears to be an ongoing competition between centrally mediated vasoconstrictor activity and local vasodilatation. The balance between these two forces sets the tonus of the smooth muscles of the terminal arterioles with the result that blood pressure is maintained.

I have stated that peak cardiac output is reduced in the elderly (see Table 18.4). The question is whether this lowering of the cardiac reserve has an impact on the output from the sympathetic nervous system. The finding of higher plasma norepinephrine values not only at rest but also during exercise may indicate that this is the case (39). Further limb blood flow during exercise in middle-aged men is less than it is in young controls (75).

It has been speculated which sensors and regulatory mechanisms contribute to this very precise adjustment of the peripheral conductance and the available blood flow (50, 58). Mechanoreceptors in the arterial system (baroreceptors) and the ventricles may be key factors in the regulation. The latter sense end-diastolic volume and thus stroke volume. The former sense the match of the ejected volume of blood and the peripheral conductance beat by beat. The question is whether a muscle reflex is part of this precise regulation. With the pronounced specificity exhibited by the various C-fibers found in the interstitium of skeletal muscle (44), it is tempting to speculate. With intense muscle contractions, substances are accumulating, activating specific groups of C-fibers that modulate the sympathetic outflow. This can be to affect both the heart and the vessels in the muscles. In the latter case, depending on signals and need, it can be either vasodilatation or vasoconstriction. Such a system has the advantage of not only sensing various levels of the metabolic status of the muscle but also mediating information of the anatomical localization precisely.

Some comparisons have been made between humans and other species, and it may be worthwhile to point out that the role of the sympathetic nervous system during exercise may be quite different in a species in which a reasonably good match exists between the cardiac output and the potential of the periphery to elevate the conductance. This relates, for example, to the dog, in which an overriding sympathetic control of vasomotor tonus in muscle may be of minimal importance, whereas it is crucial for maintaining blood pressure in exercising humans.

Conclusion

Different links in the oxygen-transporting system of the body have quite different capacities for oxygen transfer (Table 18.8). In sedentary humans the heart is clearly the variable with the lowest potential, which, with physical activity, can be brought to a level approaching the capacity of the lungs, the latter being more resistant to adaptive changes with training. Untrained and trained muscles in whole-body exercise can receive a blood flow and extract the offered oxygen.

Table 18.8   Summary of Maximal Values of the Oxygen Volume That Can Be Transferred by the Lungs and Heart and Extracted and Consumed by the Muscles

	Sedentary	Endurance athletes
Lungs	70-90	80-100
Heart	50-60	90-110
Periphery (skeletal muscle)	200-300	> 400

Note. Data expressed as ml $\cdot$ kg^{-1} $\cdot$ min^{-1}.

Another approach to analyze the role of relative links of oxygen transport is attempted in Table 18.9, in which the observed values for some variables in healthy sedentary subjects are compared with a theoretical, or obtainable, trained value. Again, the conclusion is similar to the one just made. Several possibilities for an adaptation to occur with training exist, but the link most responsive is cardiac output, which then must be viewed as the one that constitutes the major functional limitation to an individual's aerobic work capacity.

It is obvious that, although our knowledge about the physiological effects of physical conditioning has been broadened, several key issues remain unanswered. Nevertheless, the actual regulatory mechanisms of the adaptive response to training and their significance need not be understood for one to enjoy physical activity or to implement exercise programs in patient groups for which physical training has been proven to be beneficial.

Acknowledgments

The original work performed in our laboratory was supported by grants from the Medical Research Council, the Danish Heart Association, and the Research Council of the Danish Sports Federation.

References

1. Andersen, L.B., P. Henckel, and B. Saltin. Maximal oxygen uptake in Danish adolescents, 16-19 years of age. *Eur. J. Appl. Physiol.* 56: 74-82, 1987.
2. Andersen, P., and B. Saltin. Maximal perfusion of skeletal muscle in man. *J. Physiol. (Lond.)* 366: 233-249, 1985.
3. Armstrong, R.B., and M.H. Laughlin. Blood flows within and among rat muscles as a function of time during high speed treadmill exercise. *J. Physiol.* 344: 189-208, 1983.
4. Åstrand, P.-O. New records in human power. *Nature* 176: 922-923, 1955.
5. Åstrand, P.-O., and K. Rodahl. *Textbook of work physiology: Physiological bases of exercise.* 3rd ed. New York: McGraw-Hill, 1986.
6. Bar-Or, O. *Pediatric sports medicine for the practitioners: Physiological principles to clinical applications.* New York: Springer-Verlag, 1983.

Table 18.9   Summary of Normal Values for Some of the Variables of the Cardiovascular System

Variable	Observed sedentary	Theoretical or observed	
		Maximum	Improvement (%)
Arterial O_2 saturation (%)	95	100	$\approx$ 5 No
Hemoglobin (g $\cdot$ L^{-1})	150	160	$\approx$ 7 No
Arterial O_2 content (ml $\cdot$ L^{-1})	190	215	$\approx$ 13 No
Cardiac output (L $\cdot$ min^{-1})	20	38	$\approx$ 90 Yes
Blood flow to noncontracting tissues (L $\cdot$ min^{-1})	4	3.5	$\approx$ 12 Yes
Skeletal muscle O_2 extraction (ml $\cdot$ L^{-1})	170	215	$\approx$ 25 Yes

7. Benestad, A.M. Trainability of old men. *Acta Med. Scand.* 178: 321, 1965.

8. Bergh, U. *"Längdlöpning,"* Idrottsfysiologi, rapport no. 11. Stockholm: Trygg-Hansa, 1974.

9. Bevegård, S., A. Holmgren, and B. Jonsson. Circulatory studies in well trained athletes at rest and during heavy exercise, with special reference to stroke volume and the influence of body position. *Acta Physiol. Scand.* 57: 26-50, 1963.

10. Blomqvist, C.G., and B. Saltin. Cardiovascular adaptations to physical training. *Annu. Rev. Physiol.* 45: 169-189, 1983.

11. Boerhave, H. *Johann Swammerdamm's Bibel der Natur.* Leipzig, 1752.

12. Borms, J. The child and exercise: An overview. *J. Sports Sci.* 4: 3-20, 1986.

13. Clausen, J.P. Muscle blood flow during exercise and its significance for maximal performance. In: Keul, J., ed. *Limiting factors of physical performance.* Stuttgart, FRG: Georg Thieme, 1973, p. 253.

14. Clausen, J.P. Circulatory adjustments to dynamic exercise and effect of physical training in normal subjects and in patients with coronary artery disease. *Prog. Cardiovasc. Dis.* 18(6): 459-495, 1976.

15. Clausen, J.P. Effect of physical training on cardiovascular adjustments to exercise in man. *Physiol. Rev.* 57: 779-815, 1977.

16. Dempsey, J.A., P. Hanson, and K. Henderson. Exercise-induced arterial hypoxemia in healthy humans at sea-level. *J. Physiol. (Lond.)* 355: 161-175, 1984.

17. Duling, B.R., and B. Klitzman. Local control of microvascular function: Role in tissue oxygen supply. *Annu. Rev. Physiol.* 42: 373-382, 1980.

18. Ekblom, B. Effect of physical training on oxygen transport system in man. *Acta Physiol. Scand. Suppl.* 328: 5-45, 1969.

19. Ekblom, B. and L. Hermansen. Cardiac output in athletes. *J. Appl. Physiol.* 25: 619-625, 1968.

20. Eriksson, B.O. Physical training, oxygen, supply and muscle metabolism in 11-13 year old boys. *Acta Physiol. Scand. Suppl.* 384, 1972.

21. Evovainio, R., and S. Sundberg. A five year follow-up study on cardiorespiratory function in adolescent elite endurance runners. *Acta Paediatr. Scand.* 72: 351-356, 1983.

22. Folkow, B. and E. Neil. *Circulation.* New York: Oxford University Press, 1971.

23. Gollnick, P.D., and B. Saltin. Significance of skeletal muscle oxidative enzyme enhancement with endurance training. *Clin. Physiol.* 2: 1-12, 1982.

24. Granath, A., and T. Strandell. Relationships between cardiac output stroke volume and intracardiac pressures at rest and during exercise in supine position and some anthropometric data in healthy old men. *Acta Med. Scand.* 176: 447-466, 1964.

25. Grimby, G. Renal clearance during prolonged supine exercise at different loads. *J. Appl. Physiol.* 20: 1264, 1965.

26. Grimby, G., N.J. Nilsson, and B. Saltin. Cardiac output during submaximal and maximal exercise in active middle-aged athletes. *J. Appl. Physiol.* 21: 1150-1156, 1966.

27. Hagberg, J.M., W.K. Allen, D.R. Seals, B.F. Hurley, A.A. Ehsani, and J.O. Holloszy. A hemodynamic comparison of young and older endurance athletes during exercise. *J. Appl. Physiol.* 58: 2041-2046, 1985.

28. Hason, J.S., B.S. Tabakin, A.M. Levy, and W. Nedde. Long-term physical training and cardiovascular dynamics in middle-aged men. *Circulation* 38: 783-794, 1968.

29. Hartley, L.H., G. Grimby, Å. Kilbom, N.J. Nilsson, I. Åstrand, J. Bjure, B. Ekblom, and B. Saltin. Physical training in sedentary middle-aged and older men. *Scand. J. Clin. Lab. Invest.* 24: 335, 1969.

30. Heath, G.W., J.M. Hagberg, A.A. Ehsani, and J.O. Holloszy. A physiological comparison of young and older endurance athletes. *J. Appl. Physiol.* 51: 634-640.

31. Henschen, E.S. Skidlöpning och skidtäfling. In: *Reports from Uppsala Universitet* (Annual report, 1897). 1-69, 1898.

32. Hermansen, L., and B. Saltin. Oxygen uptake during maximal treadmill and bicycle exercise. *J. Appl. Physiol.* 26: 31-37, 1969.

33. Holmgren, A., F. Mossfeldt, T. Sjöstrand, et al. Effect of training on work capacity, total hemoglobin, blood volume, heart volume, and pulse rate in recumbent and upright positions. *Acta Physiol. Scand.* 50: 72, 1960.

34. Hoppeler, H., and S.L. Lindstedt. Malleability of skeletal muscle in overcoming limitations: Structural elements. *J. Exp. Biol.* 115: 355-364, 1985.

35. Hopper, M.K., A.R. Coggan, and E.F. Coyle. Exercise stroke volume relative to plasma-volume expansion. *J. Appl. Physiol.* 64(1): 404-408, 1988.

36. Kanstrup, I.-L., and B. Ekblom. Acute hypervolemia, cardiac performance and aerobic

power during exercise. *J. Appl. Physiol.* 52(5): 1186-1191, 1982.

37. Kasch, F., and J.P. Wallace. Physiological variables during 10 years of endurance exercise. *Med. Sci. Sports* 8: 5-8, 1976.

38. Keul, J., H.-H. Dickhuth, G. Simon, and M. Lehmann. Effect of static and dynamic exercise on heart volume, contractility, and left ventricular dimensions. *Cir. Res.* 48(6): I162-I170, 1981.

39. Kjaer, M. *Epinephrine and some other hormonal responses to exercise in man.* Unpublished master's thesis, Copenhagen University, Copenhagen, Denmark, 1988.

40. Knuttgen, H.G., L.-O. Nordesjö, B. Ollander, and B. Saltin. Physical conditioning through interval training with young male adults. *Med. Sci. Sports* 5: 220-226, 1973.

41. Krogh, A. *The anatomy and physiology of capillaries.* New Haven, CT: Yale University Press, 1922.

42. Lakatta, E. Hemodynamic adaptations to stress with advancing age. *Acta Med. Scand. Suppl.* 771: 39-52, 1986.

43. Mellander, S., and B. Johansson. Control of resistance, exchange, and capacitance functions in the peripheral circulation. *Pharmacol. Rev.* 20: 117, 1968.

44. Mitchell, J.H., and R.F. Schmidt. Cardiovascular reflex control by afferent fibers from skeletal muscle receptors. In: Shepherd, J.T., F.M. Abboud, and S.R. Geiger, eds. *Handbook of physiology. The cardiovascular system. Peripheral circulation and organ blood flow.* Bethesda, MD: American Physiological Society, 1983, vol. 3, sect. 2, p. 623-658.

45. Nordesjö, L. The effect of quantitated training on the capacity for short and prolonged work. *Acta Phys. Scand. Suppl.* 405: 1974.

46. Renkin, E.M. Control of microcirculation and exchange. In: Shepherd, J.T., F.M. Abboud, and S.R. Geiger, eds. *Handbook of physiology.* Bethesda, MD: American Physiological Society, 1984, sect. 2, p. 627-687.

47. Robinson, S. Experimental studies of physical fitness in relation to age. *Arbeitsphysiologie* 10: 251-323, 1938.

48. Robinson, S., H.T. Edwards, and D.B. Dill. New records in human power. *Science* 85: 409-410, 1937.

49. Rowell, L.B. *Factors affecting the prediction of the maximal oxygen intake from measurements made during submaximal work.* Unpublished doctoral dissertation, University of Minnesota, Minneapolis, 1962.

50. Rowell, L.B. *Human circulation regulation during physical stress.* New York: Oxford University Press, 1986.

51. Rowell, L.B., G.L. Brengelmann, J.R. Blackmon, R.D. Twiss, and F. Kusumi. Splanchnic blood flow and metabolism in heat-stressed humans. *J. Appl. Physiol.* 24: 475-484, 1968.

52. Rowell, L.B., B. Saltin, B. Kiens, and N.J. Christensen. Is peak quadriceps blood flow in humans even higher during exercise with hypoxemia? *Am. J. Physiol. (Heart Circ. Physiol.)* 251: H1038-H1044, 1986.

53. Saltin, B. Physiological effects of physical conditioning. *Med. Sci. Sport* 1: 50-56, 1969.

54. Saltin, B. Physiological effects of physical conditioning. In: Tybjaerg-Hansen, A., P. Schnohr, and G. Rose, eds. *Ischaemic heart disease. The strategy of postponement.* The Danish Heart Foundation, FADL's forlag: 1977, p. 104-115.

55. Saltin, B. Malleability of the system in overcoming limitations: Functional elements. *J. Exp. Biol.* 115: 345-354, 1985.

56. Saltin, B. The aging endurance athlete. In: Sutton, J.R., and R.M. Brock, ed. *Sports medicine for the mature athlete.* Indianapolis: Benchmark Press, 1986, p. 59-80.

57. Saltin, B. Fysisk arbejdsevne—før og nu. In: *Københavns Universitets Almanak*, p. 143-153, 1988.

58. Saltin, B. The capacity of blood flow delivery to exercising skeletal muscle in humans. *Am. J. Cardiol.* 62: 30E-35E, 1988.

59. Saltin, B., G. Blomqvist, J.H. Mitchell, R.L. Johnson, Jr., K. Wildenthal, and C.B. Chapman. Response to exercise after bed rest and after training. *Circulation* 38(7): 1-78, 1968.

60. Saltin, B., and B. Ollander. *Fysisk arbetsförmåga hos värnpliktiga* (Report to the chief of the Swedish Army). 1970.

61. Saltin, B., and B. Ollander. *Fysisk arbetsförmåga hos värnpliktiga* (Report to the chief of the Swedish Army). 1972.

62. Saltin, B., K. Nazar, P.L. Costill, E. Stein, E. Jansson, B. Essen, and P.D. Gollnick. The nature of the training response; peripheral and central adaptations to one-legged exercise. *Acta Physiol. Scand.* 96: 289-305, 1976.

63. Saltin, B., and P.D. Gollnick. Skeletal muscle adaptability: Significance for metabolism and performance. In: Peachey, L.D., P.H. Adrian, and S.R. Geiger, eds. *Handbook of physiology: Skeletal muscle.* Bethesda, MD: American Physiology Society, 1983, p. 555-631.

64. Savard, G.K., E.A. Richter, S. Strange, B. Kiens, N.J. Christensen, and B. Saltin. *Norepinephrine spillover from skeletal muscle during dynamic exercise in man: Role of muscle mass.* Manuscript submitted for publication, 1989.

65. Seals, D.R., J.M. Hagberg, B.F. Harley, A.A. Ehsani, and J.O. Holloszy. Endurance training in older men and women. I. Cardiovascular responses to exercise. *J. Appl. Physiol.* 57: 1024-1029, 1984.

66. Seals, D., J.M. Hagberg, J.E. Yerg II, R. Biello, C. Yamamoto, and A. Ehsani. Left ventricular systolic function during exercise in older endurance athletes. *Circulation* (in press).

67. Secher, N.H., J.P. Clausen, K. Klausen, I. Nore, and J. Trap-Jensen. Central and regional circulatory effects of adding arm exercise to leg exercise. *Acta Physiol. Scand.* 100: 288-297, 1977.

68. Secher, N.H. The physiology of rowing. *J. Sports Sci.* 1: 23, 1983.

69. Sjøgaard, G. Capillary supply and cross-sectional area of slow and fast twitch muscle fibres in man. *Histochemistry* 76: 547-555, 1982.

70. Skinner, J.S. Age and performance. In: Keul, J., ed. *Limiting factors of physical performance.* Stuttgart, FRG: Georg Thieme, 1973, p. 271-282.

71. Stray-Gundersen, J., T.I. Musch, G.C. Haidet, D.P. Swain, G.A. Ordway, and J.H. Mitchell. The effect of pericardiectomy on maximal oxygen consumption and maximal cardiac output in untrained dogs. *Circ. Res.* 58: 523-530, 1986.

72. Terrados, N., M. Mizuno, and H. Andersen. Reduction in maximal oxygen uptake at low altitudes: Role of training status and lung function. *Clin. Physiol.* 5(3): 75-79, 1985.

73. Valløe, L., and J. Wesche. The time course and magnitude of blood flow changes in the human quadriceps muscle during and following rhythmic contractions. *J. Physiol.* 405: 257-273, 1988.

74. Wagner, P.D., J.T. Reeves, J.R. Sutton, A. Cymerman, B.M. Groves, M.K. Calconian, and P.M. Young. Possible limitations of maximal O_2 uptake by peripheral tissue diffusion. *Annu. Rev. Respir. Dis.* 133: A202, 1986.

75. Wahren, J., B. Saltin, L. Jorfeldt, and B. Pernow. Influence of age on the local circulatory adaptation to leg exercise. *Scand. J. Clin. Lab. Invest.* 33: 79-86, 1974.

76. Wesche. J. The time course and magnitude of blood flow changes in the human quadriceps muscles following isometric contraction. *J. Physiol.* 44: 151-164, 1986.

Chapter 19

Discussion: Cardiovascular and Pulmonary Adaptation to Physical Activity

Jerome A. Dempsey
Scott K. Powers
Norman Gledhill

Dr. Saltin correctly analyzes central and peripheral components to the cardiovascular system as critical contributors to maximum oxygen delivery and to the determination of $\dot{V}O_2$max in all healthy persons. My only problem with this point of view is that he dismisses the pulmonary system response to exercise in health as an adequate one in terms of homeostasis of systemic arterial oxygenation and thus concludes that this organ system response offers no significant threat to the provision of maximum gas transport. In this regard he singles out some of our published findings as extreme and, by implication, nonrepresentative of highly trained athletes. We believe that these conclusions are oversimplified and incomplete. We attempt to clarify the complexities of this problem.

Imperfections in the Normal (Untrained) Response

A healthy lung and chest wall do show a remarkably precise and efficient response to exercise and even to very heavy exercise. Hallmarks of this response have been adequately chronicled, and Dr. Saltin emphasizes the end point of this response by pointing to the homeostasis of arterial oxygenation during maximum exercise in health. We and others have pointed out elsewhere the near-ideal anatomy of the lung and chest wall to subserve the requirements imposed by maximum exercise (1, 25). At the same time, this pulmonary system response is far from perfect, and its anatomical and regulatory capacities are not limitless. The following examples are provided.

- Alveolar hyperventilation occurs during heavy exercise commensurate with the onset of metabolic acidosis, but this compensatory response is far from complete, as the P_aCO_2 usually falls only to the range of 25-32 mmHg, and arterial pH becomes progressively more acid as exercise load increases from heavy to maximum intensities. In excess of 200 L · min^{-1} ventilation would be required even at normal $\dot{V}O_2$max in the untrained to elicit sufficient CO_2 elimination to compensate metabolic acidosis completely. The result is that the system "chooses" to accept some error in its acid-base regulation in lieu of expending the resources to provide the extra alveolar ventilation to achieve complete compensation.

- The ventilatory response, regardless of its magnitude, requires energy consumption by the respiratory muscles and also their share of the total cardiac output. Although the energy cost of exercise hyperventilation is not precisely known, it is estimated that during maximum exercise requiring V_E 150 L · min^{-1}, respiratory muscle $\dot{V}O_2$ may approximate as much as 10% of the total $\dot{V}O_2$ and 10%-15% of the total cardiac output (1).

- Gas exchange is not perfect. This is most readily documented by the fact that a rising alveolar PO_2 during moderate through maximum exercise (as V_A increases are greater than the increases in $\dot{V}O_2$) is not matched Torr for Torr by a coincident rise in arterial PO_2; thus, the difference between alveolar and arterial PO_2 increases to 3 or more times the resting level. The major reason for this has been documented, namely, that the distribution of alveolar ventilation to perfusion ($V_A:Q_C$) throughout the lung becomes significantly less uniform during exercise (16). More recently, similar findings concerning the $V_A:Q_C$ distribution have been interpreted to mean that alveolar-capillary diffusion is incomplete during even moderately heavy exercise (18).

So, in all healthy persons, regardless of their maximum metabolic demands, there is clear and unanimous evidence that as exercise increases in intensity and metabolic demands are rising (a) ventilation becomes less capable of providing a complete compensatory response; (b) the metabolic and circulatory cost of ventilation "steals" a significant, although as yet undetermined, amount of total available blood flow and O_2 transport from working locomotor muscles; and (c) alveolar-to-arterial gas exchange becomes less complete as $\dot{V}O_2$ increases, and the mixed venous O_2 content falls and CO_2 content rises.

We reemphasize that, despite the appearance of these indicators of imperfection, arterial PO_2 at $\dot{V}O_2$max is maintained within 5 mmHg of resting levels, and a brisk compensatory hyperventilation is accomplished with P_aCO_2 commonly in the range of 25-32 mmHg and alveolar PO_2 in excess of 110-115 mmHg. During steady-state submaximal work loads, some CO_2 retention may occur in some subjects (usually those with sluggish ventilatory responses to chemical stimuli), and P_aO_2 will decline 5-10 mmHg or so, but these "errors" are quickly removed as work load increases and the hyperventilatory response ensues (5, 7, 8).

End-Point "Failure"?

What factors determine whether these imperfections will actually result in an end-point failure of pulmonary gas exchange? Simply put, the answer is the net effect of demand versus capacity (of the lung and chest wall). By *demand* we mean the maximum metabolic requirement dictated by the (whole-body) $\dot{V}O_2$ and $\dot{V}CO_2$. Thus, the higher this metabolic requirement, the more the following consequences will be imparted to the pulmonary system: (a) Mixed venous O_2 content would be lower and CO_2 content higher. (b) A greater rate of alveolar-capillary diffusion will be required as $\dot{V}O_2$ increases. (c) Pulmonary blood flow (Q_C) is higher, and mean transit time in the pulmonary capillaries available for oxygenation of the blood cell will shorten, the exact amount depending on the relationship of increased Q to expansion of the

pulmonary capillary blood volume (V_c) (mean transit time in s = V_c/Q_c). (d) The increase in blood flow also presents the threat of generating excessive pulmonary vascular pressures and (theoretically) causing excessive accumulation of extravascular lung water (35). (e) Ventilatory requirement is related to $\dot{V}CO_2$ in a curvilinear fashion so that optimal regulation of alveolar PCO_2 and PO_2 requires ever-increasing levels of minute and alveolar ventilation. For example, in the trained subject at $\dot{V}CO_2 \approx 6$ L $\cdot$ min^{-1}, 200 L $\cdot$ min^{-1} ventilation is required to achieve the same alveolar PO_2 and PCO_2 obtained by the untrained subject ($\dot{V}CO_2 \approx 3.5$ L $\cdot$ min^{-1}) at only 150 L $\cdot$ min^{-1} ventilation.

The other side of this equation (i.e., the *regulatory capacity* of the pulmonary system) is defined both structurally and functionally by such factors as (a) the lung surface area for gas exchange and the maintenance of very short diffusion distances; (b) the capability of the pulmonary capillary blood volume for recruitment and volume expansion and for pulmonary vascular resistance to be reduced as Q increases; (c) capability for regulation of $V_A:Q_c$ distribution as each of these components increases; (d) strength and endurance of inspiratory muscles of the chest wall as pressure generators; (e) capability to achieve very high flow rates during expiration (i.e., avoiding dynamic compression of airways as lung volume decreases); and (f) minimization of ventilatory work and therefore the metabolic requirement of respiratory muscles by means of the maintenance or enlargement of intra- and extrathoracic airway diameter during exercise and the selective activation of respiratory muscles and optimization of diaphragmatic length (17, 19).

Given these two opposing forces, the question now becomes: Can in fact maximum metabolic requirement be elevated sufficiently to cause incomplete gas exchange and insufficient hyperventilatory response to such an extent that arterial PO_2 is not maintained near resting control levels? The answer is clearly yes! The evidence for these failures or inadequacies in gas exchange has accumulated in the past several years, although older studies also contain examples of exercise-induced arterial hypoxemia (see following discussion). Our working definition of clear evidence of an absence of homeostasis in this regard is a reduction of P_aO_2 below resting levels in excess of 15-20 mmHg accompanied by a widening of the (A-a)DO_2 in excess of 30-35 mmHg, an absence of an effective hyperventilatory response in very heavy exercise (whereby P_aCO_2 remains greater than 35-37 mmHg and alveolar PO_2 less than 110-115 mmHg), or both.

Incidence of Occurrence
of Inadequacies

To date, arterial blood gases have not been measured in a sufficient number of highly trained subjects during maximal exercise to determine with certainty the true incidence of exercise-induced arterial hypoxemia. We summarize the published mean values in Figure 19.1. It seems fairly safe to conclude that $\dot{V}O_2$max must be in excess of about 65 ml · kg^{-1} · min^{-1} to experience significant hypoxemia; however, there are some exceptions to this (20, 28), and on occasion a very highly trained runner will show significant arterial hypoxemia during submaximal exercise (7). In some studies, including our own, the incidence is in the range of 40%-50% (7, 27, 28, 31), whereas in other studies no or little hypoxemia occurred (12). Marked variability in P_aO_2 among subjects of similar $\dot{V}O_2$max was especially evident in studies with very high $\dot{V}O_2$max (7, 12). In general, subjects with significant hypoxemia usually showed a combination of excessively wide (A-a)DO_2 (> 30-35 mmHg) in combination with minimal hyperventilation (P_aCO_2 > 37 mmHg and P_AO_2 < 115 mmHg). There were exceptions in which sufficient hyperventilation existed in the face of a markedly widened (A-a)DO_2. We also note that the level of hyperventilation at $\dot{V}O_2$max, even among the untrained, does vary considerably.

Three studies showed that training-induced increases in $\dot{V}O_2$max may result in an increase (29), no change (6), or a reduction (28) in P_aO_2 or S_aO_2; but the levels of $\dot{V}O_2$max were less than 50 ml · kg^{-1} · min^{-1} in the first two studies cited and 55-60 ml · kg^{-1} · min^{-1} in the third. Infusions of packed red cells caused a small increase in $\dot{V}O_2$max in already extremely fit athletes and also caused a reduced level of hyperventilation, a widened (A-a)DO_2, and a lower P_aO_2 (30); these changes were not reported in a similar study using subjects with slightly lower $\dot{V}O_2$max (32).

Estimating incidence also has the problem of differences in techniques among reported studies. Significant differences among studies exist in the accuracy with which blood gases are measured, for example, the use of tonometered blood for calibration and the correction of measurements to actual blood temperatures. Furthermore, the truly maximal work loads to which subjects are taken may differ markedly among studies. This is a problem because we often observed that P_aO_2 is well maintained throughout all submaximal work loads and was precipitously reduced only at the very peak work load achieved.

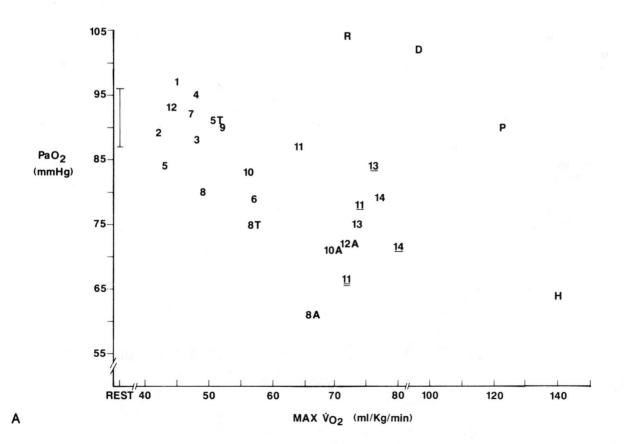

A

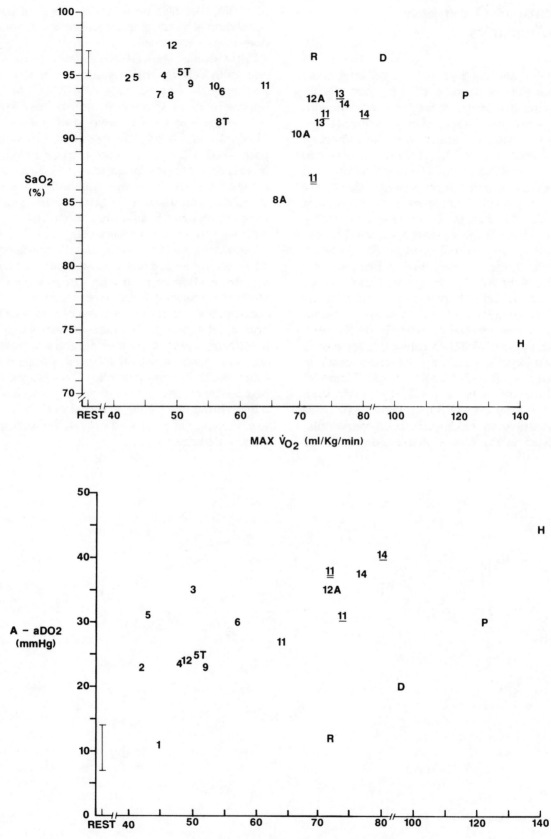

B

C

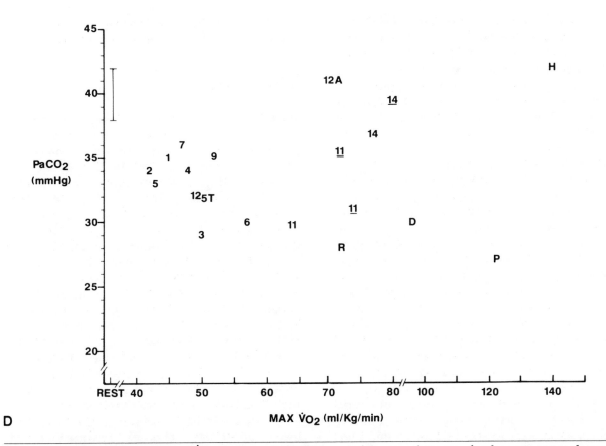

Figure 19.1: A-D.   Relationship of $\dot{V}O_2$max to various measures of the completeness of pulmonary gas exchanges—P_aO_2, S_aO_2, (A-a)DO_2, and P_aCO_2—in healthy young human adult untrained, trained, and highly trained athletic subjects exercising at sea level. All data points are mean values and are taken from the following references: 1 (35); 2 (9); 3 (2); 4 (10); 5 and 5_T (trained) (29); 6 (20); 7 (23); 8 and 8_T (trained) and 8_A (athlete) (28); 9 (18); 10 and 10_A (27); 11, 11, and 11 (7) (athletes divided into three groups according to change in P_aO_2 with maximal exercise); 12 and 12A (31); 13 and 13 (12) (athletes divided into two groups according to change in S_aO_2); 14 and 14 (30) (athletes before and after red-cell infusion). Animal studies are also shown for rats (14), dogs (24), ponies (26), and horses (3). Values for P_aO_2 were derived from reported S_aO_2 in some cases (12, 27, 28).

Sources of Variability

A puzzling feature of all these data is the high degree of interindividual variability. Although it is true that the demands of a substantially greater than normal $\dot{V}O_2$max are usually required to produce arterial hypoxemia, within these groups of athletes the correlation between $\dot{V}O_2$max and P_aO_2 (or S_aO_2) is sometimes but not always highly significant. Why should one athlete at virtually the same $\dot{V}O_2$max as another athlete show a brisk hyperventilatory response and only a moderately widened (A-a)DO_2 and therefore a P_aO_2 that is maintained within 10-15 mmHg of resting levels; whereas another equally capable runner at similar $\dot{V}O_2$ shows much less ventilatory compensation

or an excessive alveolar-to-arterial PO_2 difference, with arterial PO_2 in some rare instances even as low as 54 mmHg or 82% S_aO_2 (7, 28)? Variability of blood gas changes within subjects on repeated trials of heavy exercise is negligible (7). A more likely explanation is that at these extraordinarily high metabolic rates very small individual differences in capacity versus demand (see previous discussion) dictate significant differences in gas exchange homeostasis. For example, 5% variations in one direction in maximal cardiac output versus the other direction in maximal pulmonary capillary blood volume expansion among athletes would make a substantial difference in transit time available at maximal work load and therefore in the completeness of alveolar-capillary diffusion equilibrium. Ten percent differences in alveolar ventilation make substantial differences in alveolar PO_2; these ventilation differences in turn might be ascribed to a number of factors, such as small interindividual variations in dead space: tidal volume, ventilatory chemosensitivity, airway diameter and resistance, or the effective maximum transpulmonary pressure at which dynamic compression of airways occurs.

Differences in the mixed venous O_2 content, as affected by even small differences in the completeness of O_2 extraction or the hemoglobin concentration, can result in marked differences in arterial PO_2 in the face of similar nonuniformities in the $V_A:Q_c$ distribution. These interindividual differences are rarely studied; some of these differences probably reside even within the noise level of many of our current measurement capabilities, and some (such as red-cell transmit time distribution throughout the lung) are not even directly measurable. Finally, we again emphasize that physical training (or the trained state) has no demonstrable significant effect on lung structure or function; thus, as maximal metabolic requirements increase with training, the athlete is dependent for arterial blood gas homeostasis solely on the inherent dimensions and capacities of the lungs and chest wall. Given these many contributory factors, perhaps it is not surprising that $\dot{V}O_2$max (alone) or metabolic demand does not always correlate precisely with the degree of exercise-induced arterial hypoxemia among the highly trained.

Do different types of exercise make a difference? For all types of steady-state exercise, unless it combines highly isometric and isotonic combinations of contractions such as in rowing, the dominant determinant of gas exchange would be the magnitude of the metabolic requirement. Thus, during prolonged heavy exercise (i.e., at < 80% $\dot{V}O_2$max for 1 hr or more), whether in the laboratory or in the field (4, 5), we found that arterial PO_2 was well maintained, even in many runners who had shown significant arterial hypoxemia during maximum exercise of 2-4 min duration. Reductions of 15-20 mmHg in arterial PO_2 were observed throughout prolonged exercise in only 3 of 18 endurance runners. The most consistent difference in this prolonged submaximal work (vs. short-term, very heavy or maximum exercise) was the greater hyperventilation (P_aCO_2 < 32 mmHg) maintained throughout exercise. We do not know whether very highly conditioned marathoners who are capable of working at or more than 90% of $\dot{V}O_2$max for very prolonged periods would demon-

strate a sustained hypoxemia or inadequate ventilation under these extreme circumstances.

Other Subjects

What is the incidence of failure of pulmonary gas exchange in subjects other than this often-studied group of young, highly trained adult humans? The aging pulmonary system shows loss of lung elastic recoil leading to airway closure or narrowing at relatively high lung volumes and expiratory flow limitation, along with a significant loss of gas exchange surface area and reduced compliances of the chest wall and pulmonary vasculature. Even at rest, a significant widening of the alveolar-to-arterial PO_2 difference has been accepted as a normal aging effect, although these data are highly variable. How might these structural changes affect airflow limitation and alveolar-to-arterial gas exchange during maximal exercise in the elderly, especially highly trained healthy elderly subjects in whom these structural changes in the lung are occurring and who yet are able to achieve very high metabolic rates? Given their reduced elastic recoil, it would be of interest to know whether these older athletes "choose" to reduce their end-expiratory lung volume during exercise or whether they avoid airway closure by increasing end-expiratory lung volume, thereby not enjoying the benefits of an increased tension development from a lengthened diaphragm. Dr. Saltin cites the limited data available on this topic in trained and untrained subjects aged 47-70, and it is clear that arterial saturation S_aO_2 is well maintained at maximum or near-maximum $\dot{V}O_2$. However, these data do not really address the question of aging in the highly trained because mean $\dot{V}O_2$max is only 24 ml $\cdot$ kg^{-1} $\cdot$ min^{-1} in the oldest group, and the younger 55-yr-old age-group had a mean $\dot{V}O_2$max that was only 8%-10% greater than the average mean value for this age-group (Table 19.1). This intriguing question of failure of pulmonary gas exchange during maximum exercise in the elderly, highly fit athlete remains unexplored.

A broad continuum of bronchiolar reactivity to exercise exists within the healthy population; indeed, almost 12% of the elite athletes participating in the 1984 Olympic Games were classified as asthmatic. Virtually no data exist concerning gas exchange during exercise in the asthmatic subject, although these subjects often show a nonuniform $V_A:Q_c$ distribution and increased airway resistance with elevated functional residual capacity at rest

Table 19.1 Effects of Preventing Exercise-Induced Arterial O_2 Desaturation in Highly Trained Runners on $\dot{V}O_2$max by Assessing the Effects of a Mildly Hyperoxic Inspirate in Three Groups of Subjects

| | $\dot{V}O_2$max (ml · kg^{-1} · min^{-1}) | | % S_aO_2 | |
	.21 F_IO_2	.26 F_IO_2	.21 F_IO_2	.26 F_IO_2
Untrained	45.0 ± 3.4	43.8 ± 2.8	95.4 ± 0.4	96.3 ± 0.7
Trained	56.5 ± 1.7	57.1 ± 1.7	94.1 ± 0.2	96.1 ± 0.3*
Highly trained	70.1 ± 1.9	74.7 ± 1.2*	90.6 ± 0.8	95.9 ± 0.4*

Note. Values are means ± *SE*. (*N*s = 7-14).

*Indicates significant differences ($p < 0.05$) from normoxic test.

and during recovery from heavy exercise. Both of these factors, if present during heavy exercise, might limit the hyperventilatory response and markedly widen the (A-a)DO_2 during heavy exercise. This represents yet another interesting group with an already compromised pulmonary system in whom the hypothesis of metabolic requirement versus capacity in the pulmonary system should be tested. Blood gas homeostasis and determinants of airflow limitation during exercise have not been studied at all in female athletes of any age.

Lessons From Other Mammalian Species

Lung and chest wall structure varies greatly among mammals, probably as do their relative susceptibilities to failure of gas exchange in maximum exercise. Dogs and rats are especially resistant to exercise-induced hypoxemia, as they tend to show little or no increase in the (A-a)DO_2 even in maximum work and consistently demonstrate a marked compensatory hyperventilation (see Figure 19.1). In the rat these responses persist even as $\dot{V}O_2$max increases 10%-15% with training; and even during exhaustive exercise in a hypoxic environment, the rat maintains arterial PO_2 near resting levels (15). Response to maximum exercise in the pony ($\dot{V}O_2$max ≈ 120 ml · kg^{-1} · min^{-1}) is more human-like as (A-a)DO_2 widens three- to fourfold and a strong compensatory hyperventilation consistently occurs ($P_aCO_2 < 30$ mmHg) (26). One sign of the pulmonary system being severely taxed in this animal is the recent evidence that blood flow to, and the (a-$\bar{v}$)O_2 difference across, the diaphragm may be truly maximum in heavy exercise (22). The elite nonhuman athlete studied to date is the gal-

loping thoroughbred horse ($\dot{V}O_2$max ≈ 150 ml · kg^{-1} · min^{-1}), and they are very consistent in showing incomplete pulmonary gas exchange: P_aO_2 60-65 mmHg, (A-a)$DO_2 > 40$ mmHg, and P_aCO_2 40-50 mmHg (3) (Figure 19.1). The absence of significant compensatory hyperventilation is attributable primarily to the excessive demand for alveolar ventilation generated by the extremely high CO_2 production by the locomotor muscles. Accordingly, the horse exceeds the pony's absolute $\dot{V}CO_2$ by about fourfold (20 L · min^{-1} vs. 80 L · min^{-1}) but exceeds its alveolar ventilation only by about twofold (700 vs. 1,500 L · min^{-1}). To achieve similar levels of alveolar PO_2 and PCO_2 and thereby avoid most of the arterial hypoxemia, the horse requires a minute ventilation in excess of 3,000 L · min^{-1} and a peak inspiratory and expiratory flow rate greater than 75 L · s^{-1} (which is just above the maximum flow available in this animal). In addition, a limiting (although we think less critical) factor to ventilation in the horse may be the obligatory one-for-one entrainment of breathing frequency to stride frequency during galloping that greatly limits the time available for inspiration and expiration.

These characteristics are much like those instances of gas exchange failure in the human highly trained athlete, with the exception that failure occurs much more frequently in the horse than in the human and begins to appear at a much lower relative work load in the horse (≈ 65%-75% of $\dot{V}O_2$max). We would attribute these differences again to the imbalance struck between metabolic demand versus pulmonary system capacity and conclude that the thoroughbred horse at $\dot{V}O_2$max probably exceeds the lung's capability for gas transport by a much greater margin than occurs in humans. Of course horses have benefitted from over 200 yr of genetic engineering in which to build the capacity of their cardiovascular systems for O_2 transport and their musculoskeletal systems for O_2 extraction. One might predict a similar trend among humans over the next century to the point where $\dot{V}O_2$max currently in the range of 70-80 ml · min^{-1} · kg^{-1} will then represent only the moderately well trained runner. It will be of interest to determine whether pulmonary gas exchange also acquires a greater incidence of failure among the trained.

Finally, some additional morphological data bearing on this question of relative organ system capabilities are recently available from the studies of Weibel et al. (33), who compared several pairs of habitually sedentary versus active mammals with similar body weight, for example, cow versus horse. The active animal had a total body $\dot{V}O_2$max that exceeded that of the sedentary by almost threefold. They found that such indices as mitochondrial volume or capillary density in skeletal and cardiac muscle in these animals were comparably enlarged in magnitude in the active animals. The gas exchange surface area of the lung was also increased, but not nearly to the same extent as these other organ systems. Thus the safety factor for pulmonary diffusion limitations was more than twofold greater in the less fit species. These data support the two concepts suggested in this paper, that is, that the morphological dimensions of the pulmonary system are relatively resistant to physical training and that the cardiovascular system may be trainable in some to the point where the lung can no longer meet its ever-increasing demands for gas transport.

Lung "Failure" and $\dot{V}O_2$max

How much does the lung have to fail for $\dot{V}O_2$max to be affected? Up to this point we have emphasized only that the pulmonary system response to heavy or maximum exercise is less than ideal. Analysis of the reasons behind these stresses and failures in the system makes for fascinating study by those of us interested in these matters of the lung. Indeed, to some of us it is mind-boggling to think that what we perceived as an almost perfectly designed organ system for exercise could actually fail in healthy people and that the fitter one is, the greater the likelihood of this imbalance being struck between capacity and demand. But to most others (including Dr. Saltin) the question is: So what? What does all this mean to the limitation of $\dot{V}O_2$max and to physical performance?

Theoretically, the answer very simply is that arterial hypoxemia will reduce $\dot{V}O_2$max to the extent that the reduced arterial O_2 saturation (S_aO_2) causes a reduction in C_aO_2, in turn compromising the capability to widen the O_2 content difference across the working skeletal muscles. We addressed this question by supplementing inspired O_2 to maintain S_aO_2 at 96%-97%, both in subjects who maintain S_aO_2 during air breathing $\dot{V}O_2$max at more than 93%, and in a group of highly trained subjects who reduced S_aO_2 to 86%-92% at $\dot{V}O_2$max (Table 19.1). The data showed that a mild increase in S_aO_2 in the untrained or trained had no measurable effect on their $\dot{V}O_2$max, whereas preventing the reduction of S_aO_2 in the highly trained caused a significant increase in $\dot{V}O_2$max.

On the average, a reduction of S_aO_2 to about 92%-93% was sufficient to exert a significant measurable effect of about 6%-8% on $\dot{V}O_2$max. Theoretically, most of this average 6%-8% decrement in $\dot{V}O_2$max can be accounted for by the approximately one volumes percent lower C_aO_2, and thus narrower (a-$\bar{v}$)O_2 content difference, during air breathing (reduced S_aO_2) versus hyperoxia (maintained S_aO_2). (This estimate assumes that maximal blood flow to working skeletal muscle and the 85% extraction of O_2 content by working muscle remain unchanged by the mild hyperoxia.) Using this same analysis, we estimated that the most severe exercise-induced arterial O_2 desaturation (84%-86% S_aO_2) observed in some athletes (7, 27, 28) would result in a sizable 12%-14% reduction in $\dot{V}O_2$max. These documented effects of preventing O_2 desaturation on $\dot{V}O_2$max represent yet another example, in the physiological state, of the already demonstrated effects on $\dot{V}O_2$max of augmenting arterial O_2 content through experimental changes in Hb concentration or F_IO_2 (13, 30, 32).

Similar levels of incomplete pulmonary gas exchange can result in quite different effects on C_aO_2 and therefore on $\dot{V}O_2$max. First, the extent to which a reduced P_aO_2 reduces S_aO_2 depends on the position of the HbO_2 dissociation curve (i.e., on the coincident changes in arterial pH and temperature). For example, with a relatively mild exercise-induced metabolic acidosis of 7.30 arterial pH and an increase in temperature of only 1.5 °C, a P_aO_2 of only 75 mmHg is sufficient to reach a critical desaturation of about 92% S_aO_2. This P_aO_2 represents only a 15-mmHg reduction below resting levels and can be accomplished in the highly trained with only slightly below normal levels of hyperventilation combined with a minimal widening of the (A-a)DO_2. If the degree of acidosis increased (to 7.20 arterial pH), then, at this same

P_aO_2, the S_aO_2 is now in the range of 88%-89% and the resultant effects on C_aO_2 will have a sizable effect on $\dot{V}O_2$max. The more severe levels of desaturation reported in the 85% S_aO_2 range (which show a 10%-15% effect on $\dot{V}O_2$max) are achieved by a combination of an arterial PO_2 reduced to the relatively steep portion of the HbO_2 dissociation curve combined with a marked metabolic acidosis with pH less than 7.25. As alluded to previously, another factor affecting C_aO_2 or any degree of arterial O_2 desaturation is the magnitude of the exercise-induced hemoconcentration, which presents a variable increase in O_2-carrying capacity to oppose the negative effects of O_2 desaturation on O_2 content. Even the variation in absolute (chronic) hemoglobin concentration is significant in the healthy population, and the relatively low levels often found in the highly trained athlete (12) present an additional effect on C_aO_2 (beyond that caused by any HbO_2 desaturation) that will limit the magnitude of the maximal $(a-\bar{v})O_2$ difference and the $\dot{V}O_2$max.

Recognition of the occurrence of exercise-induced HbO_2 desaturation among the highly trained provides an explanation for the marked variation among subjects in their relative susceptibilities of $\dot{V}O_2$max to environmental hypoxia. The higher the $\dot{V}O_2$max (at sea level in normoxia), the greater the decline in $\dot{V}O_2$max at high altitudes (27, 31). This is most likely explained by the much greater effect of environmental hypoxia on S_aO_2 in the highly trained at their higher levels of $\dot{V}O_2$max (21, 31). Even acute exposure to increases in altitude of only 900-1,000 m above sea level are sufficient to lower P_aO_2 to 60 mmHg ($S_aO_2 < 90$%) in some highly trained persons (31), and at 1,200 m, P_aO_2 will be reduced as low as 45 mmHg (< 80% S_aO_2) (7). This marked effect of mild environmental hypoxia on P_aO_2 during heavy exercise in the highly trained was observed even in those athletes in whom P_aO_2 was fairly well maintained during heavy work in sea-level normoxia. We would further predict that the well-documented marked variability in high-altitude effects on $\dot{V}O_2$max, even among the highly trained, may be explained by differing susceptibilities to exercise-induced desaturation in this group. Similar explanations based on differences in S_aO_2 would logically apply to the highly variable effect of breathing hyperoxic gas mixtures (13), or of red-cell infusions (30, 32) on increasing $\dot{V}O_2$max.

Finally, another potential source of significant limitation to $\dot{V}O_2$max provided by the pulmonary system is the share of total O_2 transport (Q and $\dot{V}O_2$) required by the chest wall muscles. This re-

quirement is often alluded to but has never been satisfactorily quantitated. Most certainly, the energy requirement of breathing must steal a significant amount of blood flow, roughly proportional to the amount of mechanical work output of respiratory muscles at all work levels and in all subjects; so this also presents a fixed steal of energy and therefore a limitation to the maximum energy available to working locomotor muscles. As judged by the apparent maximum vasodilation achieved in the diaphragm in the maximally exercising pony, this requirement may be a substantial one (22). Perhaps the highly trained human athlete who "chooses" to hyperventilate during maximal exercise and thereby avoids arterial hypoxemia expends a considerable energy cost to achieve this compensatory hyperventilation. These ideas are pure speculations until the basic unknown quantity of the actual metabolic cost of the exercise hyperpnea is solved.

Conclusion

Our message is that the capacity of the healthy pulmonary system for gas transport is not always equal to or greater than the capacity of the cardiovascular system for O_2 delivery or the metabolic capacity of the skeletal muscle for O_2 uptake and CO_2 output. In many highly trained athletes, this imbalance results in significant arterial hypoxemia. The resultant effect on the maximal $(a-\bar{v})O_2$ difference and on $\dot{V}O_2$max approximates 5%-15%. This is a small effect relative to the commanding control over total systemic O_2 transport exerted by the cardiovascular system; but at the same time this effect is relatively large in terms of the small changes in $\dot{V}O_2$max that can be caused by physical training, especially in the already well-trained subject. Among the implications of these findings (as outlined previously), one wonders whether some of the additional capacity for increasing O_2 delivery obtained through increased training of the cardiovascular system in the highly trained may not be obviated by the introduction of a significant limitation at the pulmonary level of gas transport. This whole question of lung and chest wall limitations to maximum gas transport to working skeletal muscle deserves further study in a variety of species and in subpopulations of healthy humans. Future studies should consider equally important questions of the metabolic cost of exercise hyperpnea. Furthermore, we need to explore more fully the triggering mechanisms and effects of impending failure in ventilatory control. For example, the inadequate hyperventilatory response to very heavy exercise may be attributed to an active reflexly induced inhibition of respiratory motor output from the central nervous system initiated by an overworked chest wall musculature attempting to avoid fatigue. Finally, there is a need for a meticulous reexamination of the functional and morphological dimensions of the airways, gas exchange surface area, and respiratory musculature among the highly trained, especially during growth.

Acknowledgments

This research was supported by a grant from NHLBI and a contract from USARDC. We thank Jane Meicher and Kathy Henderson for manuscript preparation and Kurt Saupe for his helpful review of the manuscript.

References

1. Anholm J., R.L. Johnson, and M. Ramanathan. Changes in cardiac output during sustained maximum ventilation in humans. *J. Appl. Physiol.* 63: 181-187, 1987.

2. Asmussen, E., and M. Mielsen. Alveolo-arterial gas exchange at rest and during work at different O_2 tensions. *Acta Physiol. Scand.* 50: 153-166, 1960.

3. Bayly, W.M., D.A. Schultz, D.R. Hodgson, and P.D. Gollnick. Ventilatory response of the horse to exercise: Effect of gas collection systems. *J. Appl. Physiol.* 63: 1210-1217, 1987.

4. Dempsey, J.A. Exercise-induced imperfections in pulmonary gas exchange. *Can. J. Sports Sci.* 12(Suppl. 1): 66-71, 1987.

5. Dempsey, J.A., E. Aaron, and B.J. Morton. Pulmonary function and prolonged exercise. In: Lamb, D.R. and R. Murray, eds. *Perspectives in exercise science and sports medicine.* Indianapolis: Benchmark Press, 1988, p. 75-124.

6. Dempsey, J.A., N. Gledhill, W.G. Reddan, H.V. Forster, P.G. Hanson, and A.D. Claremont. Pulmonary adaptation to exercise: Effects of exercise type and duration, chronic hypoxia and physical training. *Ann. N.Y. Acad. Sci.* 301: 243-261, 1978.

7. Dempsey, J.A., P. Hanson, and K. Henderson. Exercise-induced arterial hypoxemia in healthy humans at sea-level. *J. Physiol. (Lond.)* 355: 161-175, 1984.

8. Dempsey, J.A., G.S. Mitchell, and G.A. Smith. Exercise and chemoreception. *Am. Rev. Respir. Dis.* 129: S31-S34, 1984.

9. Dempsey, J.A., W.G. Reddan, J. Rankin, and B. Balke. Alveolar-arterial gas exchange during muscular work in obesity. *J. Appl. Physiol.* 21: 1807-1814, 1966.

10. Dempsey, J.A., W.G. Reddan, J. Rankin, M.L. Birnbaum, H.V. Forster, J.S. Thoden, and R.F. Grover. Effects of acute through lifelong hypoxic exposure on exercise pulmonary gas exchange. *Respir. Physiol.* 13: 62-89, 1971.

11. Dempsey, J.A., E.H. Vidruk, and G.S. Mitchell. Pulmonary control systems in exercise: Update. *Fed. Proc.* 44: 2260-2270, 1985.

12. Ekblom, B., and L. Hermansen. Cardiac output in athletes. *J. Appl. Physiol.* 25: 619-625, 1968.

13. Ekblom, B., R. Huot, E.M. Stein, and A.T. Thorstensson. Effects of changes in arterial oxygen content on circulation and physical performance. *J. Appl. Physiol.* 39: 71-75, 1975.

14. Fregosi, R.F., and J.A. Dempsey. Arterial blood acid-base regulation during exercise in rats. *J. Appl. Physiol.* 57: 396-402, 1984.

15. Fregosi, R., and J.A. Dempsey. The effects of exercise in normoxia and acute hypoxia on respiratory muscle metabolites. *J. Appl. Physiol.* 60: 1274-1283, 1986.

16. Gledhill, N., A.B. Froese, F.J. Buick, and A.C. Bryan. V_A/Q_c inhomogeneity and $AaDO_2$ in man during exercise: Effect of SF_6 breathing. *J. Appl. Physiol.* 45: 512-515, 1978.

17. Grimby, G., M. Goldman, and J. Mead. Respiratory muscle actions inferred from rib cage and abdominal V-P partitioning. *J. Appl. Physiol.* 41: 739-751, 1976.

18. Hammond, M., G.E. Gale, K. Kapitan, A. Ries, and P.D. Wagner. Pulmonary gas exchange in humans during exercise at sea-level. *J. Appl. Physiol.* 60: 1590-1598, 1986.

19. Henke, H.G., M. Sharratt, D. Pegelow, and J. Dempsey. Regulation of end-expiratory lung volume during exercise. *J. Appl. Physiol.* 64: 135-146, 1988.

20. Holmgren, A., and H. Linderholm. Oxygen and carbon dioxide tensions of arterial blood during heavy and exhaustive exercise. *Acta Physiol. Scand.* 44: 203-215, 1958.

21. Lawler, J., S.K. Powers, and D. Thompson. Relationship between $\dot{V}O_2$max and $\dot{V}O_2$max decrement during exposure to acute hypoxia. *J. Appl. Physiol.* 64: 1486-1492, 1988.

22. Manohar, M. Vasodilator reserve in respiratory muscles during maximal exertion in ponies. *J. Appl. Physiol.* 60: 1571-1577, 1986.

23. Mitchell, J.H., B.J. Sproule, and C.B. Chapman. Factors influencing respiration during heavy exercise. *J. Clin. Invest.* 37: 1693-1701, 1958.

24. Musch, T.I., D.B. Friedman, G.C. Haidet, J. Stray-Gundersen, T.E. Waldrop, and G.A. Ordway. Arterial blood gases and acid-base states of dogs during graded dynamic exercise. *J. Appl. Physiol.* 61: 1914-1919, 1986.

25. Pardy, R.L., S.H. Hussain, and P.T. Macklem. The ventilatory pump in exercise. *Clin. Chest Med.* 5: 35-49, 1984.

26. Parks, C.M., and M. Monohar. Blood gas tensions and acid-base status in ponies during treadmill exercise. *Am. J. Vet. Res.* 45: 15-19, 1984.

27. Powers, S., J. Lawler, S. Dodd, G. Landry, and J. Dempsey. Effects of incomplete pulmonary gas exchange on $\dot{V}O_2max$. *J. Appl. Physiol.* (in press).

28. Rowell, L.B., H.L. Taylor, Y. Wang, and W.B. Carlson. Saturation of arterial blood with oxygen during maximal exercise. *J. Appl. Physiol.* 19: 284-286, 1964.

29. Saltin, B., G. Blomqvist, J.H. Mitchell, R.L. Johnson, Jr., K. Wildenthal, and C.B. Chapman. Response to exercise after bed rest and after training: A longitudinal study of oxygen transport and body composition. *Circulation* 38(Suppl. 7): 1-78, 1968.

30. Spriet, L.L., N. Gledhill, A. Froese, and D. Wiltes. Effect of graded erythrocythemia on cardiovascular and metabolic responses to exercise. *J. Appl. Physiol.* 61: 1942-1948, 1986.

31. Terrados, N., M. Mizuno, and H. Andersen. Reduction in maximal oxygen uptake at low altitudes; role of training status and lung function. *Clin. Physiol.* 5(3): 75-79, 1985.

32. Thomson, J.M., J.A. Stone, A.D. Ginsberg, and P. Hammett. O_2 transport during exercise following blood reinfusion. *J. Appl. Physiol.* 53: 1213-1214, 1982.

33. Weibel, E.R., L.B. Marques, M. Constantinopol, F. Doffey, P. Gehr, and C.R. Taylor. The pulmonary gas exchanger. *Respir. Physiol.* 69: 81-100, 1987.

34. Whipp, B.J., and K.A. Wasserman. Alveolar-arterial gas tension differences during graded exercise. *J. Appl. Physiol.* 27: 361-365, 1969.

35. Younes, M., Z. Bshouty, and J. Ali. Longitudinal distribution of pulmonary vascular resistance with very high pulmonary blood flow. *J. Appl. Physiol.* 62: 344-358, 1987.

Chapter 20

Hormonal Adaptation to Physical Activity

John R. Sutton
Peter A. Farrell
Victoria J. Harber

The effect of exercise on endocrine function is a relatively recent area of research. Its success has depended largely on the development of the radioimmunoassay (RIA) by Yalow and Berson in 1960 (319), which enabled the measurement of circulating hormones in nanogram and picogram quantities. Studies examining the hormonal adaptations to exercise have escalated. In addition, a vast number of hormones have been identified; however, the physiological role of many of these during exercise is unclear as yet.

Interpreting hormonal changes in the periphery requires consideration of several variables. Our knowledge of endocrine responses to prolonged exercise comes from laboratory studies and field studies during competitions. Logistical considerations may limit field sampling to only before and after exercise. This restricts one's ability to interpret changes that may be related causally. Laboratory studies allow a more detailed analysis of the endocrine responses, because indwelling intravenous or arterial catheters are used and blood sampling may be performed frequently to measure hormonal responses and related metabolic changes.

Changes in hormonal plasma concentrations must be interpreted in light of the total physiological exercise response. Increased plasma concentrations of a hormone during exercise may not always reflect increased hormonal secretion in response to physical activity. Exercise usually causes a significant shift of fluid from the circulating compartment, resulting in a reduced plasma volume. Consequently, with the onset of exercise, there will be a significantly increased plasma concentration of all substrates and hormones, without any hormone being added to the blood compartment or leaving it at a different rate. This change may be as great as 10% to 15% and dehydration would increase it further. Even so, this basic physiological phenomenon is often overlooked.

It is important to understand the physiological characteristics of various hormones. There is a dramatic increase in total blood flow with exercise; however, blood flow through specific endocrine target tissues is not completely established. Hence, the rate of delivery of a hormone to its end organ and its resulting biological effectiveness is an area requiring further research (230).

Other characteristics that must be considered when interpreting the literature include the pulsatile secretion of most pituitary hormones and diurnal and menstrual cycle variations of several hormones. The addition of exercise often complicates interpretation. Therefore, these variables must be considered when determining the timing of experiments.

Finally, those studies that use pharmacological intervention (e.g., receptor-blocking/stimulating agents) to observe the endocrine response to exercise must usually be performed in a laboratory. Their results must be interpreted cautiously because the drugs often have effects other than the one being studied.

Recent reviews of the hormonal responses to exercise include those of Bunt (32), Fotherby and Pal (83), Galbo (92), Harber and Sutton (119), Richter and Galbo (219), Sutton (260), Sutton and Heyes (263), Terjung (280), Viru (290, 291) and Wade et al. (297). The following hormonal systems will be examined in this chapter:

- Hormones and energy metabolism during exercise

  Glucagon
  Insulin
  Catecholamines
  Cortisol
  Growth Hormone

- Reproductive hormones

  Gonadotropins (luteinizing hormone [LH], follicle-stimulating hormone [FSH])

  Gonadal steroid hormones (estradiol, progesterone, testosterone)

- Endogenous opioid peptides (endorphins and enkephalins)
- Fluid and electrolyte balance (renin, angiotensin, vasopressin, atrial natriuretic hormone)

Hormones and Energy Substrates During Exercise

High-energy phosphates stored in muscle in the form of adenosine triphosphate (ATP) or creatine phosphate (CP) will allow muscle contraction to continue for only a number of seconds. The continuous production of ATP is essential for prolonged exercise; for exercise of longer duration, ATP production is derived from the metabolism of fat or carbohydrate and, to a smaller extent, protein. Gollnick reviewed the specific regulation of muscle metabolism (102); our focus is on hormonal changes as they relate to energy supply.

Intracellular and extracellular energy sources are illustrated in Figure 20.1. Fat and carbohydrate are present in muscle; glucose is transported from the liver following glycogenolysis, which is under hormonal regulation (222). Free fatty acids (FFA) are released by lipolysis in adipose tissue and transported to muscle in combination with albumin. The major hormonal effectors of these metabolic changes are also illustrated in Figure 20.1. FFA provide the major fuel for muscle in the fasting state (1). The contribution of carbohydrates as an energy source increases with increasing exercise intensity (298, 299). As exercise is prolonged, the contribution of intramuscular energy sources decreases, with increasing dependence on bloodborne sources, probably FFA (11).

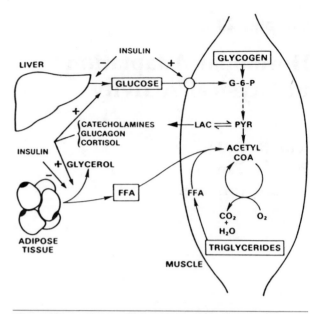

Figure 20.1. Intracellular and extracellular fuel sources during exercise. Fat and carbohydrate are present in muscle; glucose is transported from the liver following glycogenolysis. Lipolysis in adipose tissue will release free fatty acids, which are transported in combination with albumin to muscle. Also illustrated are the effects of hormones such as catecholamines, glucagon, and cortisol (which enhance hepatic glycogenolysis and adipose tissue lipolysis) and insulin (which enhances muscle glucose uptake but inhibits hepatic glycogenolysis and lipolysis in adipose tissue). (Modified from ref. 222.)

Glucose Transport Into Muscle: Insulin Receptors

The human organism possesses redundant systems that regulate glucose during exercise. Nevertheless, the precise basis for the stimulation of glucose transport into muscle during exercise is unknown. At rest, glucose transport occurs by facilitated diffusion and is modulated by insulin. Species differ greatly in the hormonal control of glucose during prolonged exercise—a point often overlooked. Dogs seem to need at least some circulating insulin during exercise (305). For example, transport is severely impaired in diabetic animals and is restored to normal by the administration of small quantities of insulin (295). It seems that insulin in some way maintains the muscle cell membrane, with the result that glucose transport increases in response to contractions. An enhanced insulin binding to receptor sites on the muscle cell may also occur, because, in most studies of exercise, insulin concentration itself is either unchanged or diminished (92, 154, 186, 201). Further support for this idea comes from the observation that, for people with euglycemic hyperinsulinism produced by an insulin-glucose clamp, exercise results in an increased glucose uptake at the same insulin concentration (246).

In the rat, the necessity of insulin for glucose transport during exercise is not so compelling. Contracting muscle is capable of significant glucose uptake in the absence of insulin (205, 300). This finding suggests that contractions and insulin work synergistically during exercise to increase glucose uptake in humans (56, 57). The binding of insulin to monocytes in response to acute exercise has been reported to both increase (149) and decrease (183). Although monocytes are easily accessible, their true physiological significance is uncertain in this setting (17, 279). To our knowledge, the only human study that measured insulin binding to human muscle during exercise was made by Bonen et al. (17), who demonstrated that insulin binding remains unchanged during mild exercise and decreases at dynamic exercise intensities requiring greater than 69% $\dot{V}O_2$max. More recently, changes in tyrosine kinase activity of the insulin receptor do not seem to be responsible for the enhanced ability of insulin to stimulate glucose uptake after exercise (283). This more complex regulatory process has been well expressed by Roth and Grunfeld (226):

> We are accustomed to the notion that hormone concentrations fluctuate widely in response to changes within the organism. With the advent of methods to measure directly the binding of hormone to its receptors, it has become evident that the concentration and affinity of receptors also change rapidly in response to signals from inside and outside the cell. Given that the receptors are at the crossroads between the interior and exterior of the cell, retrospectively it is not surprising that they are so responsive to the environment.

Plasma Glucose and Prolonged Exercise

Circulating concentrations of glucose during exercise remain relatively constant over a wide range of exercise intensities and durations and are due to a balance between peripheral uptake of glucose into muscle and output from the liver (40). This ability to maintain glucose is due to a remarkable redundancy in controllers of glucose production. The stability of circulating glucose belies the fact that exercise requires significant increases in glucose utilization (Rd), which must be matched by increased hepatic glucose production (Ra) (139). In some circumstances, Ra is greater than Rd, and circulating glucose increases. Using trained and untrained subjects, Kjaer et al. (144) demonstrated that glucose concentrations were elevated during and after supramaximal exercise and stayed elevated for approximately 30 min postexercise. Thus, hyperglycemia may occur during high-intensity work. The converse is true for prolonged moderate intensity exercise, which may result in hypoglycemia (79). However, when exercise is even more prolonged (e.g., 24 hr) and at a lower intensity, there is no further decrease in plasma glucose after the first 10 to 12 hr (320). In general, however, exercise does not cause major perturbations in circulating concentrations of glucose for well-nourished humans.

The initial signals to increase hepatic glucose production are not fully understood; however, both feed-forward (248) and feedback mechanisms probably exist (94, 95). Feed-forward mechanisms have been demonstrated in rats (247), where Ra increased prior to any change in circulating glucose. Feedback mechanisms have long been known to exist, because any persistent hypoglycemia results in significant mobilization of counterregulatory hormones such as the catecholamines and glucagon; if the hypoglycemia persists, cortisol and growth hormone may become important.

Levine et al. (162) first reported hypoglycemia during prolonged competitive exercise in the Boston Marathon. By contrast, Sutton et al. (275) showed normal and elevated plasma glucose concentrations following a marathon (Figure 20.2). Since then, hypoglycemia has been described in

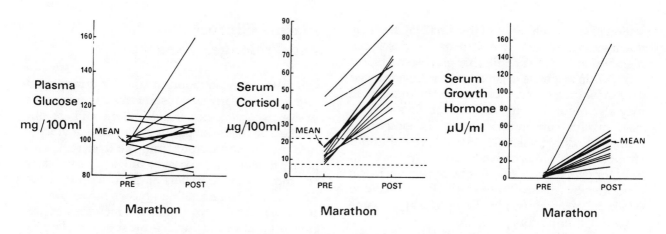

GLUCOSE, CORTISOL AND GROWTH HORMONE – PRE AND POST MARATHON

Figure 20.2. Blood glucose, plasma cortisol, and serum growth hormone before and after the marathon in trained athletes. (Reprinted by permission from ref. 260, p. 191.)

joggers entering "fun runs." With mass participation in such runs and marathons, the incidence of hypoglycemia could be significant (270).

In a comprehensive study, Felig et al. demonstrated that hypoglycemia (plasma glucose < 45 mg · dl⁻¹) was present in a significant number of subjects during prolonged laboratory exercise (79). Furthermore, when oral glucose was given to maintain plasma glucose at euglycemic levels, the time to exhaustion was unaltered. This should be contrasted with the early work of Christensen and Hansen (43), who increased performance in exhausted subjects with oral glucose. This result was supported by Coggan and Coyle (44, 45), who demonstrated clearly that glucose ingestion or infusion during hard exercise in well-trained men can help maintain glucose homeostasis and prolong exercise before exhaustion. In these studies, a large bolus of glucose (4 g) given during exercise had no effect on circulating insulin.

During exercise, plasma glucose concentration depends on a balance between peripheral glucose uptake and hepatic glucose output. Glucose disposal or peripheral glucose uptake will be determined by the following:

- Muscle contractions and insulin concentration
- Concentrations of the counterregulatory hormones—catecholamine (may affect blood flow to active muscle), cortisol, and growth hormone
- Insulin receptor site changes, both insulin binding and receptor number
- Changes in postreceptors, including those of cyclic adenosine monophosphate (cAMP) and rate-limiting enzymes in the glycolytic path-

way (e.g., hexokinase, glycogen phosphorylase, phosphofructokinase, and pyruvate dehydrogenase) (301)

Hepatic glucose is perfectly matched to peripheral glucose uptake under steady-state conditions of moderate intensity exercise and independent of insulin and the counterregulatory hormones, at least in short-term exercise (40, 296). That hepatic glucose output always increases in response to increased glucose utilization has recently been challenged. Using both rat (136, 247) and human (144) models, it has been suggested that glucoregulation may follow a feed-forward rather than a feedback mechanism (i.e., increases in glucose production may precede exercise-induced increases in glucose utilization). Neural and hormonal regulators of this proposed mechanism are not yet understood but may involve central nervous system and muscle effects (145).

Hormonal Control of Glucose Homeostasis

If it were not for the complex interaction among the counterregulatory hormones and insulin during exercise, the greatly increased glucose metabolism would quickly render humans hypoglycemic. The redundancy of these protective mechanisms has been demonstrated in several laboratories, using glucose clamp techniques (126, 174, 305). The following is a brief discussion of how glucagon, insulin, catecholamines, and the sympathetic nervous system interact to maintain glucose homeostasis during exercise.

Glucagon

This hormone is secreted by the alpha cells of the pancreas, and its actions result in increased hepatic glucose production. The importance of this action is underlined by the fact that the liver is the only tissue that can significantly replace circulating glucose. An early study by Sutton et al. (275) demonstrated that circulating glucagon increased during maximal exercise. Later reports confirmed this finding (13). The glucagon response, however, seems to occur only after a delay that, in many cases, is around 40 min after the beginning of moderate intensity exercise (95). The stimulus to this increase is not entirely clear; however, in humans, adrenergic stimulation does not seem to be important (93). Reductions in glucose may act as the primary stimulus to elevated glucagon during exercise because the rise in glucagon can be diminished greatly by glucose infusions during exercise (94). Tarnopolsky et al. (278) showed no difference between responses of females and males to exercise when they worked at the same percentage of $\dot{V}O_2$max.

The importance of glucagon to glucose homeostasis has been studied extensively by Wasserman et al. (305, 306). This group has shown that the increase in glucagon during exercise is necessary both to prevent hypoglycemia (294, 305) and to increase ketogenesis (306). Giving antibodies to glucagon to rats prior to moderate exercise leads to a hypoglycemic response during exercise (221). These studies show that glucagon is important to the normal glucose homeostasis during exercise in several species. However, the increase in glucagon concentration during exercise is considerably delayed following the onset of exercise in humans; hence, Bjorkman et al. suggested that glucagon may not be important in hepatic glycogenolysis (10).

Insulin

Since Banting and Best isolated pancreatic insulin in 1922 (6), 41 years elapsed before measurements were made of insulin during exercise. These initial bioassay studies of supposedly insulin-like activity conducted by Devlin in 1963 (60) demonstrated decreased insulin activity during exercise. Detailed studies of plasma insulin concentration during prolonged work were performed by Pruett (210, 211), who has also reviewed the topic of insulin and exercise in diabetic and nondiabetic humans (212, 307), as have Vranic and Berger (293).

Schalch (237) reported no change in serum insulin levels during exercise, a finding confirmed by several other investigators (134, 197, 218) the following year. Studies by Sutton (258) and Sutton et al. (275) revealed different insulin responses between fit and unfit subjects during exercise. Fit subjects tended to have lower fasting levels of insulin and, when exercised at the same absolute work load, showed little change in insulin. However, for the same absolute work load, there was a greater depression in plasma insulin in the unfit subjects, who were working at a higher intensity of exercise (percentage of $\dot{V}O_2$max). Exercise intensity has also been shown to influence insulin metabolism (13). Pruett (210, 211) examined the effect of prolonged exercise on serum insulin concentrations and demonstrated a decrease.

This fact makes insulin almost unique among the hormones, concentrations of most hormones are increased in almost all types of exercise. The reduction allows lipolysis and hepatic glucose production to increase while it inhibits hepatic glycogen synthesis. These actions are necessary for a normal substrate availability. It has been suggested that the decrease in circulating insulin is due to reduced secretion, because connecting peptide (C-peptide) also decreases with exercise (315). Because C-peptide is not appreciably catabolized by the liver, as is insulin, it may be a better reflection of beta-cell secretion than of insulin.

Although insulin secretion appears to decrease during exercise, some competitors in fun runs or marathons ingest glucose orally prior to exercise to augment insulin secretion when exercise begins. Glucose uptake by muscle will be facilitated and hypoglycemia may occur (50). In addition, when males and females exercise at the same percentage of $\dot{V}O_2$max, it has been demonstrated that males have a greater decrease in serum insulin concentrations when exercise is continued for 90 min (278). Wright and Malaisse (317) injected rats with guinea pig anti-insulin serum and reported a decreased insulin secretion rate following prolonged swimming.

Other studies using radiolabeled insulin have either failed to show a change in insulin secretion with exercise (197) or showed a decrease (88). Due to its greatly reduced rate of degradation, C-peptide, which is cosecreted with insulin, probably serves (with the recognition of specific limitations [206]) as a better marker of beta-cell secretion than does a change in circulating insulin concentration (67). Several studies have demonstrated reductions in C-peptide during prolonged exercise (153). It has been suggested that reduced circulating insulin concentrations during exercise may allow hepatic glucose production and lipolysis to proceed at faster rates (174, 316).

The mechanism of decreased insulin secretion is not fully understood; however, it is doubtful that the adrenal glands play a significant role, because Jarhult and Holst (138) demonstrated normal decreases in circulating insulin in biadrenalectomized humans. This finding was confirmed later (127). A more likely candidate for the primary regulator of insulin secretion may be sympathetic and parasympathetic nerves innervating the pancreas. As an example, alpha- but not beta-adrenergic blockade abolishes the exercise-induced decrease in circulating insulin (28, 93). Because peripheral norepinephrine concentrations are only a crude estimate of sympathetic nervous system activity, direct neural input to the pancreas may have a greater inhibitory influence on insulin secretion during exercise than does circulating norepinephrine (42). Miller (191) has reviewed the extensive nonexercise data that show the importance of these neural influences to pancreatic function. Neuropeptides are also important to beta-cell function (2), and the possible role of the endogenous opioid peptides in insulin secretion is beginning to receive attention since Farrell et al. have showed that naloxone reduced the glucose-stimulated insulin secretion immediately after exercise in rats (77).

The decrease in insulin could signal a malfunction if it were not for the fact that exercise also results in a concomitant increase in the ability of a given amount of insulin to stimulate glucose uptake. The precise mechanism of exercise-stimulated increases in glucose uptake remains a mystery; however, much is known concerning insulin action at its receptor and postreceptor event and about the influence of insulin on muscle enzymology.

Although there is little doubt that both insulin and muscle contractions stimulate glucose uptake and are synergistic in this capability, the interplay between them presents a fascinating area for speculation and future work. Many years ago, Defronzo et al. (57) demonstrated that glucose uptake was increased by both exercise and insulin, and when insulin infusions accompanied exercise their independent effects were additive. These in vivo findings have since been supported in in situ studies using the hind-limb perfusion model (205). Controversy exists in this area, however, because dogs may need at least some insulin to increase glucose uptake during exercise (293). Once insulin binds to the receptor complex, intracellular events begin, including the activation of receptor tyrosine kinase activity and the mobilization of glucose transporters.

Treadway et al. (283) recently demonstrated in rat muscle that the exercise-induced increase in insulin action is not due to changes in insulin receptor kinase activity. Glucose transporters are a family of proteins of immense current interest, because more than one type of transporter may be affected by exercise (253) and acute exercise may increase the number of glucose transporters within the cell (62). This facilitated diffusion process is being studied currently with in situ hind-limb preparations as well as in vitro methods, and it is probable that our knowledge of the importance of these glucose transporter proteins will increase dramatically in the near future.

Insulin Sensitivity

The following is a brief review of the consequences of chronic exercise on insulin sensitivity. A vast literature exists concerning the effects of acute and chronic exercise on insulin sensitivity, and the reader is referred to reviews (93, 219, 291).

Much has been learned about exercise training and glucose control using transient glucose challenges (160, 247); however, steady-state conditions (glucose clamp techniques) are probably more revealing in terms of identifying relationships between insulin and glucose (8). Burstein et al. (33) found that the metabolic glucose clearance rate was higher at comparable concentrations of hyperinsulinemia in trained subjects 12 hr after prolonged exercise than it was in sedentary controls. After 60 hr of inactivity in trained subjects, this difference was reduced, and no differences between groups were found after 7 d of inactivity. Sato et al. (235) found similar increases in insulin sensitivity using a glucose clamp procedure, although no mention was made of the time after the last bout of exercise. James et al. (135) demonstrated that exercise training in rats results in an increased insulin sensitivity that lasts at least 48 hr postexercise, and several reports (135, 192) have shown that muscle glucose uptake accounts for most of this adaptation.

The long-lasting effects of exercise and exercise training on insulin action have recently been assessed using the hyperinsulinemic, euglycemic, and hyperglycemic glucose clamp techniques. These studies used steady-state dose response relationships between insulin and glucose to provide the following insights into insulin sensitivity and pancreatic hormone secretion:

- A single bout of moderate exercise (1 hr of 64% $\dot{V}O_2$max) in untrained men increases insulin sensitivity and responsiveness, and this effect lasts for 48 hr (187; Figure 20.3a).
- A single bout of moderate exercise (2 or 48 hr before the glucose clamp) in untrained men did not affect glucose-stimulated insulin secretion as judged by circulating concentrations of insulin, pro-insulin, or C-peptide (185).
- A single bout of exercise in untrained men increased insulin sensitivity to values similar to those found in trained men; however, insulin responsiveness in the untrained was lower than it was in the trained (188; Figure 20.3b).
- In trained men (in contrast to untrained men), a single bout of hard exercise (1 hr at 75% $\dot{V}O_2$max) did not affect insulin sensitivity or responsiveness; however, after 5 d of detraining (no regular exercise), insulin sensitivity decreased, whereas insulin responsiveness remained unchanged and was higher than the values obtained for untrained subjects (189; Figure 20.3c).

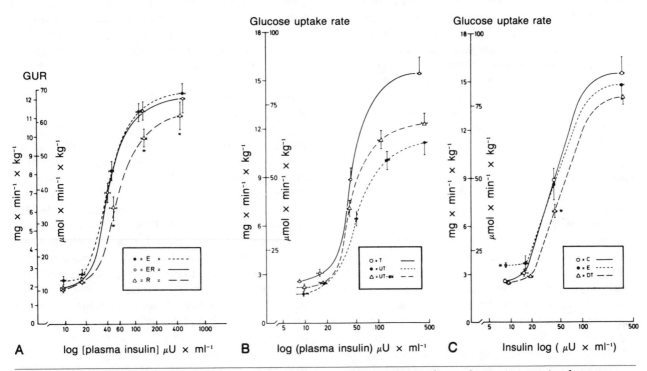

Figure 20.3. (a) Dose-response curve for insulin action on glucose uptake from plasma in untrained men. Values represent higher of either isotopically determined glucose utilization rate or steady-state glucose infusion rate during the last 30 min of each of four sequential euglycemic clamps. Experiments were carried out after prior rest (R) as well as immediately after (E) and 48 hr after (EW) 1 hr of ergometer exercise at 150 W. *Points are significantly ($p < 0.05$) different from corresponding points in E and ER curves. (Reprinted by permission from ref. 187, p. E254.) (b) Dose-response curve for insulin action on glucose uptake from plasma. Values (means ± SE) represent higher of either isotopically determined glucose utilization rate or steady-state glucose infusion rate during last 30 min of each of sequential, hyperinsulinemic euglycemic clamps. Experiments were carried out in trained subjects studied 12 to 16 hr after the last training session (T) as well as in untrained subjects studied after prior rest (UT) and 2 hr after 1 hr of ergometer exercise at 150 W (UT-ex). Values in T are always significantly higher than corresponding values in UT and UT-ex. (Reprinted by permission from ref. 188, p. 697.) (c) Dose-response curve for insulin action on glucose uptake from plasma. Values represent higher of either isotopically determined glucose utilization rate or steady-state glucose infusion rate during last 30 min of each of sequential, hyperinsulinemic euglycemic clamps. Experiments were carried out in trained subjects studied 12 to 16 hr after last training session (C) as well as after 1 hr of ergometer exercise at 72 ± 3 W carried out 12 to 16 hr (E) and 5 hr (DT) after the last training session. Glucose uptake rate is the higher of steady-state glucose infusion rate and glucose utilization calculated from isotope dilution. Curves were drawn under the assumption that glucose uptake rate at insulin concentrations of 100 μU/ml were 90% of maximal values, as was previously found (169). Values are means ± SE. *Significantly different from C day ($p < 0.05$). (Reprinted by permission from ref. 187, p. E254, and from ref. 189, p. 706).

These studies demonstrated that differences in insulin sensitivity between trained and untrained men disappeared after a brief period of inactivity and yet that insulin action at high concentrations of insulin was not altered by 5 d of inactivity.

Additionally, a single bout of exercise (in untrained men) increased insulin sensitivity but repeated bouts of exercise (training) were required to alter pancreatic sensitivity to hyperglycemia. Finally, a single bout of moderate exercise did not influence glucose-stimulated insulin secretion, and yet trained men had markedly lower insulin responses to glucose than did untrained men (11). This last observation is important because, with the exception of prolonged starvation, exercise training is the only physiological treatment (to our knowledge) that reduces glucose-stimulated insulin secretion. This meaningful observation has implications for Type II diabetics whose basal hyperinsulinemia is the result of both hypersecretion and hypocatabolism of insulin (202).

Catecholamines

Catecholamines were first investigated by measuring urinary excretion of epinephrine and norepinephrine (292). In the 1960s, Vendsalu (286) reported increases in plasma catecholamines with exercise. Subsequent studies indicated that epinephrine and norepinephrine secretion are stimulated with exercise and that the increase is best fitted to an exponential function with exercise intensity (13, 91, 95). Exercise duration is also important in determining the magnitude of the catecholamine responses; under field conditions, an inverse relationship was noted between plasma epinephrine and norepinephrine and the number of miles run (302). Another factor that influences the catecholamine responses to exercise is age. Fleg et al. (82) demonstrated that older individuals show a greater catecholamine response to any relative intensity of work than younger subjects. Males may have greater epinephrine responses than females performing the same relative intensity of work, but the norepinephrine responses seem to be identical (278). In females, there is a greater catecholamine (especially epinephrine) response to exercise in the luteal rather than in the follicular phase of the menstrual cycle (273; Figure 20.4a), an observation confirmed in 1987 by Lavoie et al. (159), which may have an impact on fat and carbohydrate metabolism and lactate production (Figure 20.4b).

The source of circulating epinephrine is mainly the adrenal medulla (220); however, some epinephrine originates from extraadrenal glands, because bilaterally adrenalectomized subjects also demonstrate increases, albeit greatly reduced (127). Circulating norepinephrine provides a "fallible index" of general sympathetic activation (65, 229).

The mechanisms of the increased plasma catecholamine concentration during exercise and the magnitude of the change with acute high-intensity exercise may be a result of increased catecholamine secretion. Kjaer et al. (143) infused tritiated epinephrine into trained and untrained males and found that the increased epinephrine was due to an increased secretion because the modest decline in epinephrine clearance could not quantitatively explain the increase in circulating epinephrine concentration.

It is not clear what physiological event causes the increases in circulating catecholamines. In 1973, Christensen and Brandsborg documented that the norepinephrine response tends to parallel the increase in heart rate rather closely (41). Christensen and Galbo (42) showed an inverse relationship between plasma norepinephrine and mixed venous oxygen saturation, which was confirmed by Sutton and coworkers (274) in "Operation Everest II" to be dependent on work load. It is possible that central command plays a major role because the epinephrine response to exercise is proportional to the effort required to perform a task. This was shown in subjects with partial neuromuscular blockade with tubocurarine (135). When subjects were required to cycle at the same absolute work load (despite a 25% reduction in handgrip strength due to curare), the circulating epinephrine and norepinephrine concentrations exceeded levels found during control exercise sessions. When the cycle work load was reduced so that the subjects performed less work but at the same relative work load as during the unblocked state, the catecholamine responses were identical to control sessions. Thus, it may be that sympathetic neural signals that excite the adrenal medulla during exercise originate in the brain and are proportional to the effort required to perform the work.

Catecholamines have a number of major metabolic effects, including the stimulation of lipolysis and hepatic glycogenolysis. Gollnick et al. (103) demonstrated that adrenomedullectomized rats with ganglion blockade failed to inhibit glycogen depletion in muscle or liver by exercise and showed an inhibition of adipose tissue lipolysis. Inhibition of beta-cell insulin secretion also occurs

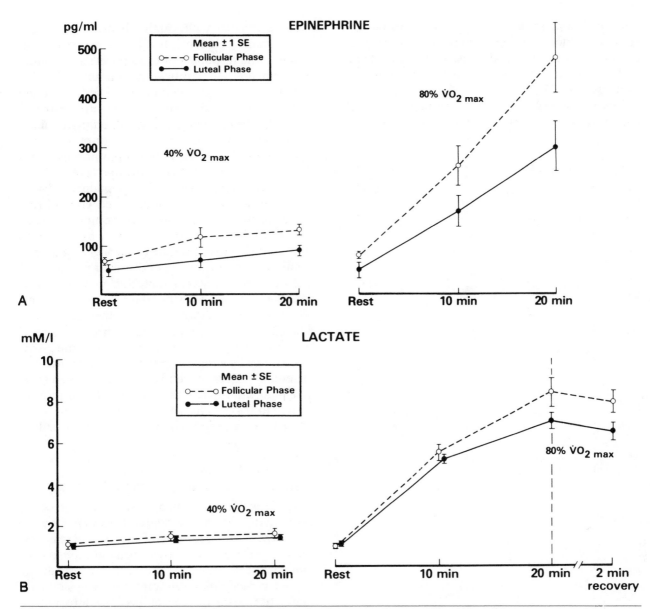

Figure 20.4. (a) The influence of the menstrual cycle phase on plasma epinephrine response to exercise. (b) The influence of the menstrual cycle phase on plasma lactate response to exercise.

and may be mediated by direct neural input to the pancreas (42, 138).

The extent of sympathetic neural activation varies from tissue to tissue (30, 65), and the tissue specificity of sympathetic stimulation may be important, as was recently demonstrated by Victor et al. (287). These workers showed that muscle sympathetic nervous activity in the peroneal nerve of the leg did not change during arm exercise. Selective neural activation to various tissues may be critical to our understanding of cardiovascular and metabolic responses to prolonged exercise (96).

Catecholamines and Their Circulatory Effects

Catecholamines have significant metabolic effects during exercise, but influence on the circulation dominates. A recent study by Rowell et al. (229) highlighted this point by exercising subjects at four intensities under two thermal conditions. Epinephrine and norepinephrine increases were related to the intensity of exercise. The increased heat load resulted in little difference in epinephrine secretion, whereas the hotter temperatures markedly increased norepinephrine secretion, with the log norepinephrine paralleling the heart rate response

(Figure 20.5). In females, norepinephrine responses tended to be higher in the follicular phase compared with the luteal phase of the menstrual cycle at the same $\dot{V}O_2$, but there was no difference in heart rate (273).

There is a reduction in norepinephrine and epinephrine with training at the same absolute exercise intensity, although when humans work at the same relative intensity of exercise post-training, the responses of epinephrine and norepinephrine are not significantly different (123, 124, 203, 313). However, when trained and untrained men exercised at the same relative supramaximal intensity, the epinephrine concentration in trained subjects was almost twice that of untrained subjects. Interestingly, the norepinephrine concentrations were similar between groups (144).

When the endogenous opioid peptide (EOP) system is antagonized, an augmented epinephrine response to prolonged exercise occurs (74, 112). Similar inhibitory effects of EOP have been demonstrated during insulin-induced hypoglycemia (21), isometric exercise (157), and a cold-pressor test (20). It therefore seems that EOP may modulate the catecholamine response (both epinephrine and norepinephrine) during times of stress so that the final response is appropriate to the imposed stress. However, two reports have contradicted the previous studies by suggesting that EOP is involved in the endocrine response to exercise. Staessen et al. (251) and Bramnert and Hokfelt (24) found little change in the plasma catecholamines during exercise when naloxone was infused at high or low concentrations.

Glucoregulation and the Prevention of Hypoglycemia During Exercise

Most of the hormonal changes with exercise, taken individually, are not essential to prevent hypoglycemia. The prevention of insulin decrease by insulin infusion (40) or the glucagon increase by somatostatin infusion (10) will not result in hypoglycemia. Beta-adrenergic responses may be somewhat more important because infusion of propranolol, not phentolamine, results in a lower plasma glucose, but not to hypoglycemic concentrations (93, 117). In addition, hypoglycemia did not develop in exercising patients who had undergone bilateral adrenalectomy and therefore had lost most of the epinephrine-secreting cells (127).

Cortisol

Early studies investigating the effects of exercise on adrenocortical secretion measured adrenal ascorbic acid cortical depletion, depression of plasma eosinophil count, and 17 ketosteroids in the urine to evaluate the response. Protein binding assays and radioimmunoassays increased the understanding of the plasma cortisol responses. Considerable variability in the cortisol responses

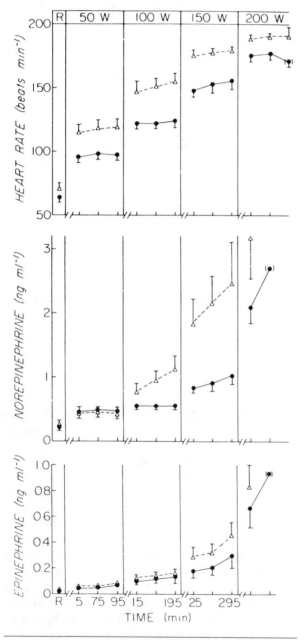

Figure 20.5. Heart rate, norepinephrine, and epinephrine responses to different intensities of exercise with body skin temperature held at 30°C (solid dots and lines, ± SE) and at 38°C (open triangles, dashed lines, ± SE). (Reprinted by permission from ref. 229, p. 647.)

was observed, depending on the nature of the study performed. Changes in plasma cortisol concentration were dependent on the intensity of exercise under most circumstances. In 1965, Cornil et al. (49) found a decrease in cortisol during short-term moderate exercise, as did Raymond et al. in 1969 (217). In 1973, Davies and Few (54) clearly demonstrated that exercise intensity was important in determining the cortisol response, an observation confirmed in 1972 by Viru (289) and in 1976 by Bloom et al. (13). However, some conflicting reports, such as those of Kuoppasalmi et al. (155) failed to show any significant increase in cortisol after short-term near-maximal work. Wade and Claybaugh (296) confirmed these findings. Duration of exercise cannot be overlooked. Some of the discrepancy in the literature may be attributed to failure to take into account the circadian rhythm of cortisol as well as the timing of the experiment after a meal. If exercise is initiated either after a meal or during an episodic secretory peak, no greater elevations of this steroid occur (26).

Sutton et al. (275) reported extremely high cortisol levels (mean of 92 μg $\cdot$ 100 ml^{-1}, range of 74-127 μg $\cdot$ 100 ml^{-1}) in 11 subjects following a marathon (Figure 20.2), findings that have been supported by the work of Dessypris et al. (59) and Newmark et al. (195). Another situation in which plasma cortisol was very elevated occurred in 5 of a group of 6 subjects who collapsed during a fun run (270). Measurements of plasma concentrations give an indication of the magnitude of the change in cortisol; however, the total integrated response is best obtained by measuring secretion rates or urinary free cortisol, as was performed by Bonen (15). The results of this study demonstrated that the magnitude of the increase in urinary free cortisol with exercise was closely related to the relative intensity of exercise. Duration of exercise was also shown to contribute to determining the cortisol response when Brandenberger and Follenius (25) found that plasma cortisol will rise, even at low work levels, provided the exercise period is sufficiently long.

Cardiorespiratory fitness was examined in 1969 by Sutton et al. (275); they showed that cortisol responses were similar in fit and unfit subjects at exercise intensities of the same relative magnitude (i.e., the same percent $\dot{V}O_2$max). By contrast, at the same absolute level of work, fit subjects showed no increase in cortisol concentration with submaximal exercise, whereas unfit subjects showed a significant increase (258). Hartley et al. (123, 124) also failed to show any significant effect

of a training program on the plasma cortisol responses to exercise.

The mechanisms of change in plasma cortisol during exercise are best understood by studies of turnover rate in which tritiated (3H) cortisol was administered and the rates of cortisol entry and removal from the plasma compartment could be quantified. At low intensities of exercise, plasma cortisol concentrations fell because the rate of removal was greater than the rate of secretion; during heavy exercise, secretion increased at a greater rate than removal, hence plasma cortisol concentrations rose (38, 80).

The release of cortisol is controlled by corticotropin-releasing hormone (CRH) from the hypothalamus and by adrenocorticotropic hormone (ACTH) from the anterior pituitary and may also be influenced by the endogenous opioids (158). Increased levels of ACTH during exercise have also been reported (36, 71, 84, 97). The hypothalamic-pituitary–adrenal axis in runners and nonrunners was examined thoroughly by Luger et al. (168), who demonstrated the importance of the relative intensity of exercise in determining cortisol and ACTH responses. Both ACTH and cortisol tended to be higher during the resting state in highly trained individuals, supporting the findings of Villanueva et al. (288), who reported an increased plasma concentration and cortisol production rate in female runners. In another study, suppression of ACTH with an injection of beta-methasone before exercise abolished the cortisol increase with exercise (259).

It seems that highly trained runners have a chronic state of hypercortisolism that is particularly heightened before a race, as demonstrated by Sutton and Casey (262) and Luger et al. (168; Figure 20.6a). The latter investigators went further in evaluating hypothalamic–pituitary–adrenal integrity by injecting ovine CRH. Compared with sedentary and moderately trained individuals, highly trained athletes had a reduced integrated response of ACTH and cortisol to the same dose of CRH (Figure 20.6b). The authors were unable to determine the mechanism whereby the increased secretion of ACTH with hypercortisolism occurred in the highly trained athletes, although they speculated that this might have been due to an increased CRH secretion, as has also been postulated in patients experiencing anorexia nervosa and depression (99, 100). The central role of CRH as it affects pituitary secretion and target organ functions has not been studied in great detail and is a new area of investigation.

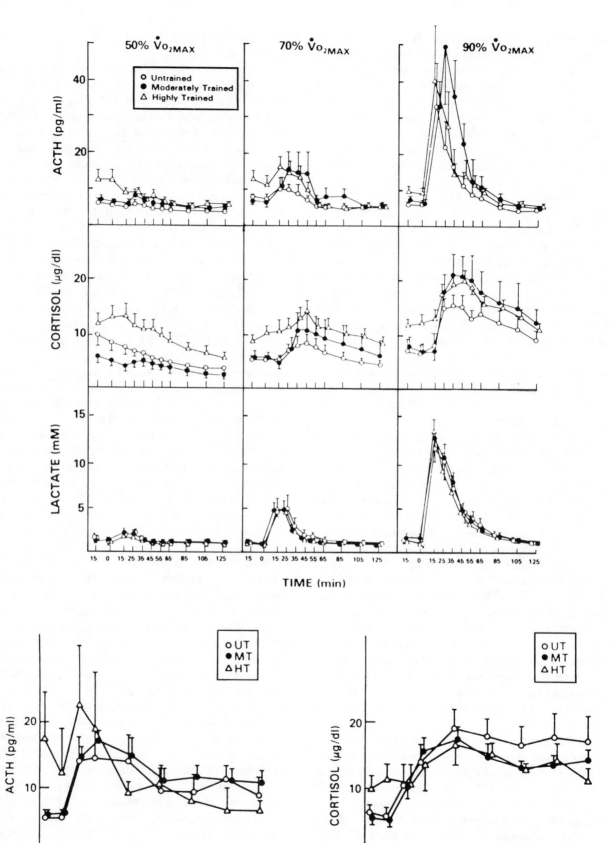

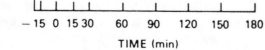

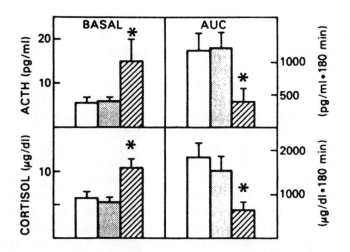

Figure 20.6. (a) Concentrations of ACTH, cortisol, and lactate (mean ± SE) in three groups of subjects (untrained, moderately trained, and highly trained) during treadmill exercise at 50%, 70%, and 90% $\dot{V}O_2$max. (b) Plasma ACTH and cortisol following administration of ovine CRH (1 μg/kg). Right panel shows basal + ovine CRH-stimulated (time-integrated stimulation above base line). UT: untrained (open bars); MT: moderately trained (stippled bars); HT: highly trained (hatched bars). (Both reprinted by permission from ref. 168, p. 1311.)

Growth Hormone

Growth hormone is released from the anterior pituitary in a pulsatile manner and responds to the physiological stimuli of sleep and exercise. It is important in human growth and has a number of other metabolic actions; including direct effects on adipose tissue to increase lipolysis. Growth hormone decreases glucose uptake in the liver, where it will stimulate RNA synthesis, protein synthesis, gluconeogenesis, and the production of somatomedin. In muscle, growth hormone increases amino acid uptake and protein synthesis, and glucose uptake decreases. The growth-promoting actions of growth hormone appear to be mediated by somatomedin. A delay of several hours is noted between the administration of growth hormone and an increase in somatomedin. Few studies have been conducted during exercise, although Stuart et al. (255; Figure 20.7) examined subjects for plasma somatomedin concentration 5 to 6 hr after a normal stimulus to growth hormone secretion such as exercise, arginine, sleep, or insulin hypoglycemia. There was a measurable increase in radioimmunoassayable growth hormone, but very little change in the biologically active somatomedin in response to this single stimulus (254).

The first studies of growth hormone responses to exercise were conducted in 1963 by Roth et al. (227) and in 1965 by Hunter and Greenwood (133). The sleep-associated increase in growth hormone

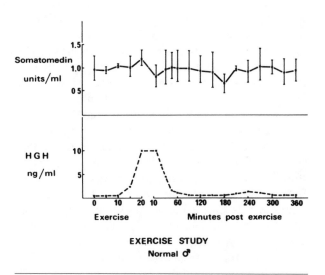

Figure 20.7. Somatomedins and serum growth hormone (HGH) with insulin hypoglycemia and exercise.

predominantly associated with the first bout of slow-wave sleep was reported in 1968 by Takahashi et al. (276). Growth hormone pulsatility and the use of 24-hr secretion studies for the assessment of growth hormone adequacy have been advocated, although it is clear that such studies involve greater effort and inconvenience for clinicians and investigators (125). Borer et al. (18) demonstrated the greatest growth in hamsters, associated with the greatest growth hormone pulse frequency and amplitude. Exercise is a great a physiological stimulus to growth hormone secretion as sleep, and it may well be a more appropriate investigation to use for growth hormone deficiency than are many of the pharmacological agents (265).

Intensity and duration of exercise are the important factors governing growth hormone secretion during exercise. When both fit and unfit subjects were exercised to exhaustion, Sutton et al. (275) noted that both groups had similar increases in growth hormone concentration. However, the unfit subjects displayed a prolonged increase in growth hormone secretion, lasting several hours after exercise. The growth hormone response during submaximal exercise was greater in the unfit subjects at the same absolute work level. Studies by Bloom et al. (13) showed similar responses in growth hormone in fit and unfit subjects who exercised at the same relative intensity. However, when the exercise was of the same absolute magnitude and therefore relatively more difficult for the unfit subjects, elevations in growth hormone were detected only in the unfit group (258). These findings were supported by Shephard and Sidney (242). Further work by these investigators (243) demonstrated a greater response in growth hormone in older men after a training program. Females were reported to have a similar response to that in males (269); however, menstrual cycle variation was apparent as a greater rise occurred in the luteal phase than in the follicular phase (207). The actual stimulation of growth hormone remains unknown, although it was postulated by Sutton et al. (275) that lactate or the acid-base alteration during exercise might be responsible. This hypothesis is supported by data from several sources, particularly the finding of an augmented growth hormone response when exercise is performed under conditions of acute hypoxia (257). However, this hypothesis was finally put to rest by a number of important observations, as discussed in the paper of Sutton et al. (272; Figure 20.8, a-c).

Hansen and colleagues examined the relationship between growth hormone and circulating levels of glucose and FFA and showed that intravenous glucose suppressed growth hormone release (115) but that Intralipid had no effect (116). Glucose infusion suppresses the growth hormone response to exercise and is greater in unfit than in fit subjects (Sutton, unpublished observations, 1969).

Various neurotransmitters influence growth hormone secretion during exercise. Adrenergic recep-

tor blockade was used by Hansen (117) and Sutton and Lazarus (264), all of whom agreed that beta blockade enhanced growth hormone secretion with exercise. Sutton and Lazarus were unable to demonstrate any significant effect of alpha blockade. In contrast, Hansen showed an inhibition of growth hormone release by exercise during alpha blockade. Serotonergic neurotransmitters regulate growth hormone secretion during exercise. Smythe and Lazarus (245) demonstrated that cyproheptadine, a serotonin antagonist, minimized growth hormone secretion.

Cholinergic neurotransmission may be the final common pathway for many of the stimuli involved in growth hormone secretion. Casanueva et al. (37) showed that injecting atropine before exercise completely suppressed the growth hormone response. These workers also indicated that many drugs (e.g., cyproheptadine and diphenhydramine) that are used to examine serotonergic and histaminergic pathways for growth hormone release are also anticholinergic. The reduction of growth hormone secretion in animals treated with reserpine to deplete the aminergic pathways may also not be specific because reserpine also reduces acetylcholine storage.

Reproductive Hormones

The pituitary gonadotropins, LH and FSH, are released from the anterior pituitary under the control of gonadotropin-releasing hormone (GnRH). Early studies by Santen and Bardin (232) showed that LH is released into the circulation in a series of pulses. In addition, pulsatile LH secretion requires pulsatile GnRH secretion from the hypothalamus (147). Without the pulsatile mode of GnRH release, gonadotropin secretion and reproductive function are disrupted. Early studies examining the reproductive hormonal response to exercise frequently accounted for the pulsatile characteristics of these hormones and often failed to identify the phase of the menstrual cycle in which female subjects were tested. These limitations in study design create difficulties in interpreting individual results.

During exercise, no significant changes were noted in gonadotropin concentration, nor were differences detected between fit and unfit subjects (275). Similar results were observed in females (269). These findings have been confirmed in both men and women on many occasions since. After a marathon, Dessypris et al. (59) found no significant

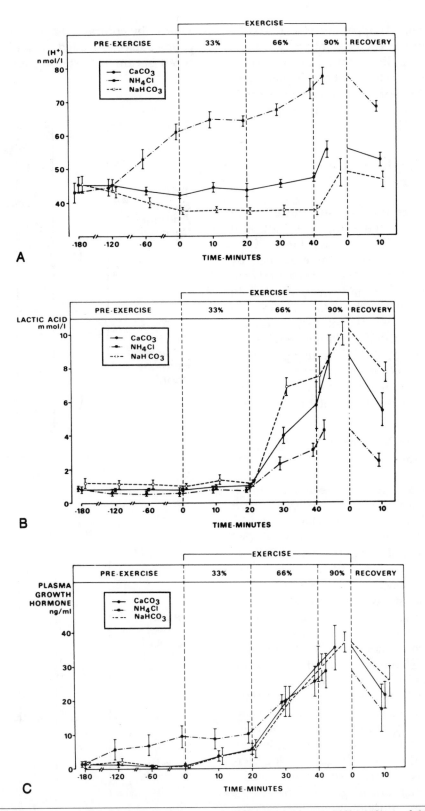

Figure 20.8. (a) Hydrogen ion concentrations at rest and during exercise at 33%, 66%, and 90% of $\dot{V}O_2$max after administration of $CaCO_3$ (solid circles), NH_4Cl (solid squares) and $NaHCO_3$ (open circles). Results are plotted as mean values ± SEM. (Reprinted by permission from ref. 272, pp. 243-244). (b) Plasma lactic acid concentrations at rest and during exercise with $CaCO_3$, NH_4Cl, and $NaHCO_3$. Other information as in (a). (c) Plasma growth hormone concentrations at rest and during exercise with $CaCO_3$, NH_4Cl, and $NaHCO_3$. Other information as in (a).

change in LH, nor did Kuoppasalmi et al. (155) find any effect of varying exercise intensity on LH secretion. Similar findings have been noted for FSH responses to exercise except that females have shown slight, but biologically minor, increases in FSH during exercise in the follicular rather than the luteal phase (141).

Gonadal Hormone Response to Exercise in Females

Results from studies investigating the effect of acute exercise on circulating estradiol and progesterone are varied. The importance of the phase of the menstrual cycle was examined by Jurkowski et al. (141), who reported elevated concentrations of estradiol and progesterone in response to a bout of exercise. Others have confirmed these findings (16). The increase in gonadal steroid hormone concentration during exercise was examined by Keizer et al. (142) infusing tritiated estradiol. Their results showed a decreased metabolic clearance of estradiol during exercise, probably as a result of decreased hepatic blood flow.

Gonadal Hormone Response to Exercise in Males

Young, exercising athletes have been noted to experience major increases in testosterone (269; Figure 20.9a), independent of any changes in LH. The more recent findings of Dessypris et al. (59) and Kuoppasalmi et al. (155, 156) support these observations. Cortisol was inhibited, but androgen responses remained unchanged with a prior injection of beta-methasone, which suppresses ACTH secretion, suggesting little androgen contribution from the adrenal cortex (267). In addition, infusions of human growth hormone (HGH) stimulating a physiological stimulus had no effect on serum androgens (Figure 20.9b; Sutton & Coleman, unpublished observations, 1969). Catecholamines stimulate the synthesis and secretion of testosterone by the testes. Alpha and beta blockade were used to investigate the role of catecholamines in causing increases in serum androgens during exercise. The result was that the plasma androgen concentration remained unchanged (Figure 20.9c; Sutton & Coleman, unpublished observations, 1972).

Sutton et al. (268) infused tritiated testosterone to demonstrate that the increase in serum androgen concentration during exercise was related to changes in metabolism of the hormone (Figure

20.9d). In contrast, Fahey et al. (69) recruited young subjects, graded them pubertally, and measured serum testosterone concentration during

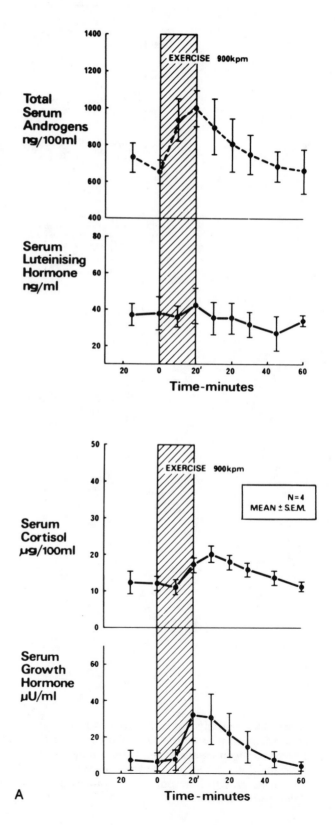

A

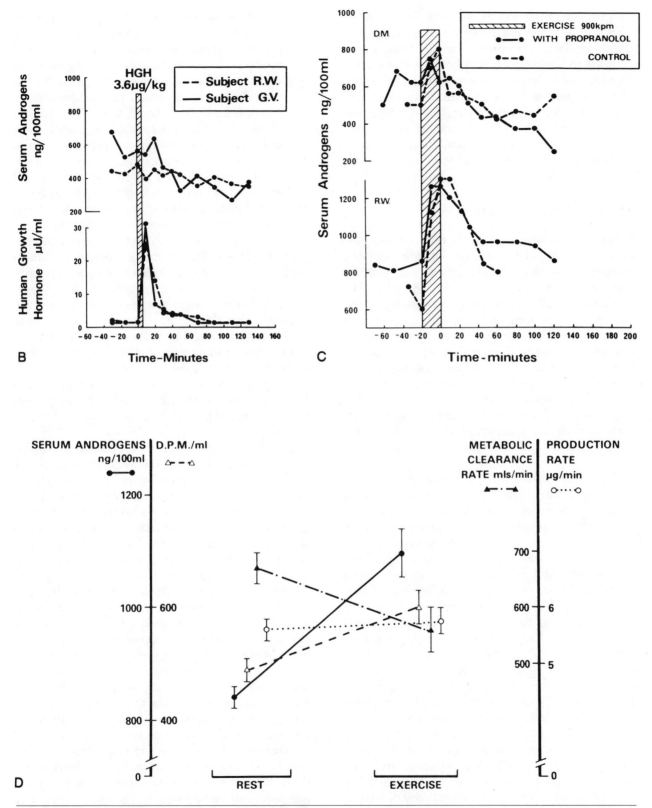

Figure 20.9. (a) Hormonal responses to 20 min exercise at 900 kpm/min (mean ± 1 SEM; *n* = 4). (b) Serum androgen responses to intravenous injection of HGH simulating the serum levels of HGH during exercise. (c) The effect of beta blockade (propranolol 3-mg bolus followed by an infusion of 0.08 mg/min) on serum androgen concentrations. (d) Serum androgens, metabolic clearance, and production rate of testosterone at rest and during exercise. (Reprinted by permission from ref. 268, p. 233.)

progressive exercise to exhaustion. Basal concentration of testosterone increased with each pubertal stage; however, only a small, insignificant increase in testosterone was noted with exercise. During very severe and strenuous exercise, a state of hypothalamic hypogonadism with decreased resting testosterone may occur (309). Endogenous opiates probably have little influence on testosterone increases with exercise, and Grossman et al. (112) showed no altered exercise response using high-dose naloxone in normal subjects.

Menstrual Dysfunction

Routine strenuous exercise is now an accepted cause of menstrual dysfunction, including delayed menarche, shortened luteal phase, and primary and secondary amenorrhea (5, 238, 303). The underlying mechanisms of exercise-assisted amenorrhea are not well understood. A number of factors have been cited that may predispose the athlete to menstrual dysfunction: age, nulliparity, history of dysfunction, intense training prior to menarche, diet, reduced body weight, reduced percentage of body fat, physical stress, or psychological stress (227, 249). The connection between these factors and the eventual disruption of the hypothalamic–pituitary–ovarian axis is unclear as yet.

The amenorrheic athlete is characterized by low gonadotropin and estrogen concentrations (5, 177), with an exaggerated LH response to exogenous GnRH (177), suggesting that amenorrhea is mediated at the hypothalamic level. Most studies investigating athletic amenorrhea are cross-sectional and are not the best designed to elicit cause-and-effect relationships between exercise and menstrual dysfunction. Few randomized prospective trials have been completed that would highlight hormonal concentration changes during training programs.

Bonen et al. (16) identified a short luteal phase (4.5 ± 0.6 d) in a group of teenage swimmers compared with a control peer group (13.4 ± 1.7 d). During the follicular phase, serum LH concentration was elevated but FSH was depressed. In the luteal phase, estradiol and progesterone were lower in the swimmers than in the inactive subjects (12; Figure 20.10). A prospective study by Prior et al. (208) demonstrated an increased frequency of cycles that were anovulatory or had an inadequate luteal phase in subjects training for a marathon. Infertility and luteal phase insufficiency were reversed in a runner who conceived 6 wk after ceasing to run (209).

Another prospective study, performed by Boyden et al. (22, 23), recruited 19 healthy and regularly menstruating women who volunteered to participate in an endurance running program designed to enable them to complete a marathon. Training duration was over 1 yr, and their mileage increased weekly from 15.1 ± 4.9 mi to 63.4 ± 6.9 mi. Changes in menstrual regularity were common; 18 of the 19 subjects had oligomenorrhea, but none had amenorrhea. There was a decrease in estradiol and a slight but insignificant reduction in LH. The most impressive finding was the impairment in LH (and to a lesser extent FSH) responsiveness to injections of GnRH (23). However, Loucks et al. (167) demonstrated an enhanced LH and FSH response to an injection of GnRH in amenorrheic athletes compared to control women. The variable response of LH to exogenous GnRH may suggest dysfunction in the pulse generator for GnRH. In response to a moderate 8-wk training program, Bullen et al. (31) showed mild ovarian impairment in 4 of 7 subjects, as evidenced by a decreased urinary excretion of estradiol, progesterone, or both. No effect of the training program on the reproductive hormonal changes (FSH, LH, and estradiol) with exercise was shown.

In 1985, Cumming et al. (52) showed almost complete abolition of GnRH, as determined by LH pulsatility in six eumenorrheic runners (Figure 20.11). In addition, LH pulse frequency and amplitude, as well as the area under the LH curve (studied in the early follicular phase), were diminished in the runners, although estradiol was not significantly different (29.9 ± 5.5 pg · ml^{-1} in runners vs. 38.5 ± 2.9 pg · ml^{-1} in controls). The authors concluded that the hypothalamic defect in athletes who were still menstruating was possibly also the mechanism involved in the more florid primary and secondary amenorrhea in the more susceptible athletes. Thus, runner's amenorrhea may be a form of hypothalamic amenorrhea with associated abnormalities of GnRH pulsatility (231). Recent evidence suggests that the inhibition of GnRH pulsatile secretion may be the result of the endogenous opioid peptide system (238). Infusion of naloxone will increase LH pulse frequency in some patients with hypothalamic amenorrhea (215). Long-term use of naloxone, which must be administered intravenously, is impractical, but studies with the oral opiate receptor antagonist naltrexone are presently under way. One such study noted that approximately 65% of athletes who train with long mileage are underweight, but

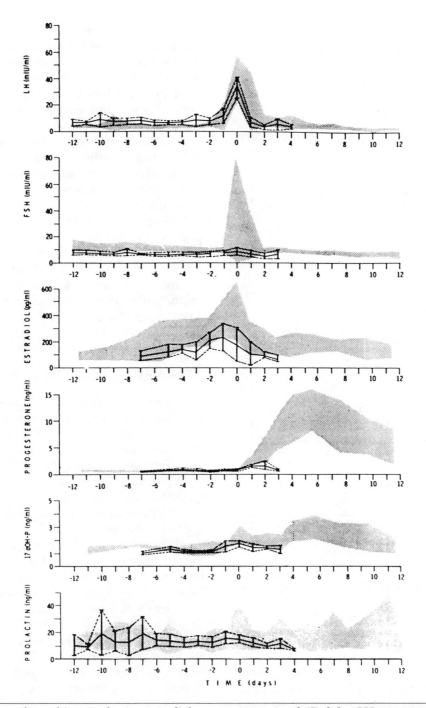

Figure 20.10. Gonadotrophins, prolactin, estradiol, progesterone, and 17 alpha-OH progesterone in swimmers with a short or inadequate luteal phase compared with normal control groups (shaded area). (Reprinted by permission from ref. 16, pp. 545-551.)

will recommence menses within 1 yr if they both gain weight and reduce their mileage (177).

Intermittent hyperprolactinemia has been suggested as a cause of athletic amenorrhea. However, prolactin responses to acute exercise are not different in amenorrheic and eumenorrheic runners (39,

166), and basal serum prolactin does not differ between the two groups (39, 285, 318). Although exercise induces prolactin output, the similarity of response in menstruating and nonmenstruating runners suggests that hyperprolactinemia by itself does not cause amenorrhea in athletes.

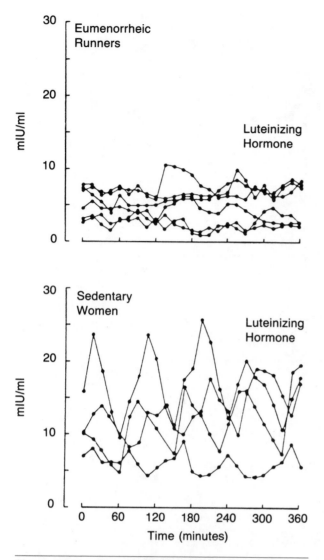

Figure 20.11. Serum LH sampled at 15-min intervals in six eumenorrheic runners showing lack of pulsatility compared with four sedentary controls. (Reproduced by permission from ref. 52, p. 810.)

Elevated testosterone levels or exercise-induced increases of testosterone have led some to suggest that excess androgens cause amenorrhea. In opposition to this, Loucks and Horvath have found normal resting levels of testosterone and no change in serum testosterone after exercise in amenorrheic runners (166).

Menstrual Dysfunction and Implications for Bone

The consequences of long-term amenorrhea in athletes were thought not to be serious at one time, but recent studies have reported reduced spinal bone density in young hypoestrogenic women, comparable to postmenopausal women (35, 63). Both studies showed a decreased bone content in the trabecular bone of the vertebrae in the amenorrheic group, whereas the predominantly cortical bone of the radius was unaffected. Harber et al. (121) found no difference in calcaneal density between eumenorrheic normally active females and either eumenorrheic or amenorrheic athletes. Using a dynamic measurement of skeletal metabolism, these investigators found body bone turnover to be greater in both groups of athletes.

Although intense exercise may reduce the impact of amenorrhea on bone mass (171), athletes may be at greater risk of premature bone loss and bone-related injuries or skeletal aberrations such as stress fractures and scoliosis (171, 304). More importantly, untreated amenorrhea of as little as 3 years' duration has been shown to lead to irreversible trabecular bone loss (34).

Reproductive Dysfunction in Males

The male equivalent of exercise-induced hypothalamic amenorrhea has become an interesting area of research. Obviously, the cessation of menses cannot be used as a measuring stick; however, intensely training male athletes have shown a suppression of spermatogenesis and testosterone (4, 309). MacConnie et al. (169) demonstrated a subtle hypothalamic–pituitary defect in endurance-trained athletes who had normal testosterone levels but decreased LH responsiveness to incremental injections of GnRH when compared with their matched nonrunning controls (Figure 20.12). These findings contrast with those of Ayers (4) and Wheeler (309); however, MacConnie et al. suggest that the differences may lie in the difference of training intensity, in that the training regimen of the latter was less severe and consequently represented an intermediate stage in the process of hypothalamic–pituitary–testicular dysfunction.

Endorphins and Enkephalins

Endogenous Opioid Peptides

Discovery of the EOP was the result of experiments designed to examine various biological and biochemical aspects of analgesia. Specific high-affinity, reversible opiate-receptor binding sites were isolated from mammalian brain and guinea pig intestines in 1975. Hughes et al. (132) used clas-

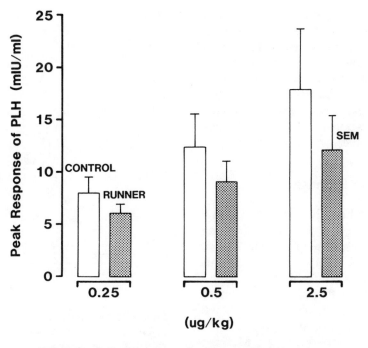

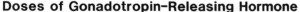

Figure 20.12. Decreased plasma LH response to GnRH in male runners compared with normal controls. (Reproduced by permission from ref. 169, pp. 411-417.)

sical pharmacological bioassays to purify and characterize two opioid pentapeptides, to be called methionine-enkephalin (Met-Enk) and leucine-enkephalon (Leu-Enk) (*enkephalin* is a Greek word meaning "in the brain"). It was soon recognized that a 91-residue peptide, isolated from the anterior pituitary gland and named beta-lipotropin by Li (163), contained the Met-Enk sequence within its structure. Furthermore, a 31-residue sequence with Met-Enk at its N-terminal was also found to have potent opiate activity. This was called beta-endorphin (endorphin: endogenous morphine) (164).

Since these early developments, a host of EOP have been isolated, purified, and sequenced. Beta-endorphin in particular has been associated with many physiological processes, including analgesia, thermoregulation (128), appetite control (27), respiratory function (179), and neuroendocrine function (110). It is known that these EOP belong to three genetically distinct peptide families designated pro-opiomelanocortin, pro-enkephalin A, and pro-dynorphin (199). Details of the complex bioassays and radioimmunoassays are discussed by Grossman and Sutton (111). Hypothalamic–pituitary function and EOP have been reviewed by Howlett and Rees (130).

Response to Acute Exercise

A detailed review of this area has been conducted by Harber and Sutton (119). Most studies to date report that serum concentrations of EOP, in particular beta-endorphin, increased in response to exercise (9, 19, 36, 46, 72, 84, 97, 131, 266). Elevations in serum concentrations ranged from slight to fivefold above recorded basal levels. Studies that have investigated men and women together (98) showed that men had greater beta-endorphin and beta-lipotropin responses to exercise than women; however, some studies showed similar responses in males and females (46, 72).

Recent studies have stressed the possibility that the EOP response to exercise may be intensity-dependent. Light to moderate aerobic activity does not significantly alter serum levels of beta-endorphin (58, 61, 76, 131); however, high intensity (i.e., 80% $\dot{V}O_2$max) and maximal exercise resulted in significant elevations of beta-endorphin (61, 76, 131, 178). In contrast, Goldfarb et al. (101) found no relationship between percent $\dot{V}O_2$max and increases in circulating beta-endorphin. The beta-endorphin response is noted to be rapid because maximal intensity exercise will lead to substantial increases in as little as 30 to 60 s (216). On the other hand, performing stationary cycling at 60% $\dot{V}O_2$max for 60 min failed to increase beta-endorphin levels (58). Time course studies have not been completed; however, investigators have reported that beta-endorphin concentrations continue rising after maximal bouts of exercise (58). Those investigators examining the enkephalin response to exercise report no change in trained subjects (73, 75, 112, 194).

Response to Chronic Exercise

Carr et al. (36) published the first study that showed an augmented effect of 8 wk of training on the beta-endorphin response to exercise. Recent data from Howlett et al. (131) conflict with this finding; they found no significant change in the beta-endorphin response to prolonged exercise when endurance training responses after 8 wk were compared with pretraining responses. This study agrees with a previous report by Metzger and Stein (182), who ran rats on a treadmill.

Recently, two reports (76, 194) support the finding of Carr et al. (36) that chronic training results in an augmented beta-endorphin response to exercise. Farrell et al. (76) compared the exercise-induced plasma beta-endorphin response of seven well-trained male athletes ($\dot{V}O_2$max = 64.6 ml • kg • min^{-1}) to that of seven untrained, age-matched, and weight-matched subjects. Trained individuals had approximately 50% greater peak beta-endorphin responses during supramaximal exercise. An enhanced endorphin output during exercise in trained individuals is debatable, and only longitudinal studies will provide additional evidence (Figure 20.13).

Endogenous Opioid Peptides and Pituitary Hormone Response to Exercise

The median eminence and hypothalamus are areas of high concentration of both EOP and their receptors. Consequently, their implication for endocrine function is not surprising (228). It has been difficult to quantify to what degree they modulate pituitary hormone secretion during exercise. Because direct measurements of hypothalamic EOP cannot be made, investigators have used the opiate receptor antagonist, naloxone, to determine the influence of EOP on pituitary hormone secretion during exercise. Interpretation is confounded by methodology: exercise protocol, type and fitness of subjects tested, and the dose or infusion regimen of naloxone. Variable results have been

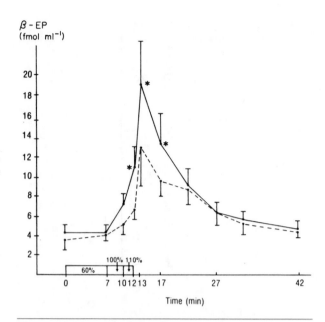

Figure 20.13. Arterialized venous plasma response of beta-endorphin (beta-EP) before, during, and after short-duration supramaximal treadmill exercise. Values are mean ± SE for seven trained (solid line) and seven untrained (dashed line) males. (Reprinted by permission from ref. 76, p. 622.)

reported. A low-dose, single-bolus injection of naloxone had virtually no effect on growth hormone, prolactin, thyroid-stimulating hormone (TSH), ACTH, or beta-lipotropin (250, 266). By contrast, a high-dose bolus injection followed by an infusion of 5.6 mg • h^{-1} resulted in major changes in all the pituitary hormones with an enhancement of prolactin, growth hormone, LH, FSH, and ACTH (112). With exception, a small but statistically significant inhibition of TSH was noted (Table 20.1). Recently, Farrell et al. (74) reported enhanced exercise-induced responses of growth hormone, cortisol, glucose, and catecholamine when 50 mg of naltrexone (a long-lasting oral opioid antagonist) was administered. Conflicting evidence is common. Several studies showed high-dose naloxone or naltrexone to augment growth hormone responses to exercise (74, 113, 175); but Moretti et al. (193) found the response to be obliterated. Experimental designs were similar; therefore, the cause of this discrepancy is unclear. Often the use of an opioid receptor antagonist further complicates the understanding of EOP and pituitary hormone function.

EOP and Mood Change During Exercise

"Runner's high" has frequently been attributed to increased circulating beta-endorphin during in-

Table 20.1 Changes in Circulating Hormones With Exercise With and Without Naloxone Infusion

Hormone	Saline (%)	Naloxone (%)
Prolactin	123	198
GH	263	802
LH	57	104
FSH	29	45
TSH	−30	−48
Testosterone	29	33
Cortisol	49	119
Renin	726	800
Aldosterone	216	298
Adrenaline	875	1,775
Noradrenaline	1,273	1,372
Met-enkephalin	32	2

Note. From Grossman et al. (112).

tense exercise. However, a correlation has not been found between measured mood alterations with exercise and peripheral EOP (72, 73, 75, 112, 266). When EOP have been antagonized during exercise, mood alterations were similar to those in control experiments (74, 172). In contrast, Janal et al. (137) found that administration of naloxone post-exercise attenuated the elevation in joy and euphoria ratings. Although plasma beta-endorphin immunoreactivity increased postexercise, these elevations were not related to mood changes. Presently available evidence does not provide a conclusive statement regarding EOP and post-exercise euphoria; indicators of central nervous system EOP must be found before the relationship of EOP and mood change during exercise is clarified.

There has been debate concerning the value of measuring peripheral EOP and whether these concentrations influence or reflect concentrations in the brain. Rossier et al. (225) showed that foot shock in rats caused increases in circulating beta-endorphin and no change in central levels. Metzger and Stein (182) reported similar findings using exercise as a stimulus. In a recent study by Sforzo et al. (239), rats exposed to prolonged swimming (2 hr) showed increased diprenorphine binding in several areas of the brain; this was interpreted as indicative of less EOP competing for opioid receptor sites. Marked increases in circulating beta-endorphin accompanied these central changes. A similar trend was observed with 1 hr of swimming but was significantly different from the control rats (204). These preliminary findings

suggest that duration of exercise influences EOP activity in the brain and that EOP measured in the periphery do not enter the central nervous system during exercise.

On the other hand, beta-endorphin has been considered impermeable to the blood/brain barrier, but a number of studies are leading investigators to reconsider peptide permeability through the blood/brain barrier. Under different experimental conditions, including stress of sufficient intensity, certain normally impermeable molecules can breach the blood/brain barrier. McArthur (176) cites an unpublished observation of Dr. Richard Bergland that rats injected intravenously with trypan blue and forced to swim to exhaustion were found to have their brains suffused with dye, whereas no such phenomenon occurred in the nonexercised control rats. Although it cannot be assumed that circulating beta-endorphin behaves in the same manner as the dye or that similar results would be observed in humans, Bergland's observation nevertheless suggests an example whereby exercise might facilitate the entry into the brain of compounds otherwise excluded.

Beta-Endorphin and Exercise-Associated Amenorrhea

Beta-endorphin has been shown to inhibit LH release in varying degrees throughout the menstrual cycle (214) and increases in response to intense exercise (131). It has been postulated that women involved in chronic exercise programs may be exposed to increased levels of beta-endorphin for prolonged periods, hence reducing the release of gonadotropins and contributing to the onset of menstrual dysfunction (36, 131). Longitudinal studies have not addressed this postulate; however, a cross-sectional study by Harber et al. (120) investigated this area. In the first part of this study, resting plasma beta-endorphin was measured in three groups during the course of a menstrual cycle: Group A, nonexercising eumenorrheic (n = 10); Group B, exercising eumenorrheic (n = 11); and Group C, exercising amenorrheic (n = 11). No significant pattern of plasma was found throughout the menstrual cycle of sedentary or exercising women. This study concluded that regardless of menstrual status, athletes had significantly higher concentrations of plasma beta-endorphin than normal menstruating sedentary women.

In a more detailed study, these same workers examined representative subjects of each group who had blood drawn at 20 intervals for 8 hr during the midfollicular and midluteal phases. Pulsatile secretion of beta-endorphin was observed in all three groups. The mean beta-endorphin pulse interval increased in the luteal phase when compared to the follicular phase in Groups A and B. The mean beta-endorphin pulse interval for Group C was similar to that seen in the follicular phase of Groups A and B, but the mean beta-endorphin pulse amplitude of Group C was significantly greater than that of Group A (p = 0.05) (Figure 20.14, a-c). Although the mean beta-endorphin pulse amplitude of Group B was greater than that of Group A, this difference did not reach significance.

The physiological significance of pulsatile secretion of beta-endorphin is yet to be determined, but the greater amplitude of beta-endorphin pulses observed in amenorrheic athletes (120) suggests that the hypothalamic regulation of GnRH release and consequent gonadotropin secretion may be inter-rupted or altered in this group. In addition, eumenorrheic athletes exhibited elevated concentrations of plasma beta-endorphin compared to sedentary subjects, but continued to have normal menstrual cycles (120), suggesting that factors other than beta-endorphin may indeed be involved in the etiology of exercise-associated amenorrhea.

Fluid and Electrolyte Balance

Fluid Regulation During Exercise

Marked changes in plasma volume (PV) occur with single bouts of exercise. The regulation of PV is complex and is influenced significantly by intensity and duration of exercise. PV is significantly reduced with exercise, whereas electrolyte and protein concentrations increase (47, 51, 108, 284,

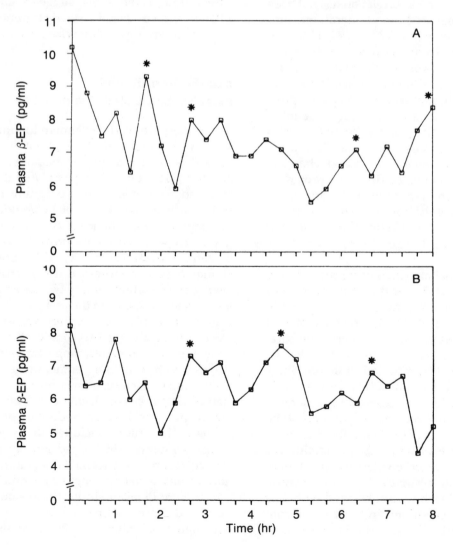

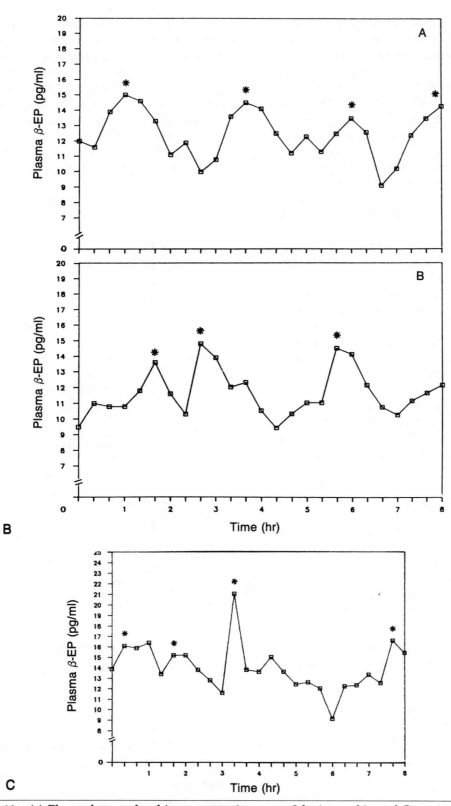

Figure 20.14. (a) Plasma beta-endorphin concentrations over 8 hr in a subject of Group A. Follicular (d.10; A), luteal (d.24; B). Asterisks indicate a beta-endorphin pulse. (b) Plasma beta-endorphin concentrations over 8 hr in a subject of Group B. Follicular (d.11; A), luteal (d.25; B). Asterisks indicate a beta-endorphin pulse. (c) Plasma beta-endorphin concentrations over 8 hr in a subject of Group C. Asterisks indicate a beta-endorphin pulse. (All reprinted by permission from *Plasma Beta-Endorphin, The Menstrual Cycle and Exercise*, doctoral thesis of V.J. Harber, McMaster University, Hamilton, ON 1988.)

311). The exception to this occurs when the single bout of exercise is prolonged for 8 to 10 hr (213).

Contrary to this, chronic training results in an increased PV (106, 129, 146, 200). In fact, training for as little as 3 d resulted in a significant elevation in PV (47). Convertino et al. postulated that the training-induced hypervolemia was more dependent on the duration of exercise bouts than on the total training program (47). In addition, Green et al. (104, 106, 107) concluded that intensity of exercise was a more important determinant of the hypervolemia than was either the length of an individual session or the total duration of the training program.

Not surprisingly, many workers have shown that athletes in a continuous state of training have greater PV than nonathletes (29, 146, 244). Such athletes also usually have an increased red cell mass, but often the increase in PV is proportionally greater, resulting in hemoglobin (HB) and hematocrit values that are low or low-normal. This finding has given rise to the spurious "disease" entity of athlete's anemia.

The mechanism of hypervolemia is not well understood. Total plasma protein increased with training, but plasma protein concentrations remained normal (47, 148, 223). This led Convertino et al. (47) to speculate that perhaps an increased plasma protein, notably albumin, may be the initial factor that gives rise to increased PV, because each gram of protein will bind 14 to 15 ml of water (236).

Recently, Green et al. (105) subjected eight untrained males to progressively heavy training of 2 hr/day, 5 to 6 times per week for 8 wk. During the initial phase of the training, hypervolemia was observed with no change in red cell mass. However, during the final 4 wk of the study, red cell mass decreased, with accompanying decreases in HB and serum ferritin concentrations. From this, the authors postulated that both anemia and pseudoanemia occurred with intensive prolonged training. A more detailed review of the various interrelationships of fluid and electrolyte balance in exercise may be found in the excellent reviews of Harrison (122) and Wade et al. (297).

Hormonal Regulation of Fluids and Electrolytes

The neuroendocrine regulation of fluid and electrolyte balance has been recently reviewed (7, 89, 297). The principal mineralocorticoid involved in sodium regulation is aldosterone, whose secretion

is closely linked with that of renin and angiotensin. Sea-level exercise results in a potent increase in renin and aldosterone secretion in both males and females (37, 151) and is demonstrated with prolonged hill walking (190). The phase of the menstrual cycle is also important—renin, angiotensin and aldosterone all increase to a greater extent in the luteal phase than in the follicular phase (140; Figure 20.15). Kotchen et al. (151) showed an excellent correlation between catecholamine and renin

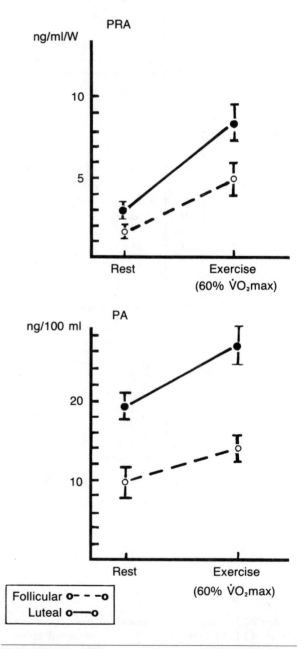

Figure 20.15. Plasma renin activity (PRA) and plasma aldosterone (PA) during 40 min exercise at 60% $\dot{V}O_2$max during the midfollicular and midluteal phases of the menstrual cycle.

concentrations. In addition, beta-receptor blockade greatly diminishes the renin increases (14, 118, 165). The renin increase is greater in circumstances of sodium restriction (68, 161); conversely, renin is reduced in response to exercise following a high sodium intake (3). The increased renin concentration results in increased angiotensin (104) and the orderly sequence of events in increased secretion of aldosterone (150, 170).

Six to 8 hr of hill walking on successive days with a fixed diet resulted in marked sodium retention, modest water retention, and expansion of the extracellular space (including plasma volume) at the expense of the intracellular space (312). Subsequent studies demonstrated that these changes were associated with activation of the renin-aldosterone system (190). Although renin is the major stimulus to aldosterone secretion during exercise, under certain circumstances increases in serum potassium were also implicated (47). Another hormone with a key role in fluid homeostasis is vasopressin (antidiuretic hormone), whose secretion is greatly attenuated by exercise (47, 48, 109, 181, 271, 296). The recently discovered and intensively studied atrial natriuretic factor (ANF) is secreted from the atria in response to atrial distention, an increase in atrial pressure, or atrial manipulation. In normal subjects, there is a significantly increased right atrial pressure (114) as well as a marked increase in ANF (198, 277, 281, 282). The increase in ANF concentration occurs progressively with exercise (274) and appears to precede the elevation of plasma renin, aldosterone, and vasopressin concentrations (277).

Under the circumstances of heat stress and states of relative dehydration, changes that might be expected to mediate internal homeostasis may be put under additional pressure. The renin response was augmented when exercise was conducted in a hot environment (109). Francesconi et al. (85, 86) showed moderate increases in renin, cortisol, aldosterone, and growth hormone during exercise in the heat. With heat acclimatization, there was expansion of the plasma volume, reduction in the physiological stress of exercise in the heat, and reduction of the hormonal response to exercise in the heat (81, 85, 86; Figure 20.16). However, these observations are in contrast to those of Davies et al. (55), who reported that heat acclimatization did not modify the renin and aldosterone responses to exercise in the heat.

The state of hydration and its effect on the hormonal responses to exercise was studied in considerable detail by Francesconi et al. (87). The authors examined volunteers under four condi-

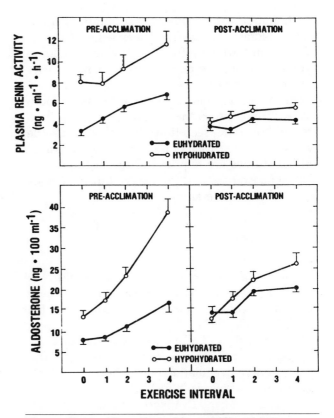

Figure 20.16. The effect of heat acclimatization on the plasma renin and aldosterone responses to exercise in normally hydrated and hypohydrated subjects. (Reprinted by permission from ref. 85, p. 1790.)

tions of hydration: euhydration and 3%, 5%, and 7% dehydration. In general, plasma renin and aldosterone increased with exercise. Also, the resting levels of renin-aldosterone, as well as cortisol levels, were higher with more severe degrees of dehydration. It seemed unusual to the authors that they found no difference in responses between 5% and 7% dehydration.

Conclusion

The endocrine system undergoes dramatic changes during acute and chronic exercise. Each system does not appear to adapt independently of another. The norepinephrine response acts primarily to preserve circulation, whereas the glucoregulatory hormones serve to prevent hypoglycemia during exercise. The chance of hypoglycemia is small because there is sufficient redundancy in the system, and several hormonal regulators participate.

Evidence is emerging of a disruption in hypothalamic messages, possibly mediated by EOP, in which hypothalamic pulsatile secretion is interrupted. Notably, active females experience several forms of menstrual dysfunction in which the long-term effects may be deleterious to bone density and skeletal formations.

Future research in the area of exercise endocrinology must consider the physiological characteristics of hormone secretion, including pulsatile features and menstrual or diurnal variation. Longitudinal studies are required to reveal the effects of chronic exercise and to observe those changes created by exercise alone.

References

1. Ahlborg, G., P. Felig, L. Hagenfeldt, R. Hendler, and J. Wahren. Substrate turnover during prolonged exercise. *J. Clin. Invest.* 53: 1080-1090, 1974.

2. Ahren, B., G.J. Taborsky, and D. Porte, Jr. Neuropeptidergic versus cholinergic and adrenergic regulation of islet hormone secretion. *Diabetologia* 29: 827-836, 1986.

3. Aurell, M., and P. Vikgren. Plasma renin activity in supine muscular exercise. *J. Appl. Physiol.* 31: 839-841, 1971.

4. Ayers, J.W., Y. Komesu, T. Romani, and R. Ansbacher. Anthropomorphic, hormonal and psychological correlates of semen quality in endurance-trained athletes. *Fertil. Steril.* 43: 917-921, 1985.

5. Baker, E.R. Menstrual dysfunction and hormonal status in athletic women: A review. *Fertil. Steril.* 36: 691-696, 1981.

6. Banting, F.G., and C.H. Best. The internal secretion of the pancreas. *J. Lab. Clin. Med.* 7: 251-266, 1922.

7. Bealer, S.L., F.J. Haddy, J.N. Diana, G.J. Grega, R.D. Manning, Jr., J.C. Rose, and D.S. Gann. Neuroendocrine mechanisms of plasma volume regulation. *Fed. Proc.* 45: 2455-2463, 1986.

8. Bergman, R.N., D.T. Finegood, and M. Ader. Assessment of insulin sensitivity in vivo. *Endocr. Rev.* 6: 45-86, 1985.

9. Berk, L.S., S.A. Tan, C.L. Anderson, and G. Reiss. Beta-EP response to exercise in athletes and non-athletes. *Med. Sci. Sports Exerc.* 13: 134, 1981.

10. Bjorkman, O., P. Felig, L. Hagenfeldt, and J. Wahren. Influence of hypoglucagonemia on splanchnic glucose output during leg exercise in man. *Clin. Physiol.* 1: 43-57, 1981.

11. Björntorp, P., M. Fahlen, G. Grimby, A. Gustafson, J. Holm, P. Renstrom, and T. Schersten. Carbohydrate and lipid metabolism in middle-aged physically well-trained men. *Metabolism* 21: 1037-1044, 1972.

12. Blankstein, J., F.I. Reyes, J.S.D. Winter, and C. Faiman. Endorphins and the regulation of the human menstrual cycle. *Clin. Endocrinol. (Oxf.)* 14: 287-294, 1981.

13. Bloom, S.R., R.H. Johnson, D.M. Park, M.J. Rennie, and W.R. Sulaiman. Differences in the metabolic and hormonal response to exercise between racing cyclists and untrained individuals. *J. Physiol. (Lond.)* 258: 1-18, 1976.

14. Bonelli, J., W. Waldhausl, D. Magometschnigg, J. Schwarzmeier, A. Korn, and G. Hitzenberger. Effect of exercise and of prolonged oral administration of propranolol on haemodynamic variables, plasma renin concentration, plasma aldosterone and c-AMP. *Eur. J. Clin. Invest.* 7: 337-343, 1977.

15. Bonen, A. Effects of exercise on excretion rates of urinary free cortisol. *J. Appl. Physiol.* 40: 155-158, 1976.

16. Bonen, A., A.N. Belcastro, W.Y. Ling, and A.A. Simpson. Profiles of selected hormones during menstrual cycles of teenage athletes. *J. Appl. Physiol.* 50: 545-551, 1981.

17. Bonen, A., M.H. Tan, P. Clune, and R.L. Kirby. Effects of exercise on insulin binding to human muscle. *Am. J. Physiol.* 248: E408, 1985.

18. Borer, K.T., D.R. Nicoski, and V. Owens. Alteration of pulsatile growth hormone secretion by growth-inducing exercise: Involvement of endogenous opiates and somatostatin. *Endocrinology* 118: 844-850, 1986.

19. Bortz, W.M., II, P. Angevin, I.N. Mefford, M.B. Boarder, N. Noyce, and J.D. Barchas. Catecholamines, dopamine and endorphin levels during extreme exercise. *N. Engl. J. Med.* 305: 466-467, 1981.

20. Bouloux, P.M.G., A. Grossman, S. Al-Damluji, T. Dailey, and G.M. Besser. Enhancement of the sympathoadrenal responses to the cold-pressor test by naloxone in man. *Clin. Sci.* 69: 365-368, 1985.

21. Bouloux, P.M.G., A. Grossman, N. Lytras, and G.M. Besser. Evidence for the participation of endogenous opioids in the sympathoadrenal response to hypoglycaemia in man. *Clin. Endocrinol.* 22: 49-56, 1985.

22. Boyden, T.W., R.W. Pamenter, P. Stanforth, T. Rotkis, and J.H. Wilmore. Sex steroids and

endurance running in women. *Fertil. Steril.* 39: 629-632, 1983.

23. Boyden, T.W., R.W. Pamenter, P. Stanforth, T. Rotkis, and J.H. Wilmore. Impaired gonadotrophin releasing hormone stimulation in endurance trained women. *Fertil. Steril.* 41: 359-363, 1984.

24. Bramnert, M., and B. Hokfelt. Effect of exercise on sympathetic activity and plasma pituitary hormones in naloxone-treated healthy subjects. In: Miller, E.E., and A.R. Genazzoni, eds. *Central and peripheral endorphins: Basic and clinical aspects.* New York: Raven Press, 1984, p. 191-194.

25. Brandenberger, G., and M. Follenius. Influence of timing and intensity of muscular exercise on temporal patterns of plasma cortisol levels. *J. Clin. Endocrinol. Metab.* 40: 845-849, 1975.

26. Brandenberger, G., M. Follenius, and B. Hietter. Feedback from meal-related peaks determines diurnal changes in cortisol response to exercise. *J. Clin. Endocrinol. Metab.* 54: 592-596, 1982.

27. Brands, B., J.B. Thornhill, M. Hirst, and C.W. Gowdey. Suppression of food intake and body weight gain by naloxone in rats. *Life Sci.* 24: 1773-1778, 1979.

28. Brisson, G.R., F. Malaisse-Lagae, and W.J. Malaisse. Effect of phentolamine upon insulin secretion during exercise. *Diabetologia* 7: 223-226, 1971.

29. Brotherhood, J., B. Brozovic, and L.G.C.E. Pugh. Haemotological status of middle- and long-distance runners. *Clin. Sci. Mol. Med.* 48: 139-145, 1975.

30. Brown, M.J., D.A. Jenner, D.J. Allison, and C.T. Dollery. Variations in individual organ release of noradrenaline measured by an improved radioenzymatic technique: Limitations of peripheral venous measurements in the assessment of sympathetic nervous activity. *Clin. Sci.* 61: 585-590, 1981.

31. Bullen, B.A., G.S. Skrinar, I.Z. Beitins, D.B. Carr, S.M. Reppert, C.O. Dotson, M. de M. Fencl, E.V. Gervino, and J.W. McArthur. Endurance training effects on plasma hormonal responsiveness and sex hormone excretion. *J. Appl. Physiol.* 56: 1453-1463, 1984.

32. Bunt, J.C. Hormonal alterations due to exercise. *Sports Med.* 3: 331-345, 1986.

33. Burstein, R., C. Polychronakos, C.J. Toews, J.D. MacDougall, H.J. Guyda, and B.I. Posner. Acute reversal of the enhanced insulin action in trained athletes: Association with insulin receptor changes. *Diabetes* 34: 756-760, 1985.

34. Cann, C.E., D.J. Cavanaugh, K. Schnurpfiel, and M.C. Martin. Menstrual history is the primary determinant of trabecular bone density in women runners. *Med. Sci. Sports Exerc.* 20: S59, 1988.

35. Cann, C.E., M.C. Martin, H.K. Genant, and R.B. Jaffe. Decreased spinal mineral content in amenorrheic women. *J.A.M.A.* 251: 626-629, 1984.

36. Carr, D.B., B.A. Bullen, G.S. Skrinar, M.A. Arnold, M. Rosenblatt, I.Z. Beitins, J.B. Martin, and J.W. McArthur. Physical conditioning facilitates the exercise-induced secretion of beta-endorphin and beta-lipotropin in women. *N. Engl. J. Med.* 305: 560-563, 1981.

37. Casanueva, F.F., L. Villanueva, J.A. Cabranes, J. Cabezas-Cerrato, and A. Fernandez-Cruz. Cholinergic mediation of growth hormone secretion elicited by arginine, clonidine, and physical exercise in man. *J. Endocrinol. Metab.* 59: 526-530, 1984.

38. Cashmore, G.C., C.T.M. Davies, and J.D. Few. Relationship between increases in plasma cortisol concentration and rate of cortisol secretion during exercise in man. *J. Endocrinol.* 72: 109-110, 1977.

39. Chang, F.E., W.G. Dodds, M. Sullivan, M.H. Kim, and W.B. Malarkey. The acute effects of exercise on prolactin and growth hormone secretion: Comparison between sedentary women and women runners with normal and abnormal menstrual cycles. *J. Clin. Endocrinol. Metab.* 62: 551-556, 1986.

40. Chisholm, D.J., A.B. Jenkins, D.E. James, and E.W. Kraegen. The effect of hyperinsulinemia on glucose homeostasis during moderate exercise in man. *Diabetes* 31: 603-608, 1982.

41. Christensen, N.J., and O. Brandsborg. The relationship between plasma catecholamine concentration and pulse rate during exercise and standing. *Eur. J. Clin. Invest.* 3: 299-306, 1973.

42. Christensen, N.J., and H. Galbo. Sympathetic nervous activity during exercise. *Annu. Rev. Physiol.* 45: 139-153, 1983.

43. Christensen, E.H., and O. Hansen. Arbeitsfahigkeit und ernahrung. *Scand. Arch. Physiol.* 81: 160-171, 1939.

44. Coggan, A.R., and E.F. Coyle. Reversal of fatigue during prolonged exercise by carbo-

hydrate infusion or ingestion. *J. Appl. Physiol.* 63: 2388-2395, 1987.

45. Coggan, A.R., and E.F. Coyle. Effect of carbohydrate feedings during high-intensity exercise. *J. Appl. Physiol.* 65: 1703-1709, 1988.

46. Colt, E.W.D., S.L. Wardlaw, and A.G. Frantz. The effect of running on plasma beta-endorphin. *Life Sci.* 28: 1637-1640, 1981.

47. Convertino, V.A., P.J. Brock, L.C. Keil, E.M. Bernauer, and J.E. Greenleaf. Exercise training-induced hypervolemia: Role of plasma albumin, renin and vasopressin. *J. Appl. Physiol.* 48: 665-669, 1980.

48. Convertino, V.A., L.C. Keil, E.M. Bernauer, and J.E. Greenleaf. Plasma volume, osmolality, vasopressin and renin activity during graded exercise in man. *J. Appl. Physiol.* 50: 123-128, 1981.

49. Cornil, A., A. DeCoster, G. Copinschi, and J.R.M. Franckson. The effect of muscular exercise on the plasma cortisol level in man. *Acta Endocrinol.* 48: 163-168, 1965.

50. Costill D.L., and J.M. Miller. Nutrition for endurance sports: Carbohydrate and fluid balance. *Int. J. Sports Med.* 1: 2-14, 1980.

51. Costill, D.L., G. Branam, W. Fink, and R. Nelson. Exercise induced sodium conservation. *Med. Sci. Sports* 8: 209-213, 1976.

52. Cumming, D.C., M.M. Vickovic, S.R. Wall, and M.R. Fluker. Defects in pulsatile LH release in normally menstruating runners. *J. Clin. Endocrinol. Metab.* 60: 810-812, 1985.

53. Dale, E., D.H. Gerlach, and A.L. Wilhite. Menstrual dysfunction in distance runners. *Obstet. Gynecol.* 54: 47-53, 1979.

54. Davies, C.T.M., and J.D. Few. Effects of exercise on adrenocortical function. *J. Appl. Physiol.* 35: 887-891, 1973.

55. Davies, J.A., M.H. Harrison, L.A. Cochrane, R.J. Edwards, and T.M. Gibson. Effect of saline loading during heat acclimation on adrenocortical hormone levels. *J. Appl. Physiol.* 50: 605-612, 1981.

56. DeFronzo, R.A., E. Ferrannini, Y. Sato, P. Felig, and J. Wahren. Synergistic interaction between exercise and insulin on peripheral glucose uptake. *J. Clin. Invest.* 68: 1468-1474, 1981.

57. DeFronzo, R.A., J.D. Tobin, and A. Reubin. Glucose clamp technique: A method for quantifying insulin secretion and resistance. *Am. J. Physiol.* 237: E214-E223, 1979.

58. DeMeirleir, K., N. Naaktgeboren, A. Van Steirteghem, F. Gorus, J. Olbrecht, and P. Block. Beta endorphin and ACTH levels in peripheral blood during and after aerobic and anaerobic exercise. *Eur. J. Appl. Physiol.* 55: 5-8, 1986.

59. Dessypris, A., K. Kuoppasalmi, and H. Adlercreutz. Plasma cortisol, testosterone, androstenedione and luteinizing hormone (LH) in a noncompetitive marathon run. *J. Steroid Biochem.* 7: 33-37, 1976.

60. Devlin, J.G. The effect of training and acute physical exercise on plasma insulin-like activity. *Irish J. Med. Sci.* 6: 423-425, 1963.

61. Donevan, R.H., and G.M. Andres. Plasma B-endorphin immunoreactivity during graded cycle ergometry. *Med. Sci. Sports Exerc.* 19: 229-230, 1987.

62. Douen, A.G., T. Ramlal, A. Klip, D.A. Young, G.D. Cartee, and J.O. Holloszy. Exercise-induced increase in glucose transporters in plasma membranes of rat skeletal muscle. *Endocrinology* 124: 449-454, 1989.

63. Drinkwater, B.L., K. Nilson, C.H. Chestnut, III, W. Bremmer, S. Shainholtz, and M. Southworth. Bone mineral content of amenorrheic and eumenorrheic athletes. *N. Engl. J. Med.* 311: 277-281, 1984.

64. Elias, A.N., K. Iyer, M.R. Pandian, P. Weathersbee, S. Stone, and J. Tobis. Beta-endorphin/beta-lipotropin release and gonadotropin secretion after acute exercise in normal males. *J. Appl. Physiol.* 61: 2045-2049, 1986.

65. Esler, M., G. Jennings, P. Korner, P. Blombery, N. Sacharias, and P. Leonard. Measurement of total and organ-specific norepinephrine kinetics in humans. *Am. J. Physiol.* 247: E21-E28, 1984.

66. Erydelyi, G. Gynecologic survey of female athletes. *J. Sports Med. Phys. Fitness* 2: 174-179, 1962.

67. Faber, O.K., C. Hagen, C. Binder, J. Markussen, V.K. Naithani, P.M. Blix, H. Kuzuya, D. Horwitz, and A.H. Rubenstein. Kinetics of human connecting peptide in normal and diabetic subjects. *J. Clin. Invest.* 62: 197-203, 1978.

68. Fagard, R., A. Amery, T. Reybrouck, P. Lijnen, E. Moerman, M. Bogaert, and A. De Schaepdryver. Effects of angiotensin antagonism on hemodynamics, renin, and catecholamines during exercise. *J. Appl. Physiol.* 43: 440-444, 1977.

69. Fahey, T.D., A. Del Valle-Zuris, G. Oehlsen, M. Trieb, and J. Seymour. Pubertal stage differences in hormonal and hematological

responses to maximal exercise in males. *J. Appl. Physiol.* 46: 823-827, 1979.

70. Faiman, C., J. Blankstein, F.I. Reyes, and J.S.D. Winter. Endorphins and the regulation of the human menstrual cycle. *Fertil. Steril.* 36: 267-268, 1981.

71. Farrell, P.A., T.L. Garthwaite, and A.B. Gustafson. Plasma adrenocorticotropin and cortisol responses to submaximal and exhaustive exercise. *J. Appl. Physiol.* 55: 1441-1444, 1983.

72. Farrell, P.A., W.K. Gates, W.P. Morgan, and M.G. Maksud. Increases in plasma beta-EP and beta-LPH immunoreactivity after treadmill running in humans. *J. Appl. Physiol.* 52: 1245-1249, 1982.

73. Farrell, P.A., W.K. Gates, W.P. Morgan, and C.B. Pert. Plasma leucine enkephalin-like radioreceptor activity and tension-anxiety before and after competitive running. In: Knuttgen, H.G., J.A. Vogel, and J. Poortmans, eds. *Biochemistry of exercise.* Champaign, IL: Human Kinetics, 1983, p. 637-644.

74. Farrell, P.A., A.B. Gustafson, T.L. Garthwaite, R.K. Kalkhoff, A.W. Cowley, Jr., and W.P. Morgan. Influence of endogenous opioids on the response of selected hormones to exercise in humans. *J. Appl. Physiol.* 61: 1051-1057, 1986.

75. Farrell, P.A., A.B. Gustafson, W.P. Morgan, and C.B. Pert. Enkephalins, catecholamines and psychological mood alterations: Effects of prolonged exercise. *Med. Sci. Sports Exerc.* (in press).

76. Farrell, P.A., M. Kjaer, F.W. Bach, and H. Galbo. Beta endorphin and adrenocorticotropin response to supramaximal treadmill exercise in trained and untrained males. *Acta Physiol. Scand.* 130: 619-625, 1987.

77. Farrell, P.A., B. Sonne, K. Mikines, and H. Galbo. Stimulatory role for endogenous opioid peptides on post-exercise insulin secretion in rats. *J. Appl. Physiol.* 65: 744-749, 1988.

78. Feicht, C.B., T.S. Johnson, B.J. Martin, K.E. Sparkes, and W.W. Wagner. Secondary amenorrhea in athletes. *Lancet* ii: 1145-1156, 1978.

79. Felig, P., A. Cherif, A. Minagawa, and J. Wahren. Hypoglycemia during prolonged exercise in normal men. *N. Engl. J. Med.* 306: 895-900, 1982.

80. Few, J.D. Effect of exercise on the secretion and metabolism of cortisol in man. *J. Endocrinol.* 62: 341-353, 1974.

81. Finberg, J.P.M., and G.M. Berlyne. Modification of renin and aldosterone: Response to heat by acclimation in man. *J. Appl. Physiol.* 42: 554-558, 1977.

82. Fleg, J.L., S.P. Tzankoff, and E.G. Lakatta. Age-related augmentation of plasma catecholamines during dynamic exercise in healthy males. *J. Appl. Physiol.* 59: 1033-1039, 1985.

83. Fotherby, K., and S.B. Pal. *Exercise endocrinology.* Berlin: de Gruyter, 1985.

84. Fraioli, F., C. Moretti, D. Paolucci, E. Alicicco, G. Crescenzi, and G. Fortunio. Physical exercise stimulates marked concomitant release of beta-endorphin and ACTH in peripheral blood in man. *Experientia* 36: 987-989, 1980.

85. Francesconi, R.P., M.N. Sawka, and K.B. Pandolf. Hypohydration and heat acclimation: Plasma renin and aldosterone during exercise. *J. Appl. Physiol.* 55: 1790-1794, 1983.

86. Francesconi, R.P., M.N. Sawka, and K.B. Pandolf. Hypohydration and acclimation: Effects on hormone responses to exercise/heat stress. *Aviat. Space Environ. Med.* 55: 365-369, 1984.

87. Francesconi, R.P., M.N. Sawka, B. Pandolf, R.W. Hubbard, A.J. Young, and S. Muza. Plasma hormone responses at graded hypohydration levels during exercise in heat stress. *J. Appl. Physiol.* 59: 1855-1860, 1985.

88. Franckson, J.R.M., R. Vanroux, R. Leclercq, H. Brunengraber, and H.A. Ooms. Labeled insulin catabolism and pancreatic responsiveness during long-term exercise in man. *Horm. Metab. Res.* 3: 366-373, 1971.

89. Freund, B.J., J.R. Claybaugh, M.S. Dice, and G.M. Hashiro. Hormonal and vascular fluid responses to maximal exercise in trained and untrained males. *J. Appl. Physiol.* 63: 669-675, 1987.

90. Frisch, R.E., G. Wyshak, and L. Vincent. Delayed menarche and amenorrhea in ballet dancers. *N. Engl. J. Med.* 303: 17-19, 1980.

91. Galbo, H. Catecholamines and muscular exercise: Assessment of sympathoadrenal activity. In Poortmans, J.R., and G. Niset, eds. *Biochemistry of exercise IVB.* Baltimore: University Park Press, 1981, p. 5-19.

92. Galbo, H. *Hormonal and metabolic adaptations to exercise.* Stuttgart: Thieme Verlag, 1983.

93. Galbo, H., N.J. Christensen, and J.J. Holst. Catecholamines and pancreatic hormones during autonomic blockade in exercising man. *Acta Physiol. Scand.* 101: 428-437, 1977.

94. Galbo, H., N.J. Christensen, and J.J. Holst. Glucose-induced decrease in glucagon and epinephrine responses to exercise in man. *J. Appl. Physiol.* 42: 525-530, 1977.

95. Galbo, H., J.J. Holst, and N.J. Christensen. Glucagon and plasma catecholamine responses to graded and prolonged exercise in man. *J. Appl. Physiol.* 38: 70-76, 1975.

96. Galbo, H., M. Kjaer, and N.H. Secher. Cardiovascular, ventilatory and catecholamine responses to maximal dynamic exercise in partially curarized man. *J. Physiol. (Lond.)* 389: 557-568, 1987.

97. Gambert, S.R., T.L. Garthwaite, C.H. Pontzer, E.E. Cook, F.E. Tristani, E.H. Duthie, D.R. Martinson, T.C. Hagen, and D.J. McCarty. Running elevates plasma beta-endorphin immunoreactivity and ACTH in untrained human subjects. *Proc. Soc. Exp. Biol. Med.* 168: 1-4, 1981.

98. Gambert, S.R., T.C. Hagen, T.L. Garthwaite, E.H. Duthie, Jr., and D.J. McCarty. Exercise and the endogenous opioids. *N. Engl. J. Med.* 305: 1590-1592, 1981.

99. Gold, P.W., H. Gwirtsman, P.C. Avgerinos, L.K. Nieman, W.T. Gallucci, W. Kaye, D. Jimerson, M. Ebert, R. Rittmaster, D.L. Loriaux, and G.P. Chrousos. Abnormal hypothalamic-pituitary-adrenal function in anorexia nervosa: Pathophysiologic mechanisms in underweight and weight-corrected patients. *N. Engl. J. Med.* 314: 1335-1342, 1986.

100. Gold, P.W., D.L. Loriaux, A. Roy, M.A. Kling, J.R. Calabrese, C.H. Kellner, L.K. Nieman, R.M. Post, D. Pickar, W. Gallucci, P. Avgerinos, S. Paul, E.H. Oldfield, G.B. Cutler, and G.P. Chrousos. Responses to corticotropin-releasing hormone on the hypercortisolism of depression and Cushing's disease: Pathophysiologic and diagnostic implications. *N. Engl. J. Med.* 314: 1329-1335, 1986.

101. Goldfarb, A.H., B.D. Hatfield, G.A. Sforzo, and M.G. Flynn. Serum B-endorphin levels during a graded exercise test to exhaustion. *Med. Sci. Sports Exerc.* 19: 78-82, 1987.

102. Gollnick, P.D. Energy metabolism and skeletal muscle function during prolonged exercise. In: Lamb, D.R., ed. *Perspectives in exercise science and sports medicine.* Indianapolis: Benchmark Press, 1988, p. 1-37.

103. Gollnick, P.D., R.G. Soule, A.W. Taylor, C. Williams, and C.D. Ianuzzo. Exercise-induced glycogenolysis and lipolysis in the rat: Hormonal influence. *Am. J. Physiol.* 219: 729-733, 1970.

104. Green, H.J., R.L. Hughson, J.A. Thomson, and M.T. Sharratt. Supramaximal exercise after training-induced hypervolemia. I. Gas exchange and acid-base balance. *J. Appl. Physiol.* 62: 1944-1953, 1987.

105. Green, H.J., J.R. Sutton, G. Coates, M. Ali, and S. Jones. Anemia and pseudo-anemia during prolonged training in man. *J. Appl. Physiol.* (in press).

106. Green, H.J., A. Thomson, M.E. Ball, R.L. Hughson, M.E. Houston, and M.T. Sharratt. Alterations in blood volume following short-term supramaximal exercise. *J. Appl. Physiol.* 56: 145-149, 1984.

107. Green, H.J., J.A. Thomson, and M.E. Houston. Supramaximal exercise after training-induced hypervolemia. II. Blood/muscle substrates and metabolites. *J. Appl. Physiol.* 62: 1954-1961, 1987.

108. Greenleaf, J.E., E.M. Bernauer, H.L. Young, J.T. Morse, R.W. Staley, L.T. Juhos, and W. Van Beaumont. Fluid and electrolyte shifts during bed rest with isometric and isotonic exercise. *J. Appl. Physiol.* 42: 59-66, 1977.

109. Greenleaf, J.E., D. Sciaraffa, E. Shvartz, L.C. Keil, and P.J. Brock. Exercise training hypotension: Implications for plasma volume, renin, and vasopressin. *J. Appl. Physiol.* 51: 298-305, 1981.

110. Grossman, A., and L.H. Rees. The neuroendocrinology of opioid peptides. *Br. Med. Bull.* 39: 83-88. 1983.

111. Grossman, A., and J.R. Sutton. Endorphins: What are they? How are they measured? What is their role in exercise? *Med. Sci. Sports Exerc.* 17: 74-81, 1985.

112. Grossman, A., P. Bouloux, P. Price, P.L. Drury, K.S.L. Lam, T. Turner, J. Thomas, G.M. Besser, and J. Sutton. The role of opioid peptides in the hormonal responses to acute exercise in man. *Clin. Sci.* 67: 483-491, 1984.

113. Grossman, A., P.J.A. Moult, H. McIntyre, J. Evans, T. Silverstone, L.H. Rees, and G.M. Besser. Opiate mediation of amenorrhea in hyperprolactinaemia and in weight-loss related amenorrhea. *Clin. Endocrinol. (Oxf.)* 17: 379-388, 1982.

114. Groves, B.M., J.T. Reeves, J.R. Sutton, P.D. Wagner, A. Cymerman, M.K. Malconian, P.B. Rock, P.M. Young, and C.S. Houston. Operation Everest II: Elevated high altitude pulmonary resistance unresponsive to oxygen. *J. Appl. Physiol.* 63: 521-530, 1987.

115. Hansen, A.P. The effect of intravenous glucose infusion on the exercise-induced serum growth hormone rise in normals and juvenile diabetics. *Scand. J. Clin. Lab. Invest.* 28: 195-205, 1971.

116. Hansen, A.P. The effect of intravenous infusion of lipids on the exercise-induced serum growth hormone rise in normals and juvenile diabetics. *Scand. J. Clin. Lab. Invest.* 28: 207-212, 1971.

117. Hansen, A.P. The effect of adrenergic receptor blockade on the exercise-induced serum growth hormone rise in normals and juvenile diabetics. *J. Clin. Endocrinol.* 33: 807-812, 1971.

118. Hansson, B.-G, and B. Hokfelt. Long-term treatment of moderate hypertension with penbutolol (Hoe 893d). I. Effects on blood pressure, pulse rate, catecholamines in blood and urine, plasma renin activity and urinary aldosterone under basal conditions and following exercise. *Eur. J. Clin. Pharmacol.* 9: 9-19, 1975.

119. Harber, V.J., and J.R. Sutton. Endorphins and exercise. *Sports Med.* 1: 154-171, 1984.

120. Harber, V.J., B.R. Bhavnani, J.R. Sutton, J.D. MacDougall, and C.A. Woolever. Pulsatility and plasma concentrations of beta-endorphin and LH in sedentary and exercising women with and without amenorrhea. *J. Clin. Endocrinol. Metab.* (in press).

121. Harber, V.J., C.E. Webber, J.R. Sutton, and J.D. MacDougall. The effect of amenorrhea on bone density and total bone turnover in runners. *Med. Sci. Sports Exerc.* (in press).

122. Harrison, M.H. Effects of thermal stress and exercise on blood volume in humans. *Physiol. Rev.* 65: 149-199, 1985.

123. Hartley, L.H., J.W. Mason, R.P. Hogan, L.G. Jones, T.A. Kotchen, E.H. Mougey, F.E. Wherry, L.L. Pennington, and P.T. Ricketts. Multiple hormonal responses to graded exercise in relation to physical training. *J. Appl. Physiol.* 33: 602-606, 1972.

124. Hartley, L.H., J.W. Mason, R.P. Hogan, L.G. Jones, T.A. Kotchen, E.H. Mougey, F.E. Wherry, L.L. Pennington, and P.T. Ricketts. Multiple hormonal responses to prolonged exercise in relation to physical training. *J. Appl. Physiol.* 33: 607-610, 1972.

125. Ho, K.Y., W.S. Evans, R.M. Blizzard, J.D. Veldhuis, G.R. Merriam, E. Samojlik, R. Furlanetto, A.D. Rogol, D.L. Kaiser, and M.O. Thorner. Effects of sex and age on the 24-hour profile of growth hormone secretion in man: Importance of endogenous estradiol concentrations. *J. Clin. Endocrinol. Metab.* 64: 51-57, 1987.

126. Hoelzer, D.R., G.P. Dalsky, W.E. Clutter, S.D. Shah, J.O. Holloszy, and P.E. Cryer. Glucoregulation during exercise: Hypoglycemia is prevented by redundant glucoregulatory systems, sympathochromaffin activation, and changes in islet hormone secretion. *J. Clin. Invest.* 77: 212-221, 1986.

127. Hoelzer, D.R., G.P. Dalsky, N.S. Schwartz, W.E. Clutter, S.D. Shah, J.O. Holloszy, and P.E. Cryer. Epinephrine is not critical to prevention of hypoglycemia during exercise in humans. *Am. J. Physiol.* 251: E104-E110, 1986.

128. Holaday, J.W., H. Loh, and C.H. Li. Unique behavioral effects of beta-endorphin and their relationship to thermoregulation and hypothalamic function. *Life Sci.* 22: 1525-1536, 1978.

129. Holmgren, A., F. Mossfeldt, T. Sjostrand, and G. Strom. Effect of training on work capacity, total hemoglobin, blood volume, heart volume and pulse rate in recumbent and upright position. *Acta Physiol. Scand.* 50: 72-83, 1960.

130. Howlett, T.A., and L.H. Rees. Endogenous opioid peptides and hypothalamo-pituitary function. In: Berne, R.M., ed. *Annual review of physiology* 48. Palo Alto, CA: Annual Reviews Inc., 1986, p. 613-623.

131. Howlett, T.A., S. Tomlin, L. Ngahfoong, L.H. Rees, B.A. Bullen, G.S. Skrinar, and J.W. McArthur. Release of beta-endorphin and met-enkephalin during exercise in normal women: Response to training. *Br. Med. J.* 288: 1950-1952, 1984.

132. Hughes, J., T.W. Smith, H.W. Kosterlitz, L.A. Fothergill, B.A. Morgan, and H.R. Morris. Identification of two related pentapeptides from the brain with potent opiate agonist activity. *Nature* 258: 577-579, 1975.

133. Hunter, W.M., and F.C. Greenwood. Studies on the secretion of human pituitary growth hormone. *Br. Med. J.* 1: 804-806, 1965.

134. Hunter, W.M., and M.Y. Sakkar. Changes in plasma insulin levels during muscular exercise. *Proc. Physiol. Soc.* (February): 110P-112P, 1968.

135. James, D.E., E.W. Kraegen, and D.J. Chisholm. Effects of exercise training on in vivo insulin action in individual tissues of the rat. *J. Clin. Invest.* 76: 657-666, 1985.

136. James, D.E., K.M. Burleigh, E.W. Kraegen, and D.J. Chisholm. Effects of acute exercise and prolonged training on insulin response

to intravenous glucose in vivo in rats. *J. Appl. Physiol.* 55: 1660-1664, 1983.

137. Janal, M.N., E.W.D. Colt, W.C. Clark, and M. Glusman. Pain sensitivity, mood and plasma endocrine levels in man following long-distance running: Effects of naloxone. *Pain* 19: 13-25, 1984.

138. Jarhult, J., and J. Holst. The role of the adrenergic innervation to the pancreatic islets in the control of insulin release during exercise in man. *Pflugers Arch.* 383: 41-45, 1979.

139. Jenkins, A.B., D.J. Chisholm, D.E. James, K.Y. Ho, and E.W. Kraegen. Exercise-induced hepatic glucose output is precisely sensitive to the rate of systemic glucose supply. *Metabolism* 34: 431-436, 1985.

140. Jurkowski, J.E., J.R. Sutton, P.M. Keane, and G.W. Viol. Plasma renin activity and plasma aldosterone during exercise in relation to the menstrual cycle. *Med. Sci. Sports* 10: 41, 1978.

141. Jurkowski, J., E. Younglai, C. Walker, N.L. Jones, and J.R. Sutton. Ovarian hormone response to exercise. *J. Appl. Physiol.* 44: 109-114, 1978.

142. Keizer, H.A., J. Poortmans, and J. Bunniks. Influence of physical exercise on sex hormone metabolism. *J. Appl. Physiol.* 50: 545-551, 1981.

143. Kjaer, M., N.J. Christensen, B. Sonne, E.A. Richter, and H. Galbo. Effect of exercise on epinephrine turnover in trained and untrained male subjects. *J. Appl. Physiol.* 59: 1061-1067, 1985.

144. Kjaer, M., P.A. Farrell, N.J. Christensen, and H. Galbo. Increased epinephrine response and inaccurate glucoregulation in exercising athletes. *J. Appl. Physiol.* 61: 1693-1700, 1986.

145. Kjaer, M., N.H. Secher, F.W. Bach, and H. Galbo. Role of motor center activity for hormonal changes and substrate mobilization in humans. *Am. J. Physiol.* 253: R687-R695, 1987.

146. Kjellberg, S.R., U. Rudhe, and T. Sjostrand. Increase of the amount of hemoglobin and blood volume in connection with physical training. *Acta Physiol. Scand.* 19: 146-151, 1949.

147. Knobil, E. The neuroendocrine control of the menstrual cycle. *Rec. Prog. Horm. Res.* 36: 53-88, 1980.

148. Koch, G., and L. Rocker. Plasma volume and intravascular protein masses in trained boys and fit young men. *J. Appl. Physiol.* 43: 1085-1088, 1977.

149. Koivisto, V.A., V.R. Soman, and P. Felig. Effects of acute exercise on insulin binding to

monocytes in obesity. *Metabolism* 29: 168-172, 1980.

150. Kosunen, K., A. Pakarinen, K. Kuoppasalmi, H. Naveri, S. Rehunen, C.G. Standerskjold-Nordenstam, M. Harkonen, and H. Adlercreutz. Cardiovascular function and the renin-angiotensin-aldosterone system in long-distance runners during various training periods. *Scand. J. Clin. Lab. Invest.* 40: 429-435, 1980.

151. Kotchen, T.A., L.H. Hartley, T.W. Rice, E.H. Mougey, L.G. Jones, and J.W. Mason. Renin, norepinephrine, and epinephrine responses to graded exercise. *J. Appl. Physiol.* 31: 178-184, 1971.

152. Kraemer, N.J., L.E. Armstrong, L.J. Marchitelli, R.W. Hubbard, and N. Leva. Plasma opioid peptide responses during heat acclimation in humans. *Peptides* 8: 715-719, 1988.

153. Krotkiewski, M., P. Björntorp, G. Holm, V. Marks, L. Morgan, V. Smith, and G.E. Glurle. Effects of physical training on insulin, connecting peptide (C-peptide), gastric inhibitory polypeptide (GIP) and pancreatic polypeptide (PP) levels in obese subjects. *Int. J. Obesity* 8: 193-199, 1984.

154. Krotkiewski, M., and J. Gorski. Effect of muscular exercise on plasma C-peptide and insulin in obese non-diabetics and diabetics, Type II. *Clin. Physiol.* 6: 499-506, 1986.

155. Kuoppasalmi, K., H. Naveri, M. Harkonen, and H. Adlercreutz. Plasma cortisol, androstenedione, testosterone and luteinizing hormone in running exercise of different intensities. *Scand. J. Clin. Lab. Invest.* 40: 403-409, 1980.

156. Kuoppasalmi, K., H. Naveri, S. Rehunen, M. Harkonen, and H. Adlercreutz. Effect of strenuous anaerobic running exercise on plasma growth hormone, cortisol, luteinizing hormone, testosterone, androstenedione, estrone and estradiol. *J. Steroid Biochem.* 7: 823-829, 1976.

157. Lam, K.S.L., A. Grossman, P. Bouloux, P.L. Drury, and G.M. Besser. Effect of an opiate antagonist on the responses of circulating catecholamines and the renin-aldosterone system to acute sympathetic stimulation by hand-grip in man. *Acta Endocrinol.* 111: 252-257, 1986.

158. Lamberts, S.W.J., E.N.W. Janssens, E.G. Bons, P. Uitterlinden, J.M. Zuiderwijk, and E. Del Pozo. The met-enkephalin analog FK 33-284 directly inhibits ACTH release by the

rat pituitary gland in vitro. *Life Sci.* 32: 1167-1173, 1983.

159. Lavoie, J.-M., N. Dionne, R. Helie, and G.R. Brisson. Menstrual cycle phase dissociation of blood glucose homeostasis during exercise. *J. Appl. Physiol.* 1084-1089, 1987.

160. LeBlanc, J., A. Nadeau, M. Boulay, and S. Rousseau-Migneron. Effects of physical training and adiposity on glucose metabolism and ^{125}I-insulin binding. *J. Appl. Physiol.* 46: 235-239, 1979.

161. Leenen, F.H.H., P. Boer, and G.G. Geyskes. Sodium intake and the effects of isoproterenol and exercise on plasma renin in man. *J. Appl. Physiol.* 45: 870-874, 1978.

162. Levine, S.A., B. Gordon, and C.L. Derick. Some changes in the chemical constituents of the blood following a marathon race. *J. Amer. Med. Assoc.* 82: 1778-1779, 1924.

163. Li, C.H. Lipotrophin, a new active peptide from pituitary glands. *Nature* 201: 924, 1964.

164. Li, C.H. Beta-endorphin: a pituitary peptide with potent morphine-like activity. *Arch. Biochem. Biophys.* 183: 592-604, 1977.

165. Lijnen, P.J., A.K. Amery, R.H. Fagard, T.M. Reybrouck, E.J. Moerman, and A.F. De Schaepdryver. The effects of beta-adrenoceptor blockade on renin, angiotensin, aldosterone and catecholamines at rest and during exercise. *Br. J. Clin. Pharmacol.* 7: 175-181, 1979.

166. Loucks, A.B., and S.M. Horvath. Exercise-induced stress responses of amenorrheic and eumenorrheic runners. *J. Clin. Endocrinol. Metab.* 59: 1109-1120, 1984.

167. Loucks, A.B., J.F. Mortola, L. Girton, and S.S.C. Yen. Alterations in the hypothalamic-pituitary-ovarian and the hypothalamic-pituitary-adrenal aces in athletic women. *J. Clin. Endocrinol. Metab.* 68: 402-411, 1989.

168. Luger, A., P.A. Deuster, S.B. Kyle, W.T. Gallucci, L.C. Montgomery, P.W. Gold, D.L. Loriaux, and G.P. Chrousos. Acute hypothalamic-pituitary-adrenal responses to the stress of treadmill exercise: Physiologic adaptations to physical training. *N. Engl. J. Med.* 316: 1309-1315, 1987.

169. MacConnie, S.E., A. Barkan, R.M. Lampman, M.A. Schork, and I.Z. Beitins. Decreased hypothalamic gonadotropin-releasing hormone secretion in male marathon runners. *N. Engl. J. Med.* 315: 411-417, 1986.

170. Maher, J.T., L.G. Jones, L.H. Hartley, G.H. Williams, and L.I. Rose. Aldosterone dynamics during graded exercise at sea level and high altitude. *J. Appl. Physiol.* 39: 18-22, 1975.

171. Marcus, R., C. Cann. P. Madvig, J. Minkoff, M. Goddard, M. Bayer, M. Martin, L. Gaudini, W. Haskell, and H. Genant. Menstrual function and bone mass in elite women distance runners. *Ann. Int. Med.* 102: 158-163, 1985.

172. Markoff, R.A., P. Ryan, and T. Young. Endorphins and mood changes in long distance running. *Med. Sci. Sports Exerc.* 14: 11-15, 1982.

173. Marshall, J.C., and R.P. Kelch. Gonadotrophin-releasing hormone: Role of pulsatile secretion in the regulation of reproduction. *N. Engl. J. Med.* 315: 1459-1468, 1986.

174. Martin, M.J., D.L. Horwitz, M. Nattrass, J.F. Granger, H. Rochman, and S. Ash. Effects of mild hyperinsulinemia on the metabolic response to exercise. *Metabolism* 30: 688-694, 1981.

175. Mayer, G., J. Wessel, and J. Kobberling. Failure of naloxone to alter exercise-induced growth hormone and prolactin release in normal men. *Clin. Endocrinol. (Oxf.)* 13: 413-416, 1980.

176. McArthur, J.W. Endorphins and exercise in females: Possible connection with reproductive dysfunction. *Med. Sci. Sports Exerc.* 17: 82-88, 1985.

177. McArthur, J.W., B.A. Bullen, I.Z. Beitins, M. Pagano, T.M. Badger, and A. Klibanski. Hypothalamic amenorrhea in runners of normal body composition. *Endocrine Res. Comm.* 7: 13-25, 1980.

178. McMurray, R.G., W.A. Forsythe, M.H. Mar, and C.J. Hardy. Exercise intensity-related responses of beta-endorphin and catecholamines. *Med. Sci. Sports Exerc.* 19: 570-574, 1987.

179. McQueen, D.S. Opioid interactions with respiratory and circulatory systems. *Br. Med. Bull.* 39: 77-82, 1983.

180. Meites, J. Relation of endogenous opioid peptides to secretion of hormones. *Fed. Proc.* 39: 2531-2532, 1980.

181. Melin, B., J.P. Eclache, G. Geelen, G. Annat, A.M. Allevard, E. Jarsaillon, A. Zebidi, J.J. Legros, and C. Gharib. Plasma AVP, neurophysin, renin activity and aldosterone during submaximal exercise performed until exhaustion in trained and untrained men. *Eur. J. Appl. Physiol.* 44: 141-151, 1980.

182. Metzger, J.M., and E.A. Stein. Beta-endorphin and sprint training. *Life Sci.* 34: 1541-1547, 1984.

183. Michel, G., T. Vocke, W. Fish, H. Weicker, W. Schwarz, and W.P. Bieger. Bidirectional alteration in insulin receptor affinity by different forms of physical exercise. *Am. J. Physiol.* 246: E153-E159, 1984.

184. Mikines, K.J., P.A. Farrell, B. Sonne, and H. Galbo. Glucose dose response curve for plasma insulin after exercise in man. *Clin. Physiol.* (Suppl. 4): 98-999, 1988.

185. Mikines, K.J., P.A. Farrell, B. Sonne, B. Tronier, and H. Galbo. Postexercise dose-response relationship between plasma glucose and insulin secretion. *J. Appl. Physiol.* 64: 988-999, 1988.

186. Mikines, K.J., B. Sonne, P.A. Farrell, and H. Galbo. Insulin sensitivity and responsiveness after acute exercise. *Med. Sci. Sports Exerc.* 17: 242, 1985.

187. Mikines, K.J., B. Sonne, P.A. Farrell, B. Tronier, and H. Galbo. Effect of physical exercise on sensitivity and responsiveness to insulin in humans. *Am. J. Physiol.* 254: E248-E259, 1988.

188. Mikines, K.J., B. Sonne, P.A. Farrell, B. Tronier, and H. Galbo. Effect of training on the dose-response relationship for insulin action in men. *J. Appl. Physiol.* 66: 695-703, 1989.

189. Mikines, K.J., B. Sonne, B. Tronier, and H. Galbo. Effects of acute exercise and detraining on insulin action in trained men. *J. Appl. Physiol.* 66: 704-711, 1989.

190. Milledge, J.S., E.I. Bryson, D.M. Catley, R. Hesp, N. Luff, B.D. Minty, M.W.J. Older, N.N. Payne, M.P. Ward, and W.R. Withey. Sodium balance, fluid homeostasis and the renin-aldosterone system during the prolonged exercise of hill walking. *Clin. Sci.* 62: 595-604, 1982.

191. Miller, R.E. Pancreatic neuroendocrinology: peripheral neural mechanism in the regulation of the islets of Langerhans. *Endocrine Rev.* 2: 471-494, 1981.

192. Mondon, C.E., C.B. Dolkas, and G.M. Reaven. Site of enhanced insulin sensitivity in exercise-trained rats at rest. *Am. J. Physiol.* 239: E169-E177, 1980.

193. Moretti, C., A. Fabbri, L. Gnessi, M. Cappa, A. Calzolari, F. Fraioli, A. Grossman, and G.M. Besser. Naloxone inhibits exercise-induced release of PRL and GH in athletes. *Clin. Endocrinol. (Oxf.)* 18: 135-138, 1983.

194. Mougin, C., A. Baulay, M.T. Henriet, D. Haton, M.C. Jacquier, D. Turnill, S. Berthelay, and R.C. Gaillard. Assessment of plasma opioid peptides, beta-endorphin and met-enkephalin, at the end of an international Nordic ski race. *Eur. J. Appl. Physiol.* 56: 281-286, 1987.

195. Newmark, S.R., T. Himathongkam, R.P. Martin, K.H. Cooper, and L.I. Rose. Adreno-cortical response to marathon running. *J. Clin. Endocrinol. Metab.* 42: 393-394, 1976.

196. Niall, H.D. Revised primary structure for human growth hormone. *Nat. N. Biol. (Lond.)* 230: 90, 1971.

197. Nikkila, E.A., M.-R. Taskinen, T.A. Meittinen, R. Pelkonen, and H. Poppius. Effect of muscular exercise on insulin secretion. *Diabetes* 17: 209-218, 1968.

198. Nishikimi, T., M. Kohno, T. Matsuura, K. Akioka, M. Teragaki, M. Yasuda, H. Oku, K. Takeuchi, and T. Takeda. Effect of exercise on circulating atrial natriuretic polypeptide in valvular heart disease. *Am. J. Cardiol.* 58: 1119-1120, 1986.

199. Numa, S., and H. Imura. ACTH and related peptides: Gene structure and biosynthesis. In: Imura, H., ed. *Pituitary gland.* New York: Raven Press, 1985, p. 83-102.

200. Oscai, L.B., B.T. Williams, and B.A. Hertig. Effect of exercise on blood volume. *J. Appl. Physiol.* 24: 622-624, 1968.

201. Pederson, O., H. Beck-Nielsen, and L. Heding. Increased insulin receptors after exercise in patients with insulin-dependent diabetes mellitus. *N. Engl. J. Med.* 302: 886-892, 1980.

202. Peiris, A., R.A. Mueller, G.A. Smith, M.F. Struve, and A.H. Kissebah. Splanchnic insulin metabolism in obesity. *J. Clin. Invest.* 78: 1648-1657, 1986.

203. Peronnet, F., J. Cleroux, H. Perrault, D. Cousineau, J. de Champlain, and R. Nadeau. Plasma norepinephrine response to exercise before and after training in humans. *J. Appl. Physiol.* 51: 812-815, 1981.

204. Pert, C.B., and D.L. Bowie. Behavioral manipulation of rats causes alterations in opiate receptor occupancy. In: Usdin, E., ed. *Endorphins in mental health research.* New York: Oxford University Press, 1979, p. 93-104.

205. Plough, T., H. Galbo, and E.A. Richter. Increased muscle glucose uptake during contractions: No need for insulin. *Am. J. Physiol.* 247: E726-E731, 1984.

206. Polonsky, K.S., and A.H. Rubenstein. C-peptide as a measure of the secretion and hepatic extraction of insulin: Pitfalls and limitations. *Diabetes* 33: 486-494, 1984.

207. Prange Hansen, A.A., and J. Weeke. Fasting serum growth hormone levels and growth hormone responses to exercise during normal menstrual cycles and cycles of oral contraceptives. *Scand. J. Clin. Lab. Invest.* 34: 199-205, 1974.

208. Prior, J.C., K. Cameron, B. Ho Yuen, and J. Thomas. Menstrual cycle changes with marathon training: Anovulation and the short luteal phase. *Can. J. Appl. Sports Sci.* 7: 173-177, 1982.

209. Prior, J.C., B. Ho Yuen, D. Clement, L. Bowie, and J. Thomas. Reversible luteal phase changes and infertility associated with marathon running. *Lancet* ii: 269-270, 1982.

210. Pruett, E.D.R. Glucose and insulin during prolonged work stress in men living on different diets. *J. Appl. Physiol.* 2: 199-208, 1970.

211. Pruett, E.D.R. Plasma insulin concentrations during prolonged work at near maximal oxygen uptake. *J. Appl. Physiol.* 29: 155-158, 1970.

212. Pruett, E.D.R. Insulin and exercise in non-diabetic and diabetic man. In: Fotherby, K., and S.B. Pal, eds. *Exercise endocrinology*. Berlin: de Gruyter, 1985, p. 1-23.

213. Pugh, L.G.C.E. Blood volume changes in outdoor exercise of 8-10 hour duration. *J. Physiol. (Lond.)* 200: 345-351, 1969.

214. Quigley, M.E., and S.S.C. Yen. The role of endogenous opiates on LH secretion during the menstrual cycle. *J. Clin. Endocrinol. Metab.* 51: 179-181, 1980.

215. Quigley, M.E., K.L. Sheehan, R.F. Casper, and S.S.C. Yen. Evidence for increased dopaminergic and opiate activity in patients with hypothalamic hypogonadotrophic amenorrhea. *J. Clin. Endocrinol. Metab.* 50: 949-954, 1980.

216. Rahkila, P., E. Hakala, K. Salminen, and T. Laatikainen. Response of plasma endorphins to running in male and female endurance athletes. *Med. Sci. Sports Exerc.* 19: 451-455, 1987.

217. Raymond, L., J. Sode, and J. Tucci. Adrenocortical responses to exercise. *Clin. Res.* 17: 523-528, 1969.

218. Reinheimer, W., P.C. Davidson, and M.J. Albrink. Effect of moderate exercise on plasma glucose, insulin and free fatty acids during oral glucose tolerance test. *J. Lab. Clin. Med.* 71: 429-437, 1968.

219. Richter, E.A., and H. Galbo. Diabetes, insulin and exercise. *Sports Med.* 3: 275-288, 1986.

220. Richter, E.A., H. Galbo, and N.J. Christensen. Control of exercise-induced muscular glycogenolysis by adrenal medullary hormones in rats. *J. Appl. Physiol.* 50: 21-26, 1981.

221. Richter, E.A., H. Galbo, J.J. Holst, and B. Sonne. Significance of glucagon for insulin secretion and hepatic glycogenolysis during exercise in rats. *Horm. Metab. Res.* 13: 323-326, 1981.

222. Richter, E.A., N.B. Ruderman, and S.H. Schneider. Diabetes and exercise. *Am. J. Med.* 70: 201-209, 1981.

223. Rocker, L., K.A. Kirsch, U. Mund, and H. Stoboy. The role of plasma proteins in the control of plasma volume during exercise and dehydration in long distance runners and cyclists. In: Howard, H., and J.R. Poortmans, eds. *Metabolic adaptation to prolonged physical exercise*. Basel: Birkhauser, 1975, p. 238-244.

224. Ropert, J.F., M.E. Quigley, and S.S.C. Yen. Endogenous opiates modulate pulsatile LH release in humans. *J. Clin. Endocrinol. Metab.* 52: 583-585, 1981.

225. Rossier, J., E.D. French, C. Rivier, N. Ling, R. Guillemia, and F.E. Bloom. Foot shock induced stress increases B-endorphin levels in blood but not the brain. *Nature* 270: 618-620, 1977.

226. Roth, J., and C. Grunfeld. Endocrine systems: Mechanisms of disease, target cells and receptors. In: Williams, R.H., ed. *Textbook of endocrinology*. Philadelphia: W.B. Saunders Co., 1981, p. 34-35.

227. Roth, J., S.M. Glick, R.S. Yalow, and S.A. Berson. Secretion of human growth hormone: Physiological and experimental modification. *Metabolism* 12: 557-559, 1963.

228. Roth, K.A., E. Weber, J.D. Barchas, D. Chang, and J.-K. Chang. Immunoreactive dynorphin-(1-8) and corticotropin-releasing factor in subpopulation of hypothalamic neurons. *Science* 219: 189-191, 1983.

229. Rowell, L.B., G.L. Brengelmann, and P.R. Freund. Unaltered norepinephrine-heart rate relationship in exercise with exogenous heat. *J. Appl. Physiol.* 62: 646-650, 1987.

230. Roy, M.W., K.C. Lee, M.S. Jones, and R.E. Miller. Neural control of pancreatic insulin and somatostatin secretion. *Endocrinology* 115: 770-775, 1984.

231. Russell, J.B., D. Mitchell, P.I. Musey, and D.C. Collins. The relationship of exercise to anovulatory cycles in female athletes: Hor-

monal and physical characteristics. *Obstet. Gynecol.* 63: 452-456, 1984.

232. Santen, B.J., and C.W. Bardin. Episodic luteinizing hormone secretion in man: Pulse analysis, clinical interpretation, physiological mechanisms. *J. Clin. Invest.* 52: 2617-2628, 1973.

233. Santen, R.J., J. Sofsky, N. Bilic, and R. Lippert. Mechanism of action of narcotics in the production of menstrual dysfunction in women. *Fertil. Steril.* 26: 538-548, 1975.

234. Santoro, N., M. Filicori, and W.F. Crowley. Hypogonadotropin disorders in men and women: Diagnosis and therapy with pulsatile gonadotropin-releasing hormone. *Endocr. Rev.* 7: 11-22, 1986.

235. Sato, Y., A. Iguchi, and N. Sakamoto. Biochemical determination of training effects using insulin clamp technique. *Horm. Metab. Res.* 16: 483-486, 1984.

236. Scatchard, G., A. Batchelder, and A. Brown. Chemical, clinical, and immunological studies on the products of human plasma fractionation. VI. The osmotic pressure of plasma and of serum albumin. *J. Clin. Invest.* 23: 458-464, 1944.

237. Schalch, D.S. The influence of physical stress and exercise on growth hormone and insulin secretion in man. *J. Lab. Clin. Med.* 69: 256-269, 1967.

238. Schwartz, B., D.C. Cumming, E. Riordan, M. Selye, S.C. Yen, and R.W. Rebar. Exercise associated amenorrhea: A distinct entity? *Am. J. Obstet. Gynecol.* 141: 662-670, 1981.

239. Sforzo, G.A., T.F. Seeger, C.B. Pert, A. Pert, and C.O. Dotson. In vivo opioid receptor occupation in the rat brain following exercise. *Med. Sci. Sports Exerc.* 18: 380-384, 1986.

240. Shangold, M., R. Freeman, B. Thysen, and M. Gatz. The relationship between long-distance running, plasma progesterone and luteal phase length. *Fertil. Steril.* 31: 130-133, 1979.

241. Shangold, M.M., M.L. Gatz, and B. Thysen. Acute effects of exercise on plasma concentrations of prolactin and testosterone in recreational women runners. *Fertil. Steril.* 35: 699-702, 1981.

242. Shephard, R.J., and K.H. Sidney. Effects of physical exercise on plasma growth hormone and cortisol levels in human subjects. *Exerc. Sport Sci. Rev.* 3: 1-30, 1975.

243. Sidney, K.H., and R.J. Shephard. Growth hormone and cortisol age differences, effects of exercise and training. *Can. J. Appl. Sports Sci.* 2: 189-193, 1977.

244. Sjostrand, T. The total quantity of hemoglobin in man and its relation to age, sex, body weight, and height. *Acta Physiol. Scand.* 18: 324-336, 1949.

245. Smythe, G.A., and L. Lazarus. Suppression of human growth hormone secretion by melatonin and cyproheptadine. *J. Clin. Invest.* 54: 116-121, 1974.

246. Soman, V.R., V.A. Koivisto, P. Grantham, and P. Felig. Increased insulin binding to monocytes after acute exercise in normal man. *J. Clin. Endocrinol. Metab.* 47: 216-219, 1978.

247. Sonne, B., and H. Galbo. Carbohydrate metabolism during and after exercise in rats: Studies with radioglucose. *J. Appl. Physiol.* 59: 1627-1639, 1985.

248. Sonne, B., and H. Galbo. Carbohydrate metabolism in fructose-fed and food-restricted running rats. *J. Appl. Physiol.* 61: 1457-1466, 1986.

249. Speroff, L., and D.B. Redwine. Exercise and menstrual function. *Phys. Sportsmed.* 8: 42-50, 1980.

250. Spiler, I.J., and M.E. Molitch. Lack of modulation of pituitary hormone stress response by neural pathways involving opiate receptors. *J. Clin. Endocrinol. Metab.* 50: 516-520, 1980.

251. Staessen, J., R. Fiocchi, R. Bouillon, R. Fagard, P. Lijnen, E. Moermon, A. DeSchaepdryver, and A. Armery. The nature of opioid involvement in the hemodynamic respiratory and humoral responses to exercise. *Circulation* 72: 982-990, 1985.

252. Starling, E. On the absorption of fluids from the connective tissue spaces. *J. Physiol.* 19: 312-328, 1986.

253. Sternlicht, E., R.J. Barnard, and G.K. Grimditch. Exercise and insulin stimulate skeletal muscle glucose transport through different mechanisms. *Am. J. Physiol.* 256: E227-E230, 1989.

254. Stuart, M.C., and L. Lazarus. Somatomedins. *Med. J. Aust.* 1: 816-820, 1975.

255. Stuart, M., L. Lazarus, and J. Sutton. Somatomedin: Changes following physiological and pharmacological stimuli to growth hormone secretion. *Proc. Endocrinol. Soc. Aust.* 15: 21, 1972.

256. Stubbs, W.A., A. Jones, C.R.W. Edwards, G. Delitala, W.J. Jeffcoate, S.J. Ratter, G.M. Besser, S.R. Bloom, and K.G.M.M. Alberti. Hormonal and metabolic responses to an enkephalin analogue in normal man. *Lancet* ii: 1225-1227, 1978.

257. Sutton, J.R. The effect of acute hypoxia on the hormonal response to exercise. *J. Appl. Physiol.* 42: 587-592, 1977.

258. Sutton, J.R. Hormonal and metabolic responses to exercise in subjects of high and low work capacities. *Med. Sci. Sports* 10: 1-6, 1978.

259. Sutton, J.R. Drugs used in metabolic disorders. *Med. Sci. Sports Exerc.* 13: 266-271, 1981.

260. Sutton, J.R. Metabolic responses to exercise in normal and diabetic individuals. In: Strauss, R.H., ed. *Sports medicine.* Philadelphia: W.B. Saunders, 1984, p. 190-204.

261. Sutton, J.R. Endorphins and the hypothalamic-pituitary-adrenal axis during exercise. In: Hales, J.R.S., and D.A.B. Richards, eds. *Heat stress.* Amsterdam: Elsevier, 1987, p. 179-192.

262. Sutton, J.R., and J.H. Casey. The adrenocortical response to competitive athletics in veteran athletes. *J. Clin. Endocrinol. Metab.* 40: 135-138, 1975.

263. Sutton, J.R., and M.P. Heyes. Endocrine responses to exercise at altitude. In: Fotherby, K., and S.B. Pal, eds. *Exercise endocrinology.* Berlin: de Gruyter, 1984, p. 239-262.

264. Sutton, J., and L. Lazarus. Effect of adrenergic blocking agents on growth hormone responses to physical exercise. *Horm. Metab. Res.* 6: 428-429, 1974.

265. Sutton, J., and L. Lazarus. Growth hormone in exercise: A comparison of physiological and pharmacological stimuli. *J. Appl. Physiol.* 41: 523-527, 1976.

266. Sutton, J.R., G.M. Brown, P. Keane, W.H.C. Walker, N.L. Jones, D. Rosenbloom, and G.M. Besser. The role of endorphins in the hormonal and psychological responses to exercise. *Int. J. Sports Med.* 3(2): 19, 1982.

267. Sutton, J.R., M.J. Coleman, and J.H. Casey. Adrenocortical contribution to serum androgens during physical exercise. *Med. Sci. Sports* 6: 72, 1974.

268. Sutton, J.R., M.J. Coleman, and J.H. Casey. Testosterone production rate during exercise. In: Landry, F., and W.A.R. Orban, eds. *3rd International symposium on biochemistry of exercise.* Miami: Symposia Specialists Inc., 1978, p. 227-234.

269. Sutton, J.R., M.J. Coleman, J. Casey, and L. Lazarus. Androgen responses during physical exercise. *Br. Med. J.* 1: 520-522, 1973.

270. Sutton, J.R., M.J. Coleman, A.P. Millar, L. Lazarus, and P. Russo. The medical problems of mass participation in athletic competition. The "City-to-Surf" race. *Med. J. Aust.* 2: 127-133, 1972.

271. Sutton, J.R., H.J. Green, P. Young, P. Rock, A. Cymerman, and C.S. Houston. Plasma vasopressin, catecholamines and lactate during exhaustive exercise at extreme simulated altitude: "Operation Everest II". *Can. J. Appl. Sports Sci.* 11: 43P, 1986.

272. Sutton, J.R., N.L. Jones, and C.J. Toews. Growth hormone secretion in acid-base alterations at rest and during exercise. *Clin. Sci. Mol. Med.* 50: 241-247, 1976.

273. Sutton, J.R., J.E. Jurkowski, P. Keane, W.H.C. Walker, N.L. Jones, and C.J. Toews. Plasma catecholamine, insulin, glucose and lactate responses to exercise in relation to the menstrual cycle. *Med. Sci. Sports* 12: 83-84, 1980.

274. Sutton, J.R., J.T. Reeves, P.D. Wagner, B.M. Groves, A. Cymerman, M.K. Malconian, P.B. Rock, P.M. Young, S.D. Walter, and C.S. Houston. Operation Everest II: Oxygen transport during exercise at extreme simulated altitude. *J. Appl. Physiol.* 64: 1309-1321, 1988.

275. Sutton, J.R., J.D. Young, L. Lazarus, J.B. Hickie, and J. Maksvytis. The hormonal response to physical exercise. *Aust. Ann. Med.* 18: 84-90, 1969.

276. Takahashi, Y., D.M. Kipnis, and W.H. Daughaday. Growth hormone secretion during sleep. *J. Clin. Invest.* 23: 2079-2090, 1968.

277. Tanaka, H., M. Shindo, J. Gutkowska, A. Kinoshita, H. Urata, M. Ikeda, and K. Arakawa. Effect of acute exercise on plasma immunoreactive-atrial natriuretic factor. *Life Sci.* 39: 1685-1693, 1986.

278. Tarnopolsky, L., M. Tarnopolsky, J.D. MacDougall, S. Atkinson, and J.R. Sutton. Differences in the hormonal and metabolic responses to prolonged exercise in males and females. *J. Appl. Physiol.* (in press).

279. Taylor, R., S.J. Proctor, O. James, F. Clark, and K.G.M.M. Alberti. The relationship between human adipocyte and monocyte insulin binding. *Clin. Sci.* 67: 139-142, 1984.

280. Terjung, R. Endocrine responses to exercise. In: Hutton, R., and D. Miller, eds. *Exercise and sports sciences reviews.* Philadelphia: Franklin Institute Press, 1979, p. 153-180, vol. 7.

281. Thamsborg, G., T. Storm, N. Keller, R. Sykulski, and J. Larsen. Changes in plasma atrial natriuretic peptide during exercise in healthy volunteers. *Acta Med. Scand.* 221: 441-444, 1987.

282. Thamsborg, G., R. Sykulski, J. Larsen, T. Storm, and N. Keller. Effect of beta-1-adrenoreceptor blockade on plasma levels of atrial natriuretic peptide during exercise in normal man. *Clin. Physiol.* 7: 313-318, 1987.

283. Treadway, J.L., D.E. James, E. Burcel, and N.B. Ruderman. Effect of exercise on insulin receptor binding and kinase activity in skeletal muscle. *Am. J. Physiol.* 255: E138-E144, 1989.

284. Van Beaumont, W., J.E. Greenleaf, and L. Juhos. Disproportional changes in hematocrit, plasma volume and proteins during exercise and bed rest. *J. Appl. Physiol.* 33: 55-61, 1972.

285. Veldhuis, J.D., W.S. Evans, L.M. Demers, M.O. Thorner, D. Wakat, and A.D. Rogol. Altered neuroendocrine regulation of gonadotropin secretion in women distance runners. *J. Clin. Endocrinol. Metab.* 61: 557-563, 1985.

286. Vendsalu, A. Studies on adrenaline and noradrenaline in human plasma. *Acta Physiol. Scand.* 49 (Suppl. 173): 1-123, 1960.

287. Victor, R.G., D.R. Seals, and A.L. Mark. Differential control of heart rate and sympathetic nerve activity during dynamic exercise. *J. Clin. Invest.* 79: 508-516, 1987.

288. Villanueva, A.L., C. Schlosser, B. Hopper, J.H. Liu, D.I. Hoffman, and R.W. Rebar. Increased cortisol production in women runners. *J. Clin. Endocrinol. Metab.* 63: 133-136, 1986.

289. Viru, A. Dynamics of blood corticoid content during and after short term exercise. *Endocrinology* 59: 61-68, 1972.

290. Viru, A. *Hormones in muscular activity: Hormonal ensemble in exercise.* Boca Raton, FL: CRC Press, 1985, vol. 1.

291. Viru, A. *Hormones in muscular activity: Adaptive effect of hormones in exercise.* Boca Raton, FL: CRC Press, 1985, vol. 2.

292. Von Euler, U.S., and S. Heller. Noradrenaline excretion in muscular work. *Acta Physiol. Scand.* 26: 183-191, 1952.

293. Vranic, M., and M. Berger. Exercise and diabetes mellitus. *Diabetes* 28: 147-163, 1979.

294. Vranic, M., and R. Kawamori. Essential roles of insulin and glucagon in regulating glucose fluxes during exercise in dogs. *Diabetes* 28 (Suppl. 1): 45-52, 1979.

295. Vranic, M., and G.A. Wrenshall. Exercise, insulin and glucose turnover in dogs. *Endocrinology* 85: 165-171, 1969.

296. Wade, C.E., and J.R. Claybaugh. Plasma renin activity, vasopressin concentration, and urinary excretory responses to exercise in men. *J. Appl. Physiol.* 49: 930-936, 1980.

297. Wade, C.E., B.J. Freund, and J.R. Claybaugh. Fluid and electrolyte homeostasis during and following exercise: Hormonal and nonhormonal factors. In: Claybaugh, J.R., and C.E. Wade, eds. *Hormonal regulation of fluids and electrolytes: Environmental effects.* New York: Plenum Publishing Co., 1989, p. 1-46.

298. Wahren, J. Glucose turnover during exercise in healthy man and in patients with diabetes mellitus. *Diabetes* 28 (Suppl. 1): 82-88, 1979.

299. Wahren, J., P. Felig, G. Ahlborg, and L. Torfeldt. Glucose metabolism during leg exercise in man. *J. Clin. Invest.* 50: 2715-2725, 1971.

300. Wallberg-Henriksson, H., and J.O. Holloszy. Contractile activity increases glucose uptake. *J. Appl. Physiol.* 57: 1045-1049, 1984.

301. Ward, G.R., J.R. Sutton, N.L. Jones, and C.J. Toews. Activation by exercise of human skeletal muscle pyruvate dehydrogenase in vivo. *Clin. Sci.* 63: 87-92, 1982.

302. Ward, M.M., I.N. Mefford, G.W. Black, and W.M. Bortz. Exercise and plasma catecholamine release. In: Fotherby, K., and S.B. Pal, eds. *Exercise endocrinology.* Berlin: de Gruyter & Co., 1985, p. 263-294.

303. Warren, M.P. The effects of exercise on pubertal progression and reproductive function in girls. *J. Clin. Endocrinol. Metab.* 51: 1150-1157, 1980.

304. Warren, M.P., J. Brooks-Gunn, L.H. Hamilton, L.F. Warren, and W.G. Hamilton. Scoliosis and fractures in young ballet dancers. *N. Engl. J. Med.* 314: 1348-1353, 1986.

305. Wasserman, D.H., H.L. Lickley, and M. Vranic. Interactions between glucagon and other counterregulatory hormones during normoglycemic and hypoglycemic exercise in dogs. *J. Clin. Invest.* 74: 1404-1413, 1984.

306. Wasserman, D.H., J.A. Spalding, D. Bracy, D. Brookslacy, and A.D. Cherrington. Exercise-induced rise in glucagon and ketogenesis during prolonged muscular work. *Diabetes* 38: 799-807, 1989.

307. Webster, B.A., S.R. Vigna, and T. Paquette. Acute exercise, epinephrine, and diabetes enhance insulin binding to skeletal muscle. *Am. J. Physiol.* 250: E186-E197, 1986.

308. Wehrenberg, W.B., S.L. Wardlaw, A.G. Frantz, and M. Ferin. Beta-endorphin in

hyophyseal portal blood: Variations throughout the menstrual cycle. *Endocrinology* 111: 879-881, 1982.

309. Wheeler, G.D., S.R. Wall, A.N. Belcastro, and D.C. Cumming. Reduced serum testosterone and prolactin levels in male distance runners. *J. Am. Med. Assoc.* 252: 514-516, 1984.

310. Wildt, L., S. Niesert, G. Wesner, and G. Layendecker. Effects of naloxone on LH, FSH and prolactin secretion in hypothalamic amenorrhea. *Acta Endocrinol.* 97 (Suppl. 243): 52, 1981.

311. Wilkerson, J.E., B. Gutin, and S.M. Horvath. Exercise-induced changes in blood, red cell and plasma volumes in man. *Med. Sci. Sports* 9: 155-158, 1977.

312. Williams, E.S., M.P. Ward, J.S. Milledge, W.R. Withey, M.W. Older, and M.L. Forsling. Effect of the exercise of seven consecutive days hill-walking on fluid homeostasis. *Clin. Sci.* 56: 305-316, 1979.

313. Winder, W.W., R.C. Hickson, J.M. Hagberg, A.A. Ehsani, and J.A. McLane. Training-induced changes in hormonal and metabolic responses to submaximal exercise. *J. Appl. Physiol.* 46: 766-771, 1979.

314. Winder, W.W., M.L. Terry, and V.M. Mitchell. Role of plasma epinephrine in fasted exercising rats. *Am. J. Physiol.* 248: R302-R307, 1985.

315. Wirth, A., C. Diehm, H. Mayer, H. Morl, I. Vogel, P. Björntorp, and G. Schlierf. Plasma C-peptide and insulin in trained and untrained subjects. *J. Appl. Physiol.* 50: 71-77, 1981.

316. Wolfe, R.R., E.R. Nadel, J.H.F. Shaw, L.A. Stephenson, and M.H. Wolfe. Role of changes in insulin and glucagon in glucose homeostasis in exercise. *J. Clin. Invest.* 77: 900-907, 1986.

317. Wright, P.H., and W.J. Malaisse. Effect of epinephrine, stress and exercise on insulin secretion in the rat. *Am. J. Physiol.* 214: 1031-1034, 1968.

318. Yahiro, J., A.R. Glass, W.B. Fears, E.W. Ferguson, and R.A. Vigersky. Exaggerated gonadotropin response to LHRH in amenorrheic runners. *Am. J. Obstet. Gynecol.* 156: 586-591, 1987.

319. Yalow, R.S., and S.A. Berson. Immunoassay of endogenous plasma insulin in man. *J. Clin. Invest.* 39: 1157-1175, 1960.

320. Young, D.R., R. Pelligra, and R.R. Adachi. Serum glucose and free fatty acids in man during prolonged exercise. *J. Appl. Physiol.* 21: 1047-1052, 1966.

321. Zinman, B., M. Vranic, A.M. Albisser, B.S. Leibel, and E.B. Marliss. The role of insulin in the metabolic response to exercise in diabetic man. *Diabetes* 28 (Suppl. 1): 76-81, 1979.

Chapter 21

Discussion: Hormonal Adaptation to Physical Activity

Henrik Galbo
Michael Kjaer
Kari J. Mikines
Flemming Dela

Niels H. Secher
Bente Stallknecht
Henrik P. Hansen

This chapter focuses on the two most prominent avenues of current research in exercise endocrinology. We describe recent findings concerning (a) the regulation of the hormonal response to acute exercise and (b) adaptations of endocrine glands to training. The wisdom characterizing the hormonal adaptation to physical activity will be readily apparent.

Accumulating evidence suggests that during exercise the control of the autonomic neuroendocrine system is exerted along the same lines as the control of circulation and respiration (2, 3, 4, 13). Feedforward as well as feedback mechanisms are involved in the regulation. We think that, from the onset of exercise, impulses from motor centers radiate within the brain as well as through afferent nerves from recruited muscles to higher endocrine centers and elicit a work-load-dependent autonomic neuroendocrine response. The need for endocrine adjustments to enhance substrate mobilization is, so to speak, anticipated (Figure 21.1). This primary setting depends on the state of the organism (e.g., as regards physical training), the hormonal response being more closely related to work load expressed in relative terms (% $\dot{V}O_2$max) than to work load expressed in absolute terms (7).

In humans the most direct evidence in favor of immediate activation of endocrine centers from motor centers (central command) has come from studies involving partial neuromuscular blockade with tubocurarine (6, 12). Tubocurarine weakens the muscles and probably makes a higher motor-center activity necessary to elicit a given absolute work intensity. In agreement with this, compared at the same absolute work load, subjects in experi-

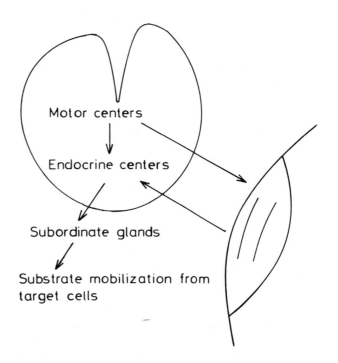

Figure 21.1. Tentative scheme for the primary control of hormonal responses to exercise. Nervous impulses from motor centers and recruited muscles modulate the activity in autonomic neuroendocrine centers in the brain.

ments with blockade had a higher perceived exertion than did those in experiments without blockade. The higher motor-center activity during curarization was accompanied by exaggerated responses of catecholamines as well as pituitary hormones to exercise, indicating that motor center activity stimulates endocrine changes rather directly (Figure 21.2). The exaggerated hormonal

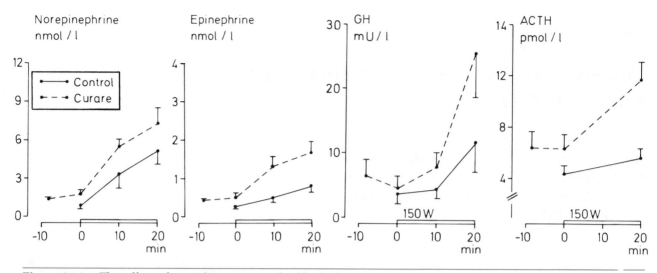

Figure 21.2. The effect of partial neuromuscular blockade on hormone concentrations in plasma measured at rest and during semisupine bicycle exercise in 7 subjects; GH means growth hormone and ACTH adrenocorticotropin. Values are means ±*SE*. Curare was administered after the -10-min sample had been drawn. Exercise responses differed significantly between the two experiments. Adapted from Kjaer et al. (12).

changes in tubocurarine compared to control experiments were accompanied by a more rapid increase in hepatic glucose production and enhanced lipolysis during exercise (12).

The interpretation of these findings in humans has been recently supported by neurophysiological studies on animals. It was shown in decorticated and paralyzed cats, as well as in those that were anesthetized, that electrical stimulation of the subthalamic locomotor region increases catecholamine secretion and glucose production (18). As motor center stimulation was not accompanied by muscle contraction, the increase in sympathoadrenal activity was not elicited by impulses in afferent nerves from muscle. However, the fact that activity in afferent nerves from working muscle participates in the regulation of the hormonal changes in exercise appears from the finding that adrenocorticotropin (ACTH) and beta-endorphin responses to submaximal bicycle exercise are abolished by epidural anesthesia of thin afferent nerve fibers from the lower body (Figure 21.3).

During continued exercise the hormonal changes may be gradually intensified due to feedback from metabolic as well as nonmetabolic error signals, the latter sensed by pressure, volume, osmolality, and temperature receptors. In humans the most important metabolic error signal is a decrease in glucose availability. The existence of the glucose feedback mechanism has most clearly been shown in experiments with different diets (5) (Figure 21.4). After intake during 4 d of a diet rich in fat, the plasma glucose concentration declined more rapidly dur-

ing prolonged running than it did after intake of a diet rich in carbohydrate. A close correlation was seen between decrease in plasma glucose and increase in epinephrine and glucagon levels, the hormonal responses to exercise being enhanced in fat compared to carbohydrate experiments. Furthermore, when late during exercise in both experiments plasma glucose concentrations were restored to preexercise levels by glucose infusion, concentrations of epinephrine and glucagon decreased markedly (Figure 21.4). When we consider the fact that a decrease in plasma glucose reflects a need for substrate supply to the working muscles and that the hormonal changes elicited by this decrease can meet the substrate demand, the depicted feedback mechanism is very appropriate.

As an illustration of the profound influence that physical training has on the body, regularly repeated exercise may change the secretory capacity of endocrine glands. Thus, recent studies indicate that prolonged endurance training increases the adrenal medullary secretory capacity and causes what might be called a sports adrenal medulla. The evidence is that—in response to similar degrees of insulin-induced hypoglycemia (11) as well as to stimulation with hypoxia, hypercapnia, glucagon (10), or caffeine (14)—athletes have higher increases in plasma epinephrine concentrations than do untrained subjects (Table 21.1). This is also the case in response to identical relative sub- and supramaximal work loads, at which similar norepinephrine levels and heart rates in trained compared to untrained subjects indicate similar

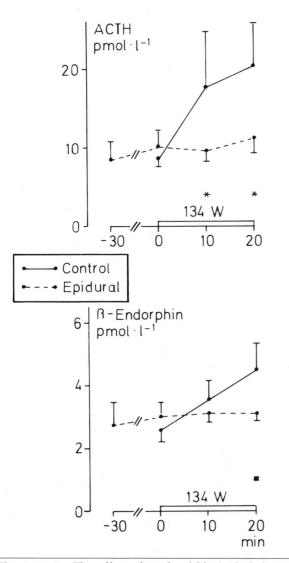

ing to note that the capacity to secrete epinephrine normally diminishes with aging. So, training causes biological rejuvenation of the adrenal medullary secretory capacity as it is the case regarding, for example, the capacities of heart and skeletal muscle.

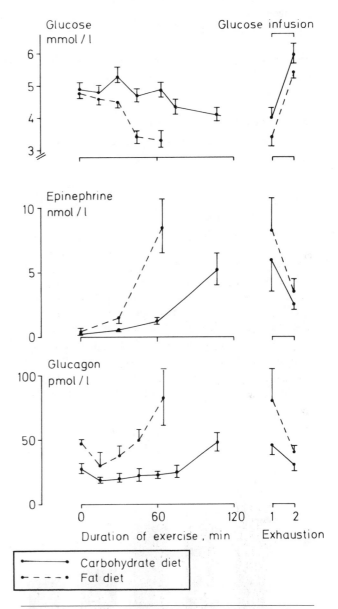

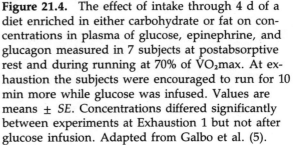

Figure 21.3. The effect of epidural blockade below Th 11-12 on plasma concentrations of ACTH and beta-endorphin measured at rest and during bicycle exercise in 6 subjects. Epidural anesthesia was administered immediately after the -30-min sample had been drawn. Values are means ± *SE*. Asterisks denote difference (*p* < 0.05) between epidural and control experiments. Square denotes time at which the beta-endorphin value in control experiment differed (*p* < 0.05) from the basal level.

Figure 21.4. The effect of intake through 4 d of a diet enriched in either carbohydrate or fat on concentrations in plasma of glucose, epinephrine, and glucagon measured in 7 subjects at postabsorptive rest and during running at 70% of VO₂max. At exhaustion the subjects were encouraged to run for 10 min more while glucose was infused. Values are means ± *SE*. Concentrations differed significantly between experiments at Exhaustion 1 but not after glucose infusion. Adapted from Galbo et al. (5).

sympathetic nervous activity (including similar input to the adrenal medulla) in the two groups (8, 9). Finally, in rats, physical training has been shown to increase the epinephrine content in the adrenal gland as well as the size of the adrenal medulla (19). When we take into account the various effects of epinephrine, it is clear that a high capacity to secrete epinephrine represents an advantage in competitive sports. It is also interest-

Table 21.1   Epinephrine Responses (nmol · L⁻¹) to Various Nonexercise Stimuli in Athletes and Sedentary Subjects

Stimulus	Untrained	Trained
Insulin-induced hypoglycemia (plasma glucose: 1.9 mmol · L⁻¹)	3.88 ± 0.40	5.78 ± 0.99*
Hypoxia (P_IO_2 = 89 mmHg for 20 min)	0 ± 0.10	0.22 ± 0.05*
Hypercapnia (F_ICO_2 = 7% for 15 min)	0.22 ± 0.05	0.38 ± 0.05*
Glucagon bolus IV (1 mg/70 kg BW)	0.38 ± 0.10	0.87 ± 0.10*
Caffeine[a] (4 mg orally/kg BW)	0.17	0.28

Note. Values are mean ± *SE* of six to eight individual differences between the catecholamine concentration in plasma after a given period of stimulation and the basal concentration. Data are from Kjaer et al. (11), Kjaer and Galbo (10), and LeBlanc et al. (14).

[a]In LeBlanc's study (14), a significant difference was found in epinephrine response integrated over a 120-min period between trained and untrained subjects.

*Significant difference in response between the two groups ($p < 0.05$).

In humans a single bout of exercise does not influence the secretory capacity of the pancreatic beta cell (16). However, studies with arginine infusion (1) as well as with the hyperglycemic clamp technique (15) have shown that the capacity to secrete insulin is lower in athletes than it is in untrained subjects. This difference is diminished, but not abolished, when athletes abstain from training for 5 d (15). Similarly, in untrained subjects 7 d of bed rest increases glucose-induced insulin secretion (15). These findings indicate that regular physical activity changes the responsiveness of the beta-cell secretion in a diabetic direction. At first this adaptation does not appear expedient. However, the average level of daily physical activity also influences the responsiveness of target tissues. Thus, the effect of insulin on glucose uptake from plasma is increased by training and reduced by inactivity (17). Accordingly, an inverse relationship exists over a wide range of daily activity levels between the beta-cell response to glucose and the effect of insulin (Figure 21.5). In other words, in trained subjects, diminished capacity to secrete insulin is justified by a lower need for insulin to handle a certain carbohydrate load. Rather than reflecting development of diabetes, the training-induced pancreatic adaptation implicates less stress on the beta cells and in turn a reduced risk

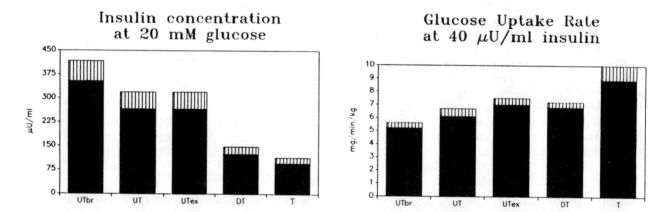

Figure 21.5. The effect of preceding level of physical activity on pancreatic beta-cell function (upper panel) and tissue sensitivity to insulin (lower panel). Hyperglycemic and euglycemic clamps respectively were applied. Insulin and glucose concentrations were measured in plasma, and glucose uptake rate is the amount of glucose infused to maintain euglycemia. Black bars represent mean values of 6-7 subjects, open bars represent *SE*, and UT means sedentary subjects. These were studied with (UTex) and without (UT) 1 h of prior exercise at 60% VO₂max as well as after 7 d of bed rest (UTbr); T means endurance-trained subjects studied 15 h after last exercise bout. The trained subjects were also studied after 5 d of detraining (DT). Adapted from Mikines et al. (15, 16, 17).

of diabetes. Future studies are needed to elucidate further the influence of training on endocrine glands in both healthy and diseased individuals and to unravel the mechanisms responsible for the development of adaptations to training within the endocrine system.

Acknowledgments

This study was supported by grants from the Danish Medical Research Council (12-7797), the Danish Sports Research Councils, the Chr. X Foundation, NOVO's Foundation, the Ib Henriksen Foundation, the Danish Heart Association, the Nordic Insulin Foundation, and the P. Carl Petersen Foundation.

References

1. Dela, F., K.J. Mikines, and H. Galbo. Arginine stimulated insulin response in trained and untrained man. *Diabetologia* 30: 513A, 1987.
2. Galbo, H. Autonomic neuroendocrine responses to exercise. *Scand. J. Sports Sci.* 8: 3-17, 1986.
3. Galbo, H. *Hormonal and metabolic adaptation to exercise.* New York: Georg Thieme, 1983.
4. Galbo, H. The hormonal response to exercise. *Proc. Nutr. Soc.* 44: 257-265, 1985.
5. Galbo, H., J.J. Holst, and N.J. Christensen. The effect of different diets and of insulin on the hormonal response to prolonged exercise. *Acta Physiol. Scand.* 107: 19-32, 1979.
6. Galbo, H., M. Kjaer, and N.H. Secher. Cardiovascular, ventilatory and catecholamine responses to maximal dynamic exercise in partially curarized man. *J. Physiol. (Lond.)* 389: 557-568, 1987.
7. Kjaer, M., J. Bangsbo, G. Lortie, and H. Galbo. Hormonal response to exercise in man: Influence of hypoxia and physical training. *Am. J. Physiol.* 254: R197-R203, 1988.
8. Kjaer, M., N.J. Christensen, B. Sonne, E.A. Richter, and H. Galbo. Effect of exercise on epinephrine turnover in trained and untrained subjects. *J. Appl. Physiol.* 59: 1061-1067, 1985.
9. Kjaer, M., P.A. Farrell, N.J. Christensen, and H. Galbo. Increased epinephrine response and inaccurate glucoregulation in exercising athletes. *J. Appl. Physiol.* 61: 1693-1700, 1986.
10. Kjaer, M., and H. Galbo. Effect of physical training on the capacity to secrete epinephrine. *J. Appl. Physiol.* 64: 11-16, 1988.
11. Kjaer, M., K.J. Mikines, N.J. Christensen, B. Tronier, J. Vinten, B. Sonne, E.A. Richter, and H. Galbo. Glucose turnover and hormonal changes during insulin-induced hypoglycemia in trained humans. *J. Appl. Physiol.* 57: 21-27, 1984.
12. Kjaer, M., N.H. Secher, F.W. Bach, and H. Galbo. Role of motor center activity for hormonal changes and substrate mobilization in humans. *Am. J. Physiol.* 253: R687-R695, 1987.
13. Kjaer, M., N.H. Secher, and H. Galbo. Physical stress and catecholamine release. *Baillières Clin. Endocrinol. Metab.* 1: 279-298, 1987.
14. LeBlanc, J., M. Jobin, J. Cote, P. Samson, and A. Labrie. Enhanced metabolic response to caffeine in exercise-trained human subjects. *J. Appl. Physiol.* 59: 832-837, 1985.
15. Mikines, K.J., F. Dela, B. Sonne, P.A. Farrell, E.A. Richter, and H. Galbo. Insulin action and secretion in man; effects of different levels of physical activity. *Can. J. Sport Sci.* 12(Suppl. 1): 113-116, 1987.
16. Mikines, K.J., P.A. Farrell, B. Sonne, B. Tronier, and H. Galbo. Postexercise dose-response relationship between plasma glucose and insulin secretion. *J. Appl. Physiol.* 64: 988-999, 1988.
17. Mikines, K.J., B. Sonne, P.A. Farrell, B. Tronier, and H. Galbo. Effect of physical exercise on sensitivity and responsiveness to insulin in man. *Am. J. Physiol.* 17: E248-E259, 1988.
18. Mitchell, J.H., J. Vissing, K.J. Rybicki, H. Galbo, and G.A. Iwamoto. Parallel activation of locomotion, metabolism and circulation from the hypothalamus. *FASEB J.* 2: A1325, 1988.
19. Stallknecht, B., M. Kjaer, T. Ploug, T. Ohkuwa, J. Vinten, and H. Galbo. Training-induced enlargement of the adrenal medulla in rats. *Acta Physiol. Scand.* 129: 50A, 1987.

Chapter 22

Adaptations of Skeletal Muscle to Physical Activity

John A. Faulkner
Timothy P. White

Human movement is characterized by individuality and diversity of expression in the arts, sports, occupational tasks, and recreational activities. The qualities that characterize the movement of a given individual arise from the properties of skeletal muscle fibers, the levers and joints through which fibers act, and the coordination of recruitment patterns of motor units in synergistic and antagonistic muscles (see chaps. 30 and 31). Specific properties of each of the approximately 660 skeletal muscles in the human body are inherited (see chaps. 13 and 14). This genetic inheritance sets unknown limits within which properties of skeletal muscle fibers are able to adapt to the habitual patterns of recruitment and loading (67, 83). Consequently, the beauty of a highly skilled movement reflects the contribution of both heredity and the adaptations that result from training.

Skeletal muscle adaptations are characterized by modifications of morphological, biochemical, and molecular variables that alter functional attributes of fibers in specific motor units. Adaptations range from a diminished capacity to generate or maintain power in response to reduced physical activity to an enhanced capacity to maintain power for long periods of time following endurance training or to develop a higher maximum power following strength training. Adaptations are readily reversible when the stimulus for adaptation is diminished or eliminated (21, 27, 54). Adaptive responses to changes in physical activity are qualitatively, and in many circumstances quantitatively, similar in skeletal muscles of humans, cats, and rodents. This review is restricted to adaptations of mammalian skeletal muscle that result from habitual patterns of physical inactivity and of physical activity. Adaptations due to other experimental interventions (35, 50, 79, 82) will be used

where these interventions provide a different perspective or insight into the mechanisms underlying adaptive responses.

Continuum of Physical Activity

Physical activity arises from the voluntary contractions of skeletal muscles. Muscle fiber contraction is defined as activation of the force-generating capacity of the actomyosin complex within fibers. Whether a fiber shortens (miometric contraction), remains at the same length (isometric contraction), or lengthens (pliometric contraction) depends on the external load applied relative to the force developed by the muscle. In nonactivated muscles, cross-bridges cycle between unbound and weakly bound states. With activation, cross-bridges execute cycles that include the states of being unbound or strongly bound or in the driving stroke (31). Only cross-bridges in the driving stroke will develop force during a shortening or isometric contraction, whereas cross-bridges in any bound state will contribute to the force that opposes the lengthening of a muscle. As a result, force during a lengthening contraction may be 1-1/2- to 2-fold greater than maximum isometric tetanic force (64).

During a single contraction, the product of the force and velocity at which muscle shortens or lengthens determines the power output or power absorption, respectively. A number of factors combine to influence the power developed by skeletal muscle fibers. Major factors include the frequency of stimulation (force); the number and size of motor units and therefore the number of cross-bridges per one-half sarcomere in parallel that are in the driving stroke (force); the length of fibers (velocity); the position of fiber length relative to the length-force relationship (force); and the myosin ATPase activity (velocity). Potential biochemical modulators of these functional determinants include the cytosolic concentrations of ATP, inorganic phosphate (31), and hydrogen ions (66). Attenuations in power will also occur due to the angles of fiber pinnation in relation to the overall longitudinal axis of the muscle and other architectural complexities (30).

The continuum of physical activity (Figure 22.1) ranges from the minimal activity associated with bed rest or immobilization to high levels of activity associated with the training regimens of world-class endurance and power performers. Volitional training occurs at the level of an intact organism, but specific adaptations can be identified in

CONTINUUM OF PHYSICAL ACTIVITY

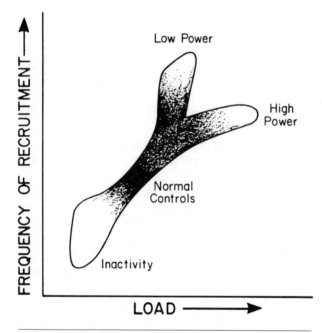

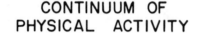

Figure 22.1. Physical activity is determined by the frequency of recruitment for contractions (ordinate) and the load on the muscle during the contraction (abscissa). Physical activity constitutes a continuum from the almost complete absence of activity through the nominal activity levels of sedentary subjects to high levels observed in physically active subjects. Toward the high end of the continuum, a dichotomy arises as endurance performers increase the frequency of recruitment cycles without increasing load significantly, whereas strength and power performers increase the load significantly without much of an increase in frequency.

skeletal muscle fibers. Determinant of the intensity of physical activity are the external load on a muscle or muscle group, the forces developed by the muscle or muscle group, and the duration and frequency of recruitment for contractions. These factors combine to provide average power and, when coupled with the total duration of the training session, lead to an estimate of total power. Additional variables include the frequency of the training sessions per week and the duration of the training sessions in months or years. The combination of these factors and variables characterizes a habitual level of physical activity and provides a potential for training stimuli of varying intensities. A training stimulus occurs when a change in the habitual level of physical activity is of sufficient magnitude and duration to produce a measurable adaptive response. Repetitive movements requiring peak power are limited by both fatigue and the possibility of injury (2). Thus, adaptive responses to peak power are difficult to evaluate.

Motor Unit Types and Muscle Power

Within skeletal muscles, fibers are organized functionally into motor units that consist of the cell body, the motor nerve and its branches, and the skeletal muscle fibers innervated by the branches (11, 12, 23). Burke et al. (12) classified the motor units in skeletal muscles of a cat as slow (S), fast fatigue resistant (FR), and fast fatigable (FF) on the basis of contraction time, a ''sag'' in the force record during unfused tetanus, and a fatigue test. Histochemical techniques for the classification of fibers in mammalian motor units are based on the activities of oxidative enzymes (75), differential sensitivity of myofibrillar ATPase activity to altered pH (7), or duration of exposure to acidic incubation (34). Markers of glycolytic capacity are ambiguous and have not been found to be particularly useful in fiber classification schemes (34, 75). Classification of fibers within motor units by the different histochemical techniques provides similar results, but the similarity is not sufficient to allow unambiguous interchange among the different classification schemes (34). For control limb muscles (11, 12, 23), a reasonable correlation has been established between the motor units classified by either of the two major histochemical techniques: Types I, IIa, and IIb (7), or slow (S), fast oxidative glycolytic (FOG), and fast glycolytic (FG) (75); and those classified by contractile properties

(S, FR, FF) (12). In each scheme of fiber classification, the primary determinants of the classification (i.e., the myosin isoform and the oxidative enzymes) constitute a continuum (34, 91). Therefore, classification of fibers into discrete types on the basis of a qualitative determination of low and high activity for these two characteristics is of limited value.

Adaptations to Physical Activity

Maximum power can increase with no adaptive changes in morphological or biochemical properties of skeletal muscles. This type of neurophysiological adaptation is observed as a large improvement in strength and power during the early stages of a strength-training program that presumably reflects neural optimization of motor unit recruitment (80). Most adaptations that occur beyond the early training sessions are characterized by measurable morphological, biochemical, and molecular changes that influence directly the contractile and metabolic properties of skeletal muscle fibers. These adaptations may be either in the muscle group directly involved in the movement, in antagonistic muscles, or in fixator muscles that provide the force platform for the movement. Later improvements in a highly coordinated task may reflect optimization of motor unit recruitment between and among these different muscle groups.

The criterion for an adaptive response is a qualitative or quantitative alteration in one or more specific muscle proteins: contractile, regulatory, structural, or metabolic. Adaptations can occur in response to a specific training stimulus, and the adaptive response is regulated at multiple sites, each of which is controlled by negative feedback (Figure 22.2). Fibers within a motor unit are relatively homogeneous as to the concentrations and

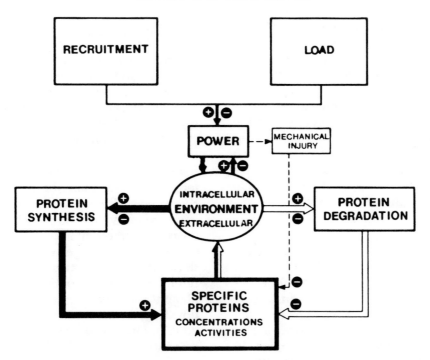

MOTOR UNIT ADAPTATION

Figure 22.2. During a training session the total power developed by a motor unit results from the frequency of recruitment for contraction of the fibers in motor units and the load against which the fibers contract. If the fibers shorten, power will be developed (+), and if the fibers are lengthened, power will be absorbed (−). Presumably, reduced power, sustained power, or high power results in acute changes in the cellular environment that then lead to altered rates of protein synthesis and degradation, leading to changes in the concentrations or activities of specific proteins and thus chronically, but not permanently, alter the cellular environment. These adaptations may increase or decrease the capability of fibers in a motor unit to develop and maintain power. The adaptive responses to some physical activities are known, but the receptors, integrating centers, and effectors involved have not been fully identified. Under certain circumstances muscle fibers are injured during contractions, and the concentration of myofibrillar proteins is decreased directly.

activities of metabolic, regulatory, and contractile proteins. As a consequence, the contractile properties of fibers within a motor unit are similar (23, 71, 76, 91). Conversely, the concentrations and activities of proteins in fibers of different motor units and the resultant contractile properties may show as much as a threefold difference (44).

The high degree of adaptive specificity results from unique modifications of morphological, biochemical, and molecular properties of skeletal muscle fibers by specific training stimuli. Fibers within motor units recruited during training will be primarily affected by the training stimulus. Furthermore, within the recruited fibers, only the organelles, enzymes, and molecules that are stimulated beyond a threshold for adaptation will undergo significant changes. The assumption is that the properties of fibers within a motor unit that adapt to a training stimulus do so in unison. Adaptations of muscle fibers appear to be mediated predominantly by the frequency and duration of stimulation and by the external load (23), with trophic factors playing at most a minor role. The enhancement of muscle growth in vitro by soluble growth factors has been documented (87, 94), but the role of growth factors in vivo has not been determined. The specificity of adaptations may result in improved performance in one physical activity with no change or even impairment in another activity (49, 65). The degree to which improved performance transfers from one physical activity to another depends on the amount of overlap in the physiological requirements of the two activities. Sufficient data are available to describe the adaptive responses to reduced activity and to endurance or strength-training activities.

Adaptations to Reduced Physical Activity

A reduction of physical activity by limb immobilization in humans leads to a decrease in muscle fiber area (57) and in the metabolic proteins that support endurance performance (59). These changes in fiber area and composition result in muscle atrophy and weakness, but little or no correlation exists between the magnitude of the atrophy and the decrease in strength (57). In rats, decreases in mass and force output of plantarflexor muscles of the foot are observed when the loading of skeletal muscles is decreased by limb casting (69, 96) or hind-limb suspension (28). Casting leads to a significant decrease in actin synthesis that likely is mediated by a change in the translation of a-actin-specific mRNA (96). Lack of weight bearing

does not affect fast myosin heavy chain significantly, but the expression of slow myosin heavy chain is depressed (92, 93). During hind-limb suspension, the EMG activity is reduced initially in plantarflexor muscles but returns to control values after 7 d (1). Conversely, the EMG activity of the dorsiflexor tibialis anterior muscle remains increased throughout the period of hind-limb suspension, yet the mass and contractile properties of this muscle are unaffected (1). Unlike the unloaded plantarflexor muscles, the dorsiflexor muscles are loaded by the mass of the foot during hind-limb suspension. These experiments emphasize the significant role of the interaction between the external load and the force of the muscle contraction in the adaptive response. Following a period of endurance training or strength training, a decrease in the habitual level of activity results in a reversal of the adaptations produced by the training (21, 27, 32, 54). The maintenance of muscle adaptations requires a sustained increase or decrease in physical activity (21, 27).

Adaptations to Endurance Activities

The primary adaptations to endurance training are metabolic and cardiovascular changes, leading to an enhanced ability to oxidize fatty acids, conserve carbohydrates, and delay metabolic acidosis during prolonged physical activity (18, 19, 45, 46, 83). With endurance training, an approximate twofold increase in the oxidative activity of whole-muscle homogenates or of markers of mitochondrial protein concentration have been reported (25, 45, 46). Kirkwood et al. (51) demonstrated the volume density of intermyofibrillar mitochondrial protein increases. Although the oxidative capacity of whole-muscle homogenates increases twofold, this does not represent a twofold increase in the maximum oxygen uptake of the total organism because of limitations in fiber recruitment and in the blood flow to fibers when a large muscle mass is activated (83). Other metabolic adaptations to physical activity, such as altered mobilization, storage, transport, and endogenous production of carbohydrates, lipids, and amino acids, are developed in chapters 24 and 26.

Following endurance training, muscle blood flow at a given submaximal level of exercise may decrease (52) or remain unchanged (3, 78). In contrast, endurance training results in higher blood flows to the active muscles during exercise at $\dot{V}O_2$max (70, 78). Armstrong, Laughlin, and associates (3, 55) demonstrated increased blood flow to the oxidative portions of skeletal muscles and lower blood flows to the glycolytic portions both in anticipation of exercise and during exercise. Thus, a major adaptive response to endurance training is the redistribution of blood flow from the glycolytic fibers to the oxidative fibers within the active muscles.

Volitional endurance-training programs of 8 to 12 wk increase the capillary-fiber ratio of human skeletal muscles by 5% to 10% (42, 48). A more dramatic increase in the capillary-fiber ratio of 55% was produced in muscles of rabbits by an 8-d program of chronic 10-Hz electrical stimulation (9), although a similar protocol in dogs produced no change in capillarity (15). Small increases in the capillary density are not likely to affect maximum blood flow significantly when compared with the changes that can be produced by recruitment of the existing capillaries by vasodilation of the vessels upstream. Increases in capillary density with endurance training may play a role in increasing the capillary transit time for red blood cells and thereby in facilitating nutrient and gas exchange (78) (see also chapt. 19).

Fibers in the soleus, medial gastrocnemius, and red portion of the vastus lateralis muscles adapt to continuous running at submaximum velocities, but fibers in the white portion of the vastus lateralis muscles require interval training at high velocities of running for adaptive responses to occur (25, 89) (Figure 22.3). During running at different velocities, the responses of the three fiber types differ and may reflect altered recruitment and power output by the motor units. Alternatively, the different velocities of running may provide stimuli of varying intensities for adaptation of a given variable, such as cytochrome c concentration (25). This experiment (25) was not designed to provide an interpretation as to whether different fiber types have inherent differences in the threshold or capacity for adaptation.

A causal relationship exists between the training stimulus and the adaptive response, but the relationship is complex and not necessarily stoichiometric. The lack of stoichiometry results from the diversity of responses elicited in skeletal muscles by a given intensity of exercise performed by a total organism. Within an individual, the diversity may arise from variations in the training stimulus or in the response. Subtle changes in recruitment and loading patterns may arise from day-to-day variations in hydration, nutrition, and fatigue and in such uncontrolled environmental factors as temperature, wind, and terrain. Among individuals, major differences in recruitment and

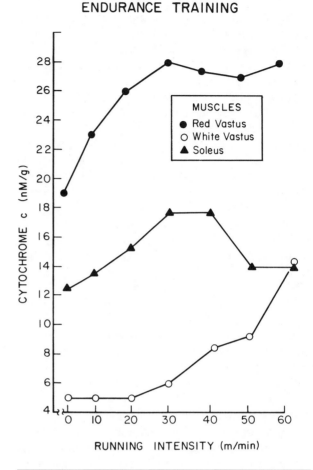

Figure 22.3. The relationship between the concentration of cytochrome c in the red and white portions of the vastus lateralis muscle and in the soleus muscle of rats following 8 w of running at different velocities. Running at velocities from 10 to 40 m/min was continuous for 60 min, whereas the velocities of 50 and 60 m/min were run for 4.5 min with 2.5 min rest and for 2.5 min with 4.5 min rest, respectively, for a duration of 15 min. *Note.* Data from "Influence of exercise intensity and duration on biochemical adaptations in skeletal muscle" by G.A. Dudley, W.A. Abraham, and R.L. Terjung, 1982, *Journal of Applied Physiology,* **53**, pp. 844-850. Reprinted by permission.

loading patterns may arise from the differences in the fiber types present in the contracting muscles (20, 33, 90). When major differences in the proportions of different fiber types in the quadriceps muscle exist even among such a homogeneous performance group as world-class marathon runners (20), the differences to be expected between physically inactive subjects and the highly trained are enormous. Consequently, a single training stimulus has the potential of eliciting a multitude of different adaptive responses due to variations in patterns of recruitment and loading as well as variations in the metabolic status of the skeletal muscle fibers recruited. In addition, physical activity is highly complex. Physical activity, or power, even for a single task, may be altered through changes of a single variable or by a number of variables, such as velocity, load, frequency, and duration. The lack of stoichiometric relationship between the training stimulus and the adaptive response constitutes a major difficulty in investigating the relationship between a training stimulus and the adaptive response in a definitive or mechanistic manner.

Considerable interest has focused on the question, Does volitional endurance training provide a sufficient stimulus for the conversion of fibers from one type to another type (6, 27, 37, 38, 83, 90)? The oxidative capacity (34) and the maximum velocity of shortening (76, 88) or myosin isoforms (76, 88) of single fibers each constitutes a continuum. Even a single fiber may express more than a single myosin isozyme profile (91). In spite of the problem of establishing discrete classification categories on a continuum, the two independent characteristics that reflect the metabolic and contractile properties of fibers have been blended into a variety of classification schemes (34). A prerequisite for meaningful interpretations of adaptations using a given classification scheme is that the fibers be classified on the basis of variables actually measured. Endurance training increases the oxidative capacity of each of the three fiber types (4, 62). If the intensity and duration of the endurance-training program is great enough, a percentage of the FG or IIb fibers may increase oxidative capacity sufficient to change their fiber classification to FOG or IIa (27, 38, 62). Such a change in the percentages of fiber types is equivocal because of the continuum (34).

The intrinsic property of velocity of shortening is a function of the myosin phenotype. This property can be assessed with validity by measurement of velocity of shortening (17), the measurement of both the heavy and light chains of myosin by quantitative electrophoretic techniques (76, 88), or an assay of myosin or myofibrillar ATPase. In most muscles the reciprocal of the contraction time correlates highly with the maximum velocity of shortening (17), but this relationship may be disturbed by experimental interventions (41). Because of the difficulty of measuring maximum velocity of shortening of motor units, contraction time has been used traditionally to classify motor units as either slow or fast (11, 12). The correlation usually observed between velocity of shortening and the histochemical demonstration of myofibrillar ATPase activity in normal adult limb muscles is not found in developing skeletal muscles (41). Consequently, under circumstances in which developmental or aging changes or experimental interventions have differential effects on different proteins, erroneous interpretations may arise from comparisons within and among classification systems.

The concept of a conversion of fibers from Type II to Type I arose initially from cross-sectional studies of different groups of athletes. Compared to the 50% Type I (low-myofibrillar ATPase) fibers normally observed in the muscles of control subjects (26), significantly greater percentages of Type I fibers (e.g., 70% to 80%) have been reported in the muscles of elite endurance athletes, whereas sprinters and power lifters have approximately 80% Type II fibers (20, 33, 90). Furthermore, the difference exists only in the muscles involved in the sport (33, 90). A strong genetic influence on the proportions of fiber types is observed in studies of twins (53) (see also chapts. 13 and 14), and none of the cross-sectional studies of elite athletes exclude the possibility that athletes who have high percentages of certain fiber types select and excel in specific activities.

An almost complete change from fast to slow or slow to fast fiber types has been shown with cross-innervation (10, 85) and cross-transplantation (24) experiments. Muscles exposed to chronic low-frequency stimulation demonstrate an increase in the percentage of Type I fibers and a decrease in the percentage of Type II (82). These experiments have established that the expression of myosin proteins can be changed from fast to slow and vice versa. A number of experiments on rats and humans have been designed to determine whether volitional recruitment can modify the type of myosin isozymes expressed in skeletal muscle fibers (83). Gregory et al. (39) trained young rats for 10 wk reaching a distance of 15 km per day, which is four-fold further than are typical endurance running protocols for rats. Myosin isozymes, reported under nondenaturing conditions, showed a significant conversion from slow (SM) to fast (FM1, FM2, and FM3), but the possibility of selective hypertrophy of existing Type I and IIa fibers rather than a true conversion of fiber type could not be ruled out.

Green et al. (37) studied 15 wk of treadmill running at a final daily distance of 5.7 km. Of four muscles studied by the histochemical demonstration of myofibrillar ATPase, only the deep portion of the vastus lateralis muscle showed a significant increase in Type I fibers and decrease in Type II fibers. Purified myosin fractions showed parallel changes in myosin light chains determined under denaturing conditions. Reiser et al. (76) have demonstrated in rabbit soleus muscle that fast and slow myosin frequently coexist in a single fiber. In these ''mixed'' fibers, the ratios of total fast to total slow light chains may be different from the ratio of fast to slow heavy chains. Under these circumstances, shortening velocities correlate highly with the proportion of fast heavy chains. Consequently, showing a change in the proportion of fast and slow light chains is not an unequivocal demonstration of the conversion from fast to slow fiber types.

The effect of 8 wk of endurance training on myosin isozymes of histochemically typed fibers in the human vastus lateralis muscle was evaluated by Baumann et al. (6). The training induced a significant decrease in Type IIb fibers from 13% to 8%, which was not balanced by a significant increase in Type I or Type IIa fibers. Fragments of single fibers that had been typed histochemically were electrophoresed under denaturing conditions. Following training, biopsies from three of four subjects showed an increase in slow light chains and heavy chains in fibers classified Type IIa histochemically. The conclusion made by these authors that the adaptations mark the beginning of a transition from Type II toward Type I fibers is not warranted. The gels were not quantified, and the differences observed were within the normal sampling variability for needle biopsies of human leg muscles (73). The issue as to whether volitional recruitment can provide the stimulus necessary to modify the expression of myosin isozymes remains unresolved and controversial.

Adaptation to Strengthening Activities

For humans, 12 wk of heavy-resistance strength training leads to a 5% increase in quadriceps muscle cross-sectional area measured by computerized tomography (49) and 5 to 6 mo of strength training of the elbow flexors results in an 11% increase in arm circumference (59). Because muscle length likely does not change appreciably, the circumference values provide an estimate of the gain in muscle mass. The increase in muscle mass following power lifting results from significant increases in the cross-sectional area of 39% for Type I and 31% for Type II muscle fibers (57). Some investigators have reported a preferential Type II hypertrophy in the muscles of power lifters

(65). Vandenburgh (95) demonstrated that when increased constant tension is applied to embryonic skeletal muscle, fibers differentiate in tissue culture through many of the same processes associated with fiber hypertrophy in vivo. These processes include sodium-dependent amino acid transport, Na^+- and K^+-ATPase activity, protein synthesis, and total protein and myosin heavy chain accumulation. The hypertrophy of single skeletal muscle fibers results from the increase in the number of myofibrils within the fiber (32).

Strength and power training has been shown to decrease mitochondrial protein concentration (58). In hypertrophied muscles of rodents, there are reports either of a decrease (14) or of no change (77) in markers of oxidative capacity. Any decrease in oxidative capacity theoretically would reduce the potential for endurance capacity. Because hypertrophied muscles in rats increase oxidative capacity in response to an endurance stimulus (77), a decreased endurance capacity with strength training is not inevitable.

Increases of approximately 5% in the number of fibers in a muscle cross section have been reported following weight-training programs for cats (36). In other than parallel-fibered muscles, the number of fibers in the muscle cross section does not necessarily provide an accurate representation of the number of fibers in the muscle (35, 61). In addition, a difference of this magnitude is not of major physiological importance and may be artifactual (35). Following increased loading of the soleus muscle by ablation of synergistic muscles, Gollnick et al. (35) used nitric acid digestion and then counted all the fibers in control and overloaded muscles. No difference in fiber number was found between the muscles overloaded by removal of the synergistic muscles and the control muscles. Kennedy et al. (50) have provided evidence of nascent muscle fibers in hypertrophied chicken anterior latissimus dorsi muscle. In spite of these observations, the predominant mechanism for adult muscle hypertrophy appears to be hypertrophy of individual fibers (83).

In studies of strength training, the gains in force development of 30% to 40% invariably exceed the increase in cross-sectional area of the muscle. This increase is due in part to the optimization of recruitment patterns (80). A change in the orientation of individual fibers within a muscle might increase the angle of fibers relative to the long axis of the muscle. Under these circumstances, the effective fiber cross-sectional area would increase more than is indicated by computerized tomography (30).

In addition to the increase in muscle mass following ablation of synergistic muscles, the myosin isoform expression shifts from the fast toward the slow isozymes of myosin (5, 39, 72). When myosin isozymes are separated electrophoretically from the soleus and plantaris muscles of rats 11 wk following ablation of the gastrocnemius muscle (39), the soleus muscle showed little or no change, whereas the plantaris muscle demonstrated a threefold increase in SM, and FM2 decreased proportionately. Peptide mapping suggested that a true transformation of myosin had occurred in the hypertrophied fibers.

Variations

Gender, age, and the nutritional state of the organism constitute variations that might result in different quantitative or qualitative adaptive responses. One problem that arises in the interpretation of the data is that the skeletal muscles of males and females, young and old, and nourished and undernourished each differ from one another at the beginning of a study and, as a consequence, are subjected to changes in physical activity that differ either relatively or absolutely. Imaginative experimental designs are required to circumvent these difficulties.

Skeletal muscles of males typically differ from those of females by having a greater mass and muscle cross-sectional area and by generating a greater maximum force and maximum power (81). Although some degree of overlap is observed, males and females constitute two distinct populations with respect to skeletal muscle attributes (60). The dichotomous populations may result in part from culturally induced differences, but this hypothesis has not been tested rigorously. The degree to which gender differences influence the adaptive response to endurance and strength training in humans has not been determined. Male and female rats do not demonstrate substantive differences in relative adaptive responses in morphological or metabolic variables to ablation of synergistic muscles (47) or absolute differences to free whole-muscle transplantation (16).

The capacity to generate maximum force decreases approximately 35% from the third to the eighth decade of human life (40). The loss in force is associated with a decrease in muscle mass explained primarily by a decrease in the cross-sectional area of individual fibers. In comparisons between skeletal muscles from young and old rats, total counts of fibers following nitric acid digestion indicate at most a 5% decline in fiber number with age, and only 25% of the total decrease in mass with age can be attributed to hypoplasia (22). With aging, the atrophy of muscle accounts for less than half the loss in maximum force, and maximum specific force is reduced by 25% (8). The degree to which the changes in skeletal muscle associated with aging constitute an adaptation to decreased physical activity is not known.

A change in the adaptive potential of skeletal muscle with aging has not been demonstrated unequivocally. The issue remains unresolved whether the difference between the adaptive response of old and young people results from an inherent difference in the potential for adaptation of skeletal muscle to a given training stimulus or to differences in the training stimuli. Men aged 60 to 72 yr demonstrated a 110% increase in force development for a 1-repetition-maximum contraction of the knee extensors following a 12-wk strength-training program (29). The increase in performance was accompanied by increases in quadriceps area (9%) and in the cross-sectional area of Type I (34%) and Type II (28%) fibers in vastus lateralis muscle. For two groups of human beings aged 18 to 26 yr and 67 to 72 yr, Moritani and deVries (68) reported comparable strength gains of 30% and 22%, respectively. The gains in performance were accompanied by an overall increase in arm girth of 9% in the young and no change in the arm girth of the elderly. These results do not resolve whether the age-associated difference in the adaptive response is due to the training stimulus or to the mechanisms underlying a gain in strength.

In terms of adaptations of skeletal muscles to endurance or strength training, neither the effects of undernutrition nor supplements beyond the daily requirements have been studied adequately. Nutritional status can have a profound, albeit secondary effect, if an organism is unable to train at the desired intensity (18). For example, lowered glycogen concentrations due to diet might prevent the performance of an endurance activity at sufficient intensity and duration to allow adaptive changes. Neither short-term starvation (74) nor lifetime dietary restriction of animals affects fiber number significantly (22), but each does cause muscle fiber atrophy. Consequently, following dietary restriction, reversal of muscle atrophy involves fiber hypertrophy rather than hyperplasia.

Relationships of Skeletal Muscle Adaptations to Fitness and Health

The adaptations that occur in skeletal muscle in response to changes in physical activity alter fitness levels (83). If the stimulus for adaptive change leads to fiber atrophy and decreased concentration of metabolic proteins, then functional capacity will be impaired. If the adaptive changes increase these variables, then the capacity to develop and sustain power will increase. Improvements in muscular endurance and power can contribute to an increase in the capability of an organism to perform different physical activities throughout its life span. Such improvements increase the potential for a higher quality of life but do not affect longevity. No data support a direct relationship between skeletal muscle adaptations and morbidity or mortality.

Substantive Issues

Many substantive issues regarding skeletal muscle adaptation have been described in previous sections of this chapter. Identification of the mechanisms that link altered physical activity levels and skeletal muscle adaptations is a major issue. The interaction of recruitment and loading with the development of force and velocity appears to be a fundamental combination in the adaptation of skeletal muscle to physical activity (1, 25, 93, 95). Neuroendocrine mechanisms in adaptive responses have been identified (86), and some of the mechanisms underlying the exercise-induced sparing of muscle atrophy have been demonstrated (43). Booth et al. have employed limb immobilization (96) and recovery from limb immobilization (69) to clarify the role of translational, pretranslational, and posttranslational mechanisms in the atrophy and regrowth of skeletal muscles. Many gaps exist in the understanding of molecular mechanisms responsible for adaptations. For example, the role of satellite cells in muscle adaptation has been implicated but not adequately resolved (50).

Although no molecular basis exists for a difference in the maximum force-generating abilities per unit cross-section of slow and fast fibers (83), data on motor units have suggested that fast fibers develop fourfold greater forces than do slow fibers

(11). Data on single-skinned fibers (56), small bundles of fibers (26), motor units, and whole muscles (83) have resolved the long-standing controversy in favor of no significant difference between slow and fast fibers in maximum specific force ($N \cdot cm^{-2}$). A value of 25 to 30 $N \cdot cm^{-2}$ appears reasonable for parallel-fibered muscles (8, 17, 26, 83). For human muscles in vivo, values of 7 to 64 $N \cdot cm^{-2}$ have been reported for maximum voluntary contraction force normalized per cross-sectional area of the whole skeletal muscle (83, 98). Under these conditions, the maximum specific force is distorted by modification of the force by levers, the contributions of synergistic and fixator muscles, and architectural differences within the muscles (30, 83). With these complexities in the evaluation of untrained muscles, the problems in the determination of any change in the maximum specific force following a strength-training program become almost unsurmountable (51, 64). Studies of hypertrophied muscles in rats produced by ablation of synergistic muscles suggest that an increase in noncontractile tissue can result in a 20% decrease in the maximum specific force of hypertrophied muscle (79).

The relationship between the pretraining status of skeletal muscle fibers and the subsequent adaptive potential needs to be determined for normal control subjects, patients with a variety of diseases, the elderly, and national and international caliber performing artists and athletes. The specific populations present unique problems because of the individuality of their existing muscle characteristics and the requirements for highly specialized training regimens. An obligatory requirement for adequate classification of the initial status of skeletal muscle fibers is the continued refinement of optimal histochemical, immunocytochemical, electrophoretic, and functional measurements for the unambiguous classification of fibers. The classification must be based on several independent variables associated with the contractile and metabolic properties of fibers.

Regenerating fibers adapt to an endurance-training stimulus (97). When exposed to atypical innervation and an atypical site, regenerating fibers adapt more rapidly than do surviving fibers (24). The role that contraction-induced injury and regeneration of skeletal muscle fibers plays in the adaptive response of fibers to training programs had not been identified. The major unresolved question is, Must a skeletal muscle fiber be injured and undergo degeneration and subsequent regeneration before the fiber is able to adapt effectively to a training stimulus? Injury to skeletal muscle fibers can occur as a result of high forces developed when muscles are lengthened during a contraction (64). In humans, contraction-induced injury is associated with physical activities of both short and long duration and of varying exercise intensities (2). Training in the specific activity that caused the injury reduces the degree of soreness, but the factors responsible for the injury and for the relief from the symptoms are unknown (2, 64).

Methodological Issues and Technical Problems

A number of methodological issues and technical problems exist for scientists investigating the adaptation of skeletal muscle fibers to decreases and increases in physical activity. A major problem stems from the lack of understanding of the interrelationships among measurements of skeletal muscle function obtained in vitro, in situ, and in vivo. A major effort should be expended by investigators making measurements of maximum force to develop appropriate equations to account for intervening variables so that measurements in vivo may be compared to those obtained in parallel bundles of fibers measured in vitro. Carefully designed experiments on skeletal muscles in vitro hold considerable promise of providing insights as to the mechanisms responsible for muscle adaptations (86). In each type of preparation, data should be checked constantly for internal consistency.

The functional significance of an increased number of capillaries per fiber is not clear, as the correlation between capillary density and maximum muscle blood flow is not significantly different from zero (63). Furthermore, electrical stimulation of latissimus dorsi muscles in dogs showed a fivefold increase in the mitochondrial fraction with no change in capillary density (15). Studies correlating capillary density and blood flows of specific portions of muscle with intravital microscopy and radioactive microspheres might clarify this controversy. The heterogeneity of muscle fiber types (4, 11, 48), even within skeletal muscles that are traditionally considered fast or slow (17), result in different adaptive responses to the same training stimulus. Under these circumstances, whole-muscle adaptations may reflect selective adaptations in only a few fibers. The development of techniques to study functional properties of single motor units (11, 12, 23) and single fibers (76) offer

unparalleled opportunities to clarify the relationship between stimulus and response.

Promising Avenues of Research

The promising avenues of research on the adaptation of skeletal muscle to physical activity involve the utilization of the techniques developed primarily in cell and molecular biology, biochemistry, physiology, and kinesiology to test hypotheses regarding skeletal muscle adaptation. These techniques include the use of monoclonal antibodies; quantitative gel electrophoresis; tissue culture; radioactive isotope tracers; and mechanics of muscles, motor units, and single fibers. These techniques, coupled to the procedure of obtaining needle biopsies of human muscle tissue before and after well-designed training programs, constitute a powerful approach to address significant problems in the understanding of the mechanisms by which exercise induces skeletal muscle fiber adaptation.

The radioactive microsphere method has the potential to resolve many problems in the cardiovascular response to changes in physical activity (3, 55). In addition, intravital microscopy has provided insights regarding the organization of blood vessels and the regulation of the microcirculation in control muscles (84) and regenerating muscles (13). Although the technique has considerable promise, intravital microscopy has not been used to study circulatory adaptations to physical activity.

Tissue imaging by computerized tomography accurately assesses the cross-sectional area of muscles (49, 98), and magnetic resonance imaging provides both muscle areas and concentrations of intracellular metabolites (15). If accurate estimates of average fiber lengths are obtained from cadaver specimens for muscles of different masses, these data may be coupled to measurements of the contractile properties of the muscle groups obtained by computerized force transducers and isokinetic ergometers. Accurate data on force and power normalized for true muscle fiber cross-sectional area would permit the design of studies to investigate significant problems regarding the mechanisms involved in the decrease or increase in skeletal muscle strength. Mathematical modeling of complex muscle groups before and after training to evaluate posture, gait, falls, and overall performance would constitute effective correlative activities.

Conclusion

The adaptation of skeletal muscle to decreases and increases in physical activity constitutes a significant field of study. The adaptive responses to altered levels of physical activity are highly complex. Research has focused primarily on the adaptive responses of whole muscles or on portions of muscles homogeneous as to fiber type. Currently, data describe the adaptive response to stimuli of reduced activity, endurance training, and strength training. Even for these interventions, the relationship between stimulus and adaptive response has not been described adequately with regard to the threshold for activation of the response or the dose-response relationship. A wide variety of important problems remain to be investigated. Most important will be an understanding of the mechanical and biochemical linkages between altered activity levels and adaptive responses. The design of definitive experiments and the utilization of a multitude of contemporary techniques could result in significant progress in this field of research that has such important implications for the quality of life.

Acknowledgments

We acknowledge the valuable contributions of our colleagues, whose names appear on joint publications. In addition, we thank James H. Sherman for his insightful review of a preliminary draft of this manuscript. Gabriele Wienert and Mary Jo Stofflet assisted in the preparation of the manuscript with skill and patience. The manuscript was written with partial grant support from National Institute of Dental Research Program Project DE-07683 and the National Institute on Aging AG-06130 and AG-06157.

References

1. Alford, E., R.R. Roy, J.A. Hodgson, and V.R. Edgerton. Electromyography of rat soleus, gastrocnemius, and tibialis anterior during hind limb suspension. *Exp. Neurol.* 96: 635-649, 1987.

2. Armstrong, R.B. Mechanisms of exercise-induced delayed onset muscular soreness: A brief review. *Med. Sci. Sports Exerc.* 16: 529-538, 1984.

3. Armstrong, R.B., and M.H. Laughlin. Exercise blood flow patterns within and among rat muscles after training. *Am. J. Physiol.* 246: H59-H68, 1984.

4. Baldwin, K.M., G.H. Klinkerfuss, R.L. Terjung, P.A. Molé, and J.O. Holloszy. Respiratory capacity of white, red and intermediate muscle, adaptive response to exercise. *Am J. Physiol.* 222: 373-378, 1972.

5. Baldwin, K.M., V. Valdez, R.E. Herrick, A.M. MacIntosh, and R.R. Roy. Biochemical properties of overloaded fast-twitch skeletal muscle. *J. Appl. Physiol.* 52: 467-472, 1982.

6. Baumann, H., M. Jaggi, F. Soland, H. Howald, and M.C. Schaub. Exercise training induces transitions of myosin isoform subunits within histochemically typed human muscle fibres. *Pflugers Arch.* 409: 349-360, 1987.

7. Brooke, M.H., and K.K. Kaiser. Three "myosin adenosine triphosphatase" systems: The nature of their pH and sulfhydryl dependence. *J. Histochem. Cytochem.* 18: 670-672, 1970.

8. Brooks, S.V., and J.A. Faulkner. Contractile properties of skeletal muscles from young, adult, and aged mice. *J. Physiol. (Lond.)* 404: 71-82, 1988.

9. Brown, M.D., M.A. Cotter, D. Hudlicka, and G. Vrbová. The effects of different patterns of muscle activity on capillary density, mechanical properties and slow and fast rabbit muscles. *Pflugers Arch.* 361: 241-250, 1976.

10. Buller, A.J., J.C. Eccles, and R.M. Eccles. Interactions between motoneurones and muscles in respect of the characteristic speeds of their responses. *J. Physiol. (Lond).* 150: 417-439, 1960.

11. Burke, R.E., and V.R. Edgerton. Motor unit properties and selective involvement in movement. In: Wilmore, J.H., and J.F. Keogh, eds. *Exercise and sport science reviews.* New York: Academic Press, 1975, vol. 3, p. 33-81.

12. Burke, R.E., D.N. Levine, F.E. Zajac III, P. Tsairis, and W.K. Engel. Physiological types and histochemical profiles in motor units of the cat gastrocnemius. *J. Physiol. (Lond.)* 234: 723-748, 1973.

13. Burton, H.W., and J.A. Faulkner. Microcirculatory adaptations to skeletal muscle transplantation. *Annu. Rev. Physiol.* 49: 439-451, 1987.

14. Carlo, J.W., S.R. Max, and D.H. Rifenberick. Oxidative metabolism of hypertrophic skeletal muscle in the rat. *Exp. Neurol.* 48: 222-230, 1975.

15. Clark, B.J., III, M.A. Acker, K. McCully, H.V. Subramanian, R.L. Hammond, S. Salmons, B. Chance, and L.W. Stephenson. In vivo ³¹P-NMR spectroscopy of chronically stimulated canine skeletal muscle. *Am. J. Physiol. (Cell Physiol. 23)* 254: C258-C266, 1988.

16. Clark, K.I., and T.P. White. Morphology of stable muscle grafts of rats: Effects of gender and muscle type. *Muscle Nerve* 8: 99-104, 1985.

17. Close, R.I. Dynamic properties of muscle. *Physiol. Rev.* 52: 129-197, 1972.

18. Conlee, R.K. Muscle glycogen and exercise endurance: A twenty-year perspective. In: Pandolf, K.B., ed. *Exercise and sport science reviews.* New York: Macmillan, 1987, vol. 15, p. 1-28.

19. Constable, S.H., R.J. Favier, J.A. McLane, R.D. Fell, M. Chen, and J.O. Holloszy. Energy metabolism in contracting rat skeletal muscle: Adaptation to exercise training. *Am. J. Physiol. (Cell Physiol. 22)* 253: C316-C322, 1987.

20. Costill, D.L., W.J. Fink, and M.L. Pollock. Muscle fiber composition and enzyme activities of elite distance runners. *Med. Sci. Sports* 8: 96-100, 1976.

21. Coyle, E.F., W.M. Martin III, D.R. Sinacore, M.J. Joyner, J.M. Hagberg, and J.O. Holloszy. Time course of loss of adaptations after stopping prolonged intense endurance training. *J. Appl. Physiol.* 57: 1857-1864, 1984.

22. Daw, C.K., J.W. Starnes, and T.P. White. Muscle atrophy and hypoplasia with aging: impact of training and food restriction. *J. Appl. Physiol.* 64: 2428-2432, 1988.

23. Desmedt, J.E., ed. *Motor unit types, recruitment and plasticity in health and disease.* New York: Karger, 1981.

24. Donovan, C.M., and J.A. Faulkner. Plasticity of skeletal muscle: Regenerating fibers adapt more readily to an atypical site. *J. Appl. Physiol.* 62: 2507-2511, 1987.

25. Dudley, G.A., W.A. Abraham, and R.L. Terjung. Influence of exercise intensity and duration on biochemical adaptations in skeletal muscle. *J. Appl. Physiol.* 53: 844-850, 1982.

26. Faulkner, J.A., D.R. Claflin, and K.K. McCully. Power output of fast and slow fibers from human skeletal muscles. In: Jones, N.L., N. McCartney, and J. McComas, eds. *Human power output.* Champaign, IL: Human Kinetics, 1986, p. 81-91.

27. Faulkner, J.A., L.C. Maxwell, and D.A. Lieberman. Histochemical characteristics of muscle fibers from trained and detrained guinea pigs. *Am. J. Physiol.* 222: 836-840, 1972.

28. Fell, R.D., L.B. Gladden, J.M. Steffen, and X.J. Musacchia. Fatigue and contraction of slow and fast muscles in hypokinetic/hypodynamic rats. *J. Appl. Physiol.* 58: 65-69, 1985.

29. Frontera, W.R., C.N. Meredith, K.P. O'Reilly, H.G. Knuttgen, and W.J. Evans. Strength conditioning in older men: Skeletal muscle hypertrophy and improved function. *J. Appl. Physiol.* 64: 1038-1044, 1988.

30. Gans, C. Fiber architecture and muscle function. In: Terjung, R.L., ed. *Exercise and sport science reviews.* Philadelphia: Franklin Institute, 1982, vol. 10, p. 160-207.

31. Goldman, Y.E. Special topic: Molecular mechanism of muscle contraction. *Annu. Rev. Physiol.* 49: 629-636, 1987.

32. Goldspink, G. Alterations in myofibril size and structure during growth, exercise and changes in environmental temperature. In: Peachey, L.D., R.H. Adrian, and S.R. Geiger, eds. *Handbook of physiology.* Baltimore: Williams & Wilkins, 1983, p. 539-554.

33. Gollnick, P.D., R.B. Armstrong, C.W. Saubert IV, K. Piehl, and B. Saltin. Enzyme activity and fiber composition in skeletal muscle of untrained and trained men. *J. Appl. Physiol.* 33: 312-319, 1972.

34. Gollnick, P.D., and D.R. Hodgson. The identification of fiber types in skeletal muscle: A continual dilemma. In: Pandolf, K.B., ed. *Exercise and sport science reviews.* New York: Macmillan, 1986, vol. 14, p. 81-103.

35. Gollnick, P.D., B.F. Timson, R.L. Moore, and M. Riedy. Muscular enlargement and number of fibers in skeletal muscles of rats. *J. Appl. Physiol.* 50: 936-943, 1981.

36. Gonyea, W.J. Role of exercise in inducing increases in skeletal muscle fiber number. *J. Appl. Physiol.* 48: 421-426, 1980.

37. Green, H.J., G.A. Klug, H. Reichmann, U. Seedorf, W. Wiehrer, and D. Petté. Exercise-induced fibre type transition with regard to myosin and sarcoplasmic reticulum in muscles of the rat. *Pflugers Arch.* 400: 432-438, 1984.

38. Green, H.J., H. Reichmann, and D. Petté. Fibre type specific transformations in the en-

zyme activity pattern of rat vastus lateralis muscle by prolonged endurance training. *Pflugers Arch.* 399: 216-222, 1983.

39. Gregory, P., R.B. Low, and W.S. Stirewalt. Changes in skeletal muscle myosin isoenzymes with hypertrophy and exercise. *Biochemistry* 238: 55-63, 1986.

40. Grimby, G., and B. Saltin. The aging muscle. *Clin. Physiol.* 3: 209-218, 1983.

41. Guth, L., and F.J. Samaha. Erroneous interpretations which may result from application of the "myofibrillar ATPase" histochemical procedure to developing muscle. *Exp. Neurol.* 34: 465-475, 1972.

42. Hermansen, L., and M. Wachtlova. Capillary density of skeletal muscle in well-trained and untrained men. *J. Appl. Physiol.* 30: 860-863, 1971.

43. Hickson, R.C., T.T. Kurowski, G.H. Andrews, J.A. Capaccio, and R.T. Chatterton Jr. Glucocorticoid cytosol building in exercise-induced sparing of muscle atrophy. *J. Appl. Physiol.* 60: 1413-1419, 1986.

44. Hintz, C.S., C.V. Lowry, K.K. Kaiser, D. McKee, and O.H. Lowry. Enzyme levels in individual rat fibers. *Am. J. Physiol. (Cell Physiol.* 8) 239: C58-C65, 1980.

45. Holloszy, J.O. Biochemical adaptations in muscle. Effects of exercise on mitochondrial oxygen uptake and respiratory enzyme activity in skeletal muscle. *J. Biol. Chem.* 242: 2278-2282, 1967.

46. Holloszy, J.O., and F.W. Booth. Biochemical adaptations to endurance exercise in muscle. *Annu. Rev. Physiol.* 38: 273-291, 1976.

47. Ianuzzo, C.D., and Y. Chen. Metabolic character of hypertrophied rat muscle. *J. Appl. Physiol.* 46: 738-742, 1979.

48. Ingjer, F. Capillary supply and mitochondrial content of different skeletal muscle fiber types in untrained and endurance trained men: A histochemical and ultrastructural study. *Eur. J. Appl. Physiol.* 40: 197-209, 1979.

49. Jones, D.A., and O.M. Rutherford. Human muscle strength training: The effects of three different regimes and the nature of the resultant changes. *J. Physiol. (Lond.)* 391: 1-11, 1987.

50. Kennedy, J.M., B.R. Eisenberg, S.K. Reid, L.J. Sweeney, and R. Zak. Nascent muscle fiber appearance in overloaded chicken slow-tonic muscle. *Am. J. Anat.* 81: 203-215, 1988.

51. Kirkwood, S.P., L. Packer, and G.A. Brooks. Effects of endurance training on a mitochon-drial reticulum in limb skeletal muscle. *Arch. Biochem. Biophys.* 255: 80-88, 1987.

52. Klausen, G.A., G.M. Andres, and M.R. Becklake. Effect of training on total and regional blood flow and metabolism in paddlers. *J. Appl. Physiol.* 28: 397-406, 1970.

53. Komi, P.V., and J. Karlsson. Physical performance, skeletal muscle enzyme activities, and fiber types in monozygous twins of both sexes. *Acta Physiol. Scand. (Suppl.)* 462: 1-28, 1979.

54. Larsson, L. Effects of long-term physical training and detraining on enzyme histochemical and functional skeletal muscle characteristics in man. *Muscle Nerve* 8: 714-722, 1985.

55. Laughlin, M.H., and J. Ripperger. Vascular transport capacity of hindlimb muscles of exercise-trained rats. *J. Appl. Physiol.* 62: 438-443, 1987.

56. Lucas, S.M., R.L. Ruff, and M.D. Binder. Specific tension measurements in single soleus and medial gastrocnemius muscle fibers of the cat. *Exp. Neurol.* 95: 142-154, 1987.

57. MacDougall, J.D., G.C.B. Elder, D.G. Sale, J.R. Moroz, and J.R. Sutton. Effects of strength training and immobilization on human muscle fibers. *Eur. J. Appl. Physiol.* 43: 25-34, 1980.

58. MacDougall, J.D., D.G. Sale, J.R. Moroz, G.C.B. Elder, J.R. Sulton, and H. Howard. Mitchondrial volume density in human skeletal muscle following heavy resistance training. *Med. Sci. Sports Exerc.* 11: 164-166, 1979.

59. MacDougall, J.D., G.R. Ward, D.G. Sale, and J.R. Sutton. Biochemical adaptation of human skeletal muscle to heavy resistance training and immobilization. *J. Appl. Physiol.* 43: 700-703, 1977.

60. Maughan, R.J., J.S. Watson, and J. Wehr. Strength and cross-sectional area of human skeletal muscle. *J. Physiol. (Lond.)* 338: 37-49, 1983.

61. Maxwell, L.C., J.A. Faulkner, and G.J. Hyatt. Estimation of the number of fibers in guinea pig skeletal muscle. *J. Appl. Physiol.* 37: 259-264, 1974.

62. Maxwell, L.C., J.A. Faulkner, and D.A. Lieberman. Histochemical manifestations of age and endurance training in skeletal muscle fibers. *Am. J. Physiol.* 224: 356-361, 1973.

63. Maxwell, L.C., T.P. White, and J.A. Faulkner. Oxidative capacity, blood flow and capillary

of skeletal muscles. *J. Appl. Physiol.* 49: 627-633, 1980.

64. McCully, K.K., and J.A. Faulkner. Injury to skeletal muscle fibers of mice following lengthening contractions. *J. Appl. Physiol.* 59: 119-126, 1985.

65. McDougall, M.J.N., and C.T.M. Davies. Adaptive response of mammalian skeletal muscle to exercise with high loads. *Eur. J. Appl. Physiol.* 52: 139-155, 1984.

66. Metzger, J.M., and R.L. Moss. Greater hydrogen ion-induced depression of tension and velocity in skinned single fibres of rat fast than slow muscles. *J. Physiol. (Lond.)* 393: 727-742, 1987.

67. Morkin, E. Chronic adaptations in contractile proteins: Genetic regulation. *Annu. Rev. Physiol.* 49: 545-554, 1987.

68. Moritani, T., and H.A. deVries. Potential for gross muscle hypertrophy in older men. *J. Gerontol.* 35: 672-682, 1980.

69. Morrison, P.R., J.A. Montgomery, T.S. Wong, and F.W. Booth. Cytochrome C protein-synthesis rates and mRNA contents during atrophy and recovery in skeletal muscle. *Biochem. J.* 241: 257-263, 1987.

70. Musch, T.I., G.C. Haidet, G.A. Ordway, J.C. Longhurst, J.H. Mitchell. Training effects on regional blood flow response to maximal exercise in fox hounds. *J. Appl. Physiol.* 62: 1724-1732, 1987.

71. Nemeth, P., D. Petté, and G. Vrbová. Malate dehydrogenase homogeneity of single fibers of the motor unit. In: Petté, D., ed. *Plasticity of muscle.* New York: de Gruyter, 1980, p. 45-54.

72. Noble, E.G., B.L. Dabrowski, and C.D. Ianuzzo. Myosin transformation in hypertrophied rat muscle. *Pflugers Arch.* 396: 260-262, 1983.

73. Nygaard, E., and J. Sanchez. Intramuscular variation of fiber types in the brachial biceps and the lateral vastus muscles of elderly men: How representative is a small biopsy sample? *Anat. Rec.* 282: 451-459, 1982.

74. Parsong, D., M. Riedy, R.L. Moore, and P.D. Gollnick. Acute fasting and fiber number in rat soleus muscle. *J. Appl. Physiol.* 53: 1234-1238, 1982.

75. Peter, J.B., R.J. Barnard, V.R. Edgerton, C.A. Gillespie, and K.E. Stemple. Metabolic profiles of three fiber types of skeletal muscle in guinea pigs and rabbits. *Biochemistry* 14: 2627-2633, 1972.

76. Reiser, P.J., R.L. Moss, G.G. Giulian, and M.L. Greaser. Shortening velocity in single fibers from adult rabbit soleus muscles is correlated with myosin heavy chain composition. *J. Biol. Chem.* 260: 9077-9080, 1985.

77. Riedy, M., R.L. Moore, and P.D. Gollnick. Adaptive response of hypertrophied skeletal muscle to endurance training. *J. Appl. Physiol.* 59: 127-131, 1985.

78. Rowell, L.B. *Human circulation.* New York: Oxford University Press, p. 257-286, 1986.

79. Roy, R.R., I.D. Meadows, K.M. Baldwin, and V.R. Edgerton. Functional significance of compensatory overload of rat fast muscle. *J. Appl. Physiol.* 52: 473-478, 1982.

80. Sale, D.G. Influence of exercise and training on motor unit activation. In: *Exercise and sport science reviews.* Pandolf, K.B., ed. New York: Macmillan, 1987, p. 95-151.

81. Sale, D.G., J.D. MacDougall, S.E. Alway, and J.R. Sutton. Voluntary strength and muscle characteristics in untrained men and women and male bodybuilders. *J. Appl. Physiol.* 62: 1786-1793, 1987.

82. Salmons, S., and J. Hendrickson. The adaptive response of skeletal muscle to increased use. *Muscle Nerve* 4: 94-105, 1981.

83. Saltin, B., and P.D. Gollnick. Skeletal muscle adaptability: Significance for metabolism and performance. In: Peachey, L.D., R.H. Adrian, and S.R. Geiger, eds. *Handbook of physiology.* Baltimore: Williams & Wilkins, 1983, Chapt. 19, p. 555-631.

84. Segal, S., and B. Duling. Flow control among microvessels coordinated by intracellular conduction. *Science* 234: 868-870, 1986.

85. Sréter, F.A., K. Pinter, F. Jolesz, and K. Mabuchi. Fast to slow transformation of fast muscles in response to long-term phasic stimulation. *Exp. Neurol.* 75: 95-102, 1982.

86. Sturek, M. Rationale for the in vitro study of neuromuscular activity. *Med. Sci. Sports Exerc.* 19: S121-S129, 1987.

87. Summers, P.J., C.R. Ashmore, Y.B. Lee, and S. Ellis. Stretch-induced growth in chicken wing muscles: Role of soluble growth-promoting factors. *J. Cell Physiol.* 125: 288-294, 1985.

88. Sweeney, H.L., M.J. Kushmerick, K. Mabuchi, J. Gergely, and F.A. Sréter. Velocity of shortening and myosin isozymes in two types of rabbit fast-twitch muscle fibers. *Am. J. Physiol. (Cell Physiol. 20)* 251: C431-C434, 1986.

89. Terjung, R.L. Muscle fiber involvement during training of different intensities and durations. *Am. J. Physiol.* 230: 946-950, 1976.

90. Tesch, P.A., and J. Karlsson. Muscle fiber types and size in trained and untrained muscles of elite athletes. *J. Appl. Physiol.* 59: 1716-1720, 1985.

91. Thomason, D.B., K.M. Baldwin, and R.E. Herrick. Myosin isozyme distribution in rodent hindlimb skeletal muscle. *J. Appl. Physiol.* 60: 1923-1931, 1986.

92. Thomason, D.B., R.E. Herrick, D. Surdyka, and K.M. Baldwin. Time course of soleus muscle myosin expression during hindlimb suspension and recovery. *J. Appl. Physiol.* 63: 130-137, 1987.

93. Tsika, R.W., R.E. Herrick, and K.M. Baldwin. Interaction of compensatory overload and hindlimb suspension on myosin isoform expression. *J. Appl. Physiol.* 62: 2180-2186, 1987.

94. Vandenburgh, H.H. Cell shape and growth regulation in skeletal muscle: Exogenous versus endogenous factors. *J. Cell. Physiol.* 116: 363-371, 1983.

95. Vandenburgh, H.H. Motion into mass: How does tension stimulate muscle growth? *Med. Sci. Sports Exerc.* 19: S142-S149, 1987.

96. Watson, P.A., J.P. Stein, and F.W. Booth. Changes in actin synthesis and a-actin-mRNA content in rat muscle during immobilization. *Am. J. Physiol.* (*Cell Physiol. 16*) 247: C39-C44, 1984.

97. White, T.P., J.F. Villanacci, P.G. Morales, S.S. Segal, and D.A. Essig. Exercise-induced adaptations of rat soleus muscle grafts. *J. Appl. Physiol.* 56: 1325-1334, 1984.

98. Young, A., M. Stokes, and M. Crowe. The size and strength of the quadriceps muscle of old and young men. *Clin. Physiol.* 5: 145-154, 1985.

Chapter 23

Discussion: Adaptations of Skeletal Muscle to Physical Activity

Howard J. Green

A primary mandate of this conference is to examine the influence of regular exercise training on the adaptations that occur in the multiple systems, tissues, and cells of the human body and the implications of these adaptations to health and well-being. Accordingly, chapters have been written on the skeletal system, the respiratory system, the cardiovascular system, the immune system, the endocrine system, and generally all systems affected either directly or indirectly by the active state. Indeed, as evidenced by Faulkner and White's authoritative and comprehensive review on skeletal muscle adaptation, impressive progress has been made and continues to be made both in the elucidation of events involved in excitation-contraction coupling and in the adaptive response that occurs in these different processes to persistent increases in contractile activity. However, another level of understanding that is of fundamental importance if we are to appreciate the role of exercise in fitness and health is the integration that occurs between the various systems and tissues as they adapt to the challenges imposed by the activity. In this context, each system is viewed as interdependent. The multiple systems of the body constantly interact so that the response in any one system is sensitively geared to a more global purpose, namely, the harmonious and efficient expression of a very specific type of behavior: physical activity. In this chapter, which serves primarily as a response to Faulkner and White's chapter, the focus is to address the role of the skeletal muscle as a determinant of the challenges imposed on other systems and the coordinated nature of the adaptations that occur between muscle and other systems of the body. To realize this objective, emphasis is placed on the adaptive strategies that occur as we ascend to the trained state and the primary role of the working muscle in eliciting these adaptations. At the very least it is hoped that this review will serve to emphasize the many gaps in our understanding and, as a result, form a prospective for future research.

The Muscular System: Characteristics and Functional Implications

Skeletal muscles in the human adult comprise the largest soft-tissue mass in the body, representing some 660 muscles and constituting approximately 25%-30% of total body weight. The individual muscles can be categorized into groups of synergists, each group being discharged with a specific functional role. For example, we can think in terms of muscles of mastication, muscles of the eye, muscles of the tongue, muscles of expression, muscles of ventilation, and muscles of locomotion. The specific functional characteristics of each group are to a considerable degree determined by the nature and composition of the individual fiber types (62). These muscle fibers are being constantly remodeled, altering their subcellular composition and character to be able to respond more appropriately to changing functional demands (6). At the most extreme level, the remodeling can include a complete transformation of muscle fiber types at all levels of organization—morphological, ultra-structural, biochemical, and molecular (43, 44). Such extensive transformations are more readily demonstrated by chronic electrical stimulation, a process that involves artificial stimulation to the motor nerve of the muscle for periods in excess of 8 h per day (43). The limits of adaptation, as determined by voluntary activity patterns in both the human and the nonhuman species, remain a matter of continuing debate.

The property of plasticity so emphasized in skeletal muscle is founded on the capability to maintain high protein turnover rates. Alterations in synthesis or degradation rates of specific proteins can lead to a rapid remodeling of the muscle (39). Indeed, protein turnovers for some of the energy metabolic enzymes in muscle have been estimated to have half-lives as short as 1 d (31a). For many of the protein components of the excitation and contraction network of the cell, the primary mechanism of altering protein levels appears to be the synthetic rate (6). How the increased contractile activity and, in particular, specific contraction histories result in different intracellular signals ultimately culminating in the expression of different protein components of the muscle cell is largely a matter of speculation (6, 44).

The large-muscle mass, combined with the high protein turnover rate, places demands on a number of systems associated with the supply and delivery of appropriate substrates and cofactors to the cell. These materials provide the cell with the essential ingredients to form new protein and to sustain the energy metabolic processes that are required to assimilate and degrade the protein. The high rates of protein degradation impose large demands on the liver and kidneys to neutralize and eliminate waste products such as ammonia and urea and on the respiratory system to eliminate the carbon dioxide arising from the oxidation of fuels (39).

Nowhere is the challenge imposed on the supporting systems more pronounced than during muscle activity, particularly large-muscle-group activity. Activities such as cycling, running, and swimming involve the activation of many groups of synergistic muscles, resulting in the need for large amounts of ATP necessary to sustain activation and force production. During exercise of increasing intensity, the increases in force production and ATP turnover rates elicit corresponding increases in respiratory and cardiovascular function (2). These systems collectively increase arterial oxygen delivery to the working muscles and remove metabolic waste products and heat. In this type of challenge, cardiovascular function (50) and in some cases gas exchange (14) appear to be incapable of responding to the increasing demands, and an inadequacy in muscle oxygen delivery occurs.

In general, the extreme requirements induced by the activation of the large-muscle mass overwhelms the capabilities of the processes involved in the uptake, transport, and delivery of substrates. At some point in the progression toward higher work intensity, the oxidation of substrates is not able to sustain the increasing energy requirements, and anaerobic glycolysis is rapidly accelerated (2).

Perhaps the most common exercise that we associate with health and fitness is expressed by large-muscle-group activity sustained at submaximal intensities for prolonged periods. Activities such as cycling, jogging, swimming, and cross-country skiing performed in this manner induce challenges that are fundamentally different from those observed in progressive exercise. In submaximal exercise the challenge is to sustain the activity in the face of a variety of different disturbances. At the level of the locomotor system, the objective is to sustain a given level of contractile behavior and force output in the face of repeated insults to the processes involved in excitation and contraction of the muscle. The functional integrity of these processes must be defended against alterations in ionic milieu (56), disruptions of membrane systems (34, 59), damage to the myofibrillar network (57), increases in heat content (47), and the direct threat to energy homeostasis as a result of reductions in endogenous and exogenous fuel reserves (4). Continued function of the locomotor system is critically dependent on a number of other systems whose functional integrity is similarly dependent on the necessity for maintaining a given level of force output. Two conspicuous examples are the respiratory system and the cardiovascular system. In the respiratory system, the sustained elevation in ventilation necessary to maintain blood gas homeostasis is provided by the recruitment of muscles involved in inspiration and expiration. The preservation of contractile function in the diaphragm is particularly important in this regard (45). Similarly, cardiac output must be sustained and an appropriate distribution of blood flow to different vascular beds facilitated. These processes are dependent on maintenance of function in the heart and the smooth-muscle cells collectively. In the case of the vascular system, increased vascular tone must occur in the splanchnic and kidney beds, accompanied by dilation in the cutaneous and working-muscle beds. The degree of tone in each bed must be sensitively geared not only to subserve the needs of the individual beds but also to maintain appropriate blood pressure characteristics (46). In the case of heavy exercise, even in a comfortable environment provision of adequate flow to the muscles, liver, and kidneys is persistently threatened by the need to increase cutaneous flow. The increasing heat content of the body occurring as a result of the increase in metabolic heat production generated primarily in the working muscles must be minimized. The primary mechanism for heat dissipation is through evaporation, and evaporation depends on increases in sweating and cutaneous blood flow (38).

Given the persistence and indeed the progression of these challenges during prolonged submaximal activity, the question is, How does the total organism adapt to facilitate function and minimize strain? Is there a well-defined hierarchy with time-dependent changes occurring at the level of specific systems? Because the locomotor system is ultimately responsible for sustaining the required force levels, it may be prudent to examine the adaptations at the level of the muscle cell and to speculate how these adaptations interact with the adaptations in other systems.

Prolonged Exercise: The Initial Insult

Perhaps the most expedient way to conceptualize the role of muscle in the ascent to fitness is to chronicle the responses that occur in a number of systems during the progression toward the trained state. This can best be accomplished by examining the time-dependent adaptations that occur

with repeated exposures to the exercise challenge.

Sustained submaximal exercise performed by the naive individual results in a major activation in a number of supporting systems. Few systems are excluded from participating in the extensive mobilization required to perform large-muscle-group activity. The locomotor muscles—and specifically those synergistic muscles and muscle fibers discharged with producing sufficient force to induce the appropriate joint torques and kinematics to insure a purposeful coordination pattern—must be recruited. At issue is the extent of involvement of specific muscles in different synergistic groups and the balance between recruitment and rate coding of the different motor units in a given muscle (Figure 23.1).

When cycling is used as the exercise modality, on the basis of electromyographic (EMG) evidence it appears as if at least seven different muscles are activated to produce the forces necessary to pedal at approximately 70% of maximal aerobic power ($\dot{V}O_2$max) (41). The interaction between recruitment and rate coding in contributing to the force generated in each of these muscles remains unknown. This is primarily because of the difficulty in monitoring single motor unit potentials during dynamic activity in large muscles. On the basis of glycogen depletion patterns in specific fiber types of one muscle—the vastus lateralis—it appears that

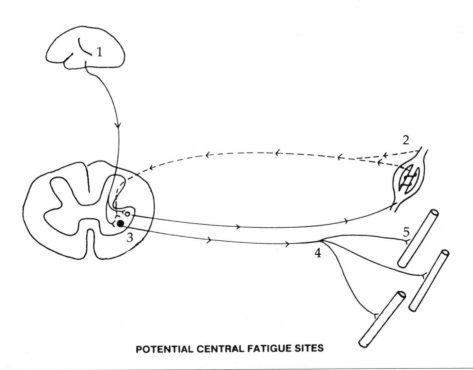

POTENTIAL CENTRAL FATIGUE SITES

Figure 23.1. Central process involved in muscle contractile behavior: supraspinal (1), afferent feedback (2), motoneuron (3), branch points (4), and neuromuscular junction (5).

slow twitch (ST), or Type I, fibers are primarily recruited at exercise intensities below 43% $\dot{V}O_2$max (61), whereas at intensities at approximately 75% or $\dot{V}O_2$max, both Type I and Type II(fast twitch) and specifically Type IIa are recruited (60). Type I and Type IIa fibers, both generally oxidative, constitute at least 90% of the fiber population in the vastus lateralis muscle of typical untrained adults (49). These results would suggests that, at least in the vastus lateralis muscle and at intensities of 60%-70% $\dot{V}O_2$max, recruitmentrepresents a primary strategy in mediating the force output at least at these submaximal levels. This is consistent with the conclusion reached by DeLuca (13) for the deltoid involved in increasing isometric force development. However, care should be taken in extrapolating these results to dynamic activity, as dynamic activity appears to be more frequency dependent at comparable levels of force (29). This is an area in which further research is urgently needed. The particular neural strategy could involve maximizing force output in selected motor unit pools such as the ST motor units to meet the criterion force or by spreading the force over a wider population of motoneurons and minimizing the contribution of each motor unit.

The particular strategy followed has important implications to both fatigue and adaptation. For example, if the neural strategy is to restrict recruitment to a specific motoneuron pool and to maximize activation at submaximal force levels, a maximal challenge will be imposed on sarcolemma function, the sarcoplasmic reticulum, and the contractile apparatus (Figure 23.2). Further, energy metabolic pathways, both aerobic and anaerobic glycolytic, will be maximally stimulated to meet the energy requirements of the maximally activated fibers. If on the other hand the strategy is to distribute the force requirement over a greater motor unit pool, lower firing frequencies, lower activation, and lower force development would occur in each motor unit and in each muscle fiber. Because the force levels in individual fibers are reduced, ATP requirements will be correspondingly reduced, resulting in less activation of the energy metabolic pathways.

From the standpoint of fatigue, a strategy that emphasizes rate coding will result in a progressive

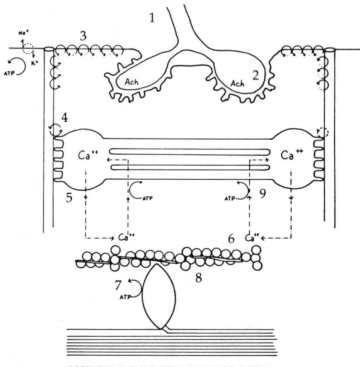

POTENTIAL FATIGUE SITES IN A MUSCLE FIBRE

Figure 23.2. Peripheral processes involved in muscle contractile behavior: motor end plate (2), sarcolemma action potential (3), coupling between T tubule and sarcoplasmic reticulum (4), calcium release from sarcoplasmic reticulum (5), binding of calcium to troponin (6), cross-bridge formation (7), cross-bridge dissociation (8), and calcium reaccumulation by sarcoplasmic reticulum. Number 1 identifies the nerve.

recruitment of the unstimulated motor neuron pool as the exercise progresses. This is apparently what happens at least at intensities below up to 60%-70% VO_2max (60, 61). As evidenced by the glycogen depletion pattern, Type IIa and Type IIb fibers are successively recruited, apparently as a result of a declining ability of the Type I motor unit pool to produce sufficient tension. At higher intensities of exercise, where there is limited opportunity for further recruitment during prolonged exercise because Type I and Type IIa fibers are recruited early, manipulative strategies are limited. Whether rate coding occurs as a desperate attempt to preserve force is uncertain, at least in dynamic prolonged exercise. If adaptation is dependent on both the imposed challenge in terms of the degree of activation of the fiber and the amount of excitation, both the intensity and the duration of activity should be of fundamental importance in eliciting specific intracellular changes.

Metabolic heat production in the muscle also rises dramatically with the onset of exercise (47). Excessive increases in the heat content of the muscle must be prevented if the activity is to be sustained. Increases in blood flow represent the primary mechanism for convecting the heat from the working muscle to the body core. The major avenue for heat loss from the core to the environment in humans is through evaporation, which depends on increases both in cutaneous blood flow and in sweat rate (38). This means that in the absence of increases in cardiac output, a direct competition is set up between the skin, the working muscle, and the splanchnic and kidney regions for available blood flow. Recent evidence (53) suggests that protection of blood flow to the working muscle remains a priority and that reductions in flow do not occur during prolonged exercise in the heat despite increases in body heat content. This means that flow is diverted away from the splanchnic and kidney areas to provide the increases in cutaneous blood flow (46). Even with the pronounced diversion of blood flow from these areas, cutaneous blood flow is inadequate, and body heat content rises (38, 46). The progressive reduction in blood flow to the kidney and splanchnic areas threatens function in both of these tissues. Increased extraction must be able to compensate for the blood flow inadequacies. The degree to which blood flow must be reduced before function is impaired is questionable.

Cardiovascular drift is a well-established phenomena during prolonged heavy exercise and is characterized by increases in heart rate and decreases in stroke volume (46). The drift has been ascribed to a reduction in central blood volume mediated either by increased cutaneous flow or by sweating (38, 46). This interpretation has recently been challenged (40). It has been suggested that the reduction in stroke volume may well be associated with an inability of the heart to maintain contractile force (53, 58). The heart rate rises to defend cardiac output. The increase in heart rate in the absence of changes in blood pressure results in an increase in the rate pressure product. This would be expected to result in an inefficient strategy to sustain the exercise cardiac output.

The ventilatory system appears capable of handling the challenge imposed by prolonged submaximal exercise, at least in the untrained (14). Provided that exercise intensities are below the threshold at which a metabolic acidosis develops and that the exercise is conducted at a neutral environment, minute ventilation and its derivates—tidal volume and frequency—remain relatively stable, and arterial blood gas homeostasis is preserved (55). Fatigue of the ventilatory muscles apparently does occur during prolonged exercise (36); however, the amount of disturbance in contractile behavior is not sufficient to affect function. Dempsey (15) has emphasized that a ventilatory drift may also be observed in prolonged heavy exercise, most notably in a hot, humid environment. The cause of the drift is unknown.

At some point during prolonged exercise, the individual becomes unable to sustain the level of work output. The cause of fatigue is a result of an inability of the locomotor muscles to act as force generators. The impairment may be peripheral, occurring as a result of a failure within the muscles to respond to the neural drive, or as a result of a central dysfunction, resulting in a reduction in motor drive (5, 21, 23). Although fatigue in this type of work has most often been attributed to a peripheral problem that occurs as a result of an energy crisis secondary to a depletion of endogenous muscle glycogen (4), experimental support for this hypothesis is not impressive. It is extremely difficult to demonstrate reductions in muscle ATP concentration at the point of fatigue in spite of low glycogen concentration (23). It is becoming extremely apparent that failure may occur at any one of a number of excitation-contraction processes, including the sarcolemma (59), the sarcoplasmic reticulum (34), and the contractile apparatus itself (57). Failure at these different sites need not be accompanied by reductions in ATP availability. Future research must address fatigue mechanisms with considerably more emphasis. Without definitive determinations of the cause of fatigue in different types of activities, it is difficult to evaluate the impact of different types of training programs on fitness.

Prolonged Exercise: Repeated Insults

With subsequent exposures to the exercise stress, a number of rapidly responding adaptations become readily apparent. Perhaps the most conspicuous adaptation is an increase in plasma volume (hypervolemia), which becomes apparent as early as 1 d following the first exposure to exercise (11, 54). With as little as 3 d of exposure to prolonged heavy exercise, an almost 20% increase in plasma volume has been reported (22). Although hypervolemia is believed to have important effects on thermoregulatory behavior by facilitating increases in cutaneous blood flow and sweat rate (12, 38), such effects have not been confirmed experimentally (28). However, it is generally acknowledged that hypervolemia has important effects on cardiac function. Exercise-induced increases in hypervolemia are accompanied by elevated cardiac output and stroke volume and a pronounced reduction in heart rate that persists throughout the exercise (27, 63). The exercise bradycardia is apparent very early in the training and is promoted by the increased ventricular filling as a result of the elevations in central blood volume. The increased ventricular filling results in an elevation of stroke volume as a result of the Frank-Starling mechanism. Heart function is now better protected against fatigue as a result of the reduction in rate pressure product and the more favorable efficiency. Hypervolemia may also serve other potentially favorable advantages, including delivery of more exogenous substrates to the working muscle, improved perfusion of kidney and splanchnic tissues, reduced resistance to capillary flow, improved blood-buffering capacity, and removal of waste products and heat from the working muscle. Several of these postulated functions are based on increased blood flow to the working muscle, a realistic probability given the reduction in arterial oxygen content that occurs with hypervolemia and the apparent desire to maintain oxygen delivery to the muscle (51). Hypervolemia would also be expected to result in attenuating a large number of hormones, many of which can effect changes in cardiovascular function, extramuscular substrate mobilization, and thermoregulatory behavior (16). For example, reductions in sympathetic drive as

determined by reductions in the exercise-induced increase in both epinephrine and norepinephrine have been found (26). The specific effect of the alteration in sympathetic behavior is not known at present. Hypervolemia appears to have a minimal effect on muscle metabolism, as energetic behavior appears unchanged (26). However, there is some evidence that a sparing of glycogen may occur, possibly as a result of increased extramuscular substrate availability (26). What appears evident is that the early adaptive response in body fluid volumes which has important physiological implications generally has been overlooked. The task now is to determine specifically specifically what the effects are on muscle function and the supporting systems.

With further exposure to the exercise stressor, additional adaptations result. Exercise cardiac output returns to pretraining levels; however, compared to pretraining levels, the cardiac output is accomplished by a reduction in heart rate and an increase in stroke volume (27, 63). Some degree of hypervolemia persists (20, 54). Thermoregulation is considerably improved as evidenced by the reduction in core temperature and the increase in sweating rate and cutaneous blood flow (11, 54). These events, which occur within the first two weeks of regular prolonged exercise training, need not be accompanied by increases in maximal aerobic power (32). During this time frame, additional adaptations result that have been characterized frequently in previous studies (30). These include a reduction in blood and muscle lactate concentration, a reduced utilization of muscle glycogen, and an increase in the utilization of free fatty acids (7). These changes are not the result of adaptations to the energy enzymatic machinery of the muscle cell or to the capillarization surrounding the muscle cell (35, 37), as has been assumed previously (18, 30). These adaptive events must be explained by some other mechanism. Although several possibilities exist, one is particularly tantalizing. Neural training has been demonstrated in high-resistance training (see chapt. 22), and the altered motor drive appears capable of explaining the early training-induced increase in strength in the absence of observable changes in muscle fiber cross-sectional area. Such a phenomenon may occur with endurance training. An increase in the recruitment of other synergistic muscles or in the recruitment of motor units within a synergist would enable the required forces to be developed with less tension generated per fiber. Stimulation frequency could be depressed in each fiber, resulting in less activation and a reduction in the ATP turnover rate.

Not only would this have the effect of increasing the safety margin and resulting in less probability of failure at different levels of excitation and contraction, it might result in less activation of anaerobic glycolysis and less of a dependency of glycogen. From the standpoint of metabolic control, this mechanism is similar to the one proposed by Holloszy and Coyle (30), Gollnick and Saltin (18), and Gollnick (19), in that the metabolic load is, in effect, spread to more mitochondria and more respiratory chains, resulting in less oxygen consumption per respiratory chain and therefore less need for an increase in the ADP-ATP ratio necessary to stimulate mitochondrial respiration. The lower ADP and Pi combined with a lower cytosolic calcium concentration (as a result of the lower activation) would be expected to reduce both glycogenolysis and glycolysis (39). In this model the adaptation results from recruiting more muscle fibers and lowering the activation and force output in each fiber. In the models used previously (18, 30), the force output per fiber is thought to remain constant; however, the metabolic adaptation occurs because of a proliferation of mitochondria with consequent increases in the number of respiratory chains within a fiber. Both of these hypotheses are speculative but represent fruitful directions for further research. During this early period of training, large increases are observed in work tolerance. Whether this increase in work tolerance is intimately associated with some energetic process associated with glycogen availability or to the adaptation in one or more of the many processes coupling motor drive to contraction, all of which may be unrelated to energetic status, is unknown.

The Trained State: The Role of the Muscle in Fitness

As regular training extends into weeks and months, pronounced adaptations are observed in the morphological, ultrastructural, and biochemical features of the cell. Increases in fiber size, capillarization, and the ratios of capillaries to fiber area also occur (1, 49). These adaptations were reported in considerable detail by Faulkner and White (see chapt. 22) and will not be repeated here. What is conspicuous about most of these training studies (particularly in humans) is that they have tended to emphasize only the cellular enzymatic adaptations. Enzymatic adaptations have been performed biochemically on samples obtained from a mixture

of the different fiber types. The limitation in these studies is that they fail to recognize the potential unique capabilities of the different fiber types to respond to an exercise stimulus. Further, without the use of ultrastructural morphometry, adaptations at least at the level of the mitochondria cannot be localized to specific regions of the cell. There is evidence to suggest that the time-dependent proliferation of mitochondria may be different in the subsarcolemmal regions as opposed to the intermyofibrillar regions (31). If this is the case, then significan improvements in sarcolemmal function or sarcoplasmic function may occur before adaptations at the level of the contractile proteins. Adaptation to these membrane systems at any level—ultrastructural, biochemical, or molecular—have generally been overlooked in exercise training studies.

Most human training studies demonstrate increases in the enzymes associated with beta-oxidation and the Krebs cycle. These changes supposedly are mediated by increases in both the size and the number of mitochondria. It is now generally accepted (at least within the range of training protocols used on humans) that no change occurs in the potential for glycogenolysis or glycolysis as measured by the lack of change in the maximal activities of the rate-limiting enzymes involved in these metabolic segments and pathways. Few studies have extended their biochemical analyses to include measurement of the enzymes involved in other metabolic functions, such as ketone body utilization and amino acid oxidation. Consequently, we have limited appreciation of how the human skeletal muscle and in particular the different fiber types respond to regular exercise. Although extensive biochemical analysis has been reported on nonhumans and in particular the rat, in muscles of different fiber composition (30), care must be taken when extrapolating these results to humans, in view of the substantial differences in fiber-type composition (21, 49). Indeed, irrespective of the species, more information is needed regarding the interrelationship between the adaptations occurring in the different metabolic segments and pathways and the significance of the types of metabolism and fuel utilized in promoting change. To a considerable extent, preferential challenges to both the type of metabolism and the type of fuel can be induced by varying the characteristics of the training session. Pette and Hoffer (42) have introduced the concept of constant proportion, and they discriminate enzyme ratios and have presented impressive evidence to suggest that the enzymes of different metabolic segments and pathways show a particular patterned response. This hypothesis needs to be investigated in considerably more detail with more creative approaches to training.

As previously indicated, the alterations in mitochondrial density and the changes in the cellular potential for beta-oxidation and aerobic end oxidation have been used to account for the depression in anaerobic glycolysis, the reduced utilization of muscle glycogen, and the increased utilization of free fatty acids during prolonged exercise following training (18, 30). However, other adaptations may also be significant in explaining these metabolic effects. Training is also accompanied by impressive increases in fiber size, fiber capillarization, and the ratio of capillaries to fiber area (1). The increase in capillarization is thought to precede the development of the fiber oxidative potential and has been suggested to be a primary adaptate necessary to explain the associated increases in aerobic power induced by training (48, 52). The increase in fiber size may have some relevance in mediating the change in muscle metabolism. Increases in fiber size result in more myofibrils and more cross-bridges; and consequently in the absence of change in neural muscular control, the tension per myofibril at constant force is reduced. This suggests that the oxidative potential appears not to be compromised during the period of fiber size increase (1). Energy exchange between the mitochondria and the myofibrils could conceivably be facilitated (19), resulting in less need for anaerobic support.

The adaptations to training in the muscle fiber also seem to be critically linked to the expression of the cardiovascular adaptations during exercise (9, 10). In experiments involving training with either the arms or the legs and testing with both trained and untrained muscle groups, it has been found that the exercise bradycardia (i.e., that beyond the lower heart rate that occurs at rest) is manifested only with the trained muscle group. This would suggest that a strong reflex originating from the working muscles and modified by some stimuli affected by training is acting to modify cardiovascular control. Because the exercise bradycardia is also evident early in exercise training and is associated with the hypervolemic response, it appears as if there is a shift in the mechanism responsible for the exercise bradycardia. At present there is no definitive evidence supporting the existence of hypervolemia with long-term training. The existence of relatively normal hematocrits in highly trained athletes would suggest that either the initial plasma volume has been lost or that red-cell volume has been increased resulting in an increase in total blood volume. Future research is needed to determine the mechanisms associated with altered cardiovascular control with endurance training, particularly with reference to the role of the working skeletal muscle and the alterations in vascular constituents. At the level of the heart, alterations in sympathetic drive, parasympathetic drive, and intrinsic rate also have been suggested to account for the resting bradycardia (33). What is apparent is that the energy enzymatic character of the running, trained heart is not different from that of the untrained heart (3).

With regard to exercise ventilation during prolonged submaximal exercise, training appears to have little effect unless the training is associated with significant reductions in blood lactate concentration (8). In such cases, exercise ventilation is lowered, an event that is probably mediated through the withdrawal of the chemoreceptor drive induced by the acidosis (8). Exercise training appears to have minimal effect in altering the character of the diaphragm (17, 24, 25) at least in the rat and at the level of enzymatic adaptation. In response to extreme daily training sessions, indications of reductions in fiber size with no alterations in capillary number were found (25). The most plausible reasons to explain the relative insensitivity of the diaphragm to adapt to exercise training is that the small change in diaphragmatic work occurring during the exercise hyperpnea (in conjunction with the relatively high oxidative potential to begin with) probably results in stimuli that is subthreshold for adaptation. It does appear, however, that in the rat the highly glycolytic intercostal muscles respond by increasing their oxidative potential (24). As in the case of the locomotor muscles, few investigations have examined the adaptability in the membrane systems and the contractile apparatus of the respiratory muscles to exercise training.

Conclusion

In summary, studies aimed at characterizing the plasticity of the skeletal muscle in response to different perturbations have received considerable emphasis in recent years. Changes in response to the perturbation of increased contractile activity induced by regular voluntary exercise programs are numerous. Although impressive progress has been made in describing the cellular adaptations, the studies are generally limited, especially in the case of humans. This is because the studies have generally focused on a limited aspect of the organization of the muscle cell and the exercise training regimens largely have been unexciting, lacking in a sound hypothetical orientation. The techniques are now available to investigate in humans a myriad of potential changes at all levels of organization in the single muscle cell. These studies should investigate each link in the chain systematically, extending from excitation of the muscle sarcolemma to the myofibrillar apparatus. Such studies should pay specific regard to the interrelationships between the different adaptates with a view to determining whether they are isolated phenomena induced by specific intracellular signals or whether they are interdependent, their expression being contingent on the development of other adaptates. At the center of these studies is the need to explain the functional significance of each adaptate in terms of its role in accounting for the considerable increase in work tolerance with training.

Appreciation of fitness and its role in health is contingent on understanding the response of the total organism to the exercise state and the interactions that occur between each system and each tissue. Subserving the needs of the large mass of skeletal muscle tissue in the typical adult, especially in the exercising state, places a major challenge on several systems. How these systems respond to the needs of the working muscle and how their function is modified by adaptations to the muscle cell remain elusive goals for future research.

Finally, we need to know more about the limits of adaptation with regards both to the general organism and to the skeletal muscle in particular. Extreme programs of contractile activity accomplished through electrical stimulation result in the extensive transformation of fast- to slow-type fibers. Whether extreme voluntary activity programs are capable of similar modifications and whether the muscle is more sensitive to change at different developmental stages or during aging is largely unknown. It is possible that the persistent nature of the involuntary activity induced by electrical stimulation is necessary for creating the proper intracellular environment, which leads to an extensive remodeling of the protein composition of the cell. Fatigue resulting either centrally or peripherally from voluntary activity may prevent establishment of a comparable extracellular environment and prevent such extensive adaptations.

Finally, all these changes, once characterized, must be evaluated not only in the context of improved function during the exercise state but also in terms of defending against disease and improving one's ability to coexist with a multitude of environmental stressors, many of which are constantly changing.

References

1. Anderson, P., and J. Henriksson. Capillary supply of the quadriceps femoris muscle in man: Adaptive response to exercise. *J. Physiol.* 270: 677-690, 1977.
2. Åstrand, P.-O., and K. Rodahl. *Textbook of work physiology.* New York: McGraw-Hill, 1986.
3. Baldwin, K.M. Effects of chronic exercise on the biochemical and functional properties of the heart. *Med. Sci. Sports Exerc.* 17(5): 522-528, 1985.
4. Bergström, J., L. Hermansen, E. Hultman, and B. Saltin. Diet, muscle glycogen and physical performance. *Acta Physiol. Scand.* 71: 140-150, 1967.
5. Bigland-Ritchie, B., and J.J. Woods. Changes in muscle contractile properties and neural control during human muscular fatigue. *Muscle Nerve* 7: 691-699, 1984.
6. Booth, F.A., and P.A. Watson. Control of adaptations in protein levels in response to exercise. *Fed. Proc.* 44: 2293-2300, 1985.
7. Burnett, M., H. Green, S. Jones, and B. Farrance. Short term endurance training: Effect on muscle glycogen, glycolytic intermediates and high energy phosphagens during exercise. *Can. J. Appl. Sports Sci.* 11(3): 1986.
8. Casaburi, R., T.W. Storer, and K. Wasserman. Mediation of reduced ventilatory response to exercise after endurance training. *J. Appl. Physiol.* 63(4): 1533-1538, 1987.
9. Clausen, J.P. Effect of physical training on cardiovascular adjustments to exercise in man. *Physiol. Rev.* 57: 779-815, 1977.
10. Clausen, J.P., K. Klausen, B. Rasmussen, and J. Trap-Jensen. Central and peripheral circulatory changes after training of the arms and legs. *Am. J. Physiol.* 225: 675-682, 1973.
11. Convertino, V.A., J.E. Greenleaf, and E.M. Bernauer. Role of thermal and exercise factors in the mechanism of hypervolemia. *J. Appl. Physiol.: Respir. Environ. Exerc. Physiol.* 48(4): 657-664, 1980.
12. Convertino, V.A. Fluid shifts and hydration state: Effects of long term exercise. *Can. J. Sport Sci.* 12(Suppl. 1): 1365-1395, 1987.

13. DeLuca, C. Control properties of motor units. *J. Exp. Biol.* 115: 125-136, 1985.

14. Dempsey, J.A., and R.F. Fregosi. Adaptability of the pulmonary system to changing metabolic requirements. *Am. J. Cardiol.* 55: 59D-67D, 1985.

15. Dempsey, J.A. Exercise-induced imperfections in pulmonary gas exchange. *Can. J. Sport Sci.* 12(Suppl. 1): 665-705, 1987.

16. Francesconi, R.P. Endocrinological responses to exercise in stressful environments. In: *Exercise and sport science reviews.* Pandolf, K.B., ed. New York: Macmillan, 1988, vol. 16, p. 255-284.

17. Fregosi, R.F., M. Sanjak, and D.J. Paulson. Endurance training does not affect diaphragm mitochondrial respiration. *Respir. Physiol.* 67: 225-237, 1987.

18. Gollnick, P.D., and B. Saltin. Significance of skeletal muscle oxidative enzyme enhancement with endurance training. *Clin. Physiol.* 2: 1-12, 1982.

19. Gollnick, P.D. Metabolic regulation in skeletal muscle: Influence of endurance training as exerted by mitochondrial protein concentration. *Acta Physiol. Scand.* 128(Suppl. 556): 53-66, 1986.

20. Green, H., J. Coates, J. Sutton, and S. Jones. Interindividual differences in the response of red cell volume to training. *Med. Sci. Sports Exerc.* 18(2): S75, 1986.

21. Green, H.J. Muscle power: Fibre type recruitment, metabolism and fatigue. In: Jones, N.L., N. MacCartney, and A.J. McComas, eds. *Human muscle power.* Champaign, IL: Human Kinetics, 1986, chapt. 5, p. 65-80.

22. Green, H.J., L.L. Jones, R.L. Hughson, D.C. Painter, and B.W. Farrance. Training-induced hypervolemia: Lack of an effect on oxygen utilization during exercise. *Med. Sci. Sports Exerc.* 19(3): 202-206, 1987.

23. Green, H.J. Neuromuscular aspects of fatigue. *Can. J. Sports Sci.* 12(Suppl. 1): 75-195, 1987.

24. Green, H.J., and H. Reichmann. Differential response of enzyme activities in rat diaphragm and intercostal muscles to exercise training. *J. Neurol. Sci.* 84: 157-165, 1988.

25. Green, H.J., M.J. Plyley, D.M. Smith, and J.G. Kile. *Extreme endurance training and fibre type adaptation in rat diaphragm.* Manuscript submitted for publication, 1988.

26. Green, H.J., L.L. Jones, M.E. Houston, M.E. Ball-Burnett, and B.W. Farrance. *Muscle energetics during prolonged cycling following exercise hypervolemia.* Manuscript submitted for publication, 1988.

27. Green, H.J., L. Jones, and D. Painter. *Effect of exercise induced hypervolemia on cardiac function during prolonged exercise.* Manuscript submitted for publication, 1988.

28. Green, H.J. *Does hypervolemia influence thermoregulation?* Manuscript submitted for publication, 1988.

29. Grimby, L. Single motor unit discharge during voluntary contraction and locomotion. In: Jones, N.L., N. McCartney, and A.J. McComas, eds. *Human muscle power.* Champaign, IL: Human Kinetics, 1986, chapt. 8, p. 111-125.

30. Holloszy, J.O., and E.F. Coyle. Adaptations of skeletal muscle to endurance exercise and their metabolic consequences. *J. Appl. Physiol.: Respir. Environ. Exerc. Physiol.* 56(4): 831-838, 1984.

31. Hoppeler, H., H. Howald, K. Conley, S.L. Lindstedt, H. Claassen, P. Vock, and E.R. Weibel. Endurance training in humans: Aerobic capacity and structure in skeletal muscle. *J. Appl. Physiol.* 59(2): 320-327, 1985.

31a. Illg, D., and D. Pette. Turnover rates of hexokinase. 1. Phosphofructokinase, pyruvate kinase and creatine kinase in slow-twitch soleus muscle and heart of the rabbit. *Eur. J. Biochem.* 97: 267-273, 1979.

32. Jones, S., H. Green, and M. Burnett. Short term endurance training: Effect on gas exchange, ventilation and circulation during exercise. *Can. J. Appl. Sports Sci.* 11(3): 1986.

33. Katona, P.G., M. McLean, D.H. Dighton, and A. Guz. Sympathetic and parasympathetic cardiac control in athletes and non athletes at rest. *J. Appl. Physiol.* 52(6): 1652-1657, 1982.

34. Klug, G.A., and G.F. Tibbits. The effect of activity on calcium-mediated events in striated muscle. In: Pandolf, K., ed. *Exercise and sport science reviews.* New York: Macmillan, 1988, vol. 16, p. 1-60.

35. Livesey, J., H. Green, S. Jones, and B. Farrance. Short term endurance training: Lack of an effect on enzymes of energy metabolism in vastus lateralis muscle. *Can. J. Appl. Sports Sci.* 11(3): 1986.

36. Martin, B.J. Limitations imposed by respiratory muscle fatigue. *Can. J. Sport Sci.* 12 (Suppl. 1): 615-625, 1987.

37. Murphy, P., H. Green, D. Smith, I. Fraser, and B. Farrance. Short term endurance train-

ing: Lack of adaptation in individual muscle cells. *Can. J. Appl. Sports Sci.* 11(3): 1986.

38. Nadel, E.R. Recent advances in temperature regulation during exercise in humans. *Fed. Proc.* 44: 2286-2292, 1985.

39. Newsholme, E.R., and A.R. Leech. *Biochemistry for the medical sciences.* New York: John Wiley & Sons, 1983, p. 382-410.

40. Nielson, B. Temperature regulation: Effects of sweat loss during prolonged exercise. *Acta Physiol. Scand.* 128(Suppl. 556): 105-109, 1986.

41. Patla, A.E. Some neuromuscular strategies characterizing adaptation process during prolonged activity in humans. *Can. J. Sport Sci.* 12(Suppl. 1): 335-445, 1987.

42. Pette, D., and H.W. Hoffer. The constant proportion enzyme group concept in the selection of reference enzymes in metabolism. In: *Trends in enzyme histochemistry and cytochemistry* (Ciba Foundation Symposium 73). Amsterdam: Excerpta Medica, 1988, p. 231-244.

43. Pette, D., and G. Vrbová. Invited review: Neural control of phenotypic expression in mammalian muscle fibers. *Muscle Nerve* 8: 676-689, 1985.

44. Pette, D. Regulation of phenotype expression in skeletal muscle by increased contractile activity. In: Saltin, B., ed. *Biochemistry of exercise VI.* Champaign, IL: Human Kinetics, 1987, p. 3-26.

45. Rochester, D.F. The diaphragm: Contractile properties and fatigue. *J. Clin. Invest.* 75: 1397-1402, 1985.

46. Rowell, L.B. *Human circulation: Regulation during physical stress.* New York: Oxford University Press, 1986, p. 213-256.

47. Saltin, B., and L. Hermansen. Esophageal, rectal and muscle temperature during exercise. *J. Appl. Physiol.* 21(6): 1757-1762, 1966.

48. Saltin, B., and L.B. Rowell. Function adaptations to physical activity and inactivity. *Fed. Proc.* 1500-1613, 1980.

49. Saltin, B., and P.D. Gollnick. Skeletal muscle adaptability: Significance for metabolism and performance. In: *Handbook of physiology: Skeletal muscle.* Bethesda, MD: American Physiological Society, 1983, sect. 10, chapt. 19, p. 555-631.

50. Saltin, B. Hemodynamic adaptations to exercise. *Am. J. Cardiol.* 55: 42D-47D, 1985.

51. Saltin, B., B. Kiens, G. Savard, and P. Pedersen. Role of hemoglobin and capillarization for oxygen delivery and extraction in muscular exercise. *Acta Physiol. Scand.* 128(Suppl. 556): 21-32, 1986.

52. Savard, G., B. Kiens, and B. Saltin. Central cardiovascular factors as limits to endurance; with a note on the distinction between maximal oxygen uptake and endurance fitness. In: MacLeod, D., R. Maughan, M. Nimmo, T. Reilly, and C. Williams, eds. *Exercise: Benefits, limits and adaptations.* New York: E. & F.N. Spon, 1987, p. 162-180.

53. Savard, G.K., B. Nielsen, J. Laszczynska, B.L. Larson, and B. Saltin. Muscle blood flow is not reduced in humans during moderate exercise and heat stress. *J. Appl. Physiol.* 64(2): 649-657, 1988.

54. Senay, L.C., D. Mitchell, and C.H. Wyndham. Acclimatization in a hot, humid environment. *J. Appl. Physiol.* 40(5): 786-796, 1976.

55. Shephard, R.J. Respiratory factors limiting prolonged effort. *Can. J. Sport Sci.* 12(Suppl. 1): 455-528, 1987.

56. Sjøgaard, G. Water and electrolyte flexes during exercise and their relation to muscle fatigue. *Acta Physiol. Scand.* 128(Suppl. 556): 129-136, 1986.

57. Sjöström, J. Friden, and B. Ekblom. Endurance, what is it? Muscle morphology after an extremely long distance run. *Acta Physiol. Scand.* 130: 513-520, 1987.

58. Tibbits, G.F. Regulation of myocardial contractility in exhaustive exercise. *Med. Sci. Sports Exerc.* 17(5): 529-537, 1985.

59. Tibbits, G.F. Cellular adaptations of skeletal muscle to prolonged work. *Can. J. Sport Sci.* 12(Suppl. 1): 265-325, 1982.

60. Vøllstad, N.K., O. Vaage, and L. Hermansen. Muscle glycogen depletion patterns in Type I and subgroups of Type II fibres during prolonged severe exercise in man. *Acta. Physiol. Scand.* 122: 441-443, 1984.

61. Vøllstad, N.K., and P.L.S. Blom. Effect of varying exercise intensity on glycogen depletion in human muscle fibres. *Acta Physiol. Scand.* 125: 395-405, 1985.

62. Vrbová , G., R. Navarrette, and M. Lowrie. Matching of muscle properties and motoneuron firing patterns during early stages of development. *J. Exp. Biol.* 115: 113-123, 1985.

63. Wyndham, C.H., G.G. Rogers, L.C. Senay, and D. Mitchell. Acclimatization in a hot, humid environment: Cardiovascular adjustments. *J. Appl. Physiol.* 40(5): 779-785, 1976.

Chapter 24

Effects of Exercise on Aspects of Carbohydrate, Fat, and Amino Acid Metabolism

Eric A. Newsholme

The physiology of exercise is a subject that has been well established for many years. It has been presented in several excellent texts and forms a part of the basic physiology that is taught to medical students. In contrast, it is only recently that the biochemistry of exercise could be considered sufficiently established to be classified as a separate subject. Perhaps not surprisingly, it is often treated as the "Cinderella" of the scientific approaches to exercise. This is unfortunate. In my opinion, knowledge of the biochemistry of exercise is of considerable importance not only for appreciating the health benefits of exercise but also to provide specific testable mechanisms to explain some, if not all, of the epidemiological observations concerning the health benefits and hazards of exercise. The enormous recent increase in the number of people who are participating in sports activities demands an answer to the question What are the *mechanisms* underlying the health benefits of exercise?

To understand the overall approaches to the question of the health benefits of exercise and exercise training in relation to carbohydrate, fat, and amino acid metabolism, the reader must be aware of the subject known as *metabolic control logic*. I believe that the application of metabolic control logic to problems and questions relating to exercise physiology, exercise biochemistry, and even exercise pathology has and will provide new insights and concepts to benefit our understanding of this fascinating subject.

The Maintenance of the ATP-ADP Concentration Ratio in Muscle

The dramatic changes that occur as a result of physical activity and training are designed primarily to maintain the constancy of the ATP-ADP level in the muscle despite dramatic changes in the rate of ATP turnover.

The energy that is required by almost every process in the cell is obtained from the hydrolysis of ATP as follows:

$$ATP^4 + H_2O \rightarrow ADP^{3-} + Pi^{2-} + H^+$$

It is, however, extremely important to appreciate that ATP does not function as a simple store of chemical energy in the cell. Its concentration in muscle is only 5-7 μ mol/g fresh muscle, which would be depleted in less than 1 s during intense muscular activity unless it were resynthesized at a rate equal to that of utilization. In combination with ADP, ATP functions as an energy transfer system in the cell. The generation of ATP from ADP during the oxidation of fuels (e.g., glucose) conserves chemical energy, which is utilized in a number of processes (including muscular contraction) (Figure 24.1). The ATP-ADP system couples the oxidative processes of the cell with the contractile process in such a way that the latter process is totally dependent on the former. Thus, when contractile activity is increased, the rate of fuel oxidation must also be increased. Furthermore, to avoid large transient changes in the ATP-ADP concentration ratio, the rate of fuel oxidation must be regulated rapidly and precisely according to the rate of ATP utilization by the contractile process. In sprinting, the rate of ATP turnover increases more than 1,000-fold, and even climbing stairs can increase it several hundred times (25, 26). However, the changes in the ATP-ADP concentration ratio during such activities are very small (Table 24.1).

The reason for this remarkable constancy of the ATP-ADP ratio may be to maintain what I call the

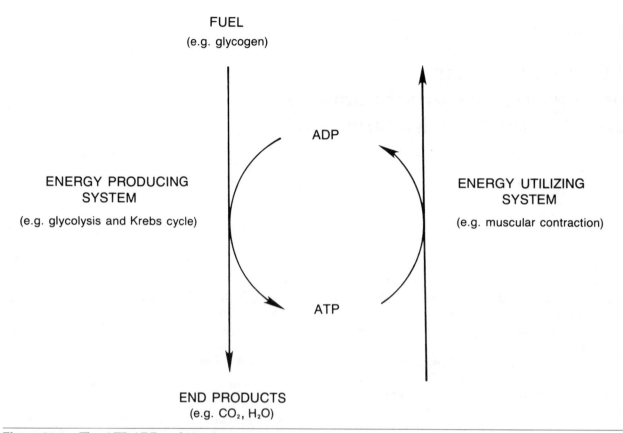

FUEL
(e.g. glycogen)

ENERGY PRODUCING
SYSTEM

(e.g. glycolysis and Krebs cycle)

ADP

ATP

ENERGY UTILIZING
SYSTEM

(e.g. muscular contraction)

END PRODUCTS
(e.g. CO_2, H_2O)

Figure 24.1. The ATP-ADP cycle in tissues.

Table 24.1 Contents of ATP, ADP, AMP, and Inorganic Phosphate After Sprinting to Exhaustion

| Metabolite | Content in muscle ($\mu mol \cdot g^{-1}$ fresh weight) | |
	Rest	After exhaustive sprinting
ATP	4.6	3.4
ADP	1.0	1.0
AMP	0.10	0.10
Pi	9.7	22.00

Note. Data are from Newsholme and Leech (26).

kinetic efficiency of the energy-producing and energy-utilizing processes in the muscle. Because ATP is chemically very similar to ADP, the catalytic site of enzymes that react with these nucleotides cannot always totally distinguish between them. This lack of complete discrimination manifests itself as competitive inhibition of the enzyme activity by one nucleotide in relation to the other. Thus, enzymes that utilize ADP as substrate are inhibited by ATP, and enzymes that utilize ATP as substrate are inhibited by ADP (Table 24.2). Consequently, if the intracellular ATP-ADP concentration ratio is increased, the activity of enzymes catalyzing the conversion of ADP into ATP would be inhibited, whereas if the ratio is decreased, the activity of enzymes catalyzing ATP utilization would be inhibited (Table 24.2). It is likely that small changes in this concentration ratio in the cell would cause only slight inhibition, but any reduction in the activity of enzymes catalyzing important regulatory reactions in the cell could reduce the rate of ATP formation, the performance of mechanical work, or both. In this way, the kinetic efficiency of energy transfer in the muscle would be reduced. If metabolic control mechanisms are ineffective for any reason, the rate of ATP production may not be controlled precisely in relation to the rate of ATP utilization, and thus changes in the ratio could occur, resulting in reduced kinetic efficiency. The significance of this can be indicated by the simple calculation that if the muscles of a sprinter understimulate glycolysis by only 10% during sprinting, in relation to the rate of ATP utilization, the concentration of ATP would be decreased by about 50% in 10 s and muscle function seriously im-

Table 24.2 Inhibition of ATP-Utilizing and ATP-Producing Enzymes by Their Nucleotide Products

Enzyme or process	Nucleotide substrate	Nucleotide inhibitor
Hexokinase	ATP	ADP
3-phosphoglycerate kinase	ADP	ATP
Pyruvate kinase	ADP	ATP
Creatine phosphokinase	ATP	ADP
Phosphoenol pyruvate carboxylase	GTP	GDP
Fatty acyl-CoA synthetase	ATP	ADP
Adenylate kinase	ATP	ADP
Actomyosin ATPase	ATP	ADP
Adenine nucleotide translocase	ADP	ATP

Note. For further information, see Newsholme and Leech (26).

paired. This is of obvious importance in the competitive athlete but is equally important in many other subjects and particularly in the elderly. An 80-yr-old may need to use almost all the maximum power output of the quadriceps to rise from a chair or a lavatory seat. Failure to generate sufficient ATP to do this will greatly affect the lifestyle of the elderly person (45).

Exercise, Exercise Training, and Carbohydrate Metabolism

Fatigue

Fatigue is the inability to maintain power output. It is as obvious in the Olympic champion running a 1,500-m race as it is in an elderly person attempting to climb stairs. Fatigue is a safety device that operates when one's conscious mind has rejected gentle hints of impending doom and switches off the power in order to prevent one's metabolic activities from causing irreversible damage to muscles and even to other organs, such as the brain. Physical fatigue affects each of us countless times during our lifetimes, and, unfortunately, the lifestyle of a patient may be dramatically influenced by fatigue. Knowledge of its basis is important therefore not only for athletics but for every aspect of life. And the question of how training influences fatigue is of obvious importance. In general, it is

possible to put forward five possible metabolic causes of fatigue:

1. A depletion of phosphocreatine in the muscle
2. An accumulation of lactic acid (protons) in muscle
3. A depletion of glycogen in the muscle
4. A depletion of the blood glucose level
5. A change in the concentration ratio of free tryptophan to branched-chain amino acids in the bloodstream

Of these points, only the second and the fifth are discussed in this chapter. Point 2 is discussed immediately below and Point 5 in the section on protein (for a detailed discussion, see refs. 25, 27).

Fatigue and the Accumulation of Lactic Acid

Lactic acid is so named because it is formed by the action of bacteria on milk sugar, or lactose. It is responsible for the sour taste of soured milk. Bacteria produce their lactic acid the same way that our muscles do and for the same reason, that is, to generate ATP in the absence of oxygen. Lactic acid causes problems because it is an acid. An acid can be defined as a compound that releases a hydrogen ion (also known as a proton) in water. This dissociation can be presented as

$$acid \rightarrow H^+ + base$$

where H^+ is the proton with the $^+$ signifying loss of an electron that is then gained by the base. In the case of lactic acid this dissociation becomes

$$lactic\ acid \rightarrow H^+ + lactate^-$$

When the athletic commentator graphically describes the sprint to the tape by saying that the athlete finishes in "a sea of lactic acid," it is not the lactic acid or the lactate but the protons that cause problems. Protons cause problems because they can associate with bases to produce acids. The bases in question are the enzymes that carry out all the chemical reactions in cells. Enzymes are proteins and, as such, bear a number of basic (as well as acidic) groups. Indeed, their catalytic activities depend on such groups, and these negative charges will disappear when they acquire protons. In a similar way, the proteins involved contraction itself (myosin and actin) may react with protons and in so doing lose their ability to form cross-bridges (i.e., lose their ability to contract).

How the acidity causes fatigue is not known, but several suggestions have been made (12, 13).

However, the mechanism of fatigue is of less importance to the athlete, the physician, or the normal subject than is how to overcome it or, more correctly, delay it. One answer to the proton problem lies in buffers. These are bases that mop protons up by combining with them but that, in so doing, cause no damage to the buffer:

$$buffer^- + H^+ \rightarrow buffer\text{-}H$$

The problem is that there is not much buffering capacity within the muscle. This is normally overcome by allowing the protons to leave the muscle and enter the blood. In athletics this is what happens in races longer than 100-200 m. Once in the blood, the protons encounter a much larger buffering system, one based on the hydrogencarbonate ion. This absorbs protons according to this equation:

$$HCO^- + H^+ \rightarrow H_2CO_3$$

Much the same happens when you take Alka-Seltzer or bicarbonate (sodium hydrogencarbonate) to reduce acidity in the stomach after overindulgence. The beauty of the hydrogencarbonate buffer is that the carbonic acid produced (H_2CO_3) readily decomposes into water and carbon dioxide, both of which are lost from the body through the lungs. This allows more carbonic acid to form and so extends the buffering capacity. An increase in blood acidity stimulates the rate of breathing so that yet more CO_2 is lost. This is the reason for the increased rate of breathing observed, for example, after running up stairs. (Hence, the rate of breathing is an excellent indication of the extent of the rate of anaerobic glycolysis; and for joggers it is advised not to run faster than a rate at which the runner can hold a conversation; that is, if breathing is too rapid to talk easily, you are relying too much on anaerobic metabolism for energy formation and should reduce the pace.) The main source of hydrogencarbonate ion in the blood is the kidneys, so that the kidneys and lungs work together in a push-pull system to rid the body of excess acid (protons).

The production of too much lactic acid is probably the cause of fatigue in many instances of normal activity. The person returning home from a job involving physical activity, the woman who has taken the dog for a walk, the man who has chopped logs for the fire, and the father who has played a few vigorous games with his children all suffer from the same cause of fatigue as does the Olympic 400-m champion: the accumulation of protons within the muscle.

Is knowledge of the cause of fatigue useful in suggesting ways of overcoming or reducing fatigue? The answer is yes. There are at least three means of decreasing the rate of proton accumulation in muscle: (a) The buffering capacity of muscle could be increased. (b) Because the oxidation of pyruvate to CO_2 and H_2O in the Krebs cycle uses protons, encouraging the oxidative processes in muscle would decrease proton accumulation. (c) The protons could be transferred more quickly from the muscles to the bloodstream, where they could be buffered by the blood bicarbonate system, which has a very high capacity. Fortunately, the latter two suggestions can be put readily into practice. An aerobic physical training program will increase not only the oxidative capacity in the muscle but also the number of capillaries; the presence of the latter will encourage the transport of protons out of the muscle into the bloodstream for extracellular buffering. A simple, gentle, but gradual and regular aerobic training program should be enormously beneficial in increasing the aerobic system of the muscle and hence reducing fatigue from proton accumulation.

There is evidence that the aerobic capacity of muscle decreases in most sedentary individuals with age, especially in early to middle old age (45). This lowers the threshold for fatigue in such individuals. If such an individual also suffered from a partial defect in one of the enzymes of the Krebs cycle or of the electron transfer chain, the effect of aging on decreasing the aerobic capacity would be most marked. This would place an even greater demand on the anaerobic system for ATP production, so that even gentle physical activity would need to utilize the anaerobic systems with the consequent rapid accumulation of protons and hence rapid fatigue. Unfortunately, if such a person repeatedly presents to the physician with a history of becoming fatigued easily but shows no signs of muscular or cardiovascular disease, he or she may well be referred to a psychiatrist. But is the patient really suffering from a psychiatric disturbance? Or is it a case of fatigue due to proton accumulation in the muscles? The patient might require a gradual and regular aerobic training program that would increase the aerobic capacity of muscle such that the energy demands of light exercise could be supported with a lower rate of lactic acid formation and hence could occur with less fatigue.

Effects of Exercise and Exercise Training on Glucose Metabolism and Its Possible Relation to Diabetes Mellitus

Exercise increases the rate of utilization of all metabolic fuels. In addition, it reduces the glycogen content of both the liver and the muscle. The latter may result in an increase in the activity of the glycogen synthase and thus reduce the requirement for insulin in the stimulation of glycogen synthesis after a carbohydrate meal (18). In addition, it has been shown that in normal subjects, endurance training markedly increases insulin sensitivity, so that very much lower concentrations of insulin are required to control the blood glucose concentration after an oral glucose load (Table 24.3). If these findings can be extrapolated to the diabetic patient (Type 1), much smaller doses of injected insulin should be adequate for control in the endurance-trained patient; moreover, any re-

maining beta-cell function could play a larger role in control of the blood glucose concentration and hence minimize the variations in blood glucose concentration. For this reason, studies are being carried out to identify a possible exercise factor that might be responsible for this improvement in sensitivity. There is no doubt that a single bout of exercise produces a factor that increases the sensitivity of glucose utilization of skeletal muscle to insulin, but the evidence in experimental animals is that it is very short-lived (possibly only for a few hours). However, exercise training increases the sensitivity of glucose utilization by isolated muscle to insulin for more than 48 hr but probably less than 72 hr (in the rat) (Table 24.4). The mechanism underlying this longer term effect may be very important. Further work regarding the identity of the factor responsible for the prolonged increase in insulin sensitivity after exercise training could provide information leading to the production of novel

Table 24.3 Effect of Training in Humans on the Response of Plasma Glucose and Insulin Levels to Oral Glucose

Subject	Compound	Time after glucose is ingested (min)	30	60	90	120	Summation
Normal middle-aged subjects	Glucose (mM)	3.5	6.7	6.0	4.7	3.8	27.7
	Insulin (μunits/ml)	10	79	95	96	55	337
Athletic middle-aged subjects	Glucose (mM)	4.0	5.9	4.4	3.8	4.2	22.3
	Insulin (μunits/ml)	22	32	34	24	21	112

The "Plasma concentration" spans the columns from "Time after glucose is ingested (min)" through "Summation".

Note. For a review of the details, see Newsholme and Leech (26).

Table 24.4 Values of EC_{50} for Insulin for Stimulation of Glucose Conversion to Lactate (Lactate Formation) and Glycogen Synthesis in Isolated Incubated Sprint-Trained and Endurance-Trained Rats

Condition	EC_{50} for insulin (μunit/ml) Endurance training		EC_{50} for insulin (μunit/ml) Sprint training	
	Lactate formation	Glycogen synthesis	Lactate formation	Glycogen synthesis
Control	122	82	122	82
24 h after exercise	3.2	24	100	70
48 h after exercise	19	20	101	132
72 h after exercise	89	72	. . .	. . .

Note. For details of this approach, see Newsholme et al. (28).

hypoglycemic agents. At present there are very few effective hypoglycemic agents.

In addition, it must be appreciated that insulin can affect control of the blood glucose level through effects other than stimulating glucose utilization by skeletal muscle, particularly through an effect on fatty acid mobilization from adipose tissue. The significance of fatty acid in relation to control of the blood sugar level follows.

Exercise and the Glucose/Fatty Acid Cycle

If the concentration of ATP in the muscle fiber falls below a preset level (as it will when muscle contraction commences), a series of events takes place to increase the catalytic activity of key enzymes in glycolysis. These are the enzymes that have previously limited the flux. Conversely, a rise in ATP concentration will reduce the flow rate. Such negative feedback serves to maintain the concentration of ATP within narrow limits despite very large changes in its rate of utilization. In the present context, the important point is that fatty acid oxidation increases the effectiveness of ATP as a feedback inhibitor of glycolysis, and hence glucose and glycogen utilization are decreased. This control interrelationship between carbohydrate and fatty acid is known as the *glucose/fatty acid cycle* (26). An important feature of this control is noteworthy. Because the rate of fatty acid oxidation is determined by the fatty acid concentration in the blood, which in turn is determined by the rate of fatty acid release from adipose tissue, it follows that this latter process can actually exert some control over the rate of carbohydrate utilization in the body. The significance of this is that exercise training may increase the sensitivity of adipose tissue lipolysis to insulin. This probably improves the ability of the subject to control the fatty acid level and therefore the blood glucose level.

Effects of Exercise and Exercise Training on Fat Metabolism

The body always has a demand for energy, which is normally met by the food we eat. However, eating is not a continuous process, so the body must store energy for use between meals, during more prolonged starvation, or when a large amount of extra energy is needed, as in endurance running. The two main energy stores in the human body are glycogen, which is stored in muscle and the liver, and fat, which is stored in adipose tissue. Each store has its own function.

The major storage fuel in humans is fat, which is composed of triglyceride molecules. A triglyceride molecule consists of glycerol, to which three fatty acid units are attached by ester links. Although several kinds of fatty acid occur in triglyceride, all have a similar structure, differing only in the number of carbon atoms (from 16 to 22) and in the number of double bonds present. Fatty acids with more than one double bond are polyunsaturated. The major store of triglyceride is in adipose tissue, which is composed of cells called *adipocytes*, each of which contains a large droplet of triglyceride that occupies about 90% of the volume of the cell. Unlike most other tissues, adipose tissue does not form a discrete organ but is widely distributed throughout the body. However, the precise significance of the distribution of the major fat reserves of the body in many different depots throughout the body is still unclear (32, 33, 34, 35).

The hydrolysis of triglyceride to glycerol and fatty acids occurs within the adipocyte and is catalyzed by the enzyme triglyceride lipase, which is present in each adipose tissue cell. The fatty acids cross the cell membrane of the adipocyte to enter the blood, in which they are carried to the muscle or other tissue. The transport of fatty acids poses a problem because they are not very soluble in the blood plasma. The problem is overcome by binding the fatty acid molecule to the plasma protein albumin. The binding is fairly tight, but, as the blood passes through a working muscle, the fatty acid-albumin complex dissociates into albumin and fatty acids, and the latter diffuse into the muscle fiber. This occurs because the concentration of fatty acids within the muscle is very low because of their being removed by the process of oxidation. A series of enzymes acting sequentially oxidize the fatty acids to form acetyl-CoA. This process is called beta-oxidation. Acetyl-CoA enters the Krebs cycle for complete oxidation.

Physical training increases the ability to hydrolyze triacylglycerol and hence the rate of release of fatty acids from the adipose tissue. But, in particular, it increases the ability of muscle to remove fatty acids from the bloodstream and increases the capacity of the beta-oxidation process (26). These effects of training have several important roles that may provide substantial health benefits.

Fatty Acids and Sudden Death

The number of reports of fatalities that occurred either during or after exercise has increased, and these are highlighted by those who are anxious to prove not only that exercise does little good but that it is positively harmful. However, a detailed investigation into deaths occurring in joggers in the state of Rhode Island indicates that jogging is not particularly dangerous (41). Unfortunately, this may not be the case for squash (29). But there is an important difference between squash and jogging. The latter depends on aerobic metabolism ("marathon" metabolism) for energy formation, whereas the former depends mainly on anaerobic metabolism ("sprinting" metabolism). The concentrations of the stress hormones adrenaline and noradrenaline are raised during exercise, and this will result in the mobilization of fatty acids from adipose tissues so that the blood fatty acid concentration increases. High concentrations of fatty acids can damage cell membranes, increase the stickiness of platelets and hence the risk of thrombosis, and (especially in the hypoxic heart) interfere with the normal electrical activity of the heart (26, 39). In addition, the catecholamines can cause metabolic changes in the heart that may also increase the risk of arrhythmias (30). In games such as squash, the plasma fatty acid concentration will be increased because of the raised levels of catecholamines, but the short bursts of explosive activity that are characteristic of this sport use mainly anaerobic metabolism to generate the ATP; hence, little fatty acid will be used. Also, the stress of competition could lead to a further elevation in the plasma fatty acid concentration. Problems arise when the concentration of plasma fatty acid exceeds that which can be transported in combination with the carrier protein albumin (about 2 mM), because then the concentration of plasma free fatty acids increases particularly and can cause the problems indicated previous (26, 39). Fatty acids are used as a fuel for muscle primarily during sustained exercise, but most ball games involve short, sharp, and explosive bursts of activity, the energy for which is obtained from the breakdown of phosphocreatine and the glycogen conversion to lactic acid. Hence, the rate of fatty acid oxidation is not increased markedly in such games and thus may increase to exceed the safe level in the blood. The stress of competition (amnifested as aggression toward the opposition) will also increase the concentrations of circulating the stress hormones, and this will further increase the fatty acid level.

It follows from this explanation that those undertaking aerobic exercise (e.g., jogging, cycling, swimming, and rowing) and especially aerobic training are not subject to the same risks because the rate of fatty acid mobilization is possibly less

rapid and the rate of fatty acid utilization by muscles greater than in games such as squash. Because aging decreases the diameter of the coronary arteries due to atherosclerosis, aerobic exercise is recommended for the middle-aged or older person and especially for the middle-aged person with Type A personality who may be very competitive in such ball games. The combination of limited coronary flow plus high levels of circulating stress hormones and fatty acids may be very dangerous in the middle-aged male (26).

The problems caused by high levels of fatty acids in the blood are not restricted to those individuals participating in sports. In primitive humans and in animals in the wild it is easy to see the benefits of increased fuel mobilization under stressful circumstances in the fight-or-flight response to stress. But in modern humans, who have recently evolved far faster socially than they have biologically, stress-inducing situations are usually very different. These may include driving in heavy traffic, discussing a contentious issue in committee, or even watching a certain television program. The important point is that although all these can raise the blood fatty acid concentration, none is followed by exercise that will consume the fuel. The concentration therefore may remain elevated for extended periods. In a normally sedentary middle-aged person, the increase in the fatty acid concentration during stress may be much greater, thus increasing the likelihood of platelet aggregation, arrhythmias, and heart failure. This provides a plausible explanation for heart attacks that strike down otherwise healthy men during or immediately after stressful situations. In some circumstances this can put others at risk, for example, if the pilot of an airliner is incapacitated by a heart attack during takeoff or landing, both of which are highly stressful conditions. Although there are a number of reports of pilots being incapacitated by a heart attack (26), perhaps the best known is the crash of the British European Airways Trident soon after takeoff on June 18, 1972. A postmortem on the pilot showed severe atherosclerosis in the coronary arteries and evidence of a previous minor infarction. Despite this, the official report indicated that, Captain Key seemed a picture of robust good health, and he was passed fit to fly after a medical examination in November 1971 (26).

Of particular relevance to the present discussion is that an hour and a half before takeoff, Captain Key had been involved in an altercation in the crew room over whether pilots should take strike action in support of a claim for higher salaries. Captain Key was directly involved in a heated argument and was reported to be very angry. I suggest that this was a stress condition that may have lasted for most of the period before takeoff and would have been extended by the preflight preparation and the takeoff itself. The official report concludes that Captain Key had a heart attack during takeoff but that the attack did not cause total incapacitation. However, it considers that Captain Key was suffering from pain and malaise, which would have impaired his judgment and his mental faculties. Thus, the aircraft failed to maintain sufficient speed, and the droops (retractable leading-edge high-lift devices) were retracted too early during the takeoff. This produced a stall and resulted in the crash. Did the stress of the preflight argument contribute to the heart attack by raising the fatty acid concentration in the blood above the safe limit of 2 mM (26)?

One of the greatest benefits of regular aerobic exercise may be to increase the capacity of skeletal muscles to use fatty acids as a fuel and so reduce the time their concentration remains elevated even when there is no opportunity for exercise. Nonetheless, my advice is that the daily run should, if possible, be delayed until after a stress period (e.g., after a difficult committee meeting). In this way, any excess fatty acids will be removed readily by the increased rate of fuel oxidation.

Exercise, Fat Mobilization, Substrate Cycles, and Weight Control

There is much controversy in scientific literature about the development of obesity and its prevention and treatment.

Garrow (10) reviewed 13 publications covering 1,481 subjects in whom weight, energy intake, and physical activity were measured. He failed to find any convincing evidence that obese people ate more or exercised less than did thin people. He concluded that there are large errors in measuring these values that make measurement incapable of identifying the reason for a small imbalance between energy intake and output necessary to cause obesity. Thus, the magnitude of energy imbalance leading to obesity is small in comparison to the range of variation of energy intake and expenditure within a group of individuals. Also, one cannot assume that alteration in any two components of the following equation will leave the third unaffected, according to Garrow (10):

$$\text{Change in energy stores} = \text{energy input} - \text{energy output}$$

Garrow provides valid criticism of investigators who fail to find the cause of obesity in the variable they are studying and then infer that it can be safely ascribed to some factor they have not measured.

Obesity is a syndrome that is characterized by an excessive amount of adipose tissue. This excess may be caused by adipocyte expansion (hypertrophy) or adipocyte hypercellularity, an example of the heterogeneity of obesity.

Adipocyte hypercellularity predisposes the individual to obesity. Sjöström (38) has cited new evidence that adipocyte hyperplasia can occur in adulthood; it may be that adipocyte numbers can only increase. This means that weight gain may irreversibly increase adipocyte numbers.

The major question to be answered is How does an excess of energy intake above energy expenditure cause obesity to develop in some subjects and not in others? Adipocytes provide the major energy storage compartment of the body. Excess dietary energy intake may be converted to triacylglycerol for storage in adipocytes causing their hypertrophy. But how is the hyperplasia stimulated? We do not know.

Energy intake is thought to be closely controlled by two antagonistic behavioral responses that originate in the hypothalamus: satiety and hunger. Garrow (10, p. 76) states that "in man control of food intake is complex, and primitive hypothalamic reflexes are so buried under so many layers of conditioning, cognitive and social factors that they are barely discernible."

It is possible that control of dietary energy intake is important in the control of body weight. But is there any evidence that this control is improved by exercise or exercise-training? Of course, there is much anecdotal evidence that exercise increases hunger, and this may lead to the ingestion of more-than-normal amounts of food. However, it is possible that a regular depletion and refilling of some energy stores during regular training may improve the sensitivity of the hunger and satiety centers with, consequently, improved control of food intake. This problem does not appear to have been examined systematically.

Energy Expenditure

The major factors responsible for energy expenditure are the basal metabolic rate; physical activity; and dietary-, exercise-, or stress-induced thermogenesis.

Basal metabolic rate undergoes a diurnal cycle. This must be remembered when carrying out experiments regarding energy expenditure at different time periods of the day. In humans, energy expenditure increases during the morning and in the early afternoon.

The basal metabolic rate represents energy expenditure under conditions of relaxation after a 12-hr fast at thermoneutrality. It represents 50%-60% of a human's daily energy expenditure and is related to the fat-free tissue mass.

Obese individuals have a higher absolute basal metabolic rate in comparison to lean individuals because they also have a larger amount of lean body mass as well as fat. There does not appear to be any alteration in the magnitude of basal metabolic rate per gram of lean body mass in the obese as opposed to the lean individual, so obesity may be dependent on changes in the response of dietary-, exercise-, or stress-induced thermogenesis. The biochemical basis for increasing thermogenesis must be determined if we are to understand the development of obesity. One important thermogenic process that until recently has largely been ignored in relation to its potential contribution to thermogenesis is substrate (so-called futile) cycling.

Substrate Cycles

Substrate cycles are composed of two nonequilibrium reactions that occur in reverse directions. They have the necessary capacity and biological variability to be responsible for considerable energy dissipation, although their primary role is considered to be metabolic regulation.

It is possible for a reaction that is nonequilibrium in the forward direction of a pathway (i.e., A → B) to be opposed by a reaction that is nonequilibrium in the reverse direction of the pathway (i.e., B → A):

$$\overset{E_1}{S} \rightarrow \overset{E_2}{A} \underset{E_5}{\overset{E_3}{\rightleftharpoons}} B \overset{E_4}{\rightarrow} P \rightarrow$$

The reactions must be chemically distinct, and consequently they will be catalyzed by different enzymes (i.e., E_2 and E_5 in the equation). It is possible that these two opposing reactions are components of two separate pathways that function under different conditions. However, the reverse reaction (E_5) may not be part of any pathway and may be present in the cell only to provide a cycle for metabolic control.

If the two enzymes are simultaneously active, A will be converted to B, and B will be converted back to A, thus constituting the substrate cycle. Thus, there are two fluxes: a linear flux converting S to P and a cyclical flux between A and B. Both fluxes are largely independent, and calculations show that the improvement in sensitivity is greatest when the cyclical flux is high but the linear flux is low (i.e., the ratio of cycling rate to flux is high) (23, 24).

The role of a cycle can best be understood when it is appreciated that, in some conditions, an enzyme activity may have to be reduced to values closely approaching zero. This would require that the concentration of an activator be reduced to almost zero or that of an inhibitor to an almost infinite level. Such enormous changes in concentration probably never occur in living organisms because they would be difficult if not impossible to achieve and would cause osmotic and ionic problems and unwanted side reactions. However, the net flux through a reaction can be reduced to very low values (approaching zero) by means of a substrate cycle. Thus, as the product of the forward enzyme (E_2) is produced (i.e., B in the previous equation), it is converted back to substrate A by the reverse enzyme (E_5). The mechanism can be viewed as a means of decreasing the concentration of B and hence the rate of E_3 to very small values, whereas the concentration of A would be higher than expected for the net flux from A to B. In other words, the net flux (i.e., A to B) is very low despite a finite activity of the forward enzyme and a moderate concentration of an activator. Now, if the concentration of this activator is increased by only a small amount above that at which the activities of the two enzymes are almost identical (and the flux is almost zero), the activity of E_2 will increase so that the net flux through the reaction will increase from almost zero to a moderate rate. Such a cycle therefore provides a large improvement in sensitivity; indeed, it can be seen as a means of producing a threshold (or almost-threshold) response with a simple metabolic system.

Because in the substrate cycle both reactions are nonequilibrium, it is not possible to operate even one turn of the cycle without conversion of chemical energy into heat. Usually, this comes about by the hydrolysis of ATP to ADP and phosphate because ATP is involved as a substrate in one reaction. Hence, the net result of the cycle is the hydrolysis of ATP. For a considerable number of years it was considered that this loss of energy was too high a price to pay and that metabolic control would ensure that such apparently energetically wasteful cycles would not occur. Such cycles are sometimes referred to as futile cycles; but there is now considerable evidence to show that these cycles do exist (28) and that the remarkable improvement in sensitivity provided by the cycles justifies the metabolic cost to the organism; that is, they are not futile! Indeed, substrate cycles may operate not only to regulate flux through metabolic pathways but also to achieve the controlled conversion of chemical energy (i.e., ATP) into heat to maintain body temperature, to raise the temperature (pyrexia), or to reduce body mass by burning off fuel (i.e., weight control) (24, 28). The advantage of such cycles may be their relative simplicity, the marked improvement in sensitivity in metabolic control they can provide, and their flexibility. Thus, a number of hormones may influence metabolic processes by changing the rate of substrate cycles.

Hormones and Substrate Cycling

It is usually considered that hormones change flux through a pathway by modifying the activity of an enzyme or a transport system that forms part of that pathway. However, rather than modifying the flux directly, some hormones may increase the sensitivity of metabolic control so that a given change in a metabolic regulator (or another secondary messenger) will have a greater (or perhaps smaller) effect on the flux. One way in which a hormone could change sensitivity is to change the rate of substrate cycling, as the sensitivity to a given change in the concentration of a regulator depends on the ratio of cycling rate to pathway flux. This change in cycling rate may be achieved by covalent modification of the two enzymes that constitute the cycle; that is, both enzymes will be regulated by an interconversion cycle (26) or the second messenger for the hormone may affect the activity of the two enzymes equally. Hormones that may be involved in changing markedly the rate of substrate cycling include catecholamines and thyroxine. Catecholamines are known to increase the rate of cycling between triacylglycerol and fatty acids in adipose and perhaps other tissues (see the following discussion).

Specific Substrate Cycles and Their Involvement in Thermogenesis

The triglyceride/fatty acid cycle consists of the processes of lipolysis of triglyceride and esterification of fatty acids (26). This cycle comprises a larger number of reactions than does the cycle described previously; and one turn of the cycle results in the hydrolysis of eight molecules of ATP to ADP and phosphate. Evidence for the existence of this cycle in adipose tissue has been recognized for many years (40). Indeed, in 1959 it was observed that adrenaline increased the rate of glucose incorporation into triglyceride-glycerol without any change in the rate of fatty acid synthesis (17). This indicates an increase in the rate of this substrate cycle. It has been established that the rate of this cycle is increased in isolated adipose tissue of the rat by both adrenaline and glucagon and furthermore that, in vivo, animals fed or injected with beta-receptor agonists show higher rates of this cycle in adipose tissue (4). Furthermore, this increase in cycling rate was inhibited by the beta blocker propranolol. It is suggested that this increase in cycling rate in vivo improves the sensitivity of the triglyceride/fatty acid cycle to changes in the insulin concentration so that the rate of lipolysis can be inhibited and the rate of esterification increased precisely to accommodate the requirements for storage of energy after feeding and for mobilization of fatty acids for provision of fuel for muscle during exercise. There is now considerable evidence that the rate of this cycle varies under different conditions (8, 11); it has also been demonstrated to be of importance in humans (42, 43, 44, R. Bahr, personal communication, July, 1989, R.R. Wolfe, personal communication, July 1988).

There is now direct evidence that the rates of at least two cycles are increased under conditions when improved metabolic sensitivity in metabolic control is considered to be required and (of importance for this review) when thermogenesis is known to be increased. The evidence is summarized as follows:

1. The rates of the fructose 6-phosphate/fructose bisphosphate (F6P/FBP) cycle in rat muscle in vitro and the triacylglycerol/fatty acid (TG/FFA) cycle in white and brown adipose tissue in the rat and mouse in vivo are increased by beta-adrenoceptor agonists. The maximum increase in the rate of the former cycle in response to adrenaline is about tenfold, and the increases in the rate of the latter cycle in white and brown adipose tissue of the mouse in response to noradrenaline are about threefold and fivefold, respectively (28).

2. Feeding increases the rate of the TG/FFA cycle in white adipose tissue of the rat and mouse by at least twofold, and this increase is completely inhibited by the beta-adreno-

ceptor antagonist propranolol; the cycling is also increased by exercise in hampsters (36); starvation of the donor animal decreases by 50% the rate of the F6P/FBP cycle in isolated muscle. In muscles isolated from exercised rats (90 min running at about 50% $\dot{V}O_2$max on a treadmill), the rate of the cycle is increased twofold in comparison to muscle isolated from sedentary animals (28).

3. Exposure to cold increases the rates of the F6P/FBP cycle in muscle and the TG/FFA cycle in white and brown adipose tissue by more than twofold (28).

4. Hyperthyroidism increases the rate of glycolytic substrate cycles in the liver of rats (14) and humans (37) and increases the sensitivity of the F6P/FBP cycle in skeletal muscle to catecholamine stimulation (6). The hypothyroid state is generally associated with reduced rates of substrate cycling.

The view that increased rates of cycling may play some part in heat generation in vivo is strongly supported by the previous findings, as increased cycling rates correlate with increased levels of catecholamines or increased sympathetic drive, both of which are known to result in increased rates of thermogenesis. Furthermore, conditions that increase thermogenesis also increase substrate cycling rates and vice versa; for example, feeding increases energy expenditure (the thermic effect of food), and starvation decreases it.

In recent systematic studies it has been demonstrated that oxygen consumption is elevated for as long as 24 hr after cessation of exercise, and it is known that the plasma level of adrenaline is elevated for a considerable period of time after exercise (19). Although it would be incorrect to assume that increased rates of substrate cycling are responsible for all the increased energy expenditure under conditions of raised catecholamine levels (i.e., feeding, postexercise, and cold exposure), the fact that rates of cycling are increased in all these conditions and are decreased in starvation does suggest that they will play some role. Furthermore, these cycles have been demonstrated in both muscle and in white and brown adipose tissue, and it has been established in both humans and experimental animals that catecholamines increase the rate of oxygen consumption in all these tissues. At present, the quantity of heat generated from increased rates of cycling cannot be precisely indicated for at least two reasons. First, many substrate cycles exist (26), and it is not known how many may be stimulated by catecholamines. Second, much higher rates of

cycling and hence thermogenesis may occur in vivo rather than in preparations such as isolated muscles and hepatocytes in vitro.

I believe that these recent findings present prima facie evidence that increased rates of substrate cycles could play a role in the increased rate of heat generation when the plasma concentrations of catecholamines, sympathetic drive, or both are raised. It is tempting to speculate that the increased metabolic rate and the elevated temperature sometimes seen after trauma may also be due to increased rates of substrate cycles. The increased cycling rate would provide improved sensitivity for control of some key processes during the increased metabolism that occurs after injury (42).

Recently, evidence has been presented that demonstrated that TG/FFA substrate cycling rate in nonobese human subjects is elevated in the fasted state (43). Furthermore, the sensitivity of lipolysis to catecholamines is increased in fasted nonobese and obese human subjects, and it has been proposed that the enhancement in sensitivity is due to increased rates of TG/FFA cycling in the fasted state (43).

In addition, evidence has been obtained for a role for the TG/FFA substrate cycle in the fasting-refeeding transition. Infusion of glucose into overnight-fasted human subjects suppressed lipolysis and significantly increased TG/FFA substrate cycling in adipose tissue (44).

The Effect of Exercise on Adipocyte Hyperplasia and Hypertrophy

Oscai et al. (31) carried out an experiment to determine the effects of exercise on adipose tissue cellularity. Male Wistar rats were used and randomly divided into three groups, each composed of rats of approximately the same starting weight. Group A swam for 23 wk and then remained sedentary for a further 34 wk. Group B were sedentary for all 62 wk but were of paired weight throughout the experiment with Group A, whereas Group C were sedentary and allowed to eat ad libitum.

The rats that had swum had a lower weight than did the sedentary, freely eating controls. This weight difference was on average 62 g and was due to a smaller body content of fat in swimming subjects. The exercised animals had significantly lighter epididymal fat pads because of a decreased cell number.

Thus, exercise may, by modifying the rate of cellular proliferation in adipose tissue, reduce the rate of fat accumulation in later life, resulting in a decreased final body weight. The mechanism by which exercise modifies adipose tissue cell numbers in animals remains unknown. Pond et al. (32) have shown that exercise of the guinea pig affects the adipose tissue cell volume in several different depots in the animal but not the number of adipocytes.

Patients with moderate obesity and with enlarged adipocytes are the group of choice for physical training as an aid for weight reduction. Sustained exercise will stimulate the catalytic activity of triacylglycerol lipase within the adipose tissue during the exercise. In addition, exercise has been shown to increase the rate of the triacylglycerol/fatty acid cycle in the adipose tissue of humans (R.R. Wolfe, personal communication, July, 1988). The quantitative significance of this cycle in expending energy after exercise, especially in subjects with enlarged adipocytes, remains to be determined.

The importance of exercise as a means of obesity treatment is controversial because there may be an associated stimulation of appetite. This causes increased energy intake and output. Consequently, energy intake restriction plus a physical activity program may well be necessary to control obesity.

Exercise, Amino Acids, Fatigue, and Mood

Most participants in endurance exercise will claim that the activity provides a feeling of well-being, an improvement in mood, and an overall feeling of tiredness and exhaustion that usually results in a good night's sleep. The improvement of mood is so much a part of the current running boom that the phenomenon of the so-called runner's high has become popular to talk about. Mandell (20) has described the runner's high graphically as follows:

Thirty minutes out, and something lifts. The fatigue goes away and the feelings of power begin. . . . Then sometime in the second hour comes the spooky time. Colours are bright and beautiful, water sparkles, clouds breathe, and my body swimming detaches from the earth. . . . A cosmic view and peace are located between six and ten miles of running.

It is interesting to compare this with the description of the feelings after transcendental meditation described by Lamott (16):

The sunlight seemed brighter. . . . The colours of the trees and of the cars driving by and the clothes of the people . . . all seemed more intense. The air seemed clearer and more invigorating. I felt as if it was the first day of spring after a long cold grey winter.

Does the similarity of these phrases suggest that there may be a common basis to the runner's high and the claimed benefits of meditation? And can a biochemical mechanism be suggested?

There is now considerable experimental evidence suggesting that exercise can lead to mood elevation in normal subjects and can have an antidepressant effect in clinically depressed patients. The extent of the improvement in mood in normal subjects after exercise correlated well with the level of physical fitness (9). A decrease in the extent of depression due to exercise has been reported both for students (5) and for older subjects (22).

In these and other studies it has been shown that exercise has a positive benefit on mood even if the subjects are exercised individually. This finding suggests that group participation is not the mechanism underlying the mood elevation. Other explanations of mood improvement include taking time away from worrisome responsibilities or increased social interaction. However, some studies (5) have demonstrated that the antidepressant effects of exercise appear to be dependent to a large extent on the intensity and duration of the physical activity, suggesting that exercise per se is responsible for the effect. Furthermore, the sports with the greatest opportunity for social interaction, such as softball, had the smallest benefit. An intriguing question, therefore, is whether the effect of exercise on mood, general tiredness, and exhaustion are biochemically related.

One hypothesis has been generally accepted by the mass media. The feeling of well-being following exercise has been linked to the increased plasma levels of endorphin (3, 21). However, there is no evidence that the level of endorphins in the brain is raised during or after exercise; because endorphins do not cross the blood-brain barrier, it is not correct to conclude that a raised plasma level is indicative of a raised brain level. Furthermore, administration of the opiate antagonist naloxone does not prevent the improvement in mood caused by exercise (21). Assuming that the naloxone had blocked all the endorphin receptors, this result suggests that changes in endorphin levels are unrelated to changes in mood. The possibility that this change in mood is related not to endorphins but to changes in the concentrations of monoamines in the brain is explored in the following discussion.

It is generally considered that none of the reactions in the pathway for formation of the neurotransmitter 5-hydroxytryptamine in the brain approach saturation with pathway substrate. These reactions include transport of tryptophan across the blood-brain barrier, transport across the cell membrane into the presynaptic nerve terminal, and hydroxylation of tryptophan by tryptophan 5-hydroxylase and finally decarboxylation by L-amino acid decarboxylase. Hence, an increase in the plasma level of tryptophan should lead to an increase in the brain concentration of tryptophan, which could lead to an increase in the rate of formation and hence an increase in the concentration of 5-hydroxytryptamine in the brain (25, 26). Furthermore, because the transport process, which is responsible for the entry of tryptophan and tyrosine across the blood-brain barrier, also transports the branched-chain amino acids into the brain, competition for entry can occur. Therefore, increases in plasma concentration ratios of tryptophan to branched-chain amino acids, tryptophan to phenylalanine, and tyrosine plus branched-chain amino acids or aromatic amino acids to branched-chain amino acids could lead to an increase in the rate of entry of tryptophan into the brain and hence in the concentration of tryptophan; the latter should cause an increase in the rate of formation and hence in the concentration of 5-hydroxytryptamine. There is evidence that an increase in this latter neurotransmitter can result in sleep (26), so that it might also cause a decrease in mental alertness or cause fatigue (central fatigue), and changes in different areas of the brain could result in mood changes. One further observation is particularly relevant to the present discussion. Whereas most amino acids are taken up and metabolized by the liver, branched-chain amino acids are taken up primarily by muscle, and their rate of removal by muscle may increase with physical activity (25, 26). Exercise may therefore increase the rate of branched-chain amino acid utilization by muscle and hence may lower the plasma concentration of branched-chain amino acids. This will therefore increase the plasma concentration ratios indicated above and hence may influence the rate of tryptophan entry into the brain.

Initial experiments to provide prima facie evidence for this hypothesis have been carried out. The concentrations of tryptophan plus the branched-chain amino acids in the plasma of human volunteers after various forms of exercise have been measured; the changes are consistent with the previously discussed hypothesis (Table 24.5).

In addition, it must be noted that a considerable part of the tryptophan in the plasma is bound to albumin, and, in my opinion, it is the free, not the total, concentration of tryptophan that controls the uptake of this amino acid by the brain (2, 15). The proportion of tryptophan that is bound to albumin can be decreased (i.e., the free concentration can be increased) by raising the concentration of long-chain fatty acids. Because the plasma fatty acid concentration is known to be increased by sustained exercise, this should lead to an increase in the plasma free concentration of tryptophan; this has been shown to occur in rats (7) and in humans (1). In volunteers in the Stockholm Marathon, the concentration ratio of free tryptophan to branched-chain amino acids is increased threefold by the 42.2-km run (Table 24.5). In my opinion, because the free concentration will compete with other amino acids for entry into the brain, the brain

Table 24.5   Effect of Marathon Run on the Plasma Levels of Glucose, Fatty Acid, Branched-Chain Amino Acids, and Free Plus Total Tryptophan

Condition	Plasma levels (μmol/L or *mmol/L)					
	Glucose*	Fatty acid	Branched-chain amino acids	Total tryptophan	Free tryptophan	Ratio of free tryptophan to branched-chain amino acids
Preexercise	4.4	380	470	55	7.7	0.016
Postexercise	4.0	1,560*	380*	57	19.0*	0.050

Note. Data are from Blomstrand et al. (1).

*Indicates a statistically significant difference.

tryptophan concentration may be increased by this change in ratio of the concentrations of amino acids.

Because this area of research is very recent, the effects of exercise training on the levels of brain neurotransmitters are not known. However, it is possible to speculate that regular aerobic exercise will maintain the capacity of muscle to take up branched-chain amino acids and hence maintain the ability of muscle to influence, perhaps markedly, the plasma amino acid concentration ratio of free tryptophan to branched-chain amino acids.

Conclusion

From this discussion, there would seem to be no doubt that exercise has beneficial effects. These effects may be particularly beneficial in a modern, stressful society. The changes in lifestyle of the last 30-40 yr in the industrialized nations have been such as to encourage the rapid development of diseases such as atherosclerosis, coronary heart disease, cancer, and diabetes mellitus. This may be due in part to misuse of our bodies by smoking, overeating, poor diet, and physical inactivity. This misuse is elegantly encapsulated in the words of Shakespeare (*Richard II*, act 3) writing about the death of kings, but his words apply equally well and directly to civilized, unfit, nonexercised, overweight, smoking, modern humans:

> for within the hollow crown
> That rounds the mortal temples of a king
> Keeps Death his court, and there the antic sits,
> Scoffing his state and grinning at his pomp,
> Allowing him a breath, a little scene,
> To monarchize, be fear'd, and kill with looks;
> Infusing him with self and vain conceit,
> As if this flesh which walls about our life
> Were brass impregnable; and, humour'd thus,
> Comes at the last, and with a little pin
> Bores through his castle wall, and farewell king!

References

1. Blomstrand, E., F. Celsing, and E.A. Newsholme. Changes in plasma concentrations of aromatic and branched chain amino acids during sustained exercise in man and their possible role in fatigue. *Acta Physiol. Scand.* 133: 115-121, 1988.
2. Bloxham, P.L., M.D. Tricklebank, A.J. Patel, and G. Curzon. Effects of albumin, amino acids and clofibrate on the uptake of tryptophan by the rat brain. *J. Neurochem.* 34: 43-49, 1980.
3. Bortz, W.M., P. Angwin, I.N. Mefford, M.R. Boarder, N. Noyle, and J.D. Barchas. Catecholamine, dopamine and endorphin levels during extreme exercise. *N. Engl. J. Med.* 305: 466-467, 1981.
4. Brooks, B.J., J.R.S. Arch, and E.A. Newsholme. Effect of some hormones on the rate of the triacylglycerol/fatty acid substrate cycle in adipose tissue of the mouse *in vivo*. *Biosci. Rep.* 3: 263-267, 1983.
5. Brown, B.S., D.E. Ramirez, and J.M. Taub. The prescription of exercise for depression. *Phys. Sportsmed.* 6: 34-35, 1978.
6. Challiss, R.A.J., A.R.S. Arch, and E.A. Newsholme. The rate of substrate cycling between fructose 6-phosphate and fructose 1,6-bisphosphate in skeletal muscle from cold-exposed, hyperthyroid or acutely exercised rats. *Biochem. J.* 231: 217-220, 1985.
7. Chaouloff, F., G.A. Kennett, B. Serrarrier, O. Morino, and G. Curzon. Amino acid analysis demonstrates that increased plasma-free tryptophan causes the increase of brain tryptophan during exercise in the rat. *J. Neurochem.* 46: 1647-1650, 1986.
8. Dobbin, S., Oxford University: 1987. Thesis.
9. Folkins, C.H., S. Lynch, and M.M. Gardner. Psychological fitness as a function of physiological fitness. *Arch. Phys. Med. Rehabil.* 53: 503-508, 1972.
10. Garrow, J.S. *Energy balance and obesity in man*. Amsterdam: Elsevier, 1978.
11. Hansson, P., E.A. Newsholme, and D.H. Williamson. Effects of lactation and removal of pups on the rate of the triacylglycerol/fatty acid substrate cycling in white adipose tissue of the rat. *Biochem. J.* 243: 267-271, 1987.
12. Hermansen, L. Effect of acidosis on skeletal muscle performance during maximal exercise in man. *Bull. Eur. Physiopathol. Respir.* 15: 220-238, 1979.
13. Hermansen, L. Effect of metabolic changes on force generation in skeletal muscle during maximal exercise. *Ciba Found. Symp.* 8: 75-88, 1981.
14. Huang, M.T., and H.A. Lardy. Effects of thyroid states on the Cori cycle, glucose-alanine cycle and futile cycling of glucose

metabolism in rats. *Arch. Biochem. Biophys.* 209: 41-47, 1981.

15. Kennett, G.A., G. Curzon, A. Hunt, and A.J. Patel. Immobilisation decreases amino acid concentrations in plasma but maintains or increases them in brain. *J. Neurochem.* 46: 208-212, 1986.

16. Lamott, K. *Escape from stress.* New York: Putnam & Sons, 1974.

17. Leboef, B., R.B. Flint, and G.F. Cahill. Effect of epinephrine on glucose uptake and glycerol release by adipose tissue *in vivo. Proc. Soc. Exp. Biol. Med.* 102: 527-537, 1959.

18. Maehlum, S., A.T. Hostmark, and L. Hermansen. Synthesis of muscle glycogen during recovery after prolonged severe exercise in diabetic subjects. Effect of insulin deprivation. *Scand. J. Clin. Lab. Invest.* 38: 35-39, 1978.

19. Maehlum, S., M. Grandmontagne, E.A. Newsholme, and O.M. Sejersted. Magnitude and duration of excess post-exercise oxygen consumption in healthy young subjects. *Metabolism* 35: 425-429, 1986.

20. Mandell, A.J. *Psychiatric Annals* 9: 57-68, 1979.

21. Markoff, R.A., P. Ryan, and T. Young. Endorphins and mood changes in long-distance running. *Med. Sci. Sports Exer.* 14: 11-15, 1982.

22. Morgan, W.P., J.A. Roberts, F.R. Brand, and A.D. Fennerman. Psychological effects of chronic physical activity. *Med. Sci. Sports Exer.* 2: 213-217, 1970.

23. Newsholme, E.A., and B. Crabtree. Substrate cycles in metabolic regulation and heat generation. *Biochem. Soc. Symp.* 41: 61-110, 1976.

24. Newsholme, E.A. A possible metabolic basis for the control of body weight. *N. Engl. J. Med.* 302: 400-405, 1980.

25. Newsholme, E.A., and A.R. Leech. *The runner: Energy and endurance.* Oxford: Fitness Books, 1983.

26. Newsholme, E.A., and A.R. Leech. *Biochemistry for the medical sciences.* Chichester: John Wiley & Sons, 1983.

27. Newsholme, E.A., A.R. Leech, and B. Tulloh. *The science behind athletic training.* Oxford: Fitness Books, 1990.

28. Newsholme, E.A., R.A.J. Challiss, B. Leighton, F.J. Lozeman, and L. Budohoski. A common mechanicm for defective thermogenesis and insulin resistance. *Nutrition* 3: 195-200, 1987.

29. Northcote, R.J., A.D.B. Evans, and D. Ballantyne. Sudden death in squash players. *Lancet* 148-150, 1984.

30. Opie, L.H., C.A. Muller, and W.F. Lubbe. Cyclic AMP and arrhythmias revisited. *Lancet* 921-923, 1978.

31. Oscai, L.B., S.P. Babirak, F.B. Dubach, J.A. McGarr, and C.N. Spirakis. Exercise or food restriction: Effect on adipose tissue cellularity. *Amer. J. Physiol.* 227: 901-904, 1974.

32. Pond, C.M., C.A. Mattacks, and D. Sadler. The effect of food restriction and exercise on site specific differences in adipocyte volume and adipose site cellularity in the guinea pig. *Br. J. Nutr.* 51: 415-424, 1974.

33. Pond, C.M., and C.A. Mattacks. Body mass and natural diet as determinants of the number and volume of adipocytes in eutherian mammals. *J. Morphol.* 185: 183-193, 1985.

34. Pond, C.M., D. Sadler, and C.A. Mattacks. Sex differences in the distribution of adipose tissue in the djungarian hampster *Phodopus sungorus. Nutr. Res.* 7: 1325-1328, 1987.

35. Pond, C.M. Fat and figures. *New Scientist* 1563: 62-66, 1987.

36. Pond, C.M., and C.A. Mattacks. Site specific differences in the rates of the triacylglycerol/fatty acid substrate cycle in adipose tissue and muscle of sedentary and exercised dwarf hampsters (*Phodopus sungorus*). *Int. J. Obes.* 12:585-597, 1988.

37. Shulman, G.I., P.W. Ladenson, M.E. Wolfe, et al. Substrate cycling between gluconeogenesis and glycolysis in euthyroid, hypothyroid and hyperthyroid man. *J. Clin. Invest.* 76: 757, 1985.

38. Sjöström, L. Fat cells and body weight. In: Stunkard, A.J., ed. *Obesity.* Philadelphia: W.B. Saunders, 1980: pp. 72-100.

39. Spector, A.A., and J.E. Fletcher. Transport of fatty acid in the circulation. In: Dietschy, J.M., A.M. Gotto, and J.A. Ontko, eds. *Disturbances in lipid and lipoprotein metabolism,* Bethesda, MD: American Physiological Society, 1978: pp. 229-250.

40. Steinberg, D. Fatty acid mobilisation: Mechanism of regulation and metabolic consequences. *Biochem. Soc. Symp.* 24: 111-144, 1963.

41. Thompson, P.D., E.J. Funk, R.A. Carleton, and W. Sturner. Incidence of death during jogging in Rhode Island from 1978 through 1980. *JAMA* 247: 2535-2538, 1982.

42. Wolfe, R.R., D.N. Herndon, R. Jahoor, H. Miyoshi, and M. Wolfe. Effect of severe burn injury on substrate cycling by glucose and fatty acids. *N. Engl. J. Med.* 371: 403-408, 1987.

43. Wolfe, R.R. The effect of short term fasting on lipolytic responsiveness in normal and obese human subjects. *Amer. J. Physiol.* 252: E189-E196, 1987.

44. Wolfe, R.R., and E.J. Peters. Lipolytic response to glucose infusion in human subjects. *Amer. J. Physiol.* 252: E218-E223.

45. Young, A. Exercise physiology in geriatric practice. *Acta Med. Scand. Suppl.* 711: 227-232, 1985.

Chapter 25

Discussion: Effects of Exercise on Aspects of Carbohydrate, Fat, and Amino Acid Metabolism

Kent Sahlin

A general feature of the human organism is its ability to adapt to functional demands. Thus, lack of physical activity will decrease the work capacity, whereas training will increase the capacity to perform work.

The physical activities in daily life normally utilize only a fraction of the maximal work capacity. However, the strain of a certain type of work is related to the relative intensity, which is determined by the maximal work capacity. Maximal work capacity is therefore of importance not only for athletic performance but also for the perceived effort during submaximal work.

Muscle contraction involves transformation of stored chemically bound energy into mechanical energy and heat. In this process, carbohydrates and fat are catabolized and oxidized to CO_2 and water in the muscle. Exercise will have a profound effect on the carbohydrate and fat metabolism both during the exercise and during the subsequent recovery period. During exercise the muscle will combust locally stored carbohydrates (muscle glycogen) and fat (muscle triglycerides) and blood-borne fuels such as glucose, free fatty acids (FFA), and, to a small extent, amino acids. Prolonged exercise will cause a decrease in the glycogen content of muscle and liver and in an increase of blood levels of FFA, ammonia, alanine, and lactate. The impact of these metabolic changes on health is to a large extent unknown.

Fitness or physical work capacity is ultimately dependent on the capacity of the biochemical processes to provide the required energy. Factors that are important for physical performance are the transport of O_2 and fuels to the muscle, the transport of waste products (CO_2 and lactate) from the muscle, the local stores of fuels, and the local metabolic capacity of the energetic processes.

During exercise with large muscle groups, the major limitation of the oxidative metabolism is not the local respiratory capacity but rather the capacity to deliver oxygen to the working muscle. The maximal oxygen uptake ($\dot{V}O_2max$) can vary from about 40 ml $\cdot$ kg^{-1} $\cdot$ min^{-1} or less in sedentary subjects to more than 70 ml $\cdot$ kg^{-1} $\cdot$ min^{-1} in well-trained athletes, and it reflects the adaptation of the cardiovascular and pulmonary function to training. Other chapters cover this topic in detail.

In addition to the adaptation of the oxygen transport system to an increased demand, there is an adaptation of the intramuscular metabolic capacity and an overall change in the metabolic pattern during exercise. This chapter focuses on carbohydrate and fat metabolism during exercise, its adaptation to training, and its relation to muscle fatigue.

Energy Sources During Exercise

The immediate energy source in the cell is the hydrolysis of ATP. The concentration of ATP is limited, however, and ATP must therefore be resynthesized at the same rate as it is utilized. This can be achieved through (a) the oxidation of carbohydrates (CHO) or fat to CO_2 and water; (b) lactate formation; and (c) the breakdown of high-energy phosphate compounds, mainly phosphocreatine (PCr). During prolonged exercise, energy is derived mainly through the oxidative processes. The choice of substrate is to a large extent determined by the intensity and the duration of the physical activity. Thus, at rest and during low-intensity exercise, the major part of the required energy is covered by fat oxidation, whereas, during strenuous exercise, oxidation of carbohydrates is the major fuel. Available data show that oxidation of

309

CHO can provide a rate of ATP formation about 2 times higher than can oxidation of fat. The reason for this is not completely understood.

Carbohydrate is stored as glycogen in the liver (500-900 mmol) and in the muscle (80-100 mmol/kg), and both of these stores are utilized as fuel during exercise. Muscle glycogen is the most important fuel during short-term exercise and is an energy source that can be mobilized immediately and at a high rate. The rate of muscle glycogen breakdown is related to the exercise intensity. During low-intensity exercise, muscle glycogen is utilized at a low rate, and the stores become only partially depleted even during prolonged work. At higher intensities (> 60% of $\dot{V}O_2$max) the rate of glycogen utilization is high, and the entire muscle glycogen contents may be depleted in certain muscle fiber types (23). It has also been shown that endurance at these intensities is dependent on the initial store of glycogen. This finding is utilized by long-distance runners who, before a competition, by certain combinations of diet and exercise ensure that their muscle glycogen store is high. The exercise-induced decrease in muscle glycogen is known to be associated with an increased post-exercise insulin sensitivity and an increased glucose tolerance (10) and could therefore be of potential benefit for the health. This is discussed in more detail elsewhere in these proceedings.

Blood-borne glucose is an important fuel during exercise at 30% to 60% of $\dot{V}O_2$max. The proportion of the oxidative metabolism that is covered by blood-borne glucose increases gradually with the duration of work and amounts to 35%-40% after 90-120 min of work during exercise at 30%-70% of $\dot{V}O_2$max (3). The glucose uptake by working skeletal muscle is corresponded by a similar release from the liver that is derived from both glycogenolysis and from glyconeogenesis. The rate of hepatic glycogen breakdown may increase fivefold above the basal level, and as much as 50% of the hepatic glycogen may therefore be mobilized during 1 h of strenuous exercise (11). Long-term exercise may therefore result in a depletion of liver glycogen and in hypoglycemia, which could impair the work capacity through an effect on the central nervous system.

Fat is an important fuel during exercise at low and moderate intensities and is to a large extent provided through an uptake of blood-borne FFA originating from the adipose tissue. The uptake of FFA has been shown to be proportional to the in-flow (i.e., plasma FFA concentration × blood flow), and is therefore to a large extent determined by the plasma concentration of FFA. The plasma concentration of FFA increases gradually during work because of an augmented rate of mobilization from the adipose tissue (12). The muscle uptake and oxidation of FFA will therefore increase in importance with the duration of the work and can contribute to 50% or more of the oxidative metabolism (1). The intramuscular store of triglycerides has been shown to decrease during exercise in some studies (6, 12) but not in others (7). The quantitative role of this fuel store for energy production is at present uncertain.

An increased availability of FFA will increase the oxidation of fat and decrease the rate of CHO utilization. This phenomenon can be explained at least in part by the glucose-FFA cycle described by Randle et al. (20). Oxidation of fat will retard the rate of glycogen utilization during exercise and will therefore prevent or delay the onset of fatigue.

During sustained exercise at low or moderate intensities the rate of pyruvate oxidation is similar to the rate of glycolysis. However, at higher intensities the catabolism of CHO is incomplete, and lactic acid is formed and accumulates in the body fluids. Accumulation of lactate in muscle and blood begins at about 50%-70% of $\dot{V}O_2$max, and at 100% of $\dot{V}O_2$max 10%-20% of the total energy production is covered by lactate formation. A slight breakdown of PCr occurs already at low exercise intensities (40% of $\dot{V}O_2$max or lower), and when the exercise intensity exceeds 80%-90% of $\dot{V}O_2$max the muscle store of PCr becomes almost completely depleted at fatigue.

Of paramount importance for the regulation of energy metabolism is the concentration of ATP and its breakdown products (ADP, AMP, and inorganic phosphate, or Pi). An increase in ADP and AMP will activate all the different pathways for ATP resynthesis, but the degree of activation at a certain ADP-AMP level will vary between the different processes. At low exercise intensities the increase in ADP and AMP in the contracting muscle cell will be low and ATP resynthesis achieved mainly through the aerobic processes. During strenuous exercise the increase in ADP-AMP will be larger, and lactate formation and PCr breakdown will occur in addition to the oxidative processes. The rate of ADP resynthesis through these different metabolic processes will be adjusted to equal the rate of ATP utilization.

Effect of Training on Energy Metabolism During Exercise

The relative rates of ATP resynthesis through the different processes will be influenced by the metabolic capacity of the tissue in addition to the exercise intensity. It has been shown that considerable increases occur in both the mitochondrial volume and the oxidative enzyme activities of muscle during both endurance training and sprint training (23). The training-induced increase in mitochondrial enzyme activity is usually larger than is the increase in $\dot{V}O_2$max. During immobilization or deconditioning there is a corresponding decrease in the activity of the mitochondrial enzymes (23). In contrast to the oxidative enzymes, glycolytic enzymes exhibit only small changes after training.

An increased aerobic capacity implies that a certain energy supply can be achieved at a lower degree of stimulation. If we accept the view that the various pathways have certain activators in common (i.e., increases in ADP, AMP, and Pi), a high aerobic capacity in the muscle would diminish the increase of the activators and consequently result in a decreased rate of anaerobic energy utilization (13). This is in analogy of the Pasteur effect, in which glycolysis is inhibited in the presence of oxygen. A vast number of studies have also shown that the increase in blood and muscle lactate after exercise at the same absolute or relative intensity is diminished after training. Thus, in a sedentary subject lactate starts to accumulate in muscle and blood at an intensity of about 50% of $\dot{V}O_2$max, whereas in a trained subject this occurs at 60%-80% of $\dot{V}O_2$max (2). An additional factor that could be important for decreased lactate formation during submaximal exercise in trained subjects is an increased capillary density, which will increase the capacity to supply the tissue with oxygen and blood-borne substrates. The finding that lactate formation is dependent on the oxygen tension in inspired air and that the muscle cell becomes reduced (increased concentration of NADH) when lactate is formed (17, 22) supports the idea that the cellular availability of O_2 is an important factor in the regulation of lactate formation.

As discussed in the previous chapter, the accumulation of lactic acid and the associated acidification of the muscle will be an important factor for the development of muscle fatigue. An increased rate of lactic acid formation will also rapidly deplete the glycogen store in the contracting muscle. Excessive lactic acid formation could therefore be associated with fatigue both through the acidification and through glycogen depletion. Training or regular physical activity will decrease the rate of lactic acid formation at a certain absolute and relative work intensity and could thereby prevent muscle fatigue. Similarly, training will decrease the degree of PCr breakdown at a certain relative work intensity (14).

Training will also have an influence on the relation between carbohydrate and fat oxidation. A trained subject will, at a certain relative exercise intensity, combust more fat than will a sedentary subject (8, 23). The mechanism for the training-induced increase in fat oxidation could at least partly be explained by the increased mitochondrial volume and the increased enzymatic capacity for catabolism of FFA that occur with training (23). The increased number of capillaries in a trained muscle could be of additional importance in facilitating the transport of FFA from the blood to the mitochondria. The increased fat oxidation after training occurs despite a lower plasma concentration of FFA, indicating that the oxidation of FFA is not solely determined by the inflow of FFA. Utilization of intramuscular triglycerides is enhanced in trained subjects (12) and might explain the training-induced increase in fat oxidation despite lower plasma FFA levels.

Muscle Fatigue

As discussed in the previous chapter accumulation of lactic acid will cause an acidification of the muscle that could impair muscle function. The major part of released H^+ will be absorbed through different buffer processes, and an increased buffer capacity would therefore be of importance for attenuating the change in pH. The buffer capacity of the thigh muscle in sprint-trained subjects has been shown to be about 15% higher than it is in sedentary control subjects (21). In another study (24) it was shown that 8 wk of sprint training resulted in a 37% increase in the muscle buffer capacity and in a higher muscle lactate concentration at fatigue. The training-induced increase in the buffer capacity of muscle will, for a given lactate accumulation, attenuate the decrease in muscle pH and thereby increase the tolerance to fatigue.

The maximal rate of ATP production is dependent on the combined rates of ATP resynthesis through PCr breakdown, glycolysis, and oxidative phosphorylation. When the maximal rates of these processes are insufficient to meet the energy demand, one would anticipate muscle fatigue. An impairment of ATP resynthesis will occur when there is

- a depletion of PCr in the contracting muscle,
- an accumulation of lactic acid in the contracting muscle, and
- a depletion of glycogen in the contracting muscle.

An insufficient rate of ADP rephosphorylation would result in increased ADP and AMP levels at the ATP-utilizing sites in the contracting muscle. However, the true increases will be difficult to determine by analytical techniques because of a high turnover rate and localized changes of the adenine nucleotides. Increases in ADP and AMP would, however, activate the breakdown of adenine nucleotides to inosine monophosphate (IMP) and ammonia (NH_3), and measurements of IMP and NH_3 in muscle and of NH_3 in blood could therefore be used as a measure of the imbalance between the rates of utilization and resynthesis of ATP. Degradation of adenine nucleotides has been shown to occur both after short-term exercise at high intensity when there is a pronounced depletion of PCr and accumulation of lactate (15, 17) and after long-term exercise at low intensity when there is a depletion of the intramuscular glycogen store (4). These data indicate that the rate of ATP resynthesis is insufficient to meet the demand at fatigue and suggest that the mechanism of fatigue could be the same during all three of the conditions depicted previously.

Ammonia is released from the muscle to the blood during exercise when the intensity exceeds 50%-70% of $\dot{V}O_2$max, resulting in increased plasma and blood NH_3 levels. Plasma NH_3, which is about 20 μ mol/L in the basal state can increase more than fivefold after exercise to fatigue. Thus plasma levels as high as 120 μ mol/L have been observed after short-term exercise to fatigue (15) and even higher values (i.e., 250 μ mol/L) have been observed during exercise at about 70% of $\dot{V}O_2$max sustained to fatigue (4). The fatigue in the latter study coincided with a depletion of the muscle glycogen store. Endurance training has been found to attenuate the increase of blood NH_3 during ex-

ercise at submaximal intensities (18). It is quite possible that the mechanism for the training-induced decrease in blood NH_3 and the decrease in lactate formation during submaximal exercise is similar (i.e., a lower ATP-ADP ratio in the contracting muscle) (see above).

It has been known for a long time that increased levels of NH_3 are toxic for the central nervous system. Detoxification of NH_3 occurs mainly in the liver through the formation of urea, and elevated blood NH_3 levels have been thought to be important in the development of coma induced by hepatic failure. It was suggested by Mutch and Banister (19) that the increase in blood NH_3 during exercise also could be of importance in the fatigue process through an effect on the central nervous system. However, central fatigue due to elevated plasma NH_3 is unlikely to be of importance during high-intensity exercise of short duration because recovery in work capacity occurs despite high plasma and blood NH_3 levels (17). The importance of elevated blood NH_3 levels during long-term exercise for the development of central fatigue remains to be elucidated.

Conclusion

Exercise will have a profound effect on carbohydrate and fat metabolism both during the exercise and during the following recovery period. Prolonged exercise will cause a decrease in the glycogen content of muscle and liver and result in elevated blood levels of FFA, NH_3, alanine, and lactate. The effect of these metabolic changes on the health is to a large extent unknown.

Physical activity and training will result in an adaptive increase not only of the $\dot{V}O_2$max, which is limited by the O_2-transporting system, but also of the metabolic capacity of the muscle. The cellular adaptation will result in increased fat oxidation (despite a lower plasma concentration of FFA) and diminished lactate formation at both an absolute and a relative submaximal work intensity. Training will also decrease ammonia formation during submaximal exercise. The adaptation with training will therefore not only increase the maximal work capacity but also diminish the metabolic perturbations during submaximal physical activity. As a consequence, the perceived effort during submaximal exercise will decrease and the tolerance to fatigue increase.

Acknowledgments

Support from the Swedish Medical Research Council (7670, 8671) and the Swedish Sports Research Council is gratefully acknowledged.

References

1. Ahlborg, G., P. Felig, L. Hagenfeldt, R. Hendler, and J. Wahren. Substrate turnover during prolonged exercise in man. *J. Clin. Invest.* 53: 1080-1090, 1974.

2. Åstrand, P.-O., and K. Rodahl. *Textbook of work physiology.* New York: McGraw-Hill, 1977.

3. Björkman, O., and J. Wahren. Glucose homeostasis during and after exercise. In: Horton, E.S., and R.L. Terjung, eds. *Exercise, nutrition and energy metabolism.* New York: Macmillan, 1988: pp. 100-115.

4. Broberg, S., and K. Sahlin. Glycogen depletion enhances adenine nucleotide degradation in human skeletal muscle during submaximal exercise. *J. Appl. Physiol.* Accepted for publication, 1989.

5. Eriksson, L.S., S. Broberg, O. Björkman, and J. Wahren. Ammonia metabolism during exercise in man. *Clin. Physiol.* 5: 325-336, 1985.

6. Essén, B., L. Hagenfeldt, and L. Kaijser. Utilization of blood-borne and intramuscular substrates during continuous and intermittent exercise in man. *J. Physiol.* 265: 489-506, 1977.

7. Gollnick, P.D., and B. Saltin. Fuel for muscular exercise: Role of fat. In: Horton, E.S., and R.L. Terjung, eds. *Exercise, nutrition and energy metabolism.* New York: Macmillan, 1988: pp. 72-88.

8. Henriksson, J. Training-induced adaptation of skeletal muscle and metabolism during submaximal exercise. *J. Physiol. (Lond.)* 270: 677-690, 1977.

9. Henriksson, J., and J.S. Reitman. Time course of changes in human skeletal muscle succinate dehydrogenase and cytochrome oxidase activities and maximal oxygen uptake with physical activity and inactivity. *Acta Physiol. Scand.* 99: 91-97, 1977.

10. Horton, E.S. Exercise and physical training: Effects on insulin sensitivity and glucose metabolism. *Diabetes Meta. Rev.* 2: 1-17, 1986.

11. Hultman, E., and L.H. Nilsson. Liver glycogen in man: Effects of different diets and muscular exercise. In: Pernow, B., and B. Saltin, eds. *Muscle metabolism during exercise.* New York: Plenum Press, 1971: pp. 143-151.

12. Hurley, B.F., P.M. Nemeth, W.H. Martin, J.M. Hagberg, G.P. Dalsky, and J.O. Holloszy. Muscle trigylceride utilization during exercise: Effect of training. *J. Appl. Physiol.* 60: 562-567, 1986.

13. Holloszy, J.O., L.B. Oscai, P.A. Molé, and I.J. Don. Biochemical adaptations to endurance exercise in skeletal muscle. In: Pernow, B., and B. Saltin, eds. *Muscle metabolism during exercise.* New York: Plenum Press, 1971: pp. 51-61.

14. Karlsson, J., L.-O. Nordesjö, L. Jorfeldt, and B. Saltin. Muscle lactate, ATP and CP levels during exercise after physical training in man. *J. Appl. Physiol.* 33: 199-203, 1972.

15. Katz, A., S. Broberg, K. Sahlin, and J. Wahren. Muscle ammonia and amino acid metabolism during dynamic exercise in man. *Clin. Physiol.* 6: 365-380, 1986.

16. Katz, A., and K. Sahlin. Effect of decreased oxygen availability on NADH and lactate contents in human skeletal muscle during exercise. *Acta Physiol. Scand.* 131: 119-120, 1987.

17. Katz, A., K. Sahlin, and J. Henriksson. Muscle NH_3 and amino acid metabolism during isometric contraction in man. *Am. J. Physiol.* 250: C834-C840, 1986.

18. Lo, P-Y., and A. Dudley. Endurance training reduces the magnitude of exercise-induced hyperammonemia in humans. *J. Appl. Physiol.* 62: 1227-1230, 1987.

19. Mutch, B.J.C., and E.W. Banister. Ammonia metabolism in exercise and fatigue: A review. *Med. Sci. Sports Exerc.* 15: 41-50, 1983.

20. Randle, P.J., P.B. Garland, C.N. Hales, and E.A. Newsholme. The glucose fatty-acid cycle: Its role in insulin sensitivity and the metabolic disturbances of diabetes mellitus. *Lancet* i: 785-789, 1963.

21. Sahlin, K., and J. Henriksson. Buffer capacity and lactate accumulation in skeletal muscle of trained and untrained men. *Acta Physiol. Scand.* 122: 331-339, 1984.

22. Sahlin, K., A. Katz, and J. Henriksson. Redox state and lactate accumulation in human skeletal muscle during dynamic exercise. *Biochem. J.* 245: 551-556, 1987.

23. Saltin, B., and P.D. Gollnick. Skeletal muscle adaptability: Significance for metabolism and performance. In: Peachey, L.D., R.H. Adrian, and S.R. Geiger, eds. *Handbook of physiology*. Baltimore: Williams & Wilkins, 1983: pp. 540-555.

24. Sharp, R.L., D.L. Costill, W.J. Fink, and D.S. King. The effects of eight weeks of bicycle ergometer sprint training on buffer capacity. *Int. J. Sports Med.* 7: 13-17, 1983.

Chapter 26

Adipose Tissue Adaptation to Exercise

Per Björntorp

Exercise requires energy. This chapter examines how the working muscles are supplied with energy for work and how this procedure is adapted to chronic, repeated bouts of work, or the physically trained condition.

The two main sources of energy for muscle contraction are carbohydrate and lipid. The former is supplied directly by muscle glycogen stores or by blood glucose, which in turn is produced by the liver during postabsorptive conditions. The major source of lipid energy is triglyceride, which is stored in adipose tissue and transported to working muscle as free fatty acids (FFA). There are also intermediate lipid energy stores in the form of triglycerides within muscle tissue, and circulating triglycerides are also used to some extent. In this review the main emphasis is on the regulation of adipose tissue mobilization of triglyceride to FFA, although the other sources of energy may be referred to for completeness when needed. Furthermore, human adipose tissue is examined specifically, unless information is available only from nonhuman species.

Lipid Mobilization From Adipose Tissue

The first step in the process of lipid mobilization from adipose tissue is the transfer of lipid from the main lipid droplet to the site of enzymatic cleavage in the cytoplasm of the adipocyte. The details of this process are incompletely known, but this transport is most likely not rate limiting for lipid mobilization. In the next step, the triglyceride is subjected to enzymatic cleavage, whereby the fatty acids esterfied in the beta (outer) positions of the

triacylglycerol are hydrolyzed. This is occurring by the action of a triglyceride lipase, which is subjected to hormonal regulation. The remaining monoacylglycerol in the alpha (middle) position is then hydrolyzed by another lipase system: a monoglyceride lipase that is much more active than is the hormone-sensitive triglyceride lipase. It is noteworthy that the liberated glycerol cannot be reutilized by the adipocyte in the absence of glycerokinase, so it provides a convenient measurement of the lipolytic process. The FFA and glycerol formed in the cytoplasm then diffuse out of the adipocyte in proportion to their formation and concentration and are transported to their peripheral utilization: the FFA bound to plasma albumin.

In this process the activity of the hormone-sensitive triglyceride lipase is the rate-limiting step. The regulation of the activity of this enzyme thus becomes of primary importance for the mobilization of lipid from adipose tissue to the exercising muscles.

There is also a possibility that blood flow through adipose tissue might contribute to the regulation of lipid mobilization, although the precise role of this factor in exercise is not well defined (58). The activity of the triglyceride lipase is dependent on stimulatory and inhibitory factors. Of the former, the sympathetic nervous system (SNS) is most probably of major importance in humans and insulin the most important inhibitory factor.

The transfer of SNS activity to the cellular level occurs through adrenergic receptors. In turn, these receptors trigger a cascade of events, starting with activation of an adenylate cyclase enzyme and a protein kinase, which activates the lipase by phosphorylation. This process is inhibited by insulin, resulting in an inactive, dephosphorylated enzyme (63).

315

Lipid Mobilization During Exercise

During exercise this chain of events is activated as follows. The increased activity of the SNS commences at the start of exercise by a regulatory process at the level of the central SNS. The regulation of this process is then of fundamental importance for this question. It probably has multifactorial causes. In principle, two types of hypotheses have been suggested for the central SNS regulation during exercise. One hypothesis states that central SNS activity is influenced by motor centers in the central nervous system. Another hypothesis says that regulation of the central SNS during exercise occurs directly by the muscle contractions, presumably by means of muscle afferents (49, 59). It is also important to emphasize here that Group III muscle afferents are known to stimulate central secretion of beta endorphins (61), which in turn probably inhibit the outflow from the central SNS (24). Such observations suggest that motor afferents also transfer signals to balance the net outflow by inhibition. It is not possible at present to state which of these mechanisms (if any) is the correct alternative, although theoretically the direct regulation by the periphery seems to be the most simple and useful. However, a number of descriptive studies suggest influences on the SNS firing, as is seen in the following discussion.

Anticipation of exercise is associated with a general activation of the SNS as measured by plasma norepinephrine concentrations. This is seen also in trained subjects who are familiar with the stress of the following exercise bout (33, 46). The activation of the SNS during exercise is dependent on the intensity of the work in relation to maximal oxygen uptake (28, 32). Arm work seems to give more activation than does leg work (11), perhaps in analogy with observations that work with small-muscle groups activates the SNS more than does work with larger-muscle groups (with SNS activity measured as heart rate) (18). The duration of work is also of importance for SNS involvement, being maximal at exhaustion (27, 44). Another factor that has been described to parallel SNS activation is oxygen availability (31). Other regulators might be body temperature (30) and hydration (25). The intense activation of the SNS by hypoglycemia is well known. It has also been suggested that glucose availability is a critical regulatory factor for SNS activation during exercise, influencing also epinephrine secretion (28, 29).

The suggested regulation of central SNS activity is then apparently influenced by a number of factors that interact and that change in parallel. Thus it has been difficult to come to a conclusion concerning the most important factors.

Another problem that makes it even more difficult to evaluate this area is the lack of specific methods. These difficulties are found at different levels. Although the methods for direct measurements of catecholamines are now specific and sensitive enough, it should be realized that circulating norepinephrine concentrations are not an adequate measurement of SNS activity. These concentrations are the result of an overflow from peripheral SNS terminals and are therefore poor indicators of the actual SNS activity for several obvious reasons. Furthermore, these concentrations parallel, at best, an average of the activity of the total SNS, and it is well known that selective stimulation occurs in one part of the SNS while other parts show low activity. Thus signs of increased SNS activity in circulatory variables might not necessarily mean, for example, a stimulation by SNS of lipolysis. Unfortunately, no available method at present can measure the direct stimulation of adipose tissue lipolysis by the SNS during exercise. Conclusions regarding lipolysis therefore have to be indirect and tentative.

The activation of lipolysis by SNS is mediated by beta-adrenergic mechanisms at the cellular level (41). As a result, FFA and free glycerol start to flow out from adipose tissue. However, an initial decrease of plasma FFA concentration is seen that may be due to an immediate increase in the uptake of FFA in muscle due to the capillary dilatation occurring in the exercising muscle. During exercise, then, FFA concentration gradually increases. Because glycerol is not utilized by the working muscle, an initial sustained increase of plasma glycerol concentration is seen. At the end of exercise the lipolytic activation is not immediately turned off but continues for some period of time. Because the dilatation of muscle capillaries seems to end immediately after the cessation of exercise, the increased outflux of FFA from plasma during exercise is no longer occurring. The net result will be a pronounced overshooting of plasma FFA concentration with a duration of about 1 h, depending on the duration and intensity of the exercise as well as the physical training state of the individual (for a more detailed review, see ref. 15).

The quantitative contribution of FFA mobilized from adipose tissue in the postabsorptive phase to the energy combustion of the exercising muscles is uncertain. Some studies suggest that only about 40% of the FFA is removed from circulation and used directly for energy purposes in the working muscles (1, 64). Direct measurements of exercising muscles show that more FFA is taken up from circulation than is possible to oxidize (53, 71). Such observations suggest that some of the FFA taken up by muscles is stored instead of oxidized. However, other studies have shown a depletion of intramuscular triglyceride during work (17, 23). Currently, the available information does not seem to allow for an evaluation of the quantitative contributions either of circulating FFA or triglycerides in circulation or of intramuscular trigylcerides to the energy need of the exercising muscle. It is of course possible that the FFA released during work is taken up in tissues other than the exercising muscle to a significant extent.

This process is balanced by inhibitory factors. As stated previously, insulin is the main inhibitory hormone. The circulating insulin concentration is also influenced by the increased SNS activity during exercise, which is followed by a decreased insulin concentration (42). Because C-peptide concentrations are also lower during exercise, it is likely that insulin secretion has actually decreased (70). This is also supported by tracer studies (26). However, hepatic clearance is probably also decreased, as suggested by a lower molar ratio of C-peptide to insulin in peripheral blood (36). The lower hepatic clearance would tend to increase peripheral insulin concentrations; but, because these concentrations are indeed lower during exercise, the inhibition of insulin secretion is probably more likely mediated by means of higher activity in the alpha-adrenergic part of the SNS (42) and is a consequence of activity in the sympathetic nerves to the pancreas (4). The inhibition of the secretion of insulin during exercise seems to be a useful event, facilitating FFA mobilization by the release of the inhibitory action of insulin.

It has also been discussed that lactate might be a regulatory factor for lipolysis during exercise. Lactate inhibits the activation of the triglyceride lipase in vitro (6) and in vivo (13, 40), and during strenuous exercise it appears that inhibitory concentrations of circulating lactate are attainable. Lipid substrate can be used by the working muscle only up to a certain degree of intensity, above which the muscle is utilizing its own glycogen depot to provide the energy required. In this situation, the lactate production due to anaerobic glycolysis in the muscle would be expected to increase. The working muscle now cannot utilize lipid substrate, and the inhibition by lactate of lipid mobilization from adipose tissue would thus be a most useful regulatory mechanism.

In spite of counterregulatory factors, the main characteristic of the lipolysis regulation mechanism during exercise seems to be that it operates at a level that provides a secure, steady flow of energy substrate to the working muscle. There seems to be much less risk of energy deficiency than of excess mobilization. As will be seen in the following discussion, this risk seems to be increased more in the sedentary than in the physically well-trained individual, particularly when lipolytically sensitive parts of adipose tissue are enlarged. When lipolysis activation is occurring more than is needed—particularly when it is not followed by a parallel exercise bout to remove excess FFA from the circulation—FFA might have harmful effects in the periphery (54).

Adipose Tissue Metabolism During Exercise in the Physically Trained Condition

After repeated bouts of exercise, the body is adapting to a physically trained condition. This occurs in the respiratory and circulatory systems as well as in the blood and the exercising muscles. Most of these adaptations lead to an improved transport of oxygen to the exercising muscles, which are now also adapted morphologically and functionally to a better capacity to utilize oxygen and energy substrate that requires oxygen for its transformation into directly accessible energy (19, 35, 37). Oxygen is mandatory for utilization of lipid energy by muscles. The lipid-mobilization process in adipose tissue has now also adapted to the physically trained condition accordingly, as will be seen in the following discussion. It seems to be possible to perform a defined submaximal exercise load with less activity from the SNS after physical training than in the sedentary condition (10, 20, 32, 39, 47). The regulation here is not known but probably occurs in the central nervous system, hypothetically by means of signals from the adapted periphery (65).

Muscle adaptations after physical training include changes in muscle fiber composition and capillarization as well as changes in muscle enzyme activity. When an adaptation to endurance-type exercise has taken place, the muscle is characterized by more oxidative enzyme activity, higher capillary density, and some change toward a higher proportion of red, slow-twitch, Type I fibers (or intermediate, Type IIa fibers) at the expense of white, fast-twitch, Type IIb fibers (2, 34). Such a muscle is now better equipped to provide work of low intensity and long duration and to use lipid substrate for this purpose.

Although capillarization is increased morphologically after physical training, it seems that total muscle blood flow is actually lower during a given absolute submaximal work load (68). In addition, there is evidence of less blood flow to nonmuscle tissues, such as the visceral tissues (64, 65). This allows cardiac output to decrease, and the body is now adapted to a better economy of circulation during submaximal work loads (67).

The lower muscle blood flow during work and the higher capillary density seem to be conflicting observations. However, the morphological observation of more capillaries per muscle fiber does not mean that these capillaries are always functioning. During submaximal work perhaps only a few are recruited, whereas the total bed of the increased number of capillaries is needed for maximal work loads.

In the physically trained condition, submaximal work loads can be performed with the combustion of more lipid. Due to the muscular adaptations of less blood flow through the working muscles, this would then mean that FFAs are more effectively extracted and utilized in such a physically trained muscle or, alternately, that intramuscular lipids can be utilized more efficiently.

There is thus evidence for important adaptations on the site of extraction and utilization of FFA after physical training. There are also changes occurring at the site of lipid mobilization in adipose tissue. These include a more sensitive trigger mechanism for activation of the hormone-sensitive lipase (3). At the level of the adrenergic receptor, it seems that the binding affinity of beta-adrenergic agonists has increased. This, along with adaptations at postreceptor sites, leads to an increased sensitivity of the lipid mobilization machinery to stimulation from the SNS (14, 38, 60). Sufficient lipid mobilization seems thus to occur at an activity level of the SNS that is lower than it was before physical training. It must be remembered, however, that a direct measurement of sympathetic flow to adipose tissue is not possible, and the reasoning here is based only on the inference that a decreased activity of the SNS occurs in the adipose tissue branches as it does in the circulatory system, such as in the regulation of cardiac function.

Another important and useful adaptation occurs in adipose tissue with physical training, now concerning the total magnitude of the adipose tissue mass. In general, the size of adipose tissue is regulated by the energy balance situation. With physical training this is kept in tight balance (48) at a level of a small amount of adipose tissue with each adipocyte containing a limited amount of lipid (7).

It should be noted that this smaller-than-average adipose tissue is by far sufficient for the lipid energy need of even an excessively protracted exercise bout. One kilogram of adipose tissue triglyceride is thus sufficient to supply the energy for about 100 km of skiing or several marathon runs. In this regard, it is more important that the total mass of adipose tissue be small, as this means that less energy is required to carry this energy depot during the work load in question. The adipose tissue in the physically well-trained individual is thus characterized by having a small total mass with small adipocytes, each containing a limited amount of triglyceride that is mobilized efficiently when needed through a sensitive lipolytic response of the trigger mechanism on which the sympathetic nervous system is acting.

As reviewed here, additional mechanisms that participate in lipolysis regulation are insulin and perhaps lactate, both of which inhibit lipolysis. In the physically trained state plasma insulin is lower (8), and plasma lactate concentration increases less on a submaximal work load because the working muscle is now capable of more complete aerobic metabolism with less lactate produced. In both cases, the inhibitory action would be diminished in the physically trained state, facilitating the mobilization of FFA from adipose tissue. However, the adipocyte, like other tissues, becomes more sensitive to insulin with physical training. Although the information is not entirely consistent, it seems that this occurs mainly by adaptations at the postreceptor level (69). The net effect of the lower circulating insulin concentrations and the antilipolytic effect of insulin on the adipocyte is not clear. It is noteworthy, however, that this is another example of the increased effectiveness of different regulatory systems after physical training that operate on a low-intensity, high-sensitivity level.

Taken together, a number of adaptations take place with physical training for endurance types of work. These adaptations occur in circulation, respiration, oxygen transport, and the effector organ (working muscle). This results in a more efficient system for oxygen transfer to the muscles, which now need oxygen so they can utilize the unlimited lipid store instead of the limited carbohydrate substrate that is available. The delivery system of lipid substrate to the working muscle also adapts and works at a higher sensitivity level of the key system for triglyceride hydrolysis, the hormone-sensitive triglyceride lipase, which can now operate at a lower level of stimulation by the SNS. In addition, adipose tissue changes to a smaller total mass by carrying less energy substrate in each adipocyte, an important mechanical adaptation for optimal long-term work.

Adaptations in the Sedentary Condition

With less physical activity and less recruitment of muscle fibers, red muscle fibers and oxidative enzymes rapidly become less abundant and eventually disappear totally when contractile activity ceases (50). Now also muscle atrophy starts, and muscle tissue becomes insulin resistant. In this condition appetite regulation is less tight, as positive caloric balance occurs. Adipose tissue is now adapted to receive excess energy by an elevated effect on the regulatory steps of both lipid uptake (activation) and lipid mobilization (inhibition), both probably results of the increased insulin concentration. This in turn is probably a result of the adaptations in muscle tissue (which is now relatively insulin resistant), and insulin concentrations are elevated as a compensatory mechanism.

In this way we see that two main conditions are prevailing: one with adaptations toward a more effective muscle machinery and the other for more effective energy storage. In an environment in which energy availability changed markedly with the seasons, this was of course very useful. However, in today's excess of energy-rich nutrients and decreasing needs for muscular work, the sedentary, energy-accumulating condition remains more or less constant. The end result of this is an excess mass of adipose tissue, or obesity.

An additional consequence, and one of a potentially harmful character, should be mentioned in this connection. As stated previously, the lipolysis machinery is adapted to work at a high level to secure an adequate availability of energy substrate for the working muscles. There is thus a risk that this system will produce unnecessarily high FFA concentrations in circulation, resulting from too much lipolysis stimulation in adipose tissue. This risk is increased further if adipose tissue is enlarged, particularly in regions where lipolytic sensitivity is very high, such as in abdominal adipose tissue (see the following discussion). In addition, if muscle is poorly adapted for lipid oxidation and lipid perhaps not even utilized, the net result might be excess concentrations of circulating FFA. This in turn will result in exposure of tissues to excess FFA concentrations, followed by uptake in the tissues and mainly esterification of FFA to triacyl-

glycerols. The liver secretes these newly synthesized triglycerides, which are then again taken up in adipose tissue. The muscle, however, seems to tend to accumulate such triglyceride (16), forming intramuscular triglyceride energy depots.

There is evidence that excessive FFA concentrations at the cellular level may result in an impairment of glucose transport and metabolism at well-defined biochemical steps (54). Although this probably should be regarded as a physiologically meaningful mechanism to save the limited carbohydrate stores of the body, a prolonged inhibitory action at this level might result in a condition with decreased sensitivity to insulin that ultimately might increase the risk for diabetes mellitus (for a more detailed review, see ref. 9).

This situation is an example of the unwanted effects of an urbanized lifestyle when imposed on an organism that was constructed for another type of life and is unmodern for our present way of life in the urbanized part of the world. Seen in this perspective it seems that the actual causal therapy is increased physical exercise, which would remove all the unwanted effects described (a) by a combination of adaptations in muscle for lipid combustion, (b) by regulating the appetite to diminish the risk of energy overconsumption, and (c) by making available lipid substrate for oxidation in adipose tissue.

Regional Variations

There is considerable evidence that lipolysis is not homogeneously active in different parts of human adipose tissue. The femoral region is less lipolytically active than are several other regions of adipose tissue, for example, the abdominal subcutaneous fat depot in studies in vitro (43, 45, 55, 62) and in vivo (51). This seems to be particularly pronounced in women and during pregnancy but, interestingly, does not seem to be the case during lactation. This suggests a specific role for this depot, namely, to provide reserve energy for the lactation process (55). Intraabdominal depots seem particularly sensitive to lipolytic stimuli (52) and are also less sensitive to the antilipolytic effect of insulin, perhaps because of a relatively low capacity of the adipocytes here to bind insulin (12). These differences in lipolytic sensitivity in various adipose tissue regions seem to be based mainly on differences in the relation between beta- and alpha-adrenergic activity (45).

There is also a marked difference in the sensitivity to different steroid hormones in adipose tissue regions. Although these effects might be most pronounced on lipid accumulation, they may also influence lipid mobilization. This is known to be the case for cortisol. Cortisol binding varies in different regions and seems to be most pronounced in intraabdominal adipose tissues, providing perhaps a background to the pronounced lipolytic sensitivity of these adipose tissue depots (56). The role of sex steroid hormones for lipolysis regulation is not clear (for a review, see ref. 57).

There seem to be differences in the adaptation of the lipolytic machinery to physical training between genders. Women have been reported to adapt their adipose tissue lipolysis less than do men (21), perhaps providing a background to the observation that men decrease body fat more efficiently during physical training than do women (22). Whether there are regional differences in this regard is currently unknown.

Conclusion

Lipid mobilization during physical exercise is regulated by a balance between stimulation and inhibition of a hormone-sensitive triglyceride lipase, which hydrolyzes triglycerides to free fatty acids and glycerol. In humans the sympathetic nervous system is the main stimulating factor and insulin (and perhaps lactate) the main inhibitor. After physical training this system for lipid mobilization is adapted to a higher sensitivity to the stimulation by the sympathetic nervous system, which now can operate at a lower level of activity. The concentrations of the inhibitory factors are lower, facilitating lipid mobilization. Furthermore, other adaptations of energy intake help in developing an adipose tissue of a limited mass and comprised of small fat cells. Physical training thus results in a relatively small adipose tissue storage of fat in adipocytes with a limited amount of triglycerides that are readily available by a lipid mobilization system that operates with high sensitivity to a limited stimulus. These are all adaptations that are useful for optimal performance after physical training. There might be regional and gender-related differences in these adaptations.

References

1. Ahlborg, G., P. Felig, L. Hagenfeldt, R. Hendler, and J. Wahren. Substrate turnover during prolonged exercise in man. *J. Clin. Invest.* 53: 1080-1090, 1974.

2. Andersen, P., and J. Henriksson. Capillary supply of the quadriceps femoris muscle of man: Adaptive response to exercise. *J. Physiol.* 270: 677-690, 1977.

3. Askew, E.W., R.L. Huston, C.G. Plopper, and A.L. Hecker. Adipose tissue cellularity and lipolysis. *J. Clin. Invest.* 56: 521-529, 1975.

4. Barwich, D., G. Klett, W. Eckert, and H. Weicker. Exercise-induced lipolysis in patients with central Cushing's disease. *Int. J. Sports Med.* 1: 120-126, 1980.

5. Berger, D., J.C. Floyd, R.M. Lampman, and S.S. Fajans. The effect of adrenergic receptor blockade on the exercise-induced rise in pancreatic polypeptide in man. *J. Clin. Endocrinol. Metab.* 50: 33-39, 1980.

6. Björntorp, P. The effect of lactic acid on adipose tissue metabolism *in vitro*. *Acta Med. Scand.* 178: 253, 1965.

7. Björntorp, P., G. Grimby, H. Sanne, L. Sjöstrom, G. Tibblin, and L. Wilhelmsen. Adipose tissue fat cell size in relation to metabolism in weight-stable physically active men. *Horm. Metab. Res.* 4: 182-186, 1972.

8. Björntorp, P., M. Fahlén, G. Grimby, A. Gustafson, J. Holm, P. Renström, and T. Scherstén. Carbohydrate and lipid metabolism in middle-aged, physically well-trained men. *Metabolism* 21: 1037-1044, 1972.

9. Björntorp, P. Classification of obese patients and complications related to the distribution of surplus fat. *Am. J. Clin. Nutr.* 45: 1120-1125, 1987.

10. Bloom, S.R., R.H. Johnson, D.M. Park, M.J. Rennie, and W.R. Sulaiman. Differences in the metabolic and hormonal response to exercise between racing cyclists and untrained individuals. *J. Physiol.* 258: 1-18, 1976.

11. Blomqvist, C.G., S.F. Lewis, W.F. Taylor, and R.M. Graham. Similarity of the hemodynamic responses to static and dynamic exercise of small muscle groups. *Circ. Res.* 48(Suppl. 1): 87-92, 1981.

12. Bolinder, J., L. Kager, J. Östman, and P. Arner. Differences at the receptor and postreceptor levels between human omental and subcutaneous adipose tissue in the action of insulin on lipolysis. *Diabetes* 32: 117-129, 1983.

13. Boyd, A.E., S.R. Giamber, M. Mager, and H.E. Lebovitz. Lactate inhibition of lipolysis in exercising man. *Metabolism* 23: 531-542, 1974.

14. Bukowiecki, L., J. Lupien, N. Follea, A. Paradis, D. Richard, and J. LeBlanc. Mechanism of enhanced lipolysis in adipose tissue of

exercise-trained rats. *Am. J. Physiol.* 239: E422-E429, 1980.

15. Carlson, L., L-G. Ekelund, and L. Orö. Studies on blood lipids during exercise. IV. Arterial concentration of plasma free fatty acids and glycerol during and after prolonged exercise in normal men. *J. Lab. Clin. Med.* 61: 724-729, 1963.

16. Carlson, L.A., S-O. Liljedahl, and C. Wirsén. Blood and tissue changes in the dog during and after excessive free fatty acid mobilization. *Acta Med. Scand.* 178: 81-102, 1965.

17. Carlson, L.A., L-G. Ekelund, and S.O. Fröberg. Concentration of triglycerides, phospholipids and glycogen in skeletal muscle and of free fatty acids and β-hydroxybutyric acid in blood in man in response to exercise. *Eur. J. Clin. Invest.* 1: 248-254, 1971.

18. Clausen, J.P. Circulatory adjustments of dynamic exercise and effect of physical training in normal subjects and in patients with coronary artery disease. *Prog. Cardiovasc. Dis.* 18: 459-495, 1976.

19. Costill, D.L., W.J. Fink, L.H. Getchell, J.L. Ivy, and F.A. Witzmann. Lipid metabolism in skeletal muscle of endurance-trained males and females. *J. Appl. Physiol.* 47: 787-791, 1979.

20. Cousineau, D., R.J. Ferguson, J. Champlain, P. deGauthier, P. Cote, and M. Bourassa. Catecholamines in coronary sinus during exercise in man before and after training. *J. Appl. Physiol.* 43: 801-806, 1977.

21. Després, J.P., C. Bouchard, R. Savard, A. Tremblay, M. Marcotte, and G. Thériault. The effect of a 20-week endurance training program on adipose tissue morphology and lipolysis in men and women. *Metabolism* 33: 235-239, 1984.

22. Després, J.P., A. Tremblay, A. Nadeau, and C. Bouchard. Physical training and changes in regional adipose tissue distribution. In: Björntorp, P., P. Lönnroth, and U. Smith, eds. *Hazards of regional obesity. Acta Med. Scand. Suppl.* 723: 205-212, 1988.

23. Essén, B., L. Hagenfeldt, and L. Kaijser. Utilization of blood-borne and intramuscular substrates during continuous and intermittent exercise in man. *J. Physiol.* 265: 489-506, 1977.

24. Feldberg, W., and E. Wei. Central cardiovascular effects of enphalins and C-fragment of lipoprotein. *J. Physiol.* 280: 18, 1978.

25. Francis, K.T. Effect of water and electrolyte replacement during exercise in the heat on biochemical indices of stress and performance. *Aviat. Space Environ. Med.* 50: 115-119, 1979.

26. Franckson, J.R.M., R. Vanroux, R. Leclercq, H. Brunengraber, and H.A. Ooms. Labelled insulin catabolism and pancreatic responsiveness during long-term exercise in man. *Horm. Metab. Res.* 3: 366-373, 1979.

27. Galbo, H., J.J. Holst, and N.J. Christensen. Glucagon and plasma catecholamine responses to graded and prolonged exercise in man. *J. Appl. Physiol.* 38: 70-76, 1975.

28. Galbo, H., N.J. Christensen, and J.J. Holst. Glucose-induced decrease in glucagon and epinephrine responses to exercise in man. *J. Appl. Physiol.* 42: 525-530, 1977.

29. Galbo, H., J.J. Holst, and N.J. Christensen. The effect of different diets and of insulin on the hormonal response to prolonged exercise. *Acta Physiol. Scand.* 107: 19-32, 1979.

30. Galbo, H., M.E. Houston, N.J. Christensen, J.J. Holst, B. Nielsen, E. Nygaard, and J. Suzuki. The effect of water temperature on the hormonal response to prolonged swimming. *Acta Physiol. Scand.* 105: 326-337, 1979.

31. Hansen, J.F., N.J. Christensen, and B. Hesse. Determinants of coronary sinus noradrenaline in patients with ischaemic heart disease: Coronary sinus catecholamine concentration in relation to arterial catecholamine concentration, pulmonary artery oxygen saturation and left ventricular end-diastolic pressure. *Cardiovasc. Res.* 12: 415-421, 1978.

32. Hartley, L.H., J.W. Mason, R.P. Hogan, L.G. Jones, T.A. Kotchen, E.H. Mougey, F.E. Wherry, L.L. Pennington, and P.T. Ricketts. Multiple hormonal responses to graded exercise in relation to physical training. *J. Appl. Physiol.* 33: 602-606, 1972.

33. Hartley, L.H., J.W. Mason, R.P. Hogan, L.G. Jones, T.A. Kotchen, E.H. Mougey, F.E. Wherry, L.L. Pennington, and P.T. Ricketts. Multiple hormonal responses to prolonged exercise in relation to physical training. *J. Appl. Physiol.* 33: 607-610, 1972.

34. Henriksson, J., and J.S. Reitman. Time course of changes in human skeletal muscle succinate dehydrogenase and cytochrome oxidase activities and maximal oxygen uptake with physical activity and inactivity. *Acta Physiol. Scand.* 99: 91-97, 1977.

35. Henriksson, J. Training induced adaptation of skeletal muscle and metabolism during submaximal exercise. *J. Physiol.* 270: 661-675, 1977.

36. Hilsted, J., H. Galbo, B. Somme, T. Schwartz, J. Fahrenberg, O.B. Schaffalitzy de Muckadell, K.B. Lauritsen, and B. Tronier. Gastroenteropancreatic hormonal changes during exercise. *Am. J. Physiol.* 239: G136-G140, 1980.

37. Holloszy, J.O., M.J. Rennie, R.C. Hickson, R.K. Conlee, and J.M. Hagberg. Physiological consequences of the biochemical adaptations to endurance exercise. *Ann. N.Y. Acad. Sci.* 301: 440-450, 1977.

38. Holm, G., B. Jacobsson, L. Toss, U. Smith, and P. Björntorp. The effect of physical exercise on the regulation of beta adrenergic receptors and adenylate cyclase in rat adipocytes [Abstract]. Paper presented at the Third International Congress of Obesity. *Alim. Nutr. Metab.* 1: 280, 1980.

39. Häggendal, L., L.H. Hartley, and B. Saltin. Arterial noradrenaline concentration during exercise in relation to the relative work levels. *Scand. J. Clin. Lab. Invest.* 26: 337-342, 1970.

40. Issekutz, B., Jr., W.A.S. Shaw, and T.B. Issekutz. Effect of lactate on FFA and glycerol turnover in resting and exercising dogs. *J. Appl. Physiol.* 39: 349-353, 1975.

41. Issekutz, B. Role of β-adrenergic receptors in mobilization of energy sources in exercising dogs. *J. Appl. Physiol.* 44: 869-876, 1978.

42. Järhult, J., and J. Holst. The role of the adrenergic innervation to the pancreatic islets in the control of insulin release during exercise in man. *Pflugers Arch.* 383: 41-45, 1979.

43. Kather, H., F. Schroeder, B. Simon, and G. Schlierf. Human fat cell adenylate cyclase: Regional differences in hormone sensitivity. *Eur. J. Clin. Invest.* 7: 595-597, 1977.

44. Koivisto, V., V. Soman, E. Nadel, and P. Felig. Exercise and insulin: Insulin binding, insulin mobilization, and counterregulatory hormone secretion. *Fed. Proc.* 39: 1481-1486, 1980.

45. LaFontan, M., L. Dang-Tran, and M. Berland. Alpha adrenergic antilipolytic effect of adrenaline responsiveness of different fat deposits. *Eur. J. Clin. Invest.* 9: 261-266, 1978.

46. Mason, J.W., L.H. Hartley, T.A. Kotchen, E.H. Mougey, P.T. Ricketts, and L.G. Jones. Plasma cortisol and norepinephrine responses in anticipation of muscular exercise. *Psychosom. Med.* 35: 406-414, 1973.

47. McCrimmon, D.R., D.A. Cunningham, P.A. Rechnitzer, and J. Griffiths. Effect of training on plasma catecholamines in post myocardial infarction patients. *Med. Sci. Sports* 8: 152-156, 1976.

48. Mayer, J., N.B. Marshall, J.J. Vitale, J.H. Christensen, M.B. Machayeken, and F.J. Stare. Exercise, food intake and body weight, in normal rats and genetically obese adult mice. *Am. J. Physiol.* 177: 544-548, 1954.

49. Mitchell, J.H., W.C. Reardon, D.I. McCloskey, and K. Wildenthal. Possible role of muscle receptors in the cardiovascular response to exercise. *Ann. N.Y. Acad. Sci.* 310: 232-242, 1977.

50. Munsat, T.L., D. McNeal, and R. Waters. Effects of nerve stimulation on human muscle. *Arch. Neurol.* 33: 608-617, 1975.

51. Marin, P., M. Rebuffé-Scrive, U. Smith, and P. Björntorp. Glucose uptake in human adipose tissue. *Metabolism* 36: 1154-1160, 1987.

52. Ostman, J., P. Arner, P. Engfeldt, and L. Kager. Regional differences in the control of lipolysis in human adipose tissue. *Metabolism* 28: 1198-1203, 1979.

53. Paul, P. Uptake and oxidation of substrates in the intact animal during exercise. In: Pernow, P., and B. Saltin, eds. *Muscle metabolism during exercise.* New York: Plenum Press, 1971: pp. 225-247.

54. Randle, P.J., P.B. Garland, C.N. Hales, and E.A. Newsholme. The glucose fatty acid cycle: Its role in insulin sensitivity and the metabolic disturbances of diabetes mellitus. *Lancet* ii: 785-789, 1963.

55. Rebuffé-Scrive, M., L. Enk, N. Crona, P. Lönnroth, L. Abahamsson, U. Smith, and P. Björntorp. Fat cell metabolism in different regions in women: Effects of menstrual cycle, pregnancy and lactation. *J. Clin. Invest.* 75: 1973-1976, 1985.

56. Rebuffé-Scrive, M., K. Lundholm, and P. Björntorp. Glucocorticoid binding of human adipose tissue. *Eur. J. Clin. Invest.* 15: 267-271, 1985.

57. Rebuffé-Scrive, M., and P. Björntorp. Regional adipose tissue metabolism in man. In: Vague, J., et al. *Metabolic complications of human obesities.* Amsterdam: Elsevier, 1985: pp. 149-159.

58. Rosell, S., and E. Belfrage. Blood circulation in adipose tissue. *Physiol. Rev.* 59: 1078-1104, 1979.

59. Shepard, R.J., and K.H. Sidney. Effects of physical exercise on plasma growth hormone and cortisol levels in human subjects: Exercise and sport. *Sci. Rev.* 3: 1-30, 1975.

60. Shepherd, R.E., E. G. Noble, G.A. Klug, and P.D. Gollnick. Lipolysis and cAMP accumulation in adipocytes in response to physical training. *J. Appl. Physiol.* 50: 143-148, 1981.

61. Shyu, B.C., S.A. Andersson, and P. Thorén. Endorphin mediated increase in pain threshold induced by long-lasting exercise in rats. *Life Sci.* 30: 833-840, 1982.

62. Smith, U., J. Hammarsten, P. Björntorp, and J. Kral. Regional differences and effect of weight reduction on human fat cell metabolism. *Eur. J. Clin. Invest.* 9: 327-333, 1979.

63. Stralfors, P., H. Olsson, and P. Belfrage. Hormone sensitive lipase. *Enzymes* 18: 147-177, 1987.

64. Terjung, R. Endocrine response to exercise. *Exer. Sport Sci. Rev.* 7: 153-180, 1979.

65. Trap-Jensen, J., N.J. Christensen, J.P. Clausen, B. Rasmussen, and K. Klausen. Arterial noradrenaline and circulatory adjustment to strenuous exercise with trained and nontrained muscle groups. In: *Physical fitness: Proceedings of a satellite symposium of the 25th International Congress of Physiological Science.* Prague: University of Karlova Press, 1973: pp. 414-418.

66. Wahren, J., L. Hagenfeldt, and P. Felig. Splanchnic and leg exchange of glucose, amino acids, and free fatty acids during exercise in diabetes mellitus. *J. Clin. Invest.* 55: 1303-1314, 1975.

67. Varnauskas, E., H. Bergman, P. Houk, and P. Björntorp. Hemodynamic effects of physical training in coronary patients. *Lancet* ii: 8-13, 1966.

68. Varnauskas, E., P. Björntorp, M. Fahlén, J. Prerovsky, and J. Stenberg. Effects of physical training on exercise blood flow and enzymatic activity in skeletal muscle. *Cardiovasc. Res.* 4: 418-421, 1970.

69. Vinten, H., and H. Galbo. Effect of physical training on transport and metabolism of glucose in adipocytes. *Am. J. Physiol.* 244: E129-134, 1983.

70. Wirth, A., C. Diehm, H. Mayer, H. Mörl, I. Vogel. P. Björntorp, and G. Schlierf. Plasma C-peptide and insulin in trained and untrained subjects. *J. Appl. Physiol.* 50: 71-77, 1981.

71. Zierler, K.L. Fatty acids as substrates for heart and skeletal muscle. *Circ. Res.* 38: 459-463, 1976.

Chapter 27

Discussion: Adipose Tissue Adaptation to Exercise

Lawrence B. Oscai
Warren K. Palmer

About 100 yr ago, adipose tissue was considered to be a form of connective tissue that was metabolically inactive. However, in 1948, Shapiro and Wertheimer (39) demonstrated fatty acid synthesis and release in vitro. This finding highlighted the functional importance of adipose tissue as a source of fuel.

Triglyceride (TG) has an important advantage over glycogen as a storage form of fuel for ATP production. Gram for gram, pure triglycerides can yield on complete oxidation nearly 2.5 times as many molecules of ATP as can pure glycogen.

Important to this discussion is the fact that oxidation of free fatty acids can provide much of the energy for prolonged exercise. In this chapter, we describe briefly the current status of the adipose tissue responses to exercise.

Effect of Exercise Training on Adipocyte Response to Insulin

It is well recognized that exercise-trained rats have a much smaller body fat content than do sedentary rats of the same age and similar body weight. This difference is due primarily to a smaller fat-cell size in the trained rats (7, 8). The smaller fat cells of the exercise-trained rats bind more insulin because of an increased number of insulin receptors (13). Further, glucose uptake and oxidation are greater in fat cells of trained rats than they are in those of sedentary rats over a wide range of insulin concentrations (13). It appears that fat cells of exercise-trained animals adapt for rapid replenishment of energy stores. For example, it has been shown that fat cells of sedentary animals had a volume 180% greater than those of the trained animals despite

only a 9% difference in body weight (14). Following cessation of training, adipocyte size increased rapidly; approximately two thirds of the initial difference in fat-cell volume between the trained and the sedentary rats had disappeared after 9 d without exercise. This notion is supported by the work of Savard et al. (37, 38), who found that basal and maximal insulin-stimulated glucose conversion to triglycerides increased significantly with endurance training. Concomitant with the increase in fat-cell size is the diminished response of glucose uptake and oxidation to insulin. Thus the effect of exercise training on the response of adipocytes to insulin is rapidly lost when exercise is stopped.

Adipose Tissue Lipolysis in Rats

Free fatty acids (FFA) can provide much of the energy to skeletal muscle during prolonged exercise (22, 35). During a long bout of submaximal exercise, plasma FFA concentration increases (12, 49). At the same time, the respiratory exchange ratio (RER) declines, indicating that a greater proportion of the energy is being supplied by the oxidation of FFA (1). One of the adaptations that characterizes the trained state is the greater reliance on FFA oxidation during submaximal exercise with the sparing of carbohydrate, reflected by the lower RER (23). In the trained individual, serum FFA and blood glycerol concentrations are unchanged or slightly lower than control concentrations when exercise is performed at a standardized work rate (20, 49). This occurs even though endurance training blunts the catecholamine response to submaximal exercise (21, 49). This finding has led numerous investigators to study the effect of lipolytic agents on adipose tissue from exercise-trained humans and animals. Parizkova and Stankova (34) were the first to report that slices of adipose tissue from trained rats released more FFA in response to epinephrine than did tissue from nontrained animals. This finding has been confirmed by other investigators (4, 9, 40, 48) using a variety of isolated tissue and cell preparations.

Regulation of Hormone-Sensitive Lipase

To determine the mechanism of the enhanced adipose tissue lipolysis induced by training, it is necessary to understand the events mediating hormone-stimulated lipolysis. In 1964, Rizack (36) found cAMP stimulation of lipolytic enzyme activity in cell free adipose tissue extracts. This activation was ATP dependent. A few years later, another piece of the puzzle was put in place when it was found that cAMP's actions were mediated through a cAMP-dependent protein kinase (47). Huttunen et al. (24) used cAMP-dependent protein kinase to activate rat adipose tissue hormone-sensitive lipase (HSL), the rate-limiting enzyme in lipolysis. Independently, Corbin et al. (11) were also able to activate HSL from adipose tissue with protein kinase. These results provided suggestive evidence that activation was mediated by protein phosphorylation. Huttunen and Steinberg (25) showed that incubation of HSL, purified approximately 100-fold from rat adipose tissue with cAMP and $[\gamma\text{-}^{32}P]$-ATP, resulted in an increase in protein-bound ^{32}P. The time course of phosphorylation closely paralleled that of lipase activation. However, because the enzyme preparation was not homogeneous, the phosphate acceptor could not be identified.

Lipase activation in rat adipose tissue was relatively small ($\leqslant$twofold). Therefore, chicken adipose tissue has been used as an enzyme source. An enzyme preparation purified three- to fivefold was activated 160% with cAMP, ATP, and theophylline. Protein kinase inhibitor reduced lipase activity about 90%. This inhibition could be reversed by the addition of protein kinase to the reaction mix (28).

The data obtained through 1974 suggested a control mechanism of adipose tissue HSL similar to that of muscle phosphorylase $\underline{b}$ kinase. As a result, a cAMP cascade system was proposed even though a pure enzyme was not available (42).

The HSL of adipose tissue is bound tightly to the endogenous tissue lipids, which float during cen-

trifugation of homogenates (45). This represented a major problem in early attempts to purify this enzyme protein. However, in 1980 a significant improvement in the purification of chicken adipose tissue was reported (6). The enzyme, when purified 300- to 500-fold, exhibited a molecular weight of 42,000 daltons on SDS polyacrylamide gel electrophoresis. This protein accepted ^{32}P from $[\gamma\text{-}^{32}P]$-ATP in the presence of cAMP-dependent protein kinase. However, although the final preparation could be phosphorylated, it could not be activated.

While Steinberg's group worked with chicken adipose tissue, the Scandinavian group headed by Belfrage continued to work on the purification of rat adipose tissue HSL. Using detergent to solubilize the enzyme and isoelectric focusing for purification, Belfrage et al. (5) obtained an enzyme that was purified 100-fold. This preparation could be phosphorylated and activated 100% with protein kinase and ATP. The protein that acted as a phosphate acceptor had an apparent molecular weight of 86,000. In a subsequent study, Fredrikson et al. (19) purified rat adipose tissue HSL 2,000-fold to 50% purity and found a specific activity 1,000-fold higher than that of chicken HSL. Activity of this preparation could be doubled using protein kinase and ATP. The rate of activation correlated with phosphate incorporation into serine residues in the protein (43). Unfortunately, these investigators were able to get only 20 μg of enzyme from adipose tissue of 100 rats (43). In subsequent work, Stralfors et al. (44) identified two phosphorylation sites on an 84,000 dalton lipase subunit. One site, phosphorylated by the cyclic AMP-independent glycogen synthase kinase 4, has been termed the *basal site*. The second has been designated the *regulatory site* and is phosphorylated by the cyclic AMP-independent protein kinase. Both sites can be dephosphorylated by specific protein phosphatases (31). The role of the phosphorylation-dephosphorylation of the basal site has yet to be determined.

The group headed by Londos (10) reported that purification of HSL from adipose tissue is hampered by the formation of aggregates comprised primarily of cytoskeletal proteins. This group has obtained a homogeneous enzyme preparation of 84,000 daltons on SDS-PAGE and was phosphorylated with the cAMP-dependent protein kinase. Enzyme yield using this preparation was approximately 60 μg from 100 g of adipose tissue. Antibodies have been prepared using this protein (J. Egan, personal communication).

It is quite evident that considerable work still needs to be done with adipose tissue HSL to determine whether the mechanism of action is mediated totally through the cAMP classical cascade proposed more than a decade ago.

Effect of Exercise Training on the Lipolytic Cascade

Studies have been designed to investigate the influence of exercise training on the various components of the lipolytic cascade scheme. The first step in the activation of adipocyte lipolysis is the binding of the hormone to the membrane receptor. Enhanced lipolysis could be mediated by a training-induced increase in receptor number or receptor binding affinity. Bukowiecki et al. (9) found that exercise training had no effect on dihydroalprenolol binding to adipocytes isolated from rat epididymal fat pads. This was supported in a study by Williams and Bishop (48). Basal adenyl cyclase activity of adipocyte ghosts from male (3, 48) and female (41) rats was not influenced by training. Shepherd et al. (41) reported that membrane adenyl cyclase activity from fat cells of trained female rats was less responsive to various doses of norepinephrine than were membrane preparations from control-rat adipose tissue cells. Unfortunately, the hormone-stimulated activity obtained was below the basal activity reported in the same study. These findings are in contrast to the results of Williams and Bishop (48), who found that peak epinephrine-stimulated adenyl cyclase activity increased by training. These authors concluded that training may increase receptor cyclase coupling, which could be modified by some modifications in the GTP-binding protein that links the receptor with the cyclase. In support of this hypothesis, Izawa et al. (27) reported that adenylate cyclase activity of adipocyte membranes of trained rats induced by Gpp(NH)p (a nonhydrolyzable guanine nucleotide) was significantly greater than that measured in membranes isolated from nontrained rats. In a subsequent study, Izawa et al. (26) reported that GTP inhibition of forskolin-stimulated adenyl cyclase activity was significantly reduced in adipocyte membranes from trained rats when compared to membranes isolated from sedentary rats. The authors suggest that exercise training may induce an attenuation of an element of the inhibitory pathway, possibly Gi itself, resulting in enhanced lipolysis. It is difficult to determine whether alterations in individual elements of a particular pathway result in a net change in pathway function. Therefore, hormone-stimulated cyclic AMP formation in whole-cell

preparations may be a more desirable indication of cyclic AMP metabolism.

Askew et al. (3), using fat pads from trained male rats, and Shepherd et al. (40), using adipocytes from trained female rats, found that less cyclic AMP was formed in the cells of trained rats at any given concentration of lipolytic agent than was produced in cells from control rats. These results could be explained by the elevated level of cyclic nucleotide phosphodiesterase activity found in the adipose tissue of trained rats (3, 40, 41). In contrast, we found that the adipose tissue cyclic AMP phosphodiesterase activity of male rats was not affected by 12 wk of treadmill running (33).

Shepherd et al. (41) reported that the cyclic AMP-dependent protein kinase activity of adipose tissue from female rats was not influenced by training. We found that the maximal adipocyte protein kinase activity is reduced with training at the same time that cyclic AMP-binding capacity is increased (32). These findings suggest a functional loss in protein kinase catalytic capacity through an alteration in the stoichiometric ratio in the subunits of protein kinase resulting from exercise training.

The final step in the hormonal activation of lipolysis is the hydrolysis of TG, a step that is catalyzed by HSL. A number of investigators claim to have measured fatty acid or glycerol release from endogenous adipocyte TG (2, 30). In only one case has endogenous TG lipase activity from fat cells of trained female rats been analyzed using an exogenous TG substrate (40). This study reported that the basal and cyclic AMP-stimulated activities of HSL from adipose tissue of trained rats were significantly reduced when compared to those of control rats. It is apparent from this discussion that no clear-cut adaptations have been identified in the enzymes involved in the regulation of adipocyte lipolysis as a result of exercise training.

Effect of Exercise Training on Adipose Tissue Lipolysis in Humans

The finding that exercise training produces an adaptation in rats that results in an increased capacity to release FFA from adipocytes has recently been confirmed in humans (15, 16, 17, 18, 29, 46). In these studies, the sensitivity of adipose tissue to the lipolytic action of catecholamines is enhanced. However, following the cessation of endurance training, the blood FFA and glycerol responses to epinephrine infusion are decreased and that of lactate increased (29). The loss of a training effect on these responses appears to be complete within 4 d of the onset of inactivity (29). These results, based on human epinephrine infusion experiments, suggest that the loss of a training effect is occurring at the level of the adipocyte.

Conclusion

An adaptation that characterizes the trained state is the greater reliance on FFA oxidation during submaximal exercise with a sparing of carbohydrate. In the trained individual, serum FFA and blood glycerol concentrations are unchanged or slightly lower than control levels when exercise is performed at a standardized work rate. This occurs even though endurance training reduces the catecholamine response to submaximal exercise.

Investigators have found that adipose tissue from trained rats releases more FFA in response to epinephrine than does tissue from untrained rats. To determine the mechanism of the enhanced adipose tissue lipolysis induced by endurance exercise, it is necessary to understand the events mediating hormone-stimulated lipolysis. Following hormone binding to a membrane receptor, adenylate cyclase is activated, promoting the formation of cAMP inside the adipocyte. Cyclic AMP activates a protein kinase that phosphorylates a hormone-sensitive lipase, the rate-limiting enzyme in adipose tissue lipolysis. Only recently has this lipase been purified to homogeneity and an antibody prepared. The protein has a molecular weight of 84,000 daltons and contains two sites of phosphorylation.

The finding that exercise training produces an adaptation in rats resulting in an increased capacity to release FFA from adipocytes has recently been confirmed in humans. In these studies, the sensitivity of adipose tissue to the lipolytic action of catecholamines is enhanced. However, following the cessation of endurance training, the blood FFA and glycerol responses to epinephrine infusion are decreased and that of lactate is increased. The loss of a training effect on these responses appears to be complete within a few days of the onset of inactivity. These results, based on human epinephrine infusion experiments, suggest that the loss of a training effect is occurring at the level of the adipocyte.

In conclusion, exercise training produces enhanced lipolysis in adipose tissue, resulting in a smaller fat cell. However, this training effect is rapidly lost after exercise training is stopped. It appears that fat cells of trained animals are adapted for an increased mobilization followed by a rapid replenishment of energy stores. The replenishment phase is facilitated by an increase in insulin binding, glucose transport, and glucose oxidation.

Acknowledgments

We wish to thank Gloria De Leon for typing the manuscript. This work was supported by National Institutes of Health research grants AM-17357 and HL-38037.

References

1. Ahlborg, G., P. Felig, L. Hagenfeldt, R. Hendler, and J. Wahren. Substrate turnover during prolonged exercise in man. *J. Clin. Invest.* 53: 1080-1090, 1974.

2. Askew, E.W., G.L. Dohm, R.L. Huston, T.W. Sneed, and R.P. Dowdy. Response of rat tissue lipases to physical training and exercise. *Proc. Soc. Exp. Biol. Med.* 141: 123-129, 1972.

3. Askew, E.W., A.L. Hecker, V.G. Coppes, and F. B. Stifel. Cyclic AMP metabolism in adipose tissue of exercise-trained rats. *J. Lipid Res.* 19: 729-736, 1978.

4. Askew, E.W., R.L. Huston, C.G. Plopper, and A.L. Hecker. Adipose tissue cellularity and lipolysis: Response to exercise and cortisol treatment. *J. Clin. Invest.* 56: 521-529, 1975.

5. Belfrage, P., B. Jergil, P. Stralfors, and H. Tornqvist. Hormone-sensitive lipase of rat adipose tissue: Identification and some properties of the enzyme protein. *FEBS Letters* 75: 259-264, 1977.

6. Berglund, L., J.C. Khoo, D. Jensen, and D. Steinberg. Resolution of hormone-sensitive triglyceride/diglyceride lipase from monoglyceride lipase of chicken adipose tissue. *J. Biol. Chem.* 255: 5420-5428, 1980.

7. Björntorp, P., and L. Sjöström. The composition and metabolism *in vitro* of adipose tissue fat cells of different sizes. *Europ. J. Clin. Invest.* 2: 78-84, 1972.

8. Booth, M.A., M.J. Booth, and A.W. Taylor. Rat fat cell size and number with exercise

training, detraining and weight loss. *Fed. Proc.* 33: 1959-1963, 1974.

9. Bukowiecki, L., J. Lupien, N. Follea, A. Paradis, D. Richard, and J. LeBlanc. Mechanism of enhanced lipolysis in adipose tissue of exercise-trained rats. *Am. J. Physiol.* 239 (*Endocrinol. Metab.* 2): E422-E429, 1980.

10. Chang, M.K., J.J. Egan, and C. Londos. Purification of adipocyte hormone-sensitive lipase and adrenal cholesterol esterase: A general protein purification strategy [Abstract]. *Fed. Proc.* 45: 1670, 1986.

11. Corbin, J.D., E.M. Reimann, D.A. Walsh, and E.G. Krebs. Activation of adipose tissue lipase by skeletal muscle cyclic adenosine $3^{1\prime}$, $5^{1\prime}$-monophosphate-stimulated protein kinase. *J. Biol. Chem.* 245: 4849-4851, 1970.

12. Costill, D.L., P.D. Gollnick, E.D. Jansson, B. Saltin, and E.M. Stein. Glycogen depletion pattern in human muscle fibers during distance running. *Acta Physiol. Scand.* 89: 374-383, 1973.

13. Craig, B.W., G.T. Hammons, S.M. Garthwaite, L. Jarett, and J.O. Holloszy. Adaptation of fat cells to exercise: Response of glucose uptake and oxidation to insulin. *J. Appl. Physiol.: Respir. Environ. Exerc. Physiol.* 51: 1500-1506, 1981.

14. Craig, B.W., K. Thompson, and J.O. Holloszy. Effects of stopping training on size and response to insulin of fat cells in female rats. *J. Appl. Physiol.: Respir. Environ. Exerc. Physiol.* 54: 571-575, 1983.

15. Crampes, F., M. Beauville, D. Riviere, and M. Garrigues. Effect of physical training in humans on the response of isolated fat cells to epinephrine. *J. Appl. Physiol.* 61: 25-29, 1986.

16. Després, J.P., C. Bouchard, R. Savard, D. Prud'homme, L. Bukowiecki, and G. Thériault. Adaptive changes to training in adipose tissue lipolysis are genotype dependent. *Int. J. Obes.* 8: 87-95, 1983.

17. Després, J.P., C. Bouchard, R. Savard, A. Tremblay, M. Marcotte, and G. Thériault. Level of physical fitness and adipocyte lipolysis in humans. *J. Appl. Physiol.: Respir. Environ, Exerc. Physiol.* 56: 1157-1161, 1984.

18. Després, J.P., C. Bouchard, R. Savard, A. Tremblay, M. Marcotte, and G. Thériault. The effect of a 20-week endurance training program on adipose-tissue morphology and lipolysis in men and women. *Metabolism* 33: 235-239, 1984.

19. Fredrikson, G., P. Stralfors, N.O. Nilsson, and P. Belfrage. Hormone-sensitive lipase of rat adipose tissue. Purification and some properties. *J. Biol. Chem.* 256: 6311-6320, 1981.

20. Gyntelberg, F., M.J. Rennie, R.C. Hickson, and J.O. Holloszy. Effect of training on the response of plasma glucagon to exercise. *J. Appl. Physiol.: Respir. Environ. Exerc. Physiol.* 43: 302-305, 1977.

21. Hartley, L.H., J.W. Mason, R.P. Hogan, L.G. Jones, T.A. Kotchen, E.H. Mougey, F.E. Wherry, L.L. Pennington, and P.T. Ricketts. Multiple hormonal responses to prolonged exercise in relation to physical training. *J. Appl. Physiol.* 33: 607-610, 1972.

22. Havel, R.J., L.A. Carlson, L-.G. Ekelund, and A. Holmgren. Turnover rate and oxidation of different free fatty acids in man during exercise. *J. Appl. Physiol.* 19: 613-618, 1964.

23. Hermansen, L., E. Hultman, and B. Saltin. Muscle glycogen during prolonged severe exercise. *Acta Physiol. Scand.* 71: 129-139, 1967.

24. Huttunen, J.K., D. Steinberg, and S.E. Mayer. ATP-dependent and cyclic AMP-dependent activation of rat adipose tissue lipase by protein kinase from rabbit skeletal muscle. *Proc. Natl. Acad. Sci. USA* 67: 290-295, 1970.

25. Huttunen, J.K., and D. Steinberg. Activation and phosphorylation of purified adipose tissue hormone-sensitive lipase by cyclic AMP-dependent protein kinase. *Biochem. Biophys. Acta* 239: 411-427, 1971.

26. Izawa, T., T. Komabayashi, S. Shinoda, K. Suda, M. Tsuboi, and E. Koshimizu. Possible mechanism of regulating adenylate cyclase activity in adipocyte membranes from exercise-trained male rats. *Biochem. Biophys. Res. Commun.* 151: 1262-1268, 1988.

27. Izawa, T., T. Komabayashi, M. Tsuboi, E. Koshimizu, and K. Suda. Augmentation of catecholamine-stimulated [³H] GDP release in adipocyte membranes from exercise-trained rats. *Jpn. J. Physiol.* 36: 1039-1045, 1986.

28. Khoo, J.C., and D. Steinberg. Reversible protein kinase activation of hormone-sensitive lipase from chicken adipose tissue. *J. Lipid Res.* 15: 602-610, 1974.

29. Martin, W.H., E.F. Coyle, M. Joyner, D. Santeusanio, A.A. Ehsani, and J.O. Holloszy. Effects of stopping exercise training on epinephrine-induced lipolysis in humans. *J. Appl. Physiol.: Respir. Environ. Exerc. Physiol.* 56: 845-848, 1984.

30. McGarr, J.A., L.B. Oscai, and J. Borensztajn. Effect of exercise on hormone-sensitive lipase activity in rat adipocytes. *Am. J. Physiol.* 230: 385-388, 1976.

31. Olsson, H., and P. Belfrage. The regulatory and basal phosphorylation sites of hormone-sensitive lipase are dephosphorylated by protein phosphatase-1, 2A and 2C but not by protein phosphatase-2B. *Euro. J. Biochem.* 168: 399-405, 1987.

32. Oscai, L.B., R.A. Caruso, A.C. Wergeles, and W.K. Palmer. Exercise and the cAMP system in rat adipose tissue. I. Lipid mobilization. *J. Appl. Physiol.* 50: 250-254, 1981.

33. Palmer, W.K., C.A. Kalina, T.A. Studney, and L.B. Oscai. Exercise and the cAMP system in rat adipose tissue. II. Nucleotide catabolism. *J. Appl. Physiol.* 50: 254-258, 1981.

34. Parizkova, J., and L. Stankova. Release of free fatty acids from adipose tissue *in vitro* after adrenalin in relation to the total body fat in rats of different age and different physical activity. *Nutr. Dieta* 9: 43-55, 1967.

35. Paul, P., and B. Issekutz, Jr. Role of extramuscular energy sources in the metabolism of the exercising dog. *J. Appl. Physiol.* 22: 615-622, 1967.

36. Rizack, M.A. Activation of an epinephrine-sensitive lipolytic activity from adipose tissue by adenosine 3', 5' Phosphate. *J. Biol. Chem.* 239: 392-395, 1964.

37. Savard, R., J.P. Després, Y. Deshaies, M. Marcotte, and C. Bouchard. Adipose tissue lipid accumulation pathways in marathon runners. *Int. J. Sports Med.* 6: 287-291, 1985.

38. Savard, R., J.P. Després, M. Marcotte, and C. Bouchard. Endurance training and glucose conversion into triglycerides in human fat cells. *J. Appl. Physiol.* 58: 230-235, 1985.

39. Shapiro, B., and E. Wertheimer. The synthesis of fatty acids in adipose tissue *in vitro*. *J. Biol. Chem.* 173: 725-728, 1948.

40. Shepherd, R.E., E.G. Noble, G.A. Klug, and P.D. Gollnick. Lipolysis and cAMP accumulation in adipocytes in response to physical training. *J. Appl. Physiol.* 50: 143-148, 1981.

41. Shepherd, R.E., W.L. Sembrowich, H.E. Green, and P.D. Gollnick. Effect of physical training on control mechanisms of lipolysis in rat fat cell ghosts. *J. Appl. Physiol.* 42: 884-888, 1977.

42. Steinberg, D. Interconvertible enzymes in adipose tissue regulated by cyclic AMP-dependent protein kinase. In: Greengard, P., and G.A. Robinson, eds. *Advances in cyclic nucleotide research*. New York: Raven Press, vol. 7, 1983: pp. 157-198.

43. Stralfors, P., and P. Belfrage. Phosphorylation of hormone-sensitive lipase by cyclic AMP-dependent protein kinase. *J. Biol. Chem.* 258: 15146-15152, 1983.

44. Stralfors, P., P. Björgell, and P. Belfrage. Hormonal regulation of hormone-sensitive lipase in intact adipocytes: Identification of phosphorylated sites and effects on the phosphorylation by lipolytic hormones and insulin. *Proc. Natl. Acad. Sci. USA* 81: 3317-3321, 1984.

45. Strand, O., M. Vaughan, and D. Steinberg. Rat adipose tissue lipases: Hormone-sensitive lipase activity against triglycerides compared with activity against lower glycerides. *J. Lipid Res.* 5: 554-562, 1964.

46. Tremblay, A., J.P. Després, and C. Bouchard. Adipose tissue characteristics of ex-obese long-distance runners. *Int. J. Obes.* 8: 641-648, 1984.

47. Walsh, D.A., J.P. Perkins, and E.G. Krebs. An adenosine 3', 5'-monophosphate-dependent protein kinase from rabbit skeletal muscle. *J. Biol. Chem.* 243: 3763-3765, 1968.

48. Williams, R.S., and T. Bishop. Enhanced receptor-cyclase coupling and augmented catecholamine-stimulated lipolysis in exercising rats. *Am. J. Physiol.* 243: E345-E351, 1982.

49. Winder, W.W., R.C. Hickson, J.M. Hagberg, A.A. Ehsani, and J.A. McLane. Training-induced changes in hormonal and metabolic responses to submaximal exercise. *J. Appl. Physiol.* 46: 766-771, 1979.

Chapter 28

Bone and Connective Tissue Adaptations to Physical Activity

Charles M. Tipton
Arthur C. Vailas

Historians responsible for summarizing the events for the last 5 decades of the 19th century in North America will certainly include the emergence, acknowledgment, and acceptance of the exercise, fitness, and health movement. Therefore, it is appropriate that we examine the past as we discuss the future.

Bone Response to Physical Activity

Although the assigned title of this chapter implies that bone is a tissue with little commonality with connective tissue, connective tissue is one of the primary tissue types (epithelial, connective, muscular, and nervous) that includes osseous, hemopoetic, fatty, ligamentous, and tendinous tissues within its domain (22). Only the central nervous system appears to lack the presence of osseous tissue within its structures. For purposes of this presentation, the primary emphasis is on the adaptations associated with bones, ligaments, and tendons. Because Everett Smith and his colleagues address the interrelationships between physical activity and osteoporosis elsewhere in these proceedings (see chapt. 43), the emphasis in the section on bone will be on exploring its adaptability and its structural importance for the integrity and function of ligaments and tendons.

In many respects, the study of connective tissue has been neglected by exercise scientists because of their interests and training and because funding opportunities have been directed toward other systems and tissues. However, more than 2,000 yr ago, Galen advanced the concept that tendons would waste away if they were idle (35). According to Akeson et al. (3), in 1892, Wolff stated that tissue would respond and adapt to the mechanical forces being placed on them. "Every change in the form and function of a bone, or of its function alone is followed by certain definite changes in its internal architecture and equally definite secondary alterations in its mathematical laws".

In 1895, Roux (47) concluded that mechanical tension was an effective stimuli for the proliferation of connective tissue, a conclusion that was brilliantly confirmed by Weiss (16) and by Stearns (57, 58) using either tissue cultures or a rabbit-ear preparation. The fact that connective tissue will exhibit stress-strain characteristics is not new, as these relationships were proposed by Wertheim in 1847 (81). Collectively, the concept that connective tissue will respond and adapt to mechanical stimuli is not an original one. What is new from the last 2 decades of research is the quantification of the adaptive responses and the investigations on the contributing mechanisms. The acquisition of our current knowledge has occurred in part by the technological advance in the testing and evaluations of connective tissues (45, 68) and by scientists with expertise in anatomy, biochemistry, bioengineering, biomechanics, histology, modeling, and physiology.

Until the use of radioisotopes became routine, many scientists concluded that the structural protein of connective tissue, collagen, was metabolically inert. Studies conducted in our laboratory have shown that the oxygen consumption and the cytochrome oxidase activity in rat or primate ligaments and/or tendons are markedly lower than they are in the liver and muscle; but, in no conceivable way can these tissues be considered inert (73).

Inherent in the acceptance of the fact that connective tissue will respond to mechanical stimuli is the concept of exercise specificity (51, 68). Although the concept has been demonstrated in many ways, for bones, ligaments, or tendons it means that exercises must be prescribed so that the resulting forces will be transmitted to these tissues. For the ligaments of the knee, we found that running on a grade significantly increased ligament junction strength by 12%, whereas running on a flat surface was associated with a 6% decrease when compared to controls even though both exercise groups significantly increased their muscle aerobic enzyme activity by 38% and 56%, respectively (68). In fact, negative findings for junction-strength and for isolated-tissue-strength results from primates (67) and swine (87) have occured, in part, because the animals were trained on flat running surfaces.

Anatomy and histology texts are replete with the fact that bone is a dynamic tissue that serves many functions for the body, the most notable being the mechanical structure for the support and locomotion of the organism. As dramatized by Wolff in 1892 (86), bone will respond to mechanical stimuli, and the classic bed-rest studies initiated by Whedon 40 yr ago (15, 83, 84) have convincingly demonstrated the importance of calcium for this effect. Of course, bones respond to genetic, nutritional, endocrinologic, and local factors (Smith addresses some of these aspects in more detail in chapter 43). As most physiologists know, responses to mechanical stimuli are site specific because bone can be classified into trabecular and cortical types. Therefore, the technological development of equipment (42) to measure bone mineral content (single- or dual-photon absorptiometry), total body calcium (neutron activation analysis), or bone density (quantitative computed tomography) has provided the means to examine these various factors as well as the influences of physical activity on bone parameters at select sites. In the past, cross-sectional studies using single-photon absorptiometry using a myriad of athletic populations (tennis and soccer players, runners, weight lifters, swimmers, track-and-field athletes, etc.) generally report that bone sites chronically experiencing the greater forces will exhibit the highest values in bone mineral content (55). Because bone mineral content is indicative of bone mass with the potential ability to resist fracture, the measurement of this parameter has experienced a virtual explosion in clinical and experimental medicine.

Even with newer and more sophisticated techniques, the evaluation of the effects of increased physical activity on bone in humans is complicated by the role and importance of the endocrine system

(42). The effects of the endocrine system are hampered by the lack of well-controlled longitudinal studies and confused by the plethora of cross-sectional studies that have not effectively standardized their subjects or the exercise histories of those subjects. When a longitudinal study (14 wk) was performed on more than 200 male army recruits whose basic training included an increased amount of physical activity (8 h/d), the bone mineral content of the tibia was significantly increased (5% for the right leg and 11% for the left leg) with no meaningful changes in bone width (33). Unfortunately, there were no controls, the incidence of stress fractures was exceedingly high, and only 60% of the population were able to complete the training without interruption. Surprisingly, no explanation was provided as to why the legs responded differently to physical activity. In a preliminary report, Dalsky et al. (14) evaluated changes in lumbar bone mineral content with 15 menopausal females who performed 40 wk of weight-bearing exercise that included walking, jogging, and stair climbing and then compared the results to those obtained from a suitable control group. The initial differences in lumbar bone mass were not statistically significant, but after 40 wk the active group had a significant increase of 14% whereas the controls exhibited a decline of 1%. Smith and Raab (54) also have longitudinal data pertaining to radius, humerus, and ulna measurements from elderly postmenopausal women that support the concept that habitual physical activity can enhance an increase in bone mineral content at select sites.

Aloia et al. (4) used neutron activation analysis procedures to study for 1 yr postmenopausal women who participated in a 1-h-per-day, 3-d-per-week physical activity program. They found a significant increase in total body calcium (4%) in the active group and a decrease (3%) in the control group. Williams et al. (85) followed runners (they called them consistent and inconsistent runners) for 4 mo before they ran their first marathon and then compared the changes with a select control group. The bone mineral content of the os calcis was significantly increased (3%), but only in the consistent runners.

Insights into how increased or compensating physical activity may alter bone mass and its remodeling process have been gained from animal studies. Chamay and Tschantz (13) removed a section of the radius from adult dogs and evaluated the effect of increased weight bearing. After 9 wk, the ulna showed a significant enlargement. Goodship et al. (21) performed a similar experiment with swine, but they removed the ulna. As expected, the cross-sectional area of the radius was significantly increased by 50%. Woo et al. (91) performed an in vitro analysis of cortical bone obtained from swine that exercised on treadmill at an intensity corresponding to 60%-85% of their maximum heart rate. As a result of this program, the cross-sectional area of the femur increased by 23% and cortical thickness by 17%. Woo et al. (92) concluded that the increased physical activity caused internal stresses in bone that resulted in increased cortical thickness and a decreased medullary cavity. During the last decade, others have creatively examined the factors that influence bone morphology in avians by attaching rosette strain gauges to bone surfaces (28, 29, 30, 48). Using a vibrational procedure, they found that physiological strain levels would either maintain or increase bone mass in immobilized ulnas from avians (see chapt. 29). These collective studies helped Marcus and Carter (32) and Wahlen et al. (82) develop a mathematical model to predict bone density that included the summation of the number of daily cycles of an effective stress magnitude, the effective stress state, and an exponent that determines the importance between the effective stress magnitude and the number of loading cycles. Although this approach uses data obtained from the calcaneous, makes generic assumptions relevant to physical activity effects, and provides no insights into hormonal or nutritional contributions, it does provide an experimental and mathematical basis on which to evaluate the prescription of physical activity for either the maintenance or the improvement of bone mass in different populations. Of course, the equation does not answer questions concerning the effects of physical activity on the growth plate. Training studies with rodents by several investigators have demonstrated that strenuous physical activity will retard the length of long bones (63). Because this issue is a profound one, studies with other species must be undertaken to resolve the uncertainty.

Insights into the effect of physical activity on the maturation of long bones have been provided by Matsuda et al. (34). Using exercise-trained chickens that were 8 and 12 wk old at sacrifice, they examined tarsometatarsal bones of runners and nonrunners. Measurements of endosteal perimeter, periosteal perimeter, medullary area, and cortical area were significantly less (17%–49%) in the younger runners than they were in the controls. In addition, their bending-stiffness averages were 40% lower than were those of the younger nonrunners.

When follow-up studies were conducted with bone collagen, the younger runners had fewer nonreducible cross-linkages. Although these results are too preliminary for extrapolation, they do raise the concern that strenuous physical activity could be producing and maintaining immature collagen in the structures of growing organisms.

The high incidence of osteoporosis and the existence of the space age has necessitated that the clinical and scientific communities also examine the hormonal, nutritional, metabolic, chemical, and mechanical factors concerned with the maintenance of bone mass. This examination requires the development of effective countermeasures and the close monitoring of calcium metabolism. To many, the rate-limiting step on the duration of future space missions is the magnitude of the loss of calcium from bones and its physiological consequences.

The advent of the space age in the *Gemini* flights (80) showed evidence of osteopenia (X-ray densitometry of the calcaneous). When single-photon-beam absorptiometry was used on the calcaneous of astronauts from *Skylab* 4 (84 d in orbit), a mean decrease of 3.9% was reported (79). In one astronaut a decrease of 7.9% was noted at this same site (83). This decrease in trabecular bone was more than that observed for the compact bone of the wrist, indicating that load-bearing sites and bone types are important considerations. Calcium studies on *Skylab* astronauts showed great variability, yet the members of *Skylab* 4 lost approximately 25 g of calcium from their total pool (83). If the calculations of Rambaut and Goode (46) are correct, in 1-yr an astronaut could lose calcium in excess of 25% of the calcium pool, which contains approximately 1,250 g. Excessive loss of calcium from bones can lead to nephrolithiasis, and sufficient anecdotal reports from spaceflight experiments suggest that this possibility must be taken seriously by NASA officials. Urinanalyses confirm not only calcium loss but also hydroxyproline increases, which imply that the collagen in bone is degraded when the mineral is lost (55). Moreover, postflight fecal calcium levels remained elevated for 20 d. At the moment it is uncertain when bone and calcium equilibriums return to baseline, and some reports suggest that it may require months or years before this state is achieved. Although more data are needed, there are results from the *Salyut* 6 and *Soyuz* 7 missions that showed significant losses in the calcaneous and tibia regions of cosmonauts. In recent unconfirmed results from the Soviet Union (70), Yuri Romanenko was quoted as saying he grew 1.25 cm in stature after 326 d in space. At this time, he had lost only 5% of his bone calcium concentration.

Studies of rats flown in space have provided insights into the effect of gravity on the properties and functions of bones. Not only are these studies inexpensive, but they also provide a means to study remodeling (9), which was one of the most strenuous arguments against their presence in space. Rats exhibit bone growth of the diaphysis and metaphysis in their long bones (26), with remodeling occurring in the secondary spongiosa of the caudal vertebrae (9). Apparently, only osteonal bone remodeling cannot be investigated in the rat (9). In the 18.5-d mission of *Cosmos 782* and *Cosmos 936*, cortical bone exhibited an inhibition of periosteal bone formation that was approximately 53% (*Cosmos 936*) of the values secured from the ground-based controls (26). As expected, this effect has not been seen in the ribs (56). In the *Cosmos 936* series, bone torque was reduced to 67% of the value noted for ground-based controls, whereas rats that were centrifuged in space (*Cosmos 936*) exhibited torque results similar to those obtained from the ground-based controls (36, 37).

Ten rats were flown on the *Cosmos 1667* biosatellite's 7-d flight during July 1984. Histomorphometric analysis of the tibia, the ilium, and the lumbar vertebrae showed osteoporosis was most marked in the spongy bone of the tibia proximal metaphysis. Moreover, the number and functional activity of the osteoblasts were depressed in all bones observed. In addition, the mechanical properties showed decreased maximum deformation and an increased modulus of elasticity.

In the *Cosmos 605* experiments, trabecular bone in the tibial and femoral metaphysis showed a decreased mass (26). In the *Cosmos 1129* mission, male rats (83 d old) were flown for 18.5 d. Trabecular bone in the tibial and humeral metaphysis were examined and exhibited an increased amount of fat in the bone marrow and a decreased number of osteoblasts near the growth plate. Because the osteoblast numbers were unchanged, bone formation may have been inhibited with bone resorption being constant (26). Most of the *Cosmos* data show that the longitudinal growth for the rat tibia, femur, and humerus was not altered by exposure to a reduced gravity (52). Interestingly, compression testing of vertebral bodies suggests a loss of stiffness and strength.

In NASA's 7-d experiments of *Spacelab 3*, the rat tibia and humerus were measured for their biomechanical properties. Few changes were statistically significant. However, 3-point bending tests indicated that the bone strength and stiffness were altered by the space environment (52). When female rats were suspended for 28 d to stimulate weightlessness (71), the most noticeable bone change was a decrease (12%) in the geometric configuration of the femur middiaphysis. There were no significant changes in femur cortical area, density, DNA, uronic acid and collagen concentration, length, and wet weight.

Response to Joint Physical Activity

The structural integrity of the body requires more than the existence of bone and cartilage; namely, it requires the presence of ligaments, tendons, and joint capsules. As noted by Frank et al. (17), the classification of ligaments, tendons, and fascia as dense connective tissue has perpetuated the concept that they were identical in structure and might be surgically interchangeable. According to Frank et al. (17) and Gelberman et al. (19), there is now sufficient anatomical, physiological, and biochemical evidence to proclaim their distinctive differences.

One could assume from the recent advances being made in the surgical approaches to bone and ligament disorders, in the knee braces for athletes, or in the testing and evaluation of limb strength and mobility (68) that similar advances have been made in the evaluation of the functions of dense connective tissues in humans. With minor exceptions, such is not the case; thus, we must continue to look to animal experiments to improve our understanding of the basic mechanisms and processes associated with the role of physical activity. Due to the high incidence of injury, aspects pertaining to the medial collateral ligament (66) are emphasized in this chapter. Although ligaments connect bone to bone, the process is not simple. In general, there are two types of insertions: direct and indirect (92). The direct is the most common type and is divided into the superficial and deep groups. These fibers meet the bone at a right angle. The deep fibers have a transition of four distinct zones: ligament, fibrocartilage, mineralized fibrocartilage, and bone. Interestingly, the four transition zones occur within a distance of 1 mm or less (92). In contrast, indirect insertions contain predominantly superficial fibers that insert by blending into the periosteum. The periosteum is composed of a superficial fibrous layer and a deep osteogenic layer that maintains its continuity with bone. The deep fibers of indirect insertions attach to bone with little or none of the transitional zone of fibrocartilage seen in direct insertions (88).

In the experimental testing of the femur–medial collateral ligament–tibia complex in rats and dogs, the failure predominantly occurred at the tibial site and between the zone of mineralized fibrocartilage and the bone (66). This result did not occur when immature and mature rabbits were tested (43). Our training studies with normal male rats and dogs indicated that an 8- to 12-wk study would significantly increase junction strength from 8% to 24%, respectively (66). Similarly, changes in rats have been noted by Adams (1) as well as by Zuckerman and Stull (94). Because trained male thyroidectomized and hypophysectomized rats exhibited increases of 13% and 19%, respectively, we believe that the repeated strains at the insertion site are as important as the presence of hormones released from the pituitary gland (66). However, in rats this effect appears to be related to gender, as we have not been able to demonstrate similar changes in normal female rats or in ovariectomized rats receiving estrogen (66) (unpublished data). When various groups of male rats were trained for 6, 12, 18, or 24 mo, the exercising groups had junction-strength means that were 10%, 11%, 12%, and 8% higher than those of their controls (68). In most comparisons, these differences were statistically significant. When rabbits were used (76), chronic physical activity also was associated with higher junction-strength values. In contrast, the junction strength of the medial collateral ligament of the nonhuman primate *Galago senegalensis* was not enhanced by a progressive training program (67). However, we believe that this lack of an exercise effect is an example of exercise specifically, as the patellar ligament is more important for the animals' locomotion and jumping actions than are the medial collateral ligaments (68).

At first approximation, one could assume that an increase in junction strength with physical activity is a reflection of osseous changes at the insertion site. Unfortunately, we have no suitable method to quantify the area of the insertion site. However, changes are also occurring in ligaments per se as reflected by in vitro biomechanical tests. When isolated ligaments are normalized by indices for cross-sectional area, chronic physical activity by rats will cause ligamentous breaking strength to be 12%–56% higher than that of their nonexercised controls (68). Because the water content of rat ligaments is not altered by training, ligamentous mass was increased. However, this change did not persist after 6 mo of physical activity, presumably because the intensity of exercise was not increased (68).

Of the dense fibrous tissues, the most specialized form are tendons, whose function is to unite muscle with bone and transmit the forces associated with muscle contractions to bone (92). As with ligaments, the insertion into bone is one that involves a transition between tendons, nonmineralized fibrocartilage, mineralized fibrocartilage, and bone. Moreover, the angle of insertion of the fibril can vary, depending on the site (92). In an early study with exercising rabbits, Viidik (77) exercised male rabbits for 40 wk and measured the tensile strength of four different tendons at the time of sacrifice. Regardless of whether the results were expressed in absolute (*N*) or in relative (*N*/area) units, no statistically significant differences were noted. Unfortunately, he had no independent data proving that the animals had been trained. Using advanced technological approaches (Figure 28.1), Woo et al. (93) measured the strength and biomechanical properties of tendons obtained from swine who had exercised for 8 mo. They found significant increases in the load at failure to range from 25% to 62% for the trained group. The cross-sectional area of the tendons from the lateral extensors of the foot was significantly increased by 21%. The slopes of the stress-strain curves showed that the trained group had more stiffness and that the curve was shifted to the left when compared to their nontrained controls. When the effects of 20 wk of endurance training by nonhuman primates were evaluated (67), the Achilles tendon showed little adaptive changes; but, the tendon from the extensor digitorium muscles exhibited significantly higher failure values (43%) for the trained group. Komi et al. (27) have developed, tested, and used a buckle transducer for the Achilles tendons of humans and recorded extremely high forces. However, to date, the effects of chronic physical activity on human tendon strength or the forces being developed have not been reported.

Interestingly, the role of increased physical activity on the mechanical properties of capsular tissue has not been systematically investigated. As will be noted in a following section, this is not the situation with physical inactivity. Until recently, the effect of physical activity on the menisci of animals has also received little experimental attention. Considered to be an extension of the tibia, menisci serve to deepen the surface of the articular fossa of the head of the tibia for placement of the condyles of the femur (8). The mensci are fibrocartilaginous tissues made up of an intermingled network of collagen fibers and cells that serve to distribute considerable physical loads being placed on the knee joints (8). They also contribute to joint stability and to the nutrition and lubrication of the articular cartilage of the knee joint. To determine

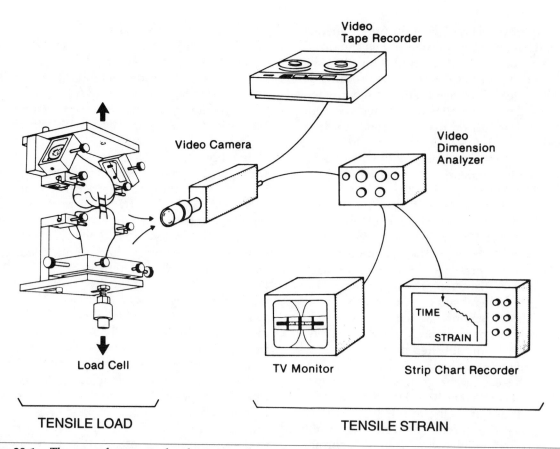

Figure 28.1. The use of newer technology to evaluate the properties of connective tissue. *Note.* From "A New Methodology to Determine the Mechanical Properties of Ligaments at High Strain Rates" by R.H. Peterson and S.L.-Y. Woo, 1986, *Journal of Biomechanical Engineering, 108,* p. 365-367. Reprinted by permission.

whether menisci were adaptable to the loads placed on them by treadmill running, Vailas et al. (75) exercised young rates for 12 wk. They found different responses in different regions of the menisci. The posterior region, which receives the higher load-bearing forces, was thicker (10%) and had higher uronic acid, hydroxyproline, and calcium concentrations than did the same region from nontrained rats. The authors interpreted these findings to mean that training had increased the concentrations of proteoglycans and collagen while increasing the stiffness properties of the collagen.

Immobilization and Inactivity

It must be appreciated that immobilization, for any reason, induces changes in the surrounding structures such as muscles, capsule, cartilage, tendons, ligaments, and bone. More than 20 yr ago, Akeson (2) developed and perfected an in vitro device to measure the contributions of the capsule to knee-

joint stability. His group found that immobilization per se increased the laxity of joint movements while causing marked changes in fiber appearance and orientation (3). Junction-strength measurements from two different groups of rats whose hind limbs were immobilized for 6 wk exhibited decreases of 21% and 24%, respectively, in the forces developed at failure, whereas dogs, immobilized for the same duration of time, demonstrated a significant decrease of 15% in their strength measures (66). Woo et al. (88) immobilized male rabbits for 9 and 12 wk and reported that tibial avulsion accounted for 100% and 90% respectively of the failures found with the two groups. Associated with these results were reductions in the load at failure of 31% and 29% at the same time periods. When Noyes et al. (39) immobilized primates for 24 mo, the load at failure was decreased by 25% when compared to the contralateral control. Although contralateral controls from the same animal are not the best controls for comparative purposes, the trend would be the same; that is, immobilization will cause a marked reduction in the strength of the junction.

These functional changes are not suprising with immobilization because gross and cellular changes are seen in capsular structures or cartilage surfaces in short periods (3). Besides marked changes in the appearance of cortical and trabecular bone, the insertion site is changed so that widespread subperiosteal bone resorption is replaced by disorganized fibrous tissue and the region exhibits increased osteoelastic activity (31, 68). We (65, 66, 68) as well as others (3, 39, 88) have followed the time course of recovery after immobilization and found that the process is extremely protracted (Figure 28.2). If the insertion site does not exhibit a transition of zones (66), then the osteoblastic activity appears greater and the junction becomes weaker. In general, 6 wk of immobilization will require 20 wk or more for recovery to occur (66, 68) (Figure 28.2). Woo et al. (88) followed the recovery profiles of 2 rabbits that had 52 wk of remobilization after 12 wk of immobilization. After 1 yr, the previously resorbed bone had undergone complete reconstruction, and its histological appearance resembled that of the controls. Rheological measurements from bone-

ligament-bone preparations from rats, dogs, rabbits, or primates that have had one limb immobilized for 6 wk or longer generally show stress-strain curves that are shifted to the right, have decreased elastic stiffness measures, show records of exaggerated tissue deformations, exhibit low failure energy values, and promote other changes that contribute to a decrement in function (3, 66, 68, 88, 89). Woo et al. (88) measured the cross-sectional area of ligaments from the legs of immobilized rabbits and noted that 9 and 12 wk of inactivity resulted in decreases of 22% and 21%, respectively.

Oakes's research on the effects of 1 mo of exercise (swimming and running) on the distribution of collagen fibril populations in cruciate ligament of young rats is summarized in chapter 29. Training was associated with an increase in the number of smaller collagen fibrils but a decrease in cross-sectional area. Ideally, a similar study should be repeated for longer durations to see whether the effects persist after maturation and aging. On the other hand, we have observed, using light microscopy, that the number and size of collagen fiber bundles were decreased in dogs (65). Interestingly,

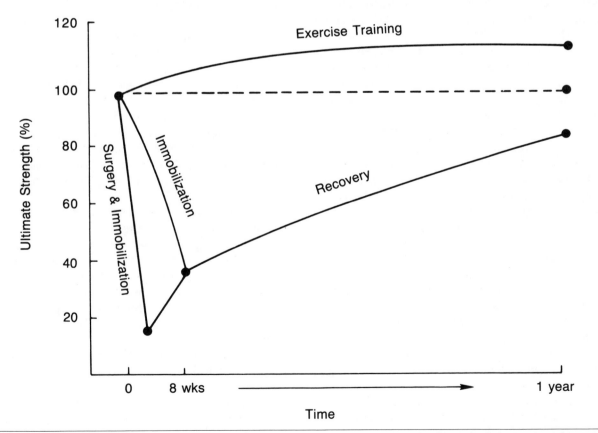

Figure 28.2. Schematic representation of the effects of physical activity on the functional properties of intact and repaired ligaments and possibly tendons. Based on conclusions of Akeson et al. (3).

Binkley and Peat (11) reported that the immobilization of rat legs for 6 wk caused a decrease in the diameter of the collagen fibrils considered to be in the small-diameter category of the medial collateral ligament. According to Akeson et al. (3), immobilization per se has more of an adverse effect on tendons than on ligaments, especially if the repair process is involved.

Biochemical Changes in Intact Structures Associated With Increased and Decreased Activity

In any discussion of the biochemical effects of physical activity on connective tissue, the importance of collagen is mentioned. This tissue protein represents approximately 25% of the total protein found in mammalian systems and exists in five major basic types, with Type I being found in tendons, ligaments, skin, and bone and Type II located in cartilage and intervertebral disks (64). However, collagen is not alone in providing structured integrity to the body, as it exists and functions with other proteins, such as elastin and the proteoglycans. In the pioneering studies of Akeson (2) and Akeson et al. (3) on changes in joint capsules with immobilization, they found decreased water content and total glycoaminoglycans concentrations as well as an increased turnover, synthesis, and degradation of collagen. Amiel et al. (5) measured the effects of immobilization on rabbit ligaments and periarticular tissues and found after 9 wk that collagen synthesis was increased, whereas after 12 wk there was a decrease in collagen degradation. However, the most striking findings by Akeson et al. (3) concerning collagen changes in immobilized limbs have been on the number of reducible cross-linkages on articular cartilage and ligaments. They found the number to be increased in select circumstances. Although these findings help to explain reduction in forces generated and changes in rheological characteristics, they do not explain how they occurred or what happened during immobilization with the nonreducible cross-linkages. When rabbits were immobilized for 24-27 d and measurements made of proteoglycan changes in articular cartilage (62), it was observed that the total amount, the type extractable, and the ability to form aggregates were reduced.

Vailas et al. (72) measured the combined effects of voluntary running and aging in rats on tendon glycoaminoglycan and collagen concentrations. After 9 mo, glycoaminoglycan concentrations had increased; but such was not the case 14 mo later, when the animals had decreased their running activity by 70%. At that age, the glycoaminoglycan concentrations had decreased and the collagen concentrations increased. In the rabbit immobilization experiments conducted by Tammi et al. (62), concerning proteoglycan changes, they found that running intermittently for 24 d increased the amount extracted and the concentrations present in cartilage.

Because of the importance of collagen to connective tissue and because collagen fibrils become smaller with immobilization and larger with increased physical activity (65, 66), investigators have measured its concentrations, type, and metabolism in a variety of experiments (10, 64). Results concerning changes in collagen concentration with increased physical activity are mixed. We have found increased concentrations in dog but not in rat ligaments (66). Viidik (77) found no increase in tendons from rabbits, whereas Woo et al. (93) observed increases in tendons from swine. Heikkinen and Vuori (25) noted in older mice that training had increased the turnover rate of collagen in tendons. It has been reported that hydroxyproline concentrations were increased in the skin of older individuals (male) who practice regular physical activity (60). Moreover, increased muscle collagen synthesis, as evaluated by prolydroxylase activity, was higher in trained populations (59) but not in subjects who trained for only 8 wk (61). To date, only Viidik (78) has evaluated whether training will alter the cross-linkages of collagen. He reported that tail collagen from trained rats had fewer cross-linkages than did the collagen obtained from non-trained animals. Because these results were obtained with older procedures, future studies using isotopes are needed to confirm these intriguing results.

Amiel et al. (6) and Harper et al. (24) are currently pursuing research on the ability of ligaments to produce collagenase enzymes and on how injury can accelerate the process. These exciting results raise intriguing questions as to whether decreased physical activity (e.g., immobilization) will facilitate its presence or whether increased physical activity will activate an inhibitor that in turn will decrease its release.

The Iowa group (43) studied on menisci changes in growing chickens who were exercised at 70% to 80% of their $\dot{V}O_2$max. Many interesting biochemical changes were observed, but one germane to this presentation was that the number of the collagen nonreducible cross-linkages was reduced.

They speculated that strenuous exercise during the periods of skeletal growth could impair the mechanical resistance of the tissue, making it more susceptible to injury. They also noted two distinct proteoglycan populations. One represented larger molecules that contained chondroitin sulfates and keratan sulfates that bind to hyaluronic acid, whereas the other represented smaller molecules that contained dermatan sulfates that do not bind to hyaluronic acid. Apparently, the ratio between the two populations are influenced by both age and exercise. To study the effect of strenuous exercise on these two populations, they exercised 3-wk-old chickens for 8, 12, 14, and 20 wk and evaluated their menisci changes. The most interesting results occurred after 5 wk, when there was a decrease in the smaller proteoglycans and an increase in the aggregation of the larger ones. Because these changes occurred when the collagen cross-linkages were reduced, strenuous exercise during growth could be a liability for the functions of the menisci.

Surprisingly, few simulated weightlessness experiments have been concerned about biochemical changes in connective tissues. One exception is the study of Vailas et al. (71), who evaluated the effects of 28 d of suspension with female rats. They noted that the collagen and proteoglycan concentrations in patellar tendons of rats were 28% lower than those found in nonsuspended rats and concluded that ground reaction forces were important in maintaining tissue homeostasis.

Physical Activity and the Repair Process With Ligaments

More than 2,400 yr ago, Hippocrates advocated exercise to assist in the healing process (66). Since that time a voluminous literature has accumulated on the subject of surgical repair and wound healing. In an early study with male dogs, we found that the strength of repaired ligaments in immobilized legs, had been reduced by 85% after 3 wk and by 65% after 6 wk (65) (Figure 28.2). In legs that were not immobilized after ligamentous repair, the repaired ligaments after 6 wk were 15% stronger than those of the repaired group with immobilized legs, indicating that activity had attenuated the expected loss in strength. When dogs were progressively exercised for 6 wk after the casts had been removed, the repaired ligaments were still 20%

weaker than was expected for normal intact structures.

Our studies (66, 68) with repaired medial collateral ligaments from rats demonstrated that training enhanced the absolute forces measured; but, when expressed on a cross-sectional basis, the forces were significantly lower because the healing process had increased the surface area of the ligament. Related results were reported in dogs by the San Diego group (90) who measured the strength of the repaired medial collateral ligament from immobilized and nonimmobilized legs. After 48 wk, the forces from the repaired ligaments were 38% lower than those of the controls. Collectively, we have used these types of information to advise athletes who have experienced surgical repair of ligaments to wait a year or more before returning to competition (Figure 28.2). Experimental investigation with repaired medial collateral ligaments from hypophysectomized rats who received replacement hormone therapy of either ICSH (interstitial cell stimulatory hormone) or testosterone significantly improved the strength of the repaired ligament (66). At that time we postulated that the increased physical activity was enhancing ligamentous repair by increasing the level of circulating anabolic steroids and by improving the capillarization and/or the distribution of blood flow to the repair site. However, it is known that the fraction of the cardiac output going to the medial collateral ligament is less than 0.1% of the total (66). When Amiel et al. (6) followed collagen synthesis, collagen degradation, and changes in collagen type for 40 wk in ligaments from rabbits whose legs were not immobilized, collagen turnover was greatest at 3-6 wk after injury (ruptures) and its concentration was decreased. The most interesting result was a shift in the percentage of Type I to Type III collagen. How a progressive physical activity recovery program would alter this shift remains to be determined.

Salter (49) and Salter et al. (50) pioneered the concept of cartilage-repair enhancement by continuous passive motion (CPM). This concept was modified by Gelberman et al. (20), who used intermittent motion to facilitate flexor tendon healing in dogs. They noted that the motion inhibited the ingrowth of granulation tissue from the tendon sheath and facilitated the rate of the repair process when compared to changes in repaired tendons that were immobilized.

The CPM concept has been extended to hospitals (18), and at the present time patients recovering from knee-joint surgery have their limbs placed in commercial units that provide passive motion to the joint for extended periods of time. Although it is too early to prove the effectiveness of the procedure, the preliminary results and prospects for extensive clinical use appear promising, as it is known that the convective flow of tissue fluid is facilitated by mechanical stimuli (23). Hence, tissue nutrition and the removal of metabolites (53) should be facilitated by light to moderate physical activity once exercise has been prescribed.

Miscellaneous Considerations

The role of physical activity in the use of connective tissue grafts is an area that is being pursued by Butler et al. (12) and Noyes et al. (40, 41). Preliminary results 6 wk later with primates show decreased ligamentous strength values when compared to preimplantation values. Physical activity could contribute to collagen synthesis and revascularization processes, although no evidence is available to support this speculation. The published data of Vailas (38), who measured plasma hydroxyproline concentrations as a marker for tissue injury, are promising. If substantiated, this would be a major advance in the diagnosis of connective tissue injuries. Because it has been reported (69) that intradermic injection of Type II collagen is arthritogenic, it becomes the responsibility of molecular biologists, immunologists, and exercise scientists to collaborate to determine whether physical activity can modify the time course of the disease.

Conclusion

The future of any area of study depends on the number of individuals interested in entering the area and the resources available for research purposes. Because of the massive consequences of bone and connective tissue diseases, departments of internal medicine, orthopedic surgery, biochemistry, and molecular biology will continue to receive funding for the investigation of clinical and basic science issues. Funding for departments of exercise science will be unlikely because of the paucity of investigators interested in these issues or because of the limited numbers of departments that have the faculty, laboratories, and courses to study the effects of physical activity on both bone and connective tissue. To change this situation, departments of exercise science, kinesiology, or physical education must include information in their curricula on biomechanics, exercise physiology, or exercise biochemistry that pertains to tissue biomechanics and to the responses of tissues to mechanical stimuli. In addition, the molecular reactions to physical forces must be addressed in such courses.

Although it is generally accepted that physical activity will modify and modulate changes in bone and connective tissue, the mechanisms remain obscure. From a theoretical standpoint, strenuous physical activity could be detrimental to growth at critical stages of the maturation process. Whether this effect is transient or permanent remains to be determined. Sufficient data are accumulating to demonstrate that physical activity will enhance the healing process, but more information is needed on when to begin, how much to prescribe, and how long it takes to enhance complete recovery.

The effects of aging on collagen metabolism have received considerable attention and funding. Yet there is a dearth of experimental information on how physical activity or a lack thereof will alter the aging process with this protein in general and with connective tissue in particular.

Finally, textbooks for exercise scientists currently devote very little space and emphasis to bone and connective tissue and to their importance to performance. It is hopeful that this conference will stimulate future authors to include this topic and readers to initiate research in these areas.

References

1. Adams, A. Effect of exercise on ligament strength. *Res. Q.* 37: 163-167, 1966.
2. Akeson, W.H. An experimental study of joint stiffness. *J. Bone Joint Surg.*, 43A: 1022-1034, 1961.
3. Akeson, W.H., C.B. Frank, D. Amiel, and S. L-Y. Woo. Ligament biology and biomechanics. In: *A.A.O.S. Symposium on Sports Medicine*, edited by G. Finnerman. St. Louis: C.V. Mosby, 1985, p. 11-51.
4. Aloia, J., S. Cohn, J. Ostuni, R. Cane, and K. Ellis. Prevention of involutional bone loss by exercise. *Ann. Int. Med.* 89: 356-358, 1987.
5. Amiel, D., W.H. Akeson, F. Harwood, and C.B. Frank. Stress deprivation effect on metabolic turnover of the medial collateral ligament. *Clin. Orthop. Rel. Res.* 172: 265-270, 1982.
6. Amiel, D., C.B. Frank, F.L. Harwood, W.H. Akeson, and J.B. Lleiner. Collagen alteration

in medial collateral ligament healing in a rabbit model. *Connect. Tissue Res.* (in press).

7. Amiel, D., K.K. Ishizue, F.L. Harwood, L. Kitabayashi, and W.H. Akeson. Injury of the anterior cruciate ligament: The role of collagenase in ligament degeneration. *J. Orthop. Res.* 7: 1989.

8. Arnoczky, S., M. Adams, K. DeHaven, D. Eyre, and V. Mow. Meniscus. In: S.L-Y. Woo and J.A. Buckwalter, eds. *Injury and repair of the musculoskeletal soft tissues*. Park Ridge, IL: American Academy of Orthopedic Surgeons, 1988: chapt. 12, pp. 487-537.

9. Baron, R., R. Tross, and A. Vignery. Evidence of sequential remodeling in the rat trabecular bone: Morphology, dynamic histomorphometry and changes during skeletal maturation. *Anat. Rec.* 208: 137-145, 1984.

10. Beyer, R.E. Regulation of connective tissue metabolism in aging and exercise. A review. In: Borer, K.T., D.W. Edington, and T.P. White, eds. *Frontiers of exercise biology*. Champaign, IL: Human Kinetics, 1983: pp. 85-99.

11. Binkley, J.M., and M. Peat. The effects of immobilization on the ultrastructure and mechanical properties of the medial collateral ligament of rats. *Clin. Orthop. Rel. Res.* 203: 301-308, 1986.

12. Butler, D.L., E.S. Grood, F.R. Noyes, and A.N. Sodd. On the interpretation of our anterior cruciate ligament data. *Clin. Orthop. Rel. Res.* 196: 26-34, 1985.

13. Chamay, A., and P. Tschantz. Mechanical influences in bone remodeling: Experimental research on Wolff's law. *J. Biomech.* 5: 173-180, 1972.

14. Dalsky, G.P., S.J. Birge, K.S. Kleinheider, and A.A. Eshani. The effect of endurance exercise training on lumbar mass in post-menopausal women [Abstract]. *Med. Sci. Sports Exerc.* 19: 5, 1987.

15. Deitrick, J.E., G.D. Whedon, and E. Schorre. Effects of immobilization upon various metabolic and physiologic functions in normal men. *Am. J. Med.* 4: 3-36, 1948.

16. Elliot, D.H. The biomechanical properties of tendon in relation to muscular strength. *Am. Phys. Med.* 9: 1-7, 1967.

17. Frank, C., S. Woo, T. Andriacchi, R. Brand, B. Oakes, L. Dahners, et al. Normal ligament: Structure, function, and composition. In: S. L-Y. Woo, and J.A. Buckwalter, eds. *Injury and repair of the musculoskeletal soft tissues*. Park Ridge, IL: American Academy of Orthopedic Surgeons, 1988, 45-101.

18. Frank, C., W.H. Akeson, S. L-Y. Woo, D. Amiel, and R.D. Coutts. Physiology and therapeutic value of passive joint motion. *Clin. Orthop. Rel. Res.* 185: 113-125. 1984.

19. Gelberman, R., K-N. Goldberg, and A. Banes. Tendon. In: *Injury and repair of the musculoskeletal soft tissues*, edited by S. L-Y. Woo and J. A. Buckwalter. Park Ridge, IL: American Academy of Orthopedic Surgeons, 1988, chapt. 1, p. 1-40.

20. Gelberman, R.H., S. L-Y. Woo, K. Lothringer, W.H. Akeson, and D. Amiel. Effects of early intermittent passive mobilization on healing canine flexor tendons. *J. Hand Surg.* 7: 170-175, 1982.

21. Goodship, A.E., L.E. Lanyon, and H. McFie. Functional adaption of bone to increased stress. *J. Bone Joint Surg.* 61A: 539-546, 1979.

22. Ham, A.W. *Textbook of histology*. 6th ed. Philadelphia: Lippincott, 1969, p. 169-187, 205-257, 374-455.

23. Hargens, A.R., and W.H. Akeson. Stress effects on tissue nutrition and viability. In: Hargens, A.R., ed. *Tissue nutrition and viability*. New York: Springer, 1986: pp. 1-24.

24. Harper, J., D. Amiel, and E. Harper. Collagenase production by rabbit ligaments and tendon. *Connect. Tissue Res.* 17: 253-259, 1988.

25. Heikkinen, E., and I. Vuori. Effect of physical activity on the metabolism of collagen in aged mice. *Acta Physiol. Scand.* 84: 543-549, 1972.

26. Jee, W.S.S., J.J. Wronski, E.R. Morey, and D.B. Kimmel. Effects of spaceflight on trabecular bone in rats. *Am. J. Physiol.* 244: R310-R314, 1983.

27. Komi, P.V., M. Salonen, M. Jarvinen, and O. Kokko. *In vivo* registration of Achilles tendon forces in man: Methodological development. *Int. J. Sports Med.* 8(Suppl.): 3-8, 1987.

28. Lanyon, L.E. Functional strain as a determinant for bone remodeling. *Calcif. Tissue Int.* 36(Suppl.): S56-S61, 1984.

29. Lanyon, L.E. Functional strain in bone as an objective, and controlling stimulus for adaptive bone remodeling. *J. Biomech.* 20: 1083-1093, 1987.

30. Lanyon, L.E., and C.T. Rubin. Static vs. dynamic loads as an influence on bone remodeling. *J. Biomech.* 17: 897-905, 1984.

31. Laros, G.S., C.M. Tipton, and R.R. Cooper. Influence of physical activity on ligament insertions. *J. Bone Joint Surg.* 53A: 275-286, 1971.

32. Marcus, R., and D.R. Carter. The role of physical activity in bone mass regulation. In: Grana, W.A., J.A. Lombardo, B.J. Sharkey,

and J.A. Stone, eds. *Advances in sports medicine and fitness.* New York: Year Book Publishers, 1988: vol. 1, pp. 63-82.

33. Margulies, J.Y., A. Simkin, I. Leichter, A. Bivas, R. Steinberg, M. Giladi, M. Stein, H. Kashtan, and C. Milgrom. Effect of intense physical activity on the bone-mineral content in the lower limbs of young adults. *J. Bone Joint Surg.* 68A: 1090-1093, 1986.

34. Matsuda, J.J., R.F. Zernicke, A.C. Vailas, V.A. Pedrini, A. Pedrini-Mille, and J.A. Maynard. Structural and mechanical adaptation of immature bone and strenuous exercise. *J. Appl. Physiol.* 60: 2028-2034, 1986.

35. May, M.T. *Galen: On the usefulness of the parts of the body.* Ithaca, NY: Cornell University Press, 1968, p. 168.

36. Morey, E.R. Spaceflight and bone turnover correlation with a new rat model of weightlessness. *Bioscience* 29: 168-170, 1979.

37. Morey, E.R., R.T. Turner, and D.J. Baylink. Quantitative analysis of selected bone parameters. In: Rosenzweig, S.N., and K.A. Souza, eds. *Final reports of U.S. experiments flown on the Soviet satellite Cosmos 936* (NASA Technical Memorandum No. 78526). Washington, D.C.: NASA; 1978: pp. 135-183.

38. Murguia, M.J., A.C. Vailas, B. Mandelbaum, J. Norton, J. Hodgson, H. Goforth, and J. Riedy. Plasma hydroxyproline: A possible predictive marker for connective tissue-related injuries. *Am. J. Sports Med.* 16: 660-664, 1988.

39. Noyes, F.R., P.J. Torvik, W.B. Hyde, and D.L. DeLucas. Biomechanics of ligament failure. *J. Bone Joint Surg.* 56A: 1406-1418, 1974.

40. Noyes, F.R., D.L. Butler, E.S. Grood, R.F. Zernicke, and M. Hefzy. Biomechanical of human ligament grafts used in knee-ligament repair and reconstruction. *J. Bone Joint Surg.* 66A: 344-352, 1984.

41. Noyes, F.R., D.R. Matthews, P.A. Mooar, and E.S. Grood. The symptomatic anterior cruciate deficient knee: II. The results of rehabilitation, activity modification and counseling on functional disability. *J. Bone Joint Surg.* 66A: 163-174, 1984.

42. Ott, S.M., R.F. Kilcoyne, and C.H. Chestnutt, III. Longitudinal changes in bone mass after one year as measured by different techniques in patients with osteoporosis. *Calcif. Tissue Int.* 39: 133-137, 1986.

43. Pedrini-Mille, A., V.A. Pedrini, J.A. Maynard, and A.C. Vailas. Response of immature chicken meniscus to strenuous exercise: Biochemical studies. *J. Orthop. Res.* 6:196-204, 1988.

44. Peterson, R.H., M.A. Gomez, and S. L-Y. Woo. The effect of strain rate on the biomechanical properties of the medial collateral ligament: A study of immature and mature rabbits [Abstract]. *Transactions of the 33rd Annual Meeting of the Orthopaedic Research Society,* 1987, p. 127.

45. Peterson, R.H. and S. L-Y. Woo. A new methodology to determine the mechanical properties of ligaments at high strain rates. *J. Biomech. Eng.* 108: 365-367, 1986.

46. Rambaut, P.C., and A.W. Goode. Skeletal changes during space flight. *Lancet* ii: 1050-1052, 1985.

47. Roux, W. *Gesammelte Abhandlung uber Entwicklungsmechanik der Organismen.* Leipzig: Engelmann, 1895, vol. 1, p. 458-460.

48. Rubin, C.T., and L.E. Lanyon. Dynamic strain simularities invertebrates: An alternative to allometric limb bone scaling. *J. Theor. Biol.* 107: 321-327, 1984.

49. Salter, R.B. Presidential address. *J. Bone Joint Surg.* 64B: 251-254, 1982.

50. Salter, R.B., D.F. Simmonds, B.W. Malcolm, E.J. Rumble, D. MacMichael, and N.D. Clements. The biological effect of continuous passive motion on the healing of full-thickness defects in articular cartilage. *J. Bone Joint Surg.* 62A: 1232-1251, 1980.

51. Scheuer J., and C.M. Tipton. Cardiovascular adaptations to training. *Annu. Rev. Physiol.* 39: 221-251, 1977.

52. Shaw, S.R., A.C. Vailas, Grindeland, and R.F. Zernicke. Effects of a one-week space flight on the morphological and mechanical properties of growing bone. *Am. J. Physiol.* 254: R78-R83, 1988.

53. Skyhar, M.J., L.A. Danzig, A.R. Hargens, and W.H. Akeson. Nutrition of the anterior cruciate ligament: Effects of continuous passive motion. *Am. J. Sports Med.* 13: 415-418, 1985.

54. Smith, E.L., and D.M. Raab. Osteoporosis and physical activity. *Acta Med. Scand. Suppl.* 711: 149-156, 1986.

55. Smith, M.C., P.C. Rambaut, J.M. Vogel, and M.M. Whittle. Bone mineral measurements— experiment M078. In: Johnson, R.S., and L.F. Dietlein, eds. *Biomedical results of Skylab* (Report No. NASA-SP-377). U.S. Govt. Printing Office; Washington, D.C.: 1977: pp. 183-190.

56. Spengler, D.M., E.R. Morey, D.R. Carter, R.T. Turner, and J.J. Baylink. Effects of space-flight on structural and material strength of growing bone. *Proc. Soc. Exp. Biol. Med.* 174: 224-228, 1983.

57. Stearns, M.L. Studies of connective tissue in transparent chambers in the rabbit's ear: I. *Am. J. Anat.* 66: 133-176, 1940.

58. Stearns, M.L. Studies on the development of connective tissue in transparent chambers in rabbit's ear: II. *Am. J. Anat.* 67: 55-97, 1940.

59. Suominen, H., and E. Heikkinen. Enzyme activities in muscle and connective tissue of M. Vastus lateralis in habitually-trained and sedentary 33- to 77-year-old men. *Eur. J. Appl. Physiol.* 34: 249-254, 1975.

60. Suominen, H., E. Heikkinen, H. Moisio, and K. Viljama. Physical and chemical properties of skin in habitually trained and sedentary 31- to 70-year-old men. *Brit. J. Dermatol.* 99: 147-154, 1978.

61. Suominen, H., E. Heikkinen, and T. Parkatti. Effect of eight weeks physical training on muscle and connective tissue of M. Vastus lateralis in 69-year-old men and women. *J. Gerontol.* 32: 33-37, 1977.

62. Tammi, M., A-M. Saamanen, A. Jauhiainen, O. Malminen, I. Kiviranta, and H. Helminen. Proteoglycan alterations in rabbit knee articular cartilage following physical exercise and immobilization. *Connect. Tissue Res.* 11: 45-55, 1983.

63. Tipton, C.M. Endocrines and the adaptations associated with exercise training. In: *Frontiers of exercise biology*, edited by K.T. Borer, D.W. Edington, and T.P. White. Champaign, IL: Human Kinetics, 1983, p. 134-151.

64. Tipton, C.M. Collagenous tissue and its responses to changes in physical activity. In: Maehlum, S., S. Nilsson, and P. Renstrom, eds. *An update on sports medicine*. Oslo: Danish and Norwegian Sports Medicine Associations and Swedish Society of Sports Medicine, 1987: pp. 79-84.

65. Tipton, C.M., S.L. James, W. Mergner, and T-K. Tcheng. Influence of exercise on strength of medical collateral knee ligaments of dogs. *Am. J. Physiol.* 218: 894-901, 1970.

66. Tipton, C.M., R.D. Matthes, J.A. Maynard, and R.A. Carey. The influence of physical activity on ligaments and tendons. *Med. Sci. Sports* 7: 165-175, 1975.

67. Tipton, C.M., R.D. Matthes, A.C. Vailas, and C.L. Schnobelen. The response of the Galago senegalensis to physical training. *Comp. Biochem. Physiol.* 63A: 29-36, 1979.

68. Tipton, C.M., A.C. Vailas, and R.D. Matthes. Experimental studies on the influences of physical activity on ligaments, tendons and joints: A brief review. *Acta Med. Scand. Suppl.* 711: 157-168, 1986.

69. Trentham, D.E. Autoimmunity to collagen as a disease mechanism. In: Weissman, J.G., ed. *Advances in inflammation research*. New York: Raven Press, 1981: pp. 149-164.

70. *U.S. News and World Report*, May 16, 1988, p. 52.

71. Vailas, A.C., D.M. Deluna, L.L. Lewis, S.L. Curwin, R.R. Roy, and E.K. Alford. Adaptation of bone and tendon to prolonged hind-limb suspension in rats. *J. Appl. Physiol.* 65: 373-376, 1988.

72. Vailas, A.C., A. Pedrini, A. Pedrini-Mille, and J.O. Holloszy. Patellar tendon matrix changes associated with aging and voluntary exercise. *J. Appl. Physiol.* 58: 1572-1576, 1986.

73. Vailas, A.C., C.M. Tipton, H.L. Laughlin, T-K. Tcheng, and R.D. Matthes. The influence of physical activity and hypophysectomy on aerobic capacity of ligaments and tendons. *J. Appl. Physiol.* 44: 542-546, 1978.

74. Vailas, A.C., C.M. Tipton, R.D. Matthes, and M. Gart. Physical activity and its influence on the repair process of medial collateral ligaments. *Connect. Tissue Res.* 9: 25-31, 1981.

75. Vailas, A.C., R.F. Zernicke, J. Matsuda, S. Curwin, and J. Durivage. Adaptation of rat knee meniscus to prolonged exercise. *J. Appl. Physiol.* 60: 1031-1034, 1986.

76. Viidik, A. Biomechanical and functional adaptation of tendons and joint ligaments. In: *Studies on the anatomy and function of bones and joints*. Evans, F.G., ed. Berlin: Springer, 1966: pp. 17-39.

77. Viidik, A. The effect of training on the tensile strength of isolated rabbit tendons. *Scand. J. Plast. Reconstr. Surg. Hand Surg.* 1: 141-147, 1967.

78. Viidik, A. Adaptability of connective tissue. In: *Biochemistry of Exercise VI*. Saltin, B., ed. 1986: vol. 16, pp. 545-562.

79. Vogel, J.M., and M.W. Whittle. Bone mineral changes: The second manned Skylab mission. *Aviat. Space Environ. Med.* 47: 396-400, 1976.

80. Vose, G.P. Review of roentgenographic bone demineralization studies of the Gemini space flights. *Am. J. Roentgenol. Rad. Therap. Nucl. Med.* 121: 1-4, 1974.

81. Wertheim, M.G. Memoire sur l'elasticite et la cohesion des principeaux tissus du corps humain. *Ann. Chim. Phys.* 21: 385-414, 1847.

82. Whalen, R.T., D.R. Carter, and C.R. Steele. The relationship between physical activity and bone density [Abstract]. *Trans. Orthop. Res. Soc.* 12: 464, 1987.

83. Whedon, G.D. Disuse osteoporosis: Physiologic aspects. *Calcif. Tissue Int.* 36(Suppl.): 146-150, 1984.

84. Whedon, G.D., J.E. Dietrick, and E. Shorr. Modification of the effects of immobilization upon metabolic and physiologic functions of normal men by the use of an oscillating bed. *Am. J. Med.* 6: 684-711, 1949.

85. Williams, J.A., J. Wagner, R. Wasnich, and L. Heilbrum. The effect of long distance running upon appendicular bone mineral content. *Med. Sci. Sports Exerc.* 16: 223-227, 1984.

86. Wolff, J. *Das Gesetz der Transformation der Knochen.* Berlin: A. Hirschwald, 1892.

87. Woo, S. L-Y., M.A. Gomez, D. Amiel, M.A. Ritter, R.H. Gelberman, and W.H. Akeson. The effect of exercise on the biomechanical and biochemical properties of swine digital flexor tendons. *J. Biomech. Eng. Trans. ASME* 103: 51-56, 1981.

88. Woo, S. L-Y., M.A. Gomez, T.J. Sites, P.O. Newton, C.A. Orlando, and W.H. Akeson. The biomechanical and morphological changes in the medial collateral ligament of the rabbit following immobilization and remobilization. *J. Bone Joint Surg.* 69A: 1200-1211, 1987.

89. Woo, S. L-Y., M.A. Gomez, and W.H. Akeson. Mechanical properties of tendons and ligaments: II. The relationship of immobilization and exercise on tissue remodeling. *Biorheology* 19: 397-408, 1982.

90. Woo, S. L-Y., M. Inone, E. McGurk-Burleson, and M.A. Gomez. Treatment of the medial collateral ligament injury: II. Structure and function of canine knees in response to differing treatment regimes. *Am. J. Sports Med.* 15: 22-29, 1987.

91. Woo, S. L-Y., S.C. Kuei, D. Amiel, M.A. Gomez, W.C. Hayes, F.C. White, and W.H. Akeson. The effect of prolonged physical training on the properties of long bone: A study of Wolff's law. *J. Bone Joint Surg.* 63A: 780-787, 1981.

92. Woo, S. L-Y., J. Maynard, D. Butler, R. Lyon, P. Torzilli, W. Akeson, et al. Ligament, tendon, and joint capsule: Insertions to bone. In: Woo, S. L-Y., and J.A. Buckwalter, eds. *Injury and repair of the musculoskeletal soft tissues.* Park Ridge, IL: American Academy of Orthopedic Surgeons, 1988: Chapter 4, pp. 133-166.

93. Woo, S. L-Y., M.A. Ritter, D. Amiel, T.M. Sanders, M.A. Gomez, S.C. Kuei et al. The biomechanical and biochemical properties of swine tendons: Long-term effects of exercise on the digital extensors. *Connect. Tissue Res.* 7: 177-183, 1980.

94. Zuckerman, J., and G.A. Stull. Effect of exercise on knee ligament separation force in rats. *J. Appl. Physiol.* 26: 716-720, 1969.

Chapter 29

Discussion: Bone and Connective Tissue Adaptations to Physical Activity

Barry W. Oakes
Anthony W. Parker

It is certainly a pleasure to discuss the excellent comprehensive review by Professor Charles Tipton and Dr. Arthur Vailas. In this chapter, we attempt to relate recent basic science data already mentioned by Tipton and Vailas and to highlight the data's relevance to clinical medicine, which is what this conference is about.

Connective tissues, be they hard (bone) or soft (ligament and tendon), obtain their load-bearing properties (compression, tension, or shear) from the appropriate mix and organization of their components. Each tissue has its own unique mix of fibers with appropriate orientation together with proteoglycans, water, and electrolytes, which determines these mechanical properties. It is still far from clear how much of the information required for tissue anlagen development in such cells as the fibroblasts of developing tendon or ligament, the osteoblasts of a newly forming long bone, or the chondroblasts of developing articular cartilage resides in the genome and how much biosynthesis is modulated by external influences such as mechanical load, hormones, and other less well-defined factors. We now have an enlarging quantitative knowledge of the effects of prolonged unloading and loading on these tissues, and we are indeed indebted to the research and endeavors of Professor Tipton and his colleagues for some of this knowledge, which has been obtained over the last 2 decades. We divide our discussion into three areas: bone, cartilage, and ligament and tendon.

Bone

Considering the high demands of the skeletal system imposed by vigorous physical activity and the high frequency of injury to components of this system (54), it is perhaps surprising that, until relatively recently, little attention has been given to skeletal adaptation to loading and the mechanisms involved.

Our capacity to monitor and prescribe activity aimed at improving the efficiency of the cardiovascular system has been well developed over a number of years using sophisticated techniques. This probably occurred out of necessity because of the increased incidence of coronary arterial disease in largely sedentary populations of the Western Hemisphere. However, until recently, techniques to assess the effect of activity on the human skeletal system were not available, and reliance was placed on extrapolation of results from animal studies or empirical clinical data to assess the positive or negative effects of various types and intensities of exercise on the morphology and mechanical properties of bones. Discrepancies in the results of animal studies that have investigated the effects of exercise on bone reflect the complexity of the relationship and the specific nature of the response depending on the type and intensity of the exercise regimen, the particular bone (or section of it), and the age of the subject.

Numerous animal experiments outlined in part by Tipton have shown that exercise will influence positively the composition and hence the mechanical properties of bone. Exercise may also have deleterious effects (54) and may retard bone growth, particularly high-intensity exercise (31).

Exercise studies are limited because of the difficulty in controlling and quantifying the precise level of mechanical loading, especially in relation to the strains imposed. The ingenious experiments of Lanyon (50) and Rubin and Lanyon (76) addressed some of these problems by using quantitative methodology. This was the first work in vivo using direct mechanical loading of bone that determined the actual strains and the frequency of their application that would prevent bone loss or encourage new periosteal bone formation. They examined the bone response using the so-called functionally isolated avian ulnar model and determined that, with an applied physiological strain of 2,050 microstrain at 4, 36, 360, and 1,800 consecutive 0.5-Hz load reversals (cycles), 4 cycles (or only 8 s of loading) per day was sufficient to prevent disuse osteoporosis; 36 cycles (or only 72 s of loading) per day was sufficient to trigger and maximize the osteogenic response. Loading times greater than 36 cycles (72 s) did not increase the osteogenic response. They also determined from a similar series of experiments, but using increasing microstrains from −500 to −4,000 microstrain at 100 consecutive 1.0-Hz reversals, that there was a distinct dose-response curve for the deposition of new endosteal and periosteal bone. Strains less than 500 microstrain were associated with bone loss and strains greater than 1,000 with an increase in osteogenic activity. Loading the functionally isolated ulnar statically with springs to induce −2,000 microstrain over 8 wk induced no new bone formation, and in fact intracortical porosis was observed. From these observations they concluded that cyclical dynamic loading rather than static loading was more effective in the transduction of the experimentally imposed mechanical strain by means of an unknown biochemical effector to surface osteoblasts. Lanyon (50) coined the term *minimum effective strain*, which is the strain magnitude required to maintain balanced remodeling and hence retain bone mass at its normal physiological level.

Lanyon (50) emphasized the importance and dependence of functional bone mass on a continuing load-related stimulus and cited the hormonally mediated bone removal that follows once functional loading is removed, as seen in paralysis (20), immobilization (44), bed rest (48), and spaceflight (86). We will not recover the ground so well outlined by Tipton on the effects of weightlessness on bone mass. However, the work of Schneider and McDonald (80) from the Kroc Foundation Conference is interesting in that attempts to prevent bone loss or disuse osteoporosis with bed rest for periods of up to 36 wk failed, using both mechanical and biochemical means that included exercise, skeletal compression, increased hydrostatic pressure to the lower body, supplemental calcium and phosphorus, calcitonin, and etidrone. The type of physical loading used in this study may not have

been enough to meet the minimal effective strain level of Lanyon to activate osteoblasts to prevent bone loss. *The important trick is to determine the type and amount of minimum activity that is required to minimize bone loss while an individual is horizontal as a patient or in space in a weightless environment.*

Rubin and Lanyon (75) also determined that normal peak physiological strains in adult weight-bearing bones were in the range of 0.002-0.003. From these observations Rubin and Lanyon (76) and Lanyon (50) suggested that osteocytes are very sensitive to the distribution, the rate of change, and the magnitude of strain within the bone matrix. Osteoblasts entombed in bone matrix seem to be able to monitor dynamic strain matrix deformation within 6 s (by means of a probable biochemical message) and to transmit this sort of mechanical information by means of their gap junctions of their long cytoplasmic extensions to the surface osteoblasts and osteoclasts to remodel the bone appropriately. Hence, the functional syncytium or network of bone cells responding to mechanical influences is critical to this concept that bone architecturally adapts to loading.

Recently, Lanyon's group (27) reported that with bone loading there was an induced birefringence using alcian blue to preserve, stain, and visualize proteoglycans, suggesting that bone matrix proteoglycans in fact may be the biochemical transducer monitoring matrix strain. This was further suggested by the use of cuprolinium blue to demonstrate proteoglycans at the ultrastructural level. With bone loading, proteoglycans were seen to reorient themselves in relation to the collagen fibers of the bone matrix. Proteoglycans would be a strong contender as a biochemical transducer of matrix strain because of their strong negative charge profile, which could inform the osteocytes by a change in charge relationships with the cell membrane. This has led to the attractive concept of the reorientation of proteoglycans being a matrix strain memory and could explain the observation that in a single period of loading the remodeling response appears to saturate after a few loading cycles. However, such a concept awaits further experimental validation. Recent results from the same group indicate that osteocytes in fact can respond to a single loading cycle by the uptake of ^{3}H-uridine into osteocytes 24 h after loading (83).

In contrast to those experiments, which have generally increased mechanical loading on developing bones and tissues, it is important to investigate the consequences of total weightlessness on the development of bone and other connective tissues. This could be done by rearing animals in space from conception and will help to determine genetic versus loading input to the genome.

Also, the understanding of bone performance in relation to fatigue failure or stress fractures has grown in the last decade. Bone fatigue failure is currently topical because of the large numbers of individuals involved in long-distance running or jogging for lifestyle benefits and who sustain stress fractures (54). Since the original observations by Rutishauser and Majno in 1951 (78) and confirmations thereof by Frost (35), little quantitative work was done in this area until relatively recently. Frost did observe cracks in nondecalcified human rib bone and noted that the cracks had a "curious predilection for the cement line planes and extra-haversian bone."

The threshold level of physical activity, or mechanical loading at which bone remodels positively or accumulates microdamage, has not been defined. In fact, the concept of microdamage is poorly defined except in terms of the status or integrity of the bone prior to a clearly diagnosable problem such as a stress fracture. Carter and Hayes (13, 14) and Carter et al. (15) have demonstrated that repetitive cyclical physiological loading in vitro can cause a progressive gradual loss of stiffness and ultimate strength due to microcracks. The total number of cycles to fatigue failure was influenced only by the total strain range and was not affected by mean strain. Bone was shown to have extremely poor fatigue resistance, and fully reversed cyclic loading to one half of the yield strain caused fatigue fracture in 1,000 cycles. Carter et al. (15) compared their strain ranges (0.005-0.010) and fatigue results and extrapolated these data to those that may occur in bone in vivo with the clinical experience with fatigue fractures in military recruits and athletes. They concluded that military recruits would within 6 wk (the earliest appearance of stress fractures) accumulate a loading history equivalent to 100-1,000 m of very rigorous exercise, which, according to them, was equivalent to 100,000-1,000,000 loading cycles. From their

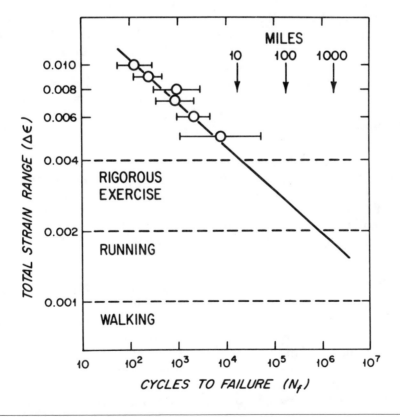

Figure 29.1. *In vitro* strain-related fatigue behavior of cortical bone compared to the levels of cyclic strain range that are expected during various *in vivo* activities. *Note.* From "Fatigue Behavior of Adult Cortical Bone: The Influence of Mean Strain and Strain Range" by D.R. Carter, W.E. Caler, D.M. Spengler, and V.H. Frankel, 1981, *Acta Orthopaedica Scandinavica*, **52**, p. 481. Reprinted by permission.

extrapolation they predicted cyclic strain ranges of 0.0029 and 0.0019, respectively, for these fatigue fractures in these recruits (Figure 29.1).

Carter et al. (15) determined that tensile fatigue caused failure at the cement lines that resulted in debonding of the osteons from surrounding interstitial bone, whereas compressive fatigue resulted in the formation of "diffuse shear microcracks throughout bone which are oblique to the loading direction". Carter (16) also estimated the fatigue strength of bone as being about 7 MPa at 10^7 cycles and suggested that this extremely low value for fatigue strength of human cortical bone would require that bones are constantly accumulating fatigue damage during everyday activities and that the processes of normal bone remodeling and repair are necessary for the long-term structural integrity of bone. The use of plasma hydroxyproline levels may be a useful marker for predicting the onset of stress fractures of bone in those who exercise vigorously (53).

Similar observations were made by Burr et al. (10) using physiological loads applied to the dog radius and also by Forwood and Parker (32) using in vitro torsional testing of the rat tibia. Burr et al. observed crack fractures across osteons that were 40 times more frequent than they were in the control radius.

In a fascinating study, Rubin et al. (77) measured the velocity of ultrasound across the patella and tibia in 98 volunteers before and after running the Boston Marathon. In summary, they found that absolute sound velocities were 2.9% higher in those runners finishing in less than 3 h than they were in those finishing after 3 h. Tibial velocities in male runners were 8.8% higher than they were in female runners. The mean velocity across the patella of three wheelchair racers was 28% lower than was the mean combined patellar velocity measures in all runners. They suggested that faster velocities were associated with bone more suited to greater functional demands. Also, a 1.6% increase in ultrasonic velocity across the tibia and a 3.5% increase across the patella between pre- and postrace velocities indicated that a change had occurred within the bone during the race. The nature of this change is speculative at the moment, but it is tempting to suggest that it could be due to fatigue fracture damage, as has been postulated by Carter et al. (15); but with fatigue fractures one would expect a marked decrease in sound velocity (77). They suggested that the increase in sound transmission observed postrace may be due to other organic mechanisms, such as proteoglycan orientation. Unfortunately, individual biomechanical profiles that may have identified structural abnormalities likely to promote a damaging overload situation were not reported.

The mechanisms by which osteocytes respond to mechanical loading have been investigated by culturing cells on deformable substrates. Harrell et al. (42) were the first to achieve this by culturing osteoblasts on petri dishes, the floor of which could be bent by using an orthodontic jackscrew bonded to the outside bottom of the flask. They demonstrated with a single deformation that the strained cells increased (PGE_2) to a maximum in 20 min, followed in minutes by an increase in intracellular cyclic AMP (84). This was confirmed by Yeh and Rodan (99), who grew embryonic rat calvarian cells on collagen ribbons subjected to strains of 5%-10% eight times over 2 h. Recently, Gross et al. (38) grew neonatal rat calvarial cells on elastic membranes and subjected them to strains of 0.02%-0.1% at 1 Hz. Cells subjected to 0.04% showed an increase in DNA synthesis and increased collagen synthesis compared to static controls at 0.02% and 0.04% strains. Buckley et al. (9) have also shown that avian osteoblastlike cells grown on an elastic substrate similarly increase their DNA synthesis within the first 72 h of stretch, and the cells aligned at 90° to the applied maximum strain field.

Recent work by Forwood and Parker (30, 31, 32) using pubescent rats showed that after an intensive 1-mo exercise, the tibia showed an increased number of haversian canals in the middle one third of the cortex, significant reductions in energy to failure, and increased bone length and width of the proximal epiphyseal plate. No change was observed in the mechanical properties of the femur, but significant reductions occurred in bone length and weight. This suggests that intensive exercise in these young rats is not beneficial for their normal growth and development. These findings are similar to those of others (6, 45, 87).

Carter et al. (17), Carter (18), and Wong and Carter (96) have recently further extended the work of Klein-Nulend et al. (46), who demonstrated that both continuous and intermittent compressive forces increased cartilage calcification in vitro. Carter et al. have demonstrated that calcification in vivo can be predicted accurately by determining strain energy density in the developing cartilage anlagen of the femur and the more complex sternum. This is the first step in the proof of Wolff's law. Julian Wolff predicted in 1892 that the internal architecture and external conformation of bone is in accordance with mathematical laws (95). His prediction is now realized in part by Carter's mathematical analyses.

Hence, at both the micro- and the macrolevels it has been demonstrated that both the cells and the matrix respond to loading in such a manner that adaptation, including calcification during development, is determined by mechanical forces. For the first time there is now strong evidence from Carter's observations that stress histories play a major role in regulating gene expression, especially during development.

Cartilage

As with bone, there have been great strides in our understanding of cartilage structure and in particular articular cartilage. The role of joint movement and articular cartilage loading for the health of articular chondrocytes is now well established. However, this was not the case 10 yr ago, when there was little quantitative information on the effect of prolonged unloading on articular cartilage, a common daily occurrence in our hospitals with major injuries from vehicle accidents.

Caterson and Lowther (19) were the first to measure the changes in proteoglycan content and metabolism under conditions of loading and unloading by immobilizing one foreleg of a sheep in a plaster cast. This prevented weight bearing on one foreleg and increased the weight bearing on the other limb. The two hind limbs served as controls. Initially, cartilage from all four major joints had similar proteoglycan content and biosynthetic rates. After 4 wk of cast immobilization, the cartilage from the immobilized ankle joint showed a signiciant reduction in proteoglycan content that apparently was due to the reduced rate of synthesis by the chondrocytes. The contralateral foreleg, which had normal movement but increased weight bearing, showed a slight increase in proteoglycan content and a marked increase in the rate of proteoglycan synthesis when compared to the control hind limb. There was no change in the collagen content. These early observations indicated that articular cartilage chondrocytes respond to load changes. Similar, but more detailed, proteoglycan analyses were reported by Tammi et al. (85) using rabbit knee articular cartilage. The animals were submitted to immobilization, running, or increased weight bearing for 24-27 d. Running increased the proteoglycan content of articular cartilage, which was the opposite to immobilization. The exercised

animals also had increased levels of nonextractable proteoglycans with 4 M GdnHCI. The ratio of keratan to chondroitin sulphate increased with loading and corresponds to the observations of others that such a ratio is highest at the sites of maximal loading or contact. The authors indicated that weight bearing rather than simple joint motion primarily determines cartilage matrix properties. These observations have also been confirmed recently for the menisci of rat knee joints that had been exercised for 12 wk (92), as outlined in chapter 28.

Recent observations by O'Driscoll et al. (59) also indicate that load bearing, coupled with joint motion, promotes chondrogenic differentiation in free autogenous periosteal grafts used to resurface whole-thickness articular cartilage defects in young-rabbit patellofemoral joints. The use of continuous passive motion (CPM) for 4 wk led to 100% of the periosteal grafts filling the defect with tissue that was identical biochemically to normal hyaline articular cartilage. However, animals that were immobilized or that had intermittent active motion (normal cage activity) or CPM for 2 wk and then were sacrificed at 4 wk had tissue very unlike normal hyaline articular cartilage and with less proteoglycan and much less Type II collagen. At present, it is unclear from this work whether movement, loading, or a combination of both is effecting the transition of the periosteal chondrogenic precursor cells to express the full chondrogenic phenotype.

In vitro culture systems have been devised to investigate mechanisms that stimulate the chondrogenic phenotype. One of the first of these systems was the use of embryonic chicken epiphyseal chondrocytes grown in high-density culture with the use of the Good buffers. This system remained differentiated for many weeks in culture as measured by both ultrastructural analysis and detailed matrix biochemistry (40, 41, 64). This system was used to investigate the effects of tensile mechanical loading on the biosynthetic capacity of these differentiated cells in culture. Cells exposed to 5.5% strain at 0.2 Hz over 24 h increased their incorporation of $^{35}SO_4$ and ^3H glucosamine into glycosaminoglycans 1.4 and 1.7, respectively. Incorporation of ^3H-thymidine increased 2.4-fold, and cAMP levels increased 2.2-fold in the mechanically loaded chondrocytes (25). Fine et al. (29) also showed recently that rabbit medial femoral condyles that are cyclically loaded during storage in vitro and then transplanted survive better as transplants than do nonloaded femoral condyles.

Handley et al. (39) and McQuillan et al. (56) developed another steady-state system using bovine cartilage in explant culture, of which the matrix formation can be maintained by using IGF-I, which can replace the serum in this system. This observation is important because it indicates that the main driving factor for continued proteoglycan biosynthesis in this system in IGF-I. These observations have recently been confirmed by others (52, 79). The use of other growth factors, such as TGF-beta and fibroblast growth factor, is also being explored by other workers (60, 91) for the role in chondrocyte metabolism.

At the macrolevel of real patients, some important studies have emerged in relation to long-distance running. It has always been intuitively expressed (usually by nonrunners!) that long-distance running or even simple jogging leads to excessive joint wear, especially in the lower-limb joints (hip, knee, and ankle joints) and that this leads to the premature onset of degenerative osteoarthrosis. There have been few studies reported on the relation between running and osteoarthritic change in the major lower-limb joints. Puranen et al. (71) examined the hip joints in 74 former champion-caliber runners. They concluded that running did not contribute to osteoarthritic development of the hip joint. Panush et al. (65) also came to the same conclusion when they compared clinical and radiological indices of joint degeneration in 17 male marathon runners (mean age = 56 yr, distance ran = 44.8 km/wk for 12 yr) with an age-, height-, and weight-matched group of 18 nonrunners. In a similar study, Lane et al. (49) compared 41 long-distance runners aged 50-72 yr with 41 matched community controls. Radiological analysis of hands, lateral lumbar spine, and knees was performed without knowledge of running status. A CT scan of the first lumbar vertebrae quantified bone mineral content. Both male and female runners had 40% more bone mineral than did matched controls. No differences were observed in joint-space narrowing, crepitation, joint stability, or symptomatic arthritis between the two groups.

These studies are at variance with animal models of arthritis, in which it has been postulated that repetitive impact loading leads to fatigue fractures of the subchondral bone, stiffens the loading response of the articular cartilage, and then, after 12-30 mo, leads to histological and biochemical manifestations of cartilage degeneration (72, 74).

Radin (73) recently reviewed the mechanisms of osteoarthrosis and concluded that it is due to an imbalance between mechanical stresses on the joint and the ability of the tissues of the joint to withstand these stresses. Effective treatment, he believes, is generally mechanical, and the progression can be halted with appropriate intervention.

Ligament and Tendon

It should be stated from the outset that ligament and tendon are quite different in their cell structures, collagen fibril population profiles, and proteoglycan content (1). This discussion centers largely on ligaments.

Tipton has comprehensively reviewed the data available for changes in ligament and ligament bone junction strength with increased and decreased levels of activity. Before discussing this in detail, however, it is useful to discuss the work of David Parry.

Parry et al. (67, 69) and Parry and Craig (70) recently completed detailed quantitative morphometric ultrastructural analyses of collagen fibrils from a large number of collagen-containing tissues in various species. They came to a number of conclusions; those that are pertinent to this disscussion can be summarized as follows:

- Type I collagen-containing tissues, such as ligament and tendon, have a bimodal distribution of collagen fibril diameters at maturity.
- The ultimate tensile strength and mechanical properties of connective tissues are positively correlated with the mass average diameter of collagen fibrils. In the context of response of ligaments to exercise, they also concluded that the collagen fibril diameter distribution is closely correlated with the magnitude and duration of the loading of the tissues. These conclusions have been confirmed (26, 62) (Figure 29.2).

Apart from the original classic work of Noyes et al. (58), in which the effects of immobilization on the anterior cruciate ligament (ACL) of the primate were examined, there have been few studies to examine the cause and mechanisms of the decreased strength and elastic stiffness of the ACL in response to immobilization. Tipton et al. (88) reported that collagen fiber bundles with light microscopy were decreased in number and size (in dogs), suggesting that this was the cause of the decreased cross-sectional area seen in immobilized medial collateral rabbit ligaments (98). The explanation for the decreased strength and elastic stiffness in these immobilized ligaments may be found at the collagen fibril level. Binkley and Peat (5)

GROWTH IN DIAMETER OF COLLAGEN FIBRES FROM RAT ANTERIOR CRUCIATE LIGAMENTS

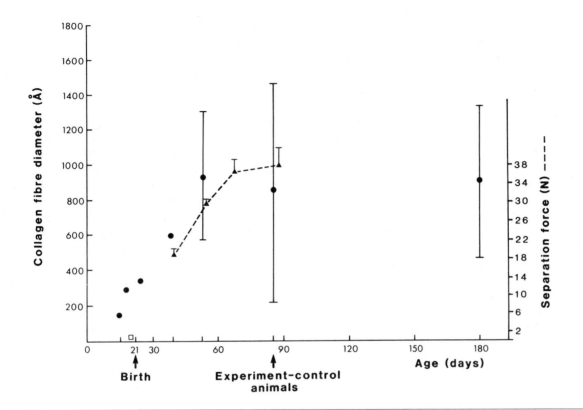

Figure 29.2.   Plot of collagen fibril diameter in the rat ACL vs. age. Also shown is the separation force for the rat ACL. *Note.* From ''Changes in Strength of Bone and Ligament in Response to Training'' by A.W. Parker and N. Larsen, 1981, in P. Russo (ed.), *Human Adaptation* (p. 211), Sydney: Cumberland College of Health Sciences. Reprinted by permission.

showed a decrease in the number of small-diameter fibrils with 6 wk of immobilization of the rat medial collateral ligament.

Oakes et al. (61, 63) and Oakes (62) quantified the collagen fibril populations in young rat anterior and posterior cruciate ligaments subjected to an intensive 1-mo exercise program. This study was performed in an attempt to explain the increased tensile strength found in these ligaments with the intensive endurance exercise program and to determine whether this could be explained at the level of the collagen fibril, which is the fundamental unit of ligament.

The observations by Tipton et al. (89), Cabaud et al. (12), Parker and Larsen (66), and others that ligament strength is dependent on physical activity prompted an ultrastructural investigation of the mechanism of this increase in tensile strength within ligaments. Increased collagen content was found in the ligaments of exercised dogs (88), and this correlated with increased cross-sectional area and larger collagen fiber bundles. This accounts for

the increased ligament tensile strength, but whether this increased collagen was due to deposition of collagen on existing fibrils or to the synthesis of new fibrils has not been investigated. Larsen and Parker (51) had already shown that with a 4-wk intensive exercise program in young male Wistar rats both the anterior and the posterior cruciate ligaments showed significant strength increases (p < .05).

Response of Collagen Fibril Populations to Intensive Exercise in Rats

Collagen fibril changes within exercised rat cruciate ligaments were investigated by placing five 30-d-old pubescent rats on a progressive 4-wk exercise program of alternating days of swimming and treadmill running. At the conclusion of the program the rats were running 60-80 min at 26 m · min⁻¹ on a 10% treadmill gradient and on alternate days swimming 60 min with a 3% body weight attached to their tails. Five caged rats of similar age and commencing body weights were controls. After 30 d the exercise and control rats underwent total body perfusion fixation, and the ACL and posterior cruciate ligaments (PCL) were removed and prepared for electron microscopy. Analysis of ultrathin transverse sections cut through collagen fibrils of the exercised ACLs revealed a larger number of fibrils per unit area examined (29% increase; p < 0.05) compared to the nonexercised caged control ACLs and a fall in mean diameter from 966 ± 30 Å in the control ACLs to 830 ± 30 Å in the exercised ACLs (p < 0.05). As a consequence, the major cross-sectional area of collagen fibrils was found in the 1,125 Å diameter group in the exercised ACLs and in the 1,500 Å diameter group in the control ACLs. However, total collagen fibril cross section per unit area examined was approximately the same in both the exercised and the nonexercised control ACLs. Similar changes occurred in the exercised and control PCLs (Figures 29.3 and 29.4). In the exercised PCL, collagen per μg DNA was almost double that

of the control, suggesting that the PCL was more loaded with this exercise regimen than was the ACL. The conclusion from this study is that ACL and PCL fibroblasts deposit tropocollagen as smaller diameter fibrils when subjected to an intense 1-mo intermittent loading (exercise). The expected accretion and increase in size of the preexisting larger diameter collagen fibrils were not observed.

The mechanism of the change to a smaller diameter fibril population is of interest and may be related to a change in the type of glycosaminoglycans (GAGs) and hence proteoglycans synthesized by ligament fibroblasts in response to the intermittent loading of exercise. It has become well recognized since the original work of Toole and Lowther (90) that GAGs have an effect on determining collagen fibril size in vitro, and this has been confirmed recently in vivo by Parry et al. (68). Merrilles and Flint (57) demonstrated a change in fibril diameters between the compression and tension regions of the flexor digitorum profundus tendon as it turns 90Å around the talus. Gillard et al.

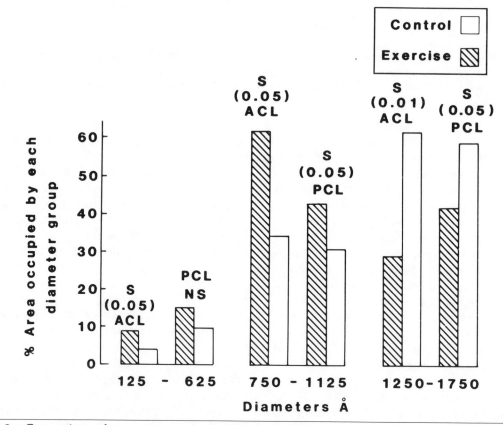

Figure 29.3. Comparison of percent area occupied by three diameter groupings of collagen fibrils used for statistical analysis for exercised and control ACL and PCL *Note. From Injury and Repair of Musculoskeletal and Soft Tissue* by S.L-Y. Woo and J.A. Buckwatter, eds. Park Ridge, IL: American Academy of Orthopedic Surgeons. Reprinted by permission.

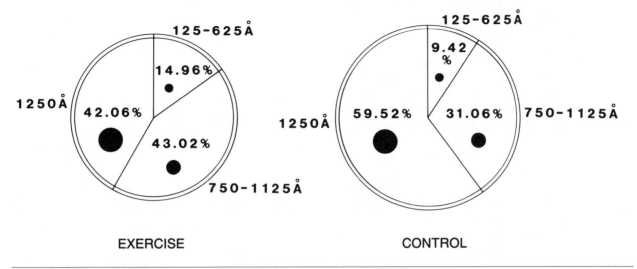

% TOTAL AREA OF DIFFERENT DIAMETER GROUPINGS (PCL)

EXERCISE   CONTROL

Figure 29.4.   Pie chart comparison of percent area occupied by the three diameter groupings of collagen fibrils used for statistical analysis in the exercised and control PCL *Note*. From *Injury and Repair of Musculoskeletal and Soft Tissue* by S.L-Y Woo and J.A. Buckwatter, eds. Park Ridge, IL: American Academy of Orthopedic Surgeons. Reprinted by permission.

(37) showed that the GAG profile for the compression and tension regions of the tendon are different and that this GAG difference may determine collagen fibril diameters. As previously mentioned, Amiel et al. (1) showed that the rabbit cruciate ligaments have more GAG than does the patellar tendon, so it is likely that GAGs also play an important role in determining collagen fibril populations in cruciate ligaments. Vogel and Evanko (94) recently showed there are two populations of proteoglycans (PG) in bovine tendons. Under compression, large proteoglycan is synsthesized in the fibrocartilage zone as a response to walking, whereas under tension in most of the tendon small proteoglycans are synthesized. Scott and Hughes (81) recently showed in tendons in three species that the growth of collagen fibrils is probably related to muscle loading in the embryonic tendon and to a dramatic fall in hyaluronate and sulphated GAG.

Collagen Fibril Populations in Human Knee Ligaments and Grafts

Biological insight into collagen repair mechanisms within human cruciate ligament grafts was gained by obtaining biopsies from autogenous ACL grafts from patients subsequently requiring arthroscopic intervention because of stiffness, problems with meniscal or articular cartilage, or removal of promi-

nent staples used for fixation of ACL grafts. Most of the ACL grafts were from the central one third of the patellar tendon as a free graft (*n* = 33). Some were left attached distally (*n* = 8), and in others the hamstrings or the iliotibial tract was used (*n* = 7). These biopsies represented approximately 20% of the total free grafts performed over the 3 yr of this study. The clinical ACL stability of the biopsy group differed little from the remainder. All had a Grade II-III pivot shift (jerk) preoperatively (10-15 mm anterior drawer neutral [ADN]) that was eliminated postoperatively in 87% of patients (0.5 mm ADN). Subsequent clinical review at 3 yr showed an increase in ADN with a return in 20% of a Grade I pivot shift.

A total of 48 biopsies have been quantitatively analyzed for collagen fibril diameter populations in patients aged 19-42 yr. These data were compared with collagen fibril populations obtained from biopsies of cadaver ACLs (*n* = 5) and from biopsies of ACLs from young (< 30 yr; *n* = 10) and old (> 30 yr; *n* = 6) patients who had sustained recent tears. Biopsies were also obtained from normal patellar tendons at operation (*n* = 7) and cadavers (*n* = 3).

The results (Figure 29.5) from the collagen fibril diameter morphometric analysis in all the ACL grafts clearly indicated a predominance of small-diameter collagen fibrils. Absence of a regular crimping of collagen fibrils was observed by both light and electron microscopy, as was a less ordered parallel arrangement of fibrils. In most biopsies, capillaries were present, and most fibroblasts appeared viable.

Quantitatively (Figure 29.5),

1. large-diameter collagen fibrils († 1,000 Å) form a large proportion (approx. 45%) of the percentage cross-sectional area in the normal human patellar tendon;
2. collagen fibrils less than 1,000 Å diameter form a large proportion (approx. 85%) of the percentage cross-sectional area in the normal human ACL; and
3. in all the ACL grafts, collagen fibrils less than 1,000 Å diameter (most 250-750 Å) are the major contributors to the collagen fibril cross-sectional area, be they young (9 mo) or old (6 yr) grafts.

Recent biochemical analysis of a human patellar tendon graft in situ for 2 yr indicated a large amount of Type III (20-30%) as well as some Type V collagen. This confirmed our suspicion morphologically that a large amount of the collagen in these remodeled grafts at this age may be Type III and not Type I, as is normally found in the patellar tendon and adult ACL (1).

Before we discuss the biopsy data, it is of interest to compare the collagen fibril profiles for the patellar tendon with the normal ACL. It can be seen that the profiles are different in that the distribution in the patellar tendon is skewed to the right, and a small number of large fibrils are not present in the normal ACL. Recent work by Butler et al. (11) showed that the patellar tendon is significantly stronger than are the human ACL, PCL, and LCL from the same knee in terms of maximum stress, linear modulus, and energy density to maximum strength. The larger fibrils observed in the patellar tendon and not found in the ACL are an obvious explanation for the stronger biomechanical properties.

The biopsies from the grafts were obtained from patients with a good-to-fair rating in terms of a moderate ADN (0-5 mm) and correction of the pivot shift, but both these tests of ACL integrity showed an increasing laxity of the ACL at the 3-yr clinical review. The length of time the grafts were in vivo before biopsy varied from 6 mo to 6 yr. The collagen fibril population did not alter much for the older grafts († 3 yr), which is not what was hoped for or expected but is in keeping with the observation clinically that the ACL grafts stretched out postoperatively.

The most striking feature of all the biopsies from the grafts irrespective of whether they were free

grafts, Jones' grafts, fascia lata grafts, or hamstring grafts was the invariable prevalence of small-diameter fibrils among a few larger fibrils that probably were the original large-diameter patellar fibrils. The packing of the small fibrils in the grafts was not as tight as is usually observed in the normal patellar tendon (compare Figures 29.5a and c). The Jones' free grafts had more large-diameter fibrils than did the Jones' grafts.

It appears from the quantitative collagen fibril observations in this study using a nonisometric surgical procedure that the large-diameter fibrils of the original graft are removed and almost entirely replaced by smaller, less well-packed and orientated fibrils rather than by the larger diameter fibrils found in the normal patellar tendon. The smaller diameter fibrils are probably recently synthesized because they are of smaller diameter than are those found in the original patellar tendon.

Is gentle mechanical loading in the ACL grafts an important stimulus to fibroblast proliferation and collagen deposition? Inadequate mechanical stimulus may occur, especially if grafts are nonisometric and are stretched out by the patient before they have adequate tensile strength. A lax ACL graft may not induce sufficient mechanical loading on graft fibroblasts to alter the ratios of GAG to collagen biosynthesis to favor large-diameter fibril formation. Certainly, in this study ACL graft laxity increased postoperatively. This would lend credence to the previous idea. However, the use of CPM in grafted primates does not increase the strength of grafts.

Another more likely possibility is that the replacement fibroblasts in the ACL grafts are derived from stem cells from the synovium and synovial perivascular cells, which are known to synthesize hyaluronate, which in turn favors small-diameter fibril formation (81).

The strong correlation of small-diameter fibrils with a lower tensile strength has been observed by Parry et al. (67), and the observations in this study confirm this and correlate with the observations of Clancy et al. (23), Arnoczky et al. (3), Shino et al. (82), and McPherson et al. (55). The recent observations by Ishizue et al. (43) indicate that collagense may play a role in the remodeling of ACL tears and grafts.

Conclusion

The conclusion from this study is that the predominance of the small-diameter collagen fibrils (< 750 Å) and their poor packing and alignment in all the ACL grafts, irrespective of the type of graft,

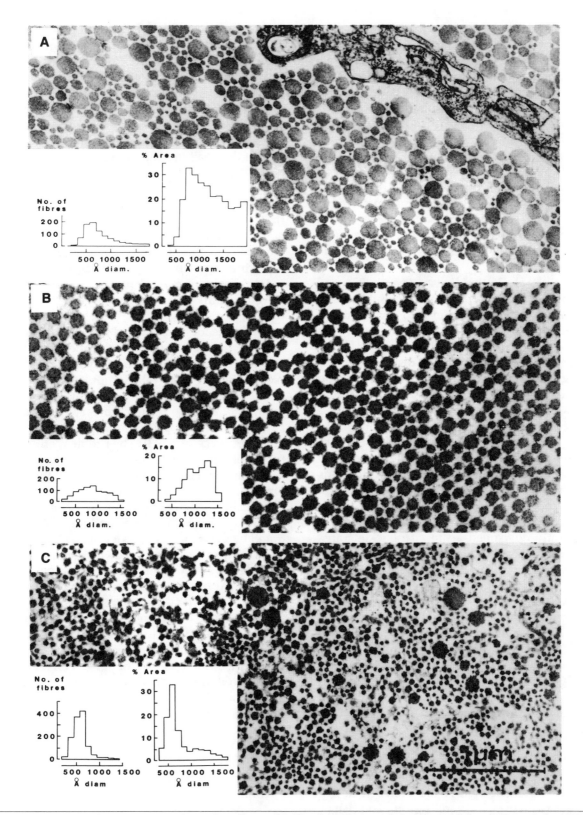

Figure 29.5. Transverse sections through collagen fibrils of (a) the normal young adult patellar tendon (PT) (mean of 6 biopsies); (b) normal young adult ACL (mean of 6 biopsies); and (c) Jones' free graft (mean of 9 biopsies) (all × 34,100). Insets: left, the number of fibrils vs. diameter; right, percent area occupied per diameter group. Note preponderance of small-diameter fibrils in the graft (c) and large fibrils in the patellar tendon (a) not seen in the normal ACL (b). *Note.* From *Injury and Repair of Musculoskeletal and Soft Tissue* by S.L-Y Woo and J.A. Buckwatter, eds. Park Ridge, IL: American Academy of Orthopedic Surgeons. Reprinted by permission.

their age, and the surgeon, may explain the clinical and experimental evidence of a decreased tensile strength in such grafts compared to the normal ACL. It appears that in the adult the replacement fibroblasts in the remodeled ACL graft cannot reform the large-diameter, regularly crimped and tightly packed fibrils seen in the normal ACL even after 6 yr (the oldest graft analyzed).

The origin of the replacement fibroblasts that remodel the ACL grafts is not known. It is our hunch that they will not come from the graft itself, although some of these cells may survive because of diffusion. However, most of the stem cells involved in the remodeling process are probably derived from the surrounding synovium and its vasculature.

Hampson et al. (36) and Engstrom et al. (28) used ultrasound to measure the cross-sectional area of the human Achilles tendon in vivo and validated this technique as a reliable method to measure the Achilles tendon cross-sectional area using cadaver Achilles tendons. Two groups of distance athletes with and without Grade I Achilles tendinitis who were age, weight, and distance matched had their Achilles tendon cross-sectional areas measured using the previously validated ultrasound technique. They demonstrated that athletes with Achilles tendinitis had about a 30% decrease in the cross-sectional areas of their Achilles tendons ($p < 0.05$). This indicates that a major mechanism in this type of common injury may simply be fatigue creep of the Achilles tendon. Komi et al. (47) recently developed an *in vivo* buckle transducer, which they located around the Achilles tendon in a number of subjects. Direct force measurements were made on several subjects who were involved in slow walking to sprinting, jumping, and hopping after calibration of the transducer. During running and jumping, forces close to the previously estimated ultimate tensile strength of the tendon were recorded, indicating that fatigue creep in a small cross-sectional tendon is a possible mechanism of injury without the need to invoke other lower-limb biomechanical pathology as has been suggested (22).

The work of Vailas et al. (93) was one of the first quantitative studies on the beneficial effects of early movement on the tensile strength of extracapsular ligament repair; it has been instrumental, as has the work of Akeson's group and Salter, in changing surgical practice from one of minimal immobilization (or "plaster is a disaster") to one of early mobilization (Frank et al., 34). Further to this point, Woo et al. (97) recently demonstrated almost complete return (98%) of structural properties of the transected canine femoral-medial collateral ligament-tibial (FMT) complex at 12 wk posttransection without immobilization. Canines immobilized for 6 wk and the FMT complex tested at 12 wk had mean loads to failure 54% that of the controls. However, the tensile strength of the medial collateral ligament (MCL) was only 62% that of controls at 48 wk. This apparent paradox was explained by the doubling in cross-sectional area of the healing MCL (and hence increased collagen deposition) during the early phases of healing. Amiel et al. (2) recently showed that maximal collagen deposition and turnover occurs during the first 3-6 wk postinjury in the rabbit. Chaudhuri et al. (21) used a Fourier domain directional filtering technique to quantify collagen fibril orientation in repairing ligaments. Results indicated that ligament collagen fibril reorientation does occur in the longitudinal axis of the ligament during remodeling.

The future for ligament and tendon healing looks exciting. The use of noninvasive methods to treat chronic tendinitis more effectively is now being explored. Binder et al. (4) used pulsed electromagnetic field therapy for persistent rotator cuff tendinitis, and the results are very encouraging. However, the use of such therapy in ligaments has not been successful (33). The problem of the poor repair of the cruciate ligaments needs to be explored and explained. The isolation and the recombinant synthesis of potent growth factors that influence connective tissues is just commencing. Wound healing is influenced and probably orchestrated by these factors. Buckley et al. (7, 8) recently showed that epidermal growth factor increases granulation tissue formation in a dose-dependent manner. Also using recombinant basic fibroblast growth factor (FGF) and transforming growth factor-beta (TGF-B), Davidson et al. (24) showed increased collagen accumulation in polyvinyl alcohol sponges implanted beneath the paniculus carnosus in adult rats. At day 14, TGF-beta was shown to double collagen content in the margins of rat wounds after a single injection, perhaps because of inhibition of metalloproteinase activity and hence attenuated collagenase activity. The tensile strength of wounds treated with both basic FGF and TGF-B were also increased. The application of growth factors to ligament repair is about to commence.

References

1. Amiel, D., C.B. Frank, F. Harwood, J. Fronek, and W.H. Akeson. Tendon and liga-

ments: A morphological and biochemical comparison. *J. Orthop. Res.* 1: 257-265, 1984.

2. Amiel, D., C.B. Frank, F. Harwood, W.H. Akeson, and J.B. Kleiner. Collagen alteration in medical collateral ligament healing in a rabbit model. *Connect. Tissue Res.* 16: 357-366, 1987.

3. Arnoczky, S.P., R.F. Warren, and M.A. Ashlock. Replacement of the anterior cruciate ligament by an allograft. *J. Bone Joint Surg.* [Am.] 63: 376-385, 1986.

4. Binder, A., G. Parr, B. Hazelman, and S. Fitton-Jackson. Pulsed electromagnetic field therapy of persistent rotator cuff tendinitis. *Lancet* 8379: Mar 31: 695-698, 1984.

5. Binkley, J.M., and M. Peat. The effects of immobilization on the ultrastructure and mechanical properties of the medial collateral ligament of rats. *Clin. Orthop. Rel. Res.* 203: 301-308, 1986.

6. Booth, F.W., and E.W. Gould. Effects of training and disuse on connective tissue. *Exer. Sports Sci. Rev.* 3: 83-112, 1975.

7. Buckley, A., J.M. Davidson, C.D. Kamerath, T.B. Wolt, and S. Woodward. Sustained release of epidermal growth factor accelerates wound repair. *Proc. Natl. Acad. Sci. USA* 82: 7340-7344, 1985.

8. Buckley, A., J.M. Davidson, C.D. Kamerath, and S.C. Woodward. Epidermal growth factor increases granulation tissue formation dose dependently. *J. Surg. Res.* 43: 322-328, 1987.

9. Buckley, M.J., A.J. Banes, L.G. Levin, B.E. Sumpio, M. Sato, R. Jordon, J. Gilbert, G.W. Link, and R. Tran Son Tay. Osteoblasts increase their rate of division and align in response to cyclic, mechanical tension *in vitro*. *Bone Miner.* (in press).

10. Burr, D.B., R.B. Martin, M.B. Schaeffer, and E.L. Radin. Bone remodelling in response to *in vivo* fatigue microdamage. *J. Biomech.* 18: 189-200, 1985.

11. Butler, D.L., M.D. Kay, and D.C. Stouffer. Comparison of material properties in fascicle-bone units from human patellar tendon and knee ligaments. *J. Biomech.* 18: 1-8, 1985.

12. Cabaud, H.E., A. Chatty, V. Gildengorin, and R.J. Feltman. Exercise effects on the strength of the rat anterior cruciate ligament. *Am. J. Sports Med.* 8: 79-86, 1980.

13. Carter, D.R., and W.C. Hayes. Compact bone fatigue damage: Residual strength and stiffness. *J. Biomech.* 10: 325-338, 1977.

14. Carter, D.R., and W.C. Hayes. Compact bone fatigue damage: A microscopic examination. *Clin. Orthop.* 127: 265-274, 1977.

15. Carter, D.R., W.E. Caler, D.M. Spengler, and V.H. Frankel. Fatigue behaviour of adult cortical bone: The influence of mean strain and strain range. *Acta Orthop. Scand.* 52: 481-490, 1981.

16. Carter, D.C. The relationships between *in vivo* bone remodelling and cortical bone remodelling. *CRC Crit. Rev. Bioeng.* 8: 1-28, 1982.

17. Carter, D.C., T.E. Orr, D.P. Fyhrie, and D.J. Schurman. Influences of mechanical stress on prenatal and postnatal skeletal development. *Clin. Orthop. Rel. Res.* 219: 237-250, 1987.

18. Carter, D.C. Mechanical loading history and skeletal biology. *J. Biomech.* 20: 1095-1109, 1987.

19. Caterson, B., and D.A. Lowther. Changes in the metabolism of the proteoglycan from sheep articular cartilage in response to mechanical stress. *Biochim. Biophys. Acta* 540: 412-422, 1978.

20. Chantraine, A., G. Heyman, and P. Franchimont. Bone metabolism, parathyroid hormone and calcitonin in paraplegia. *Calcif. Tissue Int.* 27: 199-204, 1979.

21. Chaudhuri, S., H. Nguyen, R.M. Rangayyan, S. Walsh, and C.B. Frank. A Fourier domain directional filtering method for analysis of collagen alignment in ligaments. *IEEE Trans. Biomed. Eng.* 34: 509-518, 1987.

22. Clement, D.B., J.E. Taunton, and G.W. Smart. Achilles tendinitis and peritendinitis: Aetiology and treatment. *Am. J. Sports Med.* 12: 179-184, 1984.

23. Clancy, W.G., R.G. Narechania, T.D. Rosenberg, D.D. Wisnefeske, and T.A. Lange. Anterior and posterior cruciate reconstruction in Rhesus monkeys: A histological, microangiographic and biochemical analysis. *J. Bone Joint Surg.* [Am.] 63: 1270-1284, 1981.

24. Davidson, J.M., A. Buckley, G.S. McGee, and A. Demetriou. Recombinant growth factors accelerate wound healing processes [Abstract c613]. *J. Cell Biochem. Suppl.* 12A: 147, 1988.

25. De Witt, M.T., C.J. Handley, B.W. Oakes, and D.A. Lowther. *In vitro* response of chondrocytes to mechanical loading: The effect of short term mechanical tension. *Connect. Tissue Res.* 12: 97-109, 1984.

26. Doillon, C.J., M.G. Dunn, and F.H. Silver. Correlation between collagen fibre network organization and mechanical properties of

wound tissues. In: Butler, D.L., and P. Torzilli, eds. *1987 biomechanics symposium*. New York: American Society of Mechanical Engineers, 1987: pp. 253-256.

27. El Haj, A.J., T.M. Skerry, B. Caterson, and L.E. Lanyon. Proteoglycan in bone tissue: Identifications and possible function in strain-related bone remodelling. *Trans. Orthop. Res. Soc.* 13: 538, 1988.

28. Engstrom, C.M., B.A. Hampson, J. Williams, and A.W. Parker. Muscle-tendon relations in runners [Abstract]. *Proc. Aust. Sports Med. Fed. (Ballarat)*, p. 56, 1985.

29. Fine, K.M., J.D. Kelly, C.T. Brighton, and S. Jimenez. Cyclic loading of stored rabbit medial femoral condyle and its effect upon articular cartilage when transplanted. *Trans. Orthop. Soc.* 13: 111, 1988.

30. Forwood, M.R., and D.A.W. Parker. Effects of exercise on bone morphology. *Acta Orthop. Scand.* 57: 204-208, 1986.

31. Forwood, M.R., and A.W. Parker. Effects of exercise on bone growth: Mechanical and physical properties studied in the rat. *Clin. Biomech.* 2: 185-190, 1987.

32. Forwood, M.R., and A.W. Parker. Microdamage in response to repetitive torsional loading in the rat tibia. (in press).

33. Frank, C., N. Schachar, D. Ditterich, N. Shrive, and W. deHaas. Electromagnetic stimulation of ligament healing in rabbits. *Clin. Orthop. Rel. Res.* 175: 263-272, 1983.

34. Frank, C., W.H. Akeson, S. L-Y. Woo, D. Amiel, and R.D. Coutts. Physiology and therapeutic value of passive joint motion. *Clin. Orthop. Rel. Res.* 185: 113-125, 1984.

35. Frost, H.M. Presence of microcracks in vivo in bone. *Henry Ford Hosp. Bull.* 8: 25-35, 1960.

36. Hampson, B.A., C.M. Engstrom, J. Williams, and A.W. Parker. Muscle strength and tendon cross-sectional area [Abstract]. *Proc. Aust. Sports Med. Fed. (Ballarat)*, p. 55, 1985.

37. Gillard, G.C., H.C. Reilly, P.G. Bell-Booth, and M.H. Flint. The influence of mechanical forces on the glycosaminoglycan content of the rabbit flexor digitorum profundus tendon. *Connect. Tissue Res.* 7: 37-46, 1979.

38. Gross, S.B., K.P. Spindle, C.T. Brighton, and R.P. Wassell. The proliferative and synthetic response of isolated bone cells to cyclical biaxial stress. *Trans. Orthop. Res. Soc.* 13: 262, 1988.

39. Handley, C.J., D.J. McQuillan, M.A. Campbell, and S. Bolis. Steady-state metabolism in cartilage explants. In: Kuettner, K. et al. *Articular cartilage metabolism*. New York: Raven Press, 1986: pp. 163-179.

40. Handley, C.J., J.F. Bateman, B.W. Oakes, and D.A. Lowther. Characterization of the collagen synthesized by cultured cartilage cells. *Biochim. Biophys. Acta* 386: 444-450, 1975.

41. Handley, C.J., and D.A. Lowther. Extracellular matrix metabolism by chondrocytes 5. The proteoglycans and glycosaminoglycans synthesized by chondrocytes in high density culture. *Biochim. Biophys. Acta* 582: 234-245, 1979.

42. Harell, A., S. Dekel, and I. Binderman. Biochemical effect of mechanical stress on cultured bone cells. *Calcif. Tissue Res. Suppl.* 22: 202-209, 1977.

43. Ishizue, K.K., D. Amiel, F.L. Harewood, and W.H. Akeson. Anterior cruciate ligament injury: The role of collagenase in early ligament degeneration. *Trans. Orthop. Res. Soc.* 13: 90, 1988.

44. Jaworski, Z.F.G., and H.K. Uhthoff. Reversibility of nontraumatic disuse osteoporosis during its active phase. *Bone* 7: 431-439, 1983.

45. Kiiskinen, A. Physical training and connective tissue, physical properties of Achilles tendons and long bones. *Growth* 41: 123-127, 1977.

46. Klein-Nulend, J., J.P. Veldhurizen, and E.H. Burge. Increased calcification of growth plate cartilage as a result of compressive force. *Arthritis Rheum.* 29: 1002-1009, 1980.

47. Komi, P.V., M. Salonen, M. Jarvinen, and O. Kokko. *In vivo* registration of Achilles tendon forces in man: Methodological development. *Int. J. Sports Med.* 8: 3-8, 1987.

48. Krolner, B., and B. Toft. Vertebral bone loss: An unheeded side effect of therapeutic bed rest. *Clin. Sci.* 64: 537-540, 1983.

49. Lane, N.E., D.A. Bloch, H.H. Jones, W.H. Marshall, P.D. Wood, and J.F. Fries. Long-distance running, bone density, and osteoarthritis. *JAMA* 9: 1147-1151, 1986.

50. Lanyon, L.E. Functional strain in bone as an objective, and controlling stimulus for adaptive bone remodelling. *J. Biomech.* 20(11/12): 1083-1093, 1987.

51. Larsen, N., and A.W. Parker. Sports medicine: Medical and scientific aspects of elitism in sport. In: Howell, M.L., and A.W. Parker. *Proc. Aust. Sports Med. Red.* 1982: vol. 8, pp. 63-73.

52. Luyten, F.P., V.C. Hascall, A.H. Reddi, T.E. Morales, and P.S. Nissley. Insulin-like

growth factors maintain steady state metabolism of proteoglycans in bovine cartilage explants. *Trans. Orthop. Res. Soc.* 13: 297, 1988.

53. Marguia, M.J., A. Vailas, B. Mendelbaum, J. Norton, J. Hodgdon, H. Goforth, and M. Riedy. Elevated plasma hydroxyproline: A possible risk factor associated with connective tissue injuries during overuse. *Amer. J. Sports Med.* 16(6): 660-664, 1988.

54. Matheson, G.O., D.B. Clement, D.C. McKenzie, J. Taunton, D.R. Lloyd-Smith, and J.G. McIntyre. Stress fractures in athletes: A study of 320 cases. *Am. J. Sports Med.* 15(1): 46-58, 1987.

55. McPherson, G.K., H.V. Mendenhall, D.F. Gibbons, H.P. Plenk, W. Rottman, J.B. Sanford, J.C. Kennedy, and J.C. Roth. Experimental mechanical and histological evaluation of the Kennedy augmentation device. *Clin. Orthop. Rel. Res.* 196: 186-195, 1985.

56. McQuillan, D.J., C.J. Handley, M.A. Campbell, S. Bolis, V.E. Milway, and A.C. Herrington. Stimulation of proteoglycan biosynthesis by serum and insulin-like growth factor-I in cultured bovine articular cartilage. *Biochem. J.* 240: 423-430, 1986.

57. Merrilles, M.J., and M.H. Flint. Ultrastructural study of the tension and pressure zones in a rabbit flexor tendon. *Am. J. Anat.* 157: 87-106, 1980.

58. Noyes, F.R, P.J. Torvik, W.B. Hyde, and J.L. De Lucas. Biomechanics of ligament failure: II. An analysis of immobilization, exercise and reconditioning effects in primates. *J. Bone Joint Surg.* [Am.] 56: 1406-1418, 1974.

59. O'Driscoll, S.W., F.W. Keeley, and R.B. Salter. The chondrogenic potential of free autogenous periosteal grafts for biological resurfacing of major full-thickness defects in joint surfaces under the influence of continuous passive motion. *J. Bone Joint Surg.* [Am.] 68(7): 1017-1035, 1986.

60. O'Keefe, R.J., J.S. Brand, J.E. Puzas, and R.N. Rosier. The response of epiphyseal chondrocytes to Transforming Growth Factor-Beta (TGF-B) is influenced by serum factors. *Trans. Orthop. Res. Soc.* 13: 299, 1988.

61. Oakes, B.W., A.W. Parker, and J. Norman. Changes in collagen fibre populations in young rat cruciate ligaments in response to an intensive one month's exercise program. In: Russo, P., and G. Gass, eds. *Human adaptation.* Sydney: Cumberland College of Health Sciences, Department of Biological Sciences, 1981: pp. 223-230.

62. Oakes, B.W. Ultrastructural studies on knee joint ligaments: Quantitation of collagen fibre populations in exercised and control rat cruciate ligaments and in human anterior cruciate grafts. In: Buckwalter, J., and S.L-Y. Woo, eds. *Injury and repair of the musculoskeletal tissues.* Park Ridge, IL: American Academy of Orthopedic Surgeons, 1988, sect. 2, p. 66-82.

63. Oakes, B.W., J. Leslie, J. Jacobsen, A.W. Parker, O. Deacon, and I. MacLean. Mechanisms of connective tissue rehabilitation. In: Howell, M.L., and A.W. Parker, eds. *Medical and scientific aspects of elitism in sport.* (*Proceedings of the Australian Sports Medicine Federation*) 1982: pp. 39-62, Vol. 8.

64. Oakes, B.W., C.J. Handley, F. Lisner, and D.A. Lowther. An ultrastructural study of high density primary cultures of embryonic chick chondrocytes. *J. Embryol. Exp. Morphol.* 38: 239-263, 1977.

65. Panush, R.S., C. Schmidt, J.R. Caldwell, N.L. Edwards, S. Longley, R. Yonker, E. Webster, J. Nauman, J. Stork, and H. Petterson. Is running associated with degenerative joint disease? *JAMA* 9: 1152-1154, 1986.

66. Parker, A.W., and N. Larsen. Changes in the strength of bone & ligament in response to training. In: Russo, P., and G. Gass, eds. *Human adaptation.* Sydney: Cumberland College of Health Sciences, Department of Biological Sciences, 1981: pp. 209-221.

67. Parry, D.A.D., G.R.G. Barnes, and A.S. Craig. A comparison of the size distribution of collagen fibrils in connective tissues as a function of age and possible relation between fibril size distribution and mechanical properties. *Proc. R. Soc. Lond.* [Biol.] 203: 305-321, 1978.

68. Parry, D.A.D., M.H. Flint, G.C. Gillard, and A.S. Craig. A role for glycosaminoglycans in the development of collagen fibrils. *FEBS Let* 149: 1-7, 1982.

69. Parry, D.A.D., A.S. Craig, and G.R.G. Barnes. Tendon and ligament from the horse: An ultrastructural study of collagen fibrils and elastic fibres as a function of age. *Proc. R. Soc. Lond.* [Biol.] 218: 894-902, 1978.

70. Parry, D.A.D. and A.S. Craig. Growth and development of collagen fibrils in connective tissue. In: Ruggeri, A., and P.M. Motta, eds. *Ultrastructure of connective tissue matrix.* New York: Elsevier, 1984: p. 34-64.

71. Puranen, J., L. Ala Ketola, P. Peltokallio, et al. Running and primary arthritis of the hip. *Br. Med. J.* 2: 424-425, 1975.

72. Radin, E.L., D. Eyre, and A.L. Schiller. Effects of prolonged walking on concrete on the joints of sheep [Abstract]. *Arthritis Rheum.* 22: 649, 1979.

73. Radin, E.L. Osteoarthrosis: What is known about prevention. *Clin. Orthop. Rel. Res.* 222: 60-65, 1987.

74. Radin, E.L., I.L. Paul, and R.M. Rose. Role of mechanical forces in pathogenesis of primary osteoarthritis. *Lancet* i: 519-522, 1972.

75. Rubin, C.T., and L.E. Lanyon. Dynamic strain similarities in vertebrates: An alternative to allometric limb bone scaling. *J. Theor. Biol.* 107: 321-327, 1984.

76. Rubin, C.T., and L.E. Lanyon. Osteoregulatory nature of mechanical stimuli: Function as a determinant for adaptive remodelling in bone. *J. Orthop. Res.* 5: 300-310, 1987.

77. Rubin, C.T., G.W. Pratt, A.L. Porter, L.E. Lanyon, and R. Poss. The use of ultrasound *in vivo* to determine acute change in the mechanical properties of bone following intense physical activity. *J. Biomech.* 20(7): 723-727, 1987.

78. Rutishauser, E., and G. Majno. Physiopathology of bone tissue: The osteocytes and fundamental substances. *Bull. Hosp. Joint Dis. (N.Y.)* 12: 468, 1951.

79. Sandell, L.J., and E. Dudek. IGF-I stimulates collagen gene expression in cultured chondrocytes. *Trans. Orthop. Res. Soc.* 13: 300, 1988.

80. Schneider, V.S., and J. McDonald. Skeletal calcium homeostasis and countermeasures to prevent disuse osteoporosis. *Calcif. Tissue Int.* 36: S151-S154, 1984.

81. Scott, J.E., and E.W. Hughes. Proteoglycan-collagen relationships in developing chick and bovine tendons: Influence on the physical environment. *Connect. Tissue Res.* 14: 267-278, 1986.

82. Shino, K., T. Kawasaki, H. Hirose, I. Gotoh, M. Inoue, and K. Ono. Replacement of the anterior cruciate ligament by an allograft. *J. Bone Joint Surg.* [*Br.*] 66: 672-681, 1984.

83. Skerry, T.M., M.J. Pead, R. Suswillo, S. Vedi, and L.E. Lanyon. Strain-related remodelling in bone tissue: Early stages of the cellular response to bone loading *in vivo*. *Trans. Orthop. Res. Soc.* 13: 97, 1988.

84. Somjen, D., I. Binderman, E. Berger, and A. Harell. Bone remodelling induced by physical stress is prostaglandin mediated. *Biochim. Biophys. Acta* 629: 91-100, 1980.

85. Tammi, M., A-M. Saamanen, A. Jauhiainen, O. Malminen, I. Kiviranta, and H. Helminen. Proteoglycan alterations in rabbit knee articular cartilage following physical exercise. *Connect. Tissue Res.* 11: 45-55, 1983.

86. Tilton, F.E., T.T.C. Degioanni, and V.S. Schneider. Long term follow-up of Skylab demineralization. *Aviat. Space Environ. Med.* 51: 1209-1213, 1980.

87. Tipton, C.M., A. Matthes, and J. Maynard. Influence of chronic exercise on rat bones. *Med. Sci. Sports Exer.* 4: 55, 1972.

88. Tipton, C.M., S.L. James, W. Mergner, and T.K. Tcheng. Influence of exercise on the strength of the medial collateral knee ligament of dogs. *Am. J. Physiol.* 218: 894-902, 1970.

89. Tipton, C.M., R.D. Matthes, J.A. Maynard, and R.A. Carey. The influence of physical activity on ligaments and tendons. *Med. Sci. Sports* 7: 165-175, 1975.

90. Toole, B.P., and D.A. Lowther. The effect of chondroitin sulphate-protein on the formation of collagen fibrils *in vitro*. *Biochem. J.* 109: 857-866, 1968.

91. Trippel, S.B., S. Doctrow, S. Klagsburn, M. Whelan, M.C. Hung, and H.J. Mankin. Effects of recombinant basic fibroblast growth factor on growth plate fibroblasts. *Trans. Orthop. Res. Soc.* 13: 298, 1988.

92. Vailas, A.C., R.F. Zernicke, J. Matsuda, S. Curwin, and J. Durivage. Adaptation of rat knee meniscus to prolonged exercise. *J. Appl. Physiol.* 60: 1031-1034, 1986.

93. Vailas, A.C., C.M. Tipton, R.D. Matthes, and M. Gart. Physical activity and its influence on the repair process of medial collateral ligaments. *Connect. Tissue Res.* 9: 25-31, 1981.

94. Vogel, K.C., and S.P. Evanko. Proteoglycan of fetal bovine tendon. *Trans. Orthop. Res. Soc.* 13: 182, 1988.

95. Wolff, J. *The law of bone remodelling* (P. Maquet and R. Furlong, Trans.). Berlin: Springer, 1986. (Original work published 1892).

96. Wong, M., and D.R. Carter. Mechanical stresses and morphogenic enchondral ossification in the sternum. *Trans. Orthop. Res. Soc.* 13: 241, 1988.

97. Woo, S. L-Y., M. Inoue, E. McGurk-Burleson, and M.A. Gomez. Treatment of the medial collateral ligament injury: II. Structure and function of canine knees in response to differing treatment regimes. *Am. J. Sports Med.* 15: 22-29, 1987.

98. Woo, S. L-Y., M.A. Gomez, T.J. Sites, P.O. Newton, C.A. Orlando, and W.H. Akeson. The biomechanical and morphological changes in the medial collateral ligament of the rabbit following immobilization and remobilization. *J. Bone Joint Surg.* (in press).

99. Yeh, C-K., and G.A. Rodan. Tensile forces enhance Prostaglandin E synthesis in osteoblastic cells grown on collagen ribbons. *Calcif. Tissue Int.* 36(Suppl. 1): S67-S71, 1984.

Chapter 30

Nervous System and Sensory Adaptation

V. Reggie Edgerton
Robert S. Hutton

The title of this chapter is indicative of our understanding of interactions of neural function and physical activity. The fact that one could (or assume to) review all or a major portion of the neural issues related to exercise, activity, and health in a single essay reflects the fact that little is known about the nervous system. On one hand, our lack of understanding is ironic, given the fact that the central nervous system carries most of the responsibility for the regulation of homeostasis of and among most organ systems. On the other hand, the complexity of the nervous system makes it so difficult to study. As an example of our meager understanding of neural compared to muscle function, there is no neuron of which the relative metabolic cost of its major cellular processes is well understood. This limitation in our understanding of neuronal functions is even more amazing because neural metabolism is relatively more simple than are other tissues in that it virtually solely depends on oxidative metabolism. A continuous supply of oxygen and blood glucose as a carbon source is essential for the central nervous system to function.

Given the reality of our limited knowledge of neural function as illustrated by the previous example, our strategy is limited to a few topics that relate to neural adaptation to exercise. These topics were selected because they are considered to be of importance and therefore should be noted as such for future scientists and because the authors have some familiarity with the topics.

Motor Control

Motor Unit Requirement

It is well recognized that motoneurons and their synaptic input are organized so that the order of recruitment within a single motor pool is relatively constant in repeated movements of the same kinematics (40, 91, 99). It is also accepted that some exceptions in the order of recruitment can and do occur, but the incidence and the physiological consequence of these exceptions do not override the general importance of the principle. Many of the motoneuronal properties that play a role in the excitability of motoneurons are known. Although most of this fundamental information has been derived almost entirely from animal experiments, many of the properties that have been tested in laboratory animals are qualitatively similar for humans. For example, relative constant recruitment order has been observed in humans (18, 71, 92) as well as in many other species (43, 100).

As has been true in experiments on many other species, motor units in humans can be categorized into types. For example, in a very general way the interrelationships of recruitment order, tension, contraction time, and fatigability within a pool of motor units are predictable in humans (92). Even the occurrence of doublets (short interpulse intervals at the initial phase of an effort) have been observed in humans at the onset of a rapid movement (36). Similarly, there is a high probability of a doublet when a high and rapid rate of current is injected into motoneurons (40). However, there is no agreement on the incidence or functional importance of this phenomenon in normal movements in humans and laboratory animals (18, 43, 92).

Can the physiological properties of motor units adapt to chronic exercise training? One of the most interesting findings illustrating that the recruitment of units can be altered by training is the enhanced incidence of synchronization of motor units within a pool after several weeks of a weight-lifting type of daily training. Milner-Brown et al. (71) and Sale (for a review, see ref. 82) showed that the probability of spikes occurring at the same time in more than one unit of the same muscle increased with weight training. Although the functional significance of this has not been verified, theoretically this adaptation could enhance the power output of a muscle independent of adaptation of the muscle tissue properties. This phenomenon has been implicated in studies in which work output increased in response to physical training without significant muscle fiber hypertrophy (17, 50).

Few studies have been directed toward the general but important goal of understanding the strategies used by the central nervous system to control movement. A step in this direction is to quantify the recruitment patterns across motor pools in a range of movement tasks. To date, the physiological issues regarding motor unit recruitment have been found within, rather than among, motor pools. A more thorough understanding and quantification of the interrelationships of synergists as well as agonists and antagonists in a range of movements is needed (42, 81).

The extent to which the neural strategies used to control movement utilize elastic strain energy in accomplishing the tasks of even routine movements remains unclear. However, there is rather direct evidence that even in relatively slow rates of running the neuromuscular system is able to utilize a significant amount of strain energy to generate propulsive power (32). Studies of in vivo muscle forces and joint kinematics of humans (56) and cats (32) suggest that the amount of elastic strain energy utilized is significant, even in conditions of low power output. Other studies of the strain characteristics of the human plantaris tendon suggest that a considerably important role could be played by the tendon when there is active force in the contractile tissue (84).

Within the last 15 years, remarkable progress has been made in understanding and rediscovering the phenomenon often referred to as *pattern generation*. Several reviews have been published that describe and document numerous aspects of pattern generation in a variety of animal species (33, 34, 35). In essence, pattern generation is the cyclic generation of motor patterns (e.g., locomotion, respiration, and chewing) without cyclic input from supraspinal centers or peripheral sensors. Neural preparations that are isolated from all apparent aspects of extrinsic, phasic input can demonstrate cyclic motor activity when stimulated continuously either pharmacologically or electrically (33, 34, 35, 36, 37). Although the fundamental source of the cyclic activity of the various generators remains unclear, it is likely that significant progress will be made

in the near future with the many studies being conducted on the simpler invertebrate systems.

A final comment on the concept of pattern generation is the assumption that the pattern generation of locomotion (as observed in invertebrates and vertebrates including a number of mammals) does not exist in human and nonhuman primates. Although there is little evidence at this time that locomotorlike steps can occur in primates without supraspinal input, it is premature at this time to conclude that the phenomenon cannot be observed under the proper experimental conditions (62). This fundamental property of neural networks seems far too prevalent and important to be allotted a minor role in human neurophysiology, and biological logic leads us to speculate that it is far too ubiquitous among the animal kingdom to have been lost in the evolution of primates.

Neuromuscular Fatigue

Neuromuscular fatigue has been defined as any decline in the maximum force-generating capacity of a muscle or synergistic muscle group in spite of the force required at any given point in time (7, 11). Hence, subjects may be able to produce successfully and repeatedly a brief force at 50% of their maximum voluntary contraction force (MVC) and yet show a significant decline in their ability to produce an MVC. Whether the force is sustained isometrically or produced intermittently, responses under conditions of maximum excitatory drive are characterized by a rapid linear decline followed by a more gradual linear decay over time. The inflection point of the characteristic force-decay responses usually occurs between 20% and 70% of the MVC after 1-2 min of muscular effort, depending on the nature of the contractions (e.g., isometric vs. concentric contractions; magnitude of target force) and the arrangement of the vasculature in the muscles tested (11, 37, 88). It is generally accepted that the initial faster decay rate in force is due to the occlusion of blood flow by compression of larger arteries (7, 88). This view is supported by the observation that occlusion of blood flow by a pressure cuff during a sustained isometric MVC produces a continuation of the initial force-time response to exhaustion, that is, a continuous decline to zero force without incurring an inflection point and a more gradual decay (89).

What are the potential neuromuscular mechanisms involved in the total capacity of these two organ systems to sustain a desired muscle force? Clearly, neuromuscular fatigue, changes in excitatory drive, and related compensatory adjustments to a decline in muscle force capacity represent a multidimensional problem. Sites involved in neuromuscular fatigue are typically addressed as factors involving the central nervous system (CNS) or as peripheral pre- and postjunctional factors involving the functional linkage (neuromuscular junction) between the neural and the muscular elements of the motor unit (3, 7, 27, 46, 47, 54, 63). In this chapter, changes associated with fatigue that are attributable to events at the premotoneuronal levels are considered to be of central origin. Those changes in the motoneuron itself, the neuromuscular junction, and the muscle are categorized as peripheral in origin. In the following discussion, emphasis is placed on human experimentation whenever possible.

Motor Unit: Muscle Element

At the level of the muscle fiber, most studies have involved animal tissues to determine the metabolic correlates of fatigue (27, 73). In single-fiber preparations of frog semitendinosus muscle, the effects produced by tetanic stimulation (10-s trains at 20 Hz) interrupted by 1-s rest periods and less than 40 s in duration are rapidly reversible, whereas a stimulation period lasting for 100-150 s requires up to 82 min to recover (73). Phosphocreatine falls logarithmically to 10% of resting values up to about 150 s of stimulation, and recovery to normal levels occurs after 90-120 min of rest. Fiber glycogen and ATP are insignificantly affected. Because posttetanic twitch potentiation (PTP) occurs in fatigued fibers (45, 51, 93), additional factors may interfere with the action of Ca^{++} in excitation-contraction coupling (e.g., pH level of the myoplasm) (73). In long-term, intense (but nonfatiguing) exercise, lysosomal enzyme activity in rat muscle does not appear to challenge muscle fiber homeostasis (83). Fatigue that is rapidly reversible in single-fiber experiments may involve a transient failure to activate myofibrils within the center of the fiber (73).

Metabolic alterations in human muscle during neuromuscular fatigue have been studied using repeated muscle biopsies (44) and, more recently, nuclear magnetic resonance spectroscopy (NMR) (21, 70). Hultman and Sjoholm (44) induced fatigue to a mean of 78% of initial maximum values in human quadriceps femoris muscles by electrical stimulation at 20 Hz over the course of 50 s. Circulation had been arrested by a pressure cuff 30 s before stimulation to create an anaerobic state. Successive biopsy samples were taken during contraction and analyzed for ATP, phosphocreatine, glucose-6-phosphate, and lactate. As in the findings reported previously for frog muscle, phosphocreatine stores decreased exponentially over the course of contraction to near depletion at 50 s. Although the concentrations of ATP decreased negligibly, the force declined. The ATP turnover rate declined during contraction (calculated to be 5.6 mmol • kg^{-1} dry wt s^{-1} initially and 4.0 mmol • kg^{-1} dry wt s^{-1} subsequently). Glycolysis began within 5 s of the onset of contraction, and lactate concentration was correlated significantly ($r = .91$) with glucose-6-phosphate concentration.

Miller et al. (70) studied neuromuscular fatigue in the human adductor pollicis muscle using NMR, which allowed noninvasive measurements of phosphocreatine, ATP, inorganic phosphates (Pi), and intracellular pH. Fatigue was induced by a sustained maximum voluntary contraction for 1-4 min. Simultaneous measurements were made of electromyographic (EMG) activity. Contraction force fell by 90%, pH declined from 7.1 to 6.4, and phosphocreatine fell to near total depletion. Inorganic phosphate concentrations rose rapidly in the first 2 min, whereas ATP dropped to 70% of control after 3-4 min of contraction. The electrically evoked M-wave was reduced in amplitude and increased in duration. Metabolic recovery occurred within 20 min, and the M-wave returned to normal within 4 min. A measure of neuromuscular efficiency (force/rectified integrated EMG) showed a decreased ratio to 40% of control at the end of contraction. Recovery to control values occurred within 60 min. These investigators concluded that there are three components of neuromuscular fatigue: (a) impaired muscle membrane excitation and propagation, (b) a reduction in maximum voluntary contraction correlated with the altered metabolic state of the muscle, and (c) a stage of probable prolonged impaired excitation-contraction coupling independent of changes in high-energy phosphates and cellular pH.

Frequency of activation in inducing fatigue has proven to be an important factor in producing different time courses in the recovery of contractile force to control values (9, 24, 31, 63, 68, 69). Low frequencies (20 Hz) of electrical stimulation in human muscle (e.g., adductor pollicis and quadriceps femoris) produce force decrements that recover over many hours, whereas higher frequencies (100 Hz) of stimulation lead to a measurable recovery of muscle force in minutes. Low-frequency fatigue appears to be due to prolonged impairment in the excitation-contraction coupling process, whereas high-frequency induced fatigue may be attributed to impaired electrical transmission across the neuromuscular junction as evidenced by a decline in the amplitude of the M-wave (70, 89).

In animal experiments, rate of fatigue occurs as a function of muscle fiber length (1) relative to its optimal sarcomere length, suggesting that the rate of fatigue is indirectly related to the number of effective cross-bridge interactions per half of sarcomere. Indirect support of this relationship has been reported in human dorsiflexor muscles (28). A greater reduction in twitch and tetanic torque during fatigue has been found at the optimum muscle length where the overlap of actin and myosin binding sites is maximal in contrast to the reductions measured at a shortened muscle position (28).

For submaximal tensions, one intrinsic compensatory mechanism in the muscle fiber to counter a decline in the force-generating capacity of muscle may be PTP, which is consistently observed as long as the percent decline in total muscle force due to fatigue is above the control twitch force (45, 51, 93); PTP has been observed in both animal and human experiments (46, 51, 93). Because potentiating conditioning stimuli can fall well within the range of activation frequencies incurred during normal contractions (13, 93), the potentiated muscle force response also has been called *postactivation potentiation*. When elicited by a series of repetitive contractions (rather than a single test stimulus) and tested over a range of frequencies, the force-time integral of a succession of contractions increases relative to the pretetanic values. This observation is particularly notable in the lower range of stimulation frequencies (13, 45, 46); therefore, PTP optimizes input-output coupling between the neural and the muscle elements in the production of force even when muscle fibers are in a fatigued state.

An interesting question is whether the fatigue-resistant metabolic properties of muscle fibers are in any way determined by their neural innervation. This question was addressed by experimenting on self- and cross-innervated muscles in cats (22). Fast- and slow-twitch muscles were found to retain their characteristic fatigue-resistant properties whether the reinnervated nerve had originally served a fatigue-resistant or a relatively fatigable muscle. These findings suggest that the basic protein expressions of enzymes regulating oxidative capacity in a muscle fiber are determined largely by factors endogenous to the cell.

Motor Unit: Neural Element

There has been considerable controversy over the years concerning the existence of propagation failure across the neuromuscular junction (10, 12, 53, 60, 61, 67, 86, 89). For example, Stephens and Taylor (90) reported decrements in the electrically evoked M-wave during voluntarily induced fatigue in the first dorsal interosseus, whereas Merton (67), Bigland-Ritchie (7), and Bigland-Ritchie and Woods (11) have reported either no changes in the amplitude of the M-wave during the course of muscle fatigue or no changes in the overall integrated waveform due to a slowing of conduction of the muscle action potential. It is clear that during the course of fatigue the rate of contraction force and relaxation is slowed, allowing greater summation of forces at lower frequencies (7, 10, 21, 27). This change in the dynamics of the contractile apparatus, in combination with PTP, probably explains a shift in the sigmoid-shaped muscle-force-stimulation frequency curve to the left of the frequency spectrum, that is, to the lower frequency range of stimulation, thereby lowering the fusion frequency of the muscle (7, 8, 27). Hence, lower frequencies of stimulation and amplitudes of the M-wave need not necessarily reflect a decrease in the force-generating capacity of the muscle.

The issue of differential susceptibilities of motor unit types to transmission failure during fatigue has been addressed (12, 15, 53, 61, 86). Motor units in the human short extensors of the toes with high threshold and higher conduction velocities show blocking of electrochemical transmission within 60 s of the onset of electrical stimulation at 20 Hz (12). Under conditions of voluntary drive, normal subjects can sustain discharge rates that cause full fusion of muscle tension for only a few seconds. With audiofeedback of the discharge rate, highly motivated subjects can maintain maximum tension for at least 20 s before the motor unit discharge frequency declines. Motor units with low excitation thresholds and conduction velocities can be maintained voluntarily throughout a 60-s period. These findings are consistent with those of Kugelberg and Lindegren (61), who showed in the rat anterior tibialis muscle that transmission failure during contraction was progressively greater in faster-contracting motor units exhibiting progressively lower fatigue resistance (for similar observations in human muscle, see ref. 15). In human experiments, electrical transmission blocking of either single motor units or the composite EMG activity often can be overcome by extraordinary motivation and training. This suggests that fatigue factors presumably of central origin are modifiable (7, 11, 12).

A consistent finding in studies of neuromuscular fatigue has been a shift in the mean EMG power spectrum frequency to a lower frequency as muscle fatigue progresses (7, 8, 57, 58). In humans there is a progressive decline in the range and mean rate of single motor unit discharge over a period of 40-120 s of a sustained MVC force. Mean single motor unit rates in the first 60 s have been reported to fall from 27 to 15 Hz (12). In a few observations, units showing the highest initial frequencies appeared to decline in firing rate more rapidly than did the units with low initial frequencies (12). This observation is in agreement with those reported by Kernell (53), who observed "late adaptation" of alpha motoneurons in cat in response to constant current intracellular excitation. When motoneurons are driven at a minimum rate of steady firing, there is a slow, progressive drop in discharge rate (late adaptation) during the first minute of constant stimulation. Late adaptation to excitatory current is much more prominent among fast-twitch motoneurons (usually exhibiting higher initial firing frequencies) than among slow-twitch motoneurons. Late adaptation appears to be related to cumulative effects of spike discharge on the electrogenic properties of the motoneuronal membrane (53, 54). Taken together, the decline over time in motoneuronal discharge during constant activation may be associated with the shift seen in the surface-EMG power frequency spectrum toward the lower-frequency range. The functional consequence of this adaptation is a closer matching between the discharge frequency of the neural element (alpha motoneuron) and the downward shift in the force–frequency of stimulation response (see previous discussion) observed in the muscle element as fatigue progresses (11, 46, 63). This remarkable pairing of acute adaptations has been referred to as the "muscular wisdom" that minimizes fatigue during prolonged effort in humans (63). It may also explain why a decrement in the M-wave amplitude is reported in some experiments but not in others. The occurrence and magnitude of late adaptation responses appear

specific to motor unit types, and therefore a corresponding decrease in frequency of muscle action potentials could be specific to the composition of the muscle tested.

Central Nervous System

A common approach adapted by Bigland-Ritchie and by others (7, 8, 11, 90) to study the issue of central drive failure during fatigue is to observe the change in rectified integrated EMG of muscle during a voluntary sustained MVC. If the MVC falls more rapidly than does the force resulting from electrical nerve stimulation, the fatigue may have a central origin. The specific site of the central fatigue could be in membrane electrogenic properties of the alpha motoneuron or at some premotoneuronal level. However, experimental observations of this type have led to mixed results. When EMG declines in parallel with force (a sign of neuromuscular transmission failure), some highly motivated subjects can increase the EMG amplitude in the face of a continued decline in force, suggesting that there may be some compensation to initial failure of central origin (7, 11, 12, 86). This observation is consistent with the interpretation that compensatory presynaptic mechanisms acting on motoneurons may occur during neuromuscular fatigue.

It is generally accepted that voluntary contractions are commonly produced by alpha-gamma coactivation with servo-assistance through the muscle spindle afferent pathways (66). Marsden et al. (64) demonstrated that the gain of the stretch reflex in humans could be increased in fatigued muscle. However, these findings were based solely on EMG measurements; therefore, selective alterations in the gain of the stretch reflex through the gamma loop could not be assessed apart from the selective enhancement of excitatory drive to alpha motoneurons. Recently, Nelson and Hutton (74) demonstrated in fatigued cat gastrocnemius muscle an enhancement of stretch sensitivity in Group Ia and II afferent pathways, thereby increasing autogenetic excitation to the motoneural pool. They also showed decreased stretch sensitivity in Group Ib pathways, thereby decreasing autogenetic inhibition and producing greater excitation through disinhibition (47). During prolonged motor unit activation, studies of post-stimulus-triggered histograms of afferent spindle discharge indicate that the gain of the subsystem-transforming force in response to afferent discharge is also increased (14, 96; see also 38, 49, 55, 85, 90). In contrast to these apparent compensatory reflex adjustments to contractile failure, Hayward et al. (39) recently reported reflex inhibition of the soleus from the medial gastrocnemius (a synergist) while the medial gastrocnemius was electrically induced to fatigue. The axonal fibers contributing to this inhibitory reflex were assumed to be Group III and Group IV afferents. Clearly, more experimentation on acute responses of spinal reflexes during neuromuscular fatigue is needed.

Preliminary evidence of changes in the polysynaptic pathway of the tonic vibration reflex indicates that the level of physical conditioning may be a significant factor in whether the EMG amplitude is increased (seen in sedentary controls and sprinters) or decreased (seen in long-distance runners) following an exhaustive exercise (48). Therefore, there is reason to believe that stretch reflex pathways may adapt acutely to the prevailing conditions in the contractile apparatus, thus providing a means of partially compensating for such factors as late adaptation occurring in some motoneuronal membranes (48, 53, 55, 74, 95). Perhaps such a compensation could prevent or offset in time the fast-twitch motoneuronal discharge from declining beyond critical levels for maintaining some minimum contractile force. The existence of inhibitory input to motoneuronal pools during fatigue from possibly Group III and IV afferent fibers awaits further investigation (39).

Little is known about supraspinal mechanisms that may come into play during the course of muscle fatigue. Electroencephalographic potentials associated with movement (the readiness potential) have been shown to increase in size with rhythmically induced fatigue involving contractions of the hand (29). Potential acute alterations in human long-latency reflexes (the so-called V_2, and V_3 responses) during conditions of muscle fatigue also remain to be investigated.

Central fatigue need not be viewed simply as a failure of excitatory motor command pathways (3). It is conceivable that, as a protective device against depletion of high-energy phosphate stores in muscle, there may be a gradual buildup of CNS inhibitory drive to motoneuronal pools (e.g., through the presynaptic inhibition of Group Ia afferent pathways). Asmussen (3) has reported greater facilitory effects of "diverting activity" (exercising other nonfatigued muscle groups) compared to rest between fatiguing work bouts on the recovery of force generation. He proposed that diverting activity may cause an increased inflow of excitatory impulses from nonfatigued parts of the body to motoneuronal pools undergoing fatigue, thus shifting the balance between inhibition and facilitation in the direction of facilitation. The reticular formation was suggested as one site wherein this shift might occur. Although this obviously is speculative, the facilitatory effects of diverting work cannot be explained simply as eradicating a peripheral mechanism of fatigue through enhanced oxygen transport, as circulation through the fatigued muscle group was shown to be unaltered by the diverting activity.

In summary, at the level of the muscle fiber, metabolic correlates of muscle fatigue have been well characterized, but no single metabolic factor has been isolated as the rate-limiting factor in sustaining muscle force. Interactions between rising hydrogen ion concentrations and the sequestering of Ca^{++} ions during excitation-contraction coupling remain major possible mechanisms to be explored by physiologists. It seems improbable, however, that these altered metabolic factors could explain the more prolonged deficits in maximal muscle force that occur over several minutes to hours. Although there is sufficient evidence to suggest that there are fatigue mechanisms of central origin, present findings reflect more on the nature of compensatory responses to a decline in excitatory drive to motor units than on potential sites of breakdown in CNS excitatory drive. In large part, the limited experimental research on the CNS and fatigue is a reflection of the technical difficulties encountered in monitoring the appropriate CNS activity during the induction of muscle fatigue.

As one reviews the research literature on neuromuscular fatigue, it is clear that the issue of central versus peripheral fatigue and the evidence that refutes or supports failure acting at either site are largely a function of the experimental design and the subsystems tested. Technical limitations have curtailed advancements in the study of potential fatigue processes acting within the CNS. Certainly, this latter focus of future research will lead us into a relatively unexplored area in the study of neural mechanisms associated with neuromuscular fatigue.

Future Issues and Challenges in the Neural Control of Movement

Only over the last decade have there been significant advances in the techniques and methods of the application of electrical stimulation of nerves and muscle to control movement, rehabilitate muscle, and control chronic pain. A major element in facilitating these advances has been the miniaturization and improvement of electronic components and the ability to control them with affordable computers of a manageable size. Given the present-day technology, it seems feasible that an appropriate sequence of activation patterns of muscle can be achieved to generate stereotypic movements (e.g., walking or riding a bike) (77).

However, there are other major biotechnical obstacles to attaining the goal of controlling complex movements in impaired neuromuscular systems. The means of stimulating muscles continues to be a major limiting factor. Direct stimulation of the surface of muscle does not activate the deep musculature. Also, the means of grading the strengths and speeds of contractions are imprecise at best. For example, it is well accepted that surface electrical activation of muscle occurs through the nerve branches within the muscle. Consequently, the normal recruitment order would be reversed because in percutaneous stimulation larger axons have lower electrical thresholds. Another limitation has been the inability to maintain a functionally constant interface for long periods of time between the electrode and the muscle or muscle nerve. Chronic adhesion of electrodes to the muscle or nerve can produce skin lesions or even burns. Further, an effective functional interface progressively decreases with time. In spite of these difficulties, encouraging improvements are being made that suggest that, with continued biotechnical development, it will be feasible to control some movements with reasonable precision by means of electrical stimulation of muscle, at least in semiacute preparations.

Another challenge in the field of neural control of movement is to determine the mechanisms responsible for the control of output of one muscle compared to another. How does the nervous system select the relative and absolute levels of activation of synergistic and antagonistic motor pools? Although in a very general sense we know how agonists versus antagonists are recruited in cyclic movements, little is known about the control strategies used by supraspinal centers to accomplish the intermuscle coordination observed in routine cycles. In contrast, considerable detail is known about selected excitatory and inhibiting effects of some specific peripheral sensors and interneurons. How these circuits are controlled in normal movements, however, is virtually unknown. For example, how much of the absence of activation of the flexors of the leg during the stance phase of a step is due to a reduction in facilitation versus greater inhibition?

A third general challenge in understanding neural control is to define the general strategies used by the nervous system to control movement. An example of a general design strategy that has been identified in considerable detail with respect to a single motor pool is Henneman's size principle (40). On one hand, this general principle of recruitment order (as noted earlier) within a pool is well defined and appears to be applicable to all motor pools. On the other hand (as noted previously), the means by which the interaction of motor pools are controlled in the execution of even the simplest motor tasks are poorly understood. Are there general strategies or principles at the inter-motor-pool levels as there are within motor pools? If so, then the task of controlling the details of a movement seems less formidable.

Responsiveness of the CNS to Chronic Perturbations

Adaption

Historically, the view has been that the CNS has little potential to reestablish or reorganize function lost, for example, to injury or disease. However, this opinion is changing rapidly. It has become quite clear that there is some potential for the regeneration of some connectivity of neurons, as limited as it may seem at this point. The responsiveness of the nervous system to elevated activity levels seems to be significant (96, 97). In complex networks the oxidative potential of neurons can be changed within days after activation levels are modified (98, 100). Neurons that are several synapses away from the source of activation can change their mitochondrial contents (99). Motoneurons can increase their oxidative potentials in response to chronic exercise training (30). However, when muscle fibers are induced to hypertrophy by eliminating synergists, the oxidative potential and size of the motoneurons constituting the muscle decreases. Reduced soma and axonal sizes have been reported also in endurance-trained animals (80). The inverse relationship between oxidative capacity and soma size is particularly interesting because of its implications to the size principle of motor unit recruitment (75).

As noted previously, it is generally recognized that the size of a motoneuron is indirectly related to its excitability (40). On the basis of the size principle of motor unit recruitment—and if the generation of action potentials represents a significant metabolic cost—it seems reasonable to assume that the smaller motoneurons would be the most active and have the highest oxidative potentials. Conversely, the larger, less active motoneuron should have the least oxidative potential. Although this has been reported to be true in some cases (53, 54, 75), this relationship has been reported to be insignificant or even the reverse of that expected on the basis of the size principle (72). Further, data based on accurate and valid measures of oxidative enzymes in motoneurons identified with respect to the muscle they innervate are necessary to determine the relationship between soma size and oxidative potential within a motor pool. Comparisons of the metabolic properties of motoneurons of different motor pools may be quite informative, or at least indicative, of strategies that may be important in controlling the relative recruitment of units among various motor pools. An inverse relationship of oxidative potential and soma size is important from other viewpoints. If small motoneurons are the most active, the the corresponding muscle unit will be active also. Consequently, the oxidative potential of the muscle fiber might be expected to correspond to the excitability of the motoneuron. This indeed appears to be the case, although direct proof of this has been shown for only a few motor units of cat muscle (65). Data based on muscle-specific populations of motoneurons and their respective muscles support the view that the oxidative potential of a motoneuron and its muscle unit are directly related (53, 54, 65). A close relationship at the motor unit level would be consistent with, although not proof of, the idea that the motoneuron controls the oxidative properties of the muscle unit by means of some function associated with the generation of action potentials.

The interaction of the motoneuron and its muscle unit may function in the reverse direction; that is, the muscle may influence the properties of the motoneuron. The best and most obvious evidence for this is the fact that the availability of

muscle to serve as a target organ is essential for the survival of motoneurons, particularly if the axon has been severed in close proximity to the cell body. However, a more subtle effect of muscle on motoneurons is suggested by the work of Czeh et al. (20). For example, following axotomy the duration of the after-hyperpolarization of an action potential is shorter. But if the denervated muscle is stimulated directly for several days to weeks (therefore without the generation of antidromic action potentials), then the reduction in the duration of after-hyperpolarization is less than it is with axotomy alone (20).

Because little is known about the relative importance of the different neural functions carried out by a motoneuron in driving the energy demands of neurons, one can only speculate on the importance of electrical activity in inducing adaptations, directing the proper development of neural systems, and facilitating repair of neural systems that have been damaged (4, 59, 86, 88). But given the fact that the metabolic properties of motoneurons can adapt to chronic exercise and given the theoretical relationship of motoneuron activity and oxidative metabolism, it is reasonable to hypothesize that neural activity plays an important role in the control and regulation of normal development and in the recovery from neural insults.

Considering adaptive CNS responses in healthy human subjects, we find that proprioceptive reflex pathways repeatedly have been shown to respond to progressive resistive exercise by showing potentiated maximum amplitudes after several weeks of training (for a review, see refs. 45, 82). Such changes are most often reported for the V_1 response, having a monosynaptic latency of approximately 30 ms, and the V_2 response, having an oligosynaptic latency of approximately 50 ms. The V_2 response is long enough in latency to involve supraspinal mediation through the motor cortex as well as through the slower-conducting Group II afferent fibers and their spinal pathways into the motoneuronal pool. One possible advantage of this adaptation is a more rapid mobilization of muscle force by an enhanced rate of rise in excitatory current when the gamma loop is co-activated during voluntary contraction against larger resistive loads. Sale (82) proposed a different explanation by suggesting that, before training, voluntary attempts to maximize muscle force may not involve recruitment of all motor units serving the muscle or muscles activated. If training produces the capability of recruiting all motor units that could potentially contribute to the desired force, then the antidromic component of the V_1 (or

V_2) maximum electrical stimulus would collide with the ongoing voluntary orthodromic impulses and clear all efferent axons for the subsequent V_1 reflex response. The assumption is that, before training and during reflex testing, some of the potential V_1 reflex responses were blocked antidromically by the test stimulus.

That central adaptations involving proprioceptive synaptic input to motoneurons do occur through training has been nicely demonstrated by an animal model introduced by Wolpaw (96, 97). Wolpaw has operantly conditioned monkeys to increase or decrease the gain of either the spinal stretch reflex or the H-reflex in elbow flexors or the triceps surae, respectively. Significant changes in the respective reflex amplitudes compared to preconditioned control responses occurred after about 3 days of conditioning involving 3,000-6,000 trials per day. Conditioned increases or decreases in the reflex amplitude begin to plateau, depending on the reflex elicited, at about 200% and 50% of control values, respectively, and occur over the course of 2-3 months. If there is a break in training for several days, the alteration in reflex gain persists at the conditioned level. If the reinforcement mode is reversed (e.g., from an increase to a decrease in reflex amplitude for reward), the conditioned reflex amplitudes likewise reverse in size over time. Because spinal transection above the trained spinal segments did not abolish the conditioned H-reflex responses over the course of 3 days of observations, Wolpaw (personal communication, 1988) speculates that the probable sites for the learned response reside in the Group Ia synapse on the alpha motoneuron, on the alpha motoneuron itself, and possibly on other oligosynaptic pathways involving Group Ia, Ib, and II afferent fibers. Findings from these studies reflect well on the possibility of central neural adaptations that may also occur through exercise undertaken over weeks and months of training.

It has been suggested that the activity patterns of motoneurons during the early stages of development of motor units play an important role in the eventual coordination of physiological and biochemical properties of muscle fibers and motoneurons. For example, the muscle fibers innervated by a motoneuron may have a wide variety of properties before innervation, and these muscle fibers become more homogeneous once functional innervation is established. However, there is evidence that the motoneuron may be able to select those muscle fibers that have similar and appropriate properties for that motoneuron (91). Recent experiments also suggest that activity levels may play

a role in determining the number of muscle fibers innervated by a motoneuron. For example, when activity was eliminated by applying tetrodotoxin to the axons, larger motor units were found than when there were normal activity levels (78). Other evidence of the effect of neuromuscular activity on motor units is that chronic exercise can enhance the degree of recovery from denervation (4, 41, 52). There is morphological evidence that changes in activity levels affect the size of end-plate regions of muscle fibers (26, 94). Further, there is experimental evidence that motoneuronal properties can by altered with exercise training (30).

When there is complete functional separation of the lumbar spinal cord from supraspinal input by spinal transection, the most familiar effects are muscle atrophy and spasticity. It is now well known that the lumbar spinal cord in quadrupeds is capable of generating remarkably normal locomotor patterns in the hind limbs without supraspinal input when the animal is assisted in maintaining its balance (6). On the basis of this observation, efforts are being made to determine the degree to which normality of the neuromuscular system of the hind limbs can be maintained by (a) training for 30 min daily on a moving treadmill belt, (b) moving the limbs passively through a locomotorlike pattern, or (c) standing continuously for 30 min (62, 79, 81). To date, the following have been demonstrated: (a) An animal spinalized at 2 or 6 wk of age or as an adult can be trained to perform excellent, but not completely normal, locomotor patterns on the treadmill. (b) This small amount of treadmill exercise (30 min/d, 5 d/wk) results in a significantly better locomotor capability than when the animals are similarly treated passively and not exercised on a treadmill. (c) It appears that the beneficial effect of training by standing is less than it is for stepping. (d) The treadmill training program for 30 min markedly reduces, but does not eliminate, the muscle atrophy that would normally occur with spinalization. (e) The physiological changes in muscle that usually occur following spinalization are reduced by treadmill training.

It has been found that the muscles of the hindlimb develop faster contractile properties following chronic spinalization. For example, many of the muscle fibers, particularly of predominantly slow muscles, convert from slow to fast contracting, as indicated by histochemical staining (79). In addition, myofibrillar ATPase activity increases in both slow and fast muscle and to some degree is independent of the changes in the qualitative histochemical types. Finally, it has become clear that as the muscle fiber properties change, so do the motoneurons (16). In fact, it appears that the muscle fibers that develop fastlike properties do so in increments of motor units. It is not clear why all muscle fibers (or all motor units) of the soleus of a cat do not respond similarly to spinalization, as all fibers are homogeneous, at least relative to the diversity seen among muscles based on qualitative histochemical characteristics (65).

The experimental results briefly summarized here provide a sound basis for the concept that neuromuscular activity can facilitate significant levels of recovery from neural injury. There are many cases in which this apparently is true in humans who are undergoing physical therapy following stroke, spinal injury, surgery, or other dysfunctional problems. However, some of the rehabilitation procedures being used are based on concepts that subsequently have proven to be questionable. Thus it is highly desirable to understand the mechanisms of neuronal adaptation to exercise and rehabilitation and subsequently to interject this new information as rapidly as possible into the clinical treatment protocols of neurologically impaired patients.

Overuse

The concept of overuse of the neuromuscular system is a recurring topic. Can excessive exercise cause neural damage? It is known that exhaustive exercise can cause a loss of nucleoproteins in motoneurons. After only 30 min of exercise of the forelimbs of guinea pigs on a treadmill, some motoneurons of the cervical spinal cord became chromophobic; that is, they fail to stain normally for Nissl substance (nucleoprotein). It was shown also that the nucleolus and nucleus enlarged with acute, exhaustive exercise (23). Gerchman et al. (30) reported similar effects in rats that were trained daily to swim, but the rats were unable to adapt successfully to the rigor of the training.

In contrast to the evidence that a single bout of exercise can induce marked neuronal changes is the view that neurons are quite resistant to failure to propagate impulses even when driven for long periods of stimulation. Some axons can propagate action potentials (with little or no failure even after stimulation procedures) that far exceed the level expected for a neuron to have to endure (25). Although similar types of data are not available on humans, there are clinical reasons to suspect that some neurons could be driven for prolonged periods of time (months to years) to the point of failure and possibly neuronal death (2).

It has been implied that amyotrophic lateral sclerosis is a neurological disease that is related to high levels of exercise training, as the incidence of this disease may be higher in professional athletes than in the normal population. During the polio epidemic of the 1940s and 1950s, parents were warned against letting children exercise vigorously for fear of increasing the probability of being afflicted by the polio virus. Today, the fear of overwork of the neuromuscular system of these same polio patients of 30-40 yr ago again is being expressed. It has been reported that the surviving motoneurons of the polio patient may become exhausted over a period of years and that a rapid deterioration of their functional capacity will result (2). It is being suggested that the motor system suddenly begins to deteriorate because of the prolonged period of overuse of the surviving motoneurons that must compensate for the sparsity of motoneurons. Others suggest that aging itself may be associated with neural plasticity (76). Obviously, the validity of the concept of overuse for prolonged periods has important implications and points to the fact that little is known about neural adaptation to prolonged exercise or inactivity.

What are the metabolic effects of high levels of exercise on motoneuron function? In considering this question, we need to ask, Which cellular processes require energy in motoneurons? It has been suggested that some of the energy requirements are related to (a) repolarization of resting membrane potential following each action potential, (b) repolarization of membrane potentials in response to the continuous bombardment from its thousands of synapses producing small excitatory postsynaptic potentials, (c) cytoplasmic flow, (d) protein regulation, and (e) resynthesis and repackaging of neurotransmitters (19, 59, 87, 88). Surprisingly, it is not known which of these cellular processes dominate the energy needs of the motoneuron at any state of development, age, or physiological load. An understanding of these energy demands seems essential to even begin to design appropriate experiments for identifying the impact of exercise and training on the nervous system in normal and neurologically impaired patients.

References

1. Aljure, E.F., and L.M. Borrero. The influence of muscle length on the development of fatigue in toad sartorius. *J. Physiol. (Lond.)* 199: 241-252, 1968.

2. Alter, M., L.T. Kurland, and C.A. Molgaard. Late progressive muscular and antecedent poliomyelitis. In: P. Rowland, ed. *Human motor neuron diseases*. New York: Raven Press: 1982, p. 303-309.

3. Asmussen, E. Muscle fatigue. *Med. Sci. Sports* 11: 313-321, 1979.

4. Badke, A., U. Carraro, A. Irintchev, H.A. Schuhmacher, and A. Wernig. Muscle effects of prolonged voluntary running on normal and denervated leg muscles in different strains of mice (in press).

5. Baker, S.L., and S.H. Chandler. Characterization of postsynaptic potentials evoked by sural nerve stimulation in hindlimb motoneurons from acute and chronic spinal cats. *Brain Res.* 420: 340-350, 1987.

6. Barbeau, H., and S. Rossignol. Recovery of locomotion after chronic spinalization in the adult cat. *Brain Res.* 412: 84-95, 1987.

7. Bigland-Ritchie, B. EMG/force relations and fatigue of human voluntary contributions. *Exerc. Sport Sci. Rev.* 9: 75-117, 1981.

8. Bigland-Ritchie, B., R. Johansson, O.C.J. Lippold, and J.J. Woods. Contractile speed and EMG changes during fatigue of sustained maximal voluntary contractions. *J. Neurophysiol.* 50: 313-324, 1983.

9. Bigland-Ritchie, B., D.A. Jones, and J.J. Woods. Excitation frequency and muscle fatigue: Electrical responses during human voluntary and stimulated contractions. *Exp. Neurol.* 64: 414-427, 1979.

10. Bigland-Ritchie, B., C.G. Kukulka, O.C.J. Lippold, and J.J. Woods. The absense of neuromuscular transmission failure in sustained maximal voluntary contractions. *J. Physiol. (Lond.)* 330: 265-278, 1982.

11. Bigland-Ritchie, B., and J.J. Woods. Changes in muscle contractile properties and neural control during human muscular fatigue. *Muscle Nerve* 7: 691-699, 1984.

12. Borg, J., L. Grimby, and J. Hannerz. The fatigue of voluntary contraction and the peripheral electrical propagation of single motor units in man. *J. Physiol. (Lond.)* 340: 435-444, 1983.

13. Burke, R.E., P. Rudwin, and F.E. Zajac. The effect of activation history on tension production by individual muscle units. *Brain Res.* 109: 515-529, 1976.

14. Christakos, C.N., and U. Windhorst. Spindle gain increase during muscle unit fatigue. *Brain Res.* 365: 333-392, 1986.

15. Clamann, H.P., and K.T. Broecker. Relation between force and fatigability of red and pale skeletal muscles in man. *Am. J. Phys. Med.* 58: 70-85, 1979.

16. Cope, T.C., S.C. Bodine, M. Fournier, and V.R. Edgerton. Soleus motor units in chronic spinal transected cats: Physiological and morphological alterations. *J. Neurophysiol.* 55: 1202-1220, 1986.

17. Costill, D.L., E.F. Coyle, W.F. Fink, G.R. Lesmes, and F.A. Witzmann. Adapations in skeletal muscle following strength training. *J. Appl. Physiol.* 46: 96-99, 1979.

18. Cremer, S., R.J. Gregor, and V.R. Edgerton. Voluntarily-induced differential alteration in force threshold of single motor units of human vastus lateralis. *Electromyogr. Clin. Neurophysiol.* 26: 627-641, 1983.

19. Creutzfeldt, O.D. Neurophysiological correlates of different functional states of the brain. In: *Brain work* (Alfred Benzon Symposium VIII), Munksgaard, 1975.

20. Czeh, G., R. Gallego, N. Kudo, and M. Kuno. Evidence for the maintenance of motoneurone properties by muscle activity. *J. Physiol. (Lond.)* 281: 239-252, 1982.

21. Dawson, M.J., D.G. Gadian, and D.R. Wilkie. Mechanical relaxation rate and metabolism studied in fatiguing muscle by phosphorus nuclear magnetic resonance. *J. Physiol. (Lond.)* 299: 465-484, 1980.

22. Edgerton, V.R., G.E. Goslow, Jr., S.A. Rasmussen, and S.A. Spector. Is resistance of a muscle to fatigue controlled by its motoneurones? *Nature* 285: 589-590, 1980.

23. Edstrom, J.E., and Y. Anderson. Motor hyperactivity resulting in diameter decrease of peripheral nerves. *Acta Physiol. Scand.* 39: 240-245, 1957.

24. Edwards, R.H.T., D.K. Hill, D.A. Jones, and P.A. Merton. Fatigue of long duration in human skeletal muscle after exercise. *J. Physiol. (Lond.)* 272: 769-778, 1977.

25. Eldred, E., and M.S. Perlmutter. Post-stimulation effects of high-frequency stimulation on sensory discharge from muscle. *Am. J. Phys. Med.* 66: 287-297, 1987.

26. Fahim, M.A., and N. Robbins. Remodelling of the neuromuscular junction after subtotal disuse. *Brain Res.* 383: 353-356, 1986.

27. Faulkner, J.A. Fatigue of skeletal muscle fibers. John R. Sutton, ed. *Hypoxia, Exercise, and Altitude: Proceedings of the Third Banff International Hypoxia Symposium*. New York: Alan R. Liss, 1983, p. 243-255.

28. Fitch, S., and A. McComas. Influence of human muscle length on fatigue. *J. Physiol. (Lond.)* 362: 205-213, 1985.

29. Freude, G., and P. Ullsperger. Changes in bereitschaftspotential during fatiguing and non-fatiguing hand movements. *Eur. J. Appl. Physiol.* 56: 105-108, 1987.

30. Gerchman, L.B., V.R. Edgerton, and R.E. Carrow. Effects of physical training on the histochemistry and morphology of ventral motor neurons. *Exp. Neurol.* 49: 790-801, 1975.

31. Gollnick, P.D., K. Piehl, and B. Saltin. Selective glycogen depletion pattern in human muscle fibers after exercise of varying intensity and at varying pedalling rates. *J. Physiol. (Lond.)* 241: 45-57, 1974.

32. Gregor, R.J, R.R. Roy, W.C. Whiting, R.G. Lovely, J.A. Hodgson, and V.R. Edgerton. Mechanical output of the cat soleus during treadmill locomotion: *In vivo* vs *in situ* characteristics. *J. Biomech.* (in press).

33. Grillner, S. Locomotion in spinal vertebrates physiology and pharmacology. In: Goldberg, M.E., A. Gorio, and M. Murray, eds. *Development and plasticity of the mammalian spinal cord*, vol. 3. Fidia Research Series. Padova: Livinia Press, 1986.

34. Grillner, S. The effect of L-Dopa on the spinal cord: Relation to locomotion and the half center hypothesis. In: Grillner, P., S.G. Stein, D.G. Stuart, H. Forssberg, and R.M. Herman, eds. *Neurobiology and motor control*. New York: Macmillan, 1986.

35. Grillner, S., P. Wallen, N. Dale, L. Brodin, J. Buchanan, and R. Hill. Transmitters, membrane properties, and network circuitry in the control of locomotion in lamprey. *TN* 10: 34-41, 1987.

36. Gurfinkel, V.S., M.L. Mirsky, A.M. Tarko, and T.D. Surguladze. Functioning of human motor units during the initiation of muscle tension. *Biophys. J.* 17: 303-310, 1971.

37. Hagberg, M. Muscular endurance and surface electromyogram in isometric and dynamic exercise. *J. Appl. Physiol.* 51: 1-7, 1981.

38. Hayes, K.C. Effects of fatiguing isometric exercise upon Achilles tendon reflex and plantar flexion reaction time components in man. *Eur. J. Appl. Physiol.* 34: 69-79, 1975.

39. Hayward, L., D. Brietbach, and W.Z. Rymer. Increased inhibitory effects on close synergists during muscle fatigue in the decerebrate cat. *Brain Res.* 440: 199-203, 1988.

40. Henneman, E., and L.M. Mendell. Nervous system. In: Brooks, V.B., ed. *Handbook of physiology: Motor control*. Bethesda, MD: American Physiological Society, 1981, vol. 2, sect. 1, chapt. 11, p. 423-507.

41. Hie, H.B., C.J. van Nie, and E. Vermeulen-van der Zee. Effects of endurance exercise on fibre type composition and muscle weight of reinnervating rat plantaris muscle. *Pflugers. Arch.* 408: 333-337, 1987.

42. Hodgson, J.A., F. Ibraham, and D.L. McLellan. The relationship between soleus muscle activity in human movements. *Physiol. Soc.* (January): 23-24, 1983.

43. Hoffer, J.A., N. Sugano, G.E. Loeb, W.B. Marks, M.-J. O'Donovan, and C.A. Pratt. Cats hindlimb motoneurons during locomotion: II. Normal activity patterns. *J. Neurophysiol.* 57: 530-553, 1987.

44. Hultman, E., and H. Sjoholm. Energy metabolism and contraction force of human skeletal muscle *in situ* during electrical stimulation. *J. Physiol. (Lond.)* 345: 525-532, 1983.

45. Hutton, R.S. Acute plasticity in spinal segmental pathways with use: Implications for training. In: Kimamoto, M., ed. *Neural and mechanical control of movement*. Kyoto, Japan: Yamaguchi Shoten, 1984.

46. Hutton, R.S. The central nervous system. In: Dirix, A., M.G. Knuttgen, and K. Tittel, eds. *Olympic book of sports medicine*. Oxford: Blackwood Scientific Publications, 1988.

47. Hutton, R.S., and D.L. Nelson. Stretch sensitivity of Golgi tendon organs in fatigued gastrocnemius muscle. *Med. Sci. Sports Exerc.* 18(1): 69-74, 1986.

48. Hutton, R.S., and T.L. Doolittle. Resting electromyographic triceps surae activity and tonic vibration reflexes in subjects with high and average-low maximum oxygen uptake capacities. *Res. Q. Exerc. Sports* 58(2): 280-285, 1987.

49. Hutton, R.S., J.L. Smith, and E. Eldred. Postcontraction sensory discharge from muscle and its source. *J. Neurophysiol.* 36: 1090-1103, 1973.

50. Ivey, J.L., R.T. Withers, G. Rose, D. Maxwell, and D. Costill. Isokinetic contractile properties of quadriceps in relation to fiber types. *Eur. J. Appl. Physiol.* 81: 247-255, 1981.

51. Jami, L., K.S.K. Murthy, J. Petit, and D. Zytnicki. After-effects of repetitive stimulation at low frequency on fast-contracting motor units of cat muscle. *J. Physiol. (Lond.)* 340: 129-143, 1983.

52. Jasmin, B.J., P.-A. Lavoie, and P.F. Gardiner. Fast axonal transport of acetylcholinesterase in rat sciatic motoneurons is enhanced following prolonged daily running, but not following swimming. *Neurosci. Lett.* 78: 156-160, 1987.

53. Kernell, D. Organization and properties of spinal motoneurons and motor units. *Prog. Br. Res.* 64: 21-30, 1986.

54. Kernell, D. Properties of motoneurons and motor units in relation to problems of sensorimotor integration. In: Struppler, A., and A. Weindl, eds. *Clinical aspects of sensory motor integration.* Berlin: Springer, 1987.

55. Kirsch, R.F., and W.Z. Rymer. Neural compensation for muscular fatigue: Evidence for significant force regulation in man. *J. Neurophysiol.* 57: 1893-1910, 1987.

56. Komi, P.V., M. Salonen, M. Jarvinen, and O. Kokko. *In vivo* registration of Achilles tendon forces in man: I. Methodological development. *Int. J. Sports Med.* 8(Suppl.): 3-8, 1987.

57. Komi, P.V., and P. Tesch. EMG frequency spectrum, muscle structure, and fatigue during dynamic contractions in man. *Eur. J. Appl. Physiol.* 42: 41-50, 1979.

58. Kranz, H., J.F. Cassell, and G.F. Inbar. Relation between electromyogram and force in fatigue. *J. Appl. Physiol.* 59: 821-825, 1985.

59. Krnjevic, K. Coupling of neuronal metabolism and electrical activity. In: *Brain work* (Alfred Benzon Symposium VIII), Munksgaard, 1975.

60. Krnjevic, K., and R. Mildi. Presynaptic failure of neuromuscular propagation in rats. *J. Physiol.* 149: 1-22, 1959.

61. Kugelberg, E., and B. Lindegren. Transmission and contraction fatigue of rat motor units in relation to succinate dehydrogenase activity of motor unit fibers. *J. Physiol. (Lond.)* 288: 285-300, 1979.

62. Lovely, R.G., R.J. Gregor, R.R. Roy, and V.R. Edgerton. Effects of training on the recovery of full weight bearing stepping in the adult spinal cat. *Exp. Neurol.* 92: 421-435, 1986.

63. Marsden, C.D., J.C. Meadows, and P.A. Merton. "Muscular wisdom" that minimizes fatigue during prolonged effort in man: Peak rates of motoneuron discharge and slowing of discharge during fatigue. In: Desmedt, J.E., ed. *Motor mechanisms in health and disease.* New York: Raven Press; 1983: 169-211.

64. Marsden, C.D., P.A. Merton, and H.B. Morton. Servo action in the human thumb. *J. Physiol. (Lond.)* 257: 1-44, 1976.

65. Martin, T.P., S. Bodine-Fowler, R.R. Roy, E. Eldred, and V.R. Edgerton. Metabolic and fiber size properties of cat tibialis anterior motor units. *Am. J. Physiol.* (in press).

66. Matthews, P.B.C. Evolving views on the internal operation and functional role of the muscle spindle. *J. Physiol. (Lond.)* 320: 1-30, 1981.

67. Merton, P.A. Problems of muscular fatigue. *Br. Med. Bull.* 12: 219-221, 1956.

68. Metzger, J.M., and R.H. Fitts. Fatigue from high- and low-frequency muscle stimulation: Role of sarcolemma action potentials. *Exp. Neurol.* 93: 320-333, 1986.

69. Metzger, J.M., and R.H. Fitts. Fatigue from high- and low-frequency muscle stimulation: Contractile and biochemical alterations. *J. Appl. Physiol.* 62: 2075-2082, 1987.

70. Miller, R.G., D. Giannini, H.S. Milner-Braun, R.B. Layzer, P. Koretsky, D. Hooper, and M.W. Weiner. Effects of fatiguing exercise on high-energy phosphates, force, and EMG: Evidence for three phases of recovery. *Muscle Nerve* 10: 810-821, 1987.

71. Milner-Brown, H.S., R.B. Stein, and R.G. Lee. Synchronization of human motor units: Possible roles of exercise and supraspinal reflexes. *Electroencephalogr. Clin. Neuro.* 38: 245-254, 1975.

72. Mjaatvedt, A.E., and M.T.T. Wong-Riley. Double-labeling of rat a-motoneurons for cytochrome oxidase and retrogradely transported [^{3}H] WGA. *Brain Res.* 368: 78-182, 1986.

73. Nassar-Gentina, V., J.V. Passonneau, J.L. Vegara, and S.E. Papoport. Metabolic correlates of fatigue and of recovery from fatigue in single frog muscle fibers. *J. Gen. Physiol.* 72: 593-606, 1978.

74. Nelson, D.L., and R.S. Hutton. Dynamic and static stretch responses in muscle spindle receptors in fatigued muscle. *Med. Sci. Sports Exerc.* 17: 445-450, 1985.

75. Penny, J.E., J.R. Kukums, J.H. Tyrer, and M.J. Eadie. Quantitative oxidative enzyme histochemistry of the spinal cord. II. Relation of cell size and enzyme activity to vulnerability to ischemia. *Neurol. Sci.* 26: 187-192, 1975.

76. Pestronk, A., B. Drachman, and J.W. Griffin. Effects of aging on nerve sprouting and regeneration. *Exp. Neurol.* 70: 65-82, 1980.

77. Petrofsky, J.S., R.M. Glaser, C.A. Phillips, and J.A. Gruner. The effect of electrically induced bicycle ergometer exercise on blood pressure and heart rate. *Physiologist* 25: 253, 1982.

78. Ribchester, R.R. Competitive elimination of neuromuscular synapses [Scientific correspondence]. *Nature* 331: 21-22, 1988.

79. Roy, R.R., R.D. Sacks, K.M. Baldwin, M. Short, and V.R. Edgerton. Interrelationships of contraction time, Vmax and myosin ATP-ase after spinal transection. *J. Appl. Physiol.: Respir. Environ. Exerc. Physiol.* 56: 1594-1601, 1984.

80. Roy, R.R., T.B. Gilliam, J.F. Taylor, and W.W Heusner. Activity-induced morphological changes in rat soleus nerve. *Exp. Neurol.* 80: 622-632, 1983.

81. Roy, R.R., W.K. Hirota, M. Kuehl, and V.R. Edgerton. Recruitment patterns in the rat hindlimb muscle during swimming. *Brain Res.* 337: 175-178, 1985.

82. Sale, D.G. Influence of exercise and training on motor units activation. *Exer. Sport Sci. Rev.* 15: 95-151, 1987.

83. Schott, L.H., and R.L. Terjung. The influence of exercise on muscle lysosomal enzymes. *Eur. J. Appl. Physiol.* 42: 175-182, 1979.

84. Simonson, E.B., V.R. Edgerton, and F. Bojsen-Møller. Energy restitution and power amplification in human plantaris tendons (in press).

85. Smith, J.L., R.S. Hutton, and E. Eldred. Postcontraction changes in sensitivity of muscle afferents to static and dynamic stretch. *Brain Res.* 78: 193-202, 1974.

86. Smith, S., and J.J. Woods. Changes in motoneuron firing rates during sustained maximal voluntary contractions. *J. Physiol. (Lond.)* 340: 335-356, 1983.

87. Sokoloff, L. Influence of functional activity on local cerebral glucose utilization. In: *Brain work* (Alfred Benzon Symposium VIII), Munksgaard, 1975.

88. Sokoloff, L. *Metabolic probes of central nervous system activity in experimental animals and man.* Magnes Lecture Series. MA: Sunderland, 1984, vol. 1.

89. Stephens, J.A., and A. Taylor. Fatigue of maintained voluntary contraction in man. *J. Physiol. (Lond.)* 220: 1-18, 1972.

90. Suzuki, S., and R.S. Hutton. Postcontractile motoneuronal discharge produced by muscle afferent activation. *Exp. Neuro.* 81: 141-152, 1983.

91. Thompson, W.J., L.A. Sutton, and D.A. Riley. Fiber type composition of single motor units during synapse elimination in neonatal rat soleus muscle. *Nature* 309: 709-711, 1984.

92. Usherwood, T.P., and L.A. Stevens. The mechanical properties of human motor units with special reference to their fatiguability and recruitment threshold. *Brain Res.* 125: 91-97, 1977.

93. Vandervoort, A.A., J. Quinlan, and A.J. McComas. Twitch potentiation after voluntary contraction. *Exp. Neurol.* 81: 141-152, 1983.

94. Wernig, A., M. Pecot-Dechavassine, and H. Stover. Sprouting and regression of the nerve at the frog neuromuscular junction in normal conditions and after prolonged paralysis with curare. *J. Neurocytol.* 9: 277-303, 1980.

95. Windhorst, U., C.N. Christakos, W. Koehler, T.M. Hamm, R.M. Enoka, and D.G. Stuart. Amplitude reduction of motor unit twitches during repetitive activation is accompanied by relative increase of hyperpolarizing membrane potential trajectories in homonymous a-motoneurons. *Brain Res.* 398: 181-184, 1986.

96. Wolpaw, J. R. Adaptive plasticity in the spinal stretch reflex: An accessible substrate of memory? *Cell. Molec. Neurobiol.* 5: 147-165, 1985.

97. Wolpaw, J.R. Operant conditioning of primate spinal reflexes: The H-reflex. *J. Neurophysiol.* 57: 443-459, 1987.

98. Wong-Riley, M., and D.A. Riley. The effect of impulse blockage on cytochrome oxidase activity in the cat visual system. *Brain Res.* 261: 185-193, 1983.

99. Wong-Riley, M.T.T., and C. Welt. Histochemical changes in cytochrome oxidase of cortical barrels after vibrissal removal in neonatal and adult mice. *Proc. Natl. Acad. Sci. USA* 77: 2333-2337, 1980.

100. Zajac, F.E., and J.L. Young. Discharge properties of hindlimb motoneurons in decerebrate cats during locomotion induced by mesencephalic stimulation. *J. Neurophysiol.* 43: 1221-1235, 1980.

Chapter 31

Discussion: Nervous System and Sensory Adaptation

Brenda Bigland-Ritchie

"Use it or lose it" is a popular maxim for retaining or improving the functional capacity of most physiological processes. The validity of this philosophy has been documented in numerous scientific studies on cardiovascular and muscle function; but for central and peripheral nervous system performance it is more difficult to test and demonstrate directly in laboratory studies. Nevertheless, numerous examples taken from life provide overwhelming evidence that, to develop highly proficient performance in a particular task, it is essential to train each of the particular neural processes that the task involves. Indeed, when we consider the impact of exercise on fitness and health, the "experiments of life" are often more convincing than any that can be designed in the laboratory.

Undoubtedly, the effectiveness with which a skill can be acquired varies, depending on an individual's genetic endowment, as does the capacity for muscular and cardiovascular performance. Breeding, as well as training, is required to create a winning racehorse. Most people will never be great artists or musicians no matter how hard they try. However, even those with the highest innate, genetic capacity must practice extensively to learn to paint or play supremely well. Fine sensory processing is also essential to learn to sense appropriately what others cannot. How far is this skill retained if practice is discontinued? Some activities that are difficult to learn initially, such as riding a bicycle or swimming, can be recalled effectively after many years of total inactivity, whereas others seem to deteriorate rapidly.

Cardiovascular and muscle function can be improved equally by many forms of exercise, such as regular weight lifting or running, to gain overall strength and endurance. But an excellent runner may be inept at ice hockey or swinging a golf club. The way each activity can be done most ef-fectively to maximize output at minimal energy expenditure must be learned either by hard experience or by experiment. No one can succeed in serious competitive sports or other skilled activities without extensive practice of the particular movements required for the selected activity. Optimal motor coordination involves improved neural processing within the central nervous system (CNS). It also requires increased awareness of, and memory for, the sensations arising from both within and outside the body to reproduce it successfully once experience has shown that the task has been well done. An important question is, How far does acquiring one motor skill improve the performance of related tasks (9)? For example, how far does practice in piano playing improve performance of other manual skills, such as typing or painting?

For CNS function, the task need not necessarily involve exercise in the usual sense because sensory and cognitive processing often requires no muscular activity. Thus, the word *fitness* may be replaced by *effectiveness* or *skill* and defined as the ease and accuracy with which a task can be performed. Similarly, *exercise* and *training* may both be synonymous with *use* or *practice*. The impact of practice on health may then be assessed by the capacity to succeed in that task and thus to influence the quality of life rather than by whether it reduces mortality or the incidence of accidents or degenerative neural diseases. In this connection one should also consider how far acquiring proficiency in neural activity can influence the performance of other physiological systems. For example, neuromuscular coordination improves motor performance partly by reducing the energy expenditure required. Thus, improved coordination not only reduces the risk of accidents but also affects the stress placed on the cardiovascular system. More important, the satisfaction of being able to do things in a skilled way influences one's motivation to exercise.

Response to Edgerton and Hutton

Edgerton and Hutton rightly point out the difficulties of reviewing such a wide topic and the lack of available data on which to draw. The decision to limit their discussion to only those topics that relate to adaptations of motor systems in response to physical exercise is wise. In general, I am in complete agreement with the substance of their views and their overall conclusions, although I do not necessarily agree with the interpretation of some of the details. However, these differences only reflect the complexity of the topics involved, the conflicting experimental results that have been seen, and the varied interpretations that can be quoted. Rather than point out our differences, in many cases I have chosen to restate the arguments as I see them, particularly those relating to the mechanisms underlying neuromuscular fatigue. I have also expanded consideration of some aspects of this topic to include more recent work (some as yet unpublished) from our laboratory. Where possible, I have quoted from review articles from which the original references can be obtained.

Neuromuscular Coordination

Motor skills depend on neural control networks that must first be established and then accessed effectively when required. Many rhythmic movements, such as locomotion and breathing, are controlled by circuits called *pattern generators*. Once set in motion, these appear to continue operating automatically without volition or further input from other centers. Rhythmic limb and breathing movements can often be recorded before birth, when they play no obvious functional role. Thus these circuits seem to be "hard wired" rather than learned. But with use the crude movements they produce get refined. Skilled movements involve complex neural processing in which the position of the limb in space must first be determined and then a strategy designed to move it precisely to another well-defined position by using the required strength and speed. Developing or accessing the necessary sensory and motor networks for learned skills is achieved through trial and error.

The behavior of these networks, once developed, must also be modifiable with exquisite sensitivity and response to small changes in sensory input arising during the movement from many sources generated both within and outside the body. This probably requires the growth of new synaptic connections between neurons (6). Typically, to learn a skilled task at first requires close visual attention to the limb. Later, watching the limb usually becomes unnecessary once the proprioceptive sensations associated with success are stored. These involve conscious and unconscious sensing of input from muscle, joint, and skin receptors. Finally, these design strategies can be accessed semi-automatically so that attention can then be paid to modifying them slightly as required. For skilled hand-eye coordination one must "keep one's eye on the ball."

One of the important difficulties when discussing the impact of human exercise on fitness and health with respect to CNS motor control (as Edgerton and Hutton point out) is that so much of the information currently available must be drawn from animal studies. Currently, much emphasis is being placed on trying to confirm and expand in conscious humans and primates conclusions previously reached on the basis of animal experiments only. But such data are still sparce. In general, we must still rely on data from lower animal experiments. Interspecies variations in control strategies must be kept in mind, particularly, for example, when considering locomotor behavior observed in quadrupeds to interpret those of human bipeds, for whom the problems of balance and coordination are quite different.

Human Motor Unit Contractile Properties and Their Recruitment

Ample evidence shows that human and animal voluntary contractions involve a similar orderly recruitment of motor units that is reestablished even after peripheral nerve injury (19). Histochemically, human motor units can be classified into three distinct types similar to those of animals. However, in humans it is not clear that these histochemical properties always correlate as well as do those of animals with corresponding differences in their contractile properties. For example, histochemical staining shows that the human soleus muscle is composed of about 80% Type I, or slow-twitch, motor units. As expected, the muscle's twitch and tetanic contractile speeds are also slow, like those of cats and rats. However, the human tibialis anterior and adductor pollicis muscles also contain similar proportions of Type I units, but these muscles contract as fast as do other muscles with much higher proportions of Type II, or fast-twitch, fibers (2, 4, 17). Nor can the fatigue properties of human muscles necessarily be deduced from their histochemical fiber-type composition. Comparable rates of force decline are found in sustained maximal contractions of the human tibialis and first dorsal interosseous muscles (4), and the human diaphragm is reported to be highly fatigue resistant despite a high proportion of Type II fibers (1, 8).

Reliable direct measurement of the contractile and fatigue properties of different human motor unit types has been hampered by the limitations and inherent errors in the only methods currently available for human study, such as spike-triggered averaging (18). Thus data on cats must usually be used to interpret human whole-muscle behavior. Recently, we introduced a new method based on microneurographic techniques that allows the contractile responses of individual human motor units to be recorded while stimulating single motor axons (12). This allows both twitch and tetanic responses to be measured from single units both before and after a variety of fatiguing protocols. The method is analogous to that used in animal studies except that the subject is conscious and can perform voluntary tasks, so that the properties of human motor units can now be compared with those of other animals. Currently, these experiments have been done only on human thenar muscles, reported to be 63% Type I and 37% Type II. However, preliminary results do not show that these units can be grouped into distinct types according to their physiological properties as they can in cats and rats (20). For example, the amplitudes of twitches recorded from 45 different units ranged from 2.9 to 34.0 mN (11.4 ± 8.1). However, unlike with cat units, no correlation was found between these values and their wide range of contraction or relaxation rates, axon conduction velocities, and fatigue indices in response to standard Burke fatigue tests (6). Moreover, all parameters varied unimodally in one continuum. This probably indicates that the parent motoneurons, which determine many of these muscle fiber properties, also cannot be grouped into distinct types. However, before definite conclusions about interspecies differences can be drawn, larger unit populations must be examined in muscles in which more detailed histochemical information is available about the distribution of Type IIa and IIb muscle fibers.

Neuromuscular Fatigue

Motor Drive

Fatigue is probably the major factor that limits exercise performance or the desire to exercise in those who acknowledge that it would benefit their health. Training obviously reduces both the rate at which performance declines as fatigue develops and the unpleasant sensations that are felt. Which neural factors contribute to these processes?

Classically, as Edgerton and Hutton point out, fatigue has been attributed to failure of central motor drive, impaired peripheral impulse propagation, or metabolic changes within the muscle fibers (principally, depletion of energy supplies or accumulation of metabolites that inhibit the contractile mechanisms). In our view a combination of all these processes may occur, the rate-limiting factors depending on the type of exercise and muscle groups employed (2). For example, for all the muscles so far examined, voluntary contractions performed by highly motivated subjects supplied with constant visual force feedback under suitable laboratory conditions show that voluntary effort can recruit and drive all motor units to respond with maximum tetanic force (2). Generally, full muscle activation by the CNS can also be retained or reachieved during and immediately following fatigue induced by either sustained maximal or intermittent submaximal exercise. Notable exceptions, in our hands, are the human diaphragm and, to a lesser extent, soleus. But maintaining sufficient motor drive clearly becomes increasingly more difficult and unpleasant as fatigue develops. We are convinced that under more normal exercise conditions the strong desire to reduce the intensity of the motor drive is a major component limiting most types of performance. Indeed, learning to "gate out" and overcome these inhibitory sensations is probably one of the most important factors in athletic training. Generally, we can all do more than we think!

The ability to maintain sufficient motor drive to generate optimal force does not necessarily require that motoneuron firing rates remain unaltered, as fatigue is normally accompanied by a slowing of muscle contractile speed that reduces the excitation rates required for tetanic fusion and optimum force generation. A progressive decline in mean motoneuron firing rate is seen in humans during sustained maximal voluntary contractions in which no force increase can be induced by supramaximal stimulation of the motor nerves at any frequency (13). Thus the muscle remains fully activated by the CNS despite the reduced firing rates. Consequently, there is also a corresponding decline in the quantified surface EMG (2). A similar fall in firing rates is also seen when recording from individual motor units during constant force submaximal contractions (13 + DeLuca). This process could result from changes with use in the intrinsic excitability of spinal motoneurons, as Kernell and Monster (14) and Kernell (15) showed that cat motoneuron properties adapt under conditions of constant excitatory drive and that their discharge rates decline when constant currents are injected intracellularly. However, we suggested that motoneuron firing rates are regulated by a reflex originating from the muscle in response to fatigue-induced changes in its contractile state, metabolic state, or both (2, 3). We found that normally full recovery of these rates is seen within 3 min after the termination of each fatiguing contraction. But if following the first fatiguing contraction the muscle is then kept in its fatigued state by occluding the blood supply, there is no recovery of MVC discharge rates until after the blood pressure cuff has been released. No evidence was found that ischemia for this period causes either failure of peripheral impulse propagation or reduced subject effort (22). So, some peripheral inhibitory feedback regulation from the fatigued muscle must be involved. At present the fatigue-induced factor that triggers this reflex is unknown, but it seems unlikely to be the mechanical changes in the muscle, as no corresponding reduction in firing rates was seen after the muscle contractile speed was reduced by cooling in the absence of fatigue (5). Thus, despite the falling motoneuron firing rates, it seems that the CNS can continue to generate sufficient motor drive to activate most muscles fully throughout exercise of either high intensity or long duration; but normally this is probably seldom done, and, when it is, the reduced force-generating capacity must be due to other causes.

Peripheral Impulse Propagation

When a motor nerve is stimulated electrically at relatively high frequencies (above about 20-30 Hz), impairment of peripheral impulse transmission de-velops at a rate proportional to the stimulus frequency (13). This transmission failure has come to be termed *high-frequency fatigue*. Impaired transmission may occur at either the neuromuscular junction or the muscle surface membrane, as similar rates of decline of both force and action potentials are seen when isolated muscles are stimulated either through the nerve or directly after full curarization. Under either condition both the EMG and force can be quickly restored by reducing the stimulus rate. However, we have never been convinced that impaired impulse propagation contributes to force loss during fatigue of human voluntary contractions executed under any of the conditions we have examined, including MVCs held for up to 5 min (2, 4). In all our experiments, whenever feasible, we monitor the amplitude and area of the muscle-mass action potential (M-wave) evoked by supramaximal shocks applied periodically to the motor nerve. Despite contrary findings by others, we generally find that whenever the M-waves appear to decline they can be restored by adjusting the position of the stimulating electrode (4).

However, even if an action potential decline is recorded, the argument that impaired impulse propagation must necessarily be responsible for force loss is not entirely persuasive. There is ample evidence that no fixed relation should be expected between the magnitude of the electrical signals and the force. For example, M-waves potentiate during the early stages of exercise at a time when the MVC force is already declining (10). Moreover, in our recent single motor unit experiments, when we repeatedly applied high stimulus rates (80-100 Hz) to single motor axons, the EMG amplitudes invariably declined substantially, whereas the force was always well maintained (unpublished data). Clearly, there is a large safety factor between muscle membrane depolarization and full activation of the fiber contractile machinery (excitation-contraction coupling). Impulse propagation can also be improved by exercise. Kernell et al. (16) showed a decrement in both force and EMG when normal cat muscles were stimulated by trains of 40-Hz stimulation during the Burke fatigue test. But after weeks of chronic nerve stimulation, no EMG decrement was seen even when the rate of force decline remained unchanged. Thus the force responses showed that the muscle was equally activated under both conditions, and no unique relationship between EMG and force should be expected. Similar improvements after training have also been seen in humans (7).

We believe that transmission block does not occur readily during voluntary contractions but is frequently seen during nerve or muscle stimulation because of differences in the excitation rates involved (13). For the slow human soleus muscle, firing rates of about 10.7 ± 2.9 Hz are elicited by steady maximum voluntary efforts. For most other muscles the rates recorded from different units range from about 15 to 50 Hz (2). It seems reasonable to assume that, in muscles of mixed fiber properties, the lower rates are recorded from the units with slower contractile speeds. Yet all were maximally activated because no additional force resulted from supramaximal tetanic stimulation at any frequency. However, because some units required up to 50 Hz, all must be excited at these rates when stimulated artificially. It is therefore not surprising that frequencies much higher than those that most units experienced normally cause propagation failure. Thus it seems unlikely that high-frequency fatigue plays any direct part in reducing the force of voluntary contractions, although the safety factor for successful high-frequency transmission is certainly eroded (2). However, this tendency is counterbalanced by the progressive reduction in motoneuron firing rates that must minimize this effect.

Metabolic Changes and Excitation-Contraction Coupling Failure

Whether or not failure of central drive or impulse propagation contributes to the overall fatigue processes, most investigators agree that the major causes of force loss reside within the muscle fibers. It probably results from either the depletion of energy supplies or the accumulation of metabolites that interfere with the contractile process. Depletions of phosphocreatine, glycogen, or both, are common candidates, together with a fall in pH from lactate accumulation. Certainly, profound changes in these constituents are normally found in sustained, high-intensity contractions in which the muscles become ischemic or in other types of exercise that are prolonged. Under these conditions metabolic substrate changes are probably sufficient to account for much of the reduced force-generating capacity. However, there is no general agreement as to which factor is rate limiting. It is also difficult to find any data that show a quantitative relationship between reduced performance and a given level of metabolic change.

Recently, we examined the rate of MVC force decline in response to brief maximal voluntary contractions injected periodically during 30 min of repeated 30% MVC static contractions of the quadriceps (our measure of fatigue), in which the contraction intensity and duty cycle apparently were such that the metabolic demands could be entirely met from aerobic sources (3, 21). Despite an almost 50% drop in force-generating capacity, sequential biopsies showed no significant changes in the metabolic composition of the muscle. Because there was also no indication of reduced muscle activation by the CNS or impaired impulse propagation, the fall in MVC force must have resulted from defective excitation-contraction coupling in the T tubules or sarcoplasmic reticulum. If the effectiveness of excitation-contraction coupling can be the rate-limiting factor in fatigue from some forms of exercise, perhaps it also is in others. The concomitant metabolic changes would be only coincidental in these other cases. However, it seems likely that in high-intensity contractions when muscles become ischemic, the profound metabolic changes themselves probably do determine force reduction.

Reflex Inhibition

During these low-intensity, intermittent contractions the metabolic demands of the task were met entirely from aerobic sources, as no metabolic changes could be detected in the muscle during this type of exercise (3, 21). We do not yet know the extent to which MVC firing rates also declined. If they behaved in the same way as did those in sustained maximal contractions, in which fatigue resulted in about the same amount of MVC force declines, then it is unlikely that reflex inhibition of motoneuron firing rates is triggered by either ischemia or changes in the metabolites we examined. A more likely candidate seems to be the extracellular K^+ that accumulates with activity and that is perhaps also responsible for excitation-contraction coupling failure in T tubules (13).

As yet we do not know by which muscle afferents inhibitory signals are transmitted to the CNS or how they are distributed within the CNS. It seems unlikely that they influence only the firing rates of motoneurons in the homonymous motoneuron pool. Indeed, Hayward et al. (11) recently showed that if a cat medial gastrocnemius is first fatigued before a stretch the magnitude of reflex inhibition induced in the soleus muscle increases.

The extent to which fatigue-induced reflex responses may also change the excitability of neurons elsewhere in the spinal cord and higher brain-stem centers is also unknown at present. However, there is evidence that the gain of this reflex regulation may vary in different neuromuscular systems. Thus it may also change under different exercise conditions or be influenced by training or disuse.

When examining fatigue of limb muscles (other than the soleus), we found that the firing-rate decline does not reduce the ability of the CNS to activate the muscle (2). However, when the same 50% reduction in MVC force was induced in human diaphragms by using the same intermittent contraction protocol, full muscle activation rapidly became impossible to achieve. At first, the behavior of this muscle appeared to be no different from that of others. However, once the contractile strength of the diaphragm had declined by about 25%, stimulation of both phrenic nerves always elicited more force than could be generated voluntarily. At this time the muscle surface EMG also dropped off sharply. (Again there was no sign of impaired impulse propagation.) We postulated that fatigue-induced reflex inhibition is stronger in the diaphragm, thus preventing the extremes of muscle fiber contractile failure that are induced easily in limb muscles. If so, this reflex inhibition appears to play an important protective role for survival, for respiratory muscles must continue to contract effectively under heavy loads at times when limb muscles may be exhausted. In all muscle groups, fatigue-induced reflex inhibition seems to keep motoneuron firing rates to the minimum that is required to achieve the task and thus also minimizes the rate at which impaired function develops at peripheral sites (impulse propagation and excitation-contraction coupling failure). This mechanism therefore seems to help optimize performance when force or power output must be generated most efficiently over extended periods of time, as is the case in many normal-life activities. If these reflexes prove to require use for their integrity, their relation to exercise, fitness, and health, as defined here, is obvious.

Conclusion

For cardiovascular, muscular, and other physiological systems, exercise clearly improves fitness if fitness is assessed only by an ability to perform and sustain exercise. However, the claims that regular exercise markedly improves health may be exaggerated if health is assessed by lowered mortality rates or reduced susceptibility to disease.

The long-term influence of exercise on the functional capacity of the nervous system is less clear. Learning motor skills clearly requires training, as does improved sensory and cognitive processing. The rate at which these skills deteriorate if practice is discontinued probably varies greatly among tasks and individuals. There is little evidence that the level of mental or physical activity influences mortality rates or the incidence of neural diseases. Conversely, in some persons, deliberately increasing the level of exercise may exacerbate the condition or at least its symptoms.

Alternatively, health may be defined in terms of the quality of life, regardless of its length or the presence or absence of diagnosable disease. The sense of well-being is clearly improved by regular exercise at an appropriate level. Indeed, exercise is increasingly prescribed to combat clinical depression. Conversely, the quality of life is much reduced if the sense of effort associated with a desired occupation or even the performance of necessary daily tasks becomes unacceptable. With advancing age or following debilitating illnesses involving prolonged periods of inactivity, patients often complain that they fatigue quickly and can no longer engage in their previous physical activities. In these cases objective tests may or may not reveal a real reduction in the fatigue resistance of their muscle fibers. However, with inactivity, the patients' muscles atrophy so that their maximum strength is reduced. Hence, performing their normal tasks now requires that a higher proportion of the available fibers in each muscle be activated and driven with higher intensity. Both the rate of reduction in force-generating capacity (fatigue) and the sensation of effort that accompanies it are proportional to the relative, not the absolute, load. In these cases persuading the patient to strengthen his or her muscles by exercise will not only reduce the unpleasant sensations but also protect his or her self-esteem by alleviating the anxiety that progressive physical deterioration may prevent him or her from continuing a chosen, independent lifestyle without outside assistance. Thus, when the quality of life is the index, exercise clearly improves both fitness and health. However, in this case the impact of the exercise is most readily demonstrated in one system (i.e., muscle strength and endurance) but may have its most important role in influencing another (e.g., relieving sensory and psychological pain).

References

1. Bellemare, F., and B. Bigland-Ritchie. Central components of diaphragmatic fatigue assessed from bilateral phrenic nerve stimulation. *J. Appl. Physiol.* 62(3): 1307-1316, 1987.

2. Bigland-Ritchie, B., F. Bellemare, and J.J. Woods. Excitation frequencies and sites of fatigue. In: McCartney, N., N. Jones, and A. McComans, eds. *Human muscle power.* Champaign, IL: Human Kinetics, 1986, p. 197-213.

3. Bigland-Ritchie, B., E. Cafarelli, and N.K. Vollestad. Fatigue of submaximal static contractions. *Acta Physiol. Scand.* 128(Suppl. 556): 137-148, 1986.

4. Bigland-Ritchie, B., and C. Thomas. Impulse propagation and muscle activation during prolonged human maximal contractions. *J. Physiol. (Lond.).* 391: 91P, 1987.

5. Bigland-Ritchie, B., J.J. Woods, F. Furbush, and D. Karrmann. Effect of muscle temperature on motor neuron MVC firing rates. *Neurosci. Abstr.* 12: 186.8, 1986.

6. Burke, R.E. Motor units: Anatomy, physiology and functional organization. In: V.B. Brooks, ed. *Handbook on physiology: The nervous system.* Bethesda, MD: American Physiological Society, 1981, vol. 11, sect. 1, chapt. 10, part 1, p. 345-422.

7. Ducheau, J., and K. Hainaut. Training effect on muscle fatigue in man. *Eur. J. Appl. Physiol.* 53: 248-252, 1984.

8. Gangevia, S.G., and D. Mckenzie. Human diaphragmatic endurance during different maximal respiratory efforts. *J. Physiol.* 395: 625-638, 1988.

9. Gangevia, S.G. Role of perceived voluntary motor commands in motor control. *Trends Neurosci.* 10: 81-85, 1987.

10. Garner, S., A. Hicks, and A.J. McComas. M-wave potentiation during muscle fatigue and recovery in man and rat. *J. Physiol.* 377: 108P, 1986.

11. Hayward, L., D. Breitbach, and W.Z. Rymer. Increased inhibitory effects on close synergists during muscle fatigue in the decerebrate cat. *Brain Res.* (in press).

12. Johansson, R.S., C. Thomas, G. Westling, and B. Bigland-Ritchie. A new method for examining the contractile properties of single human motor units. *Eur. J. Physiol.* (in press).

13. Jones, D.A., and B. Bigland-Ritchie. Electrical and contractile changes in muscle fatigue. In: Saltin, B., ed. *Biochemistry of exercise, IV.* Champaign, IL: Human Kinetics, 1985, vol. 16, p. 377-392.

14. Kernell, D., and A.W. Monster. Time course and properties of late adaptation in spinal motoneurones of the cat. *Exp. Brain Res.* 46: 191-196, 1982.

15. Kernell, D. The limits of firing frequency in cat lumbrosacral motoneurones possessing different time course of after-hyperpolarization. *Acta Physiol. Scand.* 65: 87-100, 1965.

16. Kernell, D., Y. Donselaar, and O. Eerbeek. Effects of physiological amounts of high- and low-rate chronic stimulation on fast-twitch muscle of the cat hindlimb: II. Endurance-related properties. *J. Neurophysiol.* 58: 614-627, 1987.

17. Round, J.M., D.A. Jones, S.J. Chapman, R.H.T. Edwaards, P.S. Ward, and D.L. Fodden. The anatomy and fibre type composition of the human adductor pollicis in relation to its contractile properties. *J. Neurol. Sci.* 66: 263-292, 1984.

18. Stein, R.B., A.S. French, D. Mannard, and R. Yemm. New methods for analysing motor function in man and animals. *Brain Res.* 40: 187-192, 1972.

19. Thomas, C.K., R.B. Stein, T. Gordon, R.G. Lee, and M.G. Elleker. Patterns of reinnervation and motor unit recruitment in human hand muscles after complete ulnar and median nerve section and resuture. *J. Neurol. Neurosurg. Psychiatry* 50: 259-268, 1987.

20. Thomas, C.K., G. Westling, R.S. Johansson, and B. Bigland-Ritchie. Contractile properties of single human motor units examined by intra-neural stimulation. *Biochemistry of Exercise* (in press).

21. Vollestad, N.K., O.M. Sejersted, R. Bahr, J.J. Woods, and B. Bigland-Ritchie. Motor drive and metabolic responses during repeated submaximal voluntary contractions in man. *J. Appl. Physiol.* 64(4): 1421-1427, 1987.

22. Woods, J.J., F. Furbush, and B. Bigland-Ritchie. Evidence for a fatigue-induced reflex inhibition of motoneuron firing rates. *J. Neurophysiol.* 58(1): 125-136, 1987.

Chapter 32

Behavioral Adaptation to Physical Activity

Steven N. Blair
Harold W. Kohl
Patricia A. Brill

Chronic diseases are the major causes of death and disability in industrialized societies (33). It is clear that health and social habits, or lifestyle, are intricately involved in multiple and interactive ways with the pathogenesis of the major chronic diseases. Tobacco smoking may be the most disastrous habit affecting health. The more prominent problems associated with tobacco use and exposure are several types of cancer, cardiovascular disease, respiratory disease, and osteoporosis (33). Other lifestyle elements associated with major health problems include a diet high in salt, fat, and cholesterol; physical inactivity; intemperate use of alcohol; abuse of other psychoactive substances; obesity; failure to use early-detection techniques and preventive health services; risk-taking behavior; poor management or adaptation to psychosocial stressors; and irregular or inadequate sleep habits (3, 21, 33). The studies linking lifestyle to disease have focused medical and lay attention on the value of preventive health behavior. Thus it appears rational in the late 1980s to recommend the adoption of good health habits, and there is some evidence that such changes may be beneficial (17, 19, 29).

Intuitively, it is appealing to assume a unitary model for the development and maintenance of preventive health behavior. The rationale for such a model is that—given appropriate information about the risks of an unhealthful lifestyle, enhanced motivation to be healthy, and development of behavioral skills to make changes—persons would identify their unhealthful lifestyle factors and make appropriate changes. If the concept of a unitary preventive health behavior model is valid, perhaps the adoption and maintenance of one particular health behavior may subsequently lead to other positive changes. Some have assumed that adoption of regular exercise could be a catalyst in initiating other beneficial lifestyle changes. The rationale for such a belief is that exercise and smoking are incompatible behaviors, that persons who start exercising become more interested in a prudent diet, and that exercise is an antidote for stress.

A better understanding of the interrelationships among health habits is important for two reasons. First, health promotion programs can be planned and implemented more efficiently. If exercise can stimulate the adoption of other beneficial health habits, physical activity programs can be the centerpiece of health promotion efforts. Second, a better understanding will enable the refinement of epidemiological studies on lifestyle and disease. The independent, interactive, or possible multiplicative associations among various habits and the pathogenesis of chronic disease are important to understand. Although statistical control of the various lifestyle elements is possible in multivariable models, a basic understanding of the interrelationships is desirable.

The purpose of this chapter is to examine whether exercise (or the adoption of exercise) promotes, or is at least associated with, beneficial changes in other health behaviors. We also address the larger issue of the validity of a unitary model of preventive health behaviors as a concept.

Methodological Issues

Advancing the understanding of the interrelatedness of health habits and their impact on disease processes is complicated. The multivariate nature

Further work is needed on the role of inactivity as an initiating factor in the development of obesity.

Regular exercise is not a universal cure for overweight, but intervention trials clearly have shown the benefit of increased caloric expenditure in weight-loss programs (34). Exercise appears to preserve lean body mass and cause acute appetite suppression (13). More work is needed on the effect of combining exercise with nutritional and behavioral interventions to produce weight loss.

Alcohol Intake

Data on physical activity and alcohol intake are equivocal (7, 8). Some studies have shown a relationship between activity or physical fitness and alcohol consumption; others have not. Sinyor et al. (31) used exercise in the treatment of alcoholism. Exercisers had higher abstinence rates after 3 mo of treatment than did nonexercising controls. About two thirds of the exercisers were abstinent compared to one third of the nonexercisers. A recent study reported an effect of exercise on heavy drinking in male college students (25). Sixty young men who consumed at least 45 drinks per month were randomly assigned to exercise, meditation, or control conditions. The exercisers met three times per week in a supervised exercise class. Meditators were trained in meditation techniques and meditated as a group three times per week. Exercise-group members reduced their alcohol intake compared to controls during an 8-wk treatment phase and a 16-wk follow-up. Meditation-group alcohol intake was intermediate between exercisers and controls during treatment but was comparable to controls during follow-up. The main conclusion from this study is that vigorous aerobic exercise is associated with lower levels of alcohol intake.

Stress Management

It is widely believed that stress (variously defined) is adversely related to health, although the data to support this hypothesis are relatively weak. Lack of data notwithstanding, stress management is a popular concept, and various approaches to managing stress exist. Generally, these techniques involve cognitive-behavioral approaches such as progressive relaxation, assertiveness training, and time management. Aerobic exercise is also frequently recommended as an antidote for stress. We found no studies that associated physical activity and other stress management techniques

(e.g., comparing relaxation practices in various physical activity groups). There are several recent studies on the value of physical activity in stress management (12, 18, 26, 28) or for treatment of depression and anxiety (23). This latter issue is dealt with in detail elsewhere in these proceedings, so we will not comment on it further here. Regarding stress management, Roth and Holmes (28) randomly assigned 55 college students who had recently experienced a high number of negative life events to exercise, progressive relaxation, or control groups. The exercise group participated for 11 wk in a supervised running program that significantly improved physical fitness. The relaxation group also met for supervised instruction and practice for 11 wk. All three groups were given standard depression rating scales periodically throughout the 11-wk intervention and 2-mo follow-up period. In general, the exercisers were less depressed throughout the study. The relaxation-group depression scores were comparable to those of the controls. These results suggest that the aerobic exercise helped ameliorate the effects of negative life events in these college students.

Brown and Lawton (12) obtained reports of stressful life events, physical and emotional well-being, and exercise habits from 220 high school girls. Stressful life events had an adverse effect on the health of the sedentary girls but not on the regular exercisers.

The role of exercise as a buffer against organizational stress was studied in a group of active-duty U.S. Navy and Marine Corps men (26). The study was conducted during a stressful period, in that the ship to which the men were assigned failed a training mission, resulting in a longer tour of sea duty than had been expected. Personnel divisions were randomly selected for exercise and control groups. Exercisers ($n = 111$) participated in a 12-wk circuit weight-training program; 134 men were in the control group. Measurements were obtained on several work-attitude and self-perception scales. Overall, the sustained high stress experienced by participants resulted in deterioration of work attitudes, but these effects were attenuated somewhat in the exercisers.

A longitudinal study of life events and somatic complaints was conducted on 278 corporate executives (18). Life events, somatic complaints, and physical activity were assessed at baseline and after 2 and 4 yr of follow-up. Multiple regression models indicated that participation in physical activity appears to moderate the impact of life events on somatic complaints.

Early Detection and Preventive Health Behavior

There is some evidence that more physically active individuals are more likely to use preventive health services. The strongest support for this concept comes from nationally representative surveys from the United States and Canada (7, 8). The Canada Health Survey was conducted in 1978-1979 on a probability sample of households. There were 17,726 noninstitutionalized adults (20 yr or older) who answered self-administered questionnaires. Stephens (32) did a factor analytic study that included data on health behaviors and the use of preventive health services. Two factors for men and three factors for women were identified. In both men and women, one of the factors included high loadings on leisure-time physical activity and recent immunizations against polio. One of the factors for women had high loadings on dental care and breast self-examination practice, but physical activity did not make an important contribution to this factor.

A survey of noninstitutionalized adults in the United States in 1979 and 1980 shows an association between physical activity and some preventive health behaviors (7, 8). More active persons were more likely to report having a physical examination or a blood pressure check during the previous 24 mo. Active women were more likely than were inactive women to have had a breast examination during the previous 24 mo, but activity was not associated with having a Pap smear.

Risk-Taking Behavior

Several multifactor studies have found positive associations between physical activity and more frequent seat-belt use, better drinking habits, and less general risk taking (7). These studies did not always control for demographic characteristics (perhaps confounding the results), although some recent analyses show similar results after control for gender, age, and educational achievement (8).

Sleep

Irregular or inadequate sleep habits, such as difficulty falling asleep, frequent waking, or insomnia, are common problems. Sleep disorders can interfere with nighttime rest and daytime alertness. Irregular or inadequate sleep habits can result in psychological and physiological hindrances to health. Changes in emotions, mood, depression, stress, and confusion, as well as decreased energy and impaired performance capabilities, can be affected (11).

Regular physical activity may improve sleep patterns, sleep habits, and the quality of sleep. Physical activity increases the amount of deep sleep, increasing alertness and helping one to feel better the next day (2). Exercise early in the day may produce relaxation and physical tiredness that encourages normal sleep. Exercise before bedtime should be avoided because it can have an arousing effect, increasing the body's metabolic rate, increasing restlessness, and making it more difficult to get to sleep (30).

Intellectual Function

Blomquist and Danner (10) studied changes in information-processing efficiency that occur when physical fitness improves. Cognitive and cycle ergometer tests were administered before and after a training program to 66 adults. Subjects were divided into two groups on the basis of percent fitness improvement (< 5% and > 15%). Improvement in memory scan rate and number of words remembered in individuals who made modest gains in fitness were reported. Greater improvements in mental efficiency occurred in the sedentary-to-low-fit subjects than in the fit subjects. Mental efficiency might have been greater if the subjects were less fit at pretest or if they increased exercise intensity. Blomquist and Danner concluded that mental efficiency is essentially genetically determined but that aerobic exercise may have some influence.

Elsayed et al. (14) studied 70 adults involved in a physical fitness program over a 4-mo period. They hypothesized that initial cardiovascular fitness level and intensity of an exercise program might have an effect on mental efficiency. The subjects were divided into four groups: high-fit young, high-fit old, low-fit young, and low-fit old. A submaximal cycle ergometer test was administered to determine pre- and postprogram cardiovascular fitness levels. Changes in fluid and crystallized intelligence were obtained through the administration of the Culture Fair Intelligence Test and the Factor B Cattell 16 PF Personality Questionnaire. Fluid intelligence reflects functioning of neurological structures and is a primary process of perceiving relations and maintaining spans of immediate awareness in concept formation. Crystallized intelligence is thought of in terms of cultural assimilation (10, 14). The subjects exercised 3 d per week for 90 min over a 4-mo period. The high-fit groups of the issue is a major problem. There are numerous health habits to consider and several different disease processes (each with multiple lifestyle, environmental, and hereditary causes) to examine. Very few controlled experiments have dealt with the interrelationships among health habits. Those that have been done rarely studied more than two habits simultaneously. The inclusion of two health habits in an intervention trial simplifies the design, but this approach cannot adequately predict how the behaviors might relate in the more complex mosaic of human behaviors and environmental factors encountered in daily living. Most of the evidence reviewed in this chapter comes from studies that do not focus on the interrelationships among health habits. For example, many exercise training studies have been done to define the exercise prescription necessary to produce given increases in physical fitness. In some of these studies, data on diet or smoking changes in the exercise and control groups are also reported, but this was not the main focus of the research. Epidemiological studies typically examine the multivariate relationships of health habits at baseline to disease outcomes during follow-up. These studies are important but do not provide much insight into how health behaviors may or may not change in concert. Cross-sectional multivariate analyses of several health habits have been published, but these studies also fail to address adequately the issue of whether change in one behavior, such as exercise, promotes change in another.

A major problem with research on lifestyle is the difficulty in obtaining valid and reliable data, primarily due to inadequate measurement techniques (7). Habitual exercise is difficult to assess, and existing measures are crude and imprecise (20). This measurement problem holds for several of the other health behaviors, notably diet and stress management practices. Intraindividual variation contributes to the problem. Measuring a behavior at a specific time may not be representative of the person's habitual behavior over longer periods of time. The large variances associated with many of the lifestyle measurements may obscure the true magnitude of relationships under study. Improved lifestyle assessment methods are urgently needed to advance research on the issues discussed in this chapter.

Materials and Methods

In this chapter, information on the associations between physical activity and other health behaviors is taken from two primary sources: (a) a review of published studies and (b) new data analyses done specifically for this report.

Literature Review

Published articles pertaining to the relationships between physical activity and smoking habits, dietary patterns, alcohol intake, weight control, substance abuse, stress management practices, risk-taking behavior, and participation in preventive health examinations were reviewed. Articles considered for review were obtained from a MEDLINE search, from known articles on the topic, and from previous reviews on physical activity and lifestyle (7, 8). Few published studies have explicitly addressed the topic of this report, and most articles reviewed were written for other purposes but had sufficient data for inclusion here. Articles were excluded from consideration if the definitions of physical activity or other lifestyle elements were uncertain or unclear.

In this chapter, definitions of physical activity, exercise and training, activity pattern, physical fitness, health, lifestyle, environment, and personal attributes are consistent with the definitions presented in other chapters. In this section we review the literature on the relationships between physical activity and lifestyle. In general, the measures of physical activity are somewhat nonspecific; but in a few cases exercise or training measures of physical activity are used. In a few instances physical fitness is used as a marker for physical activity. In addition to examining the relationships among physical activity and lifestyle factors such as smoking and diet, we include somewhat more tangential issues. Items such as intellectual achievement, work performance, and family and friend relationships commonly are not included as health behaviors; but they are considered here as important lifestyle components.

Smoking

Of all lifestyle factors, one might expect smoking behavior to be most closely associated with physical activity. It seems logical to assume that smoking might impair exercise performance and perhaps participation. Conversely, regular and vigorous exercisers may be somewhat health conscious and decide not to smoke. Published studies do not support these commonsense assumptions. Previous reviews concluded that several studies reported no association between leisure-time physical activity and smoking habits, and other cross-sectional studies showed negative but weak associations (7, 8). Two recent studies showed a more pronounced gradient of smoking prevalence across physical activity groups. Approximately 1,000 white Zimbabwean men and women were classified into five leisure-time physical activity groups (24). Prevalence of current smoking was 43%, 31%, 22%, 20%, and 17% across the activity groups from low to high, respectively. These data show a strong inverse dose-response relationship; but overlap remains between the two behaviors, and the correlation is relatively low (r = .24).

A study of 5,044 men and 3,044 women in Canada also examined smoking status in activity groups (15). Men and women under 40 yr of age classified as active were less likely to smoke than were their moderately active or inactive peers. Smoking prevalence in active men was about 40% of that in inactive men. The gradient was somewhat less in the younger women: 16% in the active and 32% in the inactive. There was no association between smoking prevalence and activity status in women over 40.

Other reports examined the issue somewhat differently. Occupational physical activity was positively associated with smoking status in several studies from Europe (7), although this finding may have been confounded by socioeconomic status. Multivariate analyses showed lower smoking rates in men and women with higher levels of physical fitness (7). These cross-sectional studies cannot determine whether smoking causes low fitness or whether low fitness predisposes one to smoke.

It might be expected that longitudinal epidemiological studies and experiments would be more likely to show an association between physical activity and smoking status, but such is not the case. Previous reviews concluded that changes in physical fitness and participation in exercise interventions did not appear to alter smoking rates (7, 8). These findings were confirmed by a recent report of a 13-yr follow-up of middle-aged men who participated in an 18-mo supervised exercise program in 1967-1968 (22). Smoking prevalence was the same in the exercise and the control groups at baseline and at follow-up.

The previous studies were not specifically designed to investigate the use of exercise as an intervention method for smoking cessation. The value of exercise as an intervention technique was directly studied by Hill (16). Smokers (N = 36) who enrolled for smoking cessation were randomly assigned to either a standard behavioral intervention or a behavioral intervention plus exercise for a 5-wk treatment. Quit rates did not differ significantly at posttreatment or at 3- or 6-mo follow-up assessments. Smoking rates were actually lower, however, in the group assigned to behavioral intervention plus exercise. This finding prompts speculation that exercise may be a useful adjunct treatment, but the statistical power of the study design was too low to detect an existing difference. This study approach probably merits further consideration with a larger sample.

Diet

Diet and physical activity are inextricably linked in the simplistic sense that all human movement is caused by energy provided by ingested food. Higher levels of activity demand higher caloric intakes to provide energy for muscular contraction. There are confounding factors such as the impact of caloric restriction on basal metabolic rate (7, 8) and the effects of weight cycling (13); but in general and over the long term, active persons will have higher caloric intakes than will inactive individuals. Beyond this generalization, little is known about the associations between habitual diet and physical activity. It is appealing to believe that the vigorous exerciser is also concerned about a healthful diet, and some cross-sectional surveys have supported that view (1, 27). Dietary assessments in these studies were crude self-reports, and their validity can be questioned. Studies in which dietary assessments were more carefully and thoroughly done showed little or no relationship between dietary composition and physical activity status (5, 7). Prospective studies and clinical trials also failed to show many significant dietary changes in groups that increased activity or physical fitness (34).

Weight Control

Weight is a physical characteristic and not a behavior, but weight control is profoundly influenced by the behaviors of diet and physical activity. Numerous epidemiological, clinical, and intervention studies have established an inverse association between physical activity and body weight (7, 8). This finding does not mean that all exercisers are lean, but in groups of individuals the more active will weigh less. Also, an individual who is physically active will likely weigh less than if he or she were sedentary. There are still many details and mechanisms to be elucidated regarding the relationship of physical activity to weight and weight control, but the general association is clear.

increased total fluid intelligence scores more than did the low-fit groups. Overall, the young group had a higher total fluid intelligence score than did the older groups. There were no differences in the crystallized intelligence scores among the groups.

Work Performance

Regular exercise habits and optimal levels of physical fitness may contribute to improved work performance. Bernacki and Baun (4) studied 3,231 white-collar workers over a 6-mo period, during which time participants recorded their exercise sessions. Job performance ratings (above average, average, and poor) were assigned by the personnel department. There was a relationship between increased physical activity and improved work performance. Possible mechanisms to improve work performance include reduced muscle tension and increased cerebral blood flow, alertness, creativeness, clear thinking, self-esteem and self-image, and job satisfaction. Physical activity also may decrease employee absenteeism and job stress (9).

Family and Friend Relationships

Limited data exist on physical activity and social life. The Gallup Organization conducted the American Health Survey for *American Health* magazine in 1984 (1). Data related to social health items were obtained from questioning 1,019 individuals aged 18 yr or older. A large group (45%) believed that exercise participation had improved their love lives, and men were more likely to report this belief than were women. One question was asked about exercise and relationships. Although most exercisers (69%) believed that exercise had no impact on their relationships with their spouses or loved ones, 20% felt that exercise made their relationships closer. Participants were asked about the association between exercise and social life. The results were about evenly split between "made no difference" and "helped make new friends." Younger participants were more inclined to believe that exercise helped them make new friends.

Data Analyses

Several new data analyses have been conducted for this review. The association of physical activity with other health behaviors was studied further in two sets of data: information collected cross-sectionally from patients of a preventive medicine center (Cooper Clinic) and a longitudinal cohort

of a subset of these patients who returned to the clinic for six examinations. Both data sets are major foundations of the Aerobics Center Longitudinal Study.

Cooper Clinic

The Cooper Clinic is a large, preventive medicine clinic located in Dallas, Texas. Nine physicians administer approximately 7,000 physical examinations annually. Since 1971, approximately 40,000 patients have been examined. Clinic patients are 99% white, 75% male, and generally well educated. They reside in upper-middle to upper socioeconomic classes. Most patients are either self-referred or sent by their employers for the examination.

The health assessment offered through the clinic is comprehensive. The examination includes medical history, lifestyle assessment, and various clinical measures, including complete blood and body fat analyses. All tests also include a maximal exercise stress test. Details of tests and procedures have been published (6).

Each patient completes an extensive medical history form before beginning the actual exam. In addition to information on prior illness there is an extensive section concerning the patient's lifestyle (exercise habits, smoking habits, alcohol intake, and dietary patterns). After all the items are completed, the physician discusses the data with the patient to clarify responses and to ensure completeness. Examination information is subsequently entered, verified, and stored on computer disks for research purposes.

Data Analyses From the Cooper Clinic

The first of the analyses in the Cooper Clinic data base utilized information collected from the medical history form to examine cross-sectional associations of physical activity habits with smoking, alcohol intake, and dietary composition. A discussion of the variables used in the analyses follows. A five-level index of exercise participation (PAI) was created from simple inquiries into the patient's exercise participation during the month before the examination: 0 = no reported exercise during the past month; 1 = reported exercise participation other than walking, jogging, or running; 2 = walking, jogging, or running 1-10 mi per week; 3 = walking, jogging, or running 11-20 mi per week; and 4 = walking, jogging, or running more than 20 mi per week. Current smoking behavior was measured by the reported number of cigarettes smoked by the patient. Nonsmokers were coded with a 0 for this variable. An index of ethanol intake was created by converting the patient's reported number of drinks per week of beer, wine, and liquor to ounces of ethanol. It was estimated that beer is 4.0% ethanol, wine 12.0%, and liquor 40.0%. Weighting factors (beer = 0.48, wine = 0.36, liquor = 0.80) based on a constant-size serving were used to obtain ounces of ethanol intake per week. Finally, several different measures of dietary composition were created. On the basis of the patient's reported number of servings per week of several food groups and types, indices of restraint of saturated fat and cholesterol intake were formed (saturated fat intake index = total number of servings per week of beef, eggs, pork, whole milk, and fried foods; unsaturated fat intake index = total number of servings per week of fish, fowl, and skim milk). A ratio of unsaturated to saturated intake (saturated index/unsaturated index) was also created. Caffeine intake was assessed by the number of cups of coffee drank per week.

One possible explanation for the lack of definitive associations among health behaviors is that assumptions of statistical techniques may have been violated in previous analyses. All measures of health behaviors were transformed to the natural log scale to counteract the severe skewness in most of the variables of interest. Moreover, because zero was a valid value for all responses but the natural log of zero is undefined, all values were increased by a constant value (1.0) before the transformation. The relationship is represented in the following equation:

$$\text{Index of health behavior} = \ln (\text{reported in times/wk} + 1)$$

The main question addressed in this analysis concerned the association of physical activity with the indices of health behavior mentioned previously. Analysis of covariance was used (adjusting for age) to identify differences among physical activity index (PAI) categories. Analyses were gender specific, and, after those subjects with incomplete records for the variables of interest were eliminated, 7,961 men and 2,289 women were available for analysis.

Results

Descriptive data for both men and women by PAI are shown in Table 32.1. In both men and women, more physical activity was associated with younger age, higher physical fitness, and a generally more favorable health profile (evidenced by mean cholesterol, blood pressure, and weight). The completely sedentary group was comprised of 28.8% of the men and 28.5% of the women.

Unadjusted means for each of the health behaviors of interest by PAI for each gender are listed in Table 32.2. Although these values may not be interpretable on the practice level, the transformation allows adherence to statistical assumptions and provides for instructive, valid comparisons among PAI groups. Within and between each gender, there is a general trend for each behavior to become more favorable as the level of physical activity increases. It should also be noted that women in general have more favorable practices of these habits than do men, for example, less saturated fat intake, higher unsaturated fat intake, lower net fat intake (bad fat to good fat), and fewer cigarettes smoked. The only variable that appears not to show a clear trend with increasing

Table 32.1 Characteristics of Cooper Clinic Patients at First Visit According to Gender and PAI

	PAI—Men					PAI—Women				
	0	1	2	3	4	0	1	2	3	4
Age	43.3	42.1	42.9	42.3	41.2	43.3	41.3	42.7	42.0	38.7
Treadmill time	821.7	965.4	1,061.7	1,249.7	1,449.5	569.5	709.7	760.6	914.3	1,101.9
Cholesterol	212.4	209.7	206.6	203.6	199.3	201.4	196.9	198.4	197.4	189.8
RSBP	120.9	118.7	119.8	120.8	120.1	112.3	110.4	111.3	111.6	108.6
RDBP	81.1	80.1	79.8	79.8	78.4	75.0	74.8	75.1	74.4	72.2
Weight	190.0	183.6	181.9	176.0	166.7	138.5	130.2	132.4	128.6	126.6
Height	70.2	70.4	70.4	70.3	70.1	64.4	64.5	64.6	64.6	64.8
n	2,381	1,727	2,723	906	521	652	499	867	196	

Note. Data from Aerobics Center Longitudinal Study.

Table 32.2   Unadjusted Mean Health Behavior Indices of Cooper Clinic Patients at First Visit

	PAI—Men					PAI—Women			
	0	1	2	3	4	0	1	2	3
Saturated fat	2.73	2.61	2.56	2.39	2.24	2.33	2.19	2.23	2.05
Unsaturated fat	1.65	1.84	1.92	1.98	2.02	1.76	1.89	1.94	2.03
Net fat intake[a]	1.62	1.36	1.24	1.10	0.97	1.20	1.00	1.00	0.84
Coffee consumption	2.28	2.07	2.05	1.97	1.86	1.95	1.83	1.76	1.65
Ethanol intake	1.30	1.39	1.27	1.23	1.24	0.84	0.93	0.76	0.84
Cigarettes smoked	1.93	1.67	1.46	1.40	1.40	1.22	1.04	0.96	0.97
n	2,381	1,727	2,723	906	521	652	499	867	196

Note. Data from Aerobics Center Longitudinal Study and expressed as natural logarithms.

[a]Saturated fat index/unsaturated fat index.

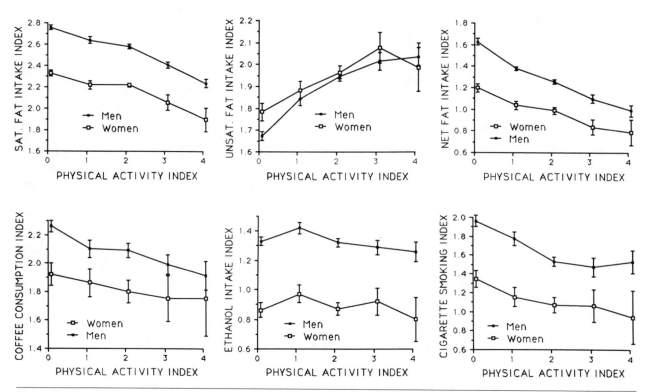

Figure 32.1.   Cross-sectional associations of health behavior indices and physical activity index for Cooper Clinic patients. Values are least squares means adjusted for age (Aerobics Center Longitudinal Study).

levels of physical activity in both men and women is ounces of ethanol consumed.

Because age appears strongly associated with the PAI, a complete analysis should include comparison of the mean values after adjustment for any effects of age. The six panels in Figure 32.1 show least squares means of each behavior index by PAI after adjusting for the effects of age. The bars around each point are 95% confidence intervals.

The results of the covariance analysis are similar to those that were unadjusted. A strong negative slope across PAI categories is evident for saturated fat intake, unsaturated fat intake, cups of coffee drank per day, and number of cigarettes smoked per day. A strong positive slope related PAI to good fat intake, and more equivocal results are seen for ounces of ethanol intake consumed per week. Also, women generally have more favorable behaviors at each PAI level than do men.

Longitudinal Tracking of Health Behaviors

The second analysis concentrated on a subset of men who had registered at least six full medical examinations at the Cooper Clinic; 2,329 men were eligible for inclusion. The purpose of this analysis was to determine the extent to which the health behavior indices examined in the first analysis track over time, depending on the individual's exercise participation. Study subjects were classified into four exercise-exposure groups on the basis of their reported exercise behavior at each of their six clinic visits. Those who reported no exercise at any visit were labeled "sedentary." If the patient reported no exercise at the first or at the first and second visits and reported that he exercised at each subsequent visit, he was labeled a "starter." Those patients who were exercisers at

each visit were labeled "continuers," and those who had no clear pattern to their behavior were labeled "cyclers."

Dependent variables of interest were all behavioral variable indices investigated in the previous analysis (saturated fat intake index, unsaturated fat intake index, net fat intake ratio, ethanol intake index, coffee consumption index, and cigarette smoking index). All transformations for minimization of variable skewness were maintained from the previous analysis.

A repeated measures analysis of variance (ANOVA) was used. Only subjects with complete information for a given health behavior index (nonmissing observations at all six visits) were included for that analysis. Six separate analyses, corresponding to the six indices, were done on the cohort, and all were done controlling for the effects of age.

The data in Table 32.3 show main effects ANOVA results for each of the six analyses. Significant

Table 32.3 Analysis of Variance Results for Main Effects of Exercise Group Status on Selected Health Behavior Indices, Six-Visit Cohort

Index	df	MS	F	p	Groups different from sedentary (p < .05)
Saturated fat intake					
Exercise group	3	4.06	7.05	< 0.001	Continuers
Age	1	11.04	19.18	< 0.001	
Residual	428	0.57			
Unsaturated fat intake					
Exercise group	3	8.01	18.06	< 0.001	Starters, cyclers, continuers
Age	1	0.65	1.47	0.225	
Residual	614	0.44			
Net fat intake					
Exercise group	3	15.30	11.96	< 0.001	Cyclers, continuers
Age	1	21.11	16.52	< 0.001	
Residual	356	1.28			
Ethanol consumption					
Exercise group	3	0.68	0.18	0.908	
Age	1	4.65	1.25	0.264	
Residual	467	3.71			
Coffee consumption					
Exercise group	3	13.76	2.58	0.052	Starters
Age	1	2.37	0.45	0.505	
Residual	661	5.33			
Cigarettes smoked					
Exercise group	3	0.69	0.07	0.977	
Age	1	9.58	0.93	0.334	
Residual	350				

Note. Data from Aerobics Center Longitudinal Study.

effects are seen by exercise group classification for each index of fat intake but not for the ethanol, coffee, or cigarette consumption indices.

The multivariate ANOVA results of the effect of time on each index are enumerated in Table 32.4. The unsaturated and net fat intake indices and the coffee consumption index showed significant time effects (i.e., a significant downward trend over the six-visit follow-up). However, no Time × Exercise Group interaction was found for these indices, meaning that each of the four exercise groups did not have statistically different alteration of the indices over time. In other words, although each group showed a significant downward trend over time, the groups did not differ among themselves. The means of the unsaturated and net fat intake indices, the saturated fat index, and the coffee consumption index are plotted for each exercise group in Figures 32.2 and 32.3.

The saturated fat index analysis had a significant Time × Exercise Group interaction. The strict interpretation of this finding is that the slopes across time are not the same among the four exercise groups. This indicates that change in saturated fat index over time is different for at least one of the groups. Inspection of the upper panel of Figure 32.2 suggests that the slope of the sedentary group may be less than that of the other exercise groups; that is, sedentary patients may be somewhat less likely to reduce their saturated fat intake over time. This conclusion is speculative because the large drop and subsequent increase in saturated fat intake at the second visit by the sedentary group makes a contribution to the significant interaction.

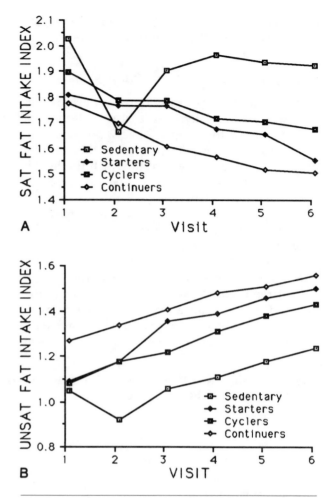

Figure 32.2. Longitudinal tracking of a) saturated and b) unsaturated fat intake indices in Cooper Clinic men by exercise group (Aerobics Center Longitudinal Study).

Table 32.4 Multivariate Analysis of Variance Repeated Measures Results for Effects of Time and Time × Exercise Groups Interaction on Selected Health Behavioral Indices, Six-Visit Cohort

Variable index	Multivariate effect of time			Multivariate effect of time × exercise group		
	df	F[a]	p	df	F[a]	p
Saturated fat intake	5,424	0.62	0.685	15,1268	2.76	< 0.001
Unsaturated fat intake	5,610	4.03	0.001	15,1826	1.39	0.143
Net fat intake	5,352	4.59	0.001	15,1052	0.98	0.476
Ethanol consumption	5,463	0.33	0.894	15,1385	1.33	0.176
Coffee consumption	5,657	2.73	0.019	15,1967	0.88	0.585
Cigarettes smoked	5,346	1.73	0.126	15,1034	1.21	0.256

Note. Data from Aerobics Center Longitudinal Study.

[a]Hotelling-Lawley trace *F*.

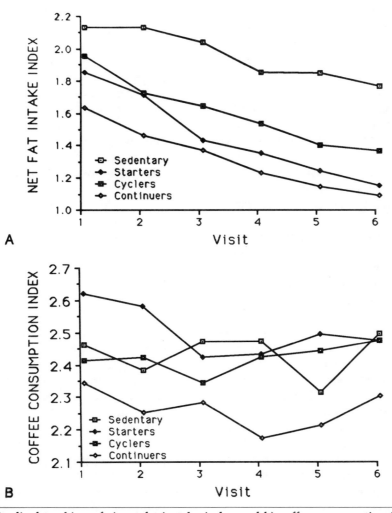

Figure 32.3. Longitudinal tracking of a) net fat in take index and b) coffee consumption index in Cooper Clinic men by exercise group (Aerobics Center Longitudinal Study).

Conclusion

This chapter addresses the association between physical activity and other health behaviors. It would be beneficial for the health educator if health behaviors and changes in health behaviors were highly related. Intervention would be simplified and less expensive. Epidemiologists studying lifestyle and disease find their work more complicated, however, if health behaviors are closely associated. The task of disentangling independent contributions of multiple health behaviors to disease processes is simpler if health behaviors are unrelated. The review presented here provides some encouragement to both health educators and epidemiologists. Physical activity is associated with several other health behaviors, but the correlations are low in most cases. This finding suggests that health educators may find that physical activity promotion is a small catalyst for other desirable lifestyle changes. The magnitude of effect is small enough that the epidemiologist can use statistical techniques to isolate attention on one health behavior while holding others constant.

Results of the new cross-sectional data analyses presented in this review are encouraging. The cross-sectional associations of saturated fat intake, unsaturated fat intake, and net fat intake indices with the physical activity index are, to our knowledge, the first to be reported. Whether this is a function of our improved method of assessing physical activity (i.e., the PAI), our statistical data transformation, or both remains to be seen. The results suggest that people who are more active are likely to have more favorable fat intake profiles, to consume less coffee, and to smoke fewer cigarettes. These results point to the need to refine further methods of assessing human health behaviors. We believe that this is the most important step in resolving the question of the degree of health behavior relationships.

The longitudinal analyses were less supportive of a unitary model for preventive health behavior. Although several of the health behaviors changed favorably over time, only one showed any evidence of differing among exercise habit groups (saturated fat intake). This was mainly because of the large variance across time in the sedentary group. Thus, although the idea of a unitary set of health behaviors remains plausible, these analyses did not provide strong evidence that behaviors of people who begin exercise programs are more likely to show beneficial alterations over the long term than are behaviors in any other group of exercisers.

The Cooper Clinic patient population is a special one. Patients are self-selected, and those who return voluntarily six times are undoubtedly more highly motivated than are their single-visit peers and the general population. We submit, however, that because of the special characteristics of the group we are more likely to identify health behavior associations, if they exist at all. The fact that the longitudinal analyses failed to find a difference in health behavior profiles over time may therefore be due to two possible explanations: (a) There actually is no effect on future health behaviors by adopting exercise habits and (b) the imprecision of our measurement instruments allows too much variance, and thus the actual relationship remains undiscovered. As we have previously stated, we believe that the latter may be the case and that future research should concentrate on methods to improve population assessment of health behaviors.

The following conclusions are based on articles reviewed and data analyses done for this review:

- Physically active persons are less likely to be overweight in spite of their having higher caloric intakes.
- Recent articles and data analyzed for this paper support the conclusion that physical activity is inversely associated with smoking habits. This conclusion differs from previous reviews (7, 8), which report little or no association.
- Published reports indicate little or no association between physical activity and dietary composition. Analyses reported here suggest

that higher levels of physical activity may be associated with a generally more healthful diet. More work is needed.
- There is some evidence in the published research that physical activity is inversely associated with alcohol intake, may help alcoholics remain abstinent, and may reduce the prevalence of heavy drinking. The results of the analyses presented here do not support this conclusion.
- More evidence is accumulating that regular exercise may have value as a stress management technique. We find no reports on the association between physical activity and other stress management practices.
- More physically active individuals may be more likely to engage in various early detection and preventive health behaviors. They may also be less likely to engage in risk-taking behaviors.
- Regular participation in physical activity has been hypothesized to be associated with better sleep habits, improved intellectual function, enhanced work performance, and more satisfying social relationships. There are very few studies on these topics, but existing reports tend to support the previous hypotheses. Much more work is needed with improved designs and better measurement before firm conclusions can be drawn.
- A major deterrent to research on the association between physical activity and other health behaviors is the lack of precise and valid assessment tools.

References

1. *American health: Public attitudes and behavior related to exercise.* Princeton, NJ: Gallup Organization, 1985.
2. Baekeland, F., and R. Lasky. Exercise and sleep patterns in college athletes. *Percept. Mot. Skills* 23: 1203-1207, 1966.
3. Berkman, L.F., and L. Breslow. *Health and ways of living.* New York: Oxford University Press, 1983.
4. Bernacki, E.J., and W.B. Baun. The relationship of job performance to exercise and adherence in a corporate fitness program. *J. Occup. Med.* 26(7): 529-531, 1984.
5. Blair, S.N., N.M. Ellsworth, W.L. Haskell, M.P. Stern, J.W. Farquhar, and P.D. Wood. Comparison of nutrient intake in middle-

aged men and women runners and controls. *Med. Sci. Sports Exer.* 13: 310-315, 1981.

6. Blair, S.N., N.N. Goodyear, L.W. Gibbons, and K.H. Cooper. Physical fitness and incidence of hypertension in healthy normotensive men and women. *JAMA* 252: 487-490, 1984.

7. Blair, S.N., D.R. Jacobs, Jr., and K.E. Powell. Relationships between exercise or physical activity and other health behaviors. *Public Health Rep.* 100: 172-180, 1985.

8. Blair, S.N., and H.W. Kohl. Measurement and evaluation of health behaviors and attitudes in relationship to physical fitness and physical activity patterns. In: Drury, T., ed. *Assessment of physical fitness and physical activity in population based surveys.* Washington, DC: U.S. Government Printing Office (in press).

9. Blair, S.N., M. Smith, T.R. Collingwood, R. Reynolds, M.C. Prentice, and C.L. Sterling. Health promotion for educators: Impact on absenteeism. *Prev. Med.* 15: 166-175, 1986.

10. Blomquist, K.B., and F. Danner. Effects of physical conditioning on information-processing efficiency. *Percept. Mot. Skills* 65: 175-186, 1987.

11. Bonnet, M.H. Sleep performance and mood after the energy expenditure equivalent of 40 hours of sleep deprivation. *Psychophysiology* 17: 56-63, 1980.

12. Brown, J.D., and M. Lawton. Stress and well-being in adolescence: The moderating role of physical exercise. *J. Hum. Stress* (Fall): 125-130, 1986.

13. Brownell, K.D. Obesity: Understanding and treating a serious, prevalent, and refractory disorder. *J. Consult. Clin. Psychol.* 50: 820-840, 1982.

14. Elsayed, M., A.H. Ismail, and R.J. Young. Intellectual differences of adult men related to age and physical fitness before and after an exercise program. *J. Gerontol.* 35: 383-387, 1980.

15. Faulkner, R.A., D.A. Bailey, and R.L. Mirwald. The relationship of physical activity to smoking characteristics in Canadian men and women. *Can. J. Public Health* 78: 155-160, 1987.

16. Hill, J.S. Effect of a program of aerobic exercise on the smoking behavior of a group of adult volunteers. *Can. J. Public Health* 76: 183-186, 1985.

17. Hjermann, I., K.V. Byre, I. Holme, and P. Leren. Effect of diet and smoking intervention on the incidence of coronary heart disease: Report from the Oslo Study Group of a randomized trial in healthy men. *Lancet* ii: 1303-1310, 1981.

18. Howard, J.H., D.A. Cunningham, and P.A. Rechnitzer. Physical activity as a moderator of life events and somatic complaints: A longitudinal study. *Can. J. Appl. Sport Sci.* 9: 195-200, 1984.

19. Kornitzer, M., G. DeBacker, M. Dramaix, F. Kittel, C. Thilly, M. Graffar, and K. Vuylsteek. Belgian Heart Disease Prevention Project: Incidence and mortality results. *Lancet* i: 1066-1070, 1983.

20. LaPorte, R.E., H.J. Montoye, and C.J. Caspersen. Assessment of physical activity in epidemiologic research: Problems and prospects. *Public Health Rep.* 100: 131-146, 1985.

21. Lewy, R. *Preventive primary medicine.* Boston: Little Brown, 1980.

22. Mackeen, P.C., J.L. Rosenberger, J.S. Slater, W.C. Nicholas, and E.R. Buskirk. A 13-year follow-up of a coronary heart disease risk factor screening and exercise program for 40- to 59-year-old men: Exercise habit maintenance and physiologic status. *J. Cardiopul. Rehabil.* 5: 510-523, 1985.

23. Martinsen, E.W. The role of aerobic exercise in the treatment of depression. *Stress Med.* 3: 93-100, 1987.

24. Morrison, J.F., S. VanMalsen, and T.D. Noakes. Leisure-time physical activity levels, cardiovascular fitness and coronary risk factors in 1015 white Zimbabweans. *S. Afr. Med. J.* 65: 250-256, 1984.

25. Murphy, T.J., R.R. Pagano, and G.A. Marlatt. Lifestyle modification with heavy alcohol drinkers: Effects of aerobic exercise and meditation. *Addict. Behav.* 11: 175-186, 1986.

26. Pavett, C.M., M. Butler, E.J. Marcinik, and J.A. Hodgdon. Exercise as a buffer against organizational stress. *Stress Med.* 3: 87-92, 1984.

27. *The Perrier Study: Fitness in America.* New York: Perrier, 1979.

28. Roth, D.L., and D.S. Holmes. Influence of aerobic exercise training and relaxation training on physical and psychologic health following stressful life events. *Psychosom. Med.* 49: 355-365, 1987.

29. Salonen, J.T., P. Puska, T.E. Kottke, J. Tuomilehto, and A. Nissinen. Decline in mortality from coronary heart disease in

Finland from 1969 to 1979. *Br. Med. J.* 286: 1857-1860, 1983.

30. Shephard, R.J. Activity and the pathology of aging. In: *Physical activity and aging*. London: Croom Helm, 1978, p. 225-267.

31. Sinyor, D., T. Brown, L. Rostant, and P. Seraganian. Aerobic fitness level and reactivity to psychosocial stress: Physiological, biochemical, and subjective measures. *Psychosom. Med.* 45: 205-217, 1983.

32. Stephens, T. Health practices and health status: Evidence from the Canada Health Survey, *Am. J. Prev. Med.* 2: 206-215, 1986.

33. U.S. Department of Health Education and Welfare. *Healthy people: 1979* (DHEW [PHS] Publication No. 79-55071A). Washington, DC: U.S. Government Printing Office, 1979.

34. Wood, P.D., W.L. Haskell, S.N. Blair, P.T. Williams, R.M. Krauss, F.T. Lindgren, J.J. Albers, P.H. Ho, and J.W. Farquhar. Increased exercise levels and plasma lipoprotein concentrations: A one-year, randomized, controlled study in sedentary, middle-aged men. *Metabolism* 32: 31-39, 1983.

Chapter 33

Discussion: Behavioral Adaptation to Physical Activity

Thomas Stephens

In their chapter on behavioral adaptation to physical activity, Blair and his colleagues provide an update of earlier reviews (4, 5) on the association between exercise and other healthful behaviors. Although behavioral adaptation is outside the mainstream of most of the topics discussed at this conference, it is an important issue with implications which are nicely described by Blair et al. They note that evidence for a behavioral adaptation or unitary conception of health behaviors will be good news for health promotion (as diverse positive outcomes can be expected from exercise adoption) but bad news for epidemiology (whose attempts to unravel the relationships between exercise and health will be confounded). As with the earlier reviews (4, 5) the authors conclude that a unitary conception of health behaviors remains a plausible hypothesis.

The assignment to Blair et al. differs from most of the others in this book in one important respect. Although there is a well-developed literature dealing with most aspects of physiological, morphological, and biochemical adaptations to physical activity, that which is relevant to behavioral adaptation is very limited in quantity and, until recently, in quality. Conceptual problems are still numerous, and methodological shortcomings abound. This discussion focuses on these aspects of the literature, identifies outstanding issues, and offers an interpretation of the evidence which is somewhat more pessimistic than that of Blair and coworkers as regards behavioral adaptation.

Conceptual Issues

As an illustration of the conceptual problems which beset a discussion of this topic, one need

look no further than the concept of behavioral adaptation. The term itself implies that behavior changes as an adaptive response to biological challenge (35), in this case from physical activity, and that the organism responds to such stress in the same fashion as does a cell or an organ. This is a dubious proposition, except perhaps within a strict stimulus-response framework, and presupposes much about the mechanisms which underlie behavioral change. Given the complexity of human behavior in the social world, it is more appropriate to speak of behavioral outcomes or consequences than adaptation, with the understanding that these are, at most, only partially influenced by physical activity.

Still at the conceptual level, it is worth nothing that the model used to develop the conference topics (8) does not easily accommodate the notion of behavioral outcomes. Rather, lifestyle is treated as a determinant of physical activity, akin to heredity or environment. If there is any validity to the concept of behavioral adaptation, the conceptual model of Bouchard et al. will need to be modified to show lifestyle as both influencing and influenced by physical activity. However, the evidence for such adaptation does not suggest that such a redrafting is an urgent task.

An important conceptual distinction must be drawn between health behaviors (or other determinants) and health outcomes. The ICEFH model achieves this by showing health (wellness, morbidity, and mortality) as the outcome of a variety of interacting determinants. Thus, it is inappropriate to treat body weight as if it were a behavior or lifestyle element, yet this has been and remains a common practice in this literature (2, 17, 24). Blair et al. correctly caution against this conception of body weight. Such caution also applies to discussions of weight control, sometimes treated as if it were a lifestyle practice when the evidence deals mainly with maintenance of appropriate body weight. With respect to weight control, the relevant behaviors are those involving caloric consumption and food selection. Happily, these are also discussed by Blair et al., who conducted some of the small amount of research so far published on these behaviors.

The study of stress management presents some conceptual difficulties similar to those that apply to weight control. *Stress management* is a somewhat loose term that may refer to either a process or an outcome. As an outcome, *distress management* might be more accurate, referring to the individual's more or less successful attempts to cope with harmful or unpleasant stressors. The four studies cited by Blair et al. (6, 12, 20, 23) describe how exercise acts as a buffer against organizational stress and life events as evidenced by fewer somatic complaints or depressive symptoms. This is undoubtedly an important outcome of exercise, but it is not behavioral adaptation so much as it is the direct effect of physical activity on physiological and psychological processes.

In a similar fashion, care is needed when discussing sleep as a health behavior. There is no doubt that regular sleep makes a positive contribution to health and that inadequate sleep is not merely or necessarily symptomatic of ill health (2). But it is apparent also that difficulty in sleeping may be a direct consequence of ill health, thus confounding the relationship between sleep and exercise, as the latter is also related to health status. Like the conceptual problems with body weight, this issue can be successfully dealt with through use of appropriate definitions and study designs.

A final conceptual matter important to this topic is the nature of physical activity. With one exception, the evidence cited by Blair et al. deals with leisure-time or discretionary activity. (The exception involves occupational activity and smoking, a relationship that is clearly confounded by the association between social status and smoking [25] and thus should be ignored here.) Given the nature of the evidence bearing on behavioral outcomes of physical activity, conclusions should properly refer to exercise (see chapt. 1) and avoid the use of the more generic term. This is more than a semantic distinction; correctly describing the nature of physical activity is essential to identifying the mechanism or mechanisms underlying behavioral adaptation.

The Evidence for Adaptation

Table 33.1 summarizes the evidence for an association between exercise and several health practices. In keeping with the earlier discussion on conceptual issues, weight control and stress management are not included here. Such topics are more properly covered in other chapters, notably those on adipose tissue adaptation (chapts. 26 and 27), obesity (chapts. 41 and 42), and mental health (chapt. 10; see also ref. 28). Quality of sleep is not included because the few reports available do not make it clear whether health status was controlled in the analysis.

The evidence is summarized under three headings according to type of study design: (a) randomized control trials or true experimental designs, (b) prospective studies (which lack random assignment to groups but benefit from data collected at two or more points in time), and (c) cross-sectional studies. These designs appear in declining order of the quality of evidence they provide for examining responses to exercise, a feature accounted for here. Cross-sectional studies account for the largest number of studies in the literature and have been ably summarized in previous reviews (4, 5). However, because the evidence for adaptation is weakest from this category of studies, only those from broad population samples are included. In Table 33.1, the following symbols are used to classify the conclusion of the studies: (+) = exercise associated with another healthy behavior, such as not smoking, quitting smoking, and reducing drinking; (−) = exercise associated with an unhealthy behavior; and (0) = a null relationship (including $r^2 < .25$) or an equivocal relationship.

As a general observation, it is apparent that there are several positive and null results but no negative ones, and that there is a fair amount of evidence from true experiments and prospective studies. On this basis it seems reasonable to conclude that exercise does not have a negative impact on other health behaviors and that the question of behavioral adaptation to exercise can be adequately examined with little recourse to cross-sectional data.

Table 33.1 also makes it plain that this is an underdeveloped area of research. The studies summarized under the first two headings are all those published since 1975 and identified through a search of MEDLINE, *Psych Abstract, Social Science*

Table 33.1 Summary of Evidence From Various Kinds of Studies Between Exercise and Other Healthful Behaviors

Exercise and	Association[a]	Randomized control trial	Prospective	Cross-sectional
Smoking	+	13, 16	31	7, 28, chapt. 32
	−			
	0	11, 22	4, 5	2, 28
Alcohol use	+	16, 19		
	−			
	0			2, 28
Diet				
Total calories	+			
	0		21	chapt. 32
Composition	+			
	−			
	0	32	4, 5	
Prevention	+			
	−			
	0			4, 28

Note. Table entries refer to reference numbers or chapter numbers.

[a]+ = exercise associated with a healthful behavior, such as quitting smoking; − = exercise associated with an unhealthful behavior; 0 = null relationship.

Citation Index, Comprehensive Dissertation Index, and the SPORT, DRUG USE, and ALCOHOL USE/ ABUSE data bases. The key words used were fairly general, and the search was not restricted regarding the type of study design or the population covered. Nor was the search confined to analyses of multiple health behaviors in relation to exercise. Such a restriction would have eliminated all but the cross-sectional studies.

Within this sparse literature there is virtually no formal replication of studies, and any substantive conclusions should therefore be regarded as tentative. Nevertheless, it is possible to take account of the quality of evidence and offer conclusions that are grouped according to the degree of certainty: (a) clearly established findings based on several studies with consistent conclusions; (b) probable findings based on a smaller number of studies with consistent findings; and (c) possible findings, where the evidence is especially sparse or there is a discernible trend within inconsistent results.

Clearly Established

• There is a paucity of good evidence from appropriate designs on the behavioral consequences of exercise or physical activity. This is especially true for randomized designs, although a start has been made with respect to alcohol and tobacco use. There are no replication studies yet published.

• For all practical purposes related to health promotion in the general population, exercise is independent of other health behaviors. There is no good reason to expect widespread and meaningful positive changes in other health behaviors because a population becomes more active; however, there is no reason to expect any degradation in other health practices either.

Probably True

• Exercise leads to a higher caloric intake, but this may be limited to individuals of normal weight. There is no consistent evidence that exercise leads to appetite suppression of any significant duration.

• Exercise can be effective in reducing alcohol use both in treatment programs and among study subjects who express no prior interest in reducing their levels of ethanol consumption. (However, exercise is not necessarily more effective than other interventions such as meditation.)

Possibly True

• Exercise can be effective in smoking cessation programs (as can meditation and other cognitive-behavioral approaches).

Outstanding Substantive Issues

Because the literature on the behavioral consequences of exercise is so limited, it is not surprising that more questions are raised than answered. Among the more important questions are those concerning underlying mechanisms, the relationship between exercise dose and behavioral response, and the generalizability of the findings.

Mechanisms

None of the research cited here or by Blair et al. was designed to examine mechanisms that might explain relationships between exercise and other health behaviors. Indeed, as Blair et al. correctly point out, many of the studies were not even intended to examine relationships between exercise and health behavior, and some do not fully describe the exercise variable. Nevertheless, there are several hypothesized mechanisms, all of which are amenable to future investigation.

A central question is whether there is one or several explanations for behavioral adaptation to exercise, and, if there are several, whether they might vary depending on the health behavior in question. This seems most plausible. For example, some researchers (14) regard exercise as a behavior that appeals to addictive personalities in much the same way as do tobacco and alcohol. If this is a valid proposition (and there is some weak evidence for it), any beneficial effects of exercise on smoking or drinking may be due to the successful substitution of one addiction for another. Because not all alcohol use represents an addiction and because not all individuals have addictive personalities, this is a limited explanation at best; but it may explain the success of those therapeutic regimens that employ exercise with individuals who have volunteered for smoking cessation programs (11) or alcohol abuse treatment (see chapt. 54), as well as the nontherapeutic and unwitting reduction of heavy alcohol consumption (16, 19).

Another mechanism possibly underlying behavioral adaptation is somatic habituation, the process whereby one learns that typical stress symptoms (i.e., rapid breathing, increased heart rate, and sweating) may be a consequence of exercise and not of stress at all. Such a mechanism could explain why exercise is useful as a stress management technique. Because somatic habituation is largely a physiological mechanism, it should apply equally well to leisure-time and occupational physical activity. However, if other job characteristics induce stress, this would confound the study of this mechanism.

Energy expenditure processes and the principles of thermodynamics are yet another mechanism underlying the increase in caloric consumption that reliably accompanies regular exercise. Although published evidence is lacking, this must be equally true of both leisure-time and occupational activity when they involve the same level of energy expenditure. However, such physiological principles cannot explain changes in food selection practices.

One mechanism that may underlie many or all of the reported relationships between exercise and health behavior is a generalized value on health, or on health as a life concern (10). Such a value orientation, coupled with the knowledge that certain health practices are conducive to good health, implicitly underlies the unitary conception of health behaviors discussed by Blair et al. Hannah (10, p. 166) has demonstrated that when health is a salient concern, that is, when health is "a sphere of your life which you . . . think about and are motivated to act upon . . . on a daily or almost daily basis," it predicts high scores on an index of health behaviors. Although this could be a plausible explanation for relationships between exercise and almost any other good health practice, it is unlikely that health is such a strong and continuing concern for most of the healthy population. The enormous challenges faced by health promoters attempting, for example, to encourage smoking cessation (8) or reduce alcohol-related problems (1) make it seem unlikely that these practices will follow more or less automatically once an exercise regimen is adopted—a practice that itself is difficult to instill in the general population (see chapt. 7).

Relationships Between Exercise Dose and Behavioral Response

As noted by Blair et al., many of the studies they reviewed did not provide a detailed description of the exercise dose, that is, the nature of physical activity and its frequency, duration, and intensity. (An exemplary exception is the scale used by Blair et al. to analyze the Cooper Clinic cross-sectional data, although this is limited to aerobic activities.)

Such descriptions of the exercise dose are essential to understanding the dose-response relationship and thus the underlying mechanism. For example, if vigorous exercise is required in an effective smoking cessation program, the mechanism may be a substitution of addictions or some form of physiological interference. If vigorous exercise is not necessary, social and psychological factors assume more importance. Whether fitness must be achieved for behavioral adaptation to occur (one of the central questions of this conference) is doubtful, but this issue cannot be addressed adequately with the information at hand. Clearly, however, it is impossible to explore this question without more complete descriptions of the exercise dose. Such descriptions would make it unnecessary to accept physical fitness as a proxy for physical activity, as Blair et al. have been forced to do with some studies in their review.

Related to the issues of exercise dose and mechanism is the effect of occupational activity. If occupational activity can be shown to have the same behavioral consequences as does leisure-time activity, this would suggest that the underlying mechanism is largely physiological. If the effects are different, however, which seems likely to be the case (28), the mechanism may be more psychological than biological. Some useful evidence on this question could be obtained by a replication of Morris et al.'s (18) classic study of London transport workers in which health practices rather than coronary disease is the dependent variable. In such a study, if the conductors were more likely than were the drivers to give up smoking and moderate their beer drinking, this would point to physiological mechanisms, although it would be necessary to ensure that the two groups were exposed to similar social and other influences outside working hours (9).

Generalizability of Findings

There are important theoretical and practical implications to the specificity or generality of the populations that may exhibit behavioral adaptation to exercise. Consistent gender differences across a range of behaviors, for example, might suggest that some mechanisms were more plausible than others as explanations of the adaptation process. On a practical level it would be useful for health promoters to know whether there are any popu-

lation groups to which a unitary model of health behaviors applies.

The most important demographic characteristics from both a theoretical and a practical point of view are age, gender, and education. Most of the literature dealing with this topic describes the age and gender composition of study subjects; only some describe education level. Even more limiting, few studies have made systematic distinctions between age groups, gender, or education levels at the intervention or analysis stage. Such refinements are essential (29), considering the covariance among these characteristics and most health behaviors (25). When gender-specific analyses are reported (e.g., Blair et al.'s cross-sectional Cooper Clinic data), women have more healthful practices but do not appear to change these in response to exercise differently than do men. Similarly, the interrelationship of health practices in a general population sample are little different for men and women, nor do they change meaningfully when age or education is controlled statistically (28, 29). Such analyses do not prove that behavioral adaptation is a universally applicable mechanism; they serve better to illustrate the need for further investigations on this issue.

Outstanding Methodological Issues

Four major methodological issues have hampered progress on the topic of behavioral adaptation to physical activity:

- A lack of randomized designs, prospective studies, and replication
- The use of small samples with the resultant lack of statistical power (see, e.g., ref. 11)
- A failure to examine systematically subjects who vary in age, gender, and education level
- A failure to vary the exercise dose systematically

Some of these problems are currently being addressed with a longitudinal follow-up to the 1981 Canada Fitness Survey (30). Of the household population sample of 23,000 Canadians who were fitness tested and questioned regarding their exercise and other habits in 1981, a sample of approximately 4,000 has recently been revisited. These individuals, age 7-69 yr, have again been tested and questioned in detail regarding their exercise habits, other health practices, and emotional and physical health status. The results of data analyses will begin to appear in 1989.

Blair et al. identify assessment problems as the major hindrance to research in this area. Accurate description of such complex behaviors as exercise and dietary consumption certainly poses a challenge but is not likely the major stumbling block in this area. Considerable progress has been made on other topics with a fairly simple characterization of activity level (e.g., relating exercise to coronary heart disease; see chapt. 54), whereas techniques are quite well standardized for assessing smoking, alcohol use, and other health practices (25). However, improvements are desirable, particularly for describing the exercise habits of subjects in prospective and cross-sectional studies. In addition, the Hawthorne effect is likely to be operating in intervention trials and prospective studies, and social desirability may affect self-reports of health practices in studies of all types.

Conclusion

The adoption of healthful behaviors in response to taking up regular exercise is an appealing prospect for those who seek to improve the health status of populations. Unfortunately, there is very little substantiation for this view in the research literature. However, there is no clear refutation of this hypothesis either.

The main distinguishing feature of the literature on behavioral adaptation to physical activity is that it is small and underdeveloped. There are few relevant studies and no replications; those studies that do pertain to the issue have usually been designed for investigating some other question. There are notable exceptions, mainly in the substance abuse area (see, e.g., refs. 11, 19), and these deserve to be repeated and extended.

The study of behavioral adaptation to exercise is important theoretically and practically. There are conceptual and methodological problems to overcome, but none is insurmountable. Further research is desirable, feasible, and likely to be rewarding.

References

1. Ashley, M.J., and J.G. Rankin. A public health approach to the prevention of alcohol-related health problems. In: Breslow, L., J.E. Fielding, and L.B. Lave, eds. *Annual review of public health*. Palo Alto, CA: Annual Reviews, Inc., 1988: vol. 9, pp. 233-271.

2. Berkman, L.F., and L. Breslow. *Health and ways of living*. New York: Oxford University Press, 1983.

3. Blair, S.N., N.N. Goodyear, K.L. Wynne, and R.P. Saunders. Comparison of dietary and smoking habit changes in physical fitness improvers and nonimprovers. *Prev. Med.* 13: 411-420, 1984.

4. Blair, S.N., D.R. Jacobs, Jr., and K.E. Powell. Relationships between exercise or physical activity and other health behaviors. *Public Health Rep.* 100: 172-180, 1985.

5. Blair, S.N., and H.W. Kohl. *Measurement and evaluation of health behaviors and attitudes in relationship to physical fitness and physical activity patterns*. Paper presented to the Workshop on Physical Fitness and Activity Assessments in NCHS General Population Surveys, Airlie House, June 1985.

6. Brown, J.D., and M. Lawton. Stress and well-being in adolescence: The moderating role of physical exercise. *J. Hum. Stress* (Fall): 125-130, 1986.

7. Faulkner, R.A., D.A. Bailey, and R.L. Mirwald. The relationship of physical activity to smoking characteristics in Canadian men and women. *Can. J. Public Health* 78: 155-160, 1987.

8. Flay, B.R. Mass media and smoking cessation: A critical review. *Am. J. Public Health* 77: 153-160, 1987.

9. Gottlieb, N.H., and J.A. Baker. The relative influence of health beliefs, parental and peer behaviors and exercise program participation on smoking, alcohol use and physical activity. *Soc. Sci. Med.* 22: 915-927, 1986.

10. Hannah, T.E. Health behaviour: The role of health as a personal life concern. *Can. J. Public Health* 78: 165-167, 1987.

11. Hill, J.S. Effect of a program of aerobic behaviour on the smoking behaviour of a group of adult volunteers. *Can. J. of Public Health* 76: 183-186, 1985.

12. Howard, J.H., D.A. Cunningham, and P.A. Rechnitzer. Physical activity as a moderator of life events and somatic complaints: A longitudinal study. *Can. J. Appl. Sport Sci.* 9: 195-200, 1984.

13. Howley, T.J. *A comparative evaluation of aerobic exercise and self-management strategies in the treatment of cigarette smoking*. Unpublished

doctoral dissertation, West Virginia University, Morgantown, 1981.

14. Kagan, D.M., and R.L. Squires. Addictive aspects of physical exercise. *J. Sports Med.* 25: 227-237, 1985.
15. Mackeen, P.C., J.L. Rosenberger, J.S. Slater, W.C. Nicholas, and E.R. Buskirk. A 13-year follow-up of a coronary heart disease risk factor screening and exercise program for 40- to 59-year-old men: Exercise habit maintenance and physiologic status. *J. Cardiopul. Rehabil.* 5: 510-523, 1985.
16. Matheson, C.M. *Exercise and meditation as a lifestyle intervention for addictive behaviours.* Unpublished doctoral dissertation, University of Washington, Seattle, 1982.
17. Milsum, J.H., and W.N. Jones. Population attributable risk for health promotion policy making: A management tool. *Can. J. Public Health* 79: 181-188, 1988.
18. Morris, J.N., A. Kagan, D.C. Pattison, M.J. Gardner, and P.A.B. Raffle. Incidence and prediction of ischaemic heart disease in London busmen. *Lancet* ii: 553-559, 1966.
19. Murphy, T.M., R.P. Pagano, and G.A. Marlatt. Lifestyle modification with heavy alcohol drinkers: Effects of aerobic exercise and meditation. *Addict. Behav.* 11: 175-186, 1986.
20. Pavett, C.M., M. Butler, E.J. Marcinik, and J.A. Hodgson. Exercise as a buffer against organization stress. *Stress Med.* 3: 87-92, 1984.
21. Pi-Sunyer, F.X., and R. Woo. Effect of exercise on food intake in human subjects. *Am. J. Clin. Nutr.* 42: 983-990, 1985.
22. Pomerleau, O.F., H.H. Scherzer, N.E. Brunberg, et al. The effects of acute exercise on subsequent cigarette smoking. *J. Behav. Med.* 10: 117-127, 1987.
23. Roth, D.L., and D.S. Holmes. Influence of aerobic exercise training on physical training and relaxation training on physical and psychologic health following stressful life events. *Psychosom. Med.* 49: 355-365, 1987.
24. Schoenborn, C.A. Health habits of U.S. adults, 1985: The "Alameda 7" revisited. *Public Health Rep.* 101: 571-580, 1986.
25. Schoenborn, C.A., and T. Stephens. Health promotion in the United States and Canada: Smoking, exercise and other health-related behaviors. *Am. J. Public Health* 78: 983-984, 1988.
26. Selye, H. *Stress without distress.* Philadelphia: Lippincott, 1974.
27. Sinyor, D., T. Brown, L. Rostant, and P. Serganian. The role of a physical fitness program in the treatment of alcoholism. *J. Stud. Alcohol* 43: 380-385, 1982.
28. Stephens, T. Health practices and health status: Evidence from the Canada Health Survey. *Am. J. Prev. Med.* 2: 209-215, 1986.
29. Stephens, T. Healthy lifestyles for all by the year 2000: How are Canadians doing? *Health Promotion* 24: 2-3, 1985.
30. Stephens, T., C.L. Craig, and B.F. Ferris. Adult physical activity in Canada: Findings from the Canada Fitness Survey I. *Can. J. Public Health* 77: 285-290, 1986.
31. Stones, M.J., A. Kozma, A.K. McNeil, and L. Stones. Smoking behaviour and participation in organized exercise. *Can. J. Public Health* 77: 153-154, 1986.
32. Wood, P.D., W.H. Haskell, S.N. Blair, et al. Increased exercise levels and plasma lipoprotein concentrations: A one-year, randomized, controlled study in sedentary, middle-aged men. *Metabolism* 32: 31-39, 1983.

PART IV

Physical Activity and Fitness in Disease

Chapter 34

Exercise, Fitness, and Atherosclerosis

Peter D. Wood
Marcia L. Stefanick

Atherosclerosis is a disease of the intima, or inner lining, of the arteries in which fatty streaks first appear, followed later by atheroma formation with an accumulation of cholesterol and cholesterol esters, scarring, and calcification (46). Atheroma encroach on the vessel channel and eventually impede blood flow significantly, causing ischemia downstream. Thrombus formation is frequently the final event leading to complete occlusion of a coronary artery and thus to a heart attack, so that the tendency of the blood to clot and its fibrinolytic activity are also important factors in the outcome of coronary atherosclerosis. Atherosclerosis, which is especially prevalent in developed countries, is the underlying cause of coronary heart disease (CHD) (the major cause of death in these countries) and of cerebral vascular disease (CVD) and peripheral vascular disease (PVD). Important manifestations of these diseases include heart attack and angina pectoris (in CHD), stroke (in CVD), and intermittent claudication (in PVD).

There is good evidence that one of the major prerequisites for the development and progression of atherosclerosis is elevated LDL-cholesterol concentrations and possibly low levels of HDL cholesterol in the blood perfusing the arteries (14). Many other factors relate importantly to the initiation and severity of atherosclerosis and its manifestations, in particular high blood pressure and cigarette smoking. These are discussed in other chapters.

In this review of exercise, fitness, and atherosclerosis, we first consider the evidence that a change in exercise (or fitness) level results in a change in the rate of progression of atherosclerosis (Hypothesis 1). Next we look at the hypothesis that a change in plasma lipoprotein concentrations leads to a change in rate of progression of atherosclerosis (Hypothesis 2) and that a change in exercise (or fitness) level leads to a change in plasma

lipoprotein concentrations (Hypothesis 3). The model under consideration is as follows:

$$\begin{array}{ccc} \text{Change in} \xrightarrow{3} & \text{Change in} \xrightarrow{2} & \text{Change in} \\ \text{exercise} & \text{plasma} & \text{rate of} \\ \text{(or fitness)} & \text{lipoprotein} & \text{progression} \\ & \text{concentrations} & \text{of atherosclerosis} \\ & 1 & \end{array}$$

We distinguish (where data are available) between the level of physical activity habitually performed and physical fitness (defined in terms of maximal oxygen uptake, or $\dot{V}O_2$max, or the ability to work at a given MET level). Some indication will be given of the effect of specific types of exercise and of frequency, intensity, and duration of exercise where possible, although much remains to be learned in these areas.

After examining the evidence to support our model, we discuss mechanisms that underlie the connections between exercise and atherosclerosis and between exercise and lipoprotein concentrations. We also consider other factors affecting lipoprotein metabolism that are modified by exercise (or fitness) level.

Exercise and Fitness in Relation to Risk of Atherosclerosis

Coronary Heart Disease

Very few studies in humans have attempted to assess directly the influence of level of physical fitness or of physical activity on the initiation or progression of coronary atherosclerosis. The work of Selvester et al. (48) in patients with angina, prior myocardial infarction, or both suggests a slowing of progression of existing coronary atherosclerosis with exercise training to endurance fitness levels.

The intriguing studies of Kramsch et al. (27) in macaque monkeys maintained on atherogenic diets indicated that long-term, regular moderate exercise substantially reduced the severity of coronary atherosclerosis in comparison to the sedentary condition. A considerable literature bears on the issue of fitness or exercise level in relation to atherosclerosis through studies in which the occurrence of manifestations of coronary atherosclerosis has been related to previously measured fitness or reported activity levels. The large-cohort studies of Morris et al. (39) and Paffenbarger et al. (41) are consistent in showing that habitually high levels of physical activity predict low rates of CHD in men even after adjustment for other major risk factors. The Framingham Study indicated a clear trend of improved coronary mortality with increased level of physical activity over 24 yr of surveillance for men at all ages (24). In a predominantly sedentary male Belgian population, physical fitness, but not reported physical activity, was an independent protective factor against CHD (51).

A recent literature survey by Powell et al. (43) reviewed 43 studies of physical activity in relation to CHD, primarily among North American and European working-aged men, paying particular attention to the quality of the investigations. It is of interest that the authors found no reports in the literature of positive associations of exercise level and CHD incidence. Rather few studies have considered women separately from men. Powell et al. (43) concluded that

> the inverse association between physical activity and incidence of CHD is consistently observed, especially in the better designed studies; this association is appropriately sequenced, biologically graded, plausible, and coherent with existing knowledge. Therefore, the observations reported in the literature support the inference that physical activity is inversely and causally related to the incidence of CHD.

The strong inverse relationship between physical activity level and incidence of CHD does not prove that exercise prevents or slows the development of atherosclerosis, although the association is consistent with this hypothesis because coronary atherosclerosis is clearly the underlying cause of CHD. Indeed, the strength of the exercise-CHD relationship is the most cogent evidence we currently have in support of the hypothesis that habitual physical activity slows the process of atherosclerosis in men. The relation of exercise level and fitness to CHD is not pursued here further because it is the subject of chapter 36.

Stroke and Cerebral Vascular Disease

The evidence for a negative relationship between CVD and physical activity level is relatively weak in comparison to the evidence for such an inverse relationship between CHD and physical activity. In the generally sedentary Framingham population, an inverse relationship for men between reported physical activity and the incidence of strokes did not reach significance after adjustment for age (23). However, for a population in eastern Finland aged 30-59, low physical activity at work (but not in leisure time) was associated with an increased risk of cerebral stroke even after controlling for serum total cholesterol, diastolic blood pressure, height, weight, and smoking (47). Furthermore, in the prospective Harvard alumni study of 16,936 men, a significant trend was seen for stroke mortality in relation to physical activity index: Stroke rates per 10,000 man-years of observation were 6.5 for participants with less than 500 Kcal/ per week of energy expenditure in leisure time; 5.2 for 500-1,999 Kcal/per week; and 2.4 for 2,000 Kcal or more per week (41). There is thus some limited evidence that cerebral atherosclerosis, as manifested by stroke, is reduced in more active people.

Peripheral Vascular Disease

Major prospective studies have shed little light on the relation of habitual physical activity level, or physical fitness, to risk of future PVD. Because CHD risk appears to be related to activity level and CHD frequently accompanies PVD, it might be reasonably hypothesized that regular physical activity reduces risk of PVD. But hard evidence appears to be lacking.

Plasma Lipid and Lipoprotein Concentrations in Relation to Risk of Atherosclerosis

The association between physical activity level and atherosclerosis is plausible, largely because of substantial evidence that habitual activity leads to lipoprotein concentrations in the blood plasma that are favorable with respect to preventing or slowing the atherosclerotic process. Before we consider this important link, the evidence that plasma lipoprotein pattern is importantly related to risk and severity of atherosclerosis is briefly reviewed. Total cholesterol, or total triglycerides, refer to the cholesterol or triglyceride content of plasma carried on all lipoprotein families combined, that is, LDL, HDL, and very low density lipoproteins (VLDL). Total cholesterol is often regarded as an acceptable surrogate for LDL cholesterol because the latter constitutes a large proportion of total cholesterol and because the two measures are usually high correlated in populations. However, this relation becomes less clear in individuals with high HDL levels.

Plasma Total Cholesterol and Triglycerides

Abundant evidence indicates that plasma total cholesterol concentration is positively associated with incidence of CHD (7, 50). The Lipid Research Clinics Coronary Primary Prevention Trial (LRC-CPPT) showed convincingly in a controlled study of asymptomatic middle-aged men with elevated cholesterol that reduction of cholesterol level by drug treatment resulted in a significant reduction in definite CHD death and definite nonfatal heart attack (34). Other indicators of coronary atherosclerosis (e.g., new positive exercise tests, development of angina, and need for coronary bypass surgery) were also reduced in the treatment group compared to the control group in this study. Total cholesterol appears to be positively associated with PVD but perhaps not with CVD (26). It is currently unclear whether total triglyceride (or the closely correlated VLDL cholesterol) is independently related to CHD incidence, and there is little evidence of associations with CVD or PVD.

Low-Density Lipoproteins

Several large, prospective studies have shown clearly that the principal carriers of cholesterol in the plasma, LDL, are positively associated with risk of CHD. In the LRC-CPPT, men who experienced an 11% (average adherers to the drug cholestyramine) or 35% (good adherers) decrease in LDL cholesterol experienced reductions of 19% and 50%, respectively, in CHD incidence in relation to untreated men (34). The Helsinki trial (10) recently reinforced the finding that reduced LDL cholesterol concentration leads to reduced CHD risk.

In high concentrations, LDL cholesterol is suspected to damage the arterial endothelium, reduce

platelet survival, and increase platelet aggregation as well as stimulate the growth of smooth-muscle cells; LDL cholesterol is also the primary source of cholesterol that is trapped in the matrix (45). A receptor mechanism whereby LDL enters peripheral cells, probably including arterial intimal cells and smooth-muscle cells, was elegantly elucidated by Brown and Goldstein (6). Factors (including certain drugs) that increase the number or activity of LDL receptors lead to decreased plasma LDL cholesterol levels and so to reduced CHD risk.

Low-density lipoprotein consists of a number of subspecies within the overall flotation interval of S_f 0-20. A simple classification separates the LDL family into small LDL (S_f 0-7), large LDL (S_f 7-12), and intermediate-density lipoprotein (IDL; S_f 12-20). There is evidence that IDL is particularly atherogenic (28).

High-Density Lipoproteins

A classic 1975 paper by Miller and Miller (37) pulled together evidence that plasma concentration of HDL cholesterol is inversely related to risk of CHD. Much subsequent work has confirmed this relationship, including the Tromso Heart Study (38) and the Israeli Ischaemic Heart Disease Study (12). Plasma HDL cholesterol concentration has also been shown to be significantly decreased in CVD and PVD patients compared to normal controls (3).

Two major intervention trials have provided support for the proposition that increasing plasma HDL cholesterol levels decreases risk of CHD. In the drug treatment group within the LRC-CPPT, each 1 mg/dl increase in HDL cholesterol from baseline levels was associated with a 4.4% reduction in risk of definite CHD death or heart attack (13). In the Helsinki Heart Study (10), the drug gemfibrozil was used in a randomized, double-blind 5-yr trial in 4,081 asymptomatic men with plasma non-HDL cholesterol levels above 199 mg/dl. The drug-treated men experienced a mean increase in plasma HDL cholesterol of more than 10% and a decrease in LDL cholesterol of 10%. The incidence of CHD was reduced by 34% compared to its incidence in the controls ($p < 0.02$).

It is suggested that HDL acts as a cholesterol acceptor in the reverse cholesterol transport system, the cholesterol in tissues being esterified under the influence of the enzyme lecithin-cholesterol acyl transferase (LCAT) before being incorporated into HDL. The enzyme lipoprotein lipase (LPL), located at the capillary endothelium of muscle and adipose tissue, is responsible for splitting VLDL and transferring surface lipids to HDL. Activity of LPL is generally positively correlated with HDL concentrations and negatively with VLDL, which is also inversely correlated with HDL.

There has been considerable interest in the role of HDL subfractions. Although there is evidence that the HDL family of lipoproteins may be quite heterogeneous in form and function, most work to date has used a simple separation (by the preparative ultracentrifuge or by precipitation techniques) into HDL_2 (larger, less dense particles in the flotation range $F_{1.20}$ 3.5-9.0) and HDL_3 (smaller, more dense particles in the flotation range $F_{1.20}$ 0-3.5). The enzyme hepatic lipase (HL) appears to be responsible for conversion of HDL_2 to HDL_3 by removing cholesterol and phospholipids in the liver. Activity of HL is often negatively correlated with HDL concentrations and particularly with HDL_2.

The HDL_2 subfraction is often considered to be protective against CHD and perhaps against the progression of atherosclerosis at any site. Most of the evidence for this is based on measurements of the cholesterol content of HDL subfractions in the plasma of individuals whose degree of atherosclerosis (usually of the coronary vessels) was estimated from coronary angiograms or from the presence or absence of symptomatic atherosclerotic disease (54). HDL_3 cholesterol concentration generally has been considered unpredictive of CHD. However, the only prospective study we are aware of that has measured both HDL_2 and HDL_3 (as total mass, using the analytical ultracentrifuge) concluded that a low serum concentration of either subfraction was significantly predictive of future CHD (11). A significant reduction of the HDL_2 and HDL_3 cholesterol concentrations was observed in 27 patients suffering from PVD compared to normal controls (36).

The accumulation or removal of cholesterol from the inner arterial lining, which influences the progression or regression of the atherosclerotic process, appears to depend on the interplay of the LDL (ingress) system and the HDL (egress) system and is clearly determined to a considerable degree by the prevailing plasma concentrations of these two major lipoprotein families. Cholesterol removed from tissues by means of HDL is eliminated in the bile as cholesterol or bile acids.

It appears that the ratio of HDL to LDL in plasma is an important predictor of risk of CHD. In the Tarahumara Indians, plasma HDL-cholesterol levels are low, yet CHD incidence is very low be-cause plasma LDL cholesterol is very low (due probably to diet and exercise levels), and the HDL-LDL ratio is high. In North American populations, in which LDL cholesterol levels tend to be high, the ratio of HDL to LDL is a strong predictor of CHD risk, and individuals with high ratios exhibit protection (14).

Apolipoproteins

The identified peptide components of the various lipoproteins are now quite numerous. Much remains to be learned about their functions, but it is clear that they are involved in the recognition of specific lipoproteins by cellular receptors and in the regulation of enzymes involved in lipoprotein catabolism. Two apolipoproteins in particular have been related to risk of CHD: apolipoprotein A-I, the major peptide component of the HDL family, and apolipoprotein B, the predominant LDL peptide. Apolipoprotein A-I has been reported to be a good discriminator of angiographically significant CHD; little coronary disease is found in individuals with high apolipoprotein A-I levels (35). Concentration of apolipoprotein B is positively associated with risk of CHD (15).

The Effects of Exercise and Fitness on Plasma Lipids and Lipoproteins

We now consider the evidence for the proposition that exercise level and fitness importantly regulate plasma lipoprotein concentrations. In evaluating studies completed to date, we emphasize that changes in many other lifestyle habits affect lipoprotein concentrations and must be controlled or adjusted for in analyzing the data. Some of these factors (to be discussed later) are alcohol consumption, cigarette smoking, dietary composition, medication with certain drugs, and fat gain or loss.

It should first be mentioned that regular exercisers have larger plasma volumes than do sedentary people and that increased exercise level leads to increased plasma volume. An increase in plasma concentration of a lipoprotein such as HDL with increased exercise represents an even greater increase in total circulating HDL because there is now more plasma. Conversely, a small decrease in a lipoprotein such as LDL with increased exercise may represent no change in total circulating LDL because there has simply been a dilution of LDL as a result of increased plasma volume. However, the evidence to date is that the LDL concentration is the important variable with respect to the functional regulation of LDL receptors. It is not clear whether this is also true of HDL, for which a specific receptor has not been identified, or whether the absolute amount of this lipoprotein is the important variable.

First, we consider evidence from cross-sectional comparisons, then evidence from longitudinal training studies, and finally the influence on lipoproteins of a variety of factors that also may vary with physical activity or fitness level.

Cross-Sectional Studies

Many comparisons of plasma lipids and lipoproteins have been made between groups of physically active individuals and sedentary controls (17, 21, 58). The consensus is that active men and women have lipoprotein patterns that predict (in comparison to sedentary controls) reduced risk of atherosclerosis and its manifestations. However, such findings alone have limited application to public health recommendations because of possible self-selection bias (e.g., people who are genetically fitter or who have advantageous lipoprotein patterns may more readily take up regular exercise) and because of potential confounding factors (e.g., regular exercisers may also be leaner and less likely to smoke cigarettes). Nonetheless, such cross-sectional data help to explain why very active people appear to enjoy some protection from atherosclerotic diseases and probably indicate the limits of beneficial lipoprotein change that might be achieved when sedentary people become active.

Table 34.1 gives mean fasting plasma lipid and lipoprotein concentrations from a comparison of 12 runners and 64 sedentary men, all middle-aged nonsmokers (54), that exemplifies results from many cross-sectional studies. Lipoprotein mass concentrations were determined on the analytical ultracentrifuge. The runners were currently running 64 ± 35 (SD) km/wk, whereas the controls were neither on programs of regular exercise nor employed in strenuous jobs.

Table 34.1   Comparison of Age, Body Mass Index, Lipids, Lipoproteins, Lipoprotein Lipase, and Hepatic Lipase Measurements in Cross-Sectional Samples of Long-Distance Runners and Sedentary Men

	Runners ($M \pm SD$)	Nonrunners ($M \pm SD$)	Difference ($M \pm SE$)	Significance (p)
Age (yr)	46.9 ± 7.5	45.7 ± 6.1	1.3 ± 2.3	0.81
Body mass index (kg/m²)	22.6 ± 2.0	25.1 ± 3.3	-2.5 ± 0.7	0.006
Lipids and lipoproteins				
Plasma total cholesterol (mg/dl)	190.9 ± 36.6	217.0 ± 31.1	-26.1 ± 11.3	0.02
Plasma total triglycerides (mg/dl)	70.8 ± 35.0	123.0 ± 59.3	-52.2 ± 12.5	0.001
Plasma HDL cholesterol (mg/dl)	64.9 ± 12.5	49.6 ± 8.7	15.3 ± 3.8	0.0001
Serum HDL mass of $F_{1.20}$ 0-1.5 (mg/dl)	70.0 ± 13.7	82.3 ± 17.5	-12.3 ± 4.5	0.02
Serum HDL mass of $F_{1.20}$ 1.5-2.0 (mg/dl)	51.2 ± 8.4	52.3 ± 7.8	-1.1 ± 2.6	0.98
Serum HDL mass of $F_{1.20}$ 2.0-9.0 (mg/dl)	213.0 ± 45.6	144.8 ± 47.9	68.2 ± 14.5	0.0002
Plasma LDL cholesterol (mg/dl)	147.0 ± 27.5	161.1 ± 30.7	-30.9 ± 9.5	0.004
Serum LDL mass of S_f 0-7 (mg/dl)	138.4 ± 45.3	227.6 ± 67.9	-89.2 ± 15.6	0.0001
Serum LDL mass of S_f 7-12 (mg/dl)	136.7 ± 39.8	134.2 ± 43.8	2.5 ± 12.7	0.85
Serum IDL mass of S_f 12-20 (mg/dl)	34.3 ± 18.2	43.8 ± 20.7	-9.5 ± 5.9	0.16
Plasma VLDL cholesterol (mg/dl)	9.1 ± 8.3	20.4 ± 11.7	-11.3 ± 2.8	0.001
Serum VLDL mass of S_f 20-400 (mg/dl)	36.8 ± 41.6	106.1 ± 72.0	-69.3 ± 15.0	0.001
Postheparin lipase activity				
Lipoprotein lipase (mEq fatty acid/ml/h)	5.0 ± 1.8	3.6 ± 1.2	1.4 ± 0.6	0.04
Hepatic lipase (mEq fatty acid/ml/h)	4.1 ± 2.1	6.5 ± 2.6	-2.4 ± 0.9	0.02

Note. From ''Lipoprotein Subfractions of Runners and Sedentary Men'' by P.T. Williams et al., 1986, *Metabolism*, **35**, p. 47. Reprinted by permission. Sample sizes are 12 runners and 64 nonrunners for all lipid and lipoprotein variables, age, and body mass index and 12 runners and 16 nonrunners for lipoprotein and hepatic lipase measurements. All significance levels are obtained from two-sample Wilcoxon sign rank tests.

Plasma Triglycerides

Plasma triglyceride levels tend to be strikingly lower in the active group (Table 34.1). As might be expected, mass levels of VLDL cholesterol and total VLDL are also significantly lower in runners. This probably relates to the fact that trained muscles utilize fat as fuel much more efficiently than do untrained muscles and that a considerable amount of fat is burned during an endurance-type exercise bout.

Plasma Total Cholesterol

Total cholesterol was lower in runners than in controls in this study, a circumstance that has been reported in some but certainly not all such comparisons. Athletes trained for speed or power tend to have total cholesterol levels that are similar to or greater than those of sedentary controls (17). In the general population, more active groups usually do not show significantly lower total cholesterol levels than do less active groups. There is a tendency for very active people compared to sedentary controls to show higher HDL cholesterol levels but lower LDL cholesterol levels, so that the net effect of regular exercise on total cholesterol level may be small (see following discussion).

Plasma LDL Cholesterol

Cross-sectional studies generally indicate that the atherogenic LDL cholesterol is not greatly different in concentration for endurance-trained athletes versus sedentary controls (58), although lower levels have been observed for groups doing very strenuous exercise. In the general population, there is no relationship between total plasma LDL cholesterol concentration and activity level in men or women (16). However, we have observed in collaboration with Drs. Krauss and Lindgren at the University of California, Berkeley, that active groups tend to have considerably lower concentrations of small LDL (S_f 0-7) than do sedentary controls despite a less pronounced difference in total LDL cholesterol (54).

Plasma HDL Cholesterol

Endurance-trained individuals (men and women, young and old) consistently show higher concentrations of plasma HDL cholesterol (58). Figure 34.1 shows plasma HDL cholesterol concentrations for trained men and women athletes versus sedentary controls of the same gender taken from 32 published cross-sectional studies (18). Values above the line of identity indicate higher concentrations for the endurance athletes in the range of 5-15 mg/dl (or 10%-30%) compared to those of sedentary controls. Such elevations have been reported for long-distance runners, tennis players, soccer players, Nordic skiers, and speed skaters (58). Weight-trained athletes and sprinters seem to have HDL cholesterol concentrations similar to those of sedentary individuals (or lower in the case of athletes taking androgenic hormones).

The elevation of HDL cholesterol in exercisers appears to be due largely to expansion of the HDL_2 region of the particle distribution, as seen for runners in Table 34.1 (HDL mass of $F_{1.20}$ 2.0-9.0 is predominantly HDL_2). However, some studies have reported elevations of both HDL_2 and HDL_3 in active groups (58).

A dose-response relationship between amount of exercise performed and plasma HDL cholesterol level has been reported, for example, across a spectrum of habitual exercise ranging from the extreme inactivity of quadriplegia to the extreme activity of marathon training (31). In several cross-sectional studies in runners, significant correlations were reported between miles run per week and HDL cholesterol concentration, ranging from .41 to .62 (58). Men and women in the general population who are more active during leisure time or on the job have only modestly higher HDL cholesterol levels than do their less active colleagues (16). This probably reflects the relatively small range of activity levels among typical U.S. populations.

Plasma Apolipoproteins

Several cross-sectional studies have reported on plasma concentrations of apolipoproteins A-I and A-II in active versus less active groups. Concentrations of apolipoprotein A-I is clearly higher in dedicated runners than in sedentary controls (58), the increase averaging about 30%. Because of the considerably increased plasma volume of runners, their actual circulating mass of apolipoprotein A-I is impressively increased to the extent of about 58% in men, as estimated by Herbert et al. (20). On the other hand, complete bed rest resulting from spinal injury is associated with a 20%-30% reduction in plasma A-I concentration in men and women in comparison to ambulatory controls (40). The latter effect may be partially due to plasma volume changes; however, in view of the stable postural status of the patients, it might be a real effect.

The association of physical activity level and the minor HDL peptide apolipoprotein A-II is less clear (58). There is very little information about the relation of physical activity to concentrations of other

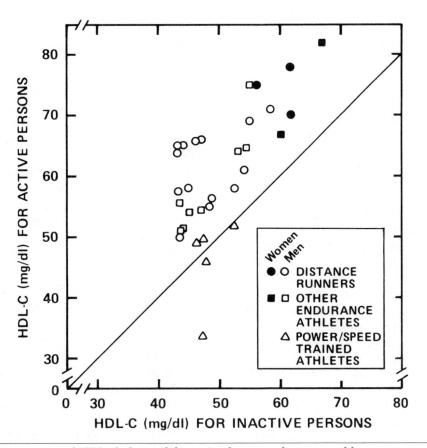

Figure 34.1. Concentrations of HDL cholesterol for trained men and women athletes versus sedentary controls of the same gender from 32 published cross-sectional studies. Reprinted with permission of Macmillan Publishing Company from "Influence of Exercise on Plasma Lipids and Lipoproteins" by W.L. Haskell, M.L. Stefanick, and R. Superko, in *Exercise, Nutrition and Energy Expenditure*, edited by E.S. Horton and R.J. Terjung. Copyright © 1988 by Macmillan Publishing Company.

lipoproteins that have been related to risk of atherosclerosis (e.g., apolipoproteins B and E). The relation of plasma apolipoprotein concentrations to physical activity level in the population at large has apparently not yet been studied.

Longitudinal Training Studies

Studies in which relatively inactive and unfit individuals joined a training program and became more active and fitter can potentially overcome many of the limitations of cross-sectional studies, particularly the problems of self-selection and simultaneity (i.e., the characteristic lipoprotein pattern of exercisers may be due to some secondary variable, such as a particular dietary intake, that also characterizes exercisers). However, in considering the results of such trials it is important to realize that a "good" trial—providing an adequate test of the hypothesis that change from a sedentary to a habitually active lifestyle results in favorable changes in lipoprotein concentrations—is both dif-

ficult and expensive to perform. A sedentary control group with random assignment to exercise or control is important. Blinding participants and investigators to the assignment status would be desirable but has never been achieved in exercise trials and is difficult to conceive. Adequate numbers of participants must be involved (as indicated by power calculations). The period of training should be as long as possible to allow time for sedentary individuals to become reasonably fit. Totally sedentary people usually cannot approach the fitness levels characteristic of many cross-sectional study participants (e.g., habitual runners) during a typical training study averaging 3 mo. Where studies have reported that participants achieved high exercise levels in relatively brief studies, the sedentary status of the participants initially may be suspect. The statistical treatment of data obtained from many trials has not been as robust as might be wished (58).

Random assignment of sedentary participants to exercise or control conditions is clearly desirable to overcome self-selection bias. However, once randomized, a participant's data should be included in the trial results regardless of the degree of change (increase or decrease) achieved in his or her exercise participation or fitness level. Herein lies the difficulty in interpreting training studies. On one hand, if participants are excluded as dropouts because they did not meet some exercise participation goal, a positive result (i.e., exercise appears to change lipoproteins favorably) may be obtained, but a self-selection bias prevails. On the other hand, if all participants are included regardless of how much exercise they did (or, indeed, of whether they did any), then self-selection is eliminated, but the average increase in exercise level achieved may be too low (especially in short trials) to test the hypothesis adequately. In this respect training studies are difficult to conduct compared to randomized drug trials because the sedentary participant's reaction to being asked to exercise, for, perhaps, several hours per week at a distant facility is likely to be quite different from his or her reaction to being asked to take one or two pills per day at home.

For these reasons, it is not surprising that the results of training studies have appeared not infrequently to contrast with cross-sectional findings. The shorter trials do not really address the question whether a permanent transformation from a sedentary to an active lifestyle results in favorable modification of lipoprotein pattern. Exercise trials that include all initially randomized participants in the final analysis are to some extent feasibility trials (Can we persuade people to exercise adequately?) as well as trials of the major hypothesis (Does exercise lead to changes in lipoprotein concentrations?).

With these cautions in mind, we attempt to summarize about 40 exercise training trials, considering group mean changes (exercisers vs. controls) reported for lipoprotein levels, associations between change in lipoprotein levels and change in exercise level (e.g., average distance run per week) in individuals assigned to training, and associations between change in lipoprotein levels and change in exercise test performance scores (fitness) with training.

Plasma Triglycerides

Exercise training lowers triglyceride levels in men who have initially elevated levels (22) but in several studies seems to have little effect on triglycerides in the normal range (5, 57). A high degree of activity and leanness may be required to produce the markedly low plasma triglyceride levels seen in very active groups (54).

Plasma Total Cholesterol

On balance, trials suggest a tendency for a reduction of total cholesterol levels with increased exercise, but this is seldom significant or independent (17, 57). In an uncontrolled long-term training study in which 14 sedentary, middle-aged men increased activity by jogging an average of 20 km per week and were followed for 2 yr, mean plasma total cholesterol decreased from 216 to 203 mg/dl ($p < .01$). During this time body fat was lost, and caloric intake increased by about 400 cal per day (59). Cholesterol reductions of this magnitude may be typical for men who become dedicated, habitual exercisers, a circumstance seldom attained in short-term trials.

Plasma LDL Cholesterol

The possibility of a beneficial effect of regular exercise or maintained high levels of fitness on plasma levels of the atherogenic LDL family of particles is of obvious public health interest. As with total cholesterol, LDL cholesterol concentration has not, on balance, been lowered importantly with exercise in trials (17, 57), although several trials have reported significant reductions in LDL cholesterol (42, 59). In 46 sedentary, middle-aged men who participated in a 1-yr running program (57), change in LDL cholesterol concentration correlated with distance run per week ($r = -.31$, $p = .04$).

It should be remembered that the plasma LDL cholesterol measurement does not necessarily tell the whole story of the relation of the LDL lipoprotein family to risk of atherosclerotic diseases. As illustrated in Table 34.1, habitual exercisers (runners) seem to differ from sedentary individuals with respect to LDL subfractions (54). Trials reported to date have not followed changes in these subfractions over prolonged periods of increased exercise in sedentary groups.

Plasma HDL Cholesterol

Review of reported training studies (17, 54) indicates at first glance rather equivocal evidence that endurance training results in increased plasma HDL cholesterol levels in spite of the clear-cut cross-sectional evidence in favor of this hypothesis. About one half of reported controlled training studies found significant HDL cholesterol increases in the exercise group. The duration of the training period is probably critical because, for 10 wk or less of training, as many studies reported a decrease in HDL cholesterol as reported an increase. But all studies of duration greater than 12 wk reported an increase in mean HDL cholesterol concentration averaging about 5 mg/dl, although not all were significant at $p < .05$ (18).

In a study of 753 middle-aged men attending the Cooper Clinic in Dallas, Texas, significant increases in treadmill time were observed over 1.6 yr. Plasma HDL cholesterol concentration rose significantly with increasing fitness level (5).

Furthermore, as indicated by a 1-yr training study, there may be a threshold at about 15 km per week of running that must be exceeded to result in a significant increase in HDL cholesterol (57). The existence of some minimum amount of exercise increase for an HDL effect, whether measured by duration of the training or by the weekly dose of exercise, would certainly help to explain the apparent lack of agreement among trials of quite diverse length and type of exercise intervention and the apparent discrepancy between the cross-sectional and longitudinal findings.

Several longitudinal studies in initially sedentary individuals have demonstrated a positive association between amount of exercise performed and HDL cholesterol change, providing stronger evidence of a dose-response relationship than can be obtained from cross-sectional correlations. For example, in the 1-yr study of 46 sedentary men assigned to exercise by running (57), distance run per week correlated significantly with change in HDL cholesterol ($r = .48$, $p < .001$).

Several uncontrolled studies of the effect of exercise in men with CHD have shown an increase in HDL cholesterol (58), but a large, controlled 1-yr study by LaRosa et al. (32) failed to confirm this effect for the exercise level that could be achieved by 110 men with CHD.

In summary, training studies of 12 wk or longer have generally indicated an increase in plasma HDL cholesterol concentration, but the increase has failed to reach significance in a proportion of trials. It seems probable that this is due to a dilution of the effect for the exercising groups by participants unable or unwilling to do enough exercise to produce substantial HDL cholesterol elevation. This belief is supported by the frequent observation that increase in physical activity level or fitness is positively and significantly correlated with increase in HDL cholesterol concentration.

Plasma HDL Subfractions

The plasma concentration of the less dense, larger HDL_2 subfraction of the HDL family appears to be more closely related to risk of atherosclerotic diseases than does the concentration of the more dense, smaller HDL_3 subfraction (54). Furthermore, in most individuals HDL_2 is the lesser com-

ponent in terms of both cholesterol carried and total particle mass. Concentration of HDL cholesterol is thus a less sensitive measure of risk of CHD and other atherosclerotic diseases than is concentration of HDL_2 cholesterol or HDL_2 mass. In a 6-mo training study, Ballantyne et al. (1) found a significantly increased mean HDL_2 cholesterol concentration (9.1-17.1 mg/dl) in exercising myocardial infarction survivors but no significant change for survivors assigned to control. The 1-yr training study by Wood et al. (57) found a correlation of .41 ($p < .01$) between distance run per week and change in plasma HDL_2 mass for 46 initially sedentary, middle-aged men. Similar findings were reported for moderately overweight men engaging in an exercise program designed to bring about weight loss (52). In both groups of men, change in fitness (measured as $\dot{V}O_2$max) was also positively correlated with change in concentration of HDL_2 mass. On the basis of reported studied (58), the effect of changed exercise or fitness level on HDL_3 concentration appears to be more variable.

Plasma Apolipoproteins

The influence of increased exercise on plasma apolipoprotein concentrations has been studied in only a few training studies. In the 12-wk study by Keins et al. (25), men increased their apolipoprotein A-I levels by 10% ($p = .02$). In the controlled 1-yr study by Wood et al. (57), there was no indication of an increase in plasma apolipoproteins A-I or A-II with exercise; however, change in apolipoprotein B (the principal apolipoprotein of LDL) was negatively correlated ($r = -.29$, $p < .05$) with distance run per week for the 46 male exercisers.

Factors Influencing Plasma Lipoprotein Levels That May Vary With Level of Physical Activity or Fitness

Numerous factors other than exercise or fitness level influence plasma lipoprotein concentrations, and these must be considered in interpreting data from both cross-sectional and longitudinal studies, especially when there is reason to believe that the factor may vary with exercise level. The more important of these factors are now briefly considered.

Gender

In the North American population, women generally have higher plasma HDL cholesterol and HDL_2 cholesterol levels and lower triglyceride levels than do men of comparable age (19, 33). This is no doubt partly because of hormonal influences and contributes to the lower CHD risk of women. Men who exercise regularly undergo a change in lipoprotein pattern toward that which is typical of females. The rather few training studies carried out in women have suggested that sedentary females elevate their HDL cholesterol with exercise less readily than do men. This may be a consequence of the higher initial HDL cholesterol level in sedentary women in relation to sedentary men; or it may reflect other preexisting gender differences, such as the general distribution of adipose tissue or differences in lipase activities that underlie lipoprotein concentrations; or it may reflect lower levels of increased physical activity that have been achievable in training studies on women.

Age

In cross-sectional studies of the adult North American population, plasma tyiglyceride, VLDL cholesterol, and LDL cholesterol tend to increase in concentration with increasing age (19). This trend is paralleled by decreasing physical activity and increasing obesity with increasing age. Men and women who exercise regularly (e.g., runners) appear to resist all these trends and maintain youthful levels of plasma lipoproteins into middle age and beyond (56). In women, a decrease in plasma estrogen in association with menopause is accompanied by changes in lipoproteins, especially HDL, that may be reversed by hormone-replacement therapy.

Race

Little is known of the race-specific effects of exercise on lipoproteins. Black men tend to have higher levels of HDL cholesterol than do white men, which may reflect a more active lifestyle among black men or differences in body composition, diet, or other factors.

Socioeconomic Status

There are now few truly strenuous occupations in North America, so that occupation and hence socioeconomic status seem today to have a relatively small influence on physical activity at work. There is a tendency for high socioeconomic status to be associated with a favorable lipoprotein pattern, which may reflect a greater tendency for better educated people with more disposable income to participate in leisure-time exercise, to pay more attention to their diets, to smoke less, or to control their weight.

Body Composition

Physical activity level and adiposity are intimately associated. Endurance athletes are generally lean, and sedentary individuals are frequently overweight. Training programs almost always result in the loss of body fat. So close is this association that exercise and weight loss might be considered a single prescription from the standpoint of public health. Exercise without weight loss is unusual within the sedentary population, and permanent weight loss without exercise, though frequently attempted, is seldom successful. Body composition in relation to lipoprotein levels is discussed in detail later in this chapter.

Diet

Endurance exercise in initially sedentary men appears to result in both body fat loss and increased caloric intake (59). Male and female runners exhibit higher caloric intakes than do heavier, age-matched sedentary controls (4). In a number of prospective population studies, higher recorded caloric intake has been predictive of lower risk of death from CHD. In a 1-yr training study in men, change in caloric intake with exercise was positively correlated ($r = .38$, $p = .03$) with change in plasma HDL cholesterol concentration (57). It should be remembered when considering how exercise relates to risk of atherosclerosis that an increased exercise level frequently results in permanently increased caloric intake and decreased body fat.

The quality of the self-selected diet may change as sedentary individuals become more active. High-carbohydrate, low-fat diets are often recommended for endurance athletes. Very little is known about this potentially important public health issue, but it may constitute another link between exercise level and risk of atherosclerotic disease.

Alcohol

Alcohol intake has pronounced effects on plasma concentrations of HDL cholesterol, HDL subfractions, and apolipoproteins A-I and A-II (2). Changes in alcohol intake accompanying changes in exercise level might potentially complicate interpretation of the influence of increased exercise on lipoproteins and indirectly on risk of atherosclerotic disease, but evidence to support this is lacking.

Smoking

Cigarette smoking is associated with a lowering of plasma HDL cholesterol levels, and abandonment of smoking results in an increase in HDL cholesterol concentration (53). Cigarette smoking appears to decrease as exercise level increases, so that adoption of an exercise program is likely to result in a reduction of smoking levels in smokers and thus an increase in HDL-cholesterol levels.

Mechanisms by Which Exercise and Fitness May Affect Atherosclerosis

Cellular and Hematologic Factors

Few studies have focused on the effects of physical activity on the progression or regression of atherosclerosis, particularly with respect to cellular interactions that underlie the development of atherosclerotic lesions, such as changes in the arterial endothelium, smooth muscle, monocytes, macrophages, or platelets. Some studies in recent years have shown physical training to have beneficial effects on fibrinolytic activity and blood coagulation (9). One study (44) demonstrated a significant inhibition of secondary platelet aggregation in men following 12 wk of regular, moderate-intensity exercise, which might have a favorable influence on the prevention of thrombosis. Whether exercise can also affect the release of mitogenic factors associated with platelets, such as platelet-derived growth factor, has not been studied to our knowledge.

Possible changes in LDL receptor or HMG-CoA reductase activity also have not been examined in association with exercise, nor have any data been gathered to determine whether genetic differences exist in any of these cellular factors between people who are fit (as demonstrated by maximum oxygen consumption) or physically active and people who are unfit and sedentary.

Vessel Wall Morphology

The effect of exercise on vessel wall morphology has not been well studied. Several investigators have found increases in arterial bore in athletes relative to sedentary subjects (8), and the progression of atherosclerosis in coronary arteries of subjects who had previous myocardial infarctions was shown to be significantly less in patients who had regular, moderate exercise programs relative to inactive and low-level exercise subjects (48). Epidemiological data also suggest that regular physical activity reduces the incidence of ECG abnormalities compatible with myocardial ischemia (48). Furthermore, in CHD where ischemia may occur with exercise, training has been shown to increase coronary arterial collateralization.

One of the well-known effects of exercise training is a decrease in resting blood pressure, presumably due to changes in the smooth-muscle tone of the arterial walls, following a reduction of circulating catecholamines (55). Epinephrine and norepinephrine also have been noted to accelerate LDL penetration into the subendothelial space of the abdominal aorta of rhesus monkeys (49), suggesting another means by which an exercise-related reduction of catecholamines could play a role in a decreased incidence of CHD.

Mechanisms by Which Exercise and Fitness Modify Plasma Concentrations of Lipoproteins and Apolipoproteins

There is a substantial literature on the effect of exercise on several mechanisms that are believed to underlie the previously described exercise-induced changes in circulating lipoprotein levels (18). The activity of at least two key enzymes in lipoprotein metabolism has been shown to be associated cross-sectionally with physical activity level and to change with increased endurance-type exercise. Specifically, lipoprotein lipase (LPL), which plays a major role in the conversion of VLDL to HDL, has been shown to be higher in runners than in sedentary persons and to be increased by exercise, whereas levels of hepatic lipase, which is believed to play a major role in the conversion of HDL_2 to HDL_3 to participate in the conversion of VLDL, IDL, and large LDL to IDL and small LDL, is lower in active people and is decreased by exercise. These changes are associated with the improved lipoprotein profile (i.e., decreased VLDL and triglycerides and elevated HDL, specifically HDL_2) seen following endurance-exercise training (52).

Increases in cardiac and skeletal muscle LPL activity with exercise seem to be specifically associated with increased muscle activity, as demonstrated by significant elevations in postheparin plasma LPL activity elevations immediately following and for days after exercise. Activity of LPL has been shown to be elevated in working versus resting muscle and to be associated with increases in HDL and HDL_2 levels in the venous blood of the working muscle relative to its arterial blood. Increased muscle LPL activity may be especially advantageous as muscle improves its ability to utilize fatty acids as fuel for endurance activities, a process that is dependent on duration and intensity of the work and on training. Activity of LPL is greater in red (slow-twitch) muscle fiber than in white (fast-twitch) fiber and may therefore account for the higher HDL levels found in people who have greater ratios of red to white fibers and who thus tend to have higher $\dot{V}O_2$max level than do people with high ratios of white to red fibers. Activity of LPL has been shown also to be positively correlated with $\dot{V}O_2$max.

The decrease in hepatic lipase activity and its association with increases in HDL and HDL_2 appear to be strongly associated with weight loss, at least in moderately overweight men who take up an exercise program, and is equally great when weight is lost by gradual caloric restriction (52). Decreased body fat therefore may be one of the most important consequences of a training program, and the relative leanness of physically active people may account for their lower hepatic lipase activity cross-sectionally and thus their higher plasma HDL and HDL_2 levels. There is evidence that hepatic lipase activity has a strong genetic component that may also underlie genetic regulation of HDL and its subfraction distribution (29).

Another means by which exercise may influence lipoprotein levels is through selective effects on adipose tissue lipolysis and distribution (18). Exercise training has been reported to increase beta-receptor sensitivity to norepinephrine, thus presumably enhancing the lipolytic effect of catecholamines. Abdominal adipocytes have been shown to be more responsive to catecholamine-induced lipolysis than are femoral adipocytes, suggesting that exercise training may result in the selective loss of abdominal fat versus femoral and gluteal fat or a reduction in the waist-to-hip ratio (WHR). The WHR has been shown to correlate strongly with HDL cholesterol and HDL_2 mass and with risk of death attributable to cardiovascular disease (30).

Conclusion

An entirely convincing test of the hypothesis that habitual physical activity prevents or reduces the rate of progression of atherosclerosis would involve the random assignment of very large numbers of young, healthy individuals (preferably male and female) to either a relatively high activity lifestyle or a relatively sedentary lifestyle, followed by adequate assessment of appearance and progression of atherosclerotic disease at a number of anatomical sites over many years. Such a study could not be conducted in a double blind manner and is most unlikely to be attempted because of the great cost and difficult ethical considerations. We are therefore obliged to draw conclusions from a mass of suggestive evidence. The foregoing sections summarize strongly suggestive, but not complete, evidence that higher compared to lower levels of habitual activity result in a slower progression of atherosclerosis and less frequent manifestations of atherosclerosis in the coronary arteries. The evidence for an exercise effect for atherosclerosis of the cerebral and peripheral arteries is less clear, in part because the manifestations of disease in these arteries are less frequent in the population than are those of CHD.

The plausibility of the exercise-CHD relationship is supported by several mechanisms in which physical activity, especially at higher levels, seems likely to inhibit the initiation and progression of atherosclerotic lesions and to lessen the probability of total occlusion of a diseased artery. Blood-clotting and fibrinolytic mechanisms are favorably influenced by exercise, reducing risk of catastrophic thrombosis. Blood pressure levels tend to be reduced by regular exercise, probably through the effect on catecholamines. Coronary artery bore appears to be considerably greater in very active than in sedentary individuals, perhaps reducing the consequences of a given degree of atherosclerotic damage to an artery.

The best-explored mechanism is the salutary effect of regular exercise on the concentration of plasma lipoproteins. This effect is seen most clearly in cross-sectional comparisons of very active individuals (often sports players) and sedentary controls, in whom HDL cholesterol, HDL_2 cholesterol, HDL_2 mass, and apolipoprotein A-I concentrations are clearly increased; triglycerides and VLDL cholesterol are decreased in the active groups. This results in plasma ratios of total cholesterol to HDL cholesterol, and of LDL cholesterol to HDL cholesterol in active individuals that are predictive of a low incidence of atherosclerotic manifestations.

Controlled trials in the exercise-lipoprotein area conducted to date have many shortcomings, notably brevity and the consequent inability to increase adequately the regular exercise level of participants. A trend toward a low-risk pattern of plasma lipoproteins is apparent in trials of durations longer than 3 mo, and significant dose-related improvements have been seen above a minimum amount of activity. Furthermore, both hepatic and lipoprotein lipase activity have been shown to be changed by exercise and to be correlated with the exercise-induced changes in lipoprotein and subfraction concentrations. It is still unclear whether there is a minimum intensity of exercise that is required to bring about these favorable lipoprotein and lipase changes.

In conclusion, much further work is needed to demonstrate truly the effect of exercise and fitness level on atherosclerosis and to determine which mechanisms underlie the beneficial changes in CHD risk that are associated with increased activity.

Acknowledgments

The authors acknowledge support from National Institutes of Health grant HL 24462 during preparation of this review.

References

1. Ballantyne, F.C., R.S. Clark, H.S. Simpson, and D. Ballantyne. The effect of moderate physical exercise on the plasma lipoprotein subfractions of male survivors of myocardial infarction. *Circulation* 65: 913-918, 1982.

2. Barboriak, J.J., and L.A. Menahan. Some implications of alcohol-induced lipid changes. In: Cappell, H.D., F.B. Glaser, Y. Israel, H. Kalant, W. Schmidt, E.M. Sellers, and R.S. Smart, eds. *Research advances in alcohol and drug problems.* New York: Plenum Press, 1986: vol. 9, Chapt. 3, pp. 127-156.

3. Bihari-Varga, M., J. Szekely, and E. Gruber. Plasma high density lipoproteins in coronary, cerebral and peripheral vascular disease. *Atherosclerosis* 40: 337-345, 1981.

4. Blair, S.N., N.M. Ellsworth, W.L. Haskell, M.P. Stern, J.W. Farquhar, and P.D. Wood. Comparison of nutrient intake in middle-aged men and women runners and controls. *Med. Sci. Sports Exer.* 13: 310-315, 1981.

5. Blair, S.N., K.H. Cooper, L.W. Gibbons, L.R. Gettman, S. Lewis, and N. Goodyear. Changes in coronary heart disease risk factors associated with increased treadmill time in 753 men. *Am. J. Epidemiol.* 118: 352-359, 1983.

6. Brown, M.S., and J.L. Goldstein. A receptor-mediated pathway for cholesterol homeostasis. *Science* 237: 32, 1986.

7. Consensus Development Conference. Lowering blood cholesterol to prevent heart disease. *JAMA* 253: 2080-2086, 1985.

8. Currens, J.H., and P.D. White. Half a century of running. Clinical, physiologic and autopsy findings in the case of Clarence DeMar (''Mr. Marathon''). *N. Engl. J. Med.* 265: 988-993, 1961.

9. Diehm, C., H. Mori, and G. Schettler. Influence of physical training on blood coagulation and fibrinolysis. *Klin. Wochenschr.* 62: 299-302, 1984.

10. Frick, M.H., O. Elo, K. Haapa, O.P. Heinonen, P. Heinsalmi, P. Helo, J.K. Huttanen, P. Kaitaniemi, P. Koskinen, V. Manninen, H. Maenpaa, M. Malkonen, M. Manttari, S. Norola, A. Pasternack, J. Pikkarainen, M. Romo, R. Sjoblom, and E.A. Nikkila. Helsinki Heart Study: Primary-prevention trial with gemfibrozil in middle-aged men with dyslipidemia. *N. Engl. J. Med.* 317: 1237-1245, 1987.

11. Gofman, J.W., W. Young, and R. Tandy. Ischemic heart disease, atherosclerosis and longevity. *Circulation* 34: 679-697, 1966.

12. Goldbourt, U., and J.H. Medalie. High density lipoprotein cholesterol and incidence of coronary heart disease: The Israeli Ischaemic Heart Disease Study. *Am. J. Epidemiol.* 109: 296-308, 1979.

13. Gordon, D.J., J. Knoke, J.L. Probstfield, R. Superko, and H.A. Tyroler. High-density lipoprotein cholesterol and coronary heart disease in hypercholesterolemic men: The Lipid Research Clinics Coronary Primary Prevention Trial. *Circulation* 74: 1217-1225, 1986.

14. Grundy, S.M. Cholesterol and coronary heart disease: A new era. *JAMA* 256: 2844-2858, 1986.

15. Hamsten, A., G. Walldius, A. Szamosi, G. Dahlen, and U. de Faire. Relationship of angiographically defined coronary disease to serum lipoproteins and apolipoproteins in young survivors of myocardial infarction. *Circulation* 73: 1097-1110, 1986.

16. Haskell, W.L., H.L. Taylor, P.D. Wood, H. Schrott, and G. Heiss. Strenuous physical activity, treadmill exercise test response and plasma high density lipoprotein cholesterol. The Lipid Research Clinic Program Prevalence Study. *Circulation* 62(Suppl. iv): 53-61, 1980.

17. Haskell, W.L. The influence of exercise training on plasma lipids and lipoproteins in health and disease. *Acta Med. Scand. Suppl.* 711: 25-37, 1986.

18. Haskell, W.L., M.L. Stefanick, and R. Superko. Influence of exercise on plasma lipids and lipoproteins. In: Horton, E.S., and R.J. Terjung, eds. *Exercise, nutrition and energy*

expenditure. Burlington, VT: The Collamore Press, 1988: Chapt. 15, pp. 213-227.

19. Heiss, G., I. Tamir, C.E. Davis, H.A. Tyroler, B.M. Rifkind, G. Schonfeld, D. Jacobs, and I.D. Frantz. Lipoprotein-cholesterol distributions in selected North American populations: The Lipid Research Clinics Program Prevalence Study. *Circulation* 61: 302-314, 1980.

20. Herbert, P.N., A.N. Bernier, E.M. Cullinane, L. Edelstein, M.A. Kantor, and P.D. Thompson. High-density lipoprotein metabolism in runners and sedentary men. *JAMA* 252: 1034-1037, 1984.

21. Hietanen, E. *Regulation of serum lipids by physical exercise.* Boca Raton, FL: CRC Press, 1982.

22. Holloszy, J.O., J.S. Skinner, G. Toro, and T.K. Cureton. Effects of a six-month program for endurance exercise on serum lipids of middle-aged men. *Am. J. Cardiol.* 14: 753-760, 1964.

23. Kannel, W.B., and P. Sorlie. Some health benefits of physical activity. *Arch. Intern. Med.* 139: 857-861, 1979.

24. Kannel, W.B., A. Belanger, R. D'Agostino, and I. Israel. Physical activity and physical demand on the job and risk of cardiovascular disease and death: The Framingham Study. *Am. Heart J.* 112: 820-825, 1986.

25. Kiens, B., I. Jorgensen, S. Lewis, G. Jensen, H. Lithell, B. Vessby, S. Hoe, and P. Schnohr. Increased plasma HDL-cholesterol and apo A-I in sedentary middle-aged men after physical conditioning. *Eur. J. Clin. Invest.* 10: 203-209, 1980.

26. Kostner, G.M., E. Marth, K.P. Pfeiffer, and H. Wege. Apolipoproteins AI, AII and HDL phospholipids but not Apo-B are risk indicators for occlusive cerebrovascular disease. *Eur. Neurol.* 25: 346-354, 1986.

27. Kramsch, D.M., A.J. Aspen, B.M. Abramowitz, T. Kreimendahl, and W.B. Hodd, Jr. Reduction of coronary atherosclerosis by moderate conditioning exercise in monkeys on an atherogenic diet. *N. Engl. J. Med.* 305: 1483-1489, 1981.

28. Krauss, R.M., P.T. Williams, P.T. Brensike, K.M. Detre, F.T. Lindgren, S.F. Kelsey, K. Vranizan, and R.I. Levy. Intermediate-density lipoproteins and progression of coronary artery disease in hypercholesterolaemic men. *Lancet* ii: 62-66, 1987.

29. Kuusi, T., Y.A. Kesaniemi, M. Vuoristo, T.A. Miettinen, and M. Koskenvuo. Inheritance of high density lipoprotein and lipoprotein

30. Lapidus, L., C. Bengtsson, B. Larsson, K. Pennert, E. Rybo, and L. Sjostrom. Distribution of adipose tissue and risk of cardiovascular disease and death: A 12-year follow-up of participants in the population study of women in Gothenburg, Sweden. *Br. Med. J.* 289: 1257-1261, 1984.

31. LaPorte, R., G. Brenes, and S. Dearwater. HDL-cholesterol across a spectrum of physical activity from quadriplegia to marathon running. *Lancet* i: 1212-1213, 1983.

32. LaRosa, J.C., P. Cleary, R.A. Muesing, P. Gorman, H.K. Hellerstein, and J. Naughton. Effect of long-term moderate physical exercise on plasma lipoproteins: The National Exercise and Heart Disease Project. *Arch. Intern. Med.* 142: 2269-2274, 1982.

33. The Lipid Research Clinics Program Epidemiology Committee. Plasma lipid distributions in selected North American populations: The Lipid Research Clinics Program Prevalence Study. *Circulation* 60: 427-439, 1979.

34. The Lipid Research Clinics Program. The Lipid Research Clinics Coronary Primary Prevention Trial Results: II. The relationship of reduction in incidence of coronary heart disease to cholesterol lowering. *JAMA* 251: 365-374, 1984.

35. Maciejko, J.J., D.R. Holmes, B.A. Kottke, A.R. Zinsmeister, D.M. Dinh, and S.J.T. Mao. Apolipoprotein A-I as a marker for angiographically assessed coronary artery disease. *N. Engl. J. Med.* 309: 385-389, 1983.

36. Mannarino, E., D. Siepi, G. Maragoni, A. Susta, and M. Ventura. HDL$_2$- and HDL$_3$-cholesterol in normolipemic patients with peripheral vascular occlusive disease. *Vasa* 15: 217-219, 1986.

37. Miller, G.J., and N.E. Miller. Plasma high-density lipoprotein concentrations and the development of ischemic heart disease. *Lancet* i: 16-19, 1975.

38. Miller, N.E., O.H. Forde, D.S. Thelle, and O.D. Mjos. The Tromso Heart Study. High-density lipoprotein and coronary heart-disease: A prospective case-control study. *Lancet* i: 965-967, 1977.

39. Morris, J.N., M.G. Everitt, R. Pollard, and S.P.W. Chave. Vigorous exercise in leisure-time: Protection against coronary heart disease. *Lancet* ii: 1207-1210, 1980.

40. Nikkila, E.A., T. Kuusi, and P. Myllynen. High-density lipoprotein and apolipoprotein

lipase and hepatic lipase activity. *Arteriosclerosis* 7: 421-425, 1987.

A-I during physical inactivity. *Atherosclerosis* 37: 457-462, 1980.

41. Paffenbarger, R.S., R.T. Hyde, A.L. Wing, and C.H. Steinmetz. A natural history of athleticism and cardiovascular health. *JAMA* 252: 491-495, 1984.

42. Peltonen, P., J. Marniemi, E. Hietanen, I. Vuori, and C. Enholm. Changes in serum lipids, lipoproteins and heparin releasable lipolytic enzymes during moderate physical training in man: A longitudinal study. *Metabolism* 30: 518-526, 1981.

43. Powell, K.E., P.D. Thompson, C.J. Caspersen, and J.S. Kendrick. Physical activity and the incidence of coronary heart disease. *Annu. Rev. Public Health* 8: 253-287, 1987.

44. Rauramaa, R., J.T. Salonen, K. Seppanen, R. Salonen, J.M. Venalainen, M. Ihanainen, and V. Rissanen. Inhibition of platelet aggregability by moderate-intensity physical exercise: A randomized clinical trial in overweight men. *Circulation* 74: 939-944, 1986.

45. Reckless, J.P.D. Hyperlipidaemia. In: Woolf, N., ed. *Biology and pathology of the vessel wall*. New York: Praeger, 1983: pp. 243-264.

46. Ross, R. The pathogenesis of atherosclerosis—an update. *N. Engl. J. Med.* 314: 488-500, 1986.

47. Salonen, J.T., P. Puska, and J. Tuomilehto. Physical activity and risk of myocardial infarction, cerebral stroke and death. *Am. J. Epidemiol.* 115: 526-537, 1982.

48. Selvester, R., J. Camp, and M. Sanmarco. Effects of exercise training on progression of documented coronary arteriosclerosis in men. *Ann. N.Y. Acad. Sci.* 301: 495-508, 1977.

49. Shimamoto, T., M. Kobayashi, and F. Numano. Immunofluorescent demonstration of plasma protein entry into arterial wall by cholesterol, epinephrine, norepinephrine and angiotensin II. *Acta Pathol. (Jpn.)* 25: 51-67, 1975.

50. Simons, L.A. Interrelations of lipids and lipoproteins with coronary artery disease mortality in 19 countries. *Am. J. Cardiol.* 57: 5G-10G, 1986.

51. Sobolski, J., M. Kornitzer, G. de Backer, M. Dramaix, M. Abramowicz, S. Degre, and H. Denolin. Protection against ischemic heart disease in the Belgian Physical Fitness Study: Physical fitness rather than physical activity? *Am. J. Epidemiol.* 125: 601-610, 1987.

52. Stefanick, M.L., R.B. Terry, W.L. Haskell, and P.D. Wood. Relationships of changes in post-heparin hepatic and lipoprotein lipase activity to HDL-cholesterol changes following weight loss achieved by dieting versus exercise. In: Gallo, L., ed. *Cardiovascular disease: Molecular and cellular mechanisms. Prevention and treatment*. New York: Plenum Press, 1988: pp. 61-69.

53. Tuomilehto, J., A. Tanskanen, J.T. Salonen, A. Nissinen, and K. Koskela. Effects of smoking and stopping smoking on serum high-density lipoprotein cholesterol levels in a representative population sample. *Prev. Med.* 15: 35-45, 1986.

54. Williams, P.T., R.M. Krauss, P.D. Wood, F.T. Lindgren, C. Giotas, and K.M. Vranizan. Lipoprotein subfractions of runners and sedentary men. *Metabolism* 35: 45-52, 1986.

55. Winder, W.W., J.M. Hagberg, R.C. Hickson, A.A. Ehsani, and J.A. McLane. Time course of sympathoadrenal adaptation to endurance exercise training in man. *J. Appl. Physiol.* 45: 370-374, 1978.

56. Wood, P.D., W.L. Haskell, M.P. Stern, S. Lewis, and C. Perry. Plasma lipoprotein distributions in male and female runners. *Ann. N.Y. Acad. Sci.* 301: 748-763, 1977.

57. Wood, P.D., W.L. Haskell, S.N. Blair, P.T. Williams, R.M. Krauss, F.T. Lindgren, J.J. Albers, P.H. Ho, and J.W. Farquhar. Increased exercise level and plasma lipoprotein concentrations: A one-year, randomized, controlled study in sedentary, middle-aged men. *Metabolism* 32: 31-39, 1983.

58. Wood, P.D., P.T. Williams, and W.L. Haskell. Physical activity and high-density lipoproteins. In: Miller, N.E., and G.J. Miller, eds. *Clinical and metabolic aspects of high-density lipoproteins*. Amsterdam: Elsevier, 1984: Chapt. 6, pp. 135-165.

59. Wood, P.D., R.B. Terry, and W.L. Haskell. Metabolism of substrates: Diet, lipoprotein metabolism, and exercise. *Fed. Proc.* 44: 358-363, 1985.

Chapter 35

Discussion: Exercise, Fitness, and Atherosclerosis

Sean Moore

The excellent summary by Peter Wood and Marcia Stefanick leaves me only the happy task of dotting some *i*'s and crossing some *t*'s. There are two topics I would like to mention. The first is the relationship between exercise, platelet aggregation, and blood coagulation. The published reports present conflicting findings regarding the effect of exercise on platelet aggregation possibly accompanied by release of platelet proteins. The question is important because in individuals with coronary heart disease any tendency to platelet aggregation and activation might lead to myocardial ischemia and possibly to sudden cardiac death. This concern is emphasized by sporadic reports of sudden death while running or just after running for those engaged in exercise programs (20), although in young athletes such deaths are more likely to be associated with structural cardiovascular disease such as hypertrophic cardiomyopathy (13). This subject is more fully discussed by Dr. Siscovick in his presentation on the risks of exercising (chapt. 61).

Platelet-specific proteins have been reported to be present in an increased amount in the plasma of patients with coronary artery disease (15), and platelet factor-4 may be considerably elevated in patients with acute myocardial infarction (9). Whether the release of platelet products occurs during exercise in subjects with myocardial ischemia is controversial (18). What seems to be better established is that in vivo platelet activation occurs when vigorous exercise is undertaken (18). The degree of activation seems to be related to the working level performed. This physiological effect needs to be considered as a possible explanation for sudden cardiac death during or following exercise. This must be balanced against the potential benefit of physical activity in relation to the risk of coronary heart disease and death (12).

Apart from the possible effects on platelet activation, the effects on the coagulability of the blood also have been examined. Reports showing an increase in blood coagulability (11) must be viewed in relation to the observation of an increase in fibrinolysis produced by exercise and adrenaline (6).

This issue is probably best summarized by the statement that more research is needed on the benefit (or otherwise) of physical activity modifying the development of thrombosis and thereby lowering the risk of developing ischemic heart disease (16).

The second topic relates to recent observations concerning the biology of the arterial wall and may go some way toward providing an explanation for the favorable effects of raised blood high-density lipoprotein (HDL) and an increased ratio of HDL to low-density lipoprotein (LDL). This involves a mechanism by which LDL entering the intima from the bloodstream is retained or trapped in the tissue. It has been known for some time that lipoproteins bind to glycosaminoglycans (GAGs), especially sulfated GAGs in vitro (4, 10). This association is broken when HDL is added (5). Human lesions of atherosclerosis contain increased amounts of proteoglycans (19), which are molecules composed of a protein core with numerous GAG side chains and some mannose-containing oligosaccharides. There is now a substantial literature indicating that positively charged amino groups on apolipoprotein B bind electrostatically to negatively charged groups of the GAG of proteoglycans (2).

Arterial smooth-muscle cells synthesize proteoglycans. In atherosclerotic lesions the GAGs are increased in content and form complexes with lipoprotein (19). Aortic GAG content is increased in pigeons that spontaneously develop atherosclerosis and are susceptible to dietarily induced disease, whereas pigeons that are resistant to atherosclerosis show no such increase (7).

Because smooth-muscle-cell proliferation occurs in most forms of experimentally induced atherosclerosis, it is likely that increased proteoglycan production may be a factor in lipid trapping in the vessel wall. We have examined these relationships extensively in relation to atherosclerotic lesions induced by injury. When the endothelium is removed from the aorta of rabbits that are fed a normal diet, a massive accumulation of lipid occurs in the neointima, which develops in response to injury. This accumulation is found exclusively in the part of the neointima that develops a covering of endothelium from the orifices of the branch vessels (14). In these areas, material that is revealed by ruthenium-red staining of the tissue is viewed by electron microscopy increases in content, whereas the areas of the neointima that remain uncovered by endothelium and that do not accumulate lipid show a less-than-normal concentration of GAGs (17).

Kinetic studies of the entry and retention of LDL into these areas show that entry is increased above that of normal intima (8) and that LDL is retained preferentially compared to the areas not covered by endothelium (1).

Changes in the GAG composition of the proteoglycan may be as important or more so than the increase in proteoglycan concentration. We have shown recently that such qualitative changes in the relative proportions of the GAG side chains of the proteoglycan molecule are important in facilitating the binding of LDL and very low density lipoprotein (3).

References

1. Alavi, M.Z., and S. Moore. Kinetics of low density lipoprotein interactions with rabbit aortic wall following balloon catheter de-endothelialization. *Arteriosclerosis* 4: 395-402, 1984.
2. Alavi, M.Z., and S. Moore. Proteoglycan composition of rabbit arterial wall under conditions of experimentally induced atherosclerosis. *Arteriosclerosis* 63: 65-74, 1987.
3. Alavi, M.Z., M. Richardson, and S. Moore. The *in vitro* interactions between serum lipoproteins and proteoglycans of the neointima of rabbit aorta after a single balloon catheter injury. *Am. J. Pathol.* 134: 287-294, 1989.
4. Bernfeld, P., J.S. Nesselbaum, B.J. Berkely, and R.W. Hamsen. Influences of the chemical and physiochemical nature of molecular polyanions and their interactions with serum β-lipoproteins. *J. Biol. Chem.* 235: 2852-2859, 1960.
5. Bihari-Varga, M., and M. Vegh. Quantitative studies on the complexes formed between aortic mucopolysaccharides and serum lipoproteins. *Biochem. Biophys. Acta* 144: 202-210, 1967.
6. Biggs, R., R.G. MacFarlane, and J. Pilling. Experimental production of increased fibrinolysis by exercise and adrenaline. *Lancet* i: 402-405, 1947.
7. Curwen, K.D., and S.C. Smith. Aortic glycosaminoglycans in atherosclerosis susceptible and resistant pigeons. *Exp. Mol. Pathol.* 27: 121-133, 1977.
8. Day, A.J., M. Alavi, and S. Moore. Influx of (^{3}H, ^{14}C) cholesterol-labelled lipoprotein into re-endothelialized and de-endothelialized areas of ballooned aortas in normal-fed and cholesterol-fed rabbits. *Artherosclerosis* 55: 339-351, 1985.
9. Handin, R.I., M. McDonough, and M. Lesch. Elevation of platelet factor 4 in acute myocardial infarction: Measurement by radioimmunoassay. *J. Lab. Clin. Med.* 91: 340-349, 1978.
10. Iverius, P.H. The interaction between human plasma lipoprotein and connective tissue glycosaminoglycans. *J. Biol. Chem.* 247: 2607-2613, 1972.
11. Korsan Bengtsen, K., L. Wilhelmsen, and G. Tibblin. Blood coagulation and fibrinolysis in relation to degree of physical activity during work and leisure time. *Acta Med. Scand.* 193: 73-77, 1973.
12. Leon, A.S., M. Cornett, D.R. Jacobs, and R. Rauramaa. Leisure time physical activity levels and risk of coronary heart disease and death: The Multiple Risk Factor Intervention Trial. *JAMA* 238: 2388-2395, 1987.
13. Maron, B.J., W.C. Roberts, H.A. McAllister, D.R. Rosing, and S.E. Epstein. Sudden death in young athletes. *Circulation* 62: 218-229, 1980.
14. Moore, S., L.W. Belbeck, M. Richardson, and W. Taylor. Lipid accumulation in the neointima formed in normal fed rabbits in response to one or six removals of the aortic endothelium. *Lab. Invest.* 47: 37-42, 1982.
15. Mulhauser, I., A.G. Scherthaner, K. Silberbauer, H. Sinzinger, and F. Kaindl. Plasma

concentration of platelet specific proteins in coronary artery disease. *Cardiology* 68: 129-139, 1981.

16. Rauramaa, R. Physical activity and prostanoids. *Acta Med. Scand. Suppl.* 711: 137-142, 1986.

17. Richardson, M., I.O. Ihnatowycz, and S. Moore. Glycosaminoglycan distribution in rabbit aortic wall following balloon catheter de-endothelialization. *Lab. Invest.* 43: 409-417, 1980.

18. Schernthaner, G., I. Mulhauser, H. Bohm, C. Seebacher, and H. Laimer. Exercise induces

in-vivo platelet activation in patients with coronary artery disease and in healthy individuals. *Haemostasis* 13: 351-357, 1983.

19. Stevens, R.L., M. Colombo, J.J. Gonzales, W. Hollander, and K. Schmid. The glycosaminoglycans of human artery and their changes in atherosclerosis. *J. Clin. Invest.* 58: 470-478, 1976.

20. Waller, B.F., and W.C. Roberts. Sudden death while running in conditioned runners aged 40 years or over. *Am. J. Cardiol.* 45: 1292-1300, 1980.

Chapter 36

Exercise, Fitness, and Coronary Heart Disease

Victor F. Froelicher

The purpose of this chapter is to describe the relationship between physical fitness and coronary heart disease. Only those references not cited in my book (15) will be given, to limit the number. This chapter begins with a discussion of animal studies. Then physiological studies in man evaluating cardiac changes and epidemiological studies regarding normals are discussed. The chapter then closes with an overview of the exercise component of cardiac rehabilitation.

Animal Studies Relating Chronic Exercise to Cardiac Changes

Animal studies provide some of the strongest evidence for the health benefits of regular exercise. The many effects listed in Table 36.1 have been demonstrated in various studies, and a review of some of these follows.

Table 36.1 Animal Studies of the Effects of Exercise on the Heart

Animal studies relating chronic exercise to cardiac changes
Myocardial hypertrophy
Myocardial microcirculatory changes
Coronary artery size changes
Coronary artery vasomotor tone
Coronary collateral circulation
Cardiac mechanical and metabolic performance
Myocardial mitochondria and respiratory enzymes
Effects on atherosclerosis and risk factors

Myocardial Hypertrophy

Numerous studies have demonstrated that vigorous exercise can induce cardiac hypertrophy in animals. Heart-to-body ratios are invariably larger in wild animals than in domestic animals. Heart hypertrophy is due to exercise in young rats, whereas in older rats exercise causes a decline in heart weight due to a loss of myocardial fibers or a decrease in fiber mass.

Myocardial Microcirculatory Changes

In comparing domestic with wild animals, we see that the density of muscle cells and capillaries is much greater in the more active, wild animals. In young animals, cardiac hypertrophy is secondary to fiber hyperplasia, whereas in older animals it is secondary to cellular hypertrophy. The capillary bed responds most markedly to growth stimuli if applied at an early age.

There is an age-related response of the ventricular capillary bed and myocardial fiber width in rats. At autopsy, the myocardial fiber width is constant, whereas the capillary-to-fiber ratio is increased in the exercised rats over the controls in all age-groups. The capillary density decreases with age and is increased over the controls only in young, exercised rats.

Rat experiments have been performed to study the effects of chronic exercise on the heart at different ages. Age-groups were subdivided into a control group, a group that swam for 1 hr daily, and a group that swam for 1 hr, 2 d per week. After 10 wk, the animals were killed. Although the response of the rat heart to chronic exercise varied with age, the capillary-to-fiber ratio increased at all ages.

Capillary proliferation in the heart and skeletal muscle by radioautography has been studied after injecting radioactive thymidine in rats exercised by swimming. Swimming led to hypertrophy of the myocardium and muscle fibers of the limbs. There was new formation of myocardial capillaries in swimming-induced cardiac hypertrophy.

429

An exercise-induced reduction in myocardial infarction size after coronary artery occlusion in the rat has been reported. When compared with sedentary controls, the ratio of capillary to muscle fiber was increased by 30% in exercised rats. Exercise training resulted in a 30% reduction of myocardial infarction size after coronary artery occlusion that was most likely due to increased vascularity. The effects of exercise on myocardial infarction in young versus old rats revealed that exercise improved the survival rates of the old rats. In addition, the old, exercised rats manifested cardiac hypertrophy, reduced infarction enzyme levels, and less evidence of arrhythmias or ECG changes.

Coronary Artery Size Changes

The effects of exercise on the coronary tree of rats have been studied by the corrosion cast technique. When the animals were killed, their hearts were weighed and the coronary arteries injected with vinyl acetate. Compared with the controls, both exercise groups had increased ratios of heart to body weight and coronary tree cast weight to heart weight. This technique has been used to ascertain the effects of exercise of different types, frequency, and duration. In the rat, forced exercise caused an increase in the coronary tree size as compared with the cardiac weight, provided the exercise was not too strenuous or frequent. Swimming in rats resulted in an increased luminal cross-sectional area of the main coronary arteries in the animals that experienced an increase in ventricular weight, that is, only the young and strenuously exercise adult rats.

Coronary Artery Vasomotor Tone

The effects of exercise on large coronary artery vasoreactivity were studied in dogs trained by treadmill running for 8 wk. The trained group showed a reduction in heart rate during submaximal exercise when compared with the controls, and resting plasma levels of norepinephrine and epinephrine were reduced in the trained group. The constriction of the coronary artery in response to serotonin infusion was not different in the two groups, but the responses to phenylephrine were attenuated in the trained dogs when compared with the nontrained dogs. The blunted constrictor response in the trained animals suggested that exercise reduces epicardial coronary vasoconstriction.

Coronary Collateral Circulation

Eckstein (12) performed the classic study of the effect of exercise and coronary artery narrowing on coronary collateral circulation. He surgically induced a constriction in the circumflex artery of approximately 100 dogs. Various degrees of narrowing were induced, but only the dogs that developed ECG changes were included in the study. After 1 wk of rest, the dogs were divided into two groups. One group was exercised on a treadmill 1 hr per day, 5 d per week, for 6-8 wk. The other group remained at rest in cages. The extent of arterial anastomoses to the circumflex artery was then determined as follows. A second thoracotomy was performed, and blood pressure was stabilized mechanically. The circumflex artery was isolated and divided beyond the surgical constriction. The flow rates through the constriction and from the distal end of the artery were measured. When these values were plotted against each other, the less the antegrade flow (or the greater the constriction), the greater the retrograde or collateral flow. Also, the exercised dogs had a greater value for retrograde flow than did the rested dogs for any degree of constriction. Moderate and severe arterial narrowing resulted in collateral development proportional to the degree of narrowing, and exercise led to even greater coronary anastomosis.

The effects of exercise training on coronary blood flow and cardiac output in rats at rest and during stress induced by breathing a mixture of 5% oxygen and 95% nitrogen for 5-7 min revealed that exercise training led to greater coronary dilation during hemodynamic stresses.

Coronary blood flow has been studied in exercised and sedentary rats using labeled microspheres during hypoxemic conditions. Although cardiac hypertrophy was found in the trained rats, this increase in perfused mass accounted for only one third of the increase in total coronary blood flow. Thus there was a greater coronary blood flow per unit mass of the myocardium in the trained rats.

The effects of endurance exercise on coronary collateral blood flow has been studied in miniature swine (4). Coronary collateral blood flow was measured in 10 sedentary control pigs and in 7 pigs that ran 20 mi per week for 10 mo. Radiolabeled microspheres were injected into the left atrium during each of three conditions: control, total occlusion of the left circumflex artery, and total occlusion plus mechanically elevated aortic pressure.

Ten months of endurance exercise training did not affect the development of coronary collaterals as assessed by microsphere blood flow measurements in the left ventricles of the pigs. When this was repeated after causing artificial partial occlusions in the coronary arteries of the pigs (i.e., ischemia was present), exercise enhanced myocardial perfusion.

The effect of physical training on collateral blood flow in 14 dogs with chronic coronary occlusions revealed that myocardial blood flow to collateral-dependent zones (measured by injecting radionuclide) was increased by 39%. In exercised beagles with occluded circumflex arteries, an isolated heart preparation revealed no increase in collaterals in the normal dogs but did reveal a doubled collateral conductance in the exercised, ischemic dogs.

The effects of exercise training on coronary collaterals developing in response to gradual coronary occlusion in dogs has been studied. Ameroid constrictors were used that initially were nonobstructive but that slowly absorbed body fluids and gradually expanded over 2-3 wk. After a constrictor was placed on the proximal left circumflex coronary artery, 33 dogs were randomly assigned to exercise or to sedentary groups. After 2 mo, the exercised dogs developed greater epicardial collateral connections to the occluded left circumflex as judged by higher blood flow and less of a drop in distal pressure. However, no difference in collaterals was found angiographically. Injected microspheres demonstrated that exercised dogs were not better protected against subendocardial ischemia induced by increased heart rate in the myocardium supplied by the collaterals. Exercise promoted coronary collateral development without improving the perfusion of the ischemic myocardium. These results raise an additional question: Even if collateral development does occur, does it significantly influence myocardial perfusion?

Cardiac Mechanical and Metabolic Performance

The effects of physical training on the mechanical and metabolic performances of the isolated rat heart have been studied. In exercised rats, the function of the heart as a pump was improved, and this effect was due at least partially to improved oxygen delivery. Other studies support the concept that the exercise-hypertrophied heart is functionally superior to the normal heart. Under controlled loading conditions, hearts of chronically exercised rats continued to perform better during ischemia than did hearts of sedentary controls.

In chronically instrumented dogs, myocardial contractility and adenosine triphosphatase activity of cardiac contractile proteins before and after exercise training have been studied. After training, maximal dp/dt was within normal limits at rest but was significantly elevated by submaximal exercise.

Using an isolated working-heart apparatus, researchers have found that a faster cardiac relaxation was a prominent effect of physical training and may foster more complete filling at high heart rates. Ten weeks of treadmill exercise on left-ventricular (LV) performance in 9 dogs chronically instrumented with LV pressure transducers revealed that at similar exercise heart rates the trained dogs had greater left contractility indices than did the sedentary dogs.

Exercise and Projection From Effects of Atherosclerosis

Kramsch et al. (23) randomly allocated 27 young adult male monkeys into three groups (23). Two groups were studied for 36 mo and one group for 42 mo. Of the groups studied for 36 mo, one was fed a vegetarian diet for the entire study and the other a vegetarian diet for 12 mo and then an isocaloric atherogenic diet for 24 mo. Both were designated as sedentary because their physical activity was limited to a single cage. The third group was fed the vegetarian diet for 18 mo and then the atherogenic diet for 24 mo. This group exercised regularly on a treadmill for the entire 42 mo. Because two of the monkeys on the atherogenic diet (one sedentary and one exercising) did not develop elevated serum cholesterol levels, they were excluded from the study. For 3 yr the animals were observed for objective evidence to support the protective value of periodic and regular exercise. Total serum cholesterol remained the same, but HDL cholesterol was higher in the exercise group. Angiographic size of coronary artery narrowing, ST depression, and sudden death were observed only in the sedentary monkeys fed the atherogenic diet. In addition, postmortem examination revealed marked coronary atherosclerosis and stenosis in this group. Exercise was associated with substantially reduced overall atherogenic involvement, lesion size, and collagen accumulation. These results demonstrate that exercise in young-adult monkeys increases the heart size, the LV mass, and the diameters of coronary arteries. Also, the subsequent experimental atherosclerosis induced by the atherogenic diet given for 2 yr was substantially reduced. Exercise before exposure to the atherogenic diet delayed the development of the manifestation of coronary heart disease. The important questions this study raises are, At what point comparable to the human life span were these studies initiated? and What percentage of that life span was represented by the 3 yr of observation? Studies in rats and dogs have found increased resistance to ventricular fibrilation after regular running, possibly through mechanisms involving cyclic adenosine monophosphate and the slow calcium channel.

Human Studies Supporting Cardiac Changes

Echocardiography Before and After an Exercise Program

Some of the longitudinal studies of exercise training using echocardiography are summarized here. Ehsani et al. (14) reported rapid changes in LV dimensions and mass in response to physical conditioning and deconditioning. Two groups of healthy, young subjects were studied. The training group consisted of 8 competitive swimmers who were studied serially for 9 wk. Mean LV end-diastolic dimension increased by 4.3 mm in the first week. A 3.3-mm increase from the pretraining value was demonstrated by the ninth week of training. Mean posterior wall thickness increased 0.7 mm by the end of the training period. There was no change in ejection fraction. The deconditioned group consisted of 6 competitive runners who stopped training for 3 wk. End-diastolic dimension decreased 4.7 mm and posterior wall thickness 2.7 mm by the end of the 3-wk period. Deconditioning did not influence ejection fraction. Exercise training induced adaptive changes in LV dimensions rapidly and mimicked the pattern of chronic volume overload, and modest degrees of exercise-induced LV enlargement were reversible. Surprisingly, changes in LV dimension occurred early during endurance training, but there was no significant increase in measured LV posterior wall thickness until the fifth week of training. Estimated LV mass significantly increased after the first week of training.

DeMaria et al. (10) reported the results of M-mode echocardiography in 24 young normals before and after 11 wk of endurance-exercise training. The subjects were participating in a program of endurance physical conditioning as part of police training and ranged in age from 20 to 34 yr. After training, they exhibited increased LV end-diastolic dimensions, decreased end-systolic dimensions, and increased stroke volumes and shortening fractions. Increases in mean fiber-shortening velocity were observed, as were increases in LV wall thickness, ECG voltage, and LV mass.

Stein et al. (52) studied the effects of exercise training on ventricular dimensions at rest and during supine submaximal exercise. Fourteen healthy students were studied by M-mode echocardiography at rest and in the third minute of 300 kp of supine bike exercise. They were studied before and after a 14-wk training program that resulted in a 30% increase in maximal oxygen consumption. The authors concluded that exercise training is associated with an increased stroke volume mediated by the Frank-Starling effect and enhanced contractility.

Parrault et al. (42) studied 14 middle-aged subjects with chest X ray, electrocardiogram, vectorcardiogram, and echocardiogram before and after 5 mo of training. Maximal oxygen consumption increased 20%. The echocardiograms showed no significant changes. This is in contrast to the studies of younger subjects. Wolfe et al. performed a similar study in 12 men with a mean age of 37 who exhibited 14% and 18% increases in aerobic capacity after 3 and 6 mo of training, respectively. They concluded that resting end-diastolic volume and stroke volume were increased but that LV structure and resting contractile status were not altered by 6 mo of jogging in healthy, previously sedentary men.

Adams et al. (1) noninvasively studied the effects of an aerobic training program on the hearts of healthy, college-age men. Compared with the control group, echocardiography after training showed an increase in LV end-diastolic dimension but no change in wall thickness or in ejection fraction. Although there was no change in myocardial wall thickness, the increase in end-diastolic dimension resulted in a calculated increase in LV mass.

Landry et al. (24) evaluated 20 sedentary subjects and 10 pairs of monozygotic twins who were submitted to a 20-wk endurance-exercise program. Maximal oxygen uptake increased significantly in both groups. Statistically significant increases in LV diameter, posterior wall and septal thicknesses, and LV end-diastolic volume and mass were observed in the sedentary subjects but not in the monozygotic twins. After training, twin pairs differed more from each other than they did at the start. Concomitantly, within-pair resemblance was greater after training than it was before. Results indicated that cardiac dimensions are amenable to significant modifications under controlled endurance-training conditions and that the extent and variability of the response of cardiac structures to training are perhaps genotype dependent.

Studies in Patients With CHD

Ehsani et al. (13) reported their results after 12 mo of intense exercise in a highly selected group of 10 patients with coronary heart disease. The patients, ranging in age from 44 to 63 yr, were the first to complete 12 mo of a high-level exercise program. Nine had sustained a single myocardial infarction, and one had severe three-vessel coronary artery disease. All 10 had asymptomatic exercise-induced ST-segment depression. Eight similar men were considered controls. After 3 mo of exercise training at a level of 50%-70% of maximal oxygen consumption, the level of training increased to 70%-80%, with two to three intervals at 80%-90% interspersed throughout the exercise session. Patients exercised three times per week during the first 3 mo and four to five times per week for the next 9 mo. The duration was initially 30 min and was later increased to 60 min.

The maximal amount of reported ST-segment depression was .30 mV, but most had .20 mV, which was less at repeat testing 1 yr later in spite of a higher double product, a greater treadmill work load, and a 38% increase in maximal oxygen consumption. In addition, 0.1 mV of ST-segment depression occurred at a higher double product after the year of training. A weight loss from a mean of 79 kg to 74 kg occurred. The sum of SV1 and RV5 increased by 15%. Both LV end-diastolic dimension and posterior wall thickness were significantly increased after training. This resulted in an increase in LV mass from 93 to 135 g $\cdot$ m^{-2} body surface area (BSA).

These results cannot be generalized to the average cardiac population. These 10 men were a highly selected group, and all had asymptomatic ST-segment depression and were able to exercise at levels that are often difficult for younger men. If applied to most patients with coronary disease, this intensity certainly could lead to a high incidence of orthopedic and cardiac complications. Rehabilitation patients with exercise-induced ST depression who exceed standard exercise prescriptions are at increased risk of cardiac events. Sub-

sequent papers described the 7-yr follow-up of these patients and the reversal of exertional hypotension in another group (27).

Ditchey et al. (11) obtained echocardiograms on 14 coronary patients before and after an average of 7 mo (range 3-14 mo) of supervised arm and leg exercise. Each echocardiogram was interpreted jointly by two blinded observers, who used three different measurement conventions and a semiautomated method of analysis to minimize errors of interpretation. Exercise training led to subjective improvement in all 14 patients and a 2-MET increase in estimated exercise capacity. However, this was not accompanied by any significant change in LV end-diastolic diameter or wall thickness. Likewise, LV cross-sectional area—an index of LV mass that corrects for altered ventricular volume and theoretically reflects directional changes in mass despite nonuniform wall thickness—did not change significantly after training by any measurement convention.

Exercise Electrocardiographic Studies

Because abnormal ST-segment shifts in coronary patients most likely are secondary to ischemia, the lessening of such shifts is consistent with improved myocardial perfusion. For purposes of comparison, only similar myocardial oxygen demands can be considered; therefore, only ST-segment measurements at matched double products should be compared. The product of heart rate and systolic blood pressure is the best noninvasive estimate of myocardial oxygen demand during exercise. The studies of the effect of an exercise program on the exercise electrocardiogram are summarized in Table 36.2. In all the studies, training produced a lower of heart rate for all submaximal exercise levels, permitting performance of more work before the onset of angina, ST-segment depression (which occurred at the same heart rate before and after training), or both.

As part of PERFEXT (PERFusion, PERFormance, EXercise Trial), 48 patients who exercised and 59 control patients had computerized exercise ECGs performed initially and 1 yr later (16). Displacement of the ST segment was analyzed 60 ms after the end of the QRS complex in the three-dimensional X, Y, and Z leads and utilizing the spatial amplitude derived from them. Analysis of variance yielded some minor differences within clinical subgroups, particularly in the spatial analysis. Obvious changes in exercise-induced ST-segment depression could not be demonstrated.

Table 36.2 Studies Performed With Exercise Electrocardiographic Analysis Before and After an Exercise Program

Principal investigator	No. trained	No. of controls	Length of exercise program	ECG lead(s) monitored	Description of subjects	Exercise ECG results
Costill	24	. . .	3 mo	CM_5	Three groups (see text)	No change in ST-segment response
Saltzman	100	None	33 mo	C_4V, CH_6	MI, angina, and/or abnormal exercise ECG	ST-segment changes correlated to changes in functional capacity
Kattus	13	15	5 mo	CA_5	Asymptomatic with abnormal exercise ECG	Similar ST-segment improvement rate in control subjects
Detry	14	None	3 mo	CB_5	MI and/or angina	No change in computerized ST-segment measurements at matched DP
Raffo	12	12	6 mo	CM_5	Angina with abnormal exercise ECG	Higher heart rate for same amount of ST depression
Watanabe	14	None	6 mo	XYZ	Mixed coronary disease	Changes only in spatial analysis
Ehsani	10	8	12 mo	V_{4-6}	9 post-MI > 4 mo; 1 with 3-VD; all with asymptomatic ST depression	Less ST-segment depression at matched DP and at maximal exercise; higher DP at ischemic ST threshold (0.1 mV flat)
PERFEXT	48	59	12 mo	XYZ	See chapter 11	No significant difference at matched DP

Note. MI = myocardial infarction; DP = double product (SBP × HR); VD = vessel disease; ECG = electrocardiogram. From Froelicher (15).

Epidemiological Studies Relating Cardiac Events to Physical Activity and Fitness

Because most animal, clinical, and pathological studies have not shown exercise to be directly related to the atherosclerotic process, it is reasonable to conclude that physical inactivity does not have a direct effect on atherosclerosis. Instead, the effects of regular exercise enable the body to better tolerate ischemia and to lessen the manifestations of coronary heart disease. In addition, it can possibly alter other risk factors for atherosclerosis. The potential beneficial actions of regular exercise are multifactorial, thus making physical inactivity a complex risk factor to assess. Some of the difficulties in studying physical inactivity as a risk factor will be discussed, as will many of the studies that have been performed.

Does exercise protect one from coronary artery disease rather than select those with less disease who are better able to tolerate being physically active? Exercise can be related to other risk factors, or markers, and studies often have not considered the selection of these factors. Particularly in a modern, industrialized society, there is usually only a small gradient of activity among different jobs. An important consideration is that people often leave active jobs at the onset of the symptoms of heart disease even without realizing the cause of the symptoms; that is, there is a premorbid transfer from an active job to a less active job that biases the relationship of inactivity to coronary heart disease. Also, individuals are often selected for active jobs or for lifestyles of physical activity. There are other difficulties in studying this question, including the uncertainty of type and quantity of exercise that is protective.

Although the most accurate way of assessing the physiological effect of an activity level is with an exercise test, few studies have had this luxury. Job title or classification has often been used and in some instances was quite accurate. However, consideration of off-the-job activity is important. Questionnaires have been used, but their reproducibility and accuracy are often doubtful. Parameters such as vital capacity, handgrip strength, and dietary assays have obvious limitations.

The methods of diagnosing coronary artery disease have included death certificates, rest and exercise electrocardiograms, medical records, medical evaluations, and autopsy. Even an autopsy has distinct limitations because it is usually not done using standardized methods. The death certificate is often coded with the most common cause of death in the community rather than with an accurate description of the cause of death. Also, multiple causes of death result in misclassification. Physicians functioning as clinicians or pathologists do not feel the need for accuracy and precision in completing these forms and records that epidemiologists do.

Many different types of populations have been used for epidemiological studies, of which there are three basic types: retrospective, prevalence, and prospective. Retrospective studies involve populations in which data have been obtained in the past not specifically for epidemiological purposes. Prevalence (or cross-sectional) studies consist of screening a population for the current manifestations of a disease. Prospective (or longitudinal) studies involve a cohort of individuals specifically chosen and studied for the purpose of following them over a period of time for the development of disease.

Physical Fitness Versus Physical Activity

The question remains whether activity level or actual maximal oxygen uptake best predicts the risk for coronary heart disease. Leon et al. (26) showed that in healthy men the results of resting measurements and a questionnaire correlate highly with treadmill time using a multivariate equation. To classify physical fitness for intervention studies, Leon et al. studied the relationship of physical characteristics and life habits to treadmill performance. Completing the questionnaire were 175 apparently healthy men, who responded to questions about habitual physical activity, smoking, beverage consumption, and sleep habits. Measured were body mass index, heart rate and blood pressure at rest and during submaximal exercise, frequency of premature ventricular beats, handgrip strength, and serum cholesterol. These characteristics were correlated with the duration of exercise using the Bruce protocol. Univariate analysis indicated that treadmill performance was significantly and positively correlated with leisure-time activity and with reports of sweating and dyspnea occurring regularly during such physical activity. Performance was negatively correlated with age, body mass index, resting heart rate, cigarette smoking, and consumption of caffeine-containing beverages. An r value of .75 was found between treadmill performance and 11 of the previously mentioned variables and increased to .81 by adding heart rate during submaximal exercise.

Retrospective Studies of Physical Inactivity

The retrospective studies include large-population studies that have utilized death certificate and population data from an entire city, state, or country. Activity level was judged from the occupation listed on the death certificate, and the end point was coronary artery disease listed on death certificates. For brevity, only the classic studies of Morris and his colleagues are reviewed here.

Morris and Crawford (34) presented data from the occupational mortality records in England and Wales, interpreting the information as support for the hypothesis that occupational physical inactivity is a risk factor for coronary artery disease. Social class, as used in these studies, was based on the grading of occupation by its level of skill, its role in production, and its general standing in the community. The level of activity was based on the independent evaluation of the occupations by several industrial experts. The activity level of the last job held was found to be inversely related to the mortality from coronary artery disease (determined from death certificates).

Morris (33) presented data from a sequence of epidemiological studies to support the hypothesis that men in physically active jobs have a lower incidence of coronary heart disease than "men in physically inactive jobs. More important, the disease is not so severe in physically active workers, tending to present first in them as angina pectoris and other relatively benign forms and to have a smaller early case fatality and a lower early mortality rate." The first study dealt with the drivers and conductors of the London transport system. They analyzed 31,000 white males, aged 35-64 yr, over a period of 18 mo from 1949 to 1950. The end points were coronary insufficiency, myocardial infarction, and angina as reported on sick-leave records, and listing of coronary artery disease on death certificates. The age-adjusted total incidence was 1.5 times higher in the driver group than in the conductor group, and the sudden and 3-mo mortality was 2 times higher.

In their original study (34), Morris and Crawford did not investigate differences in selection in the two groups but proceeded to a similar study with postmen and clerks that also resulted in numbers that agreed with their hypothesis. Morris subtitled the article "The Epidemiology of Uniforms," which reported that the drivers had greater girths (i.e., larger uniform sizes were considered because weight was not recorded) than did the conductors. In 1966, Morris also showed that the drivers had higher serum cholesterols and higher blood pressures than did the conductors. Also, a study by Oliver (36) documented that, for some unknown reason, even the recruits for the two jobs differed in lipid level and in weight. These differences put the drivers at increased risk of coronary artery disease for reasons other than an approximated difference in physical activity.

Prevalence Studies of Physical Inactivity as a Risk Factor

Prevalence (cross-sectional) studies represent a modification of the retrospective (case history) approach. The main advantage of prevalence studies is that the statistics on the studied disease are gathered at the time of the study. Thus the end points can be defined well and the methods for diagnosis standardized. Unfortunately, selecting end points is a problem, so they are not presented here.

Prospective Studies of Physical Inactivity as a Risk Factor

In 1958, Stamler et al. (51) began a prospective study of 1,241 apparently healthy male employees of the Peoples Gas Company in Chicago. By 1965 there were 39 deaths due to coronary disease among the groups. They found that the coronary disease mortality was higher in the blue-collar workers (37 deaths per 1,000 men), who had an estimated higher habitual activity at work, than in the white-collar workers (20 deaths per 1,000). However, the population in general had a low level of physical activity, and the lack of a gradient of physical activity limits the possibility of demonstrating an association of mortality and physical activity.

From 1956 to 1960, 687 healthy London bus men were examined for risk factors and coronary disease. In 1965 they were reexamined, and 47 cases of coronary disease were diagnosed, including sudden deaths, myocardial infarction (MI), ECG changes, and angina. Incidence rates per 100 men over 5 yr were 4.7 for conductors and 8.5 for drivers. However, the drivers had significantly higher blood pressure and serum cholesterol than did the conductors.

The Seven Countries Coronary Artery Disease Study included Japan, Yugoslavia, United States, Finland, Italy, the Netherlands, and Greece (3). This study minimized self-selection by complete coverage of all men aged 40-59 yr in the geographically defined areas. Individuals were classified as sedentary, moderately active, or very active as determined by a questionnaire for evaluating total physical activity. Data from the 200,000 man-years observed showed no difference in coronary disease incidence between physically active and sedentary men.

Epstein et al. (33) studied the relationship of vigorous exercise during leisure-time cardiac events in approximately 17,000 middle-aged male executive civil servants on a randomly selected Monday morning and recorded their leisure-time activities over the previous weekend. The work was sedentary. An 8-1/2-year follow-up of this population demonstrated a 50% lower incidence of coronary events in those maintaining rigorous activity on the weekend. Morris et al. reported the results of following 337 healthy middle-aged Englishmen. During 1956-1966, these men participated in a 7-d dietary survey. Men with high-caloric intakes, as assessed by diet, had lower rates of disease. A high-caloric intake can be considered to be related directly to physical activity.

Costas et al. (9) reported a prospective study involving 8,171 urban and rural men aged 45-64 yr who were participating in the Puerto Rico Heart Program. A physical activity index was based on the number of hours spent at five different levels of physical activity as assessed by questionnaire. A slight increase in risk of coronary heart disease was found in the least active group of urban men. The level of physical activity was not related to the incidence of coronary heart disease.

Paffenbarger et al. (37) reported numerous analyses of epidemiological data from San Francisco longshoremen. Work on the waterfront has been performed at relatively high activity levels under conditions that were well governed and documented by the longshoremen union. Paffenbarger analyzed a 22-yr follow-up of the longshoremen (1951-1972) for 59,401 man-years of energy expenditure on the job. One third of this experience was classified as high-energy work and the rest as low-energy work by analyzing the energy output for various longshoremen jobs. An annual accounting was taken of job transfers so that the data on energy expenditures could be correlated to the occurrence of fatal MI. Deaths from MIs were assigned to the category in which the deceased had been employed 6 mo prior to death to avoid selective bias due to premorbid job transfers. Age-adjusted frequencies of other risk factors among longshoremen were compared between the two energy expenditure groups, and little difference was found. Three parameters were associated with increased risk for fatal MI: low-energy work output, smoking cigarettes, and an elevated systolic blood pressure (SBP). Each of these factors posed an approximate twice-normal risk. Paffenbarger concluded that physical activity is protective. The threshold of 5 kcal $\cdot$ min^{-1} seemed to hold for strenuous bursts rather than for sustained activity.

Paffenbarger et al. (38) studied 36,000 Harvard University alumni who entered college between 1916 and 1950. Records of their physical activity were gathered from their student days and from middle age. Alumni offices and questionnaires were used to obtain information on adult exercise habits, morbidity, and mortality. A 6- to 10-yr follow-up during the period 1961-1972 totaled 117,680 man-years of observation after the first questionnaire, and apparently healthy men were classified with specific measures of energy expenditure. They remained under study until the occurrence of heart attack, death from any cause, age 75, or the end of observation in 1972. Weekly updating of death lists by the alumni office provided the means to obtain official death certificates. A physical activity index was devised to provide a composite estimate of total energy expenditure from stairs climbed, blocks walked, and sports played. This index was scaled in kilocalories per week and was divided at 2,000 kcal/per week, producing a 60%-40% division of man-years of observation into low- and high-energy categories.

During the follow-up, 572 men had their first MI. Men with a physical activity index below 2,000 kcal/per week were at 64% higher risk than were classmates with a higher activity index. Varsity athletic status implied selective cardiovascular fitness, and such selection alone was insufficient to explain a lower heart attack risk in later adult years. Former varsity athletes retained a lower risk only if they maintained a high physical activity index as alumni. Three high-risk characteristics were identified in this study: low physical activity index (less than 2,000 kcal/wk), cigarette smoking, and hypertension. The presence of any one characteristic was accompanied by a 50% increase in risk, and the presence of two characteristics tripled the risk. Maintenance of a high physical activity index could possibly have reduced heart attack risk by 26%.

Physical Activity and Longevity of College Alumni

In a second analysis of Harvard alumni, Paffenbarger et al. (38) examined the physical activity and other lifestyle characteristics of 16,936 alumni aged 35-74 yr for relations to rates of mortality from all causes and for influences on length of life. A total of 1,413 alumni died during 12-16 yr to follow-up (1962-1978). Exercise reported as walking, stair climbing, and sports play related inversely to total mortality, primarily to death due to cardiovascular or respiratory causes. Death rates declined steadily as energy expended on such activity increased from less than 500 to 3,500 kcal per week, beyond which rates increased slightly. Rates were one-quarter to one-third lower among alumni expending 2,000 kcal or more per week during exercise than among less active men. Alumni mortality rates were significantly lower among the physically active whether or not consideration was given to hypertension, cigarette smoking, extremes or gains in body weight, and early parental death. The relative risks of death were highest among smokers and sedentary men. By the age of 80 the amount of additional life attributable to adequate exercise, as compared with sedentariness, was 1 to more than 2 yr.

In the Framingham Study (20), approximately 5,000 men and women aged 30-62 yr and free of clinical evidence of coronary disease at the onset have been examined regularly since 1949. Coronary disease mortality was subsequently found to be higher in cohorts with indices or measurements consistent with a sedentary lifestyle. However, physical inactivity did not have the predictive power of the three cardinal risk factors. Kannel and Sorlie reanalyzed the Framingham data for the effects of physical activity on overall mortality and cardiovascular disease mortality. The effect on mortality of being sedentary was rather modest compared with the other risk factors but persisted when these other factors were taken into account.

A low correlation was noted between physical activity level and the major risk factors.

Investigations at the Cooper Aerobic Center in Dallas, Texas, have used treadmill performance to quantify physical fitness. In a cross-sectional study of 3,000 men, treadmill performance was found to be inversely related to body weight, percent body fat, lipids, glucose, and systolic blood pressure. In a longitudinal study, men who were tested on treadmills both before and after an exercise program were analyzed to determine whether their performance had improved. Those men who reached the upper quartile of improved aerobic fitness exhibited decreases in lipids, diastolic blood pressure, serum glucose, uric acid, and weight. Regular exercise resulting in increased aerobic capacity was associated with decreased risk factors.

The prospective study of Peters et al. (43) suggests that poor physical work capacity as measured by bicycle ergometry in apparently healthy Los Angeles County workers is related to subsequent MIs. This is one of the few follow-up studies that measured exercise capacity directly rather than estimating activity level. An adjusted relative risk of 2.2 was found only in men with certain other risk factors present, namely, above-median cholesterol, smoking, above-median SBP, or a combination of these. Similar findings were demonstrated by data from the Lipid Research Clinic with exercise capacity measured by treadmill testing.

Buring et al. (5) evaluated data on a series of 568 married men who died of coronary heart disease and an equal number of controls matched for age, sex, and neighborhood of residence. Information was collected from the wives of both cases and controls on a large number of variables, including usual occupation, job-related and leisure-time physical activity, medical history, and lifestyle. Usual occupation was dichotomized into blue-collar and white-collar work. White-collar workers had a statistically significant 30% decreased risk of fatal coronary heart disease compared with blue-collar workers once the effects of reported coronary risk factors were considered. These data suggest that occupation is significantly associated with fatal coronary heart disease.

The relation of self-selected leisure-time physical activity (LTPA) to first major coronary disease events and overall mortality was studied in 12,138 middle-aged men participating in the Multiple Risk Factor Intervention Trial (25). Total LTPA over the preceding year was quantified in mean minutes per day at baseline by questionnaire, and subjects were classified into tertiles (low, moderate, and high LTPA). During 7 yr of follow-up, moderate LTPA was associated with 63% as many fatal CHD events and sudden deaths and with 70% as many total deaths as was low LTPA ($p < .01$). Mortality rates with high LTPA were similar to those in moderate LTPA; however, combined fatal and nonfatal major CHD events were 20% lower with high than with low LTPA. In middle-aged men at high risk for CHD, LTPA had a modest inverse relation to CHD and overall mortality.

In the most extensive review to date, Powell et al. (44) reviewed 43 such studies and concluded that an inverse relationship between physical activity and the incidence of CHD was observed in over two thirds of the studies. Also, the relationship was strongest in those studies that best measured physical activity.

Intervention in Healthy Individuals

Bly et al. (6) reported the relationship between exposure to a comprehensive work-site health promotion program and health care costs and utilization. The experience of two groups of Johnson & Johnson employees ($n = 5,192$ and $n = 3,259$) exposed to Live for Life (a comprehensive program of healthy screens, lifestyle improvement programs, and work-site changes to support healthful lifestyles) was compared with that of a control group ($n = 2,955$) over a 5-yr period. Changes in maximal oxygen consumption were inversely associated with changes in risk factors.

As part of the multifactorial 6-yr randomized trial of risk factor intervention, 60,881 men in 80 factories located in Belgium, Italy, Poland, and the United Kingdom aged 40-59 yr were randomized (22). The treatment group received advice regarding diet, smoking, weight, blood pressure, and exercise. The intervention group had a 6.9% reduction in fatal CHD, a 14.8% reduction in nonfatal MI, and a 10.2% reduction in total CHD. These benefits were related to risk factor change and the change being sustained.

Postmortem Studies of Physical Inactivity as a Risk Factor

Mitrani et al. (32) reported the results of consecutive specialized cardiovascular autopsies on 172 European-born Jews who were victims of traumatic death. Each coronary artery was cross-sectioned at 1-cm distances to measure internal and external diameters. The percentage of vessel narrowing was calculated using these measurements. There was no significant difference between the active and the inactive groups. The results of numerous other autopsy studies have failed to demonstrate a relationship between physical activity and atherosclerosis.

National Exercise Health Objectives Regarding Exercise

In 1980, the United States Public Health Service published a report titled *Promoting Health/Preventing Disease: Objectives for the Nation*. Specific objectives (46) for the exercise and physical fitness priority area for 1990 included the following:

- *Improved health status.*
  Although increased levels of physical fitness may contribute to reduced disease rates, no specific objectives were developed.

- *Reduced risk factors.*
  (a) The proportion of children and adolescents (ages 10-17) participating regularly in appropriate activities that can be carried into adulthood (sports other than baseball and football) should be greater than 90%. (b) More than 60% of children and adolescents should be participating in daily physical education programs in school. (c) More than 60% of adults aged 18-65 yr should be participating regularly in vigorous exercise (in 1978 the estimate was 35%). (d) Half the adults 65 yr and older should be engaging in regular physical exercise (in 1975 about 36% took regular walks).

- *Increased public awareness.*
  (a) More than 70% of adults should be able to identify the appropriate type of exercise needed. (b) More than 50% of primary care doctors should include an exercise history as part of their initial exams (the specific activity scale or some similar tool).

- *Improved services/protection.*
  (a) More than 25% of companies with more than 500 employees should offer sponsored physical fitness programs (in 1979 it was 2.5%).

- *Improved surveillance and evaluation services.*
  Regarding the methodology for assessing physical fitness of 70% of our children, data should be available (a) to evaluate the health effects (positive and negative) of exercise programs, (b) to evaluate effects on job performance and health care costs, and (c) to monitor natural trends and patterns of participation in physical activity.

Intervention With Exercise in Patients With Coronary Artery Disease

Cardiac rehabilitation has been defined as the process concerned with the full development of each person's physical, mental, and social potential after a cardiac event. The following objectives should be achieved: (a) reversal of the effects of deconditioning; (b) education of the individual and family regarding risk factors for heart disease; (c) assistance in returning to activities that are important to him or her; (d) reduction of psychological disorders; (e) reduction of the cost of health care by shortening treatment time and reducing medications; and (f) preventing premature disability and lessening the need for the institutional care of elderly patients.

Much of what was known as cardiac rehabilitation has been accepted today as complete, proper patient care. It includes a multidisciplinary approach, and the health team led by the physician should include individuals with formal training in nursing, occupational and physical therapy, vocational rehabilitation, dietetics, and psychology. Although not needed in the inpatient program, an exercise physiologist can be very helpful in the out-of-hospital phases. Cardiac rehabilitation is not just an exercise program, but because of the importance of avoiding deconditioning and returning to activity and full exercise capacity, that is all that is covered in this chapter.

Phases of Cardiac Rehabilitation Post-MI

The typical constituents of the program are Phase 1: coronary care unit and inpatient care; Phase 2: convalescence—outpatient or home programs; and Phase 3: recovery—long-term community-based or home programs.

Phase 1: In the Hospital

Patient education activities during the acute phase usually consist of explanations about the coronary care unit (CCU), cardiac rehabilitation program, symptoms, and routine diagnostic and therapeutic management. The patient should be educated about the nature of the limitations imposed by the disease, the potential for improvement, and the precautions to be observed. The program must be individualized for the patient depending on his or her psychosocial and medical status. The medical status is determined largely by the severity of the MI, but the medical history should be considered.

Complicated Versus Uncomplicated MI. Morbidity and mortality in postinfarction patients who have complicated courses are much higher than they are in those with uncomplicated MIs. The criteria for a complicated MI are presented in Table 36.3. Other indices of infarction severity have been based on clinical and hemodynamic measurements (Norris, Peel, Kilip indices). The most important clinical predictors have been prior MI and the presence of CHF, cardiogenic shock, or both. The progressive ambulation program should be delayed until such individuals reach an uncomplicated status, and even then progressive ambulation should be slower.

Table 36.3   Criteria for Classification of Complicated MI

Continued cardiac ischemia (pain, late enzyme rise)

Left-ventricular failure (congestive heart failure, new murmurs, X-ray changes)

Shock (blood pressure drop, pallor, oliguria)

Important cardiac dysrhythmias (PVCs greater than 6/min, atrial fibrillation)

Conduction disturbances (bundle branch block, A-V block, hemiblock)

Severe pleurisy or pericarditis

Complicating illnesses

Marked creatinine kinase rise without a noncardiac explanation

Note. From Froelicher (15).

It is possible to assess risk at different temporal points from presentation in the emergency room, through the CCU and predischarge time, and during later follow-up. However, the clinical picture changes over time, and a low-risk patient can become a high-risk patient and vice versa. This changing risk is partially due to the vicissitudes of the atherosclerotic process, the re-formation of thrombus, interventions, and disease-host interactions. For example, a patient may present with premature ventricular contractions (PVCs) that can then disappear or worsen; in addition, chest pain may come and go, the ECG may change, or the enzymes may have a late peak. This makes it difficult to classify a patient strictly as a high or a low risk; it is only the patient's physician, aided by the nursing staff, who can determine the relative risk. However, this can lead to a great deal of frustration for the patient and the nurses. Promises by the

doctor of discharge from the CCU or other changes signifying progress often must be superseded by the day's findings. The progressive steps often must be adjusted, sometimes even several times a day.

Early Ambulation. Before 1960, patients with acute MI were thought to require prolonged restriction of physical activity. Patients were often kept at strict bed rest for 2 mo. The concern was that physical activity could lead to complications such as ventricular aneurysm formation, cardiac rupture, congestive heart failure, dysrhythmias, reinfarction, or sudden death. Hospitalization could last for months and limitations of activities for at least a year.

After prolonged bed rest, tachycardia and hypotension are common on standing. A bedside commode should be recommended because using it is less of a hemodynamic stress than is using a bedpan. The Valsalva maneuver, common when an individual is straining with a bowel movement, can lead to elevations of systolic blood pressure. However, in the sitting position it is less forceful. Controlled clinical studies of early mobilization have not found a greater incidence of death or other complications in patients mobilized early compared to patients who remain at bed rest longer. The spontaneous hemodyamic improvement usually seen is due both to improving function (scar formation and possibly compensatory hypertrophy) and to a return to normal activities.

The Effects of Bed Rest Versus the Lack of Gravitational Stress. Are the deleterious hemodynamic effects of bed rest, including decreased exercise capacity, due to inactivity or to the loss of the upright exposure to gravity (8)? Four reasons support the concept that much of these alterations are due to loss of the upright exposure to gravity: (a) Supine exercise does not prevent the deconditioning effects of being in bed. (b) There is less, and a slower decline in, maximal oxygen consumption with chair rest than with bed rest. (c) There is a greater decrease in maximal oxygen consumption after a period of bed rest measured during upright exercise versus supine exercise. (d) A lower-body positive-pressure device decreases the deconditioning effect of bed rest. Early sitting and walking may obviate much of the deterioration in cardiovascular performance.

Patient activity is regulated according to the protocol of the specific institution. Initially, it usually includes doing range-of-motion exercises, sitting with the legs dangling, and later moving on to progressive ambulation and calisthenics. Before the patient is allowed to exercise, he or she must be medically stable. There should be no evidence of congestive heart failure, dangerous arrhythmias, or unstable angina. Blood pressure should remain within 20 mmHg of the resting level. Heart rate should stay within 10-15 beats/min of the resting level initially and around 20 beats/min in the convalescent stage. If complications arise, the activity should be stopped and then restarted later at a lower level. The patient should be able to walk stairs before being discharged and by the time of discharge should be able to perform activities of daily living independently (MET level of 3-4).

A consideration often forgotten when dealing with an older patient or one with complicating illnesses is the level of activity that was maintained before the MI. If a patient was physically limited before the event, the plan for progressive ambulation must be modified. It is unlikely that a patient will be more physically active after an MI than before, unless he or she was previously limited by angina that disappeared.

In addition to the oxygen cost and heart rate achieved during activity, the duration of the activity must be considered. The effect of prolonged exercise on myocardial scar formation has not been carefully studied, but it is known that during prolonged steady-state dynamic exercise, heart rate increases, myocardial contractility declines, and LV volume increases. Although certain oxygen cost levels can be achieved by a patient, they should not be maintained for long periods of time. Probably the safest recommendation is to tell patients not to fatigue themselves and to limit the duration of exercise by their fatigue level and perceived exertion.

Exercise Testing Before Hospital Discharge. The exercise test after an acute MI has been shown to be safe. Before discharge it should be submaximal (5 METs or less). Later, when return to full activities is intended, it can be symptom and sign limited. This test has many benefits, including clarification of the response to exercise and the work capacity, determination of an exercise prescription, and recognition of the need for medications or surgery. It appears to have a beneficial psychological impact on recovery and is an effective part of rehabilitation. However, there is much debate over whether results from exercise testing can be used to identify patients who should undergo coronary angiography (17).

Postdischarge activity recommendations have had little basis for their enforcement. The patient's return to work, to driving, and to sexual activity have been based on clinical judgments rather than physiological assessments. Because of this, physicians often leave much of this up to the patient, allowing the patient to see how he or she responds symptomwise. Too conservative an approach can foster invalidism. These decisions should be made in consideration of the consequence of the coronary event (e.g., ischemia, symptoms of congestive failure, or dysrhythmias) and the nature of the activities (e.g., desk work vs. manual labor, light driving vs. congested freeway driving, or sex with an established partner vs. other relationships) as well as the response to the exercise test.

Phase 2: Out of Hospital

Hospital admission for an acute MI is a stressful experience with a powerful impact. However, hospital discharge can be equally stressful after relying on the highly protective hospital support systems. Discharge into an uncertain future and to home and work settings in which one is considered a helpless invalid can be as damaging to one's self-esteem as the acute event itself. The physician is faced with the difficult task not only of supervising the physical recovery of the patient but also of maintaining morale, providing education, helping the family cope and provide support, and facilitating the return to a gratifying lifestyle.

Contraindications to Exercise Training. Absolute contraindications are those known or suspected conditions that eliminate the patient from participating in exercise programs. Some of the absolute contraindications are unstable angina pectoris, dissecting aortic aneurysm, complete heart block, uncontrolled hypertension, coronary heart failure (dysrhythmias), and thrombophlebitis and other complicating illnesses. In some conditions, contraindications are relative; that is, the benefits outweigh the risks involved if the patient exercises cautiously. The relative contraindications include frequent PVCs, controlled dysrhythmias, intermittent claudication, metabolic disorders, and moderate anemia or pulmonary disease. If these contraindications are followed, studies show that the incidence of exertion-related cardiac arrest in cardiac rehabilitation programs is small and that, because of the availability of rapid defibrillation, death rarely occurs.

Position Statement of American College of Cardiology Regarding Phases 2 and 3. In an aging population with a high prevalence of cardiovascular disorders, the demand for cardiovascular rehabilitation programs is escalating at a time when dollar support is declining. In response to efforts by health insurances to decrease payments for out-of-hospital programs, the American College of Cardiology has taken the following position (41). Because ECG monitoring is the most costly of the services provided by these programs, it becomes imperative to redefine the role of the services provided. To achieve the goals of posthospital rehabilitation, programs can be formal or informal, supervised or unsupervised, and ECG monitored or not ECG monitored. All patients should have access to patient education with regard to risk factor modification, and dietary and psychological counseling if indicated.

The posthospital rehabilitation program should be physician prescribed and can vary greatly from patient to patient. Most patients, following a cardiovascular event, will not require formal rehabilitation services to restore them to their previous levels. Not all patients requiring rehabilitation services may have been hospitalized, and rehabilitation services for these patients should begin at the discretion of the physician.

Only a percentage of patients will require supervised, continuous ECG-monitored exercise programs in addition to the counseling services. The major expense of rehabilitation programs is the supervised ECG-monitored exercise portion, which requires trained personnel and expensive equipment. However, programs can take various forms. The program could be informal and involve patient counseling by the primary physician, who may or may not prescribe exercise to be carried out unsupervised at home or in a health facility. It could involve patient counseling by a specialist in the absence of a primary physician (if the physician is unable to provide this service) or at the physician's request. Formal programs can include patient counseling by a primary physician or counseling services plus a supervised exercise prescription without continuous ECG monitoring. They can also include counseling plus supervised continuous ECG-monitored exercise. Exercise training should be considered a dynamic rather than a uniform prescription and may be subject to change.

Duration of Programs. The exercise prescription and education programs can usually be achieved over a 12-wk period three times per week for 25-30 min per session at an appropriate intensity. Those identified as high-risk patients should be supervised, monitored, or both as prescribed by the physician.

Termination Guidelines Set Forth by the American College of Cardiology. Exit criteria are not well defined. Most patients exit a program after the 12-wk period. Obviously, some who are properly motivated could exit earlier and continue the program outside the formal setting. Others might not reach defined goals and would benefit from a longer, more formal process. Measurement of improvement should be obtained by comparing exercise performance at the end of the rehabilitation period with that at entry. Patients should be encouraged to maintain the exercise, nutritional, and psychological gains achieved in the program that provide long-term benefits. A work evaluation or activity summary should be available.

The Exercise Prescription. Stationary cycling is of equal value to both walking and jogging programs. Initially, stationary cycling usually can be tolerated at 100-300 kpm/min. If one work load cannot be tolerated for the required time span, then the interval-training method should be used. For patients with low fitness levels, this may include some zero-resistance pedaling.

Swimming can be introduced in Phase 2 but is not recommended until after the 6- to 8-wk exercise test. A swimming program has many advantages, including the fact that it is a nongravity situation. It keeps the heart rate lower and causes fewer musculoskeletal injuries. However, there is a problem in regulating swimming programs due to the wide variation in skill levels and energy costs.

Along with the range of motion exercises, strength training can also be emphasized at this stage of recovery. The strength training recommended should be dynamic (with as little an isometric component as possible) and should use large-muscle groups (i.e., arms, legs, shoulders, and back). Activities such as push-ups and sit-ups, which have a large isometric component, are not recommended.

Phase 3: Recovery

The purpose of this phase of a cardiac rehabilitation program is to prevent recurrence and to maintain working capacity. Exercises include endurance activities such as walking, jogging, cycling, or swimming, and isotonic arm exercises. A patient is admitted to the Phase 3 program after undergoing a physical examination and an exercise test and completing a medical history questionnaire.

The intensity of training is based on the patient's medical and physical status and on the results of the entry exercise test. The initial intensity prescribed is usually 70% of the heart rate maximum reserve. As a patient progresses in the program (1-6 mo), the intensity can be adjusted upward and in some participants may reach 85% of maximum. The duration of training is between 30 and 60 min and depends on available time and intensity of training. Patients should train 3-5 d per week. Once the patient has participated satisfactorily in the Phase 3 program and can easily attain the MET requirement to take part in a specific activity, other activities can be encouraged. Usually, an exercise capacity of 8-10 METs is sufficient to be placed into a jogging or biking regimen.

Monitoring the patient during the Phase 3 program can be accomplished through systematic checks of heart rate, blood pressure, and rhythm. Heart rate strips are determined before, approximately halfway through, at the end of the training session, and before the patient leaves the exercise area. Heart rate is usually checked by the patient using the palpation technique. However, in many patients, intensity can be adequately monitored by subjective personal assessments, including the Borg scale. The cost for this phase often must be borne by the patient, as most types of health insurance do not cover it.

Cardiac Changes in Coronary Heart Disease Patients. Many favorable physiological changes have been documented in patients with coronary heart disease who have undertaken an aerobic exercise program. These include lower submaximal and resting heart rates, decreased symptoms, and increased maximal oxygen consumption. Peripheral adaptations are at least partially responsible for these changes, and controversy exists as to the effects of chronic exercise on the heart. However, it is unclear whether these changes actually increase perfusion or protect the heart during ischemia. Nuclear medicine procedures to assess myocardial perfusion and performance noninvasively were employed before and after exercise training in a yearlong trial called PERFEXT (PERFusion, PERFormance, EXercise Trial) (16). There was no significant difference at rest during the three stages of exercise or the percent change from rest to exercise between the control and the trained groups at 1 yr in ejection fraction, end-diastolic volume, stroke volume, or cardiac output. An improvement in the thallium scores, particularly in the angina patients, was consistent with animal studies, suggesting that ischemia is the best inducer of collateral flow and that exercise can increase this stimulus. Changes in ST-segment depression did not occur. One of the only changes in ventricular function or volume was the significantly lower percent change end-systolic volume in the exercise intervention patients. It appears that the trained heart uses the

Frank-Starling mechanism less than does the untrained heart probably because of lessened ischemia, improved contractility, or both.

Ehsani et al. (13) have reported impressive cardiac changes in a highly selected small group of cardiac patients with asymptomatic ST-segment depression exercised at very high levels (48). However, there is an increased risk for exercise-induced events in such patients. The question remains whether the usual cardiac patient can be exercised safely at higher levels and, if so, whether more definite cardiac changes can be demonstrated.

The Effect of Beta Blockers on Exercise Training. There is evidence that a functioning sympathetic nervous system may be necessary to achieve the beneficial hemodynamic alterations of training. In addition, the limitation in cardiac output due to beta blockade may result in fatigue and reduce the intensity of training or compliance to exercise. Also, if ischemia (the major stimulus for collateral development) is lessened by beta blockade, this potential benefit of training could also be impeded. However, most studies including PERFEXT have found no preferential difference between those patients trained on or those trained off beta blockers.

Predicting Outcome in PERFEXT Patients. Cardiac rehabilitation programs are expensive and carry a risk. If a patient's likelihood of improving his or her work capacity could be predicted on the basis of initial data, much time and money could be saved. A very detailed initial evaluation did not allow accurate prediction of who would train and who would not. Even those patients whose characteristics suggested that they had the most ischemia or scarring showed as much improvement from training as did patients without such characteristics. Because many of the benefits obtained from an exercise program are intangible, it seems inappropriate to eliminate any patient from an exercise program on the basis of clinical, treadmill, or radionuclide data.

Intervention Studies With a Follow-Up (Table 36.4)

Kallio et al. were part of a project coordinated by the World Health Organization (19). The study included 375 consecutive patients under the age of 65 yr who were treated for acute MI from two urban areas in Finland between 1973 and 1975. On discharge, the patients from both urban areas were randomly allocated and then followed for 3 yr. The program for the intervention group was started

Table 36.4 Summary of the Randomized Trials of Cardiac Rehabilitation

| | | Population randomized | | | | % Women | Mean no. months entry post MI | Mean age | Length of study (yr) | Dropouts (%) | | Return to (%) | | RE-MI (%) | | Percent mortality | | | | | |
| | | | | | | | | | | | | | | | | Sudden | | Cardiac | | Total | |
Investigator	Year	Total	Controls	Exercised	Exclusions					Cont.	Exer.	Cont.	Exer.	Cont.	Exer.	Cont.	Exer.	Cont.	Exer.	Cont.	Exer.
Kentala	1972	158	81	77	150		2	53	1			5	8							22	17
Palatsi	1976	380	200	180	> 65	19	2.5	52	2.5		35	33	36	15	12	3	6	14	10	14	10
Wilhelmsen	1977	313	157	158	27 > 57	10	3	51	4		46					18	16			22	18
Kallio	1979	375	187	183	> 65	19	3	55	3					13	20	14	6	29	19	30	22
NEHDP	1981	651	328	323	280	0	14	52	3	31	23			7	5			6	4	7	5
Ontario	1982	733	354	379	28 > 54	0	6	48	4	45	46			13	14					7	10
Bengtsson	1983	171	90	81	45 > 65	0	1.5	56	1			73	75	4	2					7	10
Carson	1983	303	152	151	> 70	0	1.5	51	3.5	6	17	81	81	7	7					14	8
Vermeulen	1983	98	51	47		0	1.5	49	5	4	4			18	9			10	4	10	4
Roman	1983	193	100	93		10	2	55	9	4				5	4	7	4	5	3	6	4
Mayou	1983	129	42	44	> 60	0	1	51	1.5	25	25	30	57								
Froelicher	1984	146	74	76		0	4	53	1	14	17			1	1					0	1
Hedback	1985	297	154	143	> 65	15	1.5	57	1		45	59	66	16.2	5.4			7.8	8.4	7.8	9.1
Averages										21	29	47	54	10	8	11	8	12	8	12	10

Note. From Froelicher (15).

2 wk after hospital discharge. The cumulative coronary mortality was significantly smaller in the intervention group than in the controls (18.6% vs. 29.4%). This difference was due mainly to a reduction of sudden deaths in the intervention group (5.8% vs. 14.4%). Two weak points of this study are that more patients in the intervention group than in the control group took antihypertensives and beta blockers and that exercise capacities after acute infarction were similar in both groups.

Kentala (21) studied 298 consecutive males under the age of 65 yr who were admitted to the University of Helsinki Hospital in 1969 with a diagnosis of acute MI. They were divided by the year of birth; that is, controls were from odd-numbered years and exercisers were from even-numbered years. Eighty-one controls and 77 exercisers were accepted for the study. The training group was also urged to increase home activities daily after the exercise program, especially walking. There were two training sessions per week (later increased to three per week), and 20-min warm-up, 20-min exertion (bicycle, rowing, stairs), and cool-down phases. The exercise heart rate was optimally set at 10 beats less than the maximal heart rate obtained from exercise testing. There was no difference in morbidity or mortality between the groups. Both groups showed clear decreases in heart rate for given work loads, and both groups showed improved maximal work load, especially those patients with greater than 70% attendance. Return to work was not influenced by training; 68% who worked before MI returned to work after 1 yr.

The study by Palatsi (40) was a nonrandomized trial of 380 patients under age 65 who were recovering from an MI. The first 100 patients were allocated to an exercise program, and the second 100 were the controls. The next 50 patients entered the exercise group, then 50 entered the control group. The final total included 180 patients for exercise (including 37 women) and 200 controls (including 34 women). Exercise training was begun 10 wk after the MI and included breathing and relaxation exercises; calisthenics of all muscle groups; and walking, which progressed to running in place. Heart rate was at least 70% of the maximum rate during the 30-min session. Patients were to do this at home every day. The patients returned once a month for progression of their exercise programs. The program had no effect on the clinical condition of the trainees. There was no group difference in symptoms, smoking habits, serum cholesterol, and return to work.

The study by Wilhelmsen et al. (55) included patients born in 1913 or later and hospitalized for an MI between 1968 and 1970 in Göteborg, Sweden. Patients were randomized to a control group ($n = 157$) or an exercise group ($n = 158$). The exercise group trained three times per week for 30 min per session. Calisthenics, cycling, and running were performed at 80% of the maximal age-predicted heart rate. After 1 yr the exercise group showed increased work capacity and lower blood pressure but no difference in blood lipids. Smoking after an MI was found to be a significant predictor of fatal recurrent MI. There was also an association between stopping smoking and attending the exercise program. No significant difference was seen with respect to cause, type, or place of death.

The National Exercise and Heart Disease Project included 651 men post-MI enrolled in five centers in the United States (50). It was a randomized 3-yr clinical trial of the effects of a prescribed supervised exercise program starting 2-36 mo after an MI (80% were more than 8 mo postinfarction). In this study 323 randomly selected patients performed exercise three times per week that was designed to increase their heart rates to 85% of their individual maximal heart rates achieved during treadmill testing; 328 patients served as controls. This study was carefully designed by experts who took 2 yr to complete the protocol. An initial session of low-level exercise in both groups to exclude the faint of heart who would not comply with an exercise program was suprisingly effective in improving performance.

The 3-yr mortality rate was 7.3% (24 deaths) in the control group versus 4.6% (15 deaths) in the exercise group. Deaths from all cardiovascular causes (acute MI, sudden death, arrhythmias, congestive heart failure, cardiogenic shock, and stroke) for the 3-yr follow-up were 6.1% (20 deaths) in the control group versus 4.3% (14 deaths) in the exercise group. Neither difference was statistically significant. However, when deaths due to acute MI were considered as a separate category, the exercise group had a significantly lower rate: one acute fatal MI per 3 yr (0.3%) in the exercise group versus eight fatal MIs (2.4%) in the control group ($p < .05$). The rate of all recurrent MIs per 3 yr (fatal and nonfatal) did not significantly differ between groups. The number of rehospitalizations for reasons other than MI were identical in the two groups. The need for coronary artery surgery was also equal in both groups: 16 controls and 17 exercisers underwent surgery in the 3-yr period. This study suggests a beneficial effect of this cardiac rehabilitation program, but having an insufficient number of participants due to financial limitations and dropouts prevented the investigators from drawing a conclusion. Unfortunately, this study could not be definitive, but it does demonstrate the feasibility of resolving this important issue. It is unfortunate that it was discontinued, especially because the results were so encouraging. Only 1,400 patients would be required to demonstrate a statistically significant reduction in mortality rate in the exercise group if the reported trend persisted. The patients in the exercise group who suffered a reinfarction had a lower mortality rate, suggesting that an exercise program increases an individual's ability to survive an MI.

The Ontario study (47) included seven Canadian centers and 733 males who underwent random stratified allocation to either a high-intensity or a low-intensity exercise group. The high-intensity group trained by walking or jogging 65%-85% of their maximal oxygen consumption twice a week for 1 hr per session. This continued for 8 wk, after which time they trained four times per week on their own. The low-intensity group trained once per week with relaxation exercises, volleyball, bowling, or swimming for 1 hr. Both groups were encouraged to stop smoking and to control their weight. Less than 5% of the low-intensity group regularly exercised vigorously. The dropout rate was 47%. The rate of reinfarction in the high-intensity group was 14% and in the low-intensity group 13%. They found that the high-intensity program had similar results to one designed to produce a minimal training effect and did not reduce the risk of reinfarction.

Bengtsson (2) reported 171 MI patients under the age of 65 who were randomized to either a control or an exercise group. The rehabilitation program consisted of an outpatient exam, exercise supervised by physical therapists, and counseling. There was no reported difference between groups. Equal percentages of the exercisers and the controls (74%) returned to work. The exercisers performed 31% heavier work at the end of training and 63% heavier work at the end of follow-up. Bengtsson concluded that at 1 yr all patients were less physically and socially active than they were before their MIs. They were more dependent on their relatives than they were before and had a poor understanding of their illness.

Carson et al. (7) performed their 3-1/2-yr study on a population of 1,311 male MI patients. Seventy percent of the original admissions remained. After exclusions, 442 patients were considered suitable, and 139 of these declined, leaving 303. These pa-

tients accepted and were randomized to either a control or an exercise group. There was no group difference. The exercise group trained in a gym two times per week for 12 wk at 85% of the maximal heart rate (determined by exercise tests) or until symptoms of angina, shortness of breath, or poor systolic blood pressure response were reported. The dropout rate was 17% in the exercise group and 6% in the controls. Return to work was 81% in both groups, and both showed a similar decrease in smoking after their MIs. There was no significant decrease in mortality for the exercise group except for those with an inferior-wall MI.

Vermeulen et al. (53) described a prospective randomized trial with a 5-yr follow-up. Approximately 1 mo after the MI patients underwent a symptom-limited exercise test. There were no total descriptions of population and of training, no dropout rates were reported, and return to work was not described. Both the control and the exercise group received the same dietary advice. Vermeulen et al. found that rehabilitation did not influence smoking habits but did lower serum cholesterol. Their 6-wk rehabilitation program was associated with a 50% decrease in progressive coronary artery disease when compared to the control group. Mortality and morbidity were 50% lower in the rehabilitation group.

Roman et al. (49) reported 139 patients, including 19 women, who took part in their cardiac rehabilitation study. The control and exercise groups were comparable for age, gender, and MI location. The exercisers trained 30 min three times per week at 70% of maximum heart rate for an average of 42 mo. The mortality rate was 5.2% for the control group and 2.9% for the rehabilitation group. There was no difference in the incidence of myocardial ischemia, severe arrhythmias, or CVAs between the two groups. There was a significant decrease in angina in the exercise group.

Mayou et al. (30) and Mayou (31) studied 129 men aged 60 yr or less who were admitted with MIs. They were sequentially allocated to normal treatment, exercise-training, or counseling groups. The control group received standard inpatient care, advice booklets, and one or two visits as outpatients. They had no other education, walking programs, or instructions for exercise. The exercise group received the normal treatment plus eight sessions (two times per week) of circuit training in groups and written reminders and reviews of their results. The "advice" group received normal treatment plus discussion groups, kept daily activity diaries, had couples' therapy, and returned for three or four follow-up sessions. The three groups were comparable socially, medically, and psychologically. Evaluation was performed after 12 wk using exercise testing and standard tests of psychological state and social adjustment. There were no differences among the groups in psychological outcome, physical activity, or satisfaction with leisure or work. The exercise patients were more enthusiastic about their treatment and achieved higher work loads on exercise testing. At 18 mo the only significant findings were a better outcome in terms of overall satisfaction, hours of work, and frequency of sexual intercourse for the counseled group. The dropout rate was 25% overall. There was no difference in exercise capacity at 6 weeks, but at 12 wk there was a nonsignificant increase in the exercise group. The groups were similar for return to work, activities, sexual activity, and ratings of quality of life. There was no group difference with compliance to advice in smoking, diet, or exercise. They concluded that exercise training increased confidence during exercise in the early stages of convalescence but that the exercise program had little value with regard to cardiac performance, daily function, or emotional state.

The study by Hedback et al. (18) in Sweden was retrospective and used a control group of 154 patients and an intervention group of 143 patients. There were no meaningful group differences. Training began 6 wk after MI following a bicycle test. Training was performed on a bicycle to a maximum heart rate of 5 beats below maximal heart rate as determined during the exercise test. If symptoms or signs occurred, heart rate was limited to 15 beats below maximal heart rate. Sessions were 25-30 min long. This was done for 4 wk and then replaced by calisthenics and jogging plus a home program. Beta blockers were administered to 60% of the patients. One year following the MI, there was no group difference in mortality, but the exercise group had a significantly lower rate of nonfatal reinfarction, fewer uncontrolled hypertensives, and fewer smokers.

May et al. (29) presented an excellent review of the long-term trials in secondary prevention after MI. Trials reported before November 1981 were considered in which both intervention and follow-up were carried out beyond the time of hospital discharge. Random assignment and at least a total sample size of 100 were required. Total mortality was used whenever possible to minimize bias. All patients randomized were included in the mortality estimates to reduce the bias of differential withdrawal. Interventions not yet properly studied include cigarette smoking, bypass surgery, percutaneous transluminal angioplasty, blood pressure reduction, fibrinolytic agents, calcium antagonists, inotropics, and after-load reduction. The number of studies presented are listed with parentheses around the ones that showed a significant difference between the control and the intervention group. The effectiveness is calculated by considering the percent reduction in deaths that would have occurred if the intervention had been applied to the control group. Although few of the interventions resulted in a significant difference, all of them (except for the antidysrhythmics) show a trend toward efficacy. For those of us who recognize the clinical value of exercise and cardiac rehabilitation, the effectiveness of the exercise programs is quite encouraging. It appears that exercise is as safe and effective as are the other available means of secondary prevention. Oldridge et al. (35) reported a meta-analysis of these studies that supports the conclusion that an exercise program decreases mortality in patients post-MI.

Conclusion

Animal studies have provided substantial evidence of the cardiovascular benefits of regular physical activity. Improved coronary circulation has been demonstrated in exercise-trained animals by increased coronary artery size, greater capillary density, reduced MI size, and maintenance of coronary flow in response to hypoxia. Whether changes in myocardial collateralization improve perfusion remains controversial, but exercise probably improves perfusion when ischemia is present. Studies utilizing various animal models have reported improvement in cardiac function secondary to exercise training. Improved intrinsic contractility, faster relaxation, enzymatic alterations, calcium availability, and enhanced autonomic and hormonal control of function have all been implicated. Compelling studies in experimental animals that clearly demonstrate increased myocardial capillary growth and enlargement of extramural vessels in response to chronic physical exercise continue to stimulate the search for proof that exercise programs in humans will increase myocardial vascularity and develop coronary collaterals. Perhaps the beneficial effects of exercise would be more apparent in humans if we were as compliant to exercise programs as are animals.

Animal studies add considerable data to our knowledge of the effects of chronic exercise on the heart. They demonstrate that there are morphological and metabolic changes that make the cardiovascular system better able to withstand stress, possibly even the stress imposed by atherosclerosis. These favorable adaptations are more marked in young animals than they are in older animals. However, the data regarding beneficial effects of chronic exercise on the atherosclerotic process or on serum cholesterol levels are only suggestive, and better studies are required to confirm this effect. The study by Kramsch et al. provides the strongest evidence for exercise having a favorable impact on the primary prevention of coronary disease. In this study, exercise lessened ischemic manifestations, but only diet stopped progression of coronary atherosclerosis. Nevertheless, the therapeutic and preventive uses of exercise are supported by animal studies, but such efforts should be adjunctive to modification of the risk factors that have a well-demonstrated influence on the atherosclerotic process.

Animal studies strongly support the benefits of regular exercise for the heart. Myocardial ischemia is a necessary stimulus for the development of collateral vessels, but exercise appears to enhance their development. Exercise does not affect the atherosclerotic process, but lesions are less of a threat to myocardium supplied by coronary arteries enlarged by exercise.

In both cross-sectional and longitudinal studies, M-mode echocardiography has been utilized to evaluate cardiac adaptations to exercise training. Reported cardiac changes secondary to endurance training in young subjects have included increased ventricular mass, wall thickness, volume, and function. The echocardiographic studies have failed to yield consistent and conclusive results, probably because of the subjective nature of echocardiographic measurements. However, increases in LV mass may not occur in younger subjects unless higher levels of exercise are used and may never occur in older subjects.

An exercise program cannot be said to lessen exercise-induced ischemia as assessed indirectly by ST-segment depression in most cardiac patients. If cardiac patients are pushed to higher levels of exercise than those usually accomplished or tolerated by middle-aged individuals, perhaps more dramatic cardiac changes can be induced. However, patients with exercise-induced ST-segment depression who exceed their usually prescribed exercise limits are known to be at higher risk of cardiac events during and immediately after bouts of exercise.

The association between physical inactivity and the underlying atherosclerotic process is modest compared with other factors such as serum cholesterol, cigarette smoking, and hypertension. An inversely proportional association between the level of activity and degree of atherosclerosis has not been demonstrated. Physical inactivity does not necessarily precede the atherosclerotic process. However, the relationship between physical inactivity and cardiac events is strong.

Recent studies of primary prevention support the lifestyle of regular physical activity. Regular exercise most likely decreases one's risk for coronary heart disease and helps to decrease other risk factors. The inclusion of regular, moderate exercise in one's lifestyle makes good sense for many reasons. It can improve the quality of life by lessening fatigue and by increasing physical performance in those to whom such goals are important. The recommendation of a moderate exercise habit can help people pay attention to their health and make the changes necessary to lessen coronary risk factors. The most significant advances in public health have been in the prevention, not the treatment, of disease. The current public interest in physical fitness may be embarrassingly more effective than is the medical profession in making the public take responsibility for maintaining its health.

There is controversy regarding the effect of exercise on the hearts of patients with established coronary heart disease. High-level exercise may result in cardiac changes, but the normally prescribed programs result in only modest changes. High-level exercise prescriptions also have resulted in a high complication rate in patients who are similar to those patients reported as benefiting the most. Meta-analysis of the controlled trials of cardiac rehabilitation demonstrates a 20% reduction in mortality in post-MI patients who are in an exercise program.

References

1. Adams, T.D., F.G. Yanowitz, A.G. Fischer, et al. Noninvasive evaluation of exercise training in college-age men. *Circulation* 64: 958, 1981.

2. Bengtsson, K. Rehabilitation after myocardial infarction. *Scand. J. Rehabil. Med.* 15: 1, 1983.

3. Blackburn, H., H.L. Taylor, and A. Keys. Coronary heart disease in seven countries. *Circulation* 41: 154, 1970.

4. Bloor, C.M., F.C. White, and T.M. Sanders. Effects of exercise on collateral development in myocardial ischemia in pigs. *J. Appl. Physiol.: Respir. Environ. Exerc. Physiol.* 56: 656-665, 1984.

5. Buring, J.E., D.A. Evans, M. Fiore, B. Rosner, and C.H. Hennekens. Occupation and risk of death from coronary heart disease. *JAMA* 258(6): 791-792, 1987.

6. Bly, J.L., R.C. Jones, and J.E. Richardson. Impact of worksite health promotion of health care costs and utilization. *JAMA* 256: 3235-3240, 1986.

7. Carson, P., R. Phillips, M. Lloyd, et al. Exercise after myocardial infarction: A controlled trial. *J. R. Coll. Physician Land.* 16: 147-151, 1982.

8. Convertino, V.A. Effect of orthostatic stress on exercise performance after bed rest: Relation to in-hospital rehabilitation. *J. Cardiac Rehabil.* 3: 660-663, 1983.

9. Costas, R., M.R. Garcia-Palmieri, E. Nazario, et al. Relation of lipids, weight and physical activity to incidence of coronary heart disease. *Am. J. Cardiol.* 42: 653, 1978.

10. DeMaria, A.N., A. Neumann, G. Lee, et al. Alterations in ventricular mass and performance induced by exercise training in man evaluated by echocardiography. *Circulation* 57: 237-244, 1978.

11. Ditchey, R.V., J. Watkins, M.D. McKirnan, et al. Effects of exercise training on left ventricular mass in patients with ischemic heart disease. *Am. Heart J.* 101: 701-706, 1981.

12. Eckstein, R.W. Effect of exercise and coronary artery narrowing on coronary collateral circulation. *Circ. Res.* 5: 230, 1957.

13. Ehsani, A.A., G.W. Heath, J.M. Hagberg, et al. Effects of 12 months of intense exercise training on ischemic ST-segment depression in patients with coronary artery disease. *Circulation* 64: 1116-1124, 1981.

14. Ehsani, A.A., J.M. Hagberg, and R.C. Hickson. Rapid changes in left ventricular dimensions and mass in response to physical conditioning and deconditioning. *Am. J. Cardiol.* 42: 52, 1978.

15. Froelicher, V.F.F. *Exercise and the heart: Clinical concepts.* 2nd ed. Chicago: Year Book Medical Publishers, 1987.

16. Froelicher, V.F.F. The effect of exercise on myocardial perfusion and function in patients with coronary heart disease. *Eur. Heart J.* 8: 1-8, 1987.

17. Froelicher, V.F., S. Perude, W. Pewen, and M. Risch. Application of meta-analysis using an electronic spread sheet to exercise testing in patients after myocardial infarction. *Am. J. Med.* 83: 1045-1054, 1987.

18. Hedback, B., J. Perk, and A. Perski. Effect of a post-myocardial infarction rehabilitation program on mortality, morbidity, and risk factors. *J. Cardiopulmonary Rehabil.* 5: 576-583, 1985.

19. Kallio, V., H. Hamalainen, J. Hakkila, et al. Reduction in sudden deaths by a multifactorial intervention programme after acute myocardial infarction. *Lancet* ii: 1091-1094, 1979.

20. Kannel, W.B., A. Belanger, R. D'Agostino, et al. Physical activity and physical demand on the job and risk of CB disease and death: The Framingham Study. *Am. Heart. J.* 112: 820-825, 1986.

21. Kentala, E. Physical fitness and feasibility of physical rehabilitation after myocardial infarction in men of working age. *Ann. Clin. Res.* 4: 1972.

22. Kovat, R. Prevention of CHD (World Health Organization Multicenter Project). *Lancet* 1986.

23. Kramsch, D.M., A.J. Aspen, B.M. Abramowitz, et al. Reduction of coronary atherosclerosis by moderate conditioning exercise in monkeys on an atherogenic diet. *N. Engl. J. Med* 305: 1483-1489, 1981.

24. Landry, F., C. Bouchard, and J. Dumesnil. Cardiac dimension changes with endurance training. *JAMA* 254: 77-80, 1985.

25. Leon, A.S, J. Connett, D.R. Jacobs, and R. Rauramaa. Leisure-time physical activity levels and risk of coronary heart disease and death. *JAMA* 258(17): 2388-2395, 1987.

26. Leon, A.S., D.R. Jacobs, G. DeBacker, et al. Relationship of physical characteristics of life habits to treadmill exercise capacity. *Am. J. Epidemiol.* 653-660, 1981.

27. Martin, W.H., and A.A Ehsani. Reversal of exertional hypotension by prolonged exercise training in selected patients with ischemic heart disease. *Circulation* 76: 548-555, 1987.

28. Martin, W.H., E.F. Coyle, S.A. Bloomfield, et al. Effects of physical deconditioning after intense endurance training on left ventricular dimensions and stroke volume. *J. Am. Coll. Cardiol.* 7: 982-989, 1986.

29. May, G.S., C.D. Furberg, K.A. Eberlein, and B.J. Geraci. Secondary prevention after myocardial infarction: A review of short-term acute phase trials. *Prog. Cardiovasc. Dis.* 25:335-359, 1983.

30. Mayou, R.A., D. MacMahon, P. Sleight, et al. Early rehabilitation after myocardial infarction. *Lancet* ii: 8260-8261, 1981.

31. Mayou, R.A. A controlled trial of early rehabilitation after myocardial infarction. *Cardiac Rehabil.* 3: 397-402, 1983.

32. Mitrani, Y., H. Karplus, and D. Brunner. Coronary atherosclerosis in cases of traumatic death. *Med. Sports* 4: 241, 1970.

33. Morris, H.J.N. *Uses of epidemiology.* New York: Churchill Livingston, 1975.

34. Morris, H.J.N., and M.D. Crawford. Coronary heart disease and physical activity of work. *Br. Med. J.* 2: 1485, 1958.

35. Oldridge, N., et al. A meta analysis of cardiac rehabilitation and cardiac mortality. *JAMA,* (in press).

36. Oliver, R.M. Physique and serum lipids of young London busmen in relation to ischemic heart disease. *Br. J. Intern. Med.* 24: 181, 1967.

37. Paffenbarger, R.S., M.E. Laughlin, A.S. Gima, et al. Work activity of longshoremen as related to death from coronary heart disease and stroke. *N. Engl. J. Med.* 282: 1109, 1970.

38. Paffenbarger, R.S., A.L. Wing, and R.T. Hyde. Chronic disease in former college students: Physical activity as an index of heart attack risk in college alumni. *Am. J. Epidemiol.* 108: 161-175, 1981.

39. Paffenbarger, R.S., A.L. Wing, and R.T. Hyde. Physical activity as an index of heart attack risk in college alumni. *Am. J. Epidemiol.* 108: 161-167, 1978.

40. Palatsi, I. Feasibility of physical training after myocardial infarction and its effect on return to work, morbidity, and mortality. *Acta Med. Scand.* 599 (Suppl.): 1976.

41. Parmley, W.W. President's page: Position report on cardiac rehabilitation. *J. Am. Coll. Cardiol.* 7: 451-453, 1986.

42. Parrault, H., F. Peronnet, J. Cleroux, et al. Electro- and echocardiographic assessment of left ventricle before and after training in man. *Can. J. Appl. Sports Sci.* 3: 180, 1978.

43. Peters, R.K., L.D. Cady, D.P. Bischoff, et al. Physical fitness and subsequent myocardial infarction in healthy workers. *JAMA* 249: 3052-3056, 1983.

44. Powell, K.E., K.G. Spain, G.M. Christenson, and M.P. Mollenkamp. The status of 1990 objectives for physical fitness and exercise. *Public Health Rep.* 101: 15-22, 1986.

45. Powell, K.E., T.D. Thompson, C.J. Caspersen, and J.S. Kendrick. Physical activity and the incidence of coronary heart disease. *Annu. Rev. Public Health* 8: 253-287, 1987.

46. Progress in chronic disease prevention: Protective effect of physical activity on coronary heart disease. *MMWR* 36(26): 426-430.

47. Rechnitzer, P.A., D.A. Cunningham, G.M. Andrew, et al. Relation of exercise to the recurrence rate of myocardial infarction in men. *Am. J. Cardiol.* 51: 65-69, 1983.

48. Rogers, M.A., C. Yamamoto, J.M. Hagberg, J.O. Holloszy, and A.A. Ehsani. The effect of 7 years of intense exercise training on patients with coronary artery disease. *JACC* 10(2): 321-326, 1987.

49. Roman, O., M. Gutierrez, I. Luksic, et al. Cardiac rehabilitation after acute myocardial infarction. *Cardiology* 70: 223-231, 1983.

50. Shaw, L.W. Effects of a prescribed supervised exercise program on mortality and cardiovascular morbidity in patients after a myocardial infarction. *Am. J. Cardiol.* 48: 39-46, 1981.

51. Stamler, J., M. Kjelsberg, and Y. Hall. Epidemiologic studies on cardiovascular-renal diseases: Analysis of mortality by age-race-sex-occupation. *J. Chron. Dis.* 12: 440, 1960.

52. Stein, R.A., D. Michielli, E.L. Fox, et al. Continuous ventricular dimensions in man during supine exercise and recovery. *Am. J. Cardiol.* 41: 655, 1978.

53. Vermeulen, A., K.I. Liew, and D. Durrer. Effects of cardiac rehabilitation after myocardial infarction: Changes in coronary risk factors and long-term prognosis. *Am. Heart J.* 105: 798-801, 1983.

54. Wiklund, I., H. Sanne, A. Vedin, and C. Wilhelmsson. Coping with myocardial infarction: A model with clinical applications, a literature review. *Intern. Rehabil. Med.* 7: 167-175, 1985.

55. Wilhelmsen, L., H. Sanne, D. Elmfeldt, et al. A controlled trial of physical training after myocardial infarction. *Prev. Med.* 4: 491-508, 1975.

56. Winslow, E.B.J. Cardiac Rehabilitation. *JAMA* 258: 1937-1938, 1987.

Chapter 37

Discussion: Exercise, Fitness, and Coronary Heart Disease

Peter A. Rechnitzer

Dr. Froelicher has given a panoramic view of the complex interrelationships between exercise and cardiovascular function in healthy animals and those with induced atherosclerosis or mechanically jeopardized coronary flow and in human subjects, both those clinically free from coronary heart disease and those with documented heart disease. What emerges from all this? The salient findings appear to be as follows.

Chronic aerobic exercise definitely produces alterations in certain aspects of cardiovascular function. The most definite of these seen in both animal models and human subjects with exercise-induced myocardial ischemia is the elevation of the ischemic threshold. By virtue of some adaptive mechanism (peripheral, central, or a mixture of both), the subject can do more work before evidence of ischemia appears, measured directly (3), inferred from electrophysiological repolarization changes, measured indirectly by the double product at a constant work load, or, more recently, measured using the radionuclide imaging technique of thallium stress testing. These changes have the practical consequence of allowing the patient with stable angina to carry out higher levels of activities in daily life without subjective or objective evidence of ischemia. In this sense, the effect is similar to beta blockade, that is, it requires a lower heart rate for a given amount of work.

Much less certain is the effect of exercise on myocardial contractility. Although Scheuer and Stezoski (9) produced persuasive evidence that exercise resulted in myocardial capillary growth and contractility, studies in humans that used radionuclide techniques have shown little or no effect. The resting or exercise ejection fraction (2, 4) has generally shown no change or slight but unimpressive improvement (10), although in the PERFEXT study the end-systolic volume was less after a year of ex-

ercise, suggesting less reliance on the Frank-Starling mechanism (4).

As far as the effect on atherogenesis is concerned, the monkey study by Kramsch et al. (5) is extremely interesting in showing that in young monkeys on an atherogenic diet regular exercise reduced the development of atherosclerosis lesions. This seems to imply that regular exercise should be lifelong and not resumed in middle age after some decades of relative inactivity.

In the clinical cardiovascular outcome, an apparent effect of exercise is suggestive and seems to differ in the dose-response relationship between the long-term studies in individuals initially clinically free of coronary heart disease and those with documented disease. Among the healthy, long-term exercise (above a threshold intensity of 2,000 kcal/per week in Paffenbarger et al.'s (7) Harvard alumni study) is associated with a significant reduction in first coronary events. Among those with established coronary disease, exercise seems in the individual trials to have a marginal effect on recurrence and death, although Oldridge et al. (6) reported a meta-analysis that showed a 20% reduction. Moreover, in the coronary population, exercise intensity seems of little importance either in short-term studies (1) or in the more prolonged trials (8).

What explanation could account for the apparent importance of exercise intensity for primary prevention and its seeming unimportance for secondary prevention?

- Exercise of high or low intensity plays no role in the prophylaxis of either primary or secondary prevention, and the lower incidence in physically active individuals is really due to other factors that are already known or perhaps unknown.

451

- High-intensity exercise is of truly significant prophylactic value, but in people with coronary disease already expressed clinically (i.e., late in the course of the disease) other factors, such as myocardial irritability, the extent of myocardial damage, and so on, override the postulated benefits of exercise of either high or low intensity; or, put another way, the medicine (i.e., exercise) must be taken in large doses (i.e., high intensity) and for a long time (i.e., a long dose-response lag) to be effective. If so, for how long? We do not know at present.

We can say categorically that exercise is not the definitive treatment for coronary heart disease that, for example, penicillin, is for pneumococcal pneumonia, nor is coronary heart surgery, a low-fat diet, or any other single therapeutic approach.

Is it then, a treatment approach with limited but definite effect rather like a mastectomy for carcinoma of the breast? Or is it a pure placebo in the guise of a specific effect, like the use of pneumothorax, which was once considered to have had limited but specific effect in the treatment of tuberculosis but is now felt to have had a placebo effect?

In my opinion, the impact of chronic exercise does not fall into either of these categories. We know that it does result in physiological changes that could be described as being in the right direction, but more important are its two other effects. The less important of these is the halo effect of exercise in encouraging beneficial effects of other changes in lifestyle to occur (e.g., smoking cessation and attention to dietary habits). But the really important effect of chronic exercise is its symbolism for undiscovered or recovered potential. The realization by the patient that his or her endurance or anginal threshold has improved through his or her own effort involving self-discipline—physically taxing him- or herself often with some attendant suffering such as the transient legacy of stiff muscles and painful ligaments as well as the earned and pleasurable fatigue—is of immense and likely incalculable benefit. Anyone who has treated cardiac patients in rehabilitation knows that the satisfaction and pride of a patient (even a severely disabled one) who after many weeks or sometimes months can walk a quarter mile or even a block without stopping because of dyspnea or pain is just as rewarding to that patient as chopping a half second or more off a 400-m run would be to a young elite athlete. Exercise, therefore, as well as the improved performance that results, is a powerful symbol for the patient and reinforces the metaphysics of hope.

Finally, a word about exercise and prognosis that has been at the core of so many of the studies reviewed by Dr. Froelicher. The only scientific basis for determining prognosis is to provide the therapeutic guidelines for advising patients, and it is here that we must carefully distinguish between our responsibilities as clinician-scientists and our responsibilities as physician-healers.

As clinician-scientists we must frame our hypotheses clearly, design the studies with great care, and analyze and interpret the data honestly. But as physician-healers our responsibilities are totally different. As a therapist, be one a physician, a physical educator, or an exercise physiologist, one cannot determine the prognosis for a given patient. As Dr. Froelicher has so nicely shown in the PERFEXT study, there was no reliable correlation between the initial parameters measured and the various physiological outcome markers at the end of 1 yr. To be a good therapist with cardiac patients, that is (among other things), to be ever mindful of the importance of keeping hope alive, we should always assume that the patient is on what I call the sunny side of the bell-shaped curve. The basic concept of cardiac rehabilitation involves the assumption that physical activity, appropriately prescribed by the therapist and conscientiously carried out by the patient, will produce restorative changes in that patient's life. Moreover, these changes, psychological and physiological, will have occurred by virtue of that patient's own effort and in this sense is unlike one's being a passive receptacle for a surgical procedure or the doctor's pill. This serves to symbolize the patient's own measure of responsibility for improvement.

Viewed from this perspective, exercise has made a unique and most important contribution to the management of patients with coronary disease and, by extension, to their still clinically healthy predecessors in the general population. It is the history of the scientific struggles of this remarkable era, now spanning 3 decades, that Dr. Froelicher has so admirably presented to us.

References

1. Blumenthal, J.A., W.J. Rejeski, M. Walsh-Riddle, et al. Comparison of high and low intensity exercise training early after acute myo-

cardial infarction. *Am. J. Cardiol.* 61: 26-30, 1988.

2. DeBusk, R.F., and J. Hung. Exercise conditioning soon after myocardial infarction: Effects on myocardial perfusion and ventricular function. *Ann. N.Y. Acad. Sci.* 382: 343-351, 1982.

3. Eckstein, R.W. Effect of exercise and coronary artery narrowing on coronary collateral circulation. *Circ. Res.* 5: 230-235, 1957.

4. Froelicher, V.F. The effect of exercise on myocardial perfusion and function in patients with coronary heart disease. *Eur. Heart J.* 8(Suppl. G): 1-8, 1987.

5. Kramsch, D.M., H.A. Aspen, B.M. Abramowitz, et al. Reduction of coronary atherosclerosis by moderate conditioning exercises in monkeys on an atherogenic diet. *New Eng. J. Med.* 305: 1480-1489, 1981.

6. Oldridge, N.B., G.H. Guyatt, M. Fisher, and A. Rimm. Cardiac rehabilitation after myocardial infarction: Combining data from randomized clinical trials. *JAMA* 206: 945-950, 1988.

7. Paffenbarger, R.S., A.L. Wing, and R.T. Hyde. Physical activity as a heart attack risk in college alumni. *Am. J. Epidemiol.* 108: 161-175, 1978.

8. Rechnitzer, P.A., D.A. Cunningham, G.M. Andrew, et al. The relationship of exercise to the recurrence rate of myocardial infarction in men—Ontario Exercise Heart Collaborative Study. *Am. J. Cardiol.* 51: 65-69, 1983.

9. Scheuer, J., and S.W. Stezoski. Effect of physical training on the mechanical and metabolic response of the rat heart to hypoxia. *Circ. Res.* 30: 418-429, 1972.

10. Verani, M.S., G.H. Hartung, J. Harris-Hoepfel, et al. Effects of exercise training on left ventricular performance and myocardial perfusion in patients with coronary artery disease. *Am. J. Cardiol.* 47: 797-803, 1981.

Chapter 38

Exercise, Fitness, and Hypertension

James M. Hagberg

Hypertension is one of the most serious health problems faced by industrialized societies around the world today. To demonstrate the significance of elevated blood pressures, men with blood pressures greater than 160/95 have a threefold elevation in their risk for developing coronary artery disease and intermittent claudication and a fourfold increase in their risk for congestive heart failure and stroke (39). Even men with blood pressures from 140/90 to 160/95 have their risk doubled for these four cardiovascular complications (39). The same trends exist for women, although their disease prevalence is lower at any level of blood pressure (39). Thus it is clear that an elevated blood pressure is associated with a markedly increased risk for numerous cardiovascular pathologies.

The Impact of Essential Hypertension on World Health

The close and undoubtedly cause-and-effect relationship between elevated blood pressure and cardiovascular disease has even greater significance when one considers that 15%-25% of the people in Western societies may have hypertension (13, 39, 40, 59, 65). If a blood pressure in excess of 160/95 is used as a definition of hypertension, there were an estimated 30 million hypertensives in the United States in 1983; if the cutoff is 140/90, the estimate increases to 60 million (40). In persons over age 60, the prevalence of hypertension may be as high as 50%-60% (13, 39, 40). Hypertension is also the leading cause of physician visits in the United States (16), and is the primary cause for the prescription of medications (6). Perhaps the worst news from the hypertension prevalence studies is that nearly 75% of individuals with hypertension either are unaware of their condition, or have not sought, have refused, or have not complied with

their treatment (40, 59). Because this disease generally has few symptoms, for many the first indication that they have hypertension will be a fatal stroke or heart attack.

Mechanisms Underlying Essential Hypertension

Numerous physiological mechanisms have been proposed to underlie essential hypertension, that is, an elevation in blood pressure of unknown cause. However, at the simplest level, for blood pressure to be elevated cardiac output, total peripheral resistance, or both must be increased. Most hemodynamic studies of individuals with essential hypertension indicate that they generally have reduced or normal cardiac outputs and elevated total peripheral resistance (23, 40, 51). This sustained elevation of peripheral resistance may be secondary to an initial increase in cardiac output; the eventual increase in peripheral resistance is proposed to be a result of whole-body autoregulation to decrease cardiac output so that tissue overperfusion does not occur (23). However, in some animal models of hypertension a transient increase in cardiac output is not necessary to precipitate a rise in blood pressure (21), and an increased cardiac output is not always observed in young, hypertensive individuals.

It is also important to bear in mind that the numerous physiological variables that determine systemic hemodynamics (i.e., blood pressure, blood and plasma volume, urinary fluid and sodium excretion, vascular constriction and dilation, cardiac output, stroke volume, heart rate, and total peripheral resistance) are virtually all functions of one another. An example of this is the viewpoint proposed by Guyton (23) and Kimura et al. (43) that all hypertension is a result of abnormal kidney function. They believe that plasma volume is

455

overly large in hypertensives, not necessarily with respect to normal values but relative to the person's blood pressure. If kidney function were normal, more sodium would be excreted; this would be followed by increased fluid excretion to lower plasma volume that in turn would reduce preload, cardiac output and eventually blood pressure. However, it is also possible that a hypertensive's cardiac output, though normal or below normal, is actually too high for his or her peripheral resistance. Therefore, though most individuals with essential hypertension have elevated peripheral resistance, it is not clear whether their elevated blood pressures are due to abnormalities in the mechanisms that regulate cardiac output or in those that control total peripheral resistance. However, as pharmacologists and physicians have shown in the past century, it is not necessary to understand completely the mechanisms that initiate and perpetuate a disease to be able to treat it with beneficial results.

The Benefits of Treating Hypertension

Numerous antihypertensive medications have become available within the past 20 yr, and new and more useful drugs are appearing continuously. Although these drugs can reduce blood pressure significantly, there are numerous side-effects associated with their use (37, 40, 49, 72). One of the least obvious is the classification of the individual as a patient; the power of this classification was demonstrated in the Veterans Administration Cooperative Study (72), in which 20%-30% of the patients reported new symptoms such as arthritis, impotence, angina pectoris, and lethargy independent of whether they were on placebo or active antihypertensive medications. In addition, although patients believed that medications either improved or did not change their quality of life, their relatives nearly unanimously agreed that the medications negatively effected the patient's quality of life (37). A recent disconcerting report also indicated that hypertensive patients with ECG abnormalities, which includes 30% of the hypertensive population, increased their cardiovascular mortality when treated with diuretics (49); other clinical trials in the United States and Norway have reported similar findings. The cost of these medications, especially a multiple-drug regimen, also contributes to the generally poor compliance patients have for pharmacological antihypertensive therapies (6).

It is clear that the pharmacological treatment of individuals with blood pressures in excess of 160/105 significantly reduces their cardiovascular mortality and morbidity (72, 73); thus the benefits far exceed the risks if the therapy is tailored to the individual. However, the benefits of drug therapy for patients with less severely elevated blood pressures are still being debated (40).

It is important to bear in mind that blood pressures from 140/90 to 160/105 do increase an individual's cardiovascular risk. Actuarial data indicate that a blood pressure of 140/90 is associated with 20%-35% excess mortality in men and women and that a blood pressure of 150/95 results in nearly 60% excess mortality (65). However, the side-effects of antihypertensive medications in individuals with mild elevations in pressure may make their risk-to-benefit ratios unfavorable.

This lack of a clear-cut advantage for drug therapy in mild hypertension has led to a search for nonpharmacological therapies to reduce blood pressure in these individuals. One potential but unproven strength of these nonpharmacological therapies is that they may reduce a person's natural blood pressure, that is, his or her blood pressure when not under pharmacological treatment. This could be important because studies have shown that a person with a blood pressure lowered by drug therapy still has a risk greater than that of an individual with the same blood pressure who is not under drug therapy (40). Among the nonpharmacological antihypertensive therapies often mentioned are weight loss, reduction of dietary sodium intake, biofeedback, relaxation, and exercise (8, 9, 20, 40, 42, 66). Exercise is unique among these nonpharmacological interventions because it has numerous benefits that reduce a person's cardiovascular risk even if blood pressure is not lowered.

Hemodynamic Rationale for the Potential Antihypertensive Effect of Exercise Training

One hemodynamic mechanism proposed to underlie the potential antihypertensive effect of endurance-exercise training is the hypokinetic circulatory state that is elicited (15, 58). Heart rate at rest generally decreases by 5-10 beats/min with exercise training. Therefore, if stroke volume does not increase to the degree that heart rate decreases and peripheral resistance remains unchanged, cardiac output and hence blood pressure must be reduced.

A second potential mechanism relates to the marked peripheral vasodilation that occurs during endurance exercise (62). Total peripheral resistance decreases by nearly 85% during high-intensity endurance exercise, and resistance within the skeletal muscle vascular beds may decrease by as much as 95% (15, 58). Thus, although the skeletal muscle vasculature provides only 10%-15% of the total conductance of the vascular system at rest (58), if vasodilation persisted after exercise, the resultant decrease in total peripheral resistance would result in a lower blood pressure.

Epidemiological Relationships Between Physical Activity and Blood Pressure

Kral et al. (46) reported that less than 1% of the sportsmen and sportswomen aged 14-37 whom they studied had blood pressures in excess of 160/100. Because the incidence of hypertension in this age-group would be expected to be 5%-10% (40), these data may indicate that training reduced the prevalence of hypertension in these individuals. However, these data may also indicate that individuals with hypertension do not become or continue to be athletes.

Montoye et al. (52) found in Tecumseh, Michigan, that in men of similar age, those with the highest daily energy expenditure had the lowest systolic and diastolic blood pressures. However, the largest difference between the highest and the lowest daily energy expenditure groups amounted to 3 mmHg of blood pressure. They also found a close relationship between body fatness and blood pressure (as others have) and found that energy expenditure levels also were related to the degree of body fatness. After eliminating the confounding effect of body fatness, only the leanest men with higher daily energy expenditure levels had significantly lower blood pressures than did those undertaking less daily activity. In the men with average or the highest levels of body fatness, no significant relationship was found between daily energy expenditure and blood pressure.

Montoye et al. (52) also reviewed the results of 15 earlier epidemiological studies and concluded that, when a difference was noted between active and inactive populations, the active group always had the lower blood pressure. However, in studies that measured body fatness, when higher activity levels were associated with lower blood pressures, the more active populations were also found to be leaner.

Cross-cultural studies have also shown that those populations that are less industrialized generally have lower blood pressures and show little or no increase in blood pressure with age (13). One potential mechanism that might explain these observations is that as societies modernize, individuals in those societies also decrease their daily physical activities; however, they also add more salt to their diets and are exposed to new environmental stressors. This relationship may also be a function of body weight and fat because those populations that remain active as they age also show little change in body weight and fat with age (13).

Thus previous epidemiological data indicate that higher levels of daily activity may result in lower systolic and diastolic blood pressures. However, this effect may also be the result of less body weight and fatness in active individuals rather than a direct result of exercise.

Endurance-Exercise Training and Essential Hypertension

One way to minimize the effect of the confounding variables evident in epidemiological studies is to use animal models of hypertension to study the effect of exercise training on blood pressure. These studies have generally shown that endurance-exercise training results in a slower rate of development of hypertension in spontaneously hypertensive and Dahl salt-sensitive rats compared to age-matched genetic controls (64, 67, 68, 69). However, in none of the animal models to date has endurance-exercise training actually resulted in a chronic reduction in blood pressure; the only effect has been to attenuate the increases in blood pressure that occur with age in these animals. Thus these studies support exercise training as a preventive modality to minimize increases in blood pressure with age in persons predisposed to hypertension rather than as a therapeutic modality for individuals with established hypertension.

Twenty-five studies examining the blood-pressure-lowering effects of endurance-exercise training on individuals with essential hypertension have also been published (1, 5, 10, 11, 12, 14, 17, 18, 19, 27, 31, 33, 34, 38, 45, 47, 48, 53, 56, 57, 60,

61, 71, 74, 75). In these studies the subjects ranged in age from 15 to 70 yr, the sample sizes were from 4 to 66 subjects, and the length of the exercise-training programs varied from 4 to 52 wk. Over half of the studies used only male subjects, only three reported data from female subjects separately, and the remainder had combined populations of men and women. Thus, because of this extensive variability in study design, summary statements from these investigations must be viewed cautiously.

The total number of subjects with systolic hypertension in these studies was 671. Two thirds of the experimental groups in these studies (22 of 33) had statistically significant decreases in systolic blood pressure with endurance-exercise training. The average initial systolic blood pressure of this population, weighted for the sample size in each study, was 150 mmHg (range 130-188). The average reduction in systolic blood pressure elicited by endurance-exercise training, again weighted for sample size, was 10.8 mmHg, or approximately 7% of the subjects' initial systolic pressure.

Seventy percent of the groups in these studies (23 of 33) reduced their diastolic blood pressures significantly as a result of endurance-exercise training. The average sample-size-weighted reduction in diastolic blood pressure in these studies was 8.2 mmHg from an initial value of 92 mmHg, or a 9% reduction. However, only 495 of the subjects in these studies initially had diastolic hypertension. Seventy percent of the groups that initially had diastolic hypertension (20 of 28) reduced their diastolic pressures significantly with endurance-exercise training. The average sample-size-weighted initial diastolic pressure of these subjects was 98 mmHg, and the average reduction elicited by endurance-exercise training was 9.9 mmHg, or 10% of their initial value.

We and others have pointed out in previous reviews that numerous design limitations in the early studies in this area made us question the conclusion that endurance-exercise training lowers blood pressure in hypertensive individuals (9, 30, 62). However, recent studies (19, 31, 34, 45, 53, 71) have eliminated most of these design deficiencies by including a nonexercising hypertensive control group, using appropriate conditions for the recording of blood pressures, and ascertaining that the subjects had persistent elevations in blood pressure before enrollment. These studies have generally shown that both the systolic and the diastolic pressures of individuals with essential hyper-

tension can be reduced by endurance-exercise training.

Therefore, it appears appropriate to conclude at this time that endurance-exercise training does result in a lowering of both systolic and diastolic blood pressure by approximately 10 mmHg in individuals with essential hypertension. However, in most studies the reduction in blood pressure elicited by endurance-exercise training did not normalize the patients' blood pressures. In addition, not all data support this conclusion, perhaps indicating that there are subsets of hypertensive individuals who may not lower their blood pressures with endurance-exercise training.

A simplified meta-analysis was used to determine whether subsets of hypertensive individuals who may not lower their blood pressures with endurance-exercise training could be identified on a demographic basis. The methods were similar to those of Tran et al. (70), who treated the mean values from each study as single, independent data points. Age was not significantly correlated to the magnitude of the reduction in either systolic or diastolic blood pressure elicited by endurance-exercise training. It appears that females may elicit greater blood pressure reductions with endurance-exercise training than do males (−7/−5 mmHg vs. −19/−14 mmHg for the changes in systolic/diastolic pressure in males and females, respectively). However, only five groups of females have been studied, and three of these groups were also encouraged to initiate a mild, salt-restrictive diet in addition to exercise, although the authors stated that the dietary changes were not accomplished in most subjects (57).

Subjects who were heavier tended to have less of a reduction in systolic pressure with training ($r = -0.43$, $p = 0.06$); however, initial weight showed no relationship to the magnitude of the reduction in diastolic blood pressure elicited by endurance-exercise training. The magnitude of the reductions of both systolic and diastolic pressures elicited by endurance-exercise training were correlated to the initial diastolic blood pressure ($r = 0.34$, $p = 0.05$, and $r = 0.46$, $p = 0.01$; respectively), although neither was related to the initial systolic pressure. Thus, it appears possible that women, individuals with higher initial diastolic pressures, and, at least with respect to systolic pressure, individuals with lower initial body weights may respond to endurance-exercise training with somewhat greater reductions in blood pressure than do other hypertensive populations.

Endurance-Exercise Training and Secondary Hypertension

Few studies have assessed the effects of exercise training on patients with secondary hypertension, undoubtedly because most of them have a pathology that is amenable to various forms of medical and pharmacological therapy. However, some end-stage renal disease (ESRD) patients requiring hemodialysis have endocrine abnormalities that cause them to remain hypertensive even after their excess fluid volume is removed by ultrafiltration, and in some this removal of fluid exacerbates their hypertension. We found that ESRD patients decreased their systolic and diastolic blood pressures by 31 and 19 mmHg, respectively, with exercise training and that these reductions in blood pressure occurred despite 75% reductions in antihypertensive medications (26). Others have reported similar findings in ESRD patients (55). Cade et al. (12) also reported that four patients with hypertension as a result of renal artery stenosis, chronic glomerulonephritis, or periarteritis decreased their systolic and diastolic blood pressures by 28 and 18 mmHg, respectively, with endurance-exercise training. Therefore, it appears that patients with some forms of secondary hypertension may also reduce their blood pressures with endurance-exercise training, perhaps to an even greater extent than may individuals with essential hypertension.

Mechanisms Underlying the Antihypertensive Effect of Endurance-Exercise Training

For blood pressure to be reduced, cardiac output, total peripheral resistance, or both must be reduced. Nine studies have assessed the systemic hemodynamic changes resulting from endurance-exercise training in essential hypertensives (17, 27, 31, 33, 38, 53, 56, 61, 71). However, five of them did not elicit reductions in blood pressure as a result of endurance-exercise training. The four studies that measured cardiac output and elicited significant reductions in blood pressure with training provide a very inconsistent hemodynamic picture of the potential mechanisms accounting for the reduction in blood pressure found with endurance-exercise training. Nelson et al. (53) found that cardiac output at rest increased by 15%-20% with training, so that the entire reduction in blood pressure was due to a decreased total peripheral resistance. We found that hypertensive adolescents with above-average levels of cardiac output decreased their cardiac output with training (27). We also recently found that moderate-intensity training in older hypertensives resulted in a significant decrease in cardiac output; however, low-intensity training in older hypertensives decreased their blood pressures, especially systolic blood pressures, more than moderate-intensity training, and the reduction was solely the result of a significant decrease in total peripheral resistance (31). Thus, the systemic hemodynamic determinant that accounts for the antihypertensive effect of endurance-exercise training is unclear.

One indirect mechanism that could underlie the antihypertensive effect of endurance-exercise training is a reduction in body fat and weight. However, the meta-analysis of previous studies found no significant relationships between the change in weight and the changes in systolic or diastolic pressure elicited by endurance-exercise training ($r = 0.13$ and -0.02, respectively). Krotkiewski et al. (47) have reported that obese hypertensive females who lost weight had less of a reduction in blood pressure with training than did a similar group that did not lose weight. However, those who reduced their blood pressures with training also had substantial improvements in their plasma glucose, insulin, and triglyceride levels although their weight did not change. Therefore, in overweight persons with essential hypertension it is possible that blood pressure reductions with training may depend on adaptations in carbohydrate and lipid metabolism rather than on a loss of body fat directly.

Urata et al. (71) and Kiyonaga et al. (45) recently reported that hypertensives with low plasma renin levels reduced their blood pressures more with endurance-exercise training than did those with higher initial renin levels. However, we were unable to confirm these results in older individuals with essential hypertension (31). Urata et al. (71) also reported that endurance-exercise training reduced plasma and blood volume in individuals with essential hypertension; however, again we could not confirm this in older hypertensives (31).

The sympathetic nervous system is believed by some to be involved in the etiology of essential hypertension, and because this system is also affected by endurance-exercise training, it has also been proposed to contribute to the blood-pressure-lowering effect of endurance-exercise training. Recently, Duncan et al. (19) reported that hypertensives who had elevated plasma norepinephrine levels decreased their blood pressures with training more than those who initially had normal plasma catecholamine levels. In addition, within the group that had high plasma catecholamine levels, the changes in blood pressure and plasma norepinephrine levels at rest elicited by training were significantly correlated. Urata et al. (71) also reported significant reductions in plasma norepinephrine levels with exercise training in their essential hypertensives, and the magnitude of the reduction in blood pressure correlated to the decreases in plasma norepinephrine levels. Kiyonaga et al. (45) also reported significant decreases in plasma norepinephrine levels in essential hypertensives with exercise training. However, we have not found reductions in plasma norepinephrine levels at rest with training in older individuals (31) and adolescents (28) with essential hypertension.

Although very little data are available, it does appear that essential hypertensives on antihypertensive medications can lower their blood pressures further with endurance-exercise training and potentially can reduce or discontinue their medications. Cade et al. (12) found that hypertensives who had never been on medications, those who went off medications, and those who stayed on medications reduced their blood pressures to the same degree with exercise training. We have also found in our older hypertensives that those who were initially on antihypertensive medications elicited the same reductions in blood pressures with training as did those who had never been or were not currently on medications (31).

Roles of Varying Exercise Intensity, Duration, and Mode on the Potential Antihypertensive Effect of Exercise Training

Most of the early studies of the effects of exercise training on the blood pressures of individuals with hypertension used high-intensity training programs and generally found no reductions in blood pressure with training. Because we and others (24, 35) have shown that very high intensity programs elicit beneficial adaptations in patients with coronary artery disease and non-insulin-dependent diabetes, it is possible that such programs may elicit larger decreases in blood pressure in hypertensives. However, Roman et al. (57) found that long-term training at 50% of maximal oxygen uptake ($\dot{V}O_2$max) had the same blood-pressure-lowering effect as did training at 70% of $\dot{V}O_2$max, even though the higher intensity training increased $\dot{V}O_2$max by over twice as much. Tipton et al. (68) recently reported that spontaneously hypertensive rats had lower blood pressures than nonexercising age-matched controls only if they trained at intensities in the range of 40%-60% of $\dot{V}O_2$max. We also found in adolescents with essential hypertension that the magnitude of the increase in $\dot{V}O_2$max elicited by endurance-exercise training was not correlated to the magnitude of their reductions in blood pressures (27). Also, in older hypertensives, low-intensity (53% of $\dot{V}O_2$max) endurance-exercise training reduced systolic blood pressure more (20 vs. 11 mmHg) and diastolic blood pressure the same (12 vs. 11 mmHg) as did moderate-intensity (73% of $\dot{V}O_2$max) training (31). Finally, in the meta-analysis of previous studies the magnitude of the reductions in both systolic and diastolic blood pressures elicited by endurance-exercise training was somewhat negatively correlated to training intensity ($r = -0.40$, $p = 0.08$ and $r = -0.37$, $p = 0.11$, respectively). Thus it is possible that lower-intensity training may elicit greater reductions in blood pressure than higher-intensity training. Also, because the magnitude of the reduction in blood pressure is not related to the increase in $\dot{V}O_2$max elicited by training, these two adaptations may be mediated by different mechanisms.

Many of the early studies also trained their subjects for only 4-10 wk. However, Roman et al. (57) reported that 3 and 12 mo of low-intensity exercise training resulted in the same reductions in both systolic and diastolic blood pressures. Urata et al. (71) and Kiyonaga et al. (45) found that blood pressure was reduced after the first 3 wk of training in their patients and did not decrease further with 7 wk more of training. However, we found that older hypertensives did not decrease their blood pressures further after 3 mo of moderate-intensity training, whereas both systolic and diastolic blood pressures continued to decrease after 3 mo of low-intensity training (31). In the meta-analysis of previous studies, the reduction in systolic blood pressure was not significantly correlated ($r = 0.18$), whereas the reduction in diastolic pressure was significantly correlated to the length of the training program ($r = 0.38$, $p = 0.05$). Thus it is not clear how long it takes for endurance training to elicit lower blood pressures or whether prolonged training results in decreases in blood pressure beyond those induced by more short-term training.

Most studies of the effects of training on hypertensive individuals have used endurance activities rather than isometrics or weight lifting as the mode of exercise. This is undoubtedly because of the well-documented pressor response that accompanies static muscle contractions. This response increases both systolic and diastolic blood pressures in an attempt to restore blood flow by overcoming the mechanical resistance to blood flow in the active muscle (3). These increases in systolic and diastolic blood pressures may place an excessive demand on the myocardium, which may be contraindicated in patients suspected of having compromised left-ventricular function. However, we found that adolescents with mild systolic hypertension who first lowered their systolic blood pressures with endurance-exercise training maintained their reductions in blood pressure or decreased their pressures further with 5 mo of weight training (25). The decrease in blood pressure with endurance-exercise training was not associated with significant decreases in either cardiac output or total peripheral resistance, but maintenance of the decreased blood pressure with weight training was associated with a decreased total peripheral resistance. With the cessation of all forms of training, peripheral resistance and systolic blood pressure returned to initial levels. Along these same lines, Kiveloff and Huber (44) found that older individuals with essential hypertension decreased their blood pressures significantly with 5-8 wk of three 6-s maximal isometric contractions per day; however, no control group was included in this study. In contrast, Baechle (4) found that borderline hypertensive college-age males did not decrease their blood pressures with 10 wk of heavy-resistance training. Also, Harris and Holly (34) found that 9 wk of circuit weight training decreased diastolic, but not systolic, blood pressure in men; this study was also included in the summary of the effects of endurance-exercise training presented earlier because the circuit training program resulted in a significant increase in $\dot{V}O_2$max.

The Antihypertensive Effect of a Single Bout of Endurance

In recent years it has become apparent that some of the improvement in such heart disease risk factors as abnormal blood lipids, glucose intolerance, and insulin insensitivity supposedly elicited by long-term endurance-exercise training may, at least in part, be a function of each individual exercise session. Such a possibility was also raised over 20 yr ago (46) for the antihypertensive effect of endurance exercise. Recently, we and others have

reported that the blood pressures of individuals with essential hypertension are reduced for 1-3 hr following a session of endurance-exercise training (7, 29, 32, 41). These studies all have reported significant decreases in systolic blood pressure following a single 30- to 45-min bout of submaximal exercise; most, but not all, studies have also found a significant reduction in diastolic pressure following exercise. Those studies with appropriate study designs reported decreases in systolic blood pressure in the range of 5-20 mmHg and either nonsignificant or, at most, 5-mmHg reductions in diastolic blood pressure. Thus, although the hypotensive effect of a single bout of exercise does not normalize the blood pressures of these individuals, the transient reduction is of the same magnitude as that elicited by training programs that, on the average, consisted of three exercise sessions per week for 5 mo.

Most studies have proposed that the blood-pressure-lowering effect of a single bout of submaximal exercise is the result of a peripheral vasodilation that persists from the exercise into the recovery period (7, 32, 41). However, we have recently shown in older men and women with hypertension that this may not be the case (29). In fact, we found total peripheral resistance to be increased for 1-3 hr following 45 min of submaximal exercise at 50% and 70% of $\dot{V}O_2$max in these subjects; thus the entire reduction in blood pressure was the result of a lower cardiac output, which in turn was mediated by a lower stroke volume. Overton et al. (54) found that, following 20 or 40 min of treadmill running, vascular resistance in the iliac, superior mesenteric, and renal arteries in SH rats returned to preexercise levels within 20 min after exercise in spite of the fact that blood pressure remained decreased for 60 min after exercise. Thus the available data suggest that the transient reduction in blood pressure following a single bout of exercise may be due to a reduction in stroke volume and cardiac output. The mechanisms underlying the reduction in stroke volume are unclear at present. A reduction in preload may play a role because of a reduction in plasma volume; however, a consistent reduction in plasma volume was not found in these studies (29).

Comparison of the Antihypertensive Effect of Endurance-Exercise Training and Other Interventions

The magnitude of the reduction in blood pressure elicited by antihypertensive drug therapy depends on the aggressiveness of the treatment and on the patient's compliance and initial blood pressure. Aggressive drug therapy in patients in the Hypertension Detection and Followup Program with diastolic blood pressures closest to those of the subjects in most exercise-training studies decreased their diastolic pressures by 13 mmHg (36), which is only slightly larger than the average reduction elicited by endurance-exercise training. Even more important, these patients reduced their diastolic blood pressures only 4-5 mmHg more than did the control group; however, this further reduction in diastolic pressure resulted in a 17% lower mortality (36). In another clinical trial, individuals in the drug-therapy group reduced their diastolic blood pressures by 16 mmHg from an initial value of 101 mmHg, and although this was only a 5-mmHg greater reduction than that evident in the control group, it resulted in a 40%-60% greater reduction in cardiovascular mortalities, cardiac deaths, myocardial infarctions, morbid cardiovascular events, and cerebrovascular events (2). Thus, a number of clinical trials have shown that individuals treated with drug therapy elicited reductions in blood pressure similar to those elicited by endurance-exercise training and that these reductions in blood pressure resulted in substantial reductions in cardiovascular mortality and morbidity.

It is also of interest to compare the effect of other proposed nonpharmacological antihypertensive therapies to that of endurance-exercise training. Eleven weight-reduction studies reviewed by Kaplan (40) found a 15- and a 10-mmHg reduction in systolic and diastolic blood pressure, respectively, as a result of a 9.8-kg average weight loss. Thus, overweight individuals who undergo a substantial weight loss elicit a reduction in blood pressure only somewhat greater than the average decrease observed with endurance-exercise training. The only exercise-training study done with markedly overweight hypertensive individuals did not attempt to have the subjects lose weight (47), so it is not known whether weight loss induced by exercise training in obese individuals with essential hypertension might combine with other training-induced adaptations to decrease blood pressure more than would either mechanism alone.

It is still somewhat debated whether the effect of caloric restriction to lose weight alters blood pressure simply by reducing sodium intake. However, in a recent review of this literature (40) it was found that an 80-meq/d reduction in urinary sodium excretion was associated with a 5- and a 3-mmHg reduction for systolic and diastolic blood

pressure, respectively. Thus sodium restriction alone does not have the same magnitude of effect as does endurance-exercise training. An increase in dietary potassium intake has also been believed to lower blood pressure by inducing natriuresis; a review of this literature indicates that adding 80 mmol/d K$^+$ to the diet resulted in average reductions of 8 and 4 mmHg for systolic and diastolic blood pressure, respectively (40).

The other major class of nonpharmacological therapies proposed to exert an antihypertensive effect are behavioral modalities, such as relaxation and biofeedback. A review of approximately 15 studies of the effect of biofeedback training indicates that it reduces systolic and diastolic blood pressure by approximately 12 and 5 mmHg on average, respectively (63). A review of the effect of various relaxation techniques on blood pressure indicates that they may be somewhat more effective, with reductions averaging 18 and 11 mmHg for systolic and diastolic blood pressure, respectively (63). It must be pointed out that in many cases these reductions were elicited by single biofeedback or relaxation sessions, and very little is known about the long-term effects of such treatments. In fact, two recent well-controlled studies elicited only minimal acute and chronic reductions in the blood pressures of essential hypertensives with relaxation, biofeedback, and combined therapeutic interventions (22, 50). Thus, although some of the earlier literature in this area appeared to provide evidence for quite marked antihypertensive effects, in reality the addition of control groups appears to have diminished the effect to levels lower than those elicited by endurance-exercise training.

In summary, aggressive drug therapy in compliant patients can elicit greater reductions in blood pressure than those elicited by exercise training. However, the blood-pressure-lowering effect of exercise training in individuals with essential hypertension compares favorably with that of other nonpharmacological therapies and with the reductions in blood pressure elicited by drug therapy such as that occurring in large clinical trials and in a physician's daily practice.

Conclusion

It appears that most individuals with essential hypertension can decrease their systolic and diastolic blood pressures by approximately 10 mmHg on the average with endurance-exercise training.

Not all individuals lower their blood pressures with endurance-exercise training, but no studies have reported that exercise training resulted in an elevation in blood pressure. Thus, in light of the benefits of endurance-exercise training that extend beyond its potential to lower blood pressure in hypertensive individuals, it would appear appropriate to recommend endurance-exercise training as one component in the nonpharmacological management of patients with moderate levels of essential hypertension. Individuals with more marked elevations in blood pressure (> 160/105) should add exercise to their treatment regimens only after initiating pharmacological therapy first to lower their pressures; in these patients exercise may well reduce their blood pressures further and allow them to decrease their antihypertensive medications.

It appears that low-intensity exercise training, at 40%-60% of $\dot{V}O_2$max, may be as (or even more) efficacious in reducing blood pressure as higher intensity training. Some data also indicate that females, individuals with lower body weights, and those with higher diastolic blood pressures may elicit greater decreases in their systolic and diastolic blood pressures with exercise training. The blood-pressure-lowering effect of endurance-exercise training appears to occur in individuals ranging in age from adolescents to the otherwise healthy elderly person. The systemic hemodynamic changes underlying the reduction in blood pressure elicited by endurance-exercise training are unclear at the present, as are the neurohumoral mechanisms that may be involved.

Some studies have addressed the blood-pressure-lowering effects of weight training and single bouts of submaximal endurance exercise; however, these studies need to be expanded in the future perhaps to provide further insights into the interrelationships of blood pressure, systemic hemodynamics, and varying types of exercise. The effects of exercise, other nonpharmacological interventions, and drug therapy must be investigated to assess potential synergistic, additive, or inhibitory interactions that may exist between these therapeutic modalities in attempting to lower the blood pressures of individuals with essential hypertension.

References

1. Adragna, N.C., J.L. Chang, M.C. Morey, and R.S. Williams. Effect of exercise on cation transport in human red cells. *Hypertension* 7: 132-139, 1985.

2. Amery, A., et al. Mortality and morbidity results from the European working party on high blood pressure in the elderly trial. *Lancet* i: 1349-1355, 1985.

3. Asmussen, E. Similarities and dissimilarities between static and dynamic exercise. *Circ. Res.* 48(Pt. II): I3-I10, 1981.

4. Baechle, T.R. Effects of heavy resistance weight training on arterial blood pressure and other selected measures in normotensive and borderline hypertensive college men. In: Landry, F., and W.A.R. Orban, eds. *Sports medicine*. Miami: Symposia Specialists, 1978: vol. 5, pp. 169-176.

5. Barry, A.C., J.W. Daly, E.D.R. Pruett, J.R. Steinmetz, H.F. Page, N.C. Birkhead, and K. Rodahl. The effects of physical conditioning on older individuals: I. Work capacity, circulatory-respiratory function, and work electrocardiogram. *J. Gerontol.* 21: 182-191, 1966.

6. Baum, C., D.L. Kennedy, M.B. Forbes, and J.K. Jones. Drug use and expenditures in 1982. *JAMA* 253: 382-386, 1985.

7. Bennett, T., R.G. Wilcox, and I.A. MacDonald. Post-exercise reduction of blood pressure in hypertensive men is not due to acute impairment of baroreflex function. *Clin. Sci.* 67: 97-103, 1984.

8. Björntorp, P. Hypertension and exercise. *Hypertension* 4(Suppl. 3): 56-59, 1982.

9. Björntorp, P. Effects of physical training on blood pressure in hypertension. *Eur. Heart J.* 8(Suppl. B): 71-76, 1987.

10. Bonnano, J.A., and J.E. Lies. Effects of physical training on coronary risk factors. *Am. J. Cardiol.* 33: 760-763, 1974.

11. Boyer, J.L., and F.W. Kasch. Exercise therapy in hypertensive men. *JAMA* 211: 1668-1671, 1970.

12. Cade, R., D. Mars, H. Wagemaker, C. Zauner, D. Packer, M. Privette, M. Cade, J. Peterson, and D. Hood-Lewis. Effect of aerobic exercise training on patients with systemic arterial hypertension. *Am. J. Med.* 77: 785-790, 1984.

13. Cassel, J. Studies of hypertension in migrants. In: Paul, O., ed. *Epidemiology and control of hypertension*. Miami: Symposia Specialists, 1975, pp. 41-62.

14. Choquette, G., and R.J. Ferguson. Blood pressure reduction in "borderline" hypertensives following physical training. *Can. Med. Assoc. J.* 108: 699-703, 1973.

15. Clausen, J.P. Circulatory adjustments to dynamic exercise and effect of physical training

in normal subjects and in patients with coronary artery disease. *Prog. Cardiovasc. Dis.* 18: 459-495, 1976.

16. Cypress, B.K. NCHS Advance Data, No. 80, July 22, 1982, Vital and Health Statistics of the National Center for Health Statistics. U.S. Department of Health and Human Services.

17. DePlaen, J.F., and J.M. Detry. Hemodynamic effects of physical training in established arterial hypertension. *Acta Cardiol.* 35: 179-188, 1980.

18. DeVries, H.A. Physiological effects of an exercise training regimen upon men aged 52 to 88. *J. Gerontol.* 25: 325-336, 1970.

19. Duncan, J.J., J.E. Farr, J. Upton, R.D. Hagan, M.E. Oglesby, and S.N. Blair. The effects of aerobic exercise on plasma catecholamines and blood pressure in patients with mild essential hypertension. *JAMA* 254: 2609-2613, 1985.

20. Fagard, R., J.R. M'Buyamba, J. Staessen, L. VanHees, and A. Amery. Physical activity and blood pressure. In: Bulpitt, C.J., ed. *Handbook of hypertension: Epidemiology of hypertension.* Amsterdam: Elsevier, 1985: vol. 6, pp. 104-130.

21. Ferrario, C.M., and I.H. Page. Current views concerning cardiac output in the genesis of experimental hypertension. *Circ. Res.* 43: 821-831, 1978.

22. Glasgow, M.S., K.R. Gaardner, and B.T. Engel. Behavioral treatment of high blood pressure: II. Acute and sustained effects of relaxation and systolic blood pressure feedback. *Psychosom. Med.* 44: 155-170, 1982.

23. Guyton, A.C. Renal function curve—a key to understanding the pathogenesis of hypertension. *Hypertension* 10: 1-6, 1987.

24. Hagberg, J.M. Central and peripheral adaptations to training in patients with coronary artery disease. In: Saltin, B., ed. *Biochemistry of exercise VI.* Champaign, IL: Human Kinetics, 1986, pp. 267-278.

25. Hagberg, J.M., A.A. Ehsani, D. Goldring, A. Hernandez, D.R. Sinacore, and J.O. Holloszy. Effect of weight training on blood pressure and hemodynamics in hypertensive adolescents. *J. Pediatr.* 104: 147-151, 1984.

26. Hagberg, J.M., A.P. Goldberg, A.A. Ehsani, G.W. Heath, J.A. Delmez, and H.R. Harter. Exercise training improves hypertension in hemodialysis patients. *Am. J. Nephrol.* 3: 209-212, 1983.

27. Hagberg, J.M., D. Goldring, A.A. Ehsani, G.W. Heath, A. Hernandez, K. Schechtman, and J.O. Holloszy. Effect of exercise training on the blood pressure and hemodynamic features of hypertensive adolescents. *Am. J. Cardiol.* 52: 763-768, 1983.

28. Hagberg, J.M., D. Goldring, G.W. Heath, A.A. Ehsani, A. Hernandez, and J.O. Holloszy. Effect of exercise training on plasma catecholamines and hemodynamics of adolescent hypertensives during rest, submaximal exercise, and orthostatic stress. *Clin. Physiol.* 4: 117-124, 1984.

29. Hagberg, J.M., S.J. Montain, and W.H. Martin. Blood pressure and hemodynamic responses after exercise in older hypertensives. *J. Appl. Physiol.* 63: 270-276, 1987.

30. Hagberg, J.M., and D.R. Seals. Exercise training and hypertension. *Acta Med. Scand.* Suppl. 711: 131-136, 1987.

31. Hagberg, J.M., S.J. Montain, W.H. Martin, and A.A. Ehsani. Effect of exercise training on 60-69 year old essential hypertensives. *Am. J. Cardiol.* In press.

32. Hannum, S.M., and F.W. Kasch. Acute postexercise blood pressure response of hypertensive and normotensive men. *Scand. J. Sports Sci.* 3: 11-15, 1981.

33. Hanson, J.S., and W.H. Nedde. Preliminary observations on physical training for hypertensive males. *Circ. Res.* 27(Suppl. 1): 49-53, 1970.

34. Harris, K.A., and R.G. Holly. Physiological response to circuit weight training in borderline hypertensive subjects. *Med. Sci. Sports Exerc.* 19: 246-252, 1987.

35. Holloszy, J.O., J. Schultz, J. Kusnierkiewicz, J.M. Hagberg, and A.A. Ehsani. Effects of exercise on glucose tolerance and insulin resistance. *Acta Med. Scand.* Suppl. 711: 55-65, 1987.

36. Hypertension Detection and Followup Program Cooperative Group. Five year findings of the Hypertension Detection and Followup Program: I. Reduction in mortality of persons with high blood pressure, including mild hypertension. *JAMA* 242: 2562-2571, 1979.

37. Jachuk, S.J., H. Brierly, S. Jachuk, and D.M. Willcox. The effect of hypotensive drugs on the quality of life. *J. Roy. Coll. Gen. Pract.* 32: 103-105, 1982.

38. Johnson, W.P., and J.A. Grover. Hemodynamic and metabolic effects of physical training in four patients with essential hypertension. *Can. Med. Assoc. J.* 96: 842-846, 1967.

39. Kannel, W.B., J.T. Doyle, A.M. Ostfeld, C.D. Jenkins, L. Kuller, R.N. Podell, and J. Stam-

ler. Original resources for primary prevention of atherosclerotic diseases. *Circulation* 70: 157A-205A, 1984.

40. Kaplan, N. *Clinical hypertension*. 4th ed. Baltimore: Williams & Wilkins, 1986.

41. Kaufman, F.L., R.L. Hughson, and J.P. Schaman. Effect of exercise on recovery blood pressure in normotensive and hypertensive subjects. *Med. Sci. Sports Exerc.* 19: 17-20, 1987.

42. Kenney, W.L., and E.J. Zambraski. Physical activity in human hypertension—a mechanisms approach. *Sports Med.* 1: 459-473, 1984.

43. Kimura, G., F. Saito, S. Kojima, H. Yoshimi, H. Abe, Y. Kawano, K. Yoshida, T. Ashida, M. Kawamura, M. Kuamochi, K. Ito, and T. Omae. Renal function curve in patients with secondary forms of hypertension. *Hypertension* 10: 11-15, 1987.

44. Kiveloff, B., and O. Huber. Brief maximal isometric exercise in hypertension. *J. Am. Geriatr. Soc.* 19: 1006-1009, 1971.

45. Kiyonaga, A., K. Arakawa, H. Tanaka, and M. Shindo. Blood pressure and hormonal responses to aerobic exercise. *Hypertension* 7: 125-131, 1985.

46. Kral, J., J. Chrastek, and J. Adamirova. The hypotensive effect of physical activity in hypertensive subjects. In: Raab, W., ed. *Prevention of ischemic heart disease: Principles and practice*. Springfield, IL: Charles C Thomas, 1966.

47. Krotkiewski, M., K. Mandroukas, L. Sjöström, L. Sullivan, H. Wetterqvist, and P. Björntorp. Effects of long-term physical training on body fat, metabolism, and blood pressure in obesity. *Metabolism* 28: 650-658, 1979.

48. Kukkonen, K., R. Rauramaa, E. Voutilainen, and E. Lansimies. Physical training of middle-aged men with borderline hypertension. *Ann. Clin. Res.* 14(Suppl. 34): 139-145, 1982.

49. Kuller, L.H., S.B. Hulley, J.D. Cohen, and J. Neaton. Unexpected effects of treating hypertension in men with ECG abnormalities: A critical analysis. *Circulation* 73: 114-123, 1986.

50. Luborsky, L., P. Crits-Christoph, J.P. Brady, R.E. Kron, T. Weiss, M. Cohen, and L. Levy. Behavioral versus pharmacological treatments for essential hypertension—a needed comparison. *Psychosom. Med.* 44: 203-213, 1982.

51. Lund-Johansen, P. Hemodynamic alterations in hypertension—spontaneous changes and effects of drug therapy: A review. *Acta Med. Scand. Suppl.* 603: 1-14, 1977.

52. Montoye, H.J., H.L. Metzner, and J.B. Keller. Habitual physical activity and blood pressure. *Med. Sci. Sports* 4: 175-181, 1972.

53. Nelson, L., M.D. Esler, G.L. Jennings, and P.I. Korner. Effect of changing levels of physical activity on blood pressure and haemodynamics in essential hypertension. *Lancet* ii: 473-476, 1986.

54. Overton, M.J., M.J. Joyner, and C.M. Tipton. Reductions in blood pressure after acute exercise by hypertensive rats. *J. Appl. Physiol.* 64: 742-747, 1988.

55. Painter, P.L., J.N. Nelson-Worrel, M.M. Hill, D.R. Thronbery, W.R. Schelp, A.R. Harrington, and A.B. Weinstein. Effects of exercise training during hemodialysis. *Nephron.* 43: 87-92, 1986.

56. Ressl, J., J. Chrastek, and R. Jandova. Haemodynamic effects of physical training in essential hypertension. *Cardiologica* 32: 121-133, 1977.

57. Roman, O., A.L. Camuzzi, E. Villalon, and C. Klenner. Physical training program in arterial hypertension: A long-term prospective follow-up. *Cardiology* 67: 230-243, 1981.

58. Rowell, L.B. *Human circulation: Regulation during physical stress*. New York: Oxford University Press, 1986.

59. Rowland, M., and J. Roberts. *Vital and health statistics of the National Center for Health Statistics* (NCHS Advance Data No. 84). Washington, DC: U.S. Department of Health and Human Services, October 8, 1982.

60. Rudd, J.L., and W.C. Day. A physical fitness program for patients with hypertension. *J. Am. Geriatr. Soc.* 15: 373-379, 1967.

61. Sannerstedt, R., H. Wasir, R. Henning, and L. Werko. Systemic haemodynamics in mild arterial hypertension before and after physical training. *Clin. Sci. Molec. Med.* 45: 145s-149s, 1973.

62. Seals, D.R., and J.M. Hagberg. The effect of exercise training on human hypertension: A review. *Med. Sci. Sports Exerc.* 16: 207-215, 1984.

63. Shapiro, A.P., G.E. Schwartz, D.C.E. Ferguson, D.P. Redmond, and S.M. Weiss. Behavioral methods in the treatment of hypertension: A review of their clinical status. *Ann. Intern. Med.* 86: 626-636, 1977.

64. Shepherd, R.E., M.L. Kuehne, K.A. Kenno, J.L. Durstine, T.W. Balon, and J.P. Rapp. Attenuation of blood pressure increases in Dahl salt-sensitive rats by exercise. *J. Appl. Physiol.* 52: 1608-1613, 1982.

65. Society of Actuaries and Association of Life Insurance Medical Directors of America. *Blood pressure study, 1979.* Chicago: Author, 1980.

66. Tipton, C.M. Exercise, training, and hypertension. In: Terjung, R., ed. *Exercise and sport science reviews.* Lexington, MA: D.C. Heath, 1984, pp. 245-306.

67. Tipton, C.M., R.D. Matthes, A. Callahan, T.-K. Tcheng, and L.T. Lais. The role of chronic exercise on resting blood pressures of normotensive and hypertensive rats. *Med. Sci. Sports* 9: 168-177, 1977.

68. Tipton, C.M., R.D. Matthes, K.D. Marcus, K.A. Rowlett, and J.R. Leininger. Influences of exercise intensity, age, and medication on resting blood pressure in SHR populations. *J. Appl. Physiol.* 55: 1305-1310, 1983.

69. Tipton, C.M., M.S. Sturek, R.A. Oppliger, R.D. Matthes, J.M. Overton, and J.G. Edwards. Responses of SHR to combinations of chemical sympathectomy, adrenal demedullation, and training. *Am. J. Physiol.* 247: H109-H118, 1984.

70. Tran, Z.V., A. Weltman, G.V. Glass, and D.P. Mood. The effects of exercise on blood lipids and lipoproteins: A meta-analysis of studies. *Med. Sci. Sports Exerc.* 15: 392-402, 1983.

71. Urata, H., Y. Tanabe, A. Kiyonaga, M. Ikeda, H. Tanaka, M. Shindo, and K. Arakawa. Antihypertensive and volume-depleting effects of mild exercise on essential hypertension. *Hypertension* 9: 245-252, 1987.

72. Veterans Administration Cooperative Study Group on Antihypertensive Agents. Effects of treatment on mortality in hypertension: III. Influence of age, diastolic pressure, and prior cardiovascular disease: Further analysis of side effects. *Circulation* 45: 991-1004, 1972.

73. Veterans Administration Cooperative Study Group on Antihypertensive Agents. Effects of treatment on morbidity in hypertension: Results in patients with diastolic blood pressures averaging 115 through 129 mmHg. *JAMA* 202: 116-122, 1967.

74. Weber, F., R.J. Barnard, and D. Roy. Effects of a high-complex-carbohydrate, low-fat diet and daily exercise on individuals 70 years and older. *J. Gerontol.* 38: 155-161, 1986.

75. Wilmore, J.H., J. Royce, and R.N. Girandola. Physiological alterations resulting from a 10 week program of jogging. *Med. Sci. Sports* 2: 7-14, 1970.

Chapter 39

Exercise, Fitness, and Diabetes

Mladen Vranic
David Wasserman

Maximizing work capacity while minimizing alterations in glucose homeostasis requires not only a quantitative matching of glucose production to its accelerated uptake at the muscle but also a specific balancing of fat and carbohydrate utilization. Control of optimal substrate balance during exercise is achieved largely by the actions of insulin, glucagon, and catecholamines, whereas the role of other hormones such as cortisol, growth hormone, and IGF 1 and 2 needs to be explored further. The decrease in plasma insulin secretion during exercise sensitizes the liver to the effects of the counterregulatory hormones and facilitates the mobilization of triglycerides and muscle glycogen. A small amount of insulin appears to be essential in controlling glucose uptake in vivo but may not be important in isolated contracting muscle when factors antagonistic to glucose uptake, such as the catecholamines or free fatty acids (FFA), are absent. Glucagon controls at least 60% of glucose output during exercise in normal dogs and at least 50% in alloxan-diabetic dogs. However, the strongest correlate to hepatic glucose output is not glucagon per se but the glucagon-to-insulin molar ratio. In contrast to glucagon, the beta-adrenergic effects of catecholamines do not have important glucoregulatory effects at the liver but are critical in the mobilization of triglycerides and muscle glycogen. By providing fats and intramuscular glycogen for fuel at an increased rate, the catecholamines decrease the reliance of muscle on blood-borne glucose and lead to impaired glucose uptake.

Because poorly controlled diabetes is accompanied by diminished basal insulin levels and exaggerated glucagon and catecholamine responses to exercise, optimal substrate balance is lost. In general, diabetes is associated with a shift in substrate utilization during exercise away from carbohydrates to increased fat metabolism. The importance of beta-adrenergic mechanisms in this fuel shift is demonstrated in diabetes by the partial normalization of substrate metabolism (increased glucose metabolic clearance and reduced plasma free fatty acids and lactate) during exercise with concurrent beta-adrenergic blockade. Thus, the glucagon-to-insulin ratio regulates the dynamics of glucose release from the liver, whereas the interaction between the catecholamines and insulin controls extrahepatic substrate mobilization in both health and diabetes.

Increased metabolic demand can uncouple these hormonal effects on substrate metabolism. Thus, a mild reduction in oxygen availability will greatly exaggerate the norepinephrine and epinephrine responses to exercise, but glucose clearance actually increases fourfold above the normal exercise increment. These observations indicate that hypoxia is able to counterbalance the effects of the catecholamines on glucose uptake by muscle effectively. Therefore, in addition to hormonal mechanisms, oxygen availability and metabolic demand must be considered in control of substrate balance during exercise. The literature quoted in this chapter has been published, for the most part, in the last 5 yr. A more complete list of references can be found in previously published studies (33, 81, 95, 96, 113, 117).

Principles of Substrate Utilization During Exercise

To provide metabolic substrate in the postabsorptive state, an organism must have the capacity to store and mobilize fuel. For this purpose, carbohydrates are stored as glycogen in muscle and liver, and fatty acids are stored mainly as triglycerides, primarily in adipose tissue but also in muscle. To a lesser extent, protein may be used as fuel, particularly when the availability of other substrates is limited. The metabolic requirement of working muscle creates an additional demand on these stores beyond that seen at rest, the extent of which depends on the intensity and duration of exercise. It has long since been known that the fuel utilized during exercise, as at rest, is a combination of different substrates. During the transition from rest to moderate-intensity exercise, the muscle shifts from using primarily FFA to using a blend of FFA, extramuscular glucose, and glycogen. During the early stages of exercise, muscle glycogen is the chief source of energy for muscular contraction. With increasing duration, the contributions of circulating glucose and particularly FFA become of increasing importance as muscle glycogen gradually depletes, and the origin of glucose shifts from hepatic glycogenolysis to gluconeogenesis (1) as intrahepatic mechanisms channel a greater portion of the ^3C molecules into glucose (111). With increasing intensity the balance of substrates used shifts to a greater oxidation of carbohydrates (46, 99). Thus, the contribution of each substrate depends on work intensity and duration as well as on the type of exercise. The relative proportion of each substrate utilized is oriented toward the three main aims that follow.

Preserving Glucose Homeostasis

Because of its essential function in the nervous system, glucose must be regulated within narrow limits. During heavy exercise, blood glucose levels tend to increase (99) and during prolonged exercise may fall gradually (1, 35). However, exercise is generally characterized by euglycemia (26). Thus, the increase in hepatic glucose production rapidly and quantitatively matches the increment in glucose uptake. The tendency for blood glucose to remain constant despite large increases in glucose uptake is central to the understanding of glucoregulation during exercise. The deviations in blood glucose observed during heavy or prolonged work may give additional insight into the function of this control system.

Metabolizing the Most Efficient Substrate (Metabolic and Storage Efficiency)

Metabolic Efficiency

During high-intensity work, when adenosine triphosphate (ATP) hydrolysis is particularly rapid and oxygen availability may be limited, carbohydrates are preferred. Generation of ATP from oxi-

dation of glucose in the cytoplasm occurs more rapidly than it does from fat oxidation in the mitochondria (61). Furthermore, because glucose carbon atoms are already partially oxidized compared to the highly saturated carbon skeleton of fats, they require less oxygen to extract the electrons that provide the energy needed for ATP formation. Hence, when oxygen availability is limited, such as during heavy exercise or in hypoxia, glucose is the most efficient fuel.

Storage Efficiency

During moderate exercise, which can be sustained for long intervals, speed and efficiency of energy transduction become secondary to fuel storage efficiency. Twice as much energy can be gained from the oxidation of 1 g of pure triglyceride as from that of 1 g of pure glycogen. In addition, whereas glycogen is stored in combination with water, fats are water insoluble and are stored in pure form. Hence, fat storage is both economical and efficient for long-duration exercise. For example, the importance of massive storage of fats is apparent in migratory birds in the weeks before spring and fall migration or in the muscle of salmon just before the spawning migration.

Delaying Exhaustion (Preserving Muscle Glycogen)

Substrate balance is adjusted during exercise to prevent muscle fatigue. Although muscle glycogen concentration is relatively small, this substrate is of great importance in work performance. High correlations exist between the time it takes to reach exhaustion and the initial amount of glycogen (2) and between glycogen depletion and exhaustion (30). Hence, intramuscular and extramuscular fat and extramuscular glucose must be utilized as alternate substrates to delay the depletion of muscle glycogen while not greatly perturbing homeostasis or sacrificing metabolic efficiency. The importance of maximizing glycogen stores to the athlete is evidenced by the practice of carbohydrate loading before an endurance race.

Hormonal Control of Substrate Metabolism During Exercise

Exercise is characterized by diverse endocrine responses as well as an increased adrenergic drive, both of which are dependent on the duration and intensity of exercise. In general, there is a fall in insulin and increases in glucagon, catecholamines, and cortisol, among other hormones. Recent work has indicated that the control of the optimal substrate balance during exercise is achieved largely by the combined action of these hormones (23, 32, 36, 37, 44, 107, 109, 116, 120). In addition to hormonal factors, other parameters, such as blood flow shifts (23), subtle changes in glycemia (44, 45), or metabolic state (19, 44, 106), play a role in the control of fuel metabolism.

Regulation of Hepatic Carbohydrate Metabolism

The Role of the Glucagon-Insulin Ratio

The presence of glucagon (15, 36, 78, 109, 116) and, more precisely, the appropriate interaction of glucagon with insulin (37, 108, 116) (Figure 39.1) are essential during exercise in regulating glucose production and, as a consequence, blood glucose. When glucagon secretion is suppressed below basal with somatostatin, hepatic glucose production is attenuated by 60% during exercise (116). In the resting state, glucagon also controls about 60% of the hepatic glucose production (17), but because the rate of glucose release is accelerated, the absolute effects of glucagon action are considerably greater during exercise (Figure 39.2). It is particularly important that the strongest correlate to glucose production is not glucagon per se but the ratio of glucagon to insulin (36, 108, 116).

Recent studies in humans (32, 83, 120) have extended previous work by trying to determine whether changes in glucagon and insulin from basal are essential for the regulation of glucose production during exercise. The endogenous releases of glucagon and insulin were prevented with somastatin, and the pancreatic hormones were replaced in a peripheral vein so that normal arterial levels of these hormones and euglycemia were achieved. Although with normal exercise glucagon increases and insulin decreases, in these studies the hormone levels were unchanged. Despite the inability of the pancreatic hormones to adapt to muscular work, hepatic glucose production responded normally to exercise (32). These results are not conclusive because the normal entry site of the pancreatic hormones (i.e., into the portal vein) is virtually inaccessible in human subjects, and replacement is therefore given into a peripheral vein. Thus the important portoperipheral insulin gradient is lost, and presumably the liver is hypoinsulinemic under these conditions. When an attempt was made to overcome this problem by replacing insulin at increased rates to create portal euinsulinemia (albeit peripheral hyperinsulinemia) and euglycemia maintained with glucose infusion, hepatic glucose production was attenuated (83, 120). It was concluded that indeed physiological changes in the pancreatic hormones are important for normal glucose kinetics during exercise.

The dog has also been used to study the metabolic role of the exercise-induced fall in insulin that

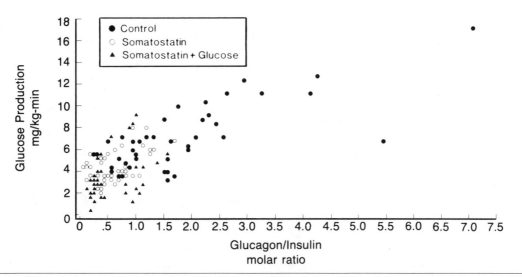

Figure 39.1. The relationship between hepatic glucose production and the glucagon-to-insulin ratio. Plotted are values from exercise alone (n = 20), exercise plus somatostatin (n = 20), and exercise plus somatostatin with euglycemic glucose replacement. Correlation coefficient for the pooled data = .86. Reproduced from *The Journal of Clinical Investigation*, 1984, **74**, 1404, by copyright permission of the American Society for Clinical Investigation.

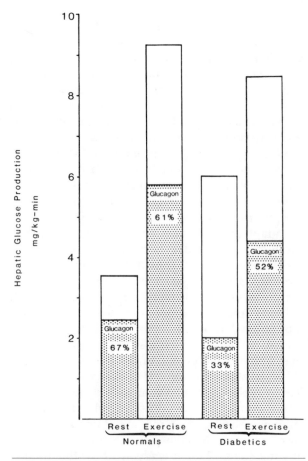

Figure 39.2. The role of glucagon in regulation of hepatic glucose production during rest and exercise in normal and alloxan-diabetic dogs. The shaded area represents the portion of the hepatic glucose production controlled by glucagon. From "Interaction Between Insulin and Counterregulatory Hormones in Control of Substrate Utilization in Health and Diabetes During Exercise" by D.H. Wasserman and M. Vranic, 1986, *Diabetes/Metabolism Reviews*, **1**(4), p. 159. Reprinted by permission of John Wiley & Sons, Inc.

is independent of glucagon (114). One advantage is that the two pancreatic hormones can be infused into the portal vein, thereby alleviating the problem caused by introducing insulin peripherally (32, 83, 120). When insulin was infused intraportally at the onset of exercise to prevent its fall, the increase in glucagon was blunted. The failure of insulin to fall and of glucagon to rise led to a 78% reduction in tracer-determined glucose output. Furthermore, the exercise-induced increase in the gluconeogenic conversion rate and efficiency was almost completely abolished. When the fall in insulin was prevented and normal exercising glucagon levels were restored by an intraportal infusion of this hormone, glucose production was still only

45% of the normal response, but the gluconeogenic conversion rate and efficiency were normalized (115). Thus the fall in insulin facilitates the rise of glucagon, and normal changes in insulin and glucagon are necessary for the control of glucose production. Furthermore, the fall in insulin controls liver glycogenolysis, whereas the rise in glucagon is critical for the increase in both gluconeogenesis and glycogenolysis.

The Role of Catecholamines

The role of catecholamines has been studied using beta- and alpha-adrenergic blockers and the effects of adrenalectomy and adrenodemedullation. Beta and alpha blockade independently (84, 107) or combined (32, 84) do not affect the increment in hepatic glucose production in humans. The role of epinephrine has been studied in subjects adrenalectomized for treatment of Cushing's disease or bilateral pheochromocytoma (31). Because hepatic glucose production increased normally, it appears that epinephrine is an unimportant determinant of glucose production during exercise. Studies in the rat have been conflicting, demonstrating either no effect of adrenodemedullation on net hepatic glycogen breakdown (4, 119) or a decrease in net hepatic glycogen breakdown and tracer-determined glucose production (85). Furthermore, hepatic denervation did not affect glucose turnover during exercise in rats (85). Recently, adrenalectomized dogs were studied during exercise with either basal replacement or epinephrine increased so as to stimulate the normal exercise response (65). Hepatic glucose output rose similarly for 120 min, irrespective of whether epinephrine was increased. However, the increment in epinephrine controlled 40% of the rise in glucose output at 120-150 min of exercise.

Regulation of Fat Metabolism

The regulation of FFA release from adipose tissue is the function primarily of insulin and catecholamines. When the exercise-induced fall in insulin was prevented in the dog by an intraportal infusion of the hormone, the FFA and glycerol increase was markedly attenuated (110). Thie led to decreases in the availability of FFA for muscle metabolism and of hepatic substrate for ketogenesis. Although the fall in insulin is important to the increase in lipolysis, no change in insulin binding (52, 102) has been observed in adipocytes biopsied from exercising humans. However, it seems that the sensitivity of postreceptor mechanisms to insulin may be enhanced in adipocytes immediately after exercise (5, 52).

The exercise-induced increase in plasma FFA in humans and dogs can be enhanced by alpha blockade and inhibited by beta blockade, presumably because of changes in lipolytic activity (84, 107). With combined alpha and beta blockade, the beta-blocking effects predominate, and the rise in FFA levels is abolished (32, 84). In a recent study, adipocytes taken from human subjects immediately after a bout of submaximal exercise had increased lipolytic responsiveness to catecholamines (102). This increase in responsiveness was mediated through beta-adrenergic mechanisms and independent of any changes in the binding of the beta-receptor-specific catecholamine ^{125}I-cyanopindolol. Thus modifications in postreceptor beta-adrenergic events may lead to an increase in catecholamine-stimulated lipolysis during muscular work.

Control of Muscle Glycogenolysis

The increase in catecholamines during exercise regulates muscle glycogenolysis, as demonstrated in muscle biopsies from humans studied during either beta blockade (16) or epinephrine infusion (43). This is supported by studies in the adrenode-medullated rat, in which an impairment in net muscle glycogen breakdown during exercise was demonstrated (4, 119). Studies in the isolated perfused rat hindquarter indicate that, in addition to epinephrine, contraction per se can stimulate muscle glycogenolysis even in the absence of catecholamines (77). Thus it appears that catecholamines and some aspect of contraction exhibit dual control over muscle glycogenolysis during exercise.

Glycogenolysis can also occur in nonworking muscle. An increased release of lactate from the resting forearm during prolonged leg exercise in excess of that which could be accounted for by the simultaneous uptake of blood glucose has been reported (3). Propranolol infusion in the brachial artery abolished this increase in lactate release, implying that beta-adrenergic mechanisms may be involved in the stimulation of glycogenolysis in the inactive muscle. Similarly, there was muscle glycogen breakdown in inactive muscle during prolonged exercise in normal rats (but not in those adrenalectomized), indicating that epinephrine is important in this process (60). Thus glycogen from inactive muscle can be mobilized by means of adrenergic mechanisms in the form of lactate for use as a fuel in working muscle or as a gluconeogenic substrate in the liver.

Regulation of Glucose Uptake

Muscle contraction per se can stimulate glucose uptake in vitro even without insulin (42, 68, 73, 76). Interestingly, the stimulatory effects of contraction can in some cases even exceed the maximal effects of insulin (42, 73). During exercise, the increase in blood flow to the muscle and the resulting increase in glucose delivery may magnify the effects of contraction. In situ experiments also support the idea that very little, if any, insulin is needed to control directly the carbohydrate metabolism in the contracting rat gastrocnemius. In streptozotocin-diabetic rats that were deprived of insulin injection for 3 d, nuclear magnetic resonance and biochemical studies indicate that all bioenergetic changes (force of contraction, energy-rich phosphorus-containing compounds, pH, and the activity of pyruvate dehydrogenase) were normal, but glycogen resynthesis was decreased during the recovery period. Only when diabetic rats were deprived of insulin treatment for 3 wk and consequently there were chronic effects of insulin deprivation was there a decrease in glucose oxidation and concentration of the energy-rich phosphoric compounds (14). Nevertheless, results in vitro cannot necessarily be extrapolated to the whole organism, in which metabolic events antagonistic to glucose uptake occur (e.g., enhanced muscle FFA oxidation and catecholamine action). In completely insulin-deprived (7, 98) or severely underinsulinized (97) depancreatized dogs there is only a small increase in whole-body glucose-metabolic clearance (Figures 39.3 and 39.4). Intraportal replacement of insulin during rest and exercise in depancreatized dogs returns metabolic glucose clearance to levels seen in normal dogs (97). It can be calculated from these studies that portal insulin replacement is responsible for 47% of the glucose cleared in depancreatized dogs during exercise.

It appears that exercise may work synergistically with insulin in regulating glucose metabolism. When a bout of exercise is superimposed on a hyperinsulinemic, euglycemic clamp, leg glucose uptake increases to a sum greater than that of the two treatments performed independently (23). Presumably, metabolic and hemodynamic changes operative during exercise sensitize the tissues to the reduced circulating insulin levels. There are at least three possibilities that could explain the increased insulin effectiveness: (a) muscle blood flow, (b) insulin binding to its receptor, or (c) postinsulin receptor mechanisms.

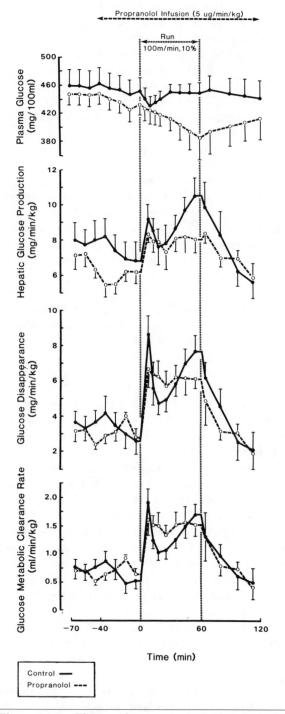

Figure 39.3. Plasma glucose concentration, hepatic glucose production, glucose disappearance, and glucose metabolic clearance during and after exercise with or without concomitant propranolol infusion during 60 min of running exercise in 6 depancreatized totally insulin-deficient dogs. Reproduced from *The Journal of Clinical Investigation*, 1988, **81**, 759, by copyright permission of the American Society for Clinical Investigation.

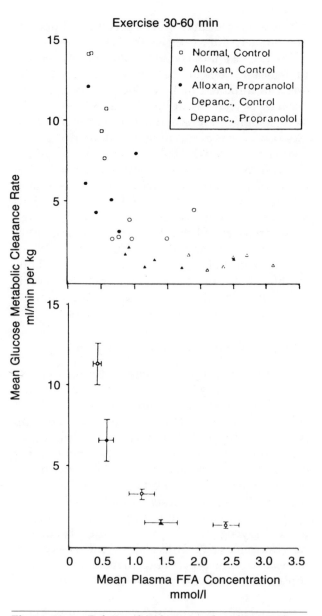

Figure 39.4. Relationship between free fatty acid levels and glucose metabolic clearance rate during 30-60 min of running exercise in dogs under the five different conditions described in the figure inset. The left panel shows individual values, and the right panel depicts mean ± *SE*. Reproduced from *The Journal of Clinical Investigation*, 1988, **81**, 759, by copyright permission of the American Society for Clinical Investigation.

Increase in Muscle Blood Flow

Exercise can be associated with a 10-fold or larger increase in blood flow to skeletal muscle. This increases the exposure of muscle, which comprises the bulk of insulin-sensitive tissue, to insulin and glucose. Indeed, a strong positive correlation exists between insulin delivery to the working muscle and insulin's action (23). Furthermore, the action of insulin in specific muscles correlates to the capillary density (58) and resting blood flow (41). Nevertheless, insulin action following exercise, when basal hemodynamic changes have been largely restored, is still increased (9, 24, 25). Thus factors besides muscle blood flow must be important.

Changes in Insulin Binding

It seems that in humans there is no increase in the binding affinity of insulin to its skeletal muscle receptor with an acute bout of exercise (11). Studies in the rat have been inconclusive and show no change (62, 128), increase (118), or, at high work intensities, decrease (62) in insulin binding. Hence, it is unclear whether insulin action during exercise is influenced by alterations in the binding of insulin to its skeletal muscle receptor. Also, the increased sensitivity to insulin is already observed at the onset of exercise, when a change in number or affinity of receptors is unlikely.

Postinsulin Receptor Modifications

In the perfused hindquarter of rats, immediately after treadmill exercise, an increase in insulin-stimulated glucose and amino acid uptake occurs without a concomitant increase in insulin binding to muscle (128). This implies that a step distal to binding must be altered. It has been proposed that a postreceptor modification may be linked to the depletion of glycogen that occurs during exercise. Indeed, glycogen depletion is correlated to the increased insulin effectiveness following exercise in many cases (9, 39, 128). However, improved insulin action after exercise persists even after preexercise glycogen levels have been restored (28). Similarly, after electrical stimulation, the increased rate of 3-0-methylglucose uptake (a measure of glucose transport) in the perfused rat hindquarter in either the presence or the absence of insulin can return promptly to baseline levels even when muscle glycogen remains depleted (73). It has also been suggested that an exercise-induced increase in maximal insulin action may rely on muscle glycogen depletion and that an increase in sensitivity could be independent of muscle glycogen levels (129).

In addition to insulin, catecholamines control glucose uptake by muscle. Epinephrine inhibits the insulin-mediated uptake of glucose in skeletal muscle through beta-adrenergic mechanisms (18). Propranolol causes an excessive increase in glucose

uptake during exercise (32, 84, 107). Oxidation of fat and glycogen in skeletal muscle initiated by an epinephrine-stimulated increase in mobilization of these fuels will result in the buildup of metabolic intermediates that can feed back to inhibit muscular glucose uptake (69). By preventing these processes, beta blockade can stimulate muscle glucose uptake. Data from the totally insulin-deprived depancreatized dog (7) (Figure 39.3) and the alloxan-diabetic dog with residual insulin secretion (107) (Figure 39.5) indicate that catecholamines

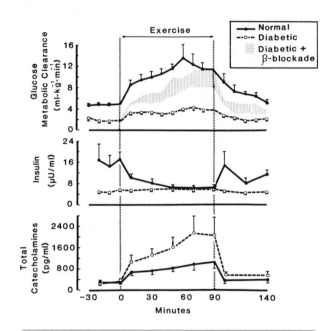

Figure 39.5. Effect of exercise on glucose metabolic clearance rate, immunoreactive insulin, and total catecholamines in normal (n = 5; solid line) and alloxan-diabetic (n = 6; dashed line) dogs. Stippled area in Panel A represents the effect of exercise with beta blockade in alloxan-diabetic dogs (n = 6). From ''Interaction Between Insulin and Counterregulatory Hormones in Control of Substrate Utilization in Health and Diabetes During Exercise'' by D.H. Wasserman and M. Vranic, 1986, *Diabetes/Metabolism Reviews*, 1(4), p. 159. Reprinted by permission of John Wiley & Sons, Inc.

may regulate glucose uptake during exercise only when sufficient insulin is available to prevent markedly elevated levels of FFA. Indeed, beta blockade does not increase glucose-metabolic clearance in exercising depancreatized dogs with excessive FFA levels. Rather, it appears that there is a threshold FFA concentration (about 1.1 mM) above which changes in FFAs do not further affect glucose clearance but below which the changes increase clearance (Figure 39.4). This would imply a significant role for the glucose/fatty acid cycle, at least in the diabetic state (69).

The importance of metabolic factors within the working muscle per se is illustrated by the excessive increments in glucose uptake when oxygen availability is limited, such as in anemia (112), when breathing a hypoxic gas mixture (19), or during severe work (46, 99). In anemic dogs, glucose utilization and clearance are markedly elevated during exercise even though insulin levels are similar and catecholamine levels excessive (112) (Figure 39.6). However, the fall in plasma glucose was only moderate, as the increment in glucose production was also exaggerated in anemic dogs, suggesting that during exercise the central nervous system is very sensitive even to small changes in oxygen. This triggers a near-maximal increase of catecholamines and glucagon, resulting in an excessive increase in hepatic glucose production. Similar results have been obtained in exercising human subjects in whom the fraction of oxygen in the inspired air was maintained at either 0.15 (hypoxia) or 0.80 (hyperoxia) during exercise (19). Exercise under hypoxic conditions resulted in a 2.5-fold greater increase in glucose uptake and clearance than when the same subjects exercised under hyperoxic conditions. As in the anemic dog, this effect of hypoxia was present despite similar insulin and excessive catecholamine levels. Also, an enhanced glucose output prevented a large fall in circulating glucose. Thus the increased metabolic demand for carbohydrates caused by tissue hypoxia clearly outweighs the peripheral counterregulatory effects of the catecholamines. The precise mechanism by which metabolic rate controls glucose uptake remains to be elucidated. However, the energy state of the muscle, as determined by the phosphocreatine concentration, correlates strongly with this process (46).

Exercise Response in Insulin-Requiring Diabetics or in Animal Models of Diabetes

It is apparent from the preceding discussion that the inability to regulate insulin secretion is a deficit for the diabetic who is faced with the enhanced metabolic requirements of muscular work. Nevertheless, during exercise, increments in glucose fluxes in the diabetic are often similar to those seen in normal subjects (100, 109); however, the mechanisms for this increase are different. For example, although the increase in glucose production is

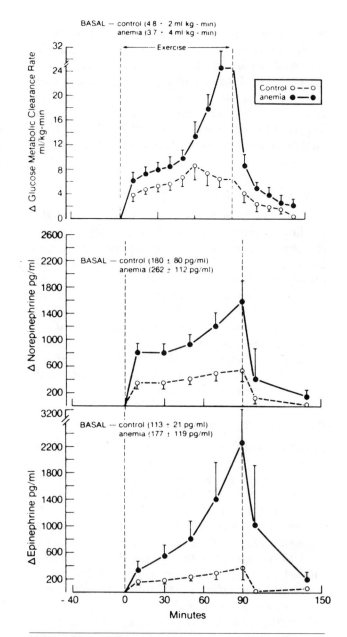

Figure 39.6. Effect of exercise on changes of glucose metabolic clearance, norepinephrine, and epinephrine in anemic (*n* = 5) and normal dogs (*n* = 5). Data expressed as mean ± SE. From "Effect of Hematocrit Reduction on Hormonal and Metabolic Responses to Exercise" by D.H. Wasserman, H.L.A. Lickley, and M. Vranic, 1986, *Journal of Applied Physiology*, **58**, p. 1257.

quantitatively similar in diabetics and healthy subjects, diabetics rely more heavily on glucose derived from gluconeogenesis (100). Glucose utilization also increases similarly in normal and diabetic subjects; however, whereas in normal subjects this is due to an increase in metabolic glucose clearance, in inadequately controlled diabetics it is a result of an increased mass action of excessive hyperglycemia (7, 97, 100) associated with a very small increment in glucose clearance (7). In addition, a smaller percentage of the glucose utilized is oxidized in diabetics, probably because of impaired pyruvate dehydrogenase activity, a key enzyme that connects the pathway of glucolysis with that of glucose oxidation (56). Increased FFA utilization can compensate, at least in part, for the reduction in energy production resulting from the diminished capacity to oxidize glucose (100). Insulin-dependent diabetes mellitus (IDDM) may also be associated with a greater availability of ketone bodies, the magnitude of which depends on the state of metabolic control (6, 100, 101). Diabetics may also exhibit differences in intramuscular substrate metabolism in response to exercise. Diabetics deprived of insulin for 24 hr exhibited a decrease in intramuscular glycogen and an increase in intramuscular fat storage, a shift in substrate storage that leads to a greater metabolism of intramuscular fat and a diminished breakdown of intramuscular glycogen (86). Although adequate insulinization is critical for physiological metabolic responses, it will be evident that insulin levels appropriate during rest can result in relative over-insulinization and hypoglycemia during exercise.

Insulin Administration and Exercise

Inadequate Insulinization

In patients or animals with severe insulin deficiency manifested by substantial hyperglycemia and ketosis, exercise can further derange the metabolic state (6, 97, 124). When IDDM patients deprived of insulin for a prolonged period (18-48 hr) exercised for 3 hr, an exaggerated counterregulatory response ensued, and, paradoxically, blood glucose rose (6). Tracer studies in the depancreatized dog indicate that this rise in glucose in severe insulin deficiency is due mainly to an inadequate increase in glucose utilization (97). In addition, underinsulinization in IDDM will further increase levels of FFA and ketone bodies with exercise (101). Thus, exercise in the poorly controlled diabetic may contribute to hyperglycemia and hyperlipidemia and lead to ketoacidosis.

The deleterious response of underinsulinized diabetics to exercise is probably not exclusively due to diminished insulin levels per se, as exercise is associated also with excessive increases in glucagon (6, 100, 101, 109), growth hormone (88, 101), catecholamines (88, 101, 109), and cortisol (6, 109),

all of which can aggravate metabolic control. Adequate insulin therapy can normalize the excessive counterregulatory response to exercise in diabetics (6, 88). Studies in the alloxan-diabetic dog deprived of exogenous insulin for 24 hr demonstrated that, as in normal dogs, the presence of glucagon was a major determinant of hepatic glucose production during exercise (109) (Figure 39.2). In this model of poorly controlled IDDM, glucagon suppression with somatostatin led to a 50% reduction in glucose production. Elevated glucagon concentrations may also play a role in liver ketogenesis in diabetes. Exercise in IDDM has been associated with strong positive correlations between splanchnic ketone body output and plasma glucagon concentrations (101), but as yet a causal relationship has not been established.

The role of catecholamines in exercise has been investigated using adrenergic blockade in well-controlled IDDM (84) and in poorly controlled alloxan-diabetic dogs (107). In well-maintained, insulin-infused diabetics (basal plasma glucose of 144 mg/dl) with normal increments in counterregulatory hormones, beta-adrenergic blockade did not appear to affect hepatic glucose output (84). However, even in the absence of beta blockade, these subjects did not show appreciable increases in glucose output during exercise. Nevertheless, hepatic glucose production during exercise in alloxan-diabetic dogs in poor metabolic control and with excessive counterregulatory hormone levels was also unaffected by beta blockade (107). In contrast, in depancreatized dogs that were totally deprived of insulin, beta blockade markedly decreased increments in glucose production during exercise (7) (Figure 39.3). It appears therefore that in the total absence of insulin the control of glucose production may be shifted from glucagon to catecholamines. This shift may be related to a catecholamine-induced mobilization of gluconeogenic substrates, hepatic insensitivity to glucagon, or both. It is interesting that in insulin-infused diabetics alpha-adrenergic blockade actually stimulated hepatic glucose output excessively during exercise (84). Although catecholamines may not be primary regulators of glucose release from the liver during exercise in most diabetics, they have potent peripheral effects. On one hand, beta blockade markedly decreased FFA levels in exercising alloxan-diabetic dogs deprived of exogenous insulin (107) and prevented the exercise-induced increment in FFA concentration in insulin-infused human diabetics (84). On the other hand, alpha blockade in insulin-infused diabetics caused a twofold increase in the FFA increment with exercise (84). Moreover, beta blockade prevented the rise in lactate in alloxan-diabetic dogs (107), offering indirect evidence that muscle glycogenolysis may be stimulated by beta-adrenergic mechanisms in insulin-deficient states.

The response to adrenergic blockade in IDDM is, in a qualitative manner, similar to the response of adrenergic blockade seen in normal subjects. However, in a quantitative sense, catecholamine action appears enhanced in diabetes (84). It is not clear whether this difference is due to a change in catecholamine sensitivity or to other abnormalities of diabetes.

Overinsulinization

It is evident that adequate insulin is important to avoid aggravating the diabetic state during exercise. However, hypoglycemia commonly occurs in individuals with IDDM during and after exercise due to hyperinsulinemia. Three factors contribute to hyperinsulinemia: (a) The absorption of insulin injected subcutaneously can be accelerated during exercise (47, 53, 126), depending on the site of the subcutaneous injection and on timing. If the rate of absorption of insulin from the depot is already very high (immediately after the injection), exercise will not be able to accelerate this rate further (48) (Figure 39.7). (b) The lack of insulin decrease during muscular work results in relative overinsulinization (114); that is, an insulin dose appropriate under resting conditions may be excessive during exercise. (c) The exercise-induced increase in insulin action contributes to the sensitivity of the individual with IDDM to relative hyperinsulinemia. The importance of factors (b) and (c) became apparent when it was shown that hypoglycemia can occur even when insulin mobilization is not accelerated (48, 87). Studies in IDDM and depancreatized dogs have shown that the exercise-induced fall in glucose levels as a result of relative or absolute overinsulinization is due primarily to an impaired rate of hepatic glucose production (Figures 39.8 and 39.9) (47, 126).

Exercise-induced hypoglycemia can be avoided by taking two precautions. First, carbohydrate ingestion in conjunction with exercise is recommended because glucose given orally during exercise is utilized promptly, as long as adequate insulin is available (56). Selection of the most appropriate meal to avoid hypoglycemia depends on the type of exercise. For example, during prolonged moderate-intensity exercise, food with a slow absorption profile taken 15 min before work has been

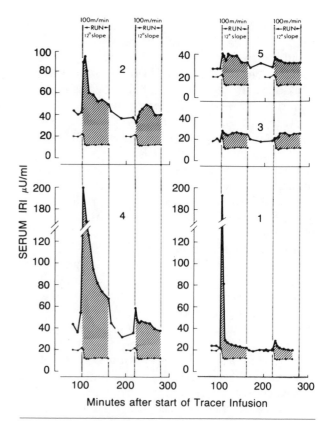

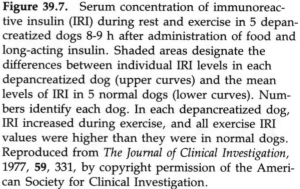

Figure 39.7. Serum concentration of immunoreactive insulin (IRI) during rest and exercise in 5 depancreatized dogs 8-9 h after administration of food and long-acting insulin. Shaded areas designate the differences between individual IRI levels in each depancreatized dog (upper curves) and the mean levels of IRI in 5 normal dogs (lower curves). Numbers identify each dog. In each depancreatized dog, IRI increased during exercise, and all exercise IRI values were higher than they were in normal dogs. Reproduced from *The Journal of Clinical Investigation*, 1977, **59**, 331, by copyright permission of the American Society for Clinical Investigation.

recommended (66). Also, a reduction in insulin dosage is an important precaution. One investigation concluded that diabetics undergoing intensive insulin therapy with fasting euglycemia can avoid hypoglycemia during 45 min of postprandial exercise at 55% maximum oxygen uptake by reducing insulin treatment by 30%-50% (80). Alternatively, hypoglycemia can be avoided by ingesting 15 g of glucose before and 15-30 g following exercise of this type. For more prolonged exercise, a greater reduction in insulin dose or a greater intake of glucose may be necessary to avoid hypoglycemia in euglycemic IDDM subjects (49). Diabetics with an 80% reduction of insulin exercised for 3 hr without hypoglycemia, whereas with

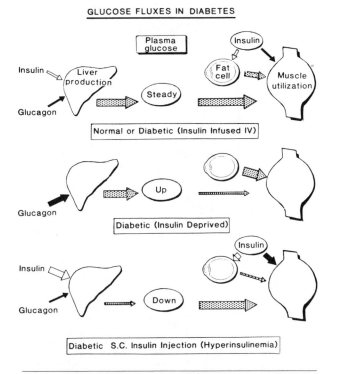

GLUCOSE FLUXES IN DIABETES

Figure 39.8. A hypothesis of the role of insulin in the regulation of glucose homeostasis in the normal and the diabetic state. Different plasma concentrations of glucose result from changes in glucose production and utilization.

a 50% reduction hypoglycemia occurred after 90 min. In contrast to tightly controlled diabetics, those with hyperglycemic IDDM need a smaller reduction in insulin (49). Exercise intensity is an important variable when assessing preexercise diet and insulin therapy (34, 124, 125). High-intensity exercise can elicit more extreme adverse effects than can moderate-intensity exercise of similar duration, whether these be the glucose-lowering effects in hyperinsulinemic patients or the hyperglycemic effects in insulin-deficient patients (124, 125). Some general guidelines for diet and insulin therapy for the physically active diabetic have been suggested (98) but with the proviso that a specific prescription cannot be uniformly applicable.

The three panels of Figure 39.8 summarize the problems related to insulinemia in physically active IDDM patients: (a) During constant IV infusion of insulin, which generates subnormal insulin concentrations in the portal vein, glucose homeostasis is preserved because glucose production and utilization are balanced as in nondiabetic subjects. (b) Due to the direct or the indirect (glucose-FFA cycle) effects of insulin deficiency (7), exercise does not stimulate glucose utilization adequately, and hence

the exercise-induced increase in hepatic glucose production leads to a rise in blood glucose levels. (c) If exercise is performed following the subcutaneous injection of insulin, the absorption of exogenous insulin into the circulation is maintained or accelerated, resulting in absolute or relative overinsulinization. Because of hyperinsulinemia, glucose production is inhibited, and the increased peripheral glucose uptake leads to a fall in blood glucose levels. This scheme reflects observations in IDDM subjects (126) (Figure 39.9) and in depancreatized dogs (7, 47, 97).

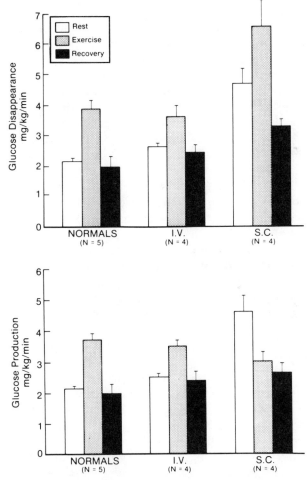

Figure 39.9. Glucose turnover: glucose disappearance (top panel) and glucose production (bottom panel) at rest at 45 min of exercise and at 60 min of recovery for normal control insulin-infused subjects (I.V.) and subcutaneous (S.C.) insulin-treated diabetic patients. From B. Zinman, F.T. Murray, M. Vranic, A.M. Albisser, B.S. Leibel, P.A. McClean, and E.B. Marliss, Glucoregulation During Moderate Exercise in Insulin Treated Diabetics, *Journal of Clinical Endocrinology and Metabolism*, **45**, p. 641, 1977, © by the Endocrine Society. Reprinted by permission.

Exercise in Non-Insulin-Dependent Diabetes Mellitus (NIDDM)

Despite the high prevalence of NIDDM, and in contrast to IDDM, few studies have examined the effects of exercise on glucose kinetics in this population. Insulin resistance in NIDDM can be due to receptor defects, postreceptor defects, or both. Furthermore, this syndrome is often characterized by obesity and hyperinsulinemia, and treatment consists of dietary prescriptions, oral hypoglycemic agents, insulin, or all these. To understand the effects of exercise in NIDDM one must take into account the specific treatment modality.

Obese NIDDM patients maintained on diet or diet plus sulfonylurea (chlorpropamide) with postabsorptive hyperglycemia (above 200 mg/dl) and normal basal insulin showed a fall in glycemia of about 50 mg/dl during a 45-min exercise (64). The fall in glucose was due to an attenuation of the normal rise in hepatic glucose production while glucose utilization increased normally (36) (Figure 39.10). This was attributed to the fact that insulin secretion was not inhibited in patients with NIDDM. These patients seem to have a defect in control of insulin secretion when challenged both with glucose (inadequate increase) and with exercise (inadequate decrease). The latter could be a consequence of hyperglycemia prevailing over the adrenergic stimulation or of neuropathy. In addition, hyperglycemia can act synergistically with insulin to suppress glucose production. During 3 h of moderate-intensity exercise in NIDDM patients with borderline fasting hyperglycemia (140 mg/dl) and hyperinsulinemia (23 μU/ml), plasma glucose fell by about 40 mg/dl (51), and with more prolonged exercise there was some decrease of the elevated plasma insulin. One recent study in NIDDM patients showed that 12-16 hr after a single bout of glycogen-depleting exercise, hepatic and peripheral insulin sensitivity increased (24). Prior exercise reduced basal hepatic glucose production by 25%, whereas a low dose of insulin infusion reduced it by 85%. The increased peripheral insulin sensitivity was due to an enhanced rate of nonoxidative glucose disposal (24). Studies demonstrating that exercise can lower plasma glucose and increase insulin sensitivity in NIDDM subjects emphasize the importance of exercise as an adjuvant therapy.

Patients with NIDDM on diet therapy should be able to exercise as normal subjects do provided

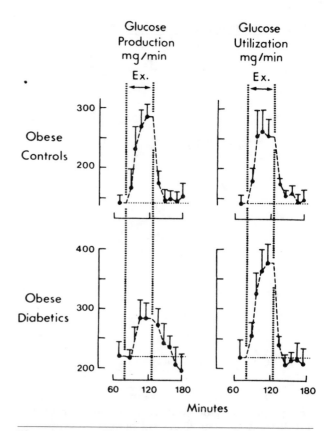

Figure 39.10. Glucose production and utilization in 7 obese controls (upper panel) and 10 obese NIDDM patients (lower panel) during rest, exercise (60% V̇O₂max), and recovery. Means and SEs are shown. From "Glucoregulatory and Metabolic Response to Exercise in Obese Noninsulin-Dependent Diabetes" by H.L. Minuk et al., 1981, *American Journal of Physiology, 240,* p. E458. Reprinted by permission.

there are no major vascular complications. However, when oral hypoglycemic drugs are used, there may be a tendency for hypoglycemia during prolonged exercise. When glyburide was given to normal subjects before exercise, insulin levels increased about twofold, and blood glucose fell to about 50 mg/dl (50). The nadir in blood glucose was deeper and occurred more promptly than it did when glyburide was administered to resting subjects. The FFA oxidation inhibitor methylpalmoxirate has been shown to accelerate glucose oxidation in the liver and to a lesser extent in muscle, resulting in a depletion of glycogen stores in the streptozotocin-diabetic rat (123). If similar compounds were to be used for therapeutic purposes, the depletion of glycogen stores, as well as the inhibition of FFA oxidation, could enhance the tendency for hypoglycemia during exercise.

Physical Training

Because this topic is so important, a consensus development conference on diet and exercise in NIDDM patients was held at the National Institutes of Health in December 1986 (67). It was recognized that, in addition to the effects of training on cardiovascular and pulmonary performance, control of lipid metabolism, and attitudes toward stresses (all of which are of such great importance for both normal and diabetic populations), the following questions concerning the aspects of training are of particular relevance to the diabetic and the prediabetic: (a) Under what conditions and in which NIDDM patients is exercise likely to be most effective in improving glucose homeostasis? (b) What is the relative effectiveness of regular physical activity and weight control in the prevention and treatment of NIDDM and its complications? (c) Can training impede the progression of atherogenic complications resulting from diabetes? We address the first two questions by summarizing the effects of training on glucose tolerance and insulin sensitivity. We then briefly assess the potential role of training in retarding the cardiovascular complications of diabetes.

Unquestionably, strenuous training in athletes increases insulin sensitivity in liver, muscle, and fat cells (79); however, such data are not available in NIDDM athletes. In NIDDM, moderate exercise that is applicable to most individuals improves glycosylated hemoglobin and insulin secretion, and these effects are independent of body weight loss (55, 91). It has been suggested that these beneficial effects are not necessarily related to training but rather reflect an integrative effect of increased insulin sensitivity after each bout of exercise (82). Although restricted caloric intake and exercise can increase insulin sensitivity, exercise appears to have a specific effect in increasing carbohydrate storage. This increase, noted in the post-exercise periods, suggests that some effects of exercise are more physiological than are those of restricted caloric intake (10, 24, 25). One epidemiological report found the prevalence of NIDDM to be two times larger in sedentary men than in active men (90). Most important, epidemiological data, animal studies, and analyses of exercise effects on atherosclerotic risk factors all suggest that physical training might retard atherosclerotic vascular disease in the general population. This is of great importance for NIDDM because a number of risk factors for atherosclerosis are accelerated in these patients (81). These main conclusions are discussed in detail in the following two sections.

Effect of Glucose Tolerance and Insulin Sensitivity

Athletes or endurance-trained subjects have normal or even increased glucose tolerance and lower fasting and glucose-stimulated insulin levels (79). Experiments using hyperinsulinemic, euglycemic clamps have demonstrated that submaximal insulin-stimulated glucose disposal is increased in aerobically trained athletes (79, 121). In an elegant study it was demonstrated that insulin action in trained distance runners was enhanced in muscle, liver, and adipose tissue (79). This was demonstrated by combining tracer methods with regional catheterization and by taking biopsies of fat tissue. The sensitivity to physiological insulin levels was assessed in trained distance runners (63 ml $\cdot$ kg^{-1} $\cdot$ min^{-1} maximal oxygen uptake) using a euglycemic clamp with insulin infusions that maintained levels of 10 and 50 μU/ml (79). At low and high insulin concentrations, respectively, trained subjects had glucose uptakes that increased 25% and 38%, whereas glucose production was 47% and 70% below what it was in controls (Figure 39.11). Furthermore, insulin-stimulated glucose uptake was 43% higher than in controls. Thus, at physiological insulin levels, trained subjects have an increased peripheral and hepatic sensitivity to insulin. Interestingly, no difference in the specific binding of insulin to its receptor on monocytes was noted between the two groups. These effects of training are probably specific for aerobic exercise. Although strength training results in a net increase in submaximal insulin-stimulated glucose disposal (121) and glucose tolerance (63), this increase is proportional to the increased muscle mass and probably does not represent an increase in insulin sensitivity per se.

Insulin sensitivity can be increased following training in IDDM patients who are on conventional (57, 105) or pump insulin therapy (122). When diabetics undergo exercise training that significantly increases their maximum oxygen consumption, glucose uptake in response to a hyperinsulinemic, euglycemic clamp is increased markedly (57, 122). Studies of streptozotocin-diabetic rats indicate that the ability to adapt to chronic exercise in insulin-deficient states may depend on the severity of the condition. Mildly diabetic rats increase insulin sensitivity in response to exercise training (89), whereas severely diabetic rats do not show this change (93).

Studies in NIDDM have shown that an exercise training program that is feasible for most individu-

als can cause an increase in glucose tolerance (55, 75, 82, 91) (Figure 39.12) and lower basal (10, 91) and glucose-stimulated insulin levels (55). Insulin sensitivity, as assessed by glucose disposal during hyperinsulinemic, euglycemic clamps, improved with exercise training (10, 51, 55, 91). By combining

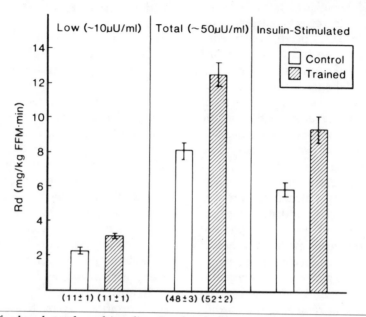

Figure 39.11. Values for basal, total, and insulin-stimulated glucose uptake (R_d) during clamp studies in control and trained individuals. Numbers in parentheses beneath bars represent plasma insulin concentrations at which R_d was measured. Data expressed as mean $\pm$ SE. From "Improved Insulin Action in Muscle, Liver, and Adipose Tissue in Physically Trained Human Subjects" by K.J. Rodnick, W.L. Haskell, A.L.M. Swislocki, J.E. Foley, and G.M. Reaven, 1987, *American Journal of Physiology*, **253**, p. E489. Reprinted by permission.

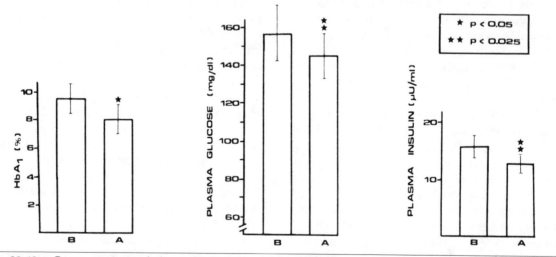

Figure 39.12. Concentrations of glycosylated hemoglobin, fasting plasma glucose, and fasting plasma insulin before (B) and after (A) 6-wk physical training in 5 NIDDM patients. Glucose and insulin values are the mean of 3 consecutive days' determinations. Data expressed as mean $\pm$ SE. From "Influence of Physical Training on Blood Glucose Control, Glucose Tolerance, Insulin Secretion, and Insulin Action in Non-Insulin Dependent Diabetic Patients" by M. Trovati, Q. Carta, F. Cavalot, S. Vitali, C. Banaudi, P. Lucchina, F., Fiocchi, G. Emanuelli, and G. Lenti, 1984, *Diabetes Care*, **7**, p. 416. Reproduced with permission from the American Diabetes Association, Inc.

euglycemic clamps, infusion of radioactive glucose, and measurement of metabolic rate, one can differentiate between glucose oxidation and glucose storage because the latter is a nonoxidative pathway. A combined exercise training and diet program increased the total glucose disposal rate during an insulin clamp in NIDDM patients by approximately 27%, primarily because of an accelerated rate of nonoxidative carbohydrate disposal (storage) (10). In contrast, diet alone did not affect glucose storage. Thus, it appears that the combination of diet and exercise has a more physiological metabolic effect than does diet alone. Basal and insulin-suppressed hepatic glucose outputs were also reduced by diet and training, but no more than by the diet program alone (10). Training programs led to an improvement in insulin sensitivity in obese subjects even with no concurrent weight loss or change in body composition (55). Nevertheless, because weight reduction by itself can also improve insulin sensitivity (8), it is likely that exercise training that results in loss of body fat will yield maximal effectiveness.

Considering the fundamental role of skeletal muscle during exercise and the fact that it represents the bulk of insulin-sensitive tissue, it is likely that muscle is the major site of the increase in insulin action that occurs with training. In trained rats, skeletal muscle is more insulin sensitive than is that from sedentary controls, mainly because of increased glucose oxidation (21, 22, 40). Hyperinsulinemic, euglycemic clamps, combined with the 2-deoxyglucose technique, demonstrated an increase in maximal insulin-stimulated glucose metabolism in soleus and red gastrocnemius and an increased insulin sensitivity in soleus, gastrocnemius, extensor digitorium longus, and diaphragm in exercise-trained rats when compared to sedentary controls (40) (Figure 39.13). These observations were confirmed in rat epitrochlearis muscle, which showed an increase in insulin-stimulated uptake and glycolytic metabolism in trained rats (22). Exercise alone does not appear to normalize muscular insulin sensitivity in insulin-resistant states (21, 38). However, diet and exercise together may correct this condition (38, 92). Insulin action was recently studied in the perfused hind limb of trained and sedentary obese Zucker rats in conjunction with dietary regimens (38) (Figure 39.14). In this model of insulin resistance, training and a high-carbohydrate diet independently increased glucose uptake above that seen in sedentary, obese Zucker rats on a high-fat diet but still below that seen in lean, control rats. A combination

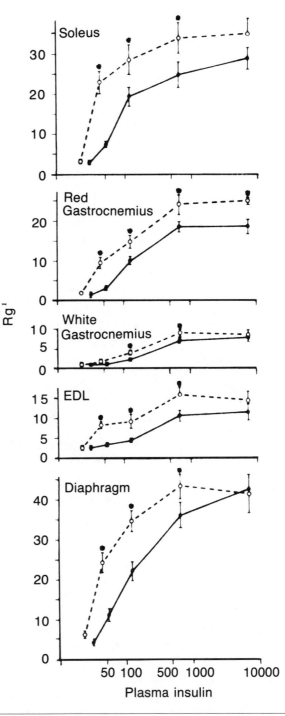

Figure 39.13. The effect of exercise training on Rg^1 (μmol [100 g $\cdot$ min]$^{-1}$), an index of glucose metabolism, in soleus, red and white gastrocnemius, extensor digitorum longus and diaphragm. Each value is the mean $\pm$ SE of 5-7 observations; o = control animals; o = exercise-trained animals. Exercise-trained animals were different from the controls at the same plasma insulin concentration ($p < 0.05$). Reproduced from *The Journal of Clinical Investigation*, 1985, **76**, 657, by copyright permission of the American Society for Clinical Investigation.

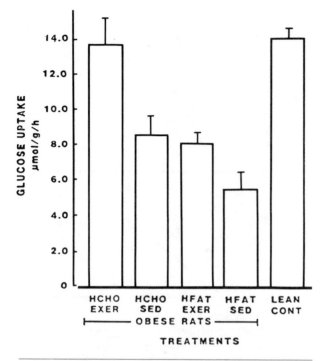

Figure 39.14. Glucose uptake in hind-limb muscles of obese and lean Zucker rats during perfusion. Perfusate contained 6 mM glucose and 1.0 μU/ml insulin. HCHO = high-carbohydrate diet; HFAT = high-fat diet; EXER = exercise trained; SED = sedentary; and CONT = control (lean littermate). From "Exercise and Diet Reduce Muscle Insulin Resistance in Obese Zucker Rat" by J.L. Ivy, W.M. Sherman, C.L. Cutler, and A.L. Katz, 1986, *American Journal of Physiology*, 251, p. E299. Reprinted by permission.

of a high-carbohydrate diet and training had a synergistic effect.

The increase in insulin action in skeletal muscle during habitual exercise may be due in part to an increase in insulin binding to its skeletal muscle receptor (12, 27). A 4-wk training program in rats resulted in a twofold increase in binding of insulin to its partially purified skeletal muscle receptor preparation at all insulin concentrations studied, suggesting an increase in the number of insulin receptors (27). In these studies training did not alter insulin receptor structure, as evidenced by electrophoretic mobility. However, it was surprising that, for similar amounts of bound insulin, trained rats had a decrease in the activity of the protein kinase.

Skeletal muscle adapts to aerobic exercise training so that it more readily uses fuel and oxygen. To enhance its metabolic capacity, muscle increases mitochondrial enzyme concentrations and capillary density in response to habitual training, and the

improved insulin sensitivity in IDDM may be due to these adaptations. Streptozotocin-diabetic rats have deficits in cytoplasmic and mitochondrial enzymes in slow- and fast-twitch muscle fibers, and these deficient enzymes can be increased by training (71). In IDDM patients, training programs can lead to increases in skeletal muscle citrate synthase and succinate dehydrogenase that parallel an increase in insulin sensitivity (105). The increase in muscle capillary density in trained nondiabetic subjects can also enhance insulin sensitivity by augmenting the exposure of muscle to insulin and glucose. In fact, in humans, muscle capillary density is strongly correlated to the total glucose disposal rate during a hyperinsulinemic, euglycemic glucose clamp (58). Indeed, in the rat, muscles with the highest blood flow are the most insulin sensitive (41). However, the evidence available so far indicates that training that increased insulin sensitivity in NIDDM and IDDM patients is not accompanied by an increase in muscle capillary density (59, 104).

In addition to skeletal muscle, adipose tissue represents another important site of adaptation to training. Regular physical activity increases insulin-stimulated glucose uptake (20, 40, 94, 106), oxidation (40, 106), and incorporation into fatty acids (40, 106) in rat adipocytes. This is consistent with the demonstration that trained rats have a greater number of glucose transporters in fat-cell membranes (94). The improvement of insulin action may also relate to the reduced fat-cell size after physical training. One such study demonstrated that insulin-stimulated 2-deoxyglucose uptake and 1-¹⁴C-glucose oxidation in adipocytes were highly correlated to fat-cell size in a population of 12- and 28-mo old exercise-trained, sedentary, and calorie-restricted sedentary rats (20). The increase in insulin action in adipocytes of trained rats occurs in the absence of any changes in insulin binding (106), indicating a modification in a postbinding event.

Although insulin sensitivity is improved and muscular metabolic capacity increased, there is no evidence that glycemic control is effectively improved in trained IDDM individuals. Indeed, there was no improvement in glycosylated hemoglobin levels, glycosuria, or fasting plasma glucose following training programs that resulted in significant increments in maximum oxidative capacity (57, 103, 105, 107, 127). In contrast, training does seem to improve glycemic control in NIDDM individuals (10, 75, 82, 91). A training program that induced a 15% increase in maximum oxygen uptake caused significant reductions in glycosylated hemoglobin and in fasting plasma glucose and insulin levels in NIDDM patients (91). It is important to note that individuals with different degrees of insulin resistance do not adapt to training in the same way. For example, training in insulin-resistant conditions characterized by high rates of insulin secretion can lead to a decrease in the release of this hormone (55), whereas, training in subjects with insulin resistance and low insulin secretion has been shown to increase the rate of insulin secretion (55). Finally, an improvement in insulin action in trained diabetic and nondiabetic subjects could be due to the accumulative effects of single exercise bouts rather than to long-term adaptations from exercise training (13, 29, 91). This is based on two lines of evidence. First, the effects of training on insulin action are rapidly reversed by inactivity, whereas the effects of training on oxygen uptake and lean body mass are more sustained (13, 29). Second, an acute bout of exercise and training share some similar effects (24, 51, 64).

Effect on the Atherogenic Complications of Diabetes

Atherosclerotic vascular disease, which affects arteries in the heart, brain, and extremities, is accelerated in patients with all forms of diabetes. Epidemiological data, animal studies, and analysis of exercise effects on atherosclerotic risk factors all suggest that physical training might retard atherosclerotic vascular disease in the general population (for a review, see ref. 81). A large number of retrospective and prospective studies are discussed in other chapters of this book and have also been reviewed previously (81). The most compelling prospective study is that of Paffenbarger et al. (72), in which 10-yr follow-ups showed that the incidence of fatal myocardial infarction among alumni with recreational energy expenditures over 2,000 kcal per week was half that of their less active classmates and was independent of other known risk factors, including hypertension, cigarette smoking, and hypercholesterolemia. The most pertinent animal study is that of Kramsch et al. (54), in which young-adult male monkeys were given a diet high in saturated fat and cholesterol, a diet that in the sedentary group produced severe atherosclerosis similar to that seen in humans. A second group on the same diet were subjected to light exercise (30-min run on treadmill three times per week) for 18 mo. The findings were dramatic: Sudden death occurred only in the sedentary group, and severity of atherosclerosis as judged by gross appearance,

light microscopy, and biochemical composition was strikingly diminished in the exercise group. Surprisingly, these improvements were not related to total plasma or LDL-cholesterol levels. Glucose intolerance, hyperinsulinemia, and insulin resistance, in addition to changes in plasma lipoproteins, have been proposed as atherogenic agents (74), and these can be present in both IDDM and NIDDM patients. Should hyperglycemia prove to be atherogenic, the possible mechanisms include the nonenzymatic glycosylation of lipoproteins, connective tissue proteins, and coagulation factors (for a review, see ref. 81).

Hyperlipidemia and disorders in lipoprotein metabolism are major risk factors for cardiovascular disease and occur with higher frequency in IDDM and particularly in NIDDM patients (70). There is an increased prevalence of hyperlipidemia and diminished HDL cholesterol in diabetics, presumably a function of metabolic control (70). Recent studies in IDDM patients (103, 105) have shown that intensive training increases the ratio of HDL cholesterol to total cholesterol. Training can reduce triglyceride levels in NIDDM patients, an effect that appears to be reversed rapidly by inactivity (82). Hypertension markedly increases the frequency of vascular disease and occurs with greater frequency in diabetics than in normal subjects (70). In general, active individuals have lower systolic and diastolic blood pressures than do sedentary controls matched for age (81).

Thus, there is evidence that the potentially beneficial effects of exercise on cardiovascular disease in normal humans applies also to those with diabetes. Hence, from the standpoint of minimizing the risk of some complications from diabetes, a regular exercise program should be part of the treatment strategy for NIDDM patients whenever possible. The problem can be that many elderly NIDDM patients may already have advanced coronary heart disease, pulmonary disease, musculoskeletal problems, and peripheral vascular insufficiency, all of which preclude all but the mildest exercise regimens. Some middle-aged individuals may already have established atherosclerosis and therefore could be at greater risk for sudden death during exercise. This is why Ruderman et al. (81) suggested that the prophylactic value of exercise may be greater in younger individuals who may be at increased risk for premature atherosclerosis. They suggested that the children of patients with premature atherosclerosis and NIDDM would represent a good target group because many of them already demonstrate some of the risk factors found in their parents.

Conclusion

Exercise has been recommended as an adjuvant therapy for diabetes mellitus for a long time. With the discovery of insulin, Joslin recommended that diet, insulin, and exercise represent the management triad in insulin-treated diabetics. In the last 15 yr, the importance of exercise in the management of both Type I and Type II diabetes has been extensively reexamined in both humans and animals. Unquestionably, it is important for both diabetics and nondiabetics to optimize cardiovascular and pulmonary parameters. In addition, in both populations improved fitness can improve one's sense of well-being and ability to cope with physical and psychological stresses that can be aggravated in diabetes. There have been a number of studies indicating that the risk of heart attack decreases in trained individuals, an observation of particular importance to diabetics, who are already at higher risk. Thus far, only experiments in animals indicate that exercise can alleviate atherosclerosis. Intense training can also improve lipoprotein profiles. In insulin-treated diabetics, there is increased insulin sensitivity and, therefore, decreased insulin requirements with exercise. Increased insulin sensitivity is of particular importance in Type II diabetics because insulin resistance is such a prominent feature of that disease. The greatest benefit can be derived in Type II diabetics if an exercise program is combined with weight loss. However, as in the nondiabetic population, there has been very little success in reducing body weight in obese Type II diabetics.

Some risks are specific to diabetics, so it is important to understand the neuroendocrinological regulations of metabolism during exercise of various intensities. Despite intense work in this area, the use of certain modern methodologies in this field has only just begun. These include the application of nuclear magnetic resonance spectroscopy (phosphorus or carbon) to monitor intracellular metabolic events continuously, modeling of C-peptide data to measure the rates of insulin secretion, and modification of tracer techniques to measure changes continuously in metabolic fluxes occurring at the onset of exercise. Some outstanding issues include discrepancies between in vitro and in vivo observations with respect to the role of insulin in regulating glucose uptake. It is also necessary to outline more precisely the acute and chronic effects of insulin on receptor and postreceptor events in the contracting muscle. In diabetes, counterregulatory responses to hypo-glycemia, exercise, or both can be abnormal; therefore, it is important to outline the neuroendocrinological defects. Specifically, the potential role of the various neuropeptides in the regulation of normal and abnormal exercise metabolism has not been assessed. More epidemiological studies are necessary to reveal the role of exercise used in conjunction with other treatment modalities that attempts to reduce diabetic complications.

In diabetes, glucoregulation is offset. With absolute or relative insulin deficiency, glucose uptake by the muscle is decreased and will be exceeded by glucose production by the liver. This results in increased hyperglycemia and excessive lipolysis, thus leading to ketosis. Clearly, under such conditions exercise is not beneficial and should not be recommended. In contrast, in hyperinsulinemic diabetics, glucose production does not increase adequately, whereas muscular glucose uptake can be excessively increased. This can lead to reactive hypoglycemia. Hypoglycemia is likely to occur when preexercise plasma glucose is high. In Type I diabetics, hyperinsulinemia occurs because the mobilization of insulin from the subcutaneous depot can be increased by exercise and because exercise cannot suppress insulin entry into the circulation as it does in normal subjects. To avoid this condition, it is recommended that the amounts of insulin injected and of additional food intake before or during exercise be reduced. Hypoglycemia generally does not occur in patients on insulin pumps, when basal infusion of insulin is slightly reduced. In Type II diabetics, hyperinsulinemia is observed during exercise of moderate duration because insulin secretion is not suppressed. This could be related to hyperglycemia, which could counterbalance the restraining effect of the adrenergic control of insulin secretion or reflect early neuropathy of these nerve fibers.

Impaired metabolic glucose clearance is related not only to absolute or relative insulin deficiency but also to the levels of counterregulatory hormones that may be excessive during exercise. Thus, adrenergic beta blockade given to diabetics during exercise can fully normalize glucose uptake by the muscle. This seems to be due primarily to a large suppression of lipolysis and hence a decrease of fatty acid oxidation in the muscle. This is known as the glucose/fatty acid cycle. Thus, a very important role for insulin in the control of glucose uptake by the muscle is not direct but indirect. The oxygen supply to the muscle and brain can greatly offset the described control mechanisms. With hypoxia there is an excessive release of counterregulatory hormones that leads to augmented glucose production. However, despite excessive counterregulation, glucose uptake by the muscle is still greatly increased. This could be of importance in diabetics with restricted blood supplies to the muscles and high levels of glycosylated hemoglobin.

Exercise cannot be regarded as an isolated modality but must be incorporated into the total program of patient treatment. An exercise prescription that could be used for Type I and Type II diabetics under a variety of metabolic states and with varying degrees of complications has not yet been developed. Some very general guidelines follow (130): (a) Before your patient starts an exercise program, perform a complete history and physical examination. Evaluate diabetes control and screening for proliferative retinopathy and cardiovascular disease. (b) Prescribe moderate work loads that increase slowly. (c) Encourage the use of self-monitoring of blood glucose to document individual glycemic responses to different circumstances, as changes in insulin or food intake before exercise may be required. (d) When possible, encourage the patient to schedule exercise that will improve post-prandial hyperglycemia. (e) Discourage the patient from exercising during peak insulin action. (f) Inform the patient that extremities that are exercised should not be used as insulin injection sites. (g) Make the patients aware of the possibility of delayed exercise-induced hypoglycemia, which may occur several hours after the completion of exercise.

Acknowledgment

We wish to thank Mrs. Linda Vranic for editing this manuscript.

References

1. Ahlborg, G., P. Felig, L. Hagenfeldt, R. Hendler, and J. Wahren. Substrate turnover during prolonged exercise in man. *J. Clin. Invest.* 53: 1080, 1974.
2. Ahlborg, B., J. Bergstrom, L.-G. Ekelund, and E. Hultman. Muscle glycogen and muscle electrolytes during prolonged exercise. *Acta Physiol. Scand.* 70: 122-142, 1967.
3. Ahlborg, G. Mechanism for glycogenolysis in non-exercising human muscle during and after exercise. *Am. J. Physiol.* 248: E540, 1985.
4. Arnall, D.A., J.C. Marker, R.K. Conlee, and W. Winder. Effect of infusing epinephrine on liver and muscle glycogenolysis during exercise in rats. *Am. J. Physiol.* 250: E641, 1986.
5. Begum, N., R. Terjung, H. Tepperman, and J. Tepperman. Effect of acute exercise on insulin generation of pyruvate dehydrogenase activator by rat liver and adipocyte plasma membranes. *Diabetes* 35: 785, 1986.
6. Berger, M., P. Berchtold, and H.J. Cuppers. Metabolic and hormonal effects of muscular exercise in juvenile type diabetics. *Diabetologia* 13: 355, 1977.
7. Bjorkman, O., P. Miles, D.H. Wasserman, L. Lickley, and M. Vranic. Regulation of glucose turnover during exercise in pancreoteconized totally insulin-deficient dogs: Effects of beta adrenergic blockade. *J. Clin. Invest.* 81: 759-767, 1988.
8. Björntorp, P., M. Fahlen, G. Grimby, A. Gustafson, J. Holm, P. Renstrom, and T. Schersten. Carbohydrate and lipid metabolism in middle aged physically well-trained men. *Metabolism* 21: 631, 1972.
9. Bogardus, C., P. Thuillez, E. Ravussin, B. Vasquez, M. Narimiga, and S. Azhar. Effect of muscle glycogen depletion on *in vivo* insulin action in man. *J. Clin. Invest.* 72: 1605, 1983.
10. Bogardus, C., E. Ravussin, D.C. Robbins, R.R. Wolfe, E.S. Horton, and E.A.H. Sims. Effects of physical training and diet therapy on carbohydrate metabolism in patients with glucose intolerance and non-insulin dependent diabetes mellitus. *Diabetes* 33: 311, 1984.
11. Bonen, A., M.H. Tan, P. Clune, and P.L. Kirby. Effects of exercise on insulin binding to human muscle. *Am. J. Physiol.* 248: E403, 1985.
12. Bonen, A., P.A. Clune, and M.H. Tan. Chronic exercise increases insulin binding in muscles but not liver. *Am. J. Physiol.* 251: E196, 1986.
13. Burstein, R., C. Polychronakos, C.J. Toews, J. MacDougall, H. Guyda, and B. Posner. Acute reversal of the enhanced insulin action in trained athletes: Association with insulin receptor changes. *Diabetes* 34: 756, 1985.
14. Challis, R.A.J., M. Vranic, and G.K. Radda. Bioenergetic changes during contraction and recovery in diabetic rat skeletal muscle. *Am. J. Physiol.* 256: E129, 1989.
15. Chalmers, R.J., S.R. Bloom, G. Duncan, R.H. Johnson, and W.R. Sulaiman. The effect of somatostatin on metabolic and hormonal

changes during and after exercise. *Clin. Endocrinol.* 10: 451, 1979.

16. Chasiostis, D., K. Sahlin, and E. Hultman. Regulation of glycogenolysis in human muscle at rest and during exercise. *J. Appl. Physiol.* 53: 708, 1982.

17. Cherrington, A.D., J.E. Liljenquist, and G.I. Shulman. Importance of hypoglycemia-induced glucose production during isolated glucagon deficiency. *Am. J. Physiol.* 236: E263, 1979.

18. Chiasson, J.L., H. Shikama, D.T.W. Chu, and J.H. Exton. Inhibitory effect of epinephrine on insulin-stimulated glucose uptake by rat skeletal muscle. *J. Clin. Invest.* 68: 706, 1981.

19. Cooper, D.M., D.H. Wasserman, M. Vranic, and K. Wasserman. Glucose turnover in response to exercise during high- and low-F_iO_2 breathing in humans. *Am. J. Physiol.* 14: E209, 1986.

20. Craig, B.W., S.M. Garthwaite, and J.O. Holloszy. Adipocyte insulin resistance: Effects of aging, obesity, exercise, and food restriction. *J. Appl. Physiol.* 62: 95, 1987.

21. Crettaz, M., E.S. Horton, L.J. Wardzala, E.D. Horton, and B. Jeanrenaud. Physical training of Zucker rats: Lack of alleviation of muscle insulin resistance. *Am. J. Physiol.* 244: E414, 1983.

22. Davis, T.A., S. Klahr, E.D. Tegtmeyer, D.F. Osborne, T.L. Howard, and I.E. Karl. Glucose metabolism in epitrochlearis muscle of acutely exercised and trained rats. *Am. J. Physiol.* 250: E137, 1986.

23. De Fronzo, R.A., E. Ferrannini, Y. Sato, P. Felig, and J. Wahren. Synergistic interaction between exercise and insulin on peripheral glucose uptake. *J. Clin. Invest.* 68: 1468, 1981.

24. Devlin, J.T., M. Hirshman, and E.S. Horton. Enhanced peripheral and splanchnic insulin sensitivity in NIDDM men after single bout of exercise. *Diabetes* 36: 434, 1987.

25. Devlin, J.T., and E.S. Horton. Effects of prior high-intensity exercise on glucose metabolism in normal and insulin-resistant men. *Diabetes* 34: 973, 1985.

26. Dill, D.B., H.T. Edwards, and S. Mead. Blood sugar regulation in exercise. *Am. J. Physiol.* 111: 21-30, 1935.

27. Dohm, G.L., M.K. Sinha, and J.F. Caro. Insulin receptor binding and protein kinase activity in muscles of trained rats. *Am. J. Physiol.* 252: E170, 1987.

28. Garetto, L.P., E.A. Richter, M.N. Goodman, and N.B. Ruderman. Enhanced muscle glucose metabolism after exercise in the rat: The two phases. *Am. J. Physiol.* 246: E471, 1984.

29. Heath, G.W., J.R. Gavin, J.R. Hinderlites, J. Hagberg, S. Bloomfield, and J.O. Holloszy. Effects of exercise and lack of exercise on glucose tolerance and insulin sensitivity. *J. Appl. Physiol.* 55: 512, 1983.

30. Hermansen, L., E. Hultman, and B. Saltin. Muscle glycogen during prolonged severe exercise. *Acta Physiol. Scand.* 71: 129-139, 1967.

31. Hoelzer, D.R., G.P. Dalsky, N.S. Schwartz, W.E. Clutter, S.D. Shah, J.O. Holloszy, and P.E. Cryer. Epinephrine is not critical to prevention of hypoglycemia during exercise in humans. *Am. J. Physiol.* 251: E104, 1986.

32. Hoelzer, D., G. Dalsky, W. Clutter, S.D. Shah, J.O. Holloszy, and P.E. Cryer. Glucoregulation during exercise: Hypoglycemia is prevented by redundant glucoregulatory systems during exercise: Sympathochromafin activation, and changes in hormone secretion. *J. Clin. Invest.* 77: 212, 1986.

33. Horton, E.S. Exercise and physical training: Effect on insulin sensitivity and glucose metabolism. *Diabetes Metab. Rev.* (1/2): 1-17, 1986.

34. Hubinger, A., I. Ridderskamp, and E. Lehmann. Metabolic response to different forms of physical exercise in Type I diabetics and the duration of the glucose lowering effect. *Eur. J. Clin. Invest.* 15: 197, 1985.

35. Issekutz, B. Effects of glucose infusion on hepatic and muscle glycogenolysis in exercising dogs. *Am. J. Physiol.* 240: E451-E457, 1981.

36. Issekutz, B., and M. Vranic. Significance of glucagon in the control of glucose production during exercise. *Am. J. Physiol.* 238: E13, 1980.

37. Issekutz, B. The role of hypoinsulinemia in exercise metabolism. *Diabetes* 29: 629, 1980.

38. Ivy, J.L., W.M. Sherman, C.L. Cutler, and A.L. Katz. Exercise and diet reduce muscle insulin resistance in obese Zucker rat. *Am. J. Physiol.* 251:E299, 1986.

39. Ivy, J.L., Frishberg, S.W. Farrell, W.J. Miller, and W.M. Sherman. Effects of elevated and exercise-reduced muscle glycogen levels on insulin sensitivity. *J. Appl. Physiol.* 59: 154, 1985.

40. James, D.E., E.W. Kraegen, and D.J. Chisholm. Effects of exercise training on in vivo insulin action in individual tissues of the rat. *J. Clin. Invest.* 76: 657, 1985.

41. James, D.E., K.M. Burleigh, L.H. Storlien, P. Bennett, and E.W. Kraegen. Heterogeneity of insulin action in muscle: Influence of blood flow. *Am. J. Physiol.* 251: E422, 1986.

42. James, D.E., E.W. Kraegen, and D.J. Chisholm. Muscle glucose metabolism in exercising rats: Comparison with insulin stimulation. *Am. J. Physiol.* 248: E575, 1985.

43. Jansson, E., P. Hjemdahl, and L. Kaijser. Epinephrine-induced changes in muscle carbohydrate metabolism during exercise in male subjects. *J. Appl. Physiol.* 60: 1466, 1986.

44. Jenkins, A.B., S.M. Furler, D.J. Chisholm, and E.W. Kraegen. Regulation of hepatic glucose output during exercise by circulating glucose and insulin in humans. *Am. J. Physiol.* 250: R411, 1986.

45. Jenkins, A.B., D.J. Chisholm, D.E. James, K.Y. Ho, and E.W. Kraegen. Exercise induced hepatic glucose output is precisely sensitive to the rate of systemic glucose supply. *Metabolism* 34: 431, 1985.

46. Katz, A., S. Brobert, K. Sahlin, and J. Wahren. Leg glucose uptake during maximal dynamic exercise in humans. *Am. J. Physiol.* 251: E65-E70, 1986.

47. Kawamori, R., and M. Vranic. Mechanism of exercise-induced hypoglycemia in depancreatized dogs maintained on long-acting insulin. *J. Clin. Invest.* 59: 331, 1977.

48. Kemmer, F.W., P. Berchtold, M. Berger, A. Starke, H.J. Cuppers, F.A. Gries, and H. Zimmerman. Exercise induced fall of blood glucose in insulin treated diabetics unrelated to alteration of insulin mobilization. *Diabetes* 28: 1131, 1979.

49. Kemmer, F.W., and M. Berger. Therapy and better quality of life: The dichotomous role of exercise in diabetes mellitus. *Diabetes Metab. Rev.* 2: 53, 1986.

50. Kemmer, F.W., M. Tacken, and M. Berger. Mechanism of exercise-induced hypoglycemia during sulfonylurea treatment. *Diabetes* 36: 1178, 1987.

51. Koivisto, V., and R. DeFronzo. Exercise in the treatment of Type II diabetes. *Acta Endocrinol.* 262(Suppl.): 107, 1984.

52. Koivisto, V.A., and H. Yki-Jarvinen. Effect of exercise on insulin binding and glucose transport in adipocytes of normal humans. *J. Appl. Physiol.* 63: 1319, 1987.

53. Koivisto, V., and P. Felig. Effects of leg exercise on insulin absorption in diabetic patients. *N. Engl. J. Med.* 298: 77, 1978.

54. Kramsch, B.M., A.J. Aspen, B.M. Abramowitz, et al. Reduction of coronary atherosclerosis by moderate conditioning exercise in monkeys on an atherogenic diet. *N. Engl. J. Med.* 305: 1483-1489, 1981.

55. Krotkiewski, M., P. Lonnroth, K. Mandroukas, Z. Wroblewski, M. Rebuffe-Scrive, G. Holm, U. Smith, and P. Björntorp. The effects of physical training on insulin secretion and effectiveness and on glucose metabolism in obesity and Type II (non-insulin dependent) diabetes mellitus. *Diabetologia* 28: 881, 1985.

56. Krzentowski, G., F. Pirnay, N. Pallikarakis, A.S. Luyckx, M. Lacroix, F. Mosora, and P. Lefebvre. Glucose utilization in normal and diabetic subjects: The role of insulin. *Diabetes* 30: 983, 1981.

57. Landt, K.W., B.N. Campaigne, F.W. James, and M. Sperling. Effects of exercise training on insulin sensitivity in adolescents with Type I diabetes. *Diabetes Care* 8: 461, 1985.

58. Lilloja, S., A.A. Young, C.L. Cutler, J.L. Ivy, W.G.H. Abbott, J. Zawadzki, H. Yki-Jarvinen, L. Christin, T.W. Secomb, and C. Bogardus. Skeletal muscle capillary density and fiber type are possible determinants of in vivo insulin resistance in man. *J. Clin. Invest.* 80: 415, 1987.

59. Lithell, H., M. Krotkiewski, and B. Kiens. Non-response of muscle capillary density and lipoprotein-lipase activity to regular training in diabetic patients. *Diabetes Res.* 2: 17, 1985.

60. McDermott, J.C., G.C. Elder, and A. Bonen. Adrenal hormones enhance glycogenolysis in non-exercising muscle during exercise. *J. Appl. Physiol.* 63: 1275, 1987.

61. McGilvery, R.W. The use of fuels for muscular work. In: Howald, H., and J.R. Poortsmans, eds. *Metabolic adaptation to prolonged physical exercise.* Basel: Birkhauser; 1975: pp. 12-30.

62. Michel, G., T. Vocke, W. Fiehn, H. Weiker, W. Schwarz, and W.P. Bieger. Bidirectional alteration on insulin receptor affinity by different forms of physical exercise. *Am. J. Physiol.* 246: E153, 1984.

63. Miller, W.J., W.M. Sherman, and J.L. Ivy. Effect of strength training on glucose tolerance and post-glucose insulin response. *Med. Sci. Sports Exerc.* 15: 539, 1984.

64. Minuk, H.L., M. Vranic, E.B. Marliss, A.K. Hanna, A.M. Albisser, and B. Zinman. Glucoregulatory and metabolic response to

exercise in obese noninsulin-dependent diabetes. *Am. J. Physiol.* 240: E458, 1981.

65. Moates, J.M., D.B. Lacy, and R.E. Goldstein. The metabolic role of the exercise-induced increment in epinephrine in the dog. *Am. J. Physiol.* 255: E428, 1988.

66. Nathan, D.M., S.F. Madnek, and L. Delahanty. Programming pre-exercise snacks to prevent post-exercise hypoglycemia in intensively treated insulin-dependent diabetics. *Ann. Intern. Med.* 1-2: 483, 1985.

67. National Institutes of Health. Consensus development conference on diet and exercise in non-insulin dependent diabetes mellitus. *Diabetes Care* 10: 639-643, 1987.

68. Nesher, R., I.E. Karl, and K.M. Kipnis. Dissociation of the effect(s) of insulin and contraction on glucose transport in rat epitrochlearis muscle. *Am. J. Physiol.* 249: C226, 1985.

69. Newsholme, E.A., and C. Start. *Regulation in metabolism.* Toronto: John Wiley & Sons, 1973.

70. Nikkila, E.A. Plasma lipid and lipoprotein abnormalities in diabetes. In: Jarrett, J.R., ed. *Diabetes and heart disease.* Amsterdam: Elsevier, 1984: pp. 133.

71. Noble, E.G., and C.D. Ianuzzo. Influence of training on skeletal muscle enzymatic adaptations in normal and diabetic rats. *Am. J. Physiol.* 249: E360, 1985.

72. Paffenbarger, R.S., A.L. Wing, R.T. Hyde, et al. Physical activity as an index of heart attack risk in college alumni. *Am. J. Epidemiol.* 108: 161-175, 1978.

73. Ploug, T., H. Galbo, J. Vinten, M. Jorgensen, and E. Richter. Kinetics of glucose transport in rat muscle: Effects of insulin and contractions. *Am. J. Physiol.* 253: E12, 1987.

74. Pyorala, K. Relationship of glucose tolerance and plasma insulin to the incidence of coronary heart disease: Results from two population studies in Finland. *Diabetes Care* 2: 131, 1979.

75. Reitman, J.S., B. Vasquez, I. Klimes, and M. Nagulesparan. Improvement of glucose homeostasis after exercise training in non-insulin dependent diabetes. *Diabetes Care* 7: 434, 1984.

76. Richter, E.A., T. Ploug, and H. Galbo. Increased muscle glucose uptake after exercise: No need for insulin during exercise. *Diabetes* 34, 1041, 1985.

77. Richter, E.A., N.B. Ruderman, H. Gavras, E. Belur, and H. Galbo. Muscle glycogenolysis during exercise: Dual control by epinephrine and contractions. *Am. J. Physiol.* 242: E25, 1982.

78. Richter, E.A., H. Galbo, J.J. Holst, and B. Sonne. Significance of glucagon for insulin secretion and hepatic glycogenolysis during exercise in rats. *Horm. Metab. Res.* 13: 323, 1981.

79. Rodnick, K.J., W.L. Haskell, A.L.M. Swislocki, J.E. Foley, and G.M. Reaven. Improved insulin action in muscle, liver, and adipose tissue in physically trained human subjects. *Am. J. Physiol.* 253: E489, 1987.

80. Schiffrin, A., and S. Parikh. Accommodating planned exercise in Type I diabetic patients on intensive treatment. *Diabetes Care* 8: 337, 1985.

81. Schneider, S.H., A. Vitug, and N.B. Ruderman. Atherosclerosis and physical activity. *Diabetes Metab. Rev.* 1: 513-553, 1986.

82. Schneider, S.H., L.F. Amorosa, A.K. Khachadurian, and N.B. Ruderman. Studies on the mechanism of improved glucose control during regular exercise in Type II (non-insulin dependent) diabetes. *Diabetologia* 25: 355, 1984.

83. Shilo, S., M. Sotsky, and H. Shamoon. Effect of plasma insulin on glucose kinetics in exercising non-diabetic and Type I diabetic man. *Diabetes* 36(Suppl. 1): 16A, 1987.

84. Simonson, D.C., V. Koivisto, R.S. Sherwin, E. Ferrannini, R. Hendler, J. Juhlin-Dannfeldt, and R. DeFronzo. Andrenergic blockade alters glucose kinetics during exercise in insulin-dependent diabetics. *J. Clin. Invest.* 73: 1648, 1984.

85. Sonne, B., K.J. Mikines, E.A. Richter, N.J. Christensen, and H. Galbo. Role of liver nerves and adrenal medulla in glucose turnover in running rats. *J. Appl. Physiol.* 59: 1650, 1985.

86. Standl, E., N. Lotz, T.H. Dexel, H. Janka, and H. Kolb. Muscle triglycerides in diabetic subjects. *Diabetologia* 18: 463, 1980.

87. Susstrunk, H., B. Morell, W.H. Ziegler, and E.R. Froesch. Insulin absorption from the abdomen and the thigh in healthy subjects during rest and exercise: Blood glucose, plasma insulin, growth hormone, adrenaline, and noradrenaline levels. *Diabetologia* 22: 171, 1982.

88. Tamborlane, W.V., R.S. Sherwin, V. Koivisto, R. Hendler, M. Genel, and P. Felig. Normalization of the growth hormone and catecholamine response to exercise in juvenile-

onset diabetic subjects treated with a portable insulin infusion pump. *Diabetes* 28: 785, 1979.

89. Tancrede, G., S. Rousseau-Migneron, and A. Nadeau. Beneficial effects of physical training in rats with a mild streptozotocin-induced diabetes mellitus. *Diabetes* 31: 406, 1982.

90. Taylor, R., P. Ram, P. Zimmet, L.R. Raper, and H. Ringrose. Physical activity and prevalence of DM in Melanesian and Indian men in Fiji. *Diabetologia* 27: 578-582, 1984.

91. Trovati, M., Q. Carta, F. Cavalot, S. Vitali, C. Banaudi, P. Lucchina, F. Fiocchi, G. Emanuelli, and G. Lenti. Influence of physical training on blood glucose control, glucose tolerance, insulin secretion, and insulin action in non-insulin dependent diabetic patients. *Diabetes Care* 7: 416, 1984.

92. Vallerand, A.L., J. Lupien, and L.J. Bukowiecki. Synergistic improvement of glucose tolerance by sucrose feeding and exercise training. *Am. J. Physiol.* 250: E607, 1986.

93. Vallerand, A.L., J. Lupien, Y. Deshaies, and L. Bukowiecki. Intensive exercise training does not improve intravenous glucose tolerance in severely diabetic rats. *Horm. Metab. Res.* 18: 79, 1986.

94. Vinten, J., L. Norgaard Petersen, B. Sonne, and H. Galbo. Effect of physical training on glucose transporters in fat cell fractions. *Biochim. Biophys. Acta* 841: 223, 1985.

95. Vranic, M., H.L.A. Lickley, and J.K. Davidson. Exercise and stress in diabetes mellitus. In: Davidson, J.K., ed. *Clinical diabetes mellitus.* New York: Thieme-Stratton; 1986: Chapt. 15, p. 172.

96. Vranic, M., F.W. Kemmer, P. Berchtold, and M. Berger. Hormonal interaction in control of metabolism during exercise in physiology and diabetes. In: Ellenberg, H., and H. Rifkin, eds. *Diabetes mellitus: Theory and practice.* 3rd ed. New York: Medical Examination Publishing/Excerpta Medica; 1983: Chapt. 27, pp. 567-590.

97. Vranic, M., R. Kawamori, S. Pek, N. Kovacevic, and G. Wrenshell. The essentiality of insulin and the role of glucagon in regulating glucose utilization and production during strenuous exercise in dogs. *J. Clin. Invest.* 57: 245, 1976.

98. Vranic, M., and G.A. Wrenshall. Exercise, insulin and glucose turnover in dogs. *Endocrinology* 85: 165-171, 1969.

99. Wahren, J., P. Felig, G. Ahlborg, and L. Jorfeldt. Glucose metabolism during leg exercise in man. *J. Clin. Invest.* 50: 2715, 1971.

100. Wahren, J., L. Hagenfeldt, and P. Felig. Splanchnic and leg exchange of glucose, amino acids, and free fatty acids during exercise in diabetes mellitus. *J. Clin. Invest.* 55: 1303, 1975.

101. Wahren, J., Y. Sato, J. Ostman, L. Hagenfeldt, and P. Felig. Turnover and splanchnic metabolism of free fatty acids and ketones in insulin-dependent diabetics during exercise. *J. Clin. Invest.* 73: 1367, 1984.

102. Wahrenberg, H., P. Engfeldt, J. Bolinder, and P. Arner. Acute adaptation in adrenergic control of lipolysis during physical exercise in humans. *Am. J. Physiol.* 253: E383, 1987.

103. Wallberg-Henriksson, H., R. Gunnarsson, S. Rossner, and J. Wahren. Long-term physical training in female Type I (insulin dependent) diabetic patients: Absence of significant effect on glycemic control and lipoprotein levels. *Diabetologia* 29: 53, 1986.

104. Wallberg-Henriksson, H., R. Gunnarsson, J. Henriksson, R. DeFronzo, P. Felig, J. Ostman, and J. Wahren. Influence of physical training on formation of muscle capillaries in Type I diabetes. *Diabetes* 34: 412, 1984.

105. Wallberg-Henriksson, H., R. Gunnarsson, J. Henriksson, R. DeFronzo, P. Felig, J. Ostman, and J. Wahren. Increased peripheral insulin sensitivity and muscle mitochondrial enzymes but unchanged blood glucose control in Type I diabetics after physical training. *Diabetes* 31: 1044, 1982.

106. Wardzala, L.J., E.S. Horton, M. Crettaz, E.D. Horton, and B. Jeanrenaud. Physical training of lean and genetically obese Zucker rats: Effect on fat cell metabolism. *Am. J. Physiol.* 243: E418, 1982.

107. Wasserman, D.H., H.L.A. Lickley, and M. Vranic. Role of beta-adrenergic mechanisms during exercise in poorly controlled insulin deficient diabetes. *J. Appl. Physiol.* 59: 1282, 1985.

108. Wasserman, D.H., and M. Vranic. Interaction between insulin, glucagon, and catecholamines in the regulation of glucose production and uptake during exercise: Physiology and diabetes. In: Saltin, B., ed. *Biochemistry of exercise VI.* Champaign, IL: Human Kinetics Publishers; 1986: p. 167.

109. Wasserman, D.H., H.L.A. Lickley, and M. Vranic. Important role of glucagon during exercise and diabetes. *J. Appl. Physiol.* 59: 1272, 1985.

110. Wasserman, D.H., S.P. Nolin, J.R. Hastings, R.E. Goldstein, and D.B. Lacy. Significance

of the exercise-induced fall in insulin to fat metabolism [Abstract]. *FASEB J.* 2: A712, 1988.

111. Wasserman, D.H., P.E. Williams, D.B. Lacy, D.R. Green, and A.D. Cherrington. Importance of intrahepatic mechanisms to gluconeogenesis from alanine during prolonged exercise and recovery. *Am. J. Physiol.* 254: E518, 1988.

112. Wasserman, D.H., H.L.A. Lickley, and M. Vranic. Effect of hematocrit reduction on hormonal and metabolic responses to exercise. *J. Appl. Physiol.* 58: 1257, 1985.

113. Wasserman, D.H., and M. Vranic. Interaction between insulin and counterregulatory hormones in control of substrate utilization in health and diabetes during exercise. In: DeFronzo, R.A., ed. *Diabetes/metabolism reviews.* New York: John Wiley & Sons; 1986: vol. 1, no. 4, pp. 159-183.

114. Wasserman, D.H., R. Goldstein, P. Donahue, S. Passalaqua, and D. Lacy. Importance of the exercise-induced fall in insulin to the regulation of hepatic carbohydrate metabolism. *Diabetes* 36(Suppl. 1): 39A, 1987.

115. Wasserman, D.H., D.B. Lacy, R. Goldstein, P. Williams, and A.D. Cherrington. Role of the exercise-induced fall in insulin independent of the effects of glucagon [Abstract]. *Med. Sci. Sports Exerc.* 20:84, 1988.

116. Wasserman, D.H., H.L.A. Lickley, and M. Vranic. Interactions between glucagon and other counterregulatory hormones during normoglycemic and hypoglycemic exercise. *J. Clin. Invest.* 74: 1404, 1984.

117. Wasserman, D.H., and M. Vranic. Exercise and diabetes. In: Alberti, K.G.M.M., and L.P. Krall, eds. *The diabetes annual/3.* Amsterdam: Elsevier, 1987, p. 527-559.

118. Webster, B., S.R. Vigna, and T. Paquette. Acute exercise, epinephrine, and diabetes enhance insulin binding to skeletal muscle. *Am. J. Physiol.* 250: E186, 1986.

119. Winder, W.W., H.T. Yang, A.W. Jaussi, and C.R. Hopkins. Epinephrine, glucose and lactate infusion in exercising adrenomedullated rats. *J. Appl. Physiol.* 62: 1442, 1987.

120. Wolfe, R.R., E.R. Nadel, J.H.F. Shaw, L.A. Stephenson, and M. Wolfe. Role of changes in insulin and glucagon in glucose homeostasis in exercise. *J. Clin. Invest.* 77: 900, 1986.

121. Yki-Jarvinen, H., and V. Koivisto. Effects of body composition on insulin sensitivity. *Diabetes* 32: 965, 1983.

122. Yki-Jarvinen, H., R. DeFronzo, and V. Koivisto. Normalization of insulin sensitivity in Type I diabetic subjects by physical training during insulin pump therapy. *Diabetes Care* 7: 520, 1984.

123. Young, J.C., J.L. Treadway, E.I. Fader, and R.F. Caslin. Effects of oral hypoglycemic agent methylpalmoxirate on exercise capacity of streptozotocin diabetic rats. *Diabetes* 35: 744, 1986.

124. Zander, E., W. Burns, P. Wulfert, W. Besch, D. Lubs, R. Chlup, and B. Schulz. Muscular exercise in Type I diabetics: I. Different metabolic reactions during heavy muscular work in dependence on actual insulin availability. *Exp. Clin. Endocrinol.* 82: 78, 1983.

125. Zander, E., B. Schulz, R. Chlup, P. Woltansky, and D. Lubs. Muscular exercise in Type I diabetics: II. Hormonal and metabolic responses to moderate exercise. *Exp. Clin. Endocrinol.* 85: 95, 1985.

126. Zinman, B., F.T. Murray, M. Vranic, A.M. Albisser, B.S. Leibel, P.A. McClean, and E.B. Marliss. Glucoregulation during moderate exercise in insulin treated diabetics. *J. Clin. Endocrinol. Metab.* 45: 641, 1977.

127. Zinman, B., S. Zuniga-Guajardo, and D. Kelly. Comparison of the acute and long-term effects of exercise on glucose control in Type I diabetes. *Diabetes Care* 7: 515, 1984.

128. Zorzano, A., T.W. Balon, L.P. Garetto, M.N. Goodman, and N.B. Ruderman. Muscle alpha aminoisobutyric acid transport after exercise: Enhanced stimulation by insulin. *Am. J. Physiol.* 248: E546, 1985.

129. Zorzano, A., T.W. Balon, M.N. Goodman, and N.B. Ruderman. Glycogen depletion and increased insulin sensitivity and responsiveness in muscle after exercise. *Am. J. Physiol.* 251: E664, 1986.

130. Zinman, B., and M. Vranic. Diabetes and exercise. *Med. Clin. N. Am.* 69: 145-157, 1985.

Chapter 40

Discussion: Exercise, Fitness, and Diabetes

Michael Berger
Friedrich W. Kemmer

Inasmuch as the physiological and pathophysiological aspects of exercise, fitness, and diabetes have been presented in depth with the utmost degree of clarity by Vranic and Wasserman in the previous chapter, this discussant paper attempts merely to highlight some related clinical issues. In this context, it appears mandatory to differentiate strictly between Type I (insulin-dependent) and Type II (non-insulin-dependent) diabetes mellitus. Whereas physical exercise and training will undoubtedly represent somatic and psychological benefits, at least to the major part of the population (with all diabetic patients included), the particular effects of physical exertion differ fundamentally between Type I and Type II diabetes. Thus the clinical implications, potential benefits, and untoward complications need to be presented separately for those two separate diseases.

Type I Diabetes Mellitus

Type I (insulin-dependent) diabetes represents a conceptually simple disorder that is due to an (initially) isolated defect of the insulin-secreting pancreatic B-cells with the development of hypoinsulinemia and the precipitation of respective acute deteriorations of many aspects of metabolic homeostasis. Depending on the varying imperfections of different strategies of insulin substitution therapy, acute complications (due to hypo- or hyperinsulinemia) and long-term complications (diabetic microangiopathy related to the long-term quality of metabolic control) are determinants of the natural history and prognosis of Type I diabetes. Patients who are metabolically well controlled by modern intensified insulin therapies (3, 17) usually do not present with lipid disorders, insulin insensitivity, or excessive risks for macrovascular disease if other cardiovascular risk factors and, in particular, diabetic nephropathy are not present.

For such patients, exercise or training programs do not need to be prescribed with the aim of maintaining or improving glycemic control. In fact, numerous studies have shown that exercise programs are not helpful when used to improve the standards of suboptimal metabolic control (12, 20, 21). However, glycemic control may very well be optimized under certain conditions by intensified treatment and teaching programs without the implementation of exercise as a part of therapy (1, 13). In fact, earlier recommendations to use physical activity intentionally (i.e., at a particular time of the day at a defined intensity and duration) to attenuate certain problems in glycemic control (e.g., the postprandial rise of blood glucose following breakfast by performing postbreakfast exercises) must be considered as a further and unnecessary burden to the patient, as such hyperglycemic excursions may be reduced effectively by revising the balance between carbohydrate intake and regular insulin dosage before the meal. Hence, the performance of regular, defined physical activity prescribed as a means to improve glycemic control to Type I patients should today be regarded as obsolete (17).

However, very much like the nondiabetic population, an ever-growing number of Type I patients intend to take up or intensify their leisure-time physical activity for a number of (mainly not health-related) motives. In fact, participation in exercises and games has become an important facet in the social development of society. It is therefore the obligation of the diabetologist-physician to enable Type I patients to perform physical activity at a minimal risk of acute complications and under optimal conditions for performance. The successes of diabetic athletes and the activities of the International Diabetic Athletes Association have impressively documented that this is very well possible (5).

Such successes need to be based on several efforts. First of all, Type I patients need to be examined carefully and specifically before exercise programs or increases in habitual physical activity are initiated. Apart from general evaluations of the cardiovascular system, particular emphasis must be placed on the retinal and neurological status of the patients. Proliferative and preproliferative retinopathy and (exercise-induced) hypertension need to be treated adequately before physical activity can be initiated safely. Of particular relevance are disturbances of the cardiovascular function (e.g., blood pressure regulation) due to autonomic neuropathy and the increased risks of severe complications associated with peripheral diabetic polyneuropathy at the level of the feet during exercise. All Type I patients need to be safeguarded against the potential metabolic deteriorations that may occur during or after exercise (i.e., further decompensation of metabolism in case of hypoinsulinemic states or, more important, exercise-induced hypoglycemia during or after physical activity).

Any effective prevention of these much-feared complications of exercise in insulin-treated diabetic patients must be attempted in the context of an intensive diabetes treatment and teaching program, the aim of which is to train the patients to perform self-treatment (including continuous autonomous amendments of insulin dosage at a very wide flexibility of diet and carbohydrate intake) based on regular and systematic blood glucose self-monitoring. The efficacy and long-term safety of such programs aiming at far-reaching independence of the patient from physicians and clinics has been documented under particular conditions, even for unselected patients, provided that comprehensive educational programs can be offered (13). Thus, patients must gain a deep insight into the various factors governing their blood glucose regulation and must understand how to manipulate glycemic control effectively and safely. Only then will they understand that during phases of substantial hyperglycemia and ketosis they should abstain from physical activity until they have corrected this metabolic deterioration by additional insulin.

For the prevention of exercise-induced hypoglycemia, the patients must know that the ultimate basis for this phenomenon is the fact that, during subcutaneous insulin therapy, circulating insulin levels do not decline in response to exercise. Hence, there is an imbalance between the increase of glucose uptake by contracting skeletal muscles and the hepatic glucose production that is suppressed by relative hyperinsulinemia and hypoglucagonemia during or after exercise, and a decrease of glycemia ensues. To prevent exercise-induced hypoglycemia, a dose reduction of insulin injections before or after exercise, the intake of additional carbohydrate, or both are mandatory. Changing the insulin injection sites before exercise to prevent any exercise-induced increase in insulinemia has no place as a recommendation to prevent exercise-induced hypoglycemia (6, 7).

For more prolonged periods of exercise, insulin dose reduction is the principle preventive measure and should be substantial, whereas shorter periods of exercise may be effectively balanced by extra carbohydrate intake. Many factors (e.g., glycemia; intensity and duration of exercise; status of the patient's training; prenutrition; degree of metabolic control; time of the day; and time elapsed since the last insulin injection, the last meal, and the last bout of exercise) play decisive roles in determining both the risk of exercise-induced hypoglycemia and the quantitative means to prevent this complication. Thus it is effectively impossible to compile concrete guidelines for advice to the patients regarding the quantity of extra carbohydrate intake or insulin dose reduction necessary in a particular exercise situation. On the basis of comprehensive training of self-control and self-treatment, the patient must be guided to identify his or her individual rules for preventing exercise-induced hypoglycemia with the help of frequent blood glucose self-monitoring. Only through a system of intensive education for self-managing his or her metabolic control can physical activity be performed safely and with optimal performance by Type I patients (8).

Offering adequate treatment and teaching programs aiming at training the patients for self-management of their metabolic control must be considered the main objective for diabetologists-physicians to enable those Type I patients who are physically able and who are for any reason motivated to participate in physical exercise programs, sports, and games to do so. The prolongation of such programs and, in particular, of long-term physical training will reduce the insulin requirements for Type I patients. Whether this lowering of insulin needs has any beneficial consequences (such as reduction in the incidence of hypoglycemia) is presently unknown.

Type II Diabetes Mellitus

Type II (non-insulin-dependent) diabetes represents a complex syndrome of hyperglycemia, insulin resistance (16), and often a variety of interrelated cardiovascular risk factors (15), as most of these patients not only are overweight but also present with hypertension and hyperlipoproteinemia. In a very high percentage of cases, macrovascular disease is already present at diagnosis of Type II diabetes. Furthermore, for most of the 3%-4% of the population presently known as Type II diabetics, this disorder develops after the age of 60 and, very often, as only one aspect of a multifaceted geriatric multimorbidity. For most of these patients, macrovascular disease and its complications are the major determinants of their prognosis; and only in those patients who manifest Type II diabetes at a younger age must the prevention of microangiopathy by the strict normalization of glycemia be regarded as a primary therapeutic goal.

Paralleling the obvious heterogeneity of Type II diabetes and the individual therapeutic goals for these patients is a diversity of treatment strategies. Whereas most cases of Type II diabetes may be effectively treated by hypocaloric diets alone, a variable percentage of patients (different from country to country and from one health care system to another) are additionally being treated with oral antidiabetic agents, insulin, or both. Despite all these aspects of heterogeneity, insulin resistance associated with a relative deficiency of insulin secretory capacity is thought to be the basic defect for all stages and subgroups of Type II diabetes. Thus, any attempt to improve the organism's insulin sensitivity should represent a most important candidate for a rational therapy of this disorder. Therefore, along with weight reduction, physical exercise and training must be regarded a priori as a crucial therapeutic approach to the treatment of Type II diabetes.

In fact, prospective studies with genetically hyperglycemic obese rodents (2) have documented that physical activity programs may be instrumental in preventing the development of insulin resistance (hyperglycemia), and epidemiological studies in Pacific populations suggest a possible role for physical inactivity in increasing the incidence of Type II diabetes in this region (11, 22). However, despite all these theoretical anticipations of the beneficial effects of physical activity and training programs on glucose tolerance in patients with Type II diabetes, the unequivocal evidence for the effectiveness of such a therapeutic approach based on prospective controlled studies remains surprisingly scarce (9, 19). In those Type II patients treated with insulin or oral sulfonylurea therapy, potential complications (e.g., exercise-induced hypoglycemia) must be taken into account (10). Although potential benefits of an exercise-training program in such patients might become readily apparent by the need or the possibility to discontinue insulin therapy or sulfonylurea treatment, no such studies have been performed to date.

In contrast, a multitude of investigations have been carried out in glucose-intolerant and Type II men that aim to demonstrate an improvement in glucose tolerance or glycemic control along with improvements in body mass index and lipidemia by regular physical exercise. Although there is essentially no indication of any difference in the hormonal or metabolic effects of acute exercise between healthy subjects and Type II patients who are well controlled on diet therapy, on the whole these studies have not rendered the anticipated beneficial effects of physical training on glucose tolerance. Difficulties in study design (e.g., the separation of dietary from exercise effects, the heterogeneity of the initial hormonal-metabolic status of the patients, and most of all the apparent lack of motivation for prolonged cooperation and physical disabilities due to age-related multimorbidity) have become major problems during these investigations. Only in a few selected subgroups of Type II patients who are few in number (e.g., the relatively healthy, the hyperinsulinemic, and the young) have clear-cut positive effects of physical activity and training on glucose tolerance been documented (4, 18). But even for those favorable circumstances the duration of the beneficial training effects remains to be elucidated. Regarding these overall rather disappointing end results from a large number of most elaborate investigations, a recent National Institutes of Health Consensus Conference (14) drew rather skeptical conclusions as to the general beneficial effects of physical training programs as part of the treatment of Type II diabetes.

Against the potential benefits (yet to be explored fully), one must balance possible risks associated with exercise-training programs in elderly populations with major cardiovascular risks and very often manifest atherosclerosis and coronary heart disease. As with other, comparable groups of patients (e.g., so-called coronary groups), the Type II patients participating in such training programs need to be screened specifically for cardiovascular risks and diseases, and particular exercise programs should be designed and carried out under professional and medical supervision. These programs also need to take into account that most of these elderly Type II patients have not participated in any physical activity for quite some time and thus are particularly vulnerable and prone to develop all kinds of injuries.

However, before more general recommendations for the use of physical activity and training programs in the context of the treatment of Type II diabetes can be made, considerably more research is needed to define, for particular subgroups of Type II diabetics, particular exercise programs that have proven to be effective in potentially improving glucose tolerance and glycemic control. These studies should be carried out with well-defined, larger groups of unselected patients and should be designed by taking into account their potential practical application for increasingly large numbers of patients. One might anticipate that the changes required for these programs to be effective and safe are considerably greater if younger age-groups of patients with shorter duration of Type II diabetes are selected for such studies and if exercise programs of sufficient intensities are combined with dietary treatment.

Of particular interest seem to be long-term studies on the efficacy of exercise-training programs in preventing Type II diabetes in individuals who are at high risk of developing this disease. On the whole, one would expect the largest potential benefits from such early interventions by physical exercise-training programs with respect to the prevention of both Type II diabetes and atherosclerotic disease.

References

1. Assal, J.P., I. Mühlhauser, A. Pernet, R. Gfeller, V. Jörgens, and M. Berger. Patient education as the basis for diabetes care in clinical practice and research. *Diabetologia* 28: 602-613, 1985.
2. Becker-Zimmerman, K., M. Berger, P. Berchtold, F.A. Gries, L. Herberg, and M. Schwenen. Treadmill training improves intravenous glucose tolerance and insulin sensitivity in fatty Zucker rats. *Diabetologia* 22: 468-474, 1982.
3. Berger, M., and V. Jörgens. *Praxis der insulintherapie.* 2nd ed. Berlin: Springer, 1986.
4. Bogardus, C., E. Ravussin, D.C. Robbins, R.R. Wolfe, E.D. Horton, and E.A.H. Sims. Effects of physical training and diet therapy on carbohydrate metabolism in patients with glucose intolerance and non-insulin-dependent diabetes mellitus. *Diabetes* 33: 311-318, 1984.
5. *International Diabetic Athletes Association Newsletter* 1: No. 2, 1986.
6. Kemmer, F.W., P. Berchtold, M. Berger, A. Starke, H.J. Cüppers, F.A. Gries, and H. Zimmerman. Exercise-induced fall of blood glucose in insulin treated diabetics unrelated to alteration in insulin mobilization. *Diabetes* 28: 1131-1137, 1979.
7. Kemmer, F.W., and M. Berger. Exercise in therapy and the life of diabetic patients. *Clin. Sci.* 67: 279-283, 1984.
8. Kemmer, F.W. *Diabetes und sport ohne probleme: Praktische hinweise für diabetische kinder und jugendliche sowie deren eltern.* Mainz: Kirchheim Verlag, 1986.
9. Kemmer, F.W., and M. Berger. Therapy and better quality of life: The dichotomous role of exercise in diabetes mellitus. *Diabetes Metab. Rev.* 2: 53-68, 1986.
10. Kemmer, F.W., M. Tacken, and M. Berger. On the mechanism of exercise induced hypoglycemia during sulfonylurea treatment. *Diabetes* 36: 1178-1187, 1987.
11. King, H., P. Zimmet, L.R. Raper, and B. Balkau. Risk factors for diabetes in three Pacific populations. *Am. J. Epidemiol.* 119: 396, 1984.
12. Landt, K.W., B.N. Campaigne, F.W. James, and M.A. Sperling. Effects of exercise training on insulin sensitivity in adolescents with Type I diabetes. *Diabetes Care* 8: 461-465, 1985.
13. Mühlhauser, I., I. Bruckner, M. Berger, D. Cheta, V. Jörgens, C. Ionescu-Tirgoviste, V. Scholz, and I. Mincu. Evaluation of an intensified insulin treatment and teaching programme as routine management of Type I (insulin dependent) diabetes: The Bucharest-Düsseldorf Study. *Diabetologia* 30: 681-691, 1987.
14. National Institutes of Health. Consensus development conference on diet and exercise in non-insulin-dependent diabetes mellitus. *Diabetes Care* 10: 639-644, 1987.
15. Panzram, G. Mortality and survival in Type 2 (non-insulin-dependent) diabetes mellitus. *Diabetologia* 30: 123-132, 1987.

16. Reaven, G.M. Insulin-dependent diabetes mellitus: Metabolic characteristics. *Metabolism* 29: 445-454, 1980.

17. Schade, D.S., J.V. Santiago, J.S. Skyler, and R.A. Rizza. *Intensive insulin therapy*. Amsterdam: Excerpta Medica, 1983.

18. Schneider, S.H., L.F. Amorosa, A.K. Khachadurian, and N.B. Ruderman. Studies on the mechanism of improved glucose control during regular exercise in Type-2 (non-insulin-dependent) diabetes. *Diabetologia* 26: 355-360, 1984.

19. Skarfors, E.T., T.A. Wegener, H. Lithell, and I. Selinus. Physical training as treatment for Type 2 (non-insulin-dependent) diabetes in elderly men: A feasibility study over 2 years. *Diabetologia* 30: 930-933, 1987.

20. Wallberg-Henriksson, H., R. Gunnarson, J. Henricksson, R.A. DeFronzo, P. Felig, J. Östman, and J. Wahren. Increased peripheral insulin sensitivity and muscle mitochondrial enzymes but unchanged blood glucose control in Type I diabetics after physical training. *Diabetes* 31: 1044-1050, 1982.

21. Yki-Järvinen, H., R.A. DeFronzo, and V.A. Koivisto. Normalization of insulin sensitivity in Type I diabetic subjects by physical training during insulin pump therapy. *Diabetes Care* 7: 520-527, 1984.

22. Zimmet, P., S. Faaiuso, J. Ainuu, S. Whitehouse, B. Milne, and W. DeBoer. The prevalence of diabetes in the rural and urban Polynesian population of Western Samoa. *Diabetes* 30: 45-51, 1981.

Chapter 41

Exercise and Obesity

G.A. Bray

Obesity is the result of a positive energy balance. The accumulation of fat is a visible manifestation that more food energy has been stored than has been expended. Correction of this imbalance can focus on either side of the equation for energy balance, but the consequences may be different. This chapter focuses on the role of physical activity and exercise in obesity. After describing the metabolic, endocrine, and cardiovascular adaptations to exercise, I review the studies that have used exercise programs in the treatment of obesity. Finally, I examine the potentially beneficial effects of exercise.

Spontaneous Movement in the Obese

One approach to detecting differences in physical activity between obese and lean subjects has been to measure spontaneous activity. This can be done by one of three methods. In the first method, people can be questioned about their habitual physical activity or can be asked to record their activities using an activity diary. A second approach is to observe activity levels directly or to record them on film or videocassette for analysis. The third group of methods are more quantitative, using pedometers, recording changes in heart rate during exercise throughout the day, or measuring oxygen consumption during given activities. In the studies on exercise and obesity, all these methods have been used, but there is no uniformity to the reports. Interpretation of some of these methods is complicated by the fact that moving a heavy body requires more energy than does moving a lighter one (10). This is shown graphically in Figure 41.1, which shows the energy expended by pedaling a bicycle with no external load. The work is the work of moving the legs and is related directly to

body weight. There is a high correlation between body weight and caloric expenditure ($r = .94$; regression line $y = 5.8 = 151$). Thus, lesser spontaneous movement by an obese person may actually result in a similar or even greater total energy expenditure than it would in a lean person with more spontaneous activity (8).

Children and Adolescents

Several studies have addressed the question of whether physical activity and body weight can be related in infancy and whether spontaneous slowing of activity precedes or follows the onset of obesity. Rose and Mayer (60) studied 6 obese infants and 25 controls by attaching an activity meter to one limb. They observed that the obese infants were significantly less active. Several studies of physical activity have also been conducted in obese children. Stunkard and Petska (68) compared 15 obese girls with 15 controls by using a pedometer from which self-reports of walking were obtained. They observed no differences between the obese and the controls. Bradfield et al. (6) also detected no significant differences in the quantity of activity recorded by teachers in 3-d records of activity in physical education classes or when using heart rate monitoring to assess physical activity in 4 obese girls and 6 controls. Using filmed activities, Corbin and Pletcher (16) found that 12 obese subjects were less active than were 30 control subjects during unorganized activity, but there were no significant differences between the groups when they participated in organized activity. However, the obese tended to spend a lesser percentage of their time in active situations than did the control subjects.

Studies of adolescents have revealed many of the same findings found in younger children. Johnson et al. (35) compared 28 obese girls with 28 controls

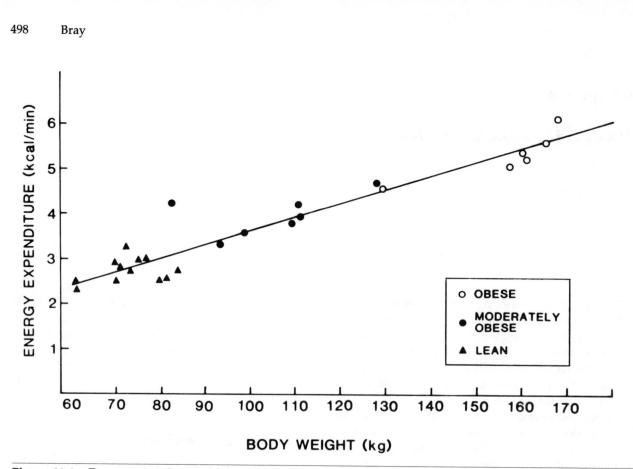

Figure 41.1. Energy expenditure of freewheeling exercise for obese, moderately obese, and lean (normal) individuals.

by using their recall of past activity and found the obese to be less active. In a follow-up study that used time-lapse photography of volleyball, tennis, and swimming, Bullen et al. (13) studied 109 obese girls in one summer camp and 72 normal-weight girls in a separate summer camp. The obese girls were less active than were the controls in all three sports and tended to spend a larger percentage of time in positions of resting. Stefanik et al. (67) used activity recall and counselor-related participation and structured activity sessions to compare 13 obese boys with 14 controls. They found no differences in the mean number of estimated hours in light, moderate, or very heavy exercise and no differences in the mean total time spent in light, moderate, and active exercise. However, the obese were less active than were the control subjects in the degree of participation in these activities. Wilkinson et al. (78) compared matched groups of 10 obese boys and 10 obese girls with appropriate controls by using a pedometer. They found no differences between obese and lean subjects.

Because physical work for any activity increases with body weight, a reduction in spontaneous activity may not reduce total energy expenditure. Griffiths and Payne (28) measured daily energy

expenditure and caloric intake in two groups of matched 5- to 7-yr-old children classified according to whether their parents were overweight or not. Children of the overweight parents expended significantly less energy at rest and also consumed significantly fewer calories during exercise than did the children of nonobese parents. Caloric intake was also significantly reduced. Finally, Roberts et al. (59) recently suggested that a lower metabolic rate in infancy may predict a higher risk of obesity at 1 yr of age.

One problem with most studies of activity is the difference related to energy costs of movement between subjects of different weights (Figure 41.1). To deal with this problem, Waxman and Stunkard (75) observed four families with an obese child and a nonobese sibling in the family setting, at school, and on the playground. The obese boys were far less active inside the home than were the lean siblings. Outside the home the obese boys were slightly less active but on the playground were equally active. The obese boys spent far more time in sedentary activities. When the energy cost of activity was used, a different picture emerged. One obese boy expended energy over a range from 1.11 to 4.10 kcal · min^{-1}, which was higher than the values ranging from 0.80 to 1.72 kcal • min⁻¹ for his lean brother. Although differences in energy expenditure or caloric intake between brothers could not be demonstrated, significant differences were detected among the four families under study.

Adults

A number of studies have also been conducted on the spontaneous activity of adults. Bloom and Eidex (5) observed that obese patients spent 15% less time each day on their feet and more time in bed than did the 6 control subjects. Chirico and Stunkard (15) compared 25 obese men and 16 obese women with an equal number of normal-weight controls matched by age and occupation. Each subject was given a pedometer. The obese females walked significantly less than did their matched controls. These differences were also observed in the males but were less striking. In a study of over- and underweight college men and women who wore actometers, Tryon (71) found no differences in spontaneous activity. Maxfield and Konishi (50) also found no differences in activity in 25 obese and 25 control women over a 48-hr period using pedometer measurements. Recently, Brownell et al. (11) recorded 45,694 observations on the frequency with which subjects spontaneously chose either an escalator or stairs. The obese used stairs significantly less frequently than did the nonobese in each of the two studies. However, in one of the two studies the frequency for the overweight individuals was similar to the rate for the lean subjects in the other study. When the subjects were encouraged to increase the use of stairs, both the obese and the lean subjects did so, but the obese still remained significantly less likely to use stairs than did the nonobese.

From these observations on physical activity it is clear that the obese subjects may be either as active or less active than are the lean ones but that they are not more active. Age may account for differences among some studies. Moreover, because the obese individuals are carrying more weight, they may indeed be doing more physical work than are lean subjects in many settings.

Physical Activity and Obesity

Muscular Adaptation to Exercise

One rationale for exercise in obese subjects is that it increases energy expenditure. The amount of energy expended during exercise is related to several factors, including the intensity and duration of the exercise and the degree of physical training. The effects of endurance training can be seen by comparing bodybuilders and weight lifters with long-distance runners. The body weight and muscle mass of the former group are large and powerful, but they are untrained for sustained physical activity. The long-distance runner has less total muscle mass and a much smaller store of body fat but has a highly conditioned cardiovascular system. Among weight lifters and bodybuilding enthusiasts and experts, the need for sustained endurance is low, and thus the muscular and cardiovascular training effects are minimal, yet muscular hypertrophy and physical strength may be very great. In contrast, long-distance runners, cross-country skiers, and other athletes who require prolonged energy expenditure need continuous training to achieve these effects (27).

The process of adapting muscles to endurance exercise involves a number of changes (1, 2, 27, 34, 51, 61, 69). There is an increase in the maximal capacity to consume oxygen. Cardiac output also increases, thus delivering more blood and oxygen to muscles. Oxygen uptake may more than double when a sedentary individual trains for endurance activities. There are concurrent increases in the activity of enzymes that can increase fat oxidation during submaximal exercise. At the cellular level these changes involve primarily the fast-twitch (or red) fibers, which have the highest capacity for oxidative metabolism. There are two types of fast-twitch fibers that have high respiratory capacities; slow-twitch fibers have only moderately high respiratory capacity. From a metabolic point of view, the energy for high-intensity, short-duration exercise is provided by utilizing intramuscular ATP obtained from creatine-phosphate and the catabolism of muscle glycogen. This energy supply is adequate for the high jump, the shot put, power lifts, and a serve in tennis. For individuals who sprint or who play on the line in football, the high-energy phosphates utilized as a source of energy also come from these sources. For more prolonged high-intensity activity the energy is provided by the metabolism of muscle glycogen and the production of ATP and lactate during rapid glycolysis.

In contrast, during adaptation for endurance exercise, the major metabolic changes involve enhancement of the ability of muscle to metabolize fatty acids and thus preserve glycogen. This metabolic change in the red muscle fibers is reflected in increases in the number of mitochondria and in the levels of the enzymes involved in the activation, transport, and beta-oxidation of long-chain fatty acids. Experimental data indicate that carnitine palmitolytransferase, cytochrome oxidase, cytochrome *c*, and acetoacetyl CoA thiolase increase in roughly the same percentage in the enlarged and numerous mitochondria. As might be expected, the quadriceps muscle of men trained to ride bicycles has an increased capacity to incorporate fatty acids in triglycerides, which can then serve as a source of oxidative fuel for the mitochondria. The rate at which carbohydrate is oxidized in trained muscles is reduced in contrast to the rate of oxidation of fatty acids. Because intramuscular glycogen stores provide a major source of energy for intense short-duration activity, the switch from the oxidation of glycogen to the utilization of fatty acids as a source of energy provides for longer half-life of muscle glycogen and thus for more endurance. At submaximal exercise in a trained individual the enhanced oxidation of fatty acids occurs at lower levels of circulating free fatty acids and is accompanied by lower levels of lactate production from glycogen, implying enhanced efficiency of the entire oxidative process. In addition to an increase in triglyceride levels there is also an increase in the level of muscle glycogen and the enzymes for glycogen synthesis.

The cardiovascular system also undergoes adaptation during endurance training. When not exercising, the physically trained person maintains a low heart rate through enhanced activity of the vagus nerve. As exercise begins there is an inhibition of the firing rate of the vagus nerve and an increase in the activity in the sympathetic nervous system, both of which participate in the rise in heart rate. The catecholamines released from the increased activity of the sympathetic nervous system increase the force of cardiac contraction. The sympathetic cholinergic vasodilator fibers dilate the arterioles in the muscle. At rest, muscles receive only about 15% of the total minute blood flow, but during exercise this rises sharply. At the same time, vasoconstrictor fibers decrease blood flow to the abdominal organs and skin so that more total blood flow reaches the muscles. The changing potassium flux in working muscle also acts locally to dilate arterioles and to open capillaries. The heat produced by muscular exercise must be dissipated through dilation of arterioles at the skin surface to maintain temperature regulation.

The potential for metabolic adaptations in the heart rate, pulmonary ventilation, and oxygen uptake during exercise is related to age. An individual aged 60 has approximately one-third less capacity for increasing maximal oxygen uptake than has an individual aged 20. A similar age-related reduction is observed on pulmonary ventilation rate during maximal exercise. A rise in blood pressure is also observed during exercise. The magnitude of the increase in systolic and diastolic blood pressures is related to the intensity of the exercise and is greater in older subjects than in younger ones. Obesity may further increase the blood pressure changes during exercise (10). To obtain the benefits of physical training on muscular activity and on the cardiovascular system, it is important to raise heart rate to a level of 120.

Effects of Physical Activity on Body Composition

It is widely held that physical training will reduce the total quantity of body fat and may be associated with a reduction in body weight in both lean and moderately obese subjects. Wilmore (79) reviewed the studies in which measurements of body composition were reported. Most of these training programs lasted from 7 to 22 wk. The changes in body composition were surprisingly small. On average, body fat decreased by only 1.6%, and 5 of the 55 studies showed a rise in body fat after training. Moreover, lean body mass also fell on average in 17 of these 55 studies.

During exercise in moderately obese subjects (as opposed to normal weight individuals), a decrease in body fat is readily demonstrated. In 12 studies on overweight men and women the mean decrease in body weight ranged between 2.6 and 14.3 kg. Most of this loss of weight is accounted for by a decrease in body fat (45). When 6 sedentary obese men expended 900-1,000 kcal per session 5 d per wk with no attention to dietary intake, body fat declined from 23.5% to 18.6% of body weight, which was greater than the decline of 5.7 kg in body weight. In an exercise program involving 23 moderately obese and 13 lean women, Franklin et al. (26) observed a decrease of 2.5 kg in body weight (75.9-73.4 kg) and a reduction of 1.8% in body fat (38%-36.2%) following 12 wk of physical conditioning. When 13 of these obese women were reevaluated 18 mo after the end of the program, both body weight and body fat had returned to the pretreatment levels (49).

An effect of physical training on body fat is more difficult to demonstrate in the massively obese. When 8 massively obese individuals initially weighing 112 kg received 3-6 mo of regular physical training three times per week, neither body weight nor body fat changed. However, a similar program of conditioning did reduce body fat and body weight in normal individuals. The degree of weight loss appeared to depend on the size of the fat cells and on the degree of cellularity of the adipose tissue. The reduction in body fat content during physical training is accompanied by a decrease in the size of individual fat cells (2). In physically trained men with a normal number of fat cells, the fat cells decreased in size from an average of 0.52 μg lipids per cell to 0.41 μg lipids per cell. This means that the extent of fat mobilization during physical training (2) was a function of the total number of cells that were present. Fat-cell size of ex-obese runners who were averaging 95 km per week can be smaller than that of elite long-distance runners, but the fat content remains higher (70).

The effects of physical training on individuals with hyperplastic obesity (i.e., individuals who have an increased total number of fat cells) differs from those of individuals with a normal number of fat cells. When the number of fat cells is increased, individuals on a regular physical training program for periods of 6 wk to 6 mo show no change both in total body fat and in the size of individual fat cells (3). The individuals with more than $80 \cdot 10^9$ fat cells gained weight during physical training (42). This weight gain occurred in spite of improved physical fitness, and this could be demonstrated not only by the lower resting heart rate but also by the improved handling of glucose and the lower levels of fasting insulin. Moreover, the muscles of these subjects showed an increase in the oxidative capacity of the fast-twitch oxidative muscle fibers and a decrease in the size and activity of the fast-twitch glycolytic fibers, both signs of physical conditioning (43). With physical training there is a significant improvement in resting systolic and diastolic blood pressures in some obese subjects. During exercise, however, there may be a significant increase of both diastolic and systolic pressures (4, 42). However, not all obese patients experience these changes. The individuals with the greatest decreases in blood pressure showed the smallest decreases in body fat during the training episode.

There are also other adaptive responses in the peripheral circulation. Obese subjects differ from lean ones in the dilation of their peripheral vessels during high levels of exercise. During the physical training of obese women resting heart rate was reduced more in the obese than in the normal-weight women (30). Oxygen consumption both before and after training in normal and obese women was related to fat-free body mass. When the obese and lean subjects were exercised at 30%, 50%, and 70% of their maximal aerobic power, the obese subjects had a significantly lower forearm blood flow

during high-intensity exercise in a hot environment than did the lean subjects. From comparisons of the changes in blood flow and core body temperatures, Vroman et al. (73) concluded that body composition may alter the balance between the two opposing sets of cutaneous vascular reflexes that regulate the competition for blood flow between skin and working muscles during exercise in a hot environment. The obese subjects showed less blood-pressure-induced vasoconstriction and more temperature-induced thermoregulatory vasodilation than did the lean subjects. When obese and lean subjects were exercised at the same percentage of their maximal oxygen uptake, there was no difference in cardiac output between the two groups (26).

Effects of Physical Training on Metabolism

Acute exercise, as well as physical training, modifies the metabolism of glucose, insulin, and lipids in obese subjects (46). Before exercise, the resting energy expenditure of obese subjects was higher than that of lean subjects, averaging 6 kJ $\cdot$ min^{-1} as compared to 4 kJ $\cdot$ min^{-1} for the lean controls (58). Because the respiratory quotient was lower in the obese individuals, this implied that the oxidation of fatty acids was higher. When exercise began, the oxidation of glucose (1^3C) rose and after the end of exercise fell. Initially, the obese subjects oxidized more fatty acids, but by the end of the first hour of exercise the obese and the lean subjects were oxidizing comparable amounts of fatty acids and carbohydrate to provide for the energy needed by the exercising muscles. In another study, Scheen et al. (62) examined the effect of 3 hr of walking on a treadmill in 9 obese males and 9 controls. The slope and rate on the treadmill produced a comparable oxygen uptake of 1.6-1.7 L $\cdot$ min^{-1} in both groups. Plasma free fatty acids, which were higher in the obese, initially rose more in the lean subjects during exercise. Blood glucose and lactate were similar initially and declined toward the end of the third hour, but there was no significant difference between the groups at the end. Insulin, which was higher in the obese subjects, fell more during exercise.

When a group of 12 obese males exercised following a 39-d fast there was a rise in serum glucose (20). This rise is contrary to the fall in glucose observed during acute exercise in obese (10) or normal-weight subjects. The expected rises in lactate, pyruvate alanine, free fatty acid, and glycerol were observed during the period of exercise, which was conducted at the level of 400-600 kpm • min⁻¹, or approximately 25%-30% of maximal aerobic capacity. Insulin levels fell in exercising fasted subjects and rebounded during recovery. Growth hormone rose with exercise, whereas glucagon behaved erratically. There was no change in the excretion of nitrogen in the urine or of the urinary concentrations of catecholamines or beta-hydroxybutyric acid.

Exercise and Lipids

The effect of exercise in a randomized yearlong study on healthy middle-aged men demonstrated that men who ran consistently were significantly fitter and leaner than were the controls. As a group these runners did not show a significant increase in high-density lipoproteins (HDLs) when compared with the sedentary controls. However, in the subgroup of men who ran at least 8 mi per week, there was a significant increase in the concentration of HDL and HDL_2 when compared to controls. As might be expected there were significant correlations between the distance run each week and the changes in plasma HDL cholesterol ($r = .48$). There was also a correlation between the changes in percent body fat and the changes in HDL cholesterol ($r = .47$). These data indicate that a significant increase in running maintained over a substantial period of time is required to produce alterations in HDLs in normal-weight subjects (82).

The changes in lipids in obese subjects are more complex. Obesity is associated with reduced circulating levels of HDL cholesterol (83), and this in turn is related to fat distribution, particularly in men (21). The levels of HDLs are of interest because they are inversely related to the risk for developing coronary artery disease (14). That is, those with higher levels of HDL cholesterol have a reduced risk of heart attack, whereas those with lower levels of HDL cholesterol have a higher risk.

Exercise has been reported to raise HDL cholesterol. Liebman et al. (48) examined the effect of dietary fiber and exercise on lipids in males who were at least 10% above ideal weight. In this group, exercise training had no significant effect on body weight or body fat, although it did tend to reduce both. However, there was a significant increase in HDL cholesterol as well as in the ratio of HDL cholesterol to low-density-lipoprotein (LDL) cholesterol by the end of 6 wk of exercise. Brownell et al. (12) found that a 10.7-kg weight loss in men was associated with a 5% increase in HDL cholesterol. There was also a 15.8% decrease in LDL cholesterol and thus a 30.1% increase in the HDL-LDL ratio. In women, in contrast, a weight loss of 8.9 kg produced no significant change in HDL cholesterol in contrast to the rise noted in the men. In a follow-up study on 24 male and 37 female volunteers who participated in a 10-wk exercise program, Brownell et al. (12) found a 5.1% increase in HDL cholesterol in the men but a 1% decrease in HDL cholesterol in the women. In a group of obese men, Leon et al. (47) observed a 5 mg/dl decrease in cholesterol. Franklin et al. (26) also noted a decrease in triglyceride and cholesterol by the third week of their 12-wk exercise program. By the end of the program, however, the cholesterol and triglycerides had returned to essentially baseline levels in spite of the continuing weight loss.

Separation of genetic and environmental factors in the control of body fat and its metabolism can be done with studies on twins. Eight pairs of twins participated in a 20-wk exercise program (22). Weight decreased significantly, but fat remained unchanged. Physical training increased basal lipolysis and epinephrine-stimulated lipolysis in isolated fat cells. Genetic factors accounted for the similarity in the epinephrine-stimulated lipolysis. However, nongenetic influences were stronger in the changes that occurred in basal lipolysis. In companion studies, Poehlman et al. (53, 55) examined the effects of overfeeding on metabolism and the function of adipose tissue. These studies are summarized in Table 41.1. Although body weight increased during the 22 d in which 6 pairs of male monozygotic twins were overfed 1,000 kcal per day, the percent body fat did not increase (53). However, fat mass did rise, as did the sum of the nine skinfolds and the skinfolds on the trunk and extremities. There was significant interaction of genetic influences and environment in all these changes and even in the percent body fat, which overall did not increase during overfeeding. Among the parameters of adipocyte function that were measured (Table 41.1), both basal lipogenesis (i.e., the incorporation of radioactivity from glucose into triglyceride) and fat-cell diameter increased (54). However, neither of these changes showed interactions between genotype and environment, whereas the other variables that were measured did. Finally, some metabolic functions were also studied (55). Resting metabolic rate did not increase, but there was a significant increase in the oxygen uptake following a meal (thermic effect of food). Glucose tolerance and the insulin response to this glucose load did not change, but the ratio of the change in insulin to the change in glucose was significantly increased.

Both serum T_3 and serum T_4 increased significantly. Of these metabolic parameters measured

Table 41.1 Effects of Short-Term Overfeeding in Monozygotic Twins

Function measured	Effect of overfeeding[a]	Genotype effect
Body weight	↑ +	< .05
Body fat (%)	→ —	< .05
Fat mass (kg)	↑ +	< .05
Sum of nine skinfolds	↑ +	< .05
Trunk skinfolds	↑ +	< .05
Extremity skinfolds	↑ +	< .05
Basal lipogenesis	↑ +	
Fat-cell diameter	↑ +	
Basal lipolysis	→ —	< .05
Stimulated lipolysis	→ —	< .05
Insulin-stimulated lipogenesis	→ —	< .05
Lipoprotein lipase (LPL)	→ —	< .05
Resting metabolic rate	→ —	
Thermic effect of food	↑↑ + +	< .05
Glucose tolerance	→ —	
Insulin response to glucose	→ —	
Ratio of insulin to glucose	↑ +	
Serum T_3	↑↑ + +	
Serum T_4	↑ +	

Note. Adapted from Poehlman et al. (53, 54, 55).

[a]+ = increase; + + = great increase; — = no change.

after overfeeding, only the thermic effect of food showed a significant genetic interaction. These elegant studies indicate that overfeeding can be a useful procedure for bringing out the interactions between underlying genetic predisposition and environmental signals in food.

Physical training in obese subjects is associated with an improvement in glucose tolerance and a marked reduction in the insulin levels during a glucose tolerance test. This falling insulin occurs during acute exercise as well as after chronic physical training (2). The training effects can be acquired rapidly and lost equally rapidly (46). This is in part related to the level of caloric intake. During 3 hr of cycle exercise, insulin binding to monocytes increased by 13% in obese subjects and by 36% in controls (40). DeFronzo et al. (18), using the glucose clamp, convincingly showed that insulin and exercise act synergistically to enhance glucose disposal in humans. In experimental studies chronic exercise has been shown to lower insulin secretion as the primary mechanism for reduced levels of insulin (80). Of note is that this improvement in glucose and insulin following an oral glucose tolerance test can occur even without a change in body fat content.

Metabolic Rate

The question of whether physical training influences metabolic rate is unsettled. It is well established that with reduced caloric intake there is a reduction in the metabolic rate (7, 39). This reduction can be up to 15%-20%. The use of physical activity to overcome this reduction is tempting, providing there is a persistent effect. With weight loss (57) or weight gain (77) the efficiency of muscular contraction is unchanged. In addition, exercise does not prevent the reduction in resting metabolic rate that is observed with dieting (31).

Effects of Physical Activity on Food Intake

The effects of exercise on food intake depend on the duration and the intensity of the exercise. In experimental animals, Katch et al. (36) showed that two different levels of exercise that produced equal caloric expenditure had significantly different effects on food consumption. The high-intensity exercise depressed the intake of food and body weight gain, whereas the low-intensity exercise, producing equal caloric expenditure, had a much smaller effect.

The data from human studies are limited. Dempsey (19) reported a study on 7 obese and 7 nonobese young men who used calisthenics, running, and isometric weight lifting over an 18-wk period. Food intake was reported daily. At the end of the first 8 wk of training, caloric intake rose from 2,003 to 2,148 kcal/d and during the second 8-wk period from 2,190 to 2,281 kcal per day. This increase of 200 kcal/d was less than the estimated 400-600 kcal per day used in these exercises. Thus, exercise did not appropriately increase food intake in this study. Other investigators have reported a small decrease in food intake following programmed exercise. Holloszy et al. (33) studied 15 middle-aged men who ran on average 3.35 times per week for 6 mo. These men recorded their caloric intakes by using 3-d dietary records and showed intakes of 2,493 kcal per day at the first month and 2,371 kcal per day during the seventh month of training. Katch et al. (37) studied 15 college women over a 16-wk period and observed almost identical caloric intakes in swimmers of 2,091 kcal per day before and 2,065 kcal per day at the end of the study and 1,811 kcal per day before and 1,797 kcal per day at the end of the study. Johnson et al. (35) evaluated 20 college women who bicycled on an ergometer at an intensity between 103 and 308 kpm for 30 min per day for 10 wk. Using 3-d dietary records, baseline caloric intake was 1,751 kcal per day. This had fallen to 1,584 kcal per day at 10 wk. Leon et al. (47) also observed a reduction in the caloric intake in 6 obese men who walked 5 d per week for 90 min at a 10% grade which was estimated to expend an additional 1,100 kcal per session. Baseline caloric intake using 3-d dietary records was 2,288 kcal per day. During the initial phase of exercise, caloric intake increased to a value of 2,459 kcal per day by the 8th week but had declined to 2,149 kcal per day by the 16th week of the program. There is thus no clear evidence of compensatory changes with exercise.

In a careful in-patient study, Woo et al. (81) reported that during graded testing in the lean subjects, there was a compensatory increase in food intake as the level of energy expenditure increased from sedentary to 10% and 25% above sedentary. In the obese subjects, however, there was no significant increase. The rise in energy intake was from 2,233 kcal per day in the sedentary state to only 2,346 kcal per day at the low level of energy expenditure (10% above sedentary) and only 2,303 kcal per day in the highest category of expenditure (25% above sedentary). As anticipated, the obese subjects lost weight during the course of the treatment program. In conclusion, this would suggest that an increase in energy expenditure of moderate degrees in obese subjects may not be accompanied by any change in their levels of food intake.

Of interest is the fact that exercise in cool water neither increases the rate of fat loss nor changes caloric intake. Sheldahl et al. (65) studied 7 obese women who performed moderate exercise for 90 min five times per week for 8 wk when immersed up to their necks in cool water (17-22 °C). Because body weight, fat-free weight, and caloric intake did not change during the exercise in cool water, the authors concluded that the heat loss incurred in the cool water must have been repaid during nonexercising time. The weight of evidence suggests that modest levels of exercise may not significantly change caloric intake. In particular, increased energy expenditure through exercise may not lead to a compensatory rise in food consumption. Thus, exercise may be useful in weight loss.

Obesity may also influence the interaction between exercise and food intake (9). At rest, the thermic effect of food was similar in obese and in lean women (63). Eating before exercising increased the metabolic rate by 11% in lean women and 4% in the obese women, and food potentiated the thermic effect of food in the lean women but not in the obese women. In a comparison study in which obese and lean men had the same mean body weight, Segal et al. (64) found that the ther-

mic effect of food was significantly greater in the lean men at rest and after exercise. There was a significant negative relationship between the thermic effect of food and body fat at rest and after exercise. These observations suggest that the reduced response to the combined stimulus of food plus exercise may be one component of the metabolic basis for the development of obesity.

Treatment of Obesity With Exercise

Studies on Hospitalized Patients

Several studies have examined the effects of adding exercise to a weight-loss program for hospitalized obese patients. Warwick and Garrow (74) compared the effects of adding exercise to a regimen of dietary restriction for 3 women living on a metabolic ward for a period of 12-13 wk, during which time they ate an 800-kcal diet each day. These authors were unable to find any increase in the rate of weight loss when subjects bicycled for 2 hr per day as compared with the periods when they did no extra exercise. Likewise, there was no effect on nitrogen balance. Using a larger number of women who were in a physical training program, Kenrick et al. (38) were able to observe an increased rate of weight loss. They compared 6 massively obese subjects who exercised while on a 1,000- to 1,500-cal diet with 6 subjects who ate the same diet but did not exercise. At the end of the 26-wk study period, the weight loss for the diet group averaged 33.9 kg compared with a weight loss of 40.3 kg in the group with diet and exercise. This extra weight loss was primarily fat. In a Swedish study of 18 obese women who ate a diet containing 500 kcal per day for 3 wk, Krotkiewski et al. (44) noted no difference between those who expended 550 kcal in exercise three times per week and those who did not. The absent or minimal effect of adding exercise to a restricted diet on the rate of weight loss is contrary to conventional wisdom, as it implies the potential for metabolic compensation in the exercising subjects during another part of the day. However, one would anticipate that if the exercise expenditure was sufficiently great, extra weight would be lost because the mechanisms of metabolic compensation would be outstripped. In a 6-wk study on a metabolic ward, 3 obese women remained sedentary, and 5 other obese women exercised regularly while ingesting a diet of 800 kcal per day (32). Weight loss was similar, and the exercise did not prevent the fall in resting metabolic rate, which is consistent with the findings of Henson et al. (31). However, the loss of protein was less and the loss of fat more in the women who exercised.

Studies of Exercise in Outpatient Settings

Studies of exercise alone as a modality for treating obesity are rather discouraging. In a study by Gwinup (29), a group of 34 subjects were enrolled in a program with exercise as the only modality for treatment. Of that group only 11 women maintained the exercise program of at least 30 min of daily exercise for a year or longer. In this group of 11, the average weight loss was 10 kg and occurred when exercise exceeded 30 min/d. There is an important difference in response to exercise between individuals with hypercellular obesity and those with normocellular obesity. Individuals with an increased number of fat cells failed to lose weight, whereas those with a normal number of fat cells were able to lose weight effectively. In a study of moderately obese subjects, Leon et al. (47) observed a significant weight loss in 6 subjects whose average initial body weight was 99.1 kg when exercising for 16 wk with an expenditure approximating 1,100 kcal per session that was obtained by walking on a 10% grade on a treadmill at 3.2 mph. This amounted to an expenditure of about 5,500 cal per week on average for the exercise time and was associated with a weight loss of 6 kg. Franklin et al. (26) observed a small reduction in body weight (2.6 kg) and body fat (2.3 kg) when 23 moderately obese women participated in a 12-wk program of aerobic conditioning carried out in four sessions per week.

Few studies are long term. In one of the best, Kukkonen et al. (45) studied the effect of exercise in 236 individuals, of whom 169 entered the program following exclusion of 26 individuals for medical contraindications to exercise and 41 people who were maintained in a separate group because of their use of medications. Of the 169 people, 41 men and 54 women trained actively for 17 mo. Seventeen percent of the men and 13% of the women lost at least 9 kg (20 lb). However, only 3 men and 6 women had attained a body mass index of less than 25 kg · m^{-2} by the end of the study. On the other hand, 4 men and 5 women showed no change in weight, and 4 men and 10 women actually gained (1-3 kg for the men and 1-5 kg for the women). Physical training significantly improved blood pressure, and triglycerides were significantly decreased after training in the women. The dropout rate and the rather low quantities of weight loss paint a disappointing picture of exercise as a primary treatment for obesity.

The addition of exercise to a weight-reduction program of dieting also has a disappointing record of short-term success. However, the longer-term impact may be more important. In a study of 12 women who were at least 40% overweight, exercise, diet alone, and diet plus exercise were compared (23). The exercise consisted of walking on a treadmill or bicycling for 1 hr per day, 4 d per week over a 6-wk period. On this regimen, weight loss in the diet-treated group was 2.9 kg (6.4 lb) compared to 4.1 kg (9.1 lb) in the exercise group. In the group receiving only exercise, weight loss was only 0.63 kg (1.4 lb), which was only slightly greater than the 0.09 kg (0.2 lb) lost by the untreated control group. Harris and Hallbauer (30) studied 35 women and 11 men who wanted to lose at least 6.8 kg. The program lasted for 12 wk and utilized various activities. The individuals treated with exercise, a contingency contract, and self-control techniques lost 1.9 kg (4.1 lb) compared to 1.4 kg (3.1 lb) for those with a contingency contract plus self-control techniques. At a 6-mo follow-up, respective weight losses were 2.7 kg (6 lb) and 1.8 kg (4 lb). Stalonas et al. (66) studied 37 women and 11 men who were at least 15% above ideal weight. The patients exercised every day for 10 wk with a variety of activities. Individuals with exercise plus behavioral tasks lost 2.7 kg (5.9 lb) during the 10 wk and at 1 yr had lost 3.4 kg (7.4 lb). Those with behavioral tasks alone lost 2.1 kg (4.7 lb) during the treatment period but had lost only 1.1 kg (2.4 lb) 12 mo later. Those with behavioral tasks plus exercise and self-reinforcement lost 1.95 kg (4.3 lb) initially and 2.7 kg (5.9 lb) at 12 mo follow-up. Dahlkoetter et al. (17) studied 44 women who were at least 6.8 kg (15 lb) above ideal weight. The group, who exercised during the 8 wk of treatment, lost 2.8 kg (6.2 lb). Those with eating habit changes lost 3.2 kg (7.0 lb), and the individuals who received the combination of exercise plus eating habit changes lost 6.1 kg (13.3 lb). When followed out to 6 mo, the numbers were, respectively, 2.5, 3.2, and 7.3 kg. Weltman et al. (76) studied 58 men who exercised for 15-45 min per day with brisk walking for 4 d per week for 10 wk. The men with diet alone lost 5.9 kg and those with diet plus moderate exercise only 5.4 kg. However, moderate exercise alone was accompanied by only a 0.9-kg weight loss and a correspondingly small loss of body fat. However, weight loss alone is not a sufficient criterion for assessing the outcome. Recently, Pavlou et al. (52) examined the effects of diet plus exercise in 72 policemen. The exercise program was instituted 3 d per week for 8 wk and consisted of a calisthenics program and aerobics at 80% of maximal heart rate. Total body fat and lean body mass were determined in these individuals. After 8 wk, the weight loss in the group treated with exercise alone was 11.8 kg, which was not significantly different than the 9.2 kg lost by the group with diet alone. However, the loss of body fat was 11.2 kg in the exercise group compared to 5.2 kg in the group without exercise. Thus, exercise led to the preservation of existing lean body mass, an increase in the maximal oxygen uptake, and an increase in strength in the participants in the exercise subgroups. However, other studies have failed to demonstrate a sparing of lean body mass by exercise during caloric restriction. For example, Van Dale et al. (72) randomly assigned 6-12 obese females who were on a 12-wk restricted diet of approximately 800 kcal/day (3.4 mJ/d) to exercise for 1 hr, 4 d per week, at 50%-60% of maximum aerobic capacity. Both groups lost 12-13 kg, but there was no difference between them in the loss of body weight, body fat, or lean body mass. Thus, it appears that exercise usually does not increase the rate of weight loss during a period of caloric restriction, but the reasons for this are not clear. However, there is a strong suggestion that exercise may reduce the loss of lean body mass during dieting, but research is contradictory on this point. Such factors as gender, age, quality and type of diet, and frequency and intensity of exercise may explain some of the discrepancies.

Concern about the long-term effectiveness of exercise was noted by MacKeen et al. (49), who evaluated 36 sedentary obese women who had previously participated in a 12-wk physical conditioning program involving walking and jogging. Eighteen months following termination of the program only 40% of the normal and 33% of the obese women were still engaged in physical activity, and none were at the frequency and duration at which they originally participated. Physical conditioning had deteriorated, and body fat returned toward preconditioning levels. The authors concluded that most of the middle-aged women who participated in the supervised program of walking and jogging tended to regress toward pretreatment status when exercise was continued on an ad libitum basis.

During caloric restriction containing 1.2 g · kg^{-1} of ideal body weight as a source of protein and calories, 6 healthy men were studied before and at 1 and 6 wk after beginning the diet. Exercise to exhaustion occurred at 80% of baseline 1 wk after starting on the diet but increased to 155% of base-line at 6 wk despite adjustments of body weight up to initial weight by adding backpacks. The resting glycogen level in the vastus lateralis muscle fell to 57% of baseline after the first week on the low-calorie protein diet but had risen to 65% after 6 wk with no decrement in muscle glycogen when measured after 4 hr of uphill walking on a treadmill. The respiratory quotient (RQ), which was .76 during baseline, fell progressively to .66 after 6 wk on the diet. Blood glucose was well maintained during exercise even when ketosis was present. The ketone bodies rose from 3.28 to 5.03 mM during exercise after 6 wk, explaining in part the low exercise rise in RQ.

Exercise may also be useful in the treatment of children with obesity (24, 25). In one study, 113 preadolescents participated in a 6-mo weight-control program involving behavioral components and exercise. Epstein et al. noted that there was a correlation between the degree of training as assessed by alterations in heart rate after a step test between those with high and low success. During the maintenance period, the fitness of the exercise group tended to deteriorate, whereas the fitness of the lifestyle group was maintained.

Two additional concerns must be added to those about the long-term benefits of exercise. The first deals with the amount of exercise required to produce satisfactory alterations in physical conditioning. In the study by Wood et al. (82) it appears that exercise must be continued with at least three and preferably four or five sessions per week to obtain the desired effect. In addition, exercise programs are associated with significant risks, particularly when running is involved (41). In a study of 1,250 randomly selected males and an equal number of female registrants (most of whom were followed 1 yr later) in a 10-km road race, 89% of the males and 79% of the females who responded were still running regularly. Weight loss was commonly associated with running and was greater in those who were overweight when they began running. More than one third of the respondents had had musculoskeletal injuries attributable to running in the year after this race, and about 1 in 7 respondents sought medical consultation for their injury. The risk of injury increased as the number of miles run each week increased. These data suggest that walking is the safest and most effective form of exercise therapy for most overweight subjects. The duration of time required to achieve its benefits may be beyond what many patients are willing to commit. Pollack et al. (56) have observed that a decrease in body fat did not occur when exercise of 30-45 min was performed 2 d per week but that a decrease was associated with a comparable intensity of exercise being performed 3 or 4 d per week.

Exercise, added to other forms of treatment for obesity, is important not so much for the extra weight lost during the treatment period but for the fact that at follow-up 3, 6, or 9 mo later there appears to be less weight gained in the individuals who exercised than in those who did not.

References

1. Åstrand, P-O., and K. Rodahl. 1970. *Textbook of work physiology*. New York: McGraw-Hill.

2. Björntorp, P. Exercise in the treatment of obesity. *Clin. Endocrinol. Metab.* 5(2): 431-453, 1976.

3. Björntorp, P., K. de Jounge, M. Krotkiewski, L. Sullivan, L. Sjöstrom, and, J. Stenberg. Physical training in human obesity. III. Effects on long-term physical training on body composition. *Metabolism* 22(12): 1467-1475, 1973.

4. Björntorp, P. Hypertension and exercise. *Hypertension* (Suppl. 3): III-56-III-59, 1982.

5. Bloom, W.L., and M.F. Eidex. Inactivity as a major factor in adult obesity. *Metabolism* 16: 679-684, 1967.

6. Bradfield, R.B., J. Paulos, and L. Grossman. Energy expenditure and heart rate of obese high school girls. *Am. J. Clin. Nutr.* 24: 1482-1488, 1971.

7. Bray, G.A. Effect of caloric restriction on energy expenditure in obese patients. *Lancet* ii: 397-398, 1969.

8. Bray, G.A. The energetics of obesity. *Med. Sci. Sports Med.* 15(1): 32-40, 1983.

9. Bray, G.A., B.J. Whipp, and S.N. Koyal. The acute effects of food intake in energy expenditure during cycle ergometry. *Am. J. Clin. Nutr.* 27: 254-259, 1974.

10. Bray, G.A., B.J. Whipp, S.N. Koyal, and K. Wasserman. Some respiratory and metabolic effects of exercise in moderately obese men. *Metabolism* 26(4): 403-412, 1977.

11. Brownell, K.D., A.J. Stundard, and J.M. Albaum. Evaluation and modification of exercise patterns in the natural environment. *Am. J. Psychiatry* 137: 1540, 1980.

12. Brownell, K.D., P.S. Bachorik, and R.S. Ayerle. Changes in plasma lipid and lipoprotein levels in men and women after a program of moderate exercise. *Circulation* 65: 477, 1982.

13. Bullen, B., R.B. Reed, and J. Mayer. Physical activity of obese and non-obese adolescent girls, appraised by motion picture sampling. *Am. J. Clin. Nutr.* 14: 211-223, 1964.

14. Castelli, W.P., J.T. Doyle, T. Gordon, C.G. Hames, M.C. Hjortland, S.B. Hulley, A. Kagan, and W.J. Zukel. HDL-cholesterol and other lipids in coronary heart disease: The cooperative lipoprotein phenotyping study. *Circulation* 55: 767-772, 1977.

15. Chirico, A.M., and A.J. Stunkard. Physical activity and human obesity. *N. Engl. J. Med.* 263: 935-940, 1960.

16. Corbin, C.B., and P. Pletcher. Diet and physical activity patterns of obese and nonobese elementary school children. *Res. Q. Am. Assoc. Health Phys. Educ.* 39: 922-928, 1968.

17. Dahlkoetter, J.A., E.J. Callahan, and J. Linton. Obesity and the unbalanced energy equation: Exercise versus eating habit change. *J. Consult. Clin. Psychol.* 47: 898-905, 1979.

18. DeFronzo, R.A., E. Ferrannini, Y. Sato, and P. Felig. Synergistic interaction between exercise and insulin on peripheral glucose uptake. *J. Clin. Invest.* 68: 1468-1474, 1981.

19. Dempsey, J.A. Relationship between obesity and treadmill performance in sedentary and active young men. *Res. Q. Am. Assoc. Health Phys. Educ.* 35: 288-297, 1964.

20. Drenick, E.J., J.S. Fisler, D.G. Johnson, and G. McGhee. Effect of exercise on substrates and hormones during prolonged fasting. *Int. J. Obes.* 1: 49-61, 1977.

21. Després, J.P., C. Allard, A. Tremblay, J. Talbot, and C. Bouchard. Evidence for a regional component of body fatness in the association with serum lipids in men and women. *Metabolism* 34(10): 967-973, 1985.

22. Després, J.P., R. Bouchard, R. Savard, D. Prud'homme, L. Bukowiecki, and G. Thériault. Adaptive changes to training in adipose tissue lipolysis are genotype dependent. *Int. J. Obes.* 8:87-95, 1984.

23. Dudleston, A.K., and M. Bennion. Effect of diet and/or exercise on obese college women. *J. Am. Diet. Assoc.* 56: 126-129, 1970.

24. Epstein, L.H., R.R. Wing, R. Koeske, D. Ossip, and S. Beck. A comparison of lifestyle change and programmed aerobic exercise on weight and fitness changes in obese children. *Behav. Ther.* 13: 651-665, 1982.

25. Epstein, L.H., R. Koeske, J. Zidansek, and R.R. Wing. Effects of weight loff on fitness

in obese children. *Am. J. Dis. Child.* 137: 654-657, 1983.

26. Franklin, B., E. Buskirk, J. Hodgson, H. Gahagan, J. Kollias, and J. Mendez. Effects of physical conditioning on cardiorespiratory function, body composition and serum lipids in relatively normal-weight and obese middle-aged women. *Int. J. Obes.* 3: 97-109, 1979.

27. Gollnick, P.D. Relationship of strength and endurances with skeletal muscles stucture and metabolic potential. *Int. J. Sports Med.* 3(Suppl. 1): 26-32, 1982.

28. Griffiths, M., and P.R. Payne. Energy expenditure in small children of obese and non-obese parents. *Nature* 260: 698-700, 1976.

29. Gwinup, G. Effect of exercise alone on the weight of obese women. *Arch. Intern. Med.* 135: 676, 1975.

30. Harris, M.B., and E.S. Hallbauer. Self-directed weight control through eating and exercise. *Behav. Res. Ther.* 11: 523-529, 1973.

31. Henson, L.C., D.C. Poole, C.P. Donahoe, and D. Heber. Effects of exercise training on resting energy expenditure during caloric restriction. *Am. J. Clin. Nutr.* 46: 893-899, 1987.

32. Hill, J.O., P.B. Sparling, T.W. Shields, and P.A. Heller. Effects of exercise and food restriction on body composition and metabolic rate in obese women. *Am. J. Clin. Nutr.* 46: 622-630, 1987.

33. Holloszy, J.O., J.S. Skinner, G. Toro, and T.K. Cureton. Effects of a six month program of endurance exercise on the serum lipids of middle-aged men. *Am. J. Cardiol.* 14: 753-760, 1964.

34. Holloszy, J.O., and F.W. Booth. Biochemical adaptations to endurance exercise in muscle. *Annu. Rev. Physiol.* 38: 273-291, 1976.

35. Johnson, R.E., J.A. Mastropaolo, and M.A. Wharton. Exercise, dietary intake, and body composition. *J. Am. Diet. Assoc.* 61: 399-403, 1972.

36. Katch, V.L., R. Martin, and J. Martin. Effects of exercise intensity on food consumption in the male rat. *Am. J. Clin. Nutr.* 32: 1401-1407, 1979.

37. Katch, F.I., E.D. Michael, and E.M. Jones. Effects of physical training on the body composition and diet of females. *Res. Q. Am. Assoc. Health Phys. Educ.* 40: 99-104, 1969.

38. Kenrick, M.M., M.F. Ball, and J.J. Canary. Exercise and weight reduction in obesity. *Arch. Phys. Med. Rehab.* 323, 1972.

39. Keys, A., J.T. Anderson, and J. Brozek. *The biology of human starvation.* Minneapolis: University of Minnesota Press, 1950.

40. Koivisto, V.A., V.R. Soman, and P. Felig. Effects of acute exercise on insulin binding to monocytes in obesity. *Metabolism* 29(2): 168-172, 1980.

41. Koplan, J.P., K.E. Powell, R.K. Sikes, R.W. Shirley, and C.C. Campbell. An epidemiologic study of the benefits and risks of running. *JAMA* 248(23): 3118-3121, 1982.

42. Krotkiewski, M.K., K. Mandroukas, L. Sjöstrom, L. Sullivan, H. Wetterqvist, and P. Björntorp. Effects of long-term physical training on body fat, metabolism and blood pressure in obesity. *Metabolism* 28(6): 650-658, 1979.

43. Krotkiewski, M., A.C. Bylund-Fallenius, J. Holm, P. Björntorp, G. Grimby, and K. Mandroukas. Relationship between muscle morphology and metabolism in obese women: The effects of long term training. *Eur. J. Clin. Invest.* 13: 5-12, 1983.

44. Krotkiewski, M., L. Toss, P. Björntorp, and G. Holm. The effect of a very low calorie diet with and without caloric exercise on thyroid and sex hormones, plasma proteins, oxygen uptake, insulin and C-peptide concentrations in obese women. *Int. J. Obes.* 5: 287-293, 1981.

45. Kukkonen, K., R. Rauramaa, O. Siitonen, and O. Hanninen. Physical training of obese middle-aged persons. *Ann. Clin. Res.* 14: 80-85, 1982.

46. LeBlanc, J., A. Nadeau, D. Richard, and A. Tremblay. Studies on the sparing effect of exercise on insulin requirements in human subjects. *Metabolism* 30(11): 1119-1124, 1981.

47. Leon, A.S., J. Conrad, D.B. Hunninghake, and R. Serfass. Effects of a vigorous walking program on body composition, and carbohydrate and lipid metabolism of obese young men. *Am. J. Clin. Nutr.* 32: 1776-1787, 1979.

48. Liebman, M., M.C. Smith, J. Iverson, F.N. Thye, D.E. Hinkle, W.G. Herbert, S.J. Ritchey, and J.A. Drishell. Effect of coarse wheat bran fiber and exercise on plasma lipids and hypoproteins in moderately overweight man. *Am. J. Clin. Nutr.* 37: 71-81, 1983.

49. MacKeen, P.C., B.A. Franklin, W.C. Nicholas, and E.R. Buskirk. Body composition, physical work capacity and physical activity habits at 18-month follow-up of middle-aged women participating in an exercise intervention program. *Int. J. Obes.* 7: 61-71, 1983.

50. Maxfield, E., and F. Konishi. Patterns of food intake and physical activity in obesity. *J. Am. Diet. Assoc.* 49: 406-408, 1966.

51. Parizkova, J. Physical training in weight reduction of obese adolescents. *Ann. Clin. Res.* 14(Suppl. 34): 63-68, 1982.

52. Pavlou, K.N., W.P. Steffee, R.H. Lerman, and B.A. Burrows. Effects of dieting and exercise on lean body mass, oxygen uptake, and strength. *Med. Sci. Sport Med.* 17: 466-471, 1985.

53. Poehlman, E.T., A. Tremblay, J.P. Després, E. Fontaine, L. Perusse, G. Thériault, and C. Bouchard. Genotype-controlled changes in body composition and fat morphology following overfeeding in twins. *Am. J. Clin. Nutr.* 43: 723-731, 1986.

54. Poehlman, E.T., J.P. Després, M. Marcotte, A. Tremblay, G. Thériault, and C. Bouchard. Genotype dependency of adaptation in adipose tissue metabolism after short-term overfeeding. *Am. J. Physiol.* 250 (*Endocrinol. Metab.* 13): E480-E485, 1986.

55. Poehlman, E.T., A. Tremblay, E. Fontaine, J.P. Després, A. Nadeau, J. Dussault, and C. Bouchard. Genotype dependency of the thermic effect of a meal and associated hormonal changes following short-term overfeeding. *Metabolism* 35(1): 30-36, 1986.

56. Pollock, M.L., H.S. Miller, A.C. Linnerud, and K.H. Cooper. Frequency of training as a determinant for improvement in cardiovascular function and body composition of middle-aged men. *Arch. Phys. Med. Rehabil.* 56: 141-145, 1975.

57. Poole, D.C., and L.C. Henson. Effect of acute caloric restriction on work efficiency. *Am. J. Clin. Nutr.* 47: 15-18, 1988.

58. Ravussin, E., P. Pahud, A. Thelin-Doerener, M.J. Arnaud, and E. Jequier. Substrate utilization during prolonged exercise after ingestion of ^{13}C-glucose in obese and control subjects. *Int. J. Obes.* 4: 235-242, 1980.

59. Roberts, S.B., J. Savage, W.A. Coward, B. Chew, and A. Lucas. Energy expenditure and intake in infant born to lean and overweight mothers. *N. Engl. J. Med.* 318: 461-466.2.

60. Rose, H.E., and J. Mayer. Activity caloric intake, fat storage, and energy balance of infants. *Pediatrics* 41: 18-29, 1968.

61. Rowell, L.B. Human cardiovascular adjustments to exercise and thermal stress. *Physiol. Rev.* 54: 75-159, 1974.

62. Scheen, A.J., F. Pirnay, A.S. Luyckx, and P.J. Lefebvre. Metabolic adaptation to prolonged exercise in severely obese subjects. *Int. J. Obes.* 7: 221-229, 1983.

63. Segal, K.R., and B. Gutin. Thermic effects of food and exercise in lean and obese women. *Metabolism* 32: 581-589, 1983.

64. Segal, K.R., B. Gutlin, A.M. Nyman, and F.X. Pi-Sunyer. Thermic effect of food at rest, during exercise, and after exercise in lean and obese men of similar body weight. *J. Clin. Invest.* 76: 1107-1112, 1985.

65. Sheldahl, L.M., E.R. Buskirk, J.L. Loomis, and J. Mendez. Effects of exercise in cool water on body weight loss. *Int. J. Obes.* 6: 29-42, 1982.

66. Stalonas, P.M., W.G. Johnson, and M. Christ. Behavior modification for obesity: The evaluations of exercise, contingency management, and program adherence. *J. Consult. Clin. Psychol.* 46: 463-469, 1978.

67. Stefanik, P.A., F.P. Heald, and J. Mayer. Calorie intake in relation to energy output of obese and non-obese adolescent boys. *Am. J. Clin. Nutr.* 7: 55-62, 1959.

68. Stunkard, A.J., and J. Petska. The physical activity of obese girls. *Am. J. Dis. Child.* 103: 812-817, 1962.

69. Sullivan, L. Obesity, diabetes mellitus and physical activity: Metabolic responses to physical training in adipose and muscle tissues. *Ann. Clin. Res.* 14(34): 51-62, 1982.

70. Tremblay, A., J.P. Després, and C. Bouchard. Adipose tissue characteristics of ex-obese long-distance runners. *Int. J. Obes.* 8: 641-648, 1984.

71. Tryon, W. Activity as a function of body weight. *Am. J. Clin. Nutr.* 46: 451-455, 1987.

72. Van Dale, D., D.H.M. Saris, P.F.M. Schoffelen, and F. Ten Hoor. Does exercise give an additional effect in weight reduction regimens? *Int. J. Obes.* 11: 367-375, 1987.

73. Vroman, N.B., E.R. Buskirk, and J.L. Hodgson. Cardiac output and skin blood flow in lean and obese individuals during exercise in the heat. *J. App. Physiol.* 55(1): 69-74, 1983.

74. Warwick, P.M., and J.S. Garrow. The effect of addition of exercise to a regime of dietary restriction on weight loss, nitrogen balance, resting metabolic rate and spontaneous physical activity in three obese women in a metabolic ward. *Int. J. Obes.* 5: 25-32, 1981.

75. Waxman, M., and A.J. Stunkard. Caloric intake and expenditure of obese boys. *J. Pediatr.* 96: 187-193, 1980.

76. Weltman, A., S. Matter, and B.A. Stamford. Caloric restriction and/or mild exercise: Effects on serum lipids and body composition. *Am. J. Clin. Nutr.* 33: 1002-1009, 1980.

77. Whipp, B.J., G.A. Bray, and S.N. Koyal. Exercise energetics in normal man following acute weight gain. *Am. J. Clin. Nutr.* 26: 1284-1286, 1973.

78. Wilkinson, P.W., J.M. Parkin, and G. Pearlson. Energy intake and physical activity in children. *Br. Med. J.* 1(6063): 756, 1977.

79. Wilmore, J.H. Body composition in sport and exercise: directions for future research. *Med. Sci. Sports Med.* 15: 21-31, 1983.

80. Wirth, A., G. Holm, B. Nilsson, U. Smith, and P. Björntorp. Insulin kinetics and insulin binding to adipocytes in physically trained and food-restricted rats. *Am. J. Physiol.* 238: E108-E115, 1980.

81. Woo, R., R. Daniels-Kush, and E.S. Horton. Regulation of energy balance. *Annu. Rev. Nutr.* 5: 411-433, 1985.

82. Wood, P.D., W.L. Haskell, S.N. Blair, P.T. Williams, R.M. Krauss, F.T. Lindgren, J.J. Albers, P.H. Ho, and J.W. Farquhar. Increased exercise level and plasma lipoprotein concentrations: A one-year, randomized, controlled study in sedentary, middle-aged men. *Metabolism* 32(1): 31-39, 1983.

83. Ylitalo, V. Treatment of obese school children. *Acta Paediatr. Scand.* 290: 1-107, 1981.

Chapter 42

Discussion: Exercise and Obesity

Paul E. Garfinkel
Donald V. Coscina

The most striking conclusion from Dr. Bray's summary is also the most disappointing. Stated simply, it is that exercise in the obese is itself not associated with weight loss. Although this is contrary to popular wisdom as well as to professional recommendations for ways in which to avoid regaining weight (e.g., 20), several recent reviews of this topic reached similar conclusions (25). A number of important considerations follow from this surprising finding, the first of which relates to methodological aspects of studies in this area.

Methodological Considerations

Today, most academics and researchers who study weight regulation accept the heterogeneous nature of obesity. Obesity may be heterogeneous with regard to its pathogenesis, degree, and type. Dr. Bray commented on important functional differences between the morphologically distinct hyperplastic and hypertrophic obesities. Those with hypertrophic obesity display a reduction in body fat following exercise in contrast to a lack of effect on body fat in the hyperplastic form. With regard to degree of obesity, there are major differences among the mild, moderate, and severely obese in many respects, including the degree of health risk. Significant morbidity develops only when the body mass index (BMI) exceeds 30 (25).

Given the significant adverse effects of dieting (26), including its role in the eating disorders, we have to begin questioning how sound it is to advise the mildly obese to reduce their weight. For these people, lifestyle changes that incorporate emphasis on moderation and acceptance of oneself are of realistic value. This contrasts with the moderately or severely obese, in whom health hazards may demand more aggressive intervention. Per-

haps related to this distinction between the treatments of different types of obesity is the degree of genetic, or constitutional, loading. As discussed by Dr. Bray, in case of strong genetic loading, the primary or secondary effects of obesity may be associated with metabolic compensations that require a very high degree of exercise to overcome.

Many studies to date have been based on relatively small sample sizes and have not taken into account the varying types of obesity alluded to previously. Attention must be given to this important variable and to others, such as duration (i.e., whether it is lifelong or very recent), age, gender, type of diet, frequency and intensity of exercise, and motivation of the subjects.

The following discussion illustrates how gender may be a significant factor in obesity. There is a well-known decline in resting metabolic rate that occurs with periods of caloric dietary restriction, and Dr. Bray noted that exercise has not been shown to reverse this effect. Lennon et al. (21) recently showed that women may benefit from exercise more than may men. Seemingly in contrast to this are recent findings by Abraham and Wynn (1), who reported that women who diet show little change in resting energy expenditure, whereas men who diet show a long-term reduction in energy expenditure that seemed to be due to the loss of lean tissue. As separate work found no decline in total energy expenditure for either gender (30), these results imply that the men in the more recent study must have increased their energy expenditure through daily activities and exercise. Clearly, the interrelationships among gender, dieting, and exercise require further study.

Another methodological issue that must be addressed is high attrition rates. One example will demonstrate this. Gwinup (17) observed 11 mildly obese women (BMI = 27) who walked for 1-3 hr per day for 1 yr while consuming an ad libitum diet. These 11 represented only one third of the original sample. Others did not complete the study.

Although a number of questions remain, the overwhelming conclusion from studies to date is that exercise does not produce weight loss in the obese. However, it has recently been suggested that different types of obesity may be associated with different physiological causes or sustaining factors, a subset of which might respond favorably to exercise (20). To determine whether this is true, future studies will need to be more methodologically vigilant. In particular, more attention will need to be given to delineating functionally distinct subtypes of obesity. Accomplishing this will require larger sample sizes than are traditionally used. This seems especially necessary in dealing with the high attrition rates that can be anticipated in this work.

Changes in Body Fat

Changes in body weight do not necessarily reflect changes in body fat. Resting metabolic rate is the major determinant of energy expenditure (16). The resting metabolic rate is most closely correlated with fat-free mass, so inactivity by reducing muscle bulk and therefore fat-free mass might have a detrimental influence on metabolic rate.

The effects of intense exercise are not consistent, but most studies have reported reductions in body fat in normal-weight subjects and in the hypertrophic obese (24). For example, Leon et al. (22) studied 6 obese men (BMI = 38) who participated in 90 min of vigorous walking daily over 16 wk. Body composition studies indicated a loss of 5.9 kg of body fat and a gain of 0.2 kg of lean tissue. The amount of body fat decreased from 23.3% to 17.4%. In another study by Woo et al. (29), 3 obese women who were engaged in treadmill exercise lost an average of 12 lb over 2 mo entirely from body fat.

Three studies published in 1987 illustrate the conflicting findings that have been seen in this research area. Hill et al. (18) studied a small group of women over 5 wk on a liquid diet of 800 cal per day; 5 subjects participated in a daily aerobic exercise program. Total weight loss did not differ between the groups, but more of the weight loss came from fat and less from fat-free mass in the exercising subjects. By contrast, Van Dale et al. (28) studied 12 obese women on a diet alone or on a diet-plus-exercise program lasting 4 hr per week. After 4 wk both groups lost very similar amounts

of weight (about 8 kg) and fat (6 kg). These losses were maintained at a 12-wk follow-up. Finally, Belko et al. (2) reported that a low-energy diet without exercise produced greater weight loss than did a moderate diet with exercise over 6 wk. As the fat loss did not differ between groups in this study, the percentage of fat lost in the exercising group was relatively greater.

Why the differences among these studies? Likely factors include the varying lengths of study periods (2-26 wk), as well as differences in the intensity and frequency of the exercise and in the level and type of macronutrients consumed. Methods of recording dietary intake are extremely variable, and those relying entirely on self-report may be subject to significant error. Subjects in the diet-plus-exercise groups may also have compensated for the extra energy expenditure produced through exercise by reducing activity in the remainder of their daily lives.

Type of diet may also be important. Pitts (25) examined the impact of exercise on body composition in young, growing animals that were eating a fat-rich diet. Fat-fed animals placed in voluntary running wheels had the same amount of body fat at 260 d as did those eating low-fat diets but about one third the level of body fat as did those animals eating the fat-rich diet and not exercising.

Practically speaking, an important issue relates to the amount of exercise needed to produce a reduction in fat stores that is clinically significant. The age and build of a person are clearly important in this regard, as are the duration and the intensity of the exercise program (5). Although a normal adult male may possess 15%-20% body fat and a female 20%-25%, highly trained athletes may have only 5% body fat, much like those with anorexia nervosa. By contrast, the obese may possess 40% more body fat. Clearly, any exercise program must be of a significant intensity and duration to have a significant clinical impact over the long term. However, the obese have a number of problems in this regard. There are physical limitations to tolerating exercise when the BMI is greater than 30. In addition, one's levels of discouragement and sense of failure are high if one does not lose weight or finds it difficult to maintain the exercise program. For example, Foss et al. (12) studied 22 extremely obese subjects who were hospitalized over a 2-mo period. Exercise involved walking 2 mi per day at each person's own pace. Despite this minimal constraint, 20% of the subjects were never able to achieve this level of activity.

Methods of increasing the physical activities of the obese are relatively unexplored (28). An attempt should be made to help patients monitor their activities by using records or pedometers. Once a baseline level has been determined, behavioral modification techniques can be used to increase this level slowly. It is important that this be done slowly so that the person does not begin to feel discouraged. Generally, this means beginning with lifestyle activities such as using the stairs more or walking an extra block to work. One has to determine those activities that appeal to the individual. Certain physical activities can also be built in. Walking and swimming are fine, but jogging should be avoided to minimize deterioration of joints (3). But even these decisions must be made within a framework of the individual's lifestyle and interests and within the context of a more complete behavioral program that includes cognitive restructuring, stimulus control, nutrition education, and reinforcement. Patients should understand the proper techniques for each exercise and should be instructed carefully as to how much physical activity they should perform.

There may be benefits to such a program for several reasons. If people can be motivated to continue the program, regular exercise may prevent regaining weight in the form of fat. Weight loss brought about by dietary restriction is composed of approximately 75% fat and 25% lean body mass (6). Combining diet and exercise can reduce the loss of lean tissue to approximately 5% of total weight loss. Because regained weight is disproportionately made up of fat (5), repeated cycles of caloric restriction and weight gain would likely increase the ratio of fat to lean tissue. Future studies should address whether continued exercise can prevent this.

Perhaps the biggest advantage to continued exercise relates to enhanced patient morale and self-esteem (11), which may be related to maintaining weight loss. For example, Marston and Criss (23) followed 47 formerly obese persons for 1 yr; about 60% of the group were able to keep off most of their weight. These "maintainers" could be differentiated on the basis of their continued exercise programs and their reduced likelihood to eat for emotional reasons.

Problems of Exercise in the Obese

Although the obese may benefit from sensible exercise programs in terms of reducing body fat and several metabolic parameters important to health, there are, nonetheless, certain risks. The limited exercise tolerance of the obese and the possibility of their feeling increased self-disparagement with failure have already been commented on. There are also a variety of complications associated with exercise, such as a worsening of osteoarthritis.

Occasionally, people develop exercise dependence (9). Although various terms have been used to describe this state (e.g., *running addiction* and *running anorexics*), exercise dependence generally refers to the development of exercise as a compulsion that can become harmful to the individual. Yates et al. (31) reported that 3 of 60 marathon runners were identified as obligatory runners on the basis of their responses to a screening questionnaire. Such individuals often use running as a strategy for the regulation of intense feeling (4). There is evidence that such runners have a high frequency of previous depression (8). These runners may well have experienced an improvement in their psychological functioning but at a cost of endangering their physical health or disrupting their family and social lives.

Of much greater clinical importance has been the huge increase in the eating disorders anorexia nervosa (AN) and bulimia nervosa (BN) over the past 15 yr. The latter disorder is particularly common in the obese (14). A number of striking similarities between the obese and people with these eating disorders include the disparagement of feelings about the body and preoccupations with foods. In the obese, Cabanac (7) documented a persistence in the perceived pleasantness of food after a meal. This contrasts with a reduction in pleasantness that occurs in normal-weight subjects. We found that people with eating disorders display responses similar to those of the obese on hedonic ratings of food pleasantness (13).

The obese are particularly vulnerable to developing BN when they begin a diet of extremes in conjunction with an exercise program. But the development of such eating disorders requires a psychological vulnerability, especially in one's sense of low self-esteem. People with BN appear to attach their sense of self-worth entirely to their weight as well as to their perception of how they look. This seems to be a response to various cognitive distortions, conflicts, and fears (15).

Several parameters of the dieting in anorexics may be relevant to this discussion of exercise in the obese. Anorexics learn to control many bodily activities rigidly to achieve the primary goal of reducing body weight and fat. Daily exercise that is inflexibile in scheduling and large in amounts is routine. Body fat and weight are greatly reduced in response to extreme dietary restrictions and purging. Glucose levels are lowered, and there is often a flattened response to an oral glucose load.

Insulin levels are very low. However, insulin sensitivity becomes high. When using the De Fronzo glucose clamp, Zuniga-Guajardo et al. (32) found a rapid clearance of insulin even in comparison with exercising women who were matched for their levels of fitness.

The role of exercise in the continued self-starvation of the anorexic is unclear. We do know that as starvation progresses these patients become locked into repetitive dieting and exercise regimens, but we do not understand why this occurs. In animals, Epling and Pierce (10) showed that a combination of rigid exercising and a fixed dietary schedule leads to further restriction of voluntary intake to the point of starvation. Whether exercising and dieting interact similarly in people is not yet known.

What seems clear is that most people who begin exercising experience a sense of increased well-being and enhanced self-esteem. For a minority of people, exercise and dieting become the sole means of feeling good about themselves. Unfortunately, this minority represents about 3% of young women. The price for such perceived control of one's world is a serious disorder that carries a 5%-10% mortality rate (15). Given these facts, our task is to develop better predictors of which individuals are vulnerable to developing these illnesses so that we can caution them about the value of moderation in both exercise and diet.

To summarize, the literature to date supports the view that exercise itself does not promote weight loss in the obese. However, a subset of the obese may be able to reduce body fat in response to exercise, and there are demonstrable benefits of exercise on various metabolic parameters that are relevant to general health. Exercise programs must be tailored to the individual and then incorporated comfortably into existing lifestyles. For most people, a benefit of exercise is an improved sense of psychological well-being. However, a minority of adolescents and young-adult women seem vulnerable to the development of serious eating disorders. In such cases, overzealous exercise may exacerbate both the physiological and the psychological risks that attend these disorders.

References

1. Abraham, R.R., and V. Wynn. Reduction in resting energy expenditure in relation to lean tissue loss in obese subjects during prolonged dieting. *Ann. Nutr. Metab.* 31: 98-108, 1987.

2. Belko, A.Z., M. VanLoan, T.F. Barbieri, and P. Mayclin. Diet, exercise, weight loss and energy expenditure in moderately overweight women. *Int. J. Obes.* 11: 93-104, 1987.

3. Blackburn, G.L., and E. St. Lezin. Obesity. In: Conn, H.F., ed. *Conn's current therapy.* Philadelphia: W.B. Saunders, 1983: pp. 444-449.

4. Blumenthal, J.H., L.C. O'Toole, and J.L. Chang. Is running an analogue of anorexia nervosa? *JAMA* 252: 520-523, 1984.

5. Blundell, J.E. Behavior modification and exercise in the treatment of obesity. *Postgrad. Med. J.* 60: 37-49, 1984.

6. Bray, G.A. *The obese patient.* Philadelphia: W.B. Saunders, 1976.

7. Cabanac, M. Physiological role of pleasure. *Science* 173: 1103-1107, 1971.

8. Colt, E.W.D., D.L. Dunner, K. Hall, and R.R. Fieve. A high prevalence of affective disorder in runners. In: Sacks, M.H., ed. *The psychology of running.* Champaign, IL: Human Kinetics, 1981: pp. 234-248.

9. Decoverley-Veale, D.M.W. Exercise dependence. *Br. J. Addiction* 82: 735-740, 1987.

10. Epling, W.F., and W.D. Pierce. Activity-based anorexia: A biobehavioral perspective. *Int. J. Eating Disorders* 7: 475-485, 1988.

11. Folkins, C.H., and W.E. Sime. Physical fitness training and mental health. *Am. Psychol.* 36: 373, 1981.

12. Foss, M.L., R.M. Lampman, and D. Schteingart. Physical training program for rehabilitating extremely obese patients. *Arch. Phys. Med. Rehabil.* 57: 425-429, 1976.

13. Garfinkel, P.E., H. Moldofsky, D.M. Garner, H.C. Stancer, and D.C. Coscina. Body awareness in anorexia nervosa: Disturbances in "body image" and "satiety." *Psychosom. Med.* 40: 487-498, 1978.

14. Garfinkel, P.E., H. Moldofsky, and D.M. Garner. The heterogeneity of anorexia nervosa: Bulimia as a distinct subgroup. *Arch. Gen. Psychiatry* 37: 1036-1040, 1980.

15. Garfinkel, P.E., and D.M. Garner. *Anorexia nervosa: A multidimensional perspective.* New York: Brunner/Mazel, 1982.

16. Garrow, J.S. *Treat obesity seriously: A clinical manual.* London: Churchill Livingstone, 1981.

17. Gwinnup, G. Effect of exercise alone on the weight of obese women. *Arch. Intern. Med.* 135: 676-680, 1975.

18. Hill, J.O., P.B. Sparling, T.W. Shields, and P.A. Heller. Effects of exercise and food

restriction on body composition and metabolic rate in obese women. *Am. J. Clin. Nutr.* 46: 622-630, 1987.

19. James, W.P.T., M.E.J. Lean, and G. McNeil. Dietary recommendations after weight loss: How to avoid relapse of obesity. *Am. J. Clin. Nutr.* 45: 1135-1141, 1987.

20. Keesey, R.E. The body-weight set point: What can you tell your patients? *Postgrad. Med.* 83: 114-132, 1988.

21. Lennon, D., F. Naghe, F. Stratman, E. Shrago, and S. Dennis. Diet and exercise training effects on resting metabolic rate. *Int. J. Obes.* 9: 39-47, 1985.

22. Leon, A.S., J. Conrad, D.B. Hunningbak, and R. Serfars. Effects of a vigorous walking program on body composition and carbohydrate and lipid metabolism of obese young men. *Am. J. Clin. Nutr.* 33: 1776, 1979.

23. Marston, A.R., and J. Criss. Maintenance of successful weight loss: Incidence and prediction. *Int. J. Obes.* 8: 435-439, 1984.

24. Pacy, P.J., J. Webster, and J.S. Garrow. Exercise and obesity. *Sports Med.* 3: 89-113, 1986.

25. Pitts, G.C. Body composition in the rat: Interactions of exercise, age, sex and diet. *Am. J. Physiol.* 246: 495-501, 1984.

26. Polivy, J., and C.P. Herman. *Breaking the diet habit*. New York: Basic Books, 1983.

27. Stunkard, A.J. Conservative treatments for obesity. *Am. J. Clin. Nutr.* 45: 1142-1154, 1987.

28. VanDale, D., W.H.M. Saris, P.F.M. Schoffelen, and F. Tenhoor. Does exercise give an additional effect in weight reduction regimens? *Int. J. Obes.* 11: 368-375, 1987.

29. Woo, R., J.S. Garrow, and F.X. Pi-Sunyer. Voluntary food intake during prolonged exercise in obese women. *Am. J. Clin. Nutr.* 36: 478-484, 1982.

30. Wynn, V., R.R. Abraham, and J.W. Densem. Studies in human obesity: I. Method for estimating rate of fat loss during treatment of obesity. *Lancet* i: 482-486, 1985.

31. Yates, A., K. Leehey, and C. Shisslak. Running: An analogue of anorexia? *N. Engl. J. Med.* 30: 251-255, 1983.

32. Zuniga-Guajardo, S., P.E. Garfinkel, and B. Zinman. Increase in insulin sensitivity and clearance of insulin in anorexia nervosa. *Metabolism* 35: 1096-1100, 1986.

Chapter 43

Exercise, Fitness, Osteoarthritis, and Osteoporosis

Everett L. Smith
Kristin A. Smith
Catherine Gilligan

Many studies have been done to determine the effects of exercise and fitness on osteoarthritis and osteoporosis. This review is an attempt to synthesize the results of those studies.

Osteoarthritis

Osteoarthritis (OA) refers to a degenerative joint disorder with a multifactorial etiology. The cartilage degeneration of OA is progressive and may not be associated with clinical symptoms in early stages. The etiology of OA is not yet clearly understood, but most agree that the following factors may contribute to the disorder: occupational and sports trauma; genetics; inflammation; and immunological, biochemical, and environmental insults. Until recently, pathological and radiological criteria for defining OA have not been uniform (51). Altman et al. (4), representing the Rheumatic Association, attempted to standardize clinical and radiological criteria. Clinical criteria include painful range of motion, morning stiffness not exceeding 30 min, bony enlargements, and crepitance. Radiological criteria include osteophytes, subchondral cysts or sclerosis, joint-space narrowing, and malalignment and attrition of normal bone formation. Early signs of OA in the articular cartilage are decreased proteoglycan content, increased water, and changes in glycosaminoglycan composition (7). In more advanced OA the cartilage surface becomes rough and develops clefts that may extend through the cartilage to the underlying bone (5). Osteoarthritis is most common in the weight-bearing knee and hip and the spine but can also occur in non-weight-bearing joints, such as distal intraphalangeal and first carpal-metacarpal joints. The symptoms are characterized as nonsystemic or inflammatory, most often presenting with pain and stiffness. The primary events in the development of OA may occur in subchondral bone (7, 10, 53). Repetitive loading of normal subchondral bone may result in microfractures that in turn lessen cartilage support, resulting in surface changes and other modifications of cartilage. The implication that repetitive loading is a major contributing factor in the development of OA has stimulated many studies of both occupational and sports activities that repetitively load specific joints. Panush and Brown (51) listed factors implicated in the development of OA that should be considered in conjunction with occupational and sports participation: (a) physical characteristics of the individual, (b) biomechanical factors, (c) biochemical factors, and (d) preventive measures taken to protect the joints being stressed.

An observed association between physically demanding jobs and the incidence of OA produced the hypothesis that repetitive loading causes OA as a result of wear and tear. Researchers have reported that incidence of OA is higher in the shoulders and elbows of pneumatic drill operators, in the hips of farm workers, and in the elbows and knees of miners. In contrast, other investigators did not observe an increased incidence of OA in the elbows of pneumatic drill operators, and foundry workers were found to have fewer cases of OA than was the general population (53). Hadler (23), after a careful review of the literature, stated that the hypothesized relationship between heavy work and OA was supported by little scientific, as opposed to anecdotal, evidence. The difference in results may lie in the selection of subjects and the presence of confounding factors. Previous injury, for example, is strongly implicated in the development of OA (51), and the incidence of injury is probably higher in physically demanding jobs or athletics. Chantraine (10) examined both knee joints of 81 veteran soccer players through clinical and X-ray examination. All players who had a meniscectomy presented with radiological signs of OA. Anatomical joint malalignment is another contributing factor in the development of OA. McDermott and Freyne (43) reported a higher prevalence of OA in runners with genu varum than in nonrunners. Bland and Cooper (7) stated that the mammalian joint does not show wear unless subjected to severe malalignment, trauma, or excessive loads, as the coefficient of joint friction is similar to that of ice sliding on ice: "Thus to describe OA as a consequence of wear and tear or aging is inappropriate" (p. 109).

If repetitive loading of well-aligned, healthy joints does not cause wear and tear, one would expect no difference between participants in noncontact sports (e.g., distance runners) and the general population in the incidence of OA. Panush et al. (52) compared 17 long-term male runners (mean age 56, mean participation length 12 yr), 53% of whom were marathon runners, to 18 nonrunners (mean age 61). The two groups did not differ significantly in age, height, or weight. Incidence of OA, evaluated by clinical and radiological examination, was not significantly different in runners and controls. Similarly, Lane et al. (38) compared 41 long-distance runners (ages 50-72) to 41 control subjects matched for age, height, weight, education, and occupation. X-ray evaluations were made of the hand, lumbar spine, and knee joints. Male runners showed no significant difference in OA from that in the control group. Female runners had significantly greater sclerosis and spur formation in the knee and sclerosis of the spine than did controls. In contrast, joint space (decreased joint space is often used as a criteria for OA) tended to be higher in both male and female runners than in controls (nonsignificant). The authors warned that this cross-sectional evidence should be evaluated cautiously because those individuals with successful running careers have probably experienced less joint pain and injury than have others who have ceased running. Correspondingly, some nonrunners are sedentary because of early incidence of OA or other conditions in which running exacerbates pain. Soh and Micheli (68) evaluated

the incidence of knee and hip OA in former college varsity runners (n = 504) and swimmers (n = 287). Subjects were surveyed 2-55 yr (mean 25 yr) after participation to determine whether running contributed to OA. The incidence of severe pain of the hip and knee was 2% in the runners and 2.4% in the swimmers. In addition, a lower proportion of runners (0.8%) than swimmers (2.4%) eventually required surgery for OA. Soh and Micheli concluded that there was no association between moderate long-distance running and the future development of OA. They further suggested that neither heavy mileage nor heavy running was implicated in the development of OA. Again, it should be noted that these subjects were elite athletes, so they were unlikely to have had poor joint alignment or body mechanics, and that these data do not represent the general population of recreational runners, which may have a greater incidence of misalignment and injury. Further prospective studies are required to delineate clearly the role of physical activity patterns in the development of OA in the general population. Fitzgerald and McLatchie (20) conducted a clinical and radiological study on the upper- and lower-limb joints of 25 experienced weight lifters (mean age 35) who had been participating at a high level for 6 yr or more. Significant degeneration was observed in 20% of the lifters, a lower incidence than the 38% reported for the general population (ages 35-44).

Osteoporosis

Osteoporosis is a major public health problem in the United States and Canada. The disease is characterized by fractures subsequent to excessive loss of bone mineral content (BMC) from both the axial and the appendicular skeleton. Bone mineral content accounts for approximately 90% of skeletal strength. The geometric structure of the tissue, determined by habitual stresses, collagen orientation, ligaments, and muscle tone, are also important factors in bone strength and resistance to fracture. The impact of osteoporosis on society is increasing. Not only are demographic trends toward an older population producing a greater percentage of the total population at risk, but the incidence among the older population is climbing. Martin et al. (42) reported that hip fracture incidence in Saskatchewan increased 75% between 1972 and 1984, whereas that of the population over age 50 increased only 12%. Osteoporosis is classified as either primary or secondary. Primary osteoporosis is related to general aging processes that promote bone involution. Secondary osteoporosis results from other diseases or disorders, such as endocrine disorders, drug-induced changes in bone metabolism, dietary deficiencies or malabsorption syndromes, organ failure, inherited disorders, and malignancies. These disorders disrupt skeletal and serum calcium homeostasis.

Bone mineral mass begins to decline at approximately the age of 35-40 in both men and women. Women lose approximately 1% per year of bone mineral mass until menopause, when bone loss increases to 2%-3% per year. Men lose bone mass at the slower rate of 0.4%-0.5% per year. The causes of the decline in bone mineral mass with age are multifactorial. The most commonly cited contributing factors are heredity, changes in hormonal function, inadequate calcium intake or calcium malabsorption, estrogen depletion in women, and decreased physical activity. Although each of these factors is important, this chapter focuses on the role that mechanical stress plays in skeletal homeostasis.

Studies of extreme states such as weightlessness or athletic training provide striking evidence of the importance of mechanical stress in maintaining bone mass. The influence of decreased or increased mechanical forces is primarily local, and the effect of the change is modulated by the habitual regimen of the skeletal segment. Patterns of bone hypertrophy in athletes reflect the patterns of activity during training for the particular sport. Greater changes occur in weight-bearing than in non-weight-bearing bones when stresses are removed. Results of cross-sectional studies of nonathletes are varied, and this may reflect confounding variables, difficulties with measurement of physical activity levels, or inappropriate bone measurement sites. Intervention studies, however, demonstrate that training can prevent or reverse bone mineral loss in a wide variety of subject populations.

Reduced Mechanical Forces

Weightlessness

The effect of weightlessness on human bone has been studied primarily through examination of the os calcis. Initial studies using densitometry showed density losses of approximately 0.5% per day in the calcaneous in spaceflights lasting 4-24 d and substantial individual diversity (58). Subsequent studies using single photon absorptiometry have indicated that earlier loss rates may have been overstated and that bone loss may gradually taper after initial loss. In spaceflights of 10-185 d, density losses averaged less than 0.1% per day (58, 67, 71). In *Apollo* flights 14-16, each lasting 10-12 d, only two of nine astronauts had significant losses in os calcis BMC; in *Skylab* flights lasting 28-84 d, only three of the nine astronauts had significant losses. Radius and ulna BMCs did not change significantly in these flights (58). On the basis of calcium balance studies, the estimated loss of total body calcium was 0.05%-1.21% for *Apollo* flights 7-11 and 0.2% for *Apollo* flight 17 (58). Studies measuring calcium metabolism reported increases in fecal and urinary calcium excretion, whereas calcium balance declined to negative values reaching -200 mg per day by 2 mo in the *Skylab* experiments (40, 58). The *Skylab* studies also reported increases in urinary hydroxyproline and hydroxylisine (58). In sum, it appears that weightlessness alters calcium metabolism and stimulates bone resorption. Non-weight-bearing bones seem less affected, but the loss of bone mineral in the calcaneous, a weight-bearing bone, may average 3% per month.

Bed Rest

Numerous studies have attempted to simulate the effect of weightlessness on humans by bed rest. During bed rest, calcium balance declines rapidly as urinary calcium output increases. Following a rapidly increasing loss for 7 wk, high urinary calcium levels gradually decrease but do not approach pre-bed-rest levels even after 36 wk. More specifically, rapid bone loss occurs in trabecular weight-bearing bones, such as the lumbar spine, iliac crest, and calcaneous. Less severe, however, is the demineralization of non-weight-bearing bones of the upper extremities (73). Deitrick et al. (15) examined 4 healthy young men immobilized for 6-7 wk in bivalved casts. Total calcium losses varied between 9 and 24 g, whereas urinary calcium increased. Nitrogen excretion also increased with extended bed rest. Goldsmith et al. (22) reported similar declines of 0.4% per month in total body calcium in bed-rested subjects with lower body immobilization. In a longer study of subjects who were not immobilized but were under strict bed-rest guidelines, Donaldson et al. (16) reported losses of approximately 4.2% in estimated total body calcium over 30-36 wk. During periods of 18-24 wk of bed rest, os calcis BMC declined 25%-45%. When normal activity resumed, the os calcis regained its bone mineral content at a rate corresponding to the rate of loss, and urinary calcium excretion returned to normal. In a similar study, os calcis bone mineral loss averaged 4% per month, but the radius demineralized at a slower rate (28). Schneider and McDonald (60) studied 90 young men at bed rest for 5-36 wk. Urinary calcium excretion increased 100 mg/d over baseline for the first 6 wk, maintained that level for several weeks, and then declined. Calcium balance decreased to about −200 mg/d within the initial 4 wk and maintained this rate throughout the study. Os calcis bone mineral content demineralized at the rate of 5% per month during the period of bed rest. Counterpoint to most bed-rest studies, urinary calcium did not elevate in 34 patients hospitalized for herniated disks (35). However, subjects were allowed to get out of bed and use bathroom facilities. Lumbar spine BMC decreased about 0.9% per week in spite of the slight weight-bearing activity but increased when bed rest was discontinued. Thirteen patients confined to strict bed rest following scoliosis surgery declined in lumbar BMC at a greater rate of approximately 2% per week (24).

Attempts have been made to reduce or prevent bone mineral loss in bed rest by inducing mechanical stresses. Hydrostatic pressure on the legs, compression, and replacement of mechanical load by supine or seated training have met with limited success. Hantman et al. (25) reported that periodic longitudinal compression did not significantly affect negative mineral balances. Issekutz et al. (29) found that quiet standing for 2-4 hr per day decreased calcium excretion. However, urinary calcium excretion was unaltered from bed-rest levels in healthy young men who trained on a bicycle ergometer for up to 4 hr per day in either a supine or a sitting position or who sat for 8 hr combined with bed rest. Nitrogen and calcium excretion declined rapidly with the resumption of normal activity. In a similar study, Schneider and McDonald (60) were unable to deter bone loss by supine training, skeletal compression, or hydrostatic pressure. In contrast, other investigators (57) reported increased calcium balance when bed-rest subjects participated in supine training.

Physical Activity and Training

Bone growth and remodeling may be significantly affected by the type, intensity, and duration of physical activity. Few studies have been able to quantify precisely the exercise necessary for bone hypertrophy or maintenance.

Athletes

Runners

Dalen and Olsson (14) studied seven skeletal sites in 15 long-term male cross-country runners between the ages of 50 and 59. Compared to age- and weight-matched controls (n = 15), BMC was increased significantly at the calcaneous, the femur shaft, the head of the humerus, and the distal ends of the radius and ulna and nonsignificantly at the third lumbar vertebra, the femur neck, and the shaft of the ulna and radius. Aloia et al. (1) reported that both potassium and total body calcium values were higher in male marathon runners than in controls. The groups, however, did not differ significantly in radius BMC. Brewer et al. (9) examined 42 female marathon runners (ages 30-49). In contrast to Dalen and Olsson's study, they reported lower os calcis mineralization in marathoners than in controls (n = 38) and attributed this to the greater body weight of controls. The BMC of the phalanx V2, as well as the density of the radius midshaft, was higher in marathoners, but distal radius BMC was identical in the two groups. For the runners, the slopes versus age were positive for the distal and midshaft radius and os calcis and significantly different at all sites from the negative slopes for the control subjects. Lane et al. (38) conducted a study of runners (8 men and 6 women from the 50+ Runners Association) and sedentary subjects matched for age, gender, education, and occupation. The female subjects were also matched for calcium intake, menopausal status, and estrogen-replacement therapy. Despite the fact that the control subjects were significantly heavier, the bone density of the lumbar spine (calculated from a CT scan of L1) was 40% greater in the runners. Previous studies have reported a smaller difference, necessitating further evaluation with a larger sampling to substantiate these results.

Other Sports

Nilsson and Westlin (47) examined distal femur bone density of world-class athletes and of controls. They reported that density varied with the sport and with the load applied to the lower limb. Participants in the control group who exercised regularly had greater bone density than did the controls who did not. Athletes had significantly greater bone density than did controls. Weight lifters had the highest hypertrophy relative to inactive controls and were followed by throwers, runners, soccer players, and finally swimmers, who were not significantly different from controls.

In a subsequent study, Nilsson et al. (46) reported that weight lifters had a greater BMC in the proximal fibula and tibia than did sedentary controls. Block et al. (8) also found that the degree of bone hypertrophy of the spine was related to the type of physical activity. Young men who reported independent, rigorous physical training (6 hr/wk) for at least 2 yr were placed into three groups: aerobic, weight lifting, and combined. Bone mineral density was evaluated through CT scans of the spine. Trabecular bone density was 14% greater in trained subjects than in controls. Integral BMC (total mass of cortical and trabecular bone in L1 and L2) was also greater in the trained subjects. The greatest trabecular bone density was found in the combined exercise group, followed by the weight lifting group, the aerobic group, and the controls. Jacobson et al. (31) found similar results on the spine in their study of intercollegiate female athletes: collegiate swim team (n = 23), tennis team (n = 11), and women not involved in any structured activity. The swimmers' and control group's spine values did not differ significantly, whereas the tennis players had significantly higher lumbar spine density than did the controls. Controls had significantly less metatarsal density and distal radius BMC and width (W) than did swimmers and tennis players.

Unilateral Sports

Sports that preferentially stress one arm provide evidence that hypertrophy in bone is modulated locally by mechanical stimuli and is not dependent entirely on hormonal or genetic variables. Athletes participating in unilateral sports have greater bone mass in their dominant arms than do controls as well as an increased disparity between the arms. Watson (72) studied 200 young baseball players (ages 8-19) and found significantly less bone mass in the nondominant humerus than in the dominant humerus. In a study of young female tennis players, the BMC of the dominant distal radius was 15% higher than was the nondominant radius (30). Jones et al. (33) and Priest et al. (56) examined radiographs of the proximal humerus of 30 female (average age 24) and 54 male (average age 27) tennis professionals. Combined cortical thickness of the dominant arm was greater than that of the nondominant arm by 34.9% for the men and by 28.4% for the women. Cortical thickness in the nondominant arm did not differ from control values. Medullary cavity diameter was smaller in the dominant arm and periosteal diameter greater. To a lesser extent, the proximal ulna and radius were also hypertrophied.

Two studies examined BMC in older male tennis players. Montoye et al. (45) studied 61 long-term male tennis players (mean age 64). The BMC of the dominant playing arm was 8% greater in the one-third distal radius and 10% greater in the humerus midshaft than in the nondominant arm. At these same sites, widths and BMC/W were also greater. The BMC/W was slightly greater in the ulna of the dominant arm, but BMC and W of the ulna did not differ significantly between arms. In the dominant hand, total cortical area was 15% greater in the second metacarpal and 7% greater in the third metacarpal. Huddleston et al. (27) also measured the one-third distal radius BMC in older male tennis participants (ages 70-84). The radius BMC of the nonplaying arm was an average of 13% less than that of the dominant arm. Although studies of older tennis players cannot be directly compared with studies of younger professional players because of differences in measurement methods and sites, relative hypertrophy in the dominant arm is less decided in older individuals. This disparity may be due to variations in duration and intensity rather than solely to age-related differences. In both studies of older men, however, BMC and age were inversely correlated.

Cross-Sectional Studies of Physical Activity Level or Fitness

Diversity in results and complications by a number of variables have limited cross-sectional studies relating bone to physical activity. Most studies have graded physical activity levels without considering the kind of activity. A wide degree of variation exists in the measurement sites selected, and studies may not measure areas affected by the activity. The variety of activities is greater, and the ranges in intensity and duration are smaller, among nonathletes than among athletes, so differences are less clearly delineated than are those between average subjects and athletes.

Self-Reported Activity Levels

Several studies have used questionnaires or interviews to evaluate physical activity levels on the basis of overall daily activities or hours of vigorous activities. Black-Sandler et al. (6) reported that radius and tibia bone mass in 59 postmenopausal women was not significantly related to physical activity level evaluated by questionnaire. However, bone mass was correlated with the level of physical activity evaluated by activity monitors worn for 3 d. A study of 45 young men and women (ages

20-25) divided into low (0 h/wk vigorous activity), moderate (2-3 h/wk), and high (6 h/wk) physical activity groups measured the bone density of the second phalange (19). Low- and moderate-activity groups did not differ significantly in bone density, but bone density was significantly greater in the high-activity group. In a similar study, Stillman et al. (69) categorized 83 women (ages 30-85) into low-, moderate-, and high-activity groups on the basis of reports of activity levels that included athletic, recreational, employment, and home-life variables. The most active group had significantly greater BMC and BMC/W (measured at the one-third distal radius) than had the less active groups even with menstrual status and age as covariates. There were no significant differences between the low- and moderate-activity groups, although BMC/W adjusted for menstrual status, and age tended to be higher in the moderate-activity group. Conversely, Frisancho et al. (21) reported no significant differences in radiographic measurements of the second metacarpal among 131 men (ages 45-64) categorized on the basis of physical activity levels. Jacobson et al. (31) measured lumbar spine and metatarsal density and distal and midshaft radius BMC and W in a study of active adult women (ages 22-70) who exercised at least three times per week compared to age-matched controls. Except for metatarsus density, the reported bone density values were higher for the active women and most differences significant. Young and old active women were less different in radius measurements than were young and old controls. Krolner et al. (37) measured BMC of the distal forearm and L2-L4 in 36 subjects (ages 50-73) who had previous Colles' fractures. Participants were categorized according to activity level on a scale of 0-6, but no participants were classified at the two lowest or the two highest levels. Results showed no relationship between activity level and age, physical fitness, or forearm or lumbar BMC. Montoye et al. (44) found that metacarpal cortical area did not differ significantly between the most active and the least active men (ages 55-64) in the Tecumseh study. Oyster et al. (50), in a study of women aged 60-69, found physical activity and estrogen usage to be highly correlated with metacarpal cortical diameter. Additionally, although they did not differ significantly in height or weight, the 10 most active women had a cortical diameter 18% greater than did the 10 least active women. Two recent studies (3, 34) reported that spine and total body bone density is correlated with physical activity level but that radius bone density is not. Yano et al. (76) studied 1,368 men (ages 61-81) and 1,098 women (ages 43-80) and

measured BMC at the proximal and the distal radius, the ulna, and the os calcis. Physical activity level (defined as hours per month of strenuous exercise) was significantly correlated with BMC of the os calcis and distal ulna in men but not in women. Zanzi et al. (78) classified 73 men (ages 20-93) and 52 women (ages 20-73) on a scale of 1-5 for occupational and recreational physical activity. The level of physical activity did not correlate with total body calcium or BMC of the 8-cm distal radius.

Physical Fitness

Bone mineral content appears to be more significantly correlated with measures of physical fitness than with estimates of physical activity levels. Krolner et al. (37) evaluated levels of physical fitness by the ability of the subjects to work at loads of 75 W and 100 W for 3 min. Lumbar spine BMC (but not forearm BMC) adjusted for age was associated with higher levels of work capacity. In the Tecumseh study (44), although reported physical activity levels were not related to percent cortical area of the metacarpal, heart rates at submaximal work loads were significantly inversely correlated. Pocock et al. (54) examined BMC in 84 women (ages 20-75) by measuring the densities of the distal radius, ulna, femoral neck, and lumbar spine. Physical fitness was assessed by the Astrand-Rhyming method for a submaximal ergometer test. Age, fitness, and weight were significant predictors of femoral and spine bone mineral density (BMD), but only age was a significant independent predictor of forearm BMC. In postmenopausal women, lumbar BMD was independently predicted by physical fitness and weight, and physical fitness was the only significant predictor of femur BMD. Chow et al. (11), in a study of healthy postmenopausal women (ages 50-59), compared bone mineral mass and physical fitness. Physical fitness was assessed by a maximum-graded treadmill exercise test and bone mass of the trunk and proximal femur by neutron activation analysis. Physical fitness correlated significantly with the calcium bone index (bone mineral adjusted for age and size). Subjects with average physical fitness had significantly lower calcium bone indices and bench-press and leg-press strength than did subjects with above-average fitness.

Muscle Mass and Strength

A number of investigators have researched the relationship between BMC and local or total muscle mass. Doyle et al. (17) found that the ash weight of L3 and the mass of the left psoas muscle from autopsy samples were significantly correlated. Ellis et al. (18) reported that normal subjects had greater total body potassium than did osteoporotic subjects of a similar age. Pogrund et al. (55) similarly found that the ratio of psoas muscle width to L3 width was significantly lower in osteoporotics. Harrison (26), in a study of 78 men and women (ages 20-80), reported that total body protein was significantly correlated with a calcium bone index. Zanzi et al. (78) also found total body calcium to be significantly correlated with total body potassium in both men and women. Sinaki et al. (63) examined BMDs of L2-L4 in 68 healthy postmenopausal women in relation to back extensor strength. The rank correlation of BMD adjusted for age and back extensor strength was significant. When age and height were used as covariates, however, back extensor strength did not significantly predict BMD. In a previous study Sinaki et al. (64) reported no relation between grip strength or elbow flexion strength and BMD of the nondominant radius in subjects ages 19-89.

Intervention

Greater training generally upgrades BMC in young subjects and upgrades BMC or retards loss in older subjects of both genders. A study by Margulies et al. (41) of 268 male recruits (ages 18-21) undergoing a vigorous physical training program for 14 wk showed an increase in tibial BMC of 11% in the left leg and 5% in the right leg. Tibial width was not affected significantly. Those subjects who ceased training ($n = 110$, most because of stress fractures) had less hypertrophy than did subjects who completed the training program. Overton et al. (49) used gamma-computed tomography to measure bone density of the distal forearm in 3 young male athletes training to develop strength in the forearm. Trabecular bone density improved by up to 3% over 1-4 mo of training, as did cortical bone density and total bone density. In another study (75) a group of 20 men (ages 35-68) participating in a 9-mo marathon training program were measured for BMC in the os calcis. The consistent runners (average 141 km/mo) improved significantly in BMC of the os calcis by 3% and the inconsistent runners (average 65 km/mo) nonsignificantly by 1%. In contrast to other studies, research by Dalen and Olsson (14) did not note a significant effect on BMC of seven skeletal sites in men who trained for 3 mo. In this study, 19 male subjects (ages 25-52) walked 3 km five times per week or ran 5 km

three times per week, a training regimen similar to that undertaken by the inconsistent runners in the study by Williams et al. (75).

The population most at risk for fractures are postmenopausal and osteoporotic women, so they have been the primary focus of most physical activity intervention studies. Total body calcium for 9 menopausal women (mean age 53) who trained three times per week for 1 yr improved relative to 9 postmenopausal control subjects (2), but radius BMC did not improve. Krolner et al. (36) also found no change in radius BMC but did report changes in lumbar spine BMC that differed significantly between training and nontraining groups. Subjects in the study were 25 women (ages 50-73) with previous Colles' fractures. Subjects who exercised 1 hr twice per week for 8 mo experienced an increased lumbar spine BMC of 3.5% compared to controls, who lost 2.7%. As neither of these exercise regimens was intended to stress the muscle and bone of the arms, the lack of radius response is not surprising. Simkin et al. (62) also evaluated BMC in the forearm but designed a training program that included dynamic loading to the forearm. Forty postmenopausal women categorized as osteoporotic on the basis of lumbar spine morphology served as subjects. The training group ($n = 14$) exercised for 5 mo three times per week for 45-50 min. Specific exercises for dynamic loading of the forearm were used for 15 min of each class session. The remainder of each session consisted of aerobic, warm-up, stretching, flexibility, and relaxation activities. Single-photon absorptiometry was used to measure distal radius BMC, and Compton scattering was used to measure trabecular BMD at the same site. The year before the programs were initiated, BMD declined 2.8% in the control group and 2.0% in the training group. During the intervention period, BMD of the control group declined 1.9%, but BMD of the training group increased 3.8%. Neither group changed significantly in BMC.

The results of this study draw attention to the necessity of designing physical activity programs that stress the bone being measured but still raise questions regarding measurement techniques. Chow et al. (12) examined osteoporotic patients treated with fluoride and studied their responses to training. The calcium bone index of the pelvis and trunk (bone mass corrected for body size) was evaluated by neutron activation analysis. The training regimen incorporated 20 min of aerobic movement and 20 min of strength training per session. Twenty subjects who trained at least three times per week had a significantly higher calcium bone index after 12.5 mo of study than did 18 subjects who trained less than three times per week (most not training at all). Smith et al. (65) reported that aerobic training combined with arm work deterred bone loss in middle-aged women. For 4 yr, 80 women (ages 35-65) trained for 45 min per session three times per week. The rate of loss in the training group was significantly less than that of the control group (n = 62) for the radius, ulna, and humerus. White et al. (74) reported changes in BMC of the distal radius with aerobic dance and walking in 73 sedentary and recently postmenopausal women who were divided into control, walking, and dancing groups. Walking participants began at 1 mi twice per week and increased their walking to 2 mi 4 d per week by the 11th wk. The aerobic dance group began with two dances twice per week and progressed to five dances 4 d per week by the 11th wk. For the following 15 wk, training continued at these levels. At the end of the study, radius BMC had decreased significantly by 1.6% in the control group and by 1.7% in the walking group, but the decrease in the dancing group was not significant. Bone widths and estimated cross-sectional moments of inertia increased significantly in both the walking and the dancing groups. The investigators suggested that the arms were loaded in aerobic dance, as evidenced by an increase of 6% in arm strength in this group. Chow et al. (13) randomly assigned healthy, postmenopausal women (ages 50-62) to two training groups (aerobic and aerobic combined with strengthening activities) and a control group. Both training groups had significantly higher calcium bone indices than did the control group by the end of the study. In addition, although the calcium bone index in controls decreased, it increased in both training groups.

Several studies have focused on bone changes with physical activity intervention in elderly subjects. Smith et al. (66), in a study of elderly women (mean age 81), compared loss rates in control and training intervention groups. Training subjects participated in a low-intensity program of chair exercises for 30 min 3 d per week. In 3 yr the BMC of the radius increased 2.3% in the training group and declined 3.3% in the control group. Changes in BMC and BMC/W differed significantly between the trained and the untrained groups. Rundgren et al. (59) measured BMC in the heels of 15 exercising subjects (mean age 72) and controls. Training subjects participated in 1 hr of training twice per week for 9 mo. Although initially the training and the control participants did not differ significantly in BMC, by the end of the study the training group had significantly higher BMC. Sidney et al. (61)

also stated that training deterred bone loss (measured by total bone calcium index), but the sample was small (n = 14), and there was no control group. Calcium bone index in the elderly, trained subjects did not change significantly over 1 yr of exercise for 1 hr four times per week.

Conclusion

Although a number of studies have shown that bone involution can be slowed or reversed by training, the optimal training program for prevention of osteoporotic fractures has not yet been defined. Training regimens aimed at preventing fractures should stress the area (i.e., hip, spine, femur, and wrist) most frequently at risk. Limited information from animal studies (39) suggests that the most effective form of mechanical stress is intermittent and compressive and that level of hypertrophy is correlated with both strain magnitude and strain rate. The repetitions of strain appear to be less important. For example, as few as 4 repetitions per day of high strain prevented bone atrophy, and bone hypertrophy did not differ between strain regimens of 36 and 1,800 repetitions per day.

Bone mineral mass is locally modulated by mechanical forces in the form of physical activity. This is most evident in extreme states, such as weightlessness or athletic training. Bone atrophies in weightlessness, bed rest, or immobilization, and the rate of bone loss is proportional to the initial bone mass and the habitual mechanical loads to the particular bone. Athletes have much greater bone mass than do sedentary controls, and the amount and sites of hypertrophy parallel the stresses placed on the bone by the sport activity. It is more difficult to establish a relationship between physical activity and bone mass in cross-sectional studies of nonathletes, partly because of methodological problems. Intervention studies, however, convincingly show that formerly sedentary individuals (whatever their age, gender, or initial bone status) can reduce bone loss or increase bone mass by physical training.

The exact forms and levels of physical activity necessary to prevent osteoporosis are unknown. Bone appears to act (like muscle) on the overload principle. Strain magnitude and strain rate appear to be important factors in the effectiveness or physical activity, and number of repetitions is relatively unimportant. Activities prescribed for preventing bone loss should stress the areas at risk for fracture with intermittent, compressive forces greater than those normally experienced by the individual. However, forces should not be traumatic, and the maximum force should be reduced when repetitions are increased to avoid fatigue fractures. The exact relation of a well-defined physical load and bone response needs to be researched further.

Most studies have evaluated bone integrity by measuring bone mass or bone mineral content. Although bone mineral content accounts for 90% of bone strength, other factors (e.g., geometric structure) are also important. Further research is needed to quantify precisely the effects of training on strength per se rather than indirectly by bone mineral content. In addition, the mechanisms by which physical activity and hormones affect bone cell activity are unknown and need further investigation.

Careful review indicates that the perceived association between athletic training and osteoarthritis is due instead to injury and joint malalignment. Physical activity programs should therefore emphasize safety to avoid inducing osteoarthritis. For the osteoarthritic, physical activities should avoid large or abrupt forces on the affected joints because these could further damage subchondral bone and cause pain. In addition, participants in physical activity should avoid extreme fatigue, as such a state may often lead to joint malalignment or injury.

References

1. Aloia, J.F., S.H. Cohn, T. Babu, C. Abesamis, N. Kalici, and K. Ellis. Skeletal mass and body composition in marathon runners. *Metabolism* 27: 1793-1796, 1978.
2. Aloia, J.F., S.H. Cohn, J. Ostuni, R. Cane, and K. Ellis. Prevention of involutional bone loss by exercise. *Ann. Intern. Med.* 89: 356-358, 1978.
3. Aloia, J.F., A.N. Vaswani, J.K. Yeh, and S.H. Cohn. Premenopausal bone mass is related to physical activity. *Arch. Intern. Med.* 148: 121-123, 1988.
4. Altman, R., R. Meenan, M. Hochberg, G. Bole, K. Brandt, et al. An approach to developing criteria for the clinical diagnosis and classification of osteoarthritis: A status report of the American Rheumatism Association diagnostic subcommittee on osteoarthritis. *J. Rheum.* 10: 180-183, 1983.
5. Beeson, P.B., and W. McDermott. *Textbook of medicine* (13th ed.). Philadelphia: W.B. Saunders, 1971.
6. Black-Sandler, R., R.E. LaPort, D. Sashin, L.H. Kuller, E. Sternglass, J.A. Cauley, and M.M. Link. Determinants of bone mass in menopause. *Prev. Med.* 11: 269-280, 1982.
7. Bland, J.H., and S.M. Cooper. Osteoarthritis: A review of the cell biology involved and evidence for reversibility, management rationally related to known genesis and pathophysiology. *Semin. Arth. Rheum.* 14: 106-133, 1984.
8. Block, J.E., H.K. Genant, and D. Black. Greater vertebral bone mineral mass in exercising young men. *West. J. Med.* 145: 39-42, 1986.
9. Brewer, V., B.M. Meyer, M.S. Keele, S.J. Upton, and R.D. Hagan. Role of exercise in prevention of involutional bone loss. *Med. Sci. Sports Exerc.* 15: 445-449, 1983.
10. Chantraine, A. Knee joint in soccer players: Osteoarthritis and axis deviation. *Med. Sci. Sports Exerc.* 17: 434-439, 1985.
11. Chow, R.K., J.E. Harrison, C.F. Brown, and V. Hajek. Physical fitness effect on bone mass in postmenopausal women. *Arch. Phys. Med. Rehabil.* 67: 231-234, 1986.
12. Chow, R.K., J.E. Harrison, and C. Notarius. Effect of two randomised exercise programmes on bone mass of healthy postmenopausal women. *Br. Med. J.* 292: 607-610, 1987.
13. Chow, R.K., J.E. Harrison, W. Sturtbridge, R. Josse, T.M. Murray, A. Bayley, J. Dornan, and T. Hammond. The effect of exercise on bone mass of osteoporotic patients on fluoride treatment. *Clin. Invest. Med.* 10: 59-63, 1987.
14. Dalen, N., and K.E. Olsson. Bone mineral content and physical activity. *Acta Orthop. Scand.* 45: 170-174, 1974.
15. Deitrick, J.E., G.D. Whedon, and E. Shorr. Effects of immobilization upon various metabolic and physiologic functions of normal men. *Am. J. Med.* 4: 3-35, 1948.
16. Donaldson, C.L., S.B. Hulley, J.M. Vogel, R.S. Hattner, J.H. Bayers, and D.E. McMillan. Effect of prolonged bed rest on bone mineral. *Metabolism* 19: 1071-1084, 1970.
17. Doyle, F., J. Brown, and C. LaChance. Relation between bone mass and muscle weight. *Lancet* i (February 21): 391-393, 1970.
18. Ellis, K.J., K.K. Shukla, S.H. Cohn, and R.N. Pierson. A predictor for total body potassium in man based on height, weight, sex and age: Applications in metabolic disorders. *J. Lab. Clin. Med.* 83: 716-727, 1974.

19. Emiola, L., and P. O'Shea. Effects of physical activity and nutrition on bone density measured by radiographic techniques. *Nutr. Rept. Int.* 17(6): 669-681, 1978.

20. Fitzgerald, B., and G.R. McLatchie. Degenerative joint disease in weight-lifters: Fact or fiction? *Br. J. Sports Med.* 14: 97-101, 1980.

21. Frisancho, A.R., H.J. Montoye, M.E. Frantz, H. Metzner, and H.J. Dodge. A comparison of morphological variables in adult males selected on the basis of physical activity. *Med. Sci. Sports* 2: 209-212, 1970.

22. Goldsmith, R.S., P. Killian, S.H. Ingbar, and D.E. Bass. Effect of phosphate supplementation during immobilization of normal men. *Metabolism* 18: 349-368, 1969.

23. Hadler, N.M. Industrial rheumatology. *Arth. Rheum.* 20: 1019-1025, 1977.

24. Hansson, T.H., B.O. Roos, and A. Nachemson. Development of osteopenia in the fourth lumbar vertebra during prolonged bed rest after operation for scoliosis. *Acta Orthop. Scand.* 46: 621-630, 1975.

25. Hantman, D.A., J.M. Vogel, C.L. Donaldson, R. Friedman, R.S. Goldsmith, and S.B. Hulley. Attempts to prevent disuse osteoporosis by treatment with calcitonin, longitudinal compression and supplementary calcium and phosphate. *J. Clin. Endocrinol. Metab.* 36: 845-858, 1973.

26. Harrison, J.E. Neutron activation studies and the effect of exercise on osteoporosis. *J. Med.* 15(4): 285-294, 1984.

27. Huddleston, A.L., D. Rockwell, D.N. Kulund, and R.B. Harrison. Bone mass in lifetime tennis athletes. *JAMA* 244: 1107-1109, 1980.

28. Hulley, S.B., J.M. Vogel, C.L. Donaldson, J.H. Bayers, R.J. Friedman, and S.N. Rosen. The effect of supplemental oral phosphate on the bone mineral changes during prolonged bed rest. *J. Clin. Invest.* 50: 2506-2518, 1971.

29. Issekutz, B., J.J. Blizzard, N.C. Birkhead, and K. Rodahl. Effect of prolonged bed rest on urinary calcium output. *J. Appl. Physiol.* 21: 1013-1020, 1966.

30. Jacobson, P., W. Beaver, D. Janeway, S. Grubb, T. Taft, and R. Talmage. Single and dual photon densitometry: Comparison of intercollegiate swimmers, tennis players, athletic adult women, and age-matched controls. *Trans. Orthop. Res. Soc.*: 202, 1984.

31. Jacobson, P.C., W. Beaver, S.A. Grubb, T.N. Taft, and R.V. Talmage. Bone density in women: College athletes and older athletic women. *J. Orthop. Res.* 2: 328-332, 1984.

32. Jenkins, D.P., and T.H. Cochran. Osteoporosis: The dramatic effect of disuse of an extremity. *Clin. Orthop.* 64: 128-134, 1969.

33. Jones, H.H., J.D. Priest, and W.C. Hayes. Humeral hypertrophy in response to exercise. *J. Bone Joint Surg. [Am.]* 59: 204-208, 1977.

34. Kanders, B., D.W. Dempster, and R. Lindsay. Interaction of calcium nutrition and physical activity on bone mass in young women. *J. Bone Miner. Res.* 3: 145-149, 1988.

35. Krolner, B., and B. Toft. Vertebral bone loss: An unheeded side effect of therapeutic bed rest. *Clin. Sci.* 64: 537-540, 1983.

36. Krolner, B., B. Toft, S.P. Nielson, and E. Tondevold. Physical exercise as prophylaxis against involutional vertebral bone loss: A controlled trial. *Clin. Sci.* 64: 541-546, 1983.

37. Krolner, B., E. Tondevold, B. Toft, B. Berthelson, and S.P. Nielsen. Bone mass of the axial and the appendicular skeleton in women with Colles' fracture: Its relation to physical activity. *Clin. Physiol.* 2: 147-157, 1982.

38. Lane, N.E., D.A. Bloch, H.H. Jones, W.H. Marshall, P.D. Wood, and J.F. Fries. Long-distance running, bone density, and osteoarthritis. *JAMA* 255(9): 1147-1151, 1986.

39. Lanyon, L.E. Functional strain as a determinant for bone remodeling. *Calcif. Tissue Int.* 36: S56-S61, 1984.

40. Lutwak, L., G.D. Whedon, P.A. LaChance, J.M. Reid, and H.S. Lipscomb. Mineral, electrolyte and nitrogen balance studies of the Gemini-VII fourteen-day orbital spaceflight. *J. Clin. Endocrinol. Metab.* 29: 1140-1156, 1969.

41. Margulies, J.Y., A. Simkin, I. Leichter, A. Bivas, R. Steinberg, M. Giladi, M. Stein, et al. Effect of intense physical activity on the bone-mineral content in the lower limbs of young adults. *J. Bone Joint Surg. [Am.]* 68(7): 1090-1093, 1986.

42. Martin, A.D., K.G. Silverthorn, and L. Roos. Hip fracture trends in Saskatchewan, 1972-1984. (Unpublished manuscript.)

43. McDermott, M., and P. Ereyne. Osteoarthrosis in runners with knee pain. *Br. J. Sports Med.* 17(2): 84-87, 1983.

44. Montoye, H.J., J.F. McCabe, H.L. Metzner, and S.M. Garn. Physical activity and bone density. *Hum. Biol.* 48: 599-610, 1976.

45. Montoye, H.J., E.L. Smith, D.F. Fardon, and E.T. Howley. Bone mineral in senior tennis players. *Scand. J. Sports Sci.* 2: 26-32, 1980.

46. Nilsson, B.E., S.M. Andersson, T. Havdrup, and N.E. Westlin. Ballet-dancing and weight-lifting—Effects on BMC. *Am. J. Roentgen.* 13: 541-542, 1978.

47. Nilsson, B.E., and N.E. Westlin. Bone density in athletes. *Clin. Orthop. Rel. Res.* 77: 177-182, 1971.

48. Nilsson, B.E.R. Post-traumatic osteopenia. *Acta Orthop. Scand.* 91: 1, 1966.

49. Overton, T.R., T.N. Hangartner, R. Heath, and J.D. Ridley. Effect of physical activity on bone: Gamma ray computed tomography. In: DeLuca, H.F., H.M. Frost, W.S.S. Jee, C.C. Johnston, and A.M. Parfitt, eds. *Osteoporosis: Recent advances in pathogenesis and treatment.* Baltimore: University Park Press, 1981, p. 147-158.

50. Oyster, N., M. Morton, and S. Linnell. Physical activity and osteoporosis in postmenopausal women. *Med. Sci. Sports Exerc.* 16(1): 44-50, 1984.

51. Panush, R.S., and D.G. Brown. Exercise and arthritis. *Sports Med.* 4: 54-64, 1987.

52. Panush, R.S., C. Schmidt, J.R. Caldwell, N.L. Edwards, S. Longley, R. Yonker, E. Webster, J. Nauman, J. Stork, and H. Pettersson. Is running associated with degenerative joint disease? *JAMA* 255: 1152-1154, 1986.

53. Peyron, J.G. Review of the main epidemiologic-etiologic evidence that implies mechanical forces as factors in osteoarthritis. *Eng. Med.* 15(2): 77-79, 1986.

54. Pocock, N.A., J.A. Eisman, M.G. Yeates, P.N. Sambrook, and S. Eberl. Physical fitness is a major determinant of femoral neck and lumbar spine bone mineral density. *J. Clin. Invest.* 78: 618-621, 1986.

55. Pogrund, H., R.A. Bloom, and H. Weinberg. Relationship of psoas width to osteoporosis. *Acta Orthop. Scand.* 57: 208-210, 1986.

56. Priest, J.D., H.H. Jones, C.J.C. Tichnor, and D.A. Nagel. Arm and elbow changes in expert tennis players. *Minn. Med.* 60: 399-404, 1977.

57. Ragan, C., and A.M. Briscoe. Effect of exercise on the metabolism of ^{40}calcium and ^{47}calcium in man. *J. Clin. Endocrinol. Metab.* 24: 385-392, 1964.

58. Rambaut, P.C. Decreased activity and bone mass: The skeleton and space flight. In: Roche, A.F., ed. *Osteoporosis: Current concepts. Report of the 7th Ross Conference on Medical Research.* Columbus, OH: Ross Laboratories, 1987, p. 38-42.

59. Rundgren, A., A. Aniansson, P. Ljungberg, and H. Wetterqvist. Effects of a training programme for elderly people on mineral content of the heel bone. *Arch. Gerontol. Geriatr.* 3: 243-248, 1984.

60. Schneider, V.S., and J. McDonald. Skeletal calcium homeostasis and countermeasures to prevent disuse osteoporosis. *Calcif. Tissue Int.* 36: S151-S154, 1984.

61. Sidney, K.H., R.J. Shephard, and J.E. Harrison. Endurance training and body composition of the elderly. *Am. J. Clin. Nutr.* 30: 326-333, 1977.

62. Simkin, A., J. Ayalon, and I. Leichter. Increased trabecular bone density due to boneloading exercises in postmenopausal osteoporotic women. *Calcif. Tissue Int.* 40: 59-63, 1986.

63. Sinaki, M., M.C. McPhee, S.F. Hodgson, J.M. Merritt, and K.P. Offord. Relationship between bone mineral density of spine and strength of back extensors in healthy postmenopausal women. *Mayo Clin. Proc.* 61: 116-122, 1986.

64. Sinaki, M., J.L. Opitz, and H.W. Wahner. Bone mineral content: Relationship to muscle strength in normal subjects. *Arch. Phys. Med. Rehabil.* 55: 508-512, 1974.

65. Smith, E.L., C. Gilligan, M.M. Shea, C.P. Ensign, and P.E. Smith. Determining bone loss by exercise intervention in premenopausal and postmenopausal women. *Calcif. Tissue Intl.* 44: 312-321, 1989.

66. Smith, E.L., W. Reddan, and P.E. Smith. Physical activity and calcium modalities for bone mineral increase in aged women. *Med. Sci. Sports Exerc.* 13(1): 60-64, 1981.

67. Smith, M.C., P.C. Rambaut, J.M. Vogel, and M.W. Whittle. Bone mineral measurement—Experiment M078. In: Johnston, R.S., and L.F. Dietlein, eds. *Biomedical Results from Skylab* (NASA Document No. SP-377). Washington, DC: NASA, 1977, p. 183-190.

68. Soh, R.S., and L.J. Micheli. The effect of running on the pathogenesis of osteoarthritis of the hips and knees. *Clin. Orthop. Rel. Res.* 198: 106-109, 1985.

69. Stillman, R.J., T.G. Lohman, M.H. Slaughter, and B.H. Massey. Physical activity and bone mineral content in women aged 30 to 85 years. *Med. Sci. Sports Exerc.* 18(5): 576-580, 1986.

70. Swezey, R.L. Low back pain in the elderly: Practical management concerns. *Geriatrics* 43: 38-44, 1988.

71. Vogel, J.M. Bone mineral measurement: Skylab experiment M078. *Acta Astronautica* 2: 129-139, 1975.

72. Watson, R.C. Bone growth and physical activity in young males. In: Mazess, R.B., ed. *International Conference on Bone Mineral Measurements* (DHEW Publication No. NIH 75-683). Washington, DC: Department of

Health, Education and Welfare, 1974, p. 380-385.

73. Whedon, G.D. Disuse osteoporosis: Physiological aspects. *Calcif. Tissue Intl.* 36: S146-S150, 1984.

74. White, M.K., R.B. Martin, R.A. Yeater, R.L. Butcher, and E.I. Radin. The effects of exercise on the bones of postmenopausal women. *Int. Orthop.* 7: 209-214, 1984.

75. Williams, J.A., J. Wagner, R. Wasnich, and L. Heilbrun. The effect of long-distance running upon appendicular bone mineral content. *Med. Sci. Sports Exerc.* 16: 223-227, 1984.

76. Yano, K., R.D. Wasnich, J.M. Vogel, and L.K. Heilbrun. Bone mineral measurements among middle-aged and elderly Japanese residents in Hawaii. *Am. J. Epidemiol.* 119: 751-764, 1984.

77. Zanzi, I., C. Colbert, R. Batchell, K. Thompson, K. Aloia, and S. Cohn. Comparison of total-body calcium with radiographic and photon absorptiometry measurements of the appendicular bone mineral content. In: Mazess, R.B., ed. *Fourth International Conference on Bone Measurement* (NIH Publication No. 80-1938). Washington, DC: National Institutes of Health, 1980, p. 393-400.

78. Zanzi, I., K.J. Ellis, J. Aloia, and S. Cohn. Effect of physical activity on body composition. In: DeLuca, H.F., H.M. Frost, W.S.S. Jee, C.C. Johnson, and A.M. Parfitt, eds. *Osteoporosis: Recent advances in pathogenesis and treatment.* Baltimore: University Park Press, 1981, p. 139-146.

Chapter 44

Discussion: Exercise, Fitness, Osteoarthritis, and Osteoporosis

Joan E. Harrison
Raphael Chow

The primary function of the skeleton is mechanical. It provides protection for vital organs and a framework for mobility. Mechanical force, through gravity and muscle pull, is the only factor known to regulate bone mass and bone strength. The skeleton also provides a reservoir for the bone minerals calcium and phosphate. A constant level of soft-tissue calcium is essential for many vital body functions, and this calcium homeostasis is therefore under tight hormonal control. These calcium-regulating hormones will, if necessary, cause bone resorption to maintain soft-tissue calcium. Their function, however, is directed to soft-tissue calcium homeostasis, whereas mechanical force is the only factor known to have a primary function of regulating bone mass and bone strength.

The profound loss of bone mass and bone strength, or osteoporosis, is a common problem of the elderly, causing recurrent fractures with little or no abnormal force. Osteoporosis can occur in both men and women of all ages, including children, but it occurs most frequently in the older population and particularly in older women. In North America, an estimated one in three women over the age of 70 have vertebral fractures. In extreme old age (over 85), one in three women and one in six men have hip fractures (3, 9). There are many diseases and some drugs that are known to cause osteoporosis, but in most cases no underlying cause can be identified. In young men and women, this idiopathic osteoporosis may be due to some primary defect of bone metabolism, perhaps a variant of the genetic abnormality of osteogenesis imperfecta. The more common osteoporosis of older subjects has been attributed to a variety of risk factors: aging, loss of female sex hormones at menopause, suboptimal nutrition, and sedentary lifestyle (3, 9). We cannot prevent the passage of time. Today, women are encouraged to delay menopause for at least 10 yr by the use of female hormones. Optimal nutrition is not well established, but attention has been given to adequate calories for ideal weight, sufficient dietary calcium, adequate intake of vitamins, and moderation in the use of protein and food drugs. The maintenance of physical fitness, however, may be the most effective measure for prevention of age-related osteoporosis. With aging, the gradual decline in physical activity may be the cause, or at least a major contributing factor, in the development of osteoporosis. With the onset of fractures, the further reduction in physical activity due to chronic pain and to fear of new fractures will accelerate bone loss. Osteoporosis associated with disease also may be partly related to loss of physical activity associated with chronic ill health. Physical fitness is of considerable importance in preserving strong bone.

Bone consists of a fibrous matrix in which the mineral hydroxyapatite is deposited. Each bone has an outer shell of dense cortical bone and a central cavity containing a varying amount of cancellous or trabecular bone within the marrow space of hematopoietic tissue and fat. Trabecular bone consists of rods or plates of bone laid down in the direction of force to give additional strength with lightness. Bones that receive multidirectional forces contain mainly trabecular bone. These include the bones of the spine, the pelvis, the ribs, and the ends of long bones. The shafts of long bones, where unidirectional force is applied, consist of a thick cortex with virtually no trabecular bone within the marrow cavity. Osteoporotic fractures usually occur at sites that are mainly trabecular bone: the vertebrae, the ribs, the distal forearm, and the proximal femur.

The skeleton is a living tissue that constantly undergoes repair and restructuring through the action of bone cells (4). During childhood growth, the bones of the skeleton increase in length and thickness, and the marrow cavity enlarges. The trabecular rods also undergo extensive restructuring to meet the demands put on the skeleton with increasing body size. At maturity, growth in bone length ceases, but throughout life the thickness of the outer cortex and the position and the amount of trabecular bone will alter in response to changes in the forces put on the bone. Bone also is continuously undergoing repair by the removal of small envelopes of old bone that are subsequently replaced with new bone. The bone-forming cell, the osteoblast, appears to be the dominant cell in controlling the amount and location of bone resorption, as well as new bone formation (12), in response to local stimuli of force and strain on bone and modified by systemic factors associated with malnutrition, disease, and drug treatment.

In general, maximum bone mass is achieved during the third or the fourth decade of life, and a gradual loss of bone mass occurs over later decades. The maximum level of bone mass and the subsequent rate of bone loss will depend, at least in part, on the level of physical activity. The importance of activity on bone mass has been reviewed by Smith and Raab (13). Athletes have greater bone mass and bone strength than do more sedentary individuals. Olympic runners and weight lifters have stronger bone than do Olympic swimmers because, with swimming, water reduces the gravitational force on bone. In tennis players, the bone in the forearm of the racket hand is stronger than it is in the other forearm. Conversely, the loss of physical activity (e.g., with paralysis or prolonged bed rest) results in profound loss of trabecular bone and a thinning of the cortex. Even healthy subjects lose bone during prolonged bed rest, and astronauts lose bone in the weightless environment of spaceflight. In experimental animals, immobilization of a limb results in profound bone loss by thinning of the cortex and by intracortical porosity. This experimental bone loss can be prevented by the daily application of cyclic forces, and the mass of bone produced following immobilization is proportional to the magnitude of the force applied (11). The same force applied continuously does not prevent bone loss. It would appear that bone mass is maintained at a level appropriate for the forces put on it during regular activity. With loss in physical activity, rapid loss of bone occurs until the mass of bone has been reduced to the level appropriate for the lower level of force applied.

There is convincing evidence that lifelong attention to physical fitness is important for the development and preservation of strong bone. The effects of improved physical fitness to increase adult bone mass substantially is less clear. In healthy, young subjects, bone loss as a result of prolonged inactivity or weightlessness in space appears to be restored on return to normal physical activity. In older women, regular exercise has decreased or prevented further postmenopausal bone loss, but only modest increases in bone mass have been observed (3). Possibly, the level of exercise was insufficient or longer periods of time were required to improve bone mass substantially. The response to exercise will vary in different parts of the skeleton. For example, aerobic exercise may not affect non-weight-bearing bone at the wrist, whereas cycling may have little effect on the bones of the wrist or spine.

Improvement in bone mass as a result of an exercise program will depend on the level of exercise that the subject can or will perform, on the site selected for bone measurement, and on the ability of bone to respond to increased activity. Cardiac function, muscle strength, and physical activity decline with age, and there is an associated loss in bone mass and bone strength. Fortunately, these older subjects cannot carry out the strenuous activity that young athletes do because the bone is not strong enough to withstand the forces applied during such intense physical activity. Furthermore, the forces applied during physical activity are taken by muscle and ligaments as well as by bone, and the poor muscle tone of older subjects puts a greater proportion of force on bone. It has been observed in horses that the maximum force on bone occurs during trotting (5). With increased speed (when the gait alters to a canter), the force on bone is actually reduced, as more force is taken by muscle. Racehorses suffer stress fractures toward the end of races, when muscle fatigue allows more force on bone.

Competitive athletes also are prone to fatigue fractures. Similarly, muscle fatigue contributes to osteoporotic fractures, although at a much lower level of activity. Patients with osteoporotic fractures have low bone mass, but some healthy subjects have bone mass values well within the osteoporotic range. The absence of fractures in these osteopenic subjects has been attributed to better bone quality and therefore greater bone strength compared to that of patients with osteoporotic fractures (3). It is possible, however, that physical fitness and muscle strength can protect against fractures in spite of osteopenic bone mass (2). In support of this idea, postmenopausal osteopenic women without fractures are, on average, 10 yr younger than patients with osteoporotic fractures and might be expected therefore to have greater muscle strength and physical fitness. Of 216 postmenopausal women whom we have investigated for osteoporosis, 71 had osteoporotic fractures. These fracture patients had low bone mass (67 $\pm$ 12% of healthy, young adults and a mean age of 69 $\pm$ 7). Twenty-three patients had no fractures but comparable osteopenic bone mass (66 $\pm$ 9%) and a mean age of 59 $\pm$ 12.

Exercise programs for the elderly and the osteoporotic must be introduced cautiously and changes in intensity made very slowly. The primary objective should be to improve muscle strength. Even without a significant increase in bone mass, greater muscle strength should reduce the force on bone during normal activity and, by increasing steadiness, reduce the risk of abnormal forces associated with accidental falls. Weight-bearing exercises may have additional value for the preservation and restoration of bone mass, but more studies are required to establish this point.

Possibly the bone of elderly and osteoporotic subjects cannot respond to increased levels of activity. It has been argued that the support rods of trabecular bone, once lost, cannot be replaced (8). In some patients, osteoporosis may be due to a primary abnormality of bone cell function. In this situation, bone cells may be unable to increase bone mass in response to increased forces on bone. For most patients, however, it is probably that bone cells can respond appropriately. For example, osteoporotic fractures heal normally with the formation of a fracture callus of bone overgrowth. Fluoride treatment for osteoporosis is also associated with substantial increases in bone mass. In our Toronto study of 61 patients treated with fluoride for 4 yr, on average almost half the bone lost with aging and with osteoporosis had been restored (1). The increases in bone mass associated with fluoride treatment were observed in the trabecular bones of the spine by X-ray, and biopsies from iliac bone showed increases in both the number and the thickness of individual trabecular support rods. Such increases in bone mass will not increase bone strength unless the new bone is of normal composition and is positioned appropriately for greater strength. Fluoride remains a research treatment until it can be established that the new bone provides the desired increase in bone strength. The data are presented here only to emphasize the fact that increases in trabecular bone of elderly and osteoporotic patients can occur.

Improvement in physical fitness should increase bone mass that is structurally positioned to provide greater bone strength. Even without substantial improvement in bone mass, exercise should increase muscle strength and postural stability and thus reduce the risk of bone and joint injuries associated with muscle fatigue. In our experience, a supervised exercise program has proven to be the most effective measure for the rehabilitation of osteoporotic patients. Much of the benefit is psychological. With social activity, group support, and regular exercise, the patient slowly gains confidence to return to a more active and interesting way of life. Regular exercise improves muscle tone, steadiness, and mobility; reduces pain and depression; and does not increase the incidence of fractures. Improvement in bone mass has been more difficult to establish, although preliminary data are encouraging.

As with all therapeutic measures, there is an optimal range for the level of physical activity, and excessive exercise can be harmful. Women marathon runners have, on average, greater bone mass than do more sedentary controls. With such maximum conditioning programs, however, some women disturb their normal sex hormone activity and lose the cyclic periods of blood flow (amenorrhea), and these athletes have lower bone mass than do runners with normal cyclical activity (6). Furthermore, about 40% of these noncyclic women develop stress fractures. The adverse effects of excessive exercise may be related to loss of sex hormone activity, but other factors also may be involved. Marathon runners tend to have very low food intakes and low body weight. Low body weight is associated with low bone mass. Patients with anorexia, for example, have low bone mass and may develop osteoporotic fractures even in early adult life (10). Of interest is that the low bone mass in patients with anorexia was found to be related to duration of starvation and to the degree of inactivity but not to loss of sex hormone activity or to low intake of dietary calcium.

Stress fractures and joint and ligament injuries are common among competitive athletes and are usually associated with prolonged activity at maximum intensity and with muscle fatigue that causes abnormal forces to be put on ligaments and bone. These athletic injuries may lead to degenerative changes of osteoarthritis in later years. Osteoarthritis causes joint pain and stiffness and is due to degenerative changes of articular surfaces and also to bone overgrowth at the insertion of ligaments and tendons (7). There is no evidence that these athletic injuries and subsequent degenerative abnormalities will occur in well-controlled exercise programs in which prolonged effort at maximum intensity is not required. As one ages and both physical fitness and bone strength progressively decline, exercise programs must be correspondingly modified to avoid undue fatigue in participants.

Many factors can contribute to bone loss and osteoporotic fractures. Physical fitness is an important factor both for prevention of osteoporosis and for rehabilitation of the osteoporotic patient. More research is required to establish optimal activity programs for each level of fitness. The programs should be attractive as well as beneficial and should avoid the possible deleterious effects of fatigue, starvation diets, or altered sex hormone activity. Prevention of osteoporosis requires attention to overall good health. Physical fitness is an important part of good health and well-being for all ages and particularly for the older population.

References

1. Bayley, T.A., J.E. Harrison, R.G. Josse, T.M. Murray, W. Sturtridge, C. Williams, N. Patt, G. Goodwin, K.P.H. Pritzker, and V. Fornasier. The relationships between fluoride effects on bone histology, bone mass and bone strength. Proceedings of the International Symposium on Osteoporosis, Copenhagen. *Osteoporosis* 2: 865-867, 1987.

2. Cummings, S.R. Are patients with hip fractures more osteoporotic? *Am. J. Med.* 78: 487-494, 1985.

3. Cummings, S.R., J.L. Kelsey, M.C. Nevitt, and K.J. O'Dowd. Epidemiology of osteoporosis and osteoporotic fractures. *Epidemiol. Rev.* 7: 178-204, 1985.

4. Kahn, R.J., J.D. Fallon, and S.L. Teitelbaum. Structure-function relationships in bone: An examination of events at the cellular level. *Bone Miner. Res.* 2: 125-174, 1984.

5. Lanyon, L.E. Functional strain as a determinant for bone remodeling. *Calcif. Tissue Int.* 23: S56-S61, 1984.

6. Marcus, R., C. Cann, P. Madvig, J. Minkoff, M. Goddard, M. Bayer, M. Martin, L. Gaudiani, W. Haskell, and H. Genant. Menstrual function and bone mass in elite women distance runners. *Ann. Intern. Med.* 102: 158-163, 1985.

7. Panush, R.S., and D.G. Brown. Exercise and arthritis. *Sports Med.* 4: 54-64, 1987.

8. Parfitt, A.M. Trabecular bone architecture in the pathogenesis and prevention of fracture. *Am. J. Med.* 82(1B): 68-72, 1987.

9. Riggs, B.L., and L.J. Melton III. Involutional osteoporosis. *N. Engl. J. Med.* 314: 1676-1686, 1986.

10. Rigotti, N.A., S.R. Nussbaum, D.B. Herzog, and R.M. Neer. Osteoporosis in women with anorexia nervosa. *N. Engl. J. Med.* 311: 1601-1606, 1984.

11. Rubin, C.T. Skeletal strain and the functional significance of bone architecture. *Calcif. Tissue Int.* 36: S11-S18, 1984.

12. Sakamoto, S., and M. Sakamoto. Bone collagenase, osteoblasts and cell-mediated bone resorption. *Bone Miner. Res.* 4: 49-102, 1986.

13. Smith, E.L., and D.M. Raab. Osteoporosis and physical activity. *Acta Med. Scand. Suppl.* 711: 149-156, 1985.

Chapter 45

Exercise, Fitness, and Back Pain

Alf L. Nachemson

This chapter discusses low-back pain and the possible benefits that can be gained from exercise and fitness. A large body of knowledge exists on the epidemiology and natural history of low-back pain. Several reports (5, 12, 52, 61) from industrialized countries have clearly delineated that low-back pain for the middle-aged subjects is the most costly disease from society's point of view. For example, sickness and disability due to low-back pain have increased in the United States by 2,500% over the last 20 yr (24) and in Sweden by 4,000% over the last 30 yr (47). It must be clearly stated that this enormous increase in sickness and disability is due neither to sudden changes in lifestyle nor to more hazardous workplaces (24). We all know that improvements have occurred in lifestyles and workplaces. Rather, the advent of specific legal and insurance issues (27) has played a role that is further increased by the general notion in the industrialized countries that any type of discomfort should be treated by rest rather than by activity. It is known (27) that low-back discomfort exists as often in nonindustrialized countries as it does in industrialized ones, but in those countries (as in our ancient ones) some personal discomfort was and is still dealt with by continuous activity. Physicians treating patients with low-back pain have the responsibility to get not only their patients but also the society at large active so that, at least partly, the issues can be resolved.

Epidemiological and Natural History

About 80% of the population have had some type of back pain when asked (19, 27, 41), and some 50%-60% must leave work on occasion because of the ailment (4). However, in a community study (12) in which all reported cases of work hindered by low-back pain were tabulated and followed with the help of the Swedish Sick Insurance Registry until they were reported to have returned to work, the recovery rate was quick for the vast majority. Within 2 wk, 67% returned to work, and within 6 wk 88% returned (Table 45.1).

In the same study (12) of 100,000 people covering an 18-mo period, a high rate of recurrence was noted, as it was in many other studies (3, 43, 52, 61). Within a year, 40%-60% reported a recurrence. Some of the risk factors for more frequent and more severe recurrences have been described (24, 43, 52, 61). Recurrences tend to taper off over a 3- to 5-yr period.

Table 45.1 Recovery Rate (%) in 7,526 Patients Reporting Low-Back Disability

Recovery to work within	Percent
1 wk	57
2 wk	67
4 wk	82
6 wk	88
12 wk	95
24 wk	98
52 wk	99

Note. Population base was 49,000 (ages 20-65). Registration period was 18 mo.

What Causes Low-Back Pain?

Despite claims by proponents of various methods of treatment, there is little scientific knowledge of what causes an acute attack of low-back pain. Only in about 2% of these patients can an established diagnosis be made (46). As the time that a patient is in pain increases, this percentage of known definable causes increases such that after 6 wk it has risen to about 15% and after 3 mo to about 30% (43, 46). For most, however, the cause of pain remains unknown.

The known pathoanatomic causes for low-back pain and sciatica include disk herniation; definite, measurable spinal stenosis; fracture; infection; rheumatic diseases; spondylolisthesis; and other types of clearly demonstrable instability (45). It is also clear from available epidemiological studies (4, 24, 52, 61, 62) that severe psychosocial disturbances, including the abuse of various drugs, should be listed here, especially in the subacute and chronic patients.

For most cases, at least to start with, some minor injury occurs in the intervertebral disk and its immediate surroundings: ligaments, intervertebral joints, or muscles or tendons. The multijointed lumbar spine has an abundance of such structures, most of which (except the disk) are richly innervated (64). The intervertebral disk, however, is the structure that is the subject of most studies despite the fact that it does not contain any free, naked nerve endings. Only the outer part of the annulus fibrosus and the longitudinal ligament contain such pain-carrying nerve endings (64). On the other hand, the integrity of the intervertebral disk plays an important mechanical role for the whole motion segment, in that biochemical or biomechanical disturbances in the disk have consequences for all the other structures in the functional spinal unit.

Looking at the natural history of low-back pain (12), it seems likely from a teleological point of view that most cases of acute low-back pain are caused by small ruptures or swelling of the myotendinous structures. Small injuries such as these, when they occur in other parts of the body, heal quickly without treatment (49, 65), as is the case for most of the patients with low-back pain.

The Importance of Exercise and Fitness for the Structures of the Functional Spinal Unit

There is an abundance of literature on the effect of exercise and fitness on muscles (8, 48, 49) and healing muscles (35, 65). This is dealt with in other chapters of these proceedings, and the reader is also referred to current textbooks on sport injuries. The beneficial effects of motion on tendons and joints are also clear (1, 30, 37, 65). There probably also exists a training effect on collagen maturation and connective tissue strength (55, 59, 65). Early graded motion on an injured part is also of proven benefit for strength and healing (1, 59). The evidence is less clear, however, regarding disks proper, although animal studies (21, 32, 56, 57, 58, 59, 60) have so demonstrated. We exercised nonchondrodystrophic dogs at various intervals and in a variety of ways and found that the nutrition to the disks was enhanced, particularly when the animals were exercised for 30 min per day compared to less exercise or just sitting in the cages (32). More frequent and more violent exercises did not enhance further the nutrition or transport of solutes into or out of the disks. Other studies showed similar results, although there seems to be a genetically determined specific difference in disk metabolism (14, 16, 25, 26). Cellularity also plays a role (40). Even more clear-cut is the evidence regarding immobilization, of which the detrimental effects have been definitely proven for disks (15, 31, 54, 60), joints (39, 59), tendons (1, 65), ligaments (55, 65), and muscles (7, 8, 33). The same is true for bone (8, 28, 29), particularly the spongy substance of the lumbar vertebrae.

Pain

Several other chapters of these proceedings deal with the effects of exercise and fitness on the production of enkephalins and other pain-reducing substances. The interrelationships between psychology and the production of endorphins, as well as the effects of depression and anxiety on endorphins, are also well known (13, 23). Perhaps less well known is that psychology must be taken into consideration when developing treatment programs for patients with low-back pain (23, 38, 41, 61, 62). Behavioral psychologists (22, 23) have used behavioral models to prove that treatment programs aimed at reducing disability by activity are beneficial. Other studies have demonstrated that a reduction of depression also clearly benefits patients with low-back pain (63).

Thus, basic scientific knowledge at least speaks in favor of the benefits of motion for all the tissues that might cause low-back pain; that is, there is some proof that tissues become mechanically stronger when exercised (65), and there is definite evidence that a lack of exercise and fitness (i.e., the result of immobilization) is detrimental (8). This is also true for the intervertebral disk (15, 31).

The minimum amount of motion that is needed to maintain or enhance the strength or healing of the various tissues involved in low-back pain is not known. However, some guidelines can be inferred from animal studies and clinical observations of the relationship between physical fitness and the occurrence of low-back pain.

For disk and cartilage the animal models suggest that about 30 min of running per day is beneficial. More violent or longer time of motion did not result in any improvement (32). Järvinen and Lehto (35) actually demonstrated that extensive running in rabbits resulted in a negative effect on the proteoglycans of their joints.

For the heart, somatic training does not have the same positive effects as does general fitness exercising (50). It seems reasonable that for the disk (which has no direct blood supply) exercises that improve the general circulation are more important than are very strong muscles.

In a prospective study (2) of 3,000 workers, those with the greatest muscular strength had an average number of reported attacks of low-back pain. The back-pain problem of elite gymnasts is also well known (24).

Do Exercise and Fitness Prevent Low-Back Pain?

Epidemiological studies in general have shown a weak correlation among less physical fitness, less activity both at work and during leisure time, and some increase of incidence prevalence and absence due to low-back pain (4, 9, 10, 11, 20, 46, 51, 53, 61). However, this relationship, when sought for as the only factor preventing low-back pain, becomes less clear. In the much-quoted studied by Cady et al. (10, 11) a clear relationship between fitness and reported low-back injury was found over a 10-yr period in a select population of firefighters in Los Angeles. The least-fit group reported 10 times more low-back-pain accidents than did the best-fit group. In a recent report, Deyo and Bass (20) demonstrated a high level of significance for the three combined factors of body weight, smoking, and decreased physical activity for the occurrence of low-back pain. Weaker associations have been found (9, 24, 34, 51, 52).

In a prospective study (2) in which cardiovascular fitness was investigated as a risk factor in industrial back pain, the subjects were workers in a large industry in the northwestern United States; however, we could not substantiate in this blue-collar population a definite relationship between cardiovascular fitness and subsequent reports of low-back pain over a 3-yr period of the 2,400 subjects who completed treadmill testing; 228 reported such back injuries. The study suggests that higher cardiovascular fitness alone does not place workers who perform a wide variety of tasks at less risk of low-back pain. However, cardiovascular fitness in that study, as well as in others (53, 61) related to the response to back injury, demonstrated that those who developed chronic disabling back pain later have a significantly lower fitness to begin with when compared to age- and gender-matched controls.

Thus, there is no absolute evidence that fitness prevents low-back pain. There are, however, several studies that have demonstrated that increased body awareness—gained in programs that promote general health and fitness and that, in cohorts that were followed for various lengths of time, exercise large-muscle groups—decreases absenteeism in general and absenteeism from low-back pain in particular (6, 11, 17, 51). Again, the contrary seems to be more convincing, that is, that low endurance of large-muscle groups, particularly the back extensors, seems to put one at a greater risk to experience long-term back pain within the next year (4, 24, 34, 36).

Treatment

There is little evidence that general fitness exercise plays a major role in the treatment of the patient with acute low-back pain. However, with increasing duration of an attack of low-back pain, some types of activity programs aimed at increased endurance have beneficial effects (3, 5, 12, 23, 37, 43). Immobilization by bed rest for more than 1 or 2 d also seems contraindicated (19).

The benefits of motion and activity can occur at multiple levels. At the tissue level, disks have been demonstrated to improve their nutritional status by motion (32). The general oxygenation process (50) probably plays a part, as does the pumping effect at the disk level per se (58). The pain level governed by endorphins is influenced by exercising large-muscle groups, and the psychological perception of pain can be manipulated by exercises (13, 41, 62).

In a study performed at the Volvo plant in Gothenburg, Sweden, in the 1970s (3), it was demonstrated that information given to a group in the form of a 4-hr back-school program that aimed at activity and return to work resulted in a 1-wk more rapid return when compared to the group that received mostly passive physical therapy, including manipulative treatment. Both these patient groups recovered from the pain as rapidly or significantly more rapidly than did the third, randomized group, which received detuned shortwave diathermia only. Most of the patients in the back-school group returned to work with some pain but also with some knowledge of how to move at the workplace. Perhaps the most interesting finding at the 1-yr follow-up was that there was no significant difference in the rate of recurrence in these three groups. There was a tendency for the back-school group, who returned 1 wk earlier than did the two other groups, to exhibit fewer and also less severe recurrences over the follow-up year. A return to work with some pain but with some knowledge of back pain does not mean that the risk of recurrence in the next year will be higher. This tendency was even more pronounced in a community-based study (12) in which health officers were asked to refer patients who did not recover within 3 wk. Overall in the community, the recurrence rate was again about 50%. In the group subjected to information and activity, the recurrence rate was only one third of that.

In another randomized study at the Volvo plant in Gothenburg (recently concluded but not yet published), we have been able to demonstrate a highly significant reduction in low-back disability when 50 subjects suffering from idiopathic low-back pain of 9-wk duration were activated to perform increasing exercises per quota according to Fordyce et al. (22, 23). The comparison was made to a control group of equal size who did not receive any particular treatment but who were allowed to continue treatment with their general practitioners or industrial health officers after the first thorough investigation and randomization. The screening, performed by an orthopedic surgeon, served to eliminate those patients from the study who exhibited signs of definite pathology, including not only back-related diseases but also obvious medical diseases such as obstructive emphysema, recent myocardiac infarction, and substance abuse. Again in acute and subacute patients Fordyce et al. (22) demonstrated that a behavioral approach to activity gives good results and less recurrence over the subsequent years.

Even in the most deconditioned patients who have demonstrable deficits in strength, endurance, and fitness, goal-oriented activity using group and behavioral psychology methods have demonstrated an astonishingly rapid return of these parameters as well as a high percentage of returns to work (41, 42). Actually, the recovery was far more rapid than was thought possible from other studies of injured individuals. This clearly points to the psychological role of deconditioning the patient with chronic low-back pain (23, 27, 62).

Biomechanically, we know which limits to set for exercise programs for patients with low-back pain (43, 45). In the beginning any vigorous muscular activities that are combined with large motions of the spine should be avoided, particularly in the upright positions. Isometric training and probably also limited eccentric muscle training should be used for leg, back, and abdominal muscles (4, 5, 12, 34, 36, 46, 49). The principal aim should be to increase the endurance of both large and small back muscles.

Backstroke swimming or pedaling in the water, bicycling, brisk walking, stair climbing (33), and jogging are exercises that I most commonly recommend. Whatever exercise the patient can perform he or she must increase at regular intervals. The physician, not the patient, dictates this increase, and the patient should be assured that even if he or she experiences some pain it is not dangerous. Such advice necessitates a thorough clinical examination to exclude contraindicated diseases, of which there are very few.

It is extremely important that, as has been demonstrated (22, 23), the physician or the physiotherapist take charge in prescribing the exercise program; that is, the patients must exercise by an increasing amount every day and should keep a record of this in a logbook that is checked every week. Continuous positive reinforcement is of paramount importance, and pain behavior (23, 62) should not be attended to.

The success of such activity programs in randomized studies for acute, subacute, and chronic patients clearly speaks in favor of the fact that exercise and fitness are likely the most important factors in the overall treatment of patients with low-back pain. In studies in which endurance, strength, and fitness have been measured, the respective increases in these factors mirror the recovery from low-back pain.

Conclusion

When all our present knowledge is viewed with some perspective, it seems suggestive that although physical fitness does not in itself prevent low-back pain, a general healthy lifestyle that includes moderate motion and exercise of the lumbar spine combined with reduction in smoking may have some preventive effects. However, it is also clear that so-called wellness programs (6, 11, 17, 18) must include organizational changes at the workplace to reduce monotony and increase worker satisfaction by other means, some of them still unknown, to obtain a significant reduction of the now epidemiologically increasing absenteeism due to low-back pain.

For those patients struck by acute attacks of low-back pain, it has also been shown in some studies (19, 44) that as little immobilization as possible is beneficial. Basic scientific experiments also underline this clinical observation. Very little proof exists of any beneficial effects of most of the many treatment modalities that otherwise exist for these patients (46). Information programs containing facts on how to move and how to exercise have demonstrated benefits in randomized and case control series of patients (3, 12, 22).

For those with 3 wk of back pain, repeat information seems to be of value (12), and in the patients with subchronic low-back pain our randomized Gothenburg study (unpublished) demonstrated clear-cut benefits from activity that was mirrored also by increased strength and fitness. The most severely deconditioned patient in the series of studies by Mayer et al. (41) also clearly benefited from increased fitness, endurance, and improved coordination. Actually, the improvement was so rapid that a psychological reduction of the activity in the strength and endurance tests performed at the beginning of such sessions must have existed; otherwise, it would be impossible, from our present knowledge of muscle physiology and training effects (35, 37, 49, 50), to account for the large increases in muscle strength that occurred, that is, a three- to fourfold increase in weight-lifting capacity within a 3-wk training program.

This last observation points to another factor that was dealt with only in the introduction to these proceedings and that will help to solve the problem of low-back pain. Fitness and exercise programs alone will not give a global solution to this problem. A cohesive effort by physicians, politicians, and employers is necessary to solve the most expensive medical problem of modern industrialized societies.

We have accepted that health, according to the World Health Organization, has more dimensions rather than only the somatic one. Health is not only the absence of sickness and handicap but also a state of complete physical, psychological, and social well-being. It is quite clear from our present knowledge that this is definitely true with regard also to low-back pain and its prevention and treatment.

References

1. Akeson, W.H., D. Amiel, M.F. Abel, S.R. Garfin, and S. L-Y. Woo. Effects of immobilization on joints. *Clin. Orthop.* 219: 28-37, 1987.

2. Batti'e, M.C., S.J. Bigos, L.D. Fisher, A.L. Nachemson, T.H. Hansson, D.M. Spengler, M.D. Wortley, and J. Zeh. Cardiovascular fitness as a risk factor in industrial back pain. (Unpublished manuscript.)

3. Bergquist-Ullman, M., and U. Larsson. Acute low back pain in industry: A controlled prospective study with special reference to therapy and confounding factors. *Acta Orthop. Scand.* 170: 1-117, 1977.

4. Biering-Sorenson, F. Physical measurements as risk indicators for low-back trouble over a one-year period. *Spine* 9: 106-119, 1984.

5. Bigos, S.J., and M.C. Batti'e. Acute care to prevent back disability: Ten years of progress. *Clin. Orthop.* 221: 121-130, 1987.

6. Blair, S.N., P.V. Oiserchia, C.S. Wilbur, and J.H. Crowder. A public health intervention model for work-site health promotion: Impact on exercise and physical fitness in a health promotion plan after 24 months. *JAMA* 255: 921-926, 1986.

7. Booth, F.W. Physiologic and biochemical effects of immobilization on muscle. *Clin. Orthop.* 219: 15-20, 1987.

8. Bortz, W.M. The disuse syndrome. *West. J. Med.* 141: 691-694, 1984.

9. Brennan, G.P., R.O. Ruhling, R.S. Hood, B.B. Schultz, S.C. Johnson, and B.C. Andrews. Physical characteristics of patients with herniated lumbar discs. *Spine* 12: 699-702, 1987.

10. Cady, L.D., D.P. Bischoff, E.R. O'Connell, P.C. Thomas, and J.H. Allan. Strength and fitness and subsequent back injuries in firefighters. *J. Occup. Med.* 4: 269-272, 1979.

11. Cady, L.D., P.C. Thomas, and R.J. Karwasky. Program for increasing health and physical fitness of firefighters. *J. Occup. Med.* 2: 111-114, 1985.

12. Chöler, U., R. Larsson, A. Nachemson, and L.-E. Peterson. Ont i ryggen. *Spri-rapport* 188: Stockholm, 1985.

13. Clark, W.C., J.C. Yang, and M.N. Janal. Altered pain and visual sensitivity in humans: The effects of acute and chronic stress. *Ann. N.Y. Acad. Sci.* 467: 116-129, 1986.

14. Cole, T.-C., P. Ghosh, N.J. Hannan, T.K.F. Taylor, and C.R. Bellenger. The response of the canine intervertebral disc to immobilization produced by spinal arthrodesis is dependent on constitutional factors. *J. Orthop. Res.* 5: 337-347, 1987.

15. Cole, T.-C., D. Burkhardt, P. Ghosh, M. Ryan, and T. Taylor. Effects of spinal fusion on the proteoglycans of the canine intervertebral disc. *J. Orthop. Res.* 3: 277-291, 1985.

16. Cole, T.-C., P. Ghosh, and T. Taylor. Variations of the proteoglycans of the canine intervertebral disc with ageing. *Biochim. Biophys. Acta* 880: 209-219, 1986.

17. Cox, M., R.J. Shephard, and P. Corey. Influence of an employee fitness programme upon fitness, productivity and absenteeism. *Ergonomics* 24: 795-806, 1981.

18. Cox, M., R.J. Shephard, and P. Corey. Absenteeism, fitness and worker satisfaction [Abstract]. *Can. J. Appl. Sports Sci.* 8: 227, 1983.

19. Deyo, R.A., et al. How many days bed rest for acute low back pain? A randomized clinical trial. *N. Engl. J. Med.* 215: 10-64, 1986.

20. Deyo, R.A., and J.E. Bass. Lifestyle and low back pain: The influence of smoking, exercise and obesity. *Clin. Res.* 35: 577A, 1987. In: Proceeding at the Annual Scientific Meeting of the American Rheumatism Association, Washington, DC, June 1987.

21. Evans, W., W. Jobe, and C. Seiberg. *A cross-sectional prevalence study of lumbar disc degeneration in a working population.* Manuscript submitted for publication, 1988.

22. Fordyce, W.E., J.A. Brockway, J.A. Bergman, and D. Spengler. Acute back pain: A control-group comparison of behavioral vs. traditional management methods. *J. Behav. Med.* 9: 127-140, 1986.

23. Fordyce, W.E., A.H. Roberts, and R.A. Sternbach. The behavioral management of chronic pain: A response to critics. *Pain* 22: 113-125, 1985.

24. Frymoyer, J.W., and W. Cats-Baril. Predictors of low back pain disability. *Clin. Orthop.* 221: 89-98, 1987.

25. Ghosh, P., T.K.F. Taylor, and K.G. Braund. Variation of the glycosaminoglycans of the canine intervertebral disc with ageing: I. Chondrodystrophoid breed. *Gerontology* 23: 87-98, 1977.

26. Ghosh, P., T.K.F. Taylor, and K.G. Braund. Variation of the glycosaminoglycans of the canine intervertebral disc with ageing: II. Non-chondrodystrophoid breed. *Gerontology* 23: 99-109, 1977.

27. Hadler, N.M. Regional musculoskeletal diseases of the low back cumulative trauma versus single incident. *Clin. Orthop.* 221: 33-41, 1987.

28. Hansson, T., B. Roos, and A. Nachemson. Development of osteopenia in the fourth lumbar vertebra during prolonged bed rest after operation for scoliosis. *Acta Orthop. Scand.* 46: 621-630, 1975.

29. Hansson, T., J. Sandström, B. Roos, R. Jonson, and G. Andersson. The bone mineral content of the lumbar spine in patients with chronic low back pain. *Spine* 2: 158-160, 1985.

30. Hitchcock, T.F., T.R. Light, W.H. Bunch, et al. The effect of immediate controlled mobilization on the strength of flexor tendon repairs. In: Goldberg, V.M., ed. *Proceedings of 32nd Annual Orthopaedic Research Society.* Chicago: Adept, 1986, p. 216.

31. Holm, S., and A. Nachemson. Nutritional changes in the canine intervertebral disc after spinal fusion. *Clin. Orthop.* 169: 234-258, 1982.

32. Holm, S., and A. Nachemson. Variations in the nutrition of the canine intervertebral disc induced by motion. *Spine* 8: 866-874, 1983.

33. Ilmarinen, J., R. Ilmarinen, A. Koskela, O. Korhonen, P. Fardy, T. Partanen, and J. Rutenfranz. Training effects of stair-climbing during office hours on female employees. *Ergonomics* 22: 507-516, 1979.

34. Jackson, C.P., and M.D. Brown. Is there a role for exercise in the treatment of low back pain patients? *Clin. Orthop.* 179: 39-45, 1983.

35. Järvinen, M.J., and M.U.K. Lehto. Biological background of the treatment of muscle injuries. A review with special reference to the effects of early mobilization or immobilization on the healing process. *Acta Othop. Scand.* (in press).

36. Kahanovitz, N., M. Nordin, R. Verderame, S. Yabut, M. Parnianpour, K. Viola, and M. Mulvihill. Normal trunk muscle strength and endurance in women and the effect of exercises and electrical stimulation and exercises to increase trunk muscle strength and endurance. *Spine* 12: 112-118, 1987.

37. Komi, P.V. Neuromuscular biomechanics: Selective correlates between structure and function. In: Maehlum, S., S. Nilsson, and P. Renström, eds. *An update on sports medicine: Proceedings of the Second Scandinavian Conference in Sports Medicine.* Syntex, Norway: 1987, p. 60-78.

38. Linton, S.J. The relationship between activity and chronic pain. *Pain* 21: 289-294, 1985.

39. Langenskiold, A., J.-E. Michelsson, and T. Videman. Osteoarthritis of the knee in the rabbit produced by immobilization: Attempts to achieve a reproducible model for studies on pathogenesis and therapy. *Acta Orthop. Scand.* 50: 1-14, 1979.

40. Maroudas, A., R.A. Stockwell, A. Nachemson, and J. Urban. Factors involved in the nutrition of the human lumbar intervertebral disc: Cellularity and diffusion of glucose in-vitro. *J. Anat.* 120: 113-130, 1975.

41. Mayer, G., R.J. Gatchel, N. Kishino, J. Keeley, P. Capra, H. Mayer, J. Barnett, and V. Mooney. Objective assessment of spine function following industrial injury. A prospective study with comparison group and one-year follow-up. *Spine* 10: 482-493, 1985.

42. Mayer, T.G. Assessment of lumbar function. *Clin. Orthop.* 221: 99-109, 1987.

43. Nachemson, A. Work for all. For those with low back pain as well. *Clin. Orthop.* 179: 77-83, 1983.

44. Nachemson, A. Recent advances in the treatment of low back pain. Current trend lecture: SICOT, London 1984. *Int. Orthop.* (SICOT) 9: 1-10, 1985.

45. Nachemson, A., and S.J. Bigos. The low back. In: Cruess, R.L., and W.R.J. Rennie, eds. *Adult orthopaedics.* New York: Churchill Livingstone, 1984, vol. 2, Chapt. 16, p. 843-937.

46. Nachemson, A., W.O. Spitzer, et al. Scientific approaches to the assessment and management of activity-related spinal disorders. A monograph for clinicians. Report of the Quebec Task Force on Spinal Disorders. *Spine* 12(75, Suppl. 1): S1-S59, 1987.

47. Nettelbladt, E. Antalet reumatikerinvalider i Sverige under en 30-årsperiod. *OPMEAR* 30: 54-56, 1985.

48. Radin, E.L. Role of muscles in protecting athletes from injury. *Acta Med. Scand.* 220 (Suppl. 711): 143-147, 1986.

49. Renström, P., and R.J. Johnsson. Overuse injuries—A great problem in sports. In: Maehlum, S, S. Nilsson, and P. Renström, eds. *An update on sports medicine: Proceedings of the Second Scandinavian Conference in Sports Medicine.* Syntex, Norway: 1987, p. 169-190.

50. Saltin, B. The physiological and biochemical basis of aerobic and anaerobic capacities in man: Effect of training and range of adapta-tion. In: Maehlum, S., S. Nilsson, and P. Renström, eds. *An update on sports medicine: Proceedings of the Second Scandinavian Conference in Sports Medicine.* Syntex, Norway: 1987, p. 16-60.

51. Saraste, H., and G. Hultman. Life conditions of persons without low-back pain. *Scand. J. Rehabil. Med.* 19: 109-115, 1986.

52. Svensson, H.-O. Low back pain in forty- to forty-seven-year-old men: A retrospective cross-sectional study [Thesis]. Göteborg, Sweden: 1981.

53. Svensson, O.H., A. Vedin, C. Wilhelmsson, and G.B.J. Andersson. Low-back pain in relation to other diseases and cardiovascular risk factors. *Spine* 8: 277-285, 1983.

54. Taylor, T.K.F., P. Ghosh, K.G. Braund, J.M. Sutherland, and A.A. Sherwood. The effect of spinal fusion on intervertebral disc composition: An experimental study. *J. Surg. Res.* 21: 91-104, 1976.

55. Tipton, C.M., A.C. Vailas, and R.D. Matthes. Experimental studies on the influences of physical activity on ligaments, tendons and joints: A brief review. *Acta Med. Scand.* 220 (Suppl. 711): 157-168, 1986.

56. Urban, J.P.G., S. Holm, A. Maroudas, and A. Nachemson. Nutrition of the intervertebral disk—An in-vivo study of solute transport. *Clin. Orthop.* 129: 101-114, 1977.

57. Urban, J.P.G., S. Holm, A. Maroudas, and A. Nachemson. Nutrition of the intervertebral disc. Effect of fluid flow on solute transport. *Clin. Orthop.* 170: 296-302, 1982.

58. Urban, J., and A. Maroudas. The chemistry of the intervertebral disc in relation to its physiological function and requirements. *Clin. Rheum. Dis.* 6: 51-76, 1980.

59. Videman, T. Connective tissue and immobilization: Key factors in musculoskeletal degeneration? *Clin. Orthop.* 221: 26-32, 1987.

60. Vuorinen, J., and P. Rokkanen. The effect of immobilization of the spine of rats. *Acta Orthop. Scand.* 58: 458, 1987.

61. Vällfors, B. Acute, subacute and chronic low back pain. *Scand. J. Rehabil. Med.* 11 (Suppl.): 1-98, 1985.

62. Waddell, G. A new clinical model for the treatment of low back pain. *Spine* 12: 632-644, 1987.

63. Ward, N.G. Tricyclic antidepressants for chronic low-back pain: Mechanisms of action and predictors of response. *Spine* 11: 661-665, 1986.

64. Wyke, B. The neurology of low back pain. In: Jayson, M.I.V., ed. *The lumbar spine and back pain*. London: Churchill Livingstone, 1987, 3rd ed., p. 56-99.

65. Woo, S. L-Y., and J.A. Buckwalter. Injury and repair of the musculoskeletal soft tissue. Paper presented at the American Academy of Orthopedic Surgeons Symposium, Park Ridge, IL, June 1988.

Chapter 46

Discussion: Exercise, Fitness, and Back Pain

Tom G. Mayer

It is a pleasure to discuss the well-organized and thorough review presented by Dr. Nachemson for this segment of the International Conference on Exercise, Fitness, and Health. His summary of the cost, epidemiology, natural history, and basic science of the problem is excellent. It clearly supports the hypothesis that exercise is necessary for the nutritional support of the structures involved in dysfunction associated with low-back pain. Moreover, it supports the view that exercise may lead to both local and systemic fitness and encourage the health of the tissues and of the whole person. It provides weak evidence for a role of exercise or fitness in preventing back incidents but suggests that those who are least fit will have the more serious, chronically disabling incidents.

Dr. Nachemson's review also cites studies showing the interrelationship between physiological and psychological aspects of disability and highlights those showing rapid restoration of function in chronically disabled patients. These rapid changes can be explained only if one considers that the initial deficits are based as much on psychological (motivational and effort) factors as on physiological ones. There can be no argument with the data summarized from the literature, or the conclusions drawn.

Although Dr. Nachemson focused to a great extent on acute and subacute problems (as well as on research efforts to find predictors of low-back outcome to provide greater prevention capabilities to industry), I will shift the emphasis somewhat to the more chronic patient. This situation has not been ignored in Dr. Nachemson's work but has received less attention than might be provided here. In the dismal statistics of the human and financial costs of low-back pain, it is clear that there is a large discrepancy between median and mean costs. This is related to the fact that, in our life-

times, almost all of us will have back incidents at some time but that most of us will resolve them in a very short time. In fact, more than 90% of disabling back pain has resulted in a return to productivity within 3 mo almost regardless of the mode of treatment applied. Many investigators have attempted to demonstrate the efficacy of one treatment modality over another for acute and subacute back pain (6), but the healing of soft tissues is generally so rapid that effects of treatment cannot be distinguished from spontaneous recovery in most cases. However, when one considers the cost of the small group of patients remaining, most of the cost is associated with this group. About 10% of the patient population ends up costing 80% of the dollars in the American system, and this group accounts for most of the disability and loss of productivity that affects society as a whole through a variety of social disability payment systems and the loss of worker skills. There is also a psychosocial multiplier effect, in that a patient's social withdrawal and litigation set an example for families, friends, and co-workers that tends to cluster such cases of long-term disability.

With the foregoing in mind, I will discuss the special considerations inherent in developing exercise, fitness, and healthy minds and bodies in this group of individuals.

Functional Capacity Measurement in the Spine: Luxury or Necessity?

In his review, Dr. Nachemson indicated that in the Volvo study those individuals who produced the greatest isometric lifting capacity (to be distinguished from greatest muscular strength) have more than the average number of attacks of low-back pain. In addition, he cited the high prevalence of low-back incidents in elite gymnasts (7) and concluded that both of the studies indicate that too much strength and motion thus probably is as detrimental as too little. This conclusion, one of the few in the review with which I disagree, is indicative of the great problem confronting both the scientist and the clinician in low-back research today: the absence of visual feedback to the small structures of the spine (as Dr. Nachemson has described). The absence of this feedback produces several quandries for the observer. The first problem is that it prevents the scientist from making simple judgments on low-back fitness by observation or palpation. For example, the anorexic female ballerina with a normal or hypermobile spine may have her deficient trunk strength go unrecognized as a possible source of her episodic low-back pain.

Absence of routine monitoring potentially prevents regular comparison of physical performance capability against work demands. This assessment deficiency potentially prevents recognition of an imbalance between trunk strength and work demands in the elite gymnast. The appropriate conclusion might be that high injury rates are related to such an imbalance, not that they are too strong. Until we have a systematized method for describing physical capacity in the spine, we will probably continue to have disputed conclusions drawn from the same data.

A second problem in this area is the failure to recognize the relevance of the various measures of physical capacity to the specific element of fitness being measured. For example, an isometric test is static, measuring strength in only one body position that may be very different from usual work position. In fact, the question of relevance has been raised as to whether any static test can adequately describe a dynamic process. Because the body consists of multiple biomechanical links, or functional units, the functional spinal unit may be held in a fixed static posture even in a dynamic total body motion such as lifting. Lifting is a compound movement in which lower extremity squatting and upper extremity reaching can substitute for back motion and positioning. Thus a worker with a weak link in the spinal functional unit might well be able to continue to lift to high capacity even when isolated trunk-strength testing shows a severe deficit of extensor strength.

A third problem is that the absence of visual feedback can prevent us from recognizing imprecision and validity defects of many of our common tests of fitness. An excellent example is the use of the Schober technique for measuring spinal range

of motion. Although this is the oldest available measurement technique for lumbar spine flexion, it suffers from multiple drawbacks that make it an invalid test for measuring range of motion. Some problems of validity with this test include the following: (a) There is a lack of standardized anatomic surface landmarks for test performance, and up to 50% of cohorts have either no landmarks or landmarks so large that they distort the test. (b) There is intersubject variance in the number of segments measured from T12 to S1 of as much as three of six segments. The variation is based on differences in subject height and surface landmarks (i.e., an examiner may be measuring motion only from L3 to S1, believing that he or she is measuring from T12 to S1). (c) There is a commonly noted lengthening of the 5-cm distance below S2 (the usual level of the landmarks), where no skeletal motion could possibly be occurring (4). Because the Schober test was assumed to be valid (32) merely because it was reproducible (these are not synonymous concepts), conclusions drawn by many investigators about the importance (or lack of it) of range-of-motion measurements are highly suspect.

As Dr. Nachemson noted in reporting on several studies of patients with chronic back pain (21, 22, 23, 24), the patients made such rapid progress in physical capacity as to surpass any known physiological phenomenon. In fact, new data presented by our group (14) demonstrated that with better education, counseling, and training there have been even more dramatic improvements in physical capacity on both entry and discharge from the comprehensive portion of the PRIDE treatment program. In fact, patients entering this treatment program currently show mean physical capacity scores on standardized tests now nearly as high as the scores of the individuals being discharged from the program in our earlier studies (21, 22). Even more astonishing is the fact that physical capacity means for the more recent group now being discharged approximate those of normal subjects. In other words, chronically disabled patients may show extremely rapid improvement in physical capacity measurements (over a 2- to 3-mo period) with vigorous, progressive-resistive exercise even after prolonged deconditioning and detraining.

As Dr. Nachemson pointed out, we should not lose sight of the fact that the extremely low physical capacity measures noted on initial testing in both the early and the recent groups are generally due to problems of *effort* and *motivation*. These are based primarily on pain, fear of injury, previous education encouraging inactivity, and psychosocial factors (e.g., depression). The motivation problem points up the third most important factor in physical capacity measurement; that is, an *effort factor* must be present to validate a standardized test. Such factors may or may not be associated with all tests, so test usefulness must also be evaluated on this basis. There are many situations (such as disability and impairment evaluation) in which patients will receive greater economic benefit if they can demonstrate *poor* work capacity. If socioeconomic disincentives can lead the clinician to misinterpret a test in impairment evaluation, work capacity evaluation, or certain worker selection situations, then the test is misleading and encourages conscious cheating by the subject.

Finally, if a test meets all the foregoing criteria—including validity and reproducibility, relevance, and presence of an effort factor—there is still the need for a normative data base. Because we cannot provide intraindividual comparisons as we can with the extremities, population norms similar to those for internal organs (such as pulse and blood pressure monitoring for cardiovascular function) must be developed. Of course, the development of a normative data base implies reaching a consensus on the methods and devices that should be used for measuring elements of fitness. Such a consensus remains unavailable, probably because of the lack of familiarity of most musculoskeletal clinicians and researchers with the need for, and evaluation of, indirect performance measures. In fact, most of the musculoskeletal system not only is amenable to visual inspection but also demonstrates bilateral comparability. As a consequence, most musculoskeletal scientists have not dealt with the unique problems imposed by inaccessible, nonvisualizable axial structures of the spine. I believe that one of our major goals over the next 10 yr should be to produce a consensus on measurement techniques for use in normal and clinical patient studies. These techniques must show sufficient sensitivity and specificity to provide data that will result in valid conclusions. Until such a consensus is reached, dubious conclusions will continue to emerge.

Current Methods of Assessing Spinal Fitness

Range of Motion

The only system of measuring range of motion that satisfies the foregoing criteria is inclinometry. Al-

though more cumbersome to use than the simple goniometer, the inclinometer is able to measure compound, as opposed to simple, joint motion. When the spine moves, particularly in the sagittal plane, causal structures also move. Traditionally, we assume that the motion occurs on a stable base. Inclinometry permits measurement of motion at both the superior and the inferior extent of the motion segment to be isolated, separating out the true lumbar motion component from the hip-motion component in the lumbar spine (11, 17, 25, 26, 27). The technique has been shown to be consistent with radiographic measurements and is reproducible (30, 31, 32, 40). Effort is documented by the comparison between straight leg raising and the hip-flexion component. Inferences can be drawn about spinal pathology from abnormal true lumbar motion in the presence of normal hip mobility. As discussed previously, other modes of measurement, such as the Schober method (33) and the simple goniometric technique (1), lack validity and the capability of assessing effort. In contrast, other valid techniques may be cumbersome or impractical for general clinical usage.

Isolated Trunk Strength and Endurance

Isokinetic measurement techniques have been utilized for clinical trunk-strength measurements for some time. Many pioneers have created innovative laboratory models of trunk-strength devices to test normal subjects and patients (5, 8, 16, 39). Commercial models have been utilized only recently (15, 23, 34, 38). Currently, at least four manufacturers make equipment that measures isokinetic trunk strength, all using different dynamometers, stabilization methods, positions, and speeds. It is not yet apparent that all the measuring dynamometers are equally accurate. It is certainly unlikely that normative data (or test data) from one machine will be subject to mathematical manipulation that would permit the use of the data on another device. Effort assessment is performed by comparing curve-consistency measurements, but accuracy of this method has been assumed by the manufacturers with only preliminary evidence (9). The sagittal plane testers examine strength in the ventral and dorsal strap muscles, whereas the rotation device measures primarily oblique muscle function.

Aerobic Capacity

This area of interest is being discussed extensively in other chapters of these proceedings. Aerobic detraining through prolonged inactivity is common and requires cardiovascular reconditioning. Low cardiovascular performance has an effect on muscular performance by decreasing the flow of nutrients and oxygen to, and removal of metabolites from, the predominantly slow-twitch paraspinal musculature.

Lifting Capacity

Competing lifting measures have been described frequently in the literature. There is much debate concerning the usefulness of isometric (2, 3, 12), isoinertial and psychophysical (19, 21, 35, 41), and isokinetic lifting (13) tests in clinical use. It is possible that no system alone may be sufficient for measuring this compound total body activity in a relevant manner. Recent work by our group suggests a poor correlation between lifting progression on isoinertial and isokinetic methodologies (20). This should not be entirely surprising because isokinetics control velocity and acceleration, both customarily used by a trained lifter. Such techniques would be unconstrained in an isoinertial lift. Lifting capacity is not the same as isolated strength testing, which measures the strength of an individual spinal functional unit. By contrast, lifting is a total body compound activity involving the interaction of multiple functional units. In this compound activity, one link of the biomechanical chain may substitute for another and thus produce different styles of lifting that make interindividual comparisons difficult. Therefore, the testing of lift strength is inadequate as a measure of trunk strength without the addition of isolated trunk-strength measurements.

Other Parameters

Other parameters of performance require measurement. Isolated trunk-strength devices have endurance protocols built into them that purport to provide a mechanical endurance test, the usefulness of which has not yet been proven. The use of a Roman chair as an endurance test has been described by Kahanovitz et al. (10). There has also been recent enthusiasm for myoelectric signal power spectrum analysis for fatigue measurements (28, 37). However, our group and others have found that this technique has very low sensitivity and specificity in discriminating endurance capacity among individuals, even in highly motivated, healthy subjects (15, 18, 36). At this point, endurance or fatigue-resistance testing is still awaiting a valid measurement technique.

Such performance elements as agility and coordination are also still awaiting a measurement technique for the low-back area. Other multiunit tasks (e.g., climbing, bending, twisting, etc.) require objective tests for identifying rehabilitation progress and work capacity. Yet without indirect objective assessment and (for the axial skeleton) in the absence of direct visual feedback, progress in correlating low-back pain to exercise, fitness, and health is unlikely to materialize. Measuring all elements of performance is, of course, a formidable task. For this reason—and because of the many measures yet to be devised and the associated sorting-out process that will be needed to find those of most significance—it will be some time before the issues of measurement are resolved.

Finally, more research is needed in the area of psychosocial assessment. Of course, psychosocial evaluation instruments have the disadvantage of relying on patient self-reports. However, as Dr. Nachemson and I agree that psychosocial aspects of low-back dysfunction generate the greatest cost, the simultaneous measurement of psychosocial and socioeconomic factors in conjunction with physical ones is of utmost importance.

References

1. *American Medical Association guide to the evaluation of permanent impairment*. Chicago: AMA, 1983.
2. Caldwell, L., D. Chaffin, F. Dukes-Dobos, K. Kroemer, L. Laubach, S. Snook, and D. Wasserman. A proposed standard procedure for static muscle strength testing. *Am. Ind. Hyg. Assoc. J.* 35: 201-206, 1974.
3. Chaffin, D., and G. Andersson. *Occupational biomechanics*. New York: John Wiley & Sons, 1984.
4. Cox, R., J. Keeley, D. Barnes, R. Gatchel, and T. Mayer. *Effects of functional restoration treatment upon Waddell impairment/disability ratings in chronic low back pain patients*. Paper presented at Transactions of the International Society for the Study of the Lumbar Spine. Miami, FL, April 1988
5. Davies, G., and J. Gould. Trunk testing using a prototype Cybex II isokinetic stabilization system. *J. Orthop. Sports Phys. Ther.* 3: 164-170, 1982.

6. Deyo, R. Conservative therapy for low back pain: Distinguishing useful from useless therapy. *JAMA* 250: 1057-1062, 1983.

7. Frymoyer, J., and W. Cats-Baril. Predictors of low back pain disability. *Clin. Orthop.* 221: 89-98, 1987.

8. Hasue, M., M. Fujuwara, and S. Kikuchi. A new method of quantitative measurement of abdominal back muscle strength. *Spine* 5: 143-148, 1980.

9. Hazard, R., S. Fenwick, V. Reeves, and B. Reid. Isokinetic trunk and lifting strength measurements: Variability as a predictor of effort. *Spine* (in press).

10. Kahanovitz, N., M. Nordin, S. Verderame, M. Yabut, R. Parnianpour, K. Viola, and M. Mulvihill. Normal trunk muscle strength and endurance in women and the effect of exercises and electrical stimulation and exercises to increase trunk muscle strength and endurance. *Spine* 12: 112-118, 1987.

11. Keeley, J., T. Mayer, R. Cox, R. Gatchel, J. Smith, and V. Mooney. Quantification of lumbar function 5: Reliability of range-of-motion measures in the sagittal plane and *in vivo* torso rotation measurement techniques. *Spine* 11: 31-35, 1986.

12. Keyserling, W., G. Herrin, and D. Chaffin. Isometric strength testing as a means of controlling medical incidents on strenuous jobs. *J. Occup. Med.* 22: 332-336, 1980.

13. Kishino, N., T. Mayer, R. Gatchel, M. Parrish, C. Anderson, L. Gustin, and V. Mooney. Quantification of lumbar function 4: Isometric and isokinetic stimulation in control subjects and low back pain patients. *Spine* 10: 921-927, 1985.

14. Kohles, S., D. Barnes, R. Gatchel, and T. Mayer. *Improved functional restoration of industrially injury CLBP patients.* Paper presented at Transactions of the International Society for the Study of the Lumbar Spine. Miami, FL, April 1988.

15. Kondraske, G., S. Deivanayagam, T. Carmichael, T. Mayer, and V. Mooney. Myoelectric spectral analysis and strategies for quantifying trunk muscular fatigue. *Arch. Phys. Med. Rehabil.* 68: 103-110, 1987.

16. Langrana, N., C. Lee, and H. Alexander. Quantitative assessment of back strength using isokinetic testing. *Spine* 9: 287-290, 1984.

17. Loebl, W. Measurements of spinal posture and range in spine movements. *Ann. Phys. Med.* 9: 103, 1967.

18. Matthusse, P., K. Hendrich, W. Runsburger, R. Woittiez, and P. Huung. Ankle angle effects on endurance time, median frequency and mean power of gastrocnemius EMG power spectrum: A comparison between individual and group analysis. *Ergonomics* 30: 1149-1159, 1987.

19. Mayer, T., D. Barnes, N. Kishino, G. Nichols, R. Gatchel, H. Mayer, and V. Mooney. Progressive isoinertial lifting evaluation: I. A standardized protocol and normative database. *Spine* (in press).

20. Mayer, T., D. Barnes, G. Nichols, N. Kishino, K. Coval, B. Piel, D. Hoshino, and R. Gatchel. Progressive isoinertial lifting evaluation. II: A comparison with isokinetic lifting in a disabled chronic low back pain industrial population. *Spine* (in press).

21. Mayer, T., R. Gatchel, N. Kishino, J. Keeley, P. Capra, H. Mayer, J. Barnett, and V. Mooney. Objective assessment of spine function following industrial accident: A prospective study with comparison group and one-year follow-up (1985 Volvo Award in Clinical Sciences). *Spine* 10: 482-493, 1985.

22. Mayer, T., R. Gatchel, H. Mayer, N. Kishino, J. Keeley, and V. Mooney. A prospective two-year study of functional restoration in industrial low back injury: An objective assessment procedure. *JAMA* 258: 1763-1767, 1987.

23. Mayer, T., S. Smith, J. Keeley, and V. Mooney. Quantification of lumbar function 2: Sagittal plane trunk strength in trunk strength in chronic low back pain patients. *Spine* 10: 765-772, 1985.

24. Mayer, T., S. Smith, G. Kondraske, R. Gatchel, T. Carmichael, and V. Mooney. Quantification of lumbar function 3: Isokinetic torso rotation testing data in normal and pathological subjects and comparison with other isokinetic strength tests. *Spine* 10: 912-920, 1985.

25. Mayer, T., A. Tencer, S. Kristoferson, and V. Mooney. Use of noninvasive techniques for quantification of sagittal range-of-motion in normal subjects and chronic low back dysfunction patients. *Spine* 9: 588-595, 1984.

26. McRae, I., and V. Wright. Measurement of back movement. *Ann. Rheum. Dis.* 28: 584, 1969.

27. Moll, J., and V. Wright. In: Jayson, M., ed. *Measurements of spinal movement in the lumbar spine and low back pain.* New York: Grune & Stratton, 1976, p. 93-112.

28. Moritani, T., M. Muro, A. Kijiama, F. Gaffney, and D. Parsons. Electromechanical changes during electrically induced and maximal voluntary contractions: Surface and intramuscular EMG responses during sustained maximal voluntary contraction. *Exp. Neurol.* 88: 484-499, 1985.

29. Nachemson, A., and M. Lindh. Measurement of abdominal and back muscle strength with and without low back pain. *Scand. J. Rehabil. Med.* 1: 60-65, 1969.

30. Pearcy, M., I. Portek, and J. Sheperd. The effect of low back pain on lumbar spine movements measured by three-dimensional X-ray analysis. *Spine* 10: 150-153, 1985.

31. Pearcy, M., and J. Sheperd. Is there instability in spondylolisthesis? *Spine* 10: 175-177, 1985.

32. Reynolds, P. Measurement of spinal mobility: A comparison of three methods. *Rheum. Rehabil.* 14: 180-185, 1975.

33. Schober, P. Lendenwirbelsaule und Kreuzschmerzen. *Munch. Med. Wschr.* 84: 336, 1937.

34. Smith, S., T. Mayer, R. Gatchel, and T. Becker. Quantification of lumbar function 1: Isometric and multispeed isokinetic trunk strength measures in sagittal and axial planes in normal subjects. *Spine* 10: 757-764, 1985.

35. Snook, S., and C. Irvine. Maximum acceptable weight of lift. *J. Amer. Ind. Hyg.* 9: 322-329, 1967.

36. Standridge, R., G. Kondraske, V. Mooney, T. Mayer, and T. Carmichael. Temporal characterization of myoelectrical spectral moment changes: Analysis of common measures. *IEEE Trans. Biomed. Eng.* (in press).

37. Stulen, F., and C. DeLuca. Frequency parameters of the myoelectrical signal as a measure of muscle conduction velocity. *IEEE Trans. Biomed. Eng.* 28: 513-523, 1981.

38. Thompson, N., J. Gould, G. Davies, D. Ross, and S. Price. Descriptive measures of isokinetic trunk testing. *J. Orthop. Sports Phys. Ther.* 7: 43-49, 1985.

39. Thorstensson, A., and J. Nilsson. Trunk muscle strength during constant and velocity movement. *Scand. J. Rehabil. Med.* 14: 61-68, 1982.

40. Tibrewal, S., J. Pearcy, I. Portek, and J. Spivey. A prospective study of lumbar spinal movements before and after discectomy using bi-planar radiography. *Spine* 10: 455-460, 1985.

41. Troup, J., T. Foreman, C. Baxter, and D. Brown. The perception of back pain and the role of psychophysical tests of lifting capacity (1987 Volvo Award in Clinical Sciences). *Spine* 7: 645-657, 1987.

Chapter 47

Exercise in Chronic Airway Obstruction

N.L. Jones
K.J. Killian

Patients with chronic airflow obstruction experience limitations in the ability to perform and sustain many activities. These limitations are most often related to the discomfort associated with the act of breathing. The quality of this sensation of dyspnea, or breathlessness, varies in description, but its severity is usually identified from the intensity of activity associated with discomfort. Thus, if discomfort occurs at a level of activity where it is unexpected, breathlessness is considered present. Breathlessness is most severe if it occurs at rest and is considered normal or physiological if it occurs at high-intensity exercise. Less commonly than dyspnea, exercise is limited by subjective muscle fatigue, a sensation that an excessive amount of muscular effort is required in tasks previously performed with much less effort.

Usually, the clinical examination and investigation of effort intolerance is directed toward heart or lung disorders to identify a specific disease process. The general assumption inherent in this approach is that the degree of organ impairment is reasonably closely related to the disability experienced (reduced capacity to perform functional activities) and the severity of symptoms experienced in everyday life (handicap) (59); thus the model used may be represented in the following scheme:

Organ impairment → Disability → Handicap

This description may caricature the diagnostic approach to disabled patients with chronic airflow limitation, but it serves to set the scene for a critical look at the relationships among organ impairment, disability, and handicap.

Organ Impairment and Disability in Chronic Airflow Limitation

Given the limitations common to the selection of any representative population, there is a close relationship between exercise capacity and the severity of airflow limitation as reflected in the FEV_1 (Figure 47.1). Although several studies have also demonstrated a decline in exercise capacity with declining FEV_1 (3, 28), Figure 47.1 illustrates the wide range of exercise capacity that is found in patients with comparable severities of airflow limitation. Were limitation of exercise ventilation the dominant single factor in limiting performance in these patients, such a wide range in responses would not be expected. Adding a measurement of the capacity to exchange gas, such as the CO transfer factor (D_{co}), explains some of the range effect; but its contribution is small (24, 28), and the accuracy of resting FEV_1 and D_{co} in predicting exercise capacity is not perfect.

Dyspnea in Airflow Limitation

As discomfort experienced during breathing (dyspnea) is generally assumed to limit exercise in patients with chronic airflow obstruction, explaining the factors that contribute to the symptom is the major goal of this chapter.

Patients readily identify specific symptoms limiting exercise. Table 47.1 illustrates the percentage of patients limited by breathlessness and leg fatigue at different severities of airflow limitation in

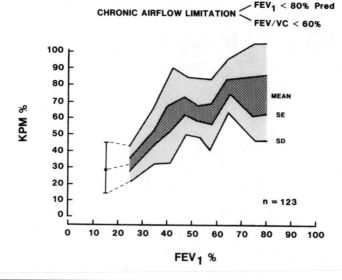

EXERCISE CAPACITY

CHRONIC AIRFLOW LIMITATION < FEV$_1$ < 80% Pred
FEV/VC < 60%

Figure 47.1. Relation between FEV$_1$, expressed as % predicted, and the maximum power output % predicted in 123 patients with chronic airflow obstruction.

Table 47.1 Symptom Limitation in 97 Patients With Chronic Airflow Limitation

	Limiting symptoms		
	Breathlessness	Leg fatigue	Both equally
FEV$_1$ 0%-40% (n = 31)	12 (39%)	11 (35%)	8 (26%)
Work capacity %	38 ± 4.9	41 ± 6.2	50 ± 3.9
FEV$_1$ 40%-60% (n = 48)	7 (14%)	22 (46%)	19 (40%)
Work capacity %	61 ± 8.1	73 ± 4.2	58 ± 5.0
FEV$_1$ 60%-80% (n = 18)	6 (33%)	10 (56%)	2 (11%)
Work capacity %	75 ± 4.4	75 ± 8.0	76

Note. FEV$_1$ and work capacity are expressed as % predicted.

the same population as that in Figure 47.1. It may be noted that an appreciable number of patients with severe airflow limitation were limited by leg fatigue and a large number of subjects with little airflow limitation by breathlessness.

Rather than limiting our examination of breathlessness to its severity at maximum exercise, we may also examine the relationship between breathlessness and exercise by asking patients to scale the intensity of breathing discomfort at each incremental step during an exercise test continued to

maximum performance (Figure 47.2). Breathlessness is increased when compared to normal subjects, but at maximum exercise the intensity of breathlessness is comparable in normal subjects and patients with airflow limitation. Breathlessness is not unique to airflow limitation but is present in normal subjects, although at a much higher absolute exercise intensity. The basis for this analysis was provided by studies in which dyspnea was quantified, and established and validated psychophysical methods were used (8, 33, 42). The application of these methods to studies of exercise and loaded breathing in healthy subjects and of patients with respiratory disorders has increased our understanding by allowing a quantitative analysis of the factors contributing to limiting symptoms.

Mechanisms Contributing to Dyspnea

Dyspnea is the dominant symptom at maximum exercise in most patients with chronic airflow obstruction and in many healthy subjects. Several studies have demonstrated a close relationship between the intensity of the sensation and the pressure generated by inspiratory muscles as a proportion of their capacity to generate pressure (17, 25, 36). The capacity to generate pressure itself is a function of the static strength and the contractile properties of the inspiratory muscles as expressed in the length-tension and force-velocity characteristics. In this analysis, tension and force

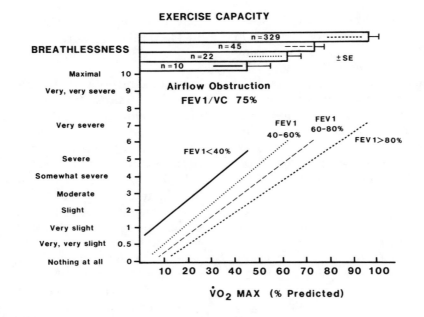

Figure 47.2. Dyspnea during exercise (Borg scale) in groups of patients with differing airflow obstruction. From Borg, Gunner, and David Ottoson (eds.), THE PERCEPTION OF EXERTION IN PHYSICAL WORK. Basingstoke: Macmillan; New York: Sheridan House, 1986. Reprinted by permission.

are reflected by maximum esophageal pressures, length by changes in volume, and velocity by inspiratory airflow.

Ventilation During Exercise

The increase in ventilation that occurs in exercise is closely correlated with the increase in metabolic demands expressed in terms of CO_2 output. For a given intensity of total body dynamic exercise, or oxygen intake, CO_2 output is influenced by a number of factors. The dietary history related to exercise exerts a strong effect by modulating the balance between fats and carbohydrates as fuel sources. If subjects fast for 24 hr fat is the predominant fuel source for exercise, and CO_2 output will be relatively low. In contrast, exercise taken shortly following a meal, when increases in plasma insulin effectively inhibit the mobilization of free fatty acids (44), is accompanied by high CO_2 output. Conditions associated with lactate production are also associated with increases in CO_2 output through their effects on acid-base variables; subjects who are poorly conditioned accumulate lactate at relatively low exercise levels, a buildup that is associated with increased CO_2 output. Similarly, patients with a cardiac impairment or severe arterial oxygen desaturation are exposed to poor oxygen delivery to exercising tissues accompanied by in-

creases in lactate production and CO_2 output (57). In contrast, trained individuals exhibit low CO_2 output during exercise due not only to their accumulating less lactate than do untrained subjects but also to their greater use of fat as an aerobic fuel (22, 55).

The efficiency of the lung as a gas exchanger also influences the ventilation at a given power output. An increase in dead space ventilation due to areas in the lung with a high ventilation-to-perfusion ($\dot{V}/\dot{Q}$) ratio is associated with increases in total ventilation ($\dot{V}_E$). Conditions associated with hypoxia are also accompanied by increases in ventilation during exercise through the effects of hypoxemia on respiratory control mechanisms (23).

Respiratory Muscle Tension

Increases in ventilation during exercise are accompanied by increases in the tension generated by the respiratory muscles, as defined by the mechanical characteristics of the lung (35). These may be expressed in terms of the pressures that are required to overcome elastic, resistive, and accelerative components in the following equation (46):

$$Pressure = (V \cdot E) + (\dot{V} \cdot R) + \ddot{V} \cdot I)$$

The intrathoracic pressures generated during exercise have been measured by several investigators (19, 20, 38, 53); pressures recorded at zero flow at the end of inspiration and expiration represent the pressures generated to achieve changes in volume (V) against the elastance (E) of the respiratory system. Pressures generated during active inspiratory and expiratory flow ($\dot{V}$), insofar as they deviate from these static characteristics, represent the pressures required to overcome flow resistance (R). Accelerative forces ($\ddot{V}$) against inertial impedance are assumed to be insignificant. During exercise, increases in inspiratory pressure occur gradually, but once tidal volume exceeds 50% of the vital capacity the change in pressure gradually increases (39). End-expiratory pressure shows little change until high levels of exercise, when an increase is observed; this represents a reduction in the end-expiratory lung volume. This may be considered an adaptive response, in that a reduction in end-inspiratory volume minimizes end-inspiratory volume and thus the end-inspiratory pressure.

The contributions of elastance and resistance to both the pressure generated by respiratory muscles and the sense of effort in breathing have been identified by studies in which breathing has been loaded by the imposition of graded resistances and elastances during inspiration (17, 25). These studies showed that the sense of effort increases with increased pressure generation by the respiratory muscles but also that the forces may be modified considerably by changes in the pattern of breathing (34). Thus, with an elastic load, inspiratory pressures may be minimized by the adoption of a smaller tidal volume and a greater frequency of breathing. Similarly, when a resistive load is imposed, inspiratory airflow may be slowed, and the time spent in inspiration is relatively lengthened (an increase in the duty cycle, T_i/T_{tot}).

Studies of loaded breathing have also allowed measurement of the oxygen cost of breathing. These studies have shown that the maximum oxygen consumption of the respiratory muscles is 100-300 ml $\cdot$ min^{-1} (25). This increase in metabolic demands theoretically may contribute to a limitation of maximal oxygen intake, but as the oxygen uptake of respiratory muscles will seldom exceed 10% of the total body $\dot{V}O_2$max, this effect is small in healthy subjects. However, in patients whose maximal oxygen uptake is severely restricted, the increased oxygen cost of breathing imposed by increases in respiratory impedance may well contribute to reductions in exercise capacity.

The Capacity of Respiratory Muscles to Generate Pressure

In the healthy population there is a wide range in respiratory muscle strength as measured by maximal inspiratory pressure (MIP) and maximal expiratory pressure (MEP) against an occluded airway. This variation may be as much as fivefold, between 60 cm H_2O to 300 cm H_2O for MIP (15, 25). Studies of loaded breathing in healthy subjects have shown that the intensity of respiratory effort for a given development of pressure is related to the respiratory muscle strength; subjects with weak muscles indicate a higher sense of effort for a given pressure generated than do subjects with a higher respiratory muscle strength (25).

In addition to the effect of static muscle strength, the dynamic characteristics of respiratory muscles influence the functional capacity under varying operational conditions. These characteristics are traditionally defined in terms of the length-tension and force-velocity characteristics of muscle (58); capacity falls as the muscle becomes shorter or contracts faster. In applying these muscle characteristics to respiratory muscles, we can use changes in volume as an indication of changes in respiratory muscle length, and changes in inspiratory flow are used to reflect changes in respiratory muscle velocity of contraction. Leblanc et al. (39) applied a similar approach to the early work of Agostoni and Fenn (1) in the context of ventilation during exercise to show that the tension-generating capacity of respiratory muscles declined linearly by 1.7% for each 1% of total lung capacity (TLC) that volume increases above functional residual capacity and by 5% for every L $\cdot$ s^{-1} increase in inspiratory flow; these authors also established the interaction between these two effects. When these findings were applied to studies of loaded breathing during exercise, the sense of respiratory effort was found to be closely related to the pressure generated by the respiratory muscles as a percentage of the pressure-generating capacity corrected for the effects of end-inspiratory volume and peak inspiratory flow (17).

In addition to quantifying the factors that contributed to the sense of effort in breathing, studies of loaded breathing in healthy subjects during exercise suggest that the pattern of breathing may be adopted to optimize the sense of effort by minimizing the tension generated in respiratory muscles and by maintaining the tension-generating capacity.

Respiratory Muscle Fatigue

In addition to isometric strength, force velocity, and length-tension, the duration of activity may influence the maximum capacity of the respiratory muscles. For any skeletal muscle the relationship between power and the length of time for which it may be sustained is a curve that declines exponentially, as described in the following general equation (58):

$$W = E + S/t$$

This equation states that below a threshold (E), power (W) may be maintained indefinitely. Above the threshold, fatigue will occur after a duration (t) that is influenced by the power output and the muscle's maximum strength (S). In this context fatigue is defined as failure to maintain a given power (16).

In the case of the respiratory muscles, the length of time for which a given ventilation may be sustained can be given with a fair degree of precision; the threshold is usually defined as the ventilation that can be maintained for 15 min: the maximum sustained ventilatory capacity (47). The form of the curve is similar to that of skeletal muscle in showing a decline from the traditional 15-s maximum breathing capacity to a threshold value that is about 60% of the maximum. Bellemare and Grassino (5) extended these findings by introducing the concept of the tension-time integral, which is obtained by multiplying the pressure generated by the respiratory muscles expressed as a percentage of a proportion of maximum by the duty cycle (T_i/T_{tot}). When the tension-time integral for the diaphragm exceeds 0.15-0.18, electromyographic signs of muscle failure are found if the pattern of breathing is continued.

The identification of fatigue in respiratory muscles is not as clear-cut as it is in skeletal muscle. An increased amplitude of the lower frequency component (20-50 Hz), a decreased amplitude of the high-frequency component (150-350 Hz), and a decreased ratio of high to low frequencies in electromyograms recorded from esophageal or chest electrodes have been used to indicate diaphragm fatigue (50). Also, the occurrence of paradoxical movement of the abdomen and rib cage during breathing has been advocated as an indication of respiratory muscle fatigue. However, it has been argued that neither the electromyographic changes (4) nor the presence of paradox (56) are necessarily indicators of muscle fatigue. It seems likely that during exercise the intensity of dyspnea that occurs as muscle tension approaches its maximum capacity will lead to the subject's stopping or reducing exercise before actual respiratory failure occurs.

Dyspnea During Exercise in Patients With Airflow Limitation

With this background we can examine the factors that contribute to the sense of respiratory effort during exercise in patients with chronic airflow obstruction.

Ventilation During Exercise

In patients with chronic airflow obstruction, the total ventilation in relation to the power output or oxygen uptake generally is within the normal range or is elevated. Although alveolar underventilation frequently occurs, this is seldom sufficiently severe to lead to a reduction in the total ventilatory response to exercise, as it is almost invariably accompanied by a high ratio of dead space to tidal volume (V_D/V_T) (26). As the capacity to increase ventilation is severely limited, any factor tending to increase ventilation at a given exercise level will contribute to a reduction in the total exercise capacity, often to a marked degree. For example, oxygen uptake at a given power output in patients with severe airflow obstruction is increased on average by about 200 ml/min (28) above that observed in healthy subjects at comparable loads. As this value is similar to the maximal increase in oxygen uptake shown in healthy subjects during loaded breathing, it seems likely that these increased metabolic costs are due to the increased tension developed by the respiratory muscles in overcoming the impedance to breathing. Increases in CO_2 output can occur following a meal or a glucose infusion and are accompanied by increases in ventilation; if ventilatory capacity is severely limited, a reduction in exercise capacity results (10). Lactate production in patients with chronic airflow obstruction is unusual (14), mainly because the maximum power output achieved by these patients is too low to require muscle glycolysis. However, in less disabled subjects who are capable of achieving relatively high exercise levels or in subjects who become severely hypoxemic or have an impaired cardiac output response to exercise, lactate production may contribute to an increase in CO_2 output and ventilation.

It might be thought that hypoxemia might lead to increases in ventilation by stimulating chemoreceptors. However, falls in arterial O_2 saturation in patients with chronic airflow limitation are the consequence of impaired ventilatory capacity, respiratory control, and gas exchange and thus have little independent effect on increasing ventilation. Studies in patients have shown correlations between arterial O_2 desaturation in exercise and the reduction in FEV_1 (severity of airflow obstruction), the reduction in D_{co} (severity of gas exchange impairment), and the intensity of exercise (O_2 demands) (26).

The efficiency of the lungs in terms of gas exchange is very frequently impaired in patients with chronic airflow obstruction (27). Marked inhomogeneity in the distribution of ventilation and perfusion leads to areas with a high ventilation-to-perfusion ratio, which act as dead space, and to areas with a low ventilation-to-perfusion ratio, which act as venous admixture and contribute to arterial oxygen desaturation. A high V_D/V_T ratio leads to a high ventilation for a given $\dot{V}CO_2$ and thus contributes to dyspnea. In some patients this effect is lessened by alveolar underventilation with increases in arterial PCO_2 by as much as 20 mmHg during exercise (26). Thus hypoventilation acts to reduce the sensation of dyspnea but at the uncertain expense of an increase in PCO_2.

Respiratory Muscle Tension

In patients with chronic airflow obstruction, the impedance to breathing is predominately resistive; indeed, in patients with emphysema the elastic components to impedance may be reduced because of the fall in elastic recoil. Airflow resistance is worse during expiration than during inspiration in most patients, and in patients with a severe reduction in elastic recoil the limitation of expiratory airflow at low lung volumes may become extreme (Figure 47.3). Ventilatory capacity is conventionally assessed by expiratory flow measurements, such as the FEV_1. Several studies have shown

correlations between the FEV_1 and maximum ventilation during exercise (28), suggesting that expiratory flow limitation leads to impaired ventilatory capacity and to limited exercise capability. Armstrong et al. (3) suggested that the FEV_1 may be used in conjunction with submaximal exercise ventilation to predict maximum exercise capacity. The data in these studies, although showing significant correlations, indicate a large residual variance. This variance may be understood when one considers first that maximum ventilation during exercise depends as much on inspiratory as on expiratory flow and second that inspiratory flow is extremely variable in patients with a given reduction in FEV_1. For example, in patients with emphysema, FEV_1 and expiratory flow rates may be very low, whereas during inspiration airflow resistance may be normal. In these patients the limitation of expiratory flow leads to a prolongation of expiratory time, in turn placing a heavy responsibility on increases in inspiratory flow and thus on reductions in inspiratory time to achieve a given tidal volume and total ventilation (9); T_i/T_{tot} may be less than .2, and relatively high levels of ventilation are obtained if the respiratory muscles are of normal strength and inspiratory resistance is low. On the other hand, in patients with severe chronic bronchitis there may be reductions in inspiratory flow due to reductions in airway caliber (Figure 47.3); this limits the increase in inspiratory flow and thus the reduction in T_i/T_{tot}. Ventilation during exercise in such patients may be very limited.

Increases in inspiratory flow may also be limited in patients with weak respiratory muscles or in patients whose respiratory muscle strength is compromised by gross increases in functional residual capacity (FRC) (Figure 47.3). If the pattern of breathing in terms of tidal volume and inspiratory and expiratory flow is considered in the context of the flow-volume loop (21), the adopted pattern of breathing may usually be explained. Also, changes in end-expiratory lung volume may be understood. Patients with airflow obstruction seldom are able to reduce end-expiratory lung volume because of the extreme reduction in airflow at low lung volumes. Thus the adaptation that is available to normal subjects in heavy exercise is not available to these patients. Some patients with airflow obstruction increase their inspiratory lung volume, but this strategy is seldom seen in any patient with poor inspiratory flow because of increases in inspiratory resistance, respiratory muscle weakness, or very high FRC (54). This is because the gains in expiratory flow achieved by an increase in end-inspiratory

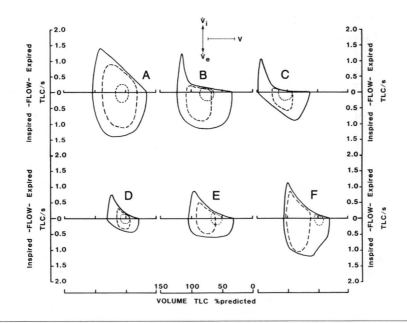

Figure 47.3. Pattern of flow-volume loop in normal subject (A) and patients with airflow obstruction (B-F), showing maximum resting loop (__), quiet breathing at rest (....), and breathing in maximum exercise (----).
A. Increase in V_T, $\dot{V}_i$, and $\dot{V}_E$ in normal subject.
B. Patient with severe expiratory flow reduction but normal inspiratory flow and respiratory muscle strength.
C. Severe obstruction with increase in FRC reducing strength and leading to marked reduction in V_i at higher lung volumes.
D. Inspiratory muscle weakness.
E. Inspiratory and expiratory obstruction with normal strength.
F. Less severe obstruction than B and C, normal strength, showing marked increase in end-expiratory volume with exercise.

lung volume are offset by the accompanying reduction in inspiratory flow capacity.

Respiratory Muscle Capacity

The strength of the respiratory muscles is compromised by both static and dynamic factors in patients with chronic airflow obstruction. Hyperinflation, associated with increases in FRC, may be marked; as this is associated with shortening of the respiratory muscles (Figure 47.3), these patients are unable to generate a normal maximum inspiratory pressure. To this effect may be added other factors that tend to weaken respiratory muscle, such as prolonged inactivity, steroid administration, and chronic hypoxemia. These effects may be quantified by the measurement of maximum inspiratory pressure corrected for the volume at which it is measured. Reductions in maximum inspiratory pressure may be shown to contribute to dyspnea during exercise independently of reductions in FEV₁ (Figure 47.4). During exercise the increase in end-inspiratory volume

associated with increasing tidal volume serves to weaken muscles further. However, the most important factor tending to weaken respiratory muscles in a dynamic sense is the increase in the velocity of inspiratory muscle contraction required to reduce inspiratory time and increase inspiratory flow. Because of the dominant effect of expiratory airflow slowing, the inspiratory muscles must contract at a much faster velocity than they do in normal subjects at comparable work loads; in addition to requiring greater muscle forces (as pointed out previously), these changes are associated with progressive functional weakening of the inspiratory muscles.

These factors were quantified by Leblanc et al. (38), who measured esophageal pressures in patients with respiratory disorders. They were able to show that the sense of effort in breathing was related to the pressure generated as a proportion of maximum static capacity (PpL/MIP), the inspiratory flow rate ($\dot{V}_i$), the tidal volume expressed as a proportion of vital capacity (V_T/VC), breathing frequency (f_b), and duty cycle (T_i/T_{tot}) in the following equation:

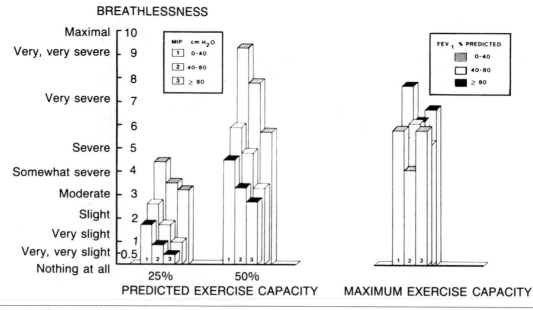

Figure 47.4. The contribution of reduction in FEV$_1$ and of maximum inspiratory pressure (MIP) on dyspnea in patients with airflow obstruction. From Borg, Gunner, and David Ottoson (eds.), THE PERCEPTION OF EXERTION IN PHYSICAL WORK. Basingstoke: Macmillan; New York: Sheridan House, 1986. Reprinted by permission.

$$\text{Borg rating} = 3.0\,\text{PpL/MIP} + 1.2\dot{V}_i + 4.5\,(V_T/VC) + 0.13f_b + 5.6\,(T_i/T_{tot}) - 6.2$$

where dyspnea is scored on a 0-10 scale as shown in Figures 47.2 and 47.4.

Although in a number of studies the sensation of dyspnea is related to indices of respiratory muscle forces and the capacity to meet them, some recent studies cast doubt on this simple interpretation. Lane et al. (37) found in a small number of subjects that changes in arterial O$_2$ saturation influenced dyspnea independently of the mechanical accompaniments. The same group found that different intensities of breathlessness occurred when the subjects voluntarily copied patterns of breathing first used in CO$_2$ breathing and exercise studies. These authors suggested that hypoxia per se may contribute to dyspnea, but this conclusion awaits the support of other studies.

Respiratory Muscle Fatigue

As already pointed out, there is no doubt that combinations of respiratory loading and exercise can lead to situations in which the forces required exceed the capacity to meet them; in healthy subjects this situation is associated with an extreme sense of dyspnea together with an elevation in PCO$_2$ and a fall in arterial O$_2$ saturation (25). Al-

though elevations of PCO$_2$ and falls in arterial O$_2$ saturation occur during exercise in patients with chronic airflow obstruction, these changes should not be construed as indicating respiratory failure; the individual tolerance to both changes is extremely variable in patients with chronic airflow obstruction. Furthermore, in some patients such changes may be accepted as part of the price paid to reduce ventilation and the sense of dyspnea.

The McGill group has shown that changes in the electromyographic frequency spectrum consistent with diaphragm fatigue occur in patients with chronic airflow obstruction during exercise (11, 50). However, Levine et al. (40) did not find such changes in exercising patients who were generating large pressures. Furthermore, Gallagher and Younes (18), in finding similar breathing patterns during recovery as were found in exercise, reasoned that respiratory muscle fatigue was unlikely to have occurred. An earlier study by Raimondi et al. (49) approached the same question by testing whether exercise duration could be prolonged by helium-oxygen breathing; as duration and ventilation were unaffected, these authors also concluded that the onset of fatigue was not responsible for exercise limitation. Although respiratory muscle fatigue seems unlikely to be a factor that limits exercise, there is little doubt that the forces generated by patients during exercise are high and that the capacity to meet these demands is reduced by a number of dynamic factors, including the time for which exercise is maintained. The sensation of dyspnea thereby increases with both the intensity and the duration of exercise and ultimately leads to the patient's stopping or reducing exertion.

Many factors are capable of contributing to dyspnea and thus to disability and handicap; exercise testing is helpful in identifying which factors may be playing roles in an individual patient to provide explanations for both symptoms and exercise intolerance (Figure 47.5).

A primary objective in the management of patients is an increase in exercise tolerance. Theoretically, in a given patient the options might include reductions in respiratory impedance (bronchodilation), reductions in ventilation (endurance training and oxygen therapy), increases in respiratory muscle strength and endurance (xanthines and ventilatory muscle training), and changes in the pattern of force deployment (education). Such strategies may be chosen on the basis of exercise studies; there is little point, for example, in instituting training of the respiratory muscles if their strength is normal and if dyspnea is solely due to severe airflow obstruction. The topic of training is briefly reviewed in the following discussion.

Other Factors That May Limit Exercise in Patients With Airflow Obstruction

Dyspnea is not the only symptom to limit exercise; many patients, while they are experiencing severe dyspnea, will indicate that they are unable to continue exercising because of severe leg-muscle effort. In a large series of patients with severe airflow obstruction, Killian (unpublished data) recently found that 31% identified leg fatigue as the main factor limiting further exercise.

Reductions in activity in the everyday lives of patients are usual accompaniments to chronic airflow limitation and may be expected to lead to impaired skeletal muscle function. The most extreme example or model for these effects is limb immobilization, which, over a period of 4-6 wk, is accompanied by marked reductions in muscle strength, muscle fiber cross-sectional area (52), energy stores, and metabolic enzyme activities (22, 41). Bed rest for a similar period, even in otherwise fit individuals, is accompanied by reductions in maximal oxygen uptake and impaired cardiovascular control (51). Differences between active and sedentary individuals in muscle strength and oxidative enzyme activities are also well known. Such effects are particularly marked in elderly individuals (2). Few studies

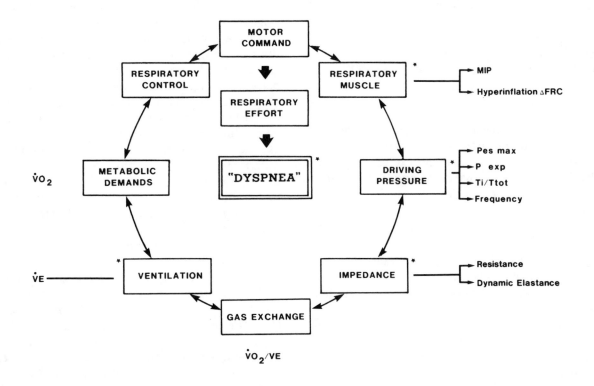

Figure 47.5. The multiple factors that contribute to dyspnea in exercise.

have been carried out in patients with disability due to heart or pulmonary disorders. Jones and McCartney (30) measured maximal quadriceps isokinetic power in patients recovering from myocardial infarction. During a 12-wk observation period, maximal power fell in patients who were inactive and increased in those who entered a rehabilitation program. Although we are unaware of published data, our own recent experience suggests that many patients who are seriously disabled by chronic respiratory disorders have weak quadriceps muscles that contribute to poor exercise performance. Apart from inactivity, steroid-induced myopathy and diuretic therapy may account for weakness in some patients, and, theoretically, hypoxemia and hypercapnia may also impair muscle function.

Among other factors contributing to exercise intolerance in patients with chronic airflow obstruction, coexisting coronary artery disease or leg atherosclerosis are usually easy to identify. Whether heart failure constitutes a limitation to exercise has been debated (43); as patients with right-heart failure usually are hypoxemic and hypercapnic and have a low ventilatory capacity, it usually is difficult to separate their individual effects. Patients with right-heart failure associated with idiopathic hypoventilation may have virtually normal exercise capacity, making it unlikely that heart failure per se limits the ability to exercise.

The Place of Exercise in the Management of Chronic Airflow Obstruction

There are a number of ways in which exercise capacity might be increased in patients. These include endurance exercise and exercises specifically designed to improve the strength and endurance of respiratory muscles.

Respiratory Muscle Training

In patients who are unable to generate adequate ventilatory pressures because of respiratory muscle weakness or those whose muscles fatigue rapidly, specific training of the muscles should increase maximum ventilation and power in exercise, reduce dyspnea, and improve one's quality of life. The principles of training regimens have been reviewed recently (7, 47) and are not detailed here. Training methods have included isocapnic hyperventilation, resistive breathing, and threshold

inspiratory loading, all of which are successful in increasing the maximal sustained ventilatory capacity and respiratory muscle strength. Recent studies have suggested that regimens that incorporate targeted flow rates and tidal volumes during training may be more effective than is unprescribed training (13). Although ventilatory capacity and endurance may be improved by as much as 50% by these means, the associated improvements in exercise tolerance and activities in everyday life are not as consistent. Keens et al. (31), in patients with cystic fibrosis, and Belman and Mittman (6), in adults with chronic airflow limitation, found improvements in exercise capacity following respiratory muscle training. However, Levine et al. (40) compared outcome measures in a control group who received intermittent positive pressure breathing and did not find a significant benefit of respiratory muscle training in terms of exercise tolerance or activities of daily living.

It is generally considered that endurance-exercise training is unlikely to benefit patients with chronic airflow limitation because they are unable to exercise at an intensity sufficient to elicit a training response. This type of training in healthy subjects and patients with coronary artery disease improves exercise capacity and reduces heart rate and blood pressure during exercise; associated with these changes are reductions in lactate accumulation in blood and in CO_2 output. Theoretically, the associated reduction in ventilation and dyspnea would be of great value to patients who are limited by dyspnea, but such benefits are likely to be limited to patients who accumulate lactate during exercise before training. In most patients exercise is limited at an intensity that is not associated with lactate production. Also theoretically, the increase in ventilation that occurs during training exercise may be associated with improvements in respiratory muscle strength if the respiratory muscles are weak to begin with. Chester et al. (12), among others, have demonstrated a reduced ventilation following training in 21 patients with moderately severe airway obstruction, and an increase in sustained ventilatory capacity has been a feature of several training studies (e.g., 31, 45).

Studies of training (both whole-body endurance and respiratory muscle) have shown variable effects in patients with chronic airflow limitation (48). The reasons for the variable responses have not been systematically investigated. In part they may be due to the experimental design, as several have not included a control group, and in some appropriate outcome measures may not have been used. More important, however, may be a poor identification of the objectives of training. By this we mean that when the mechanisms that underlie limiting symptoms are clarified, treatment measures may be tailored specifically to an individual. Thus, on the one hand, if respiratory muscle weakness is identified, respiratory muscle training is likely to help; on the other hand, a patient who shows increased CO_2 output and ventilation during exercise may be helped more by a general exercise program. In such a program it may prove difficult to prescribe an appropriate exercise intensity by using guidelines developed for cardiac patients. In respiratory patients the usual aerobic program in which exercise is maintained for a prolonged period of time may be associated with an unacceptable intensity of dyspnea; in such patients improvements in muscle function may be achieved by high-intensity muscle forces sustained for only short periods but repeated frequently. This type of exercise has proved helpful in cardiac patients (32).

In both the understanding of exercise limitation and the approach to treatment, quantitative information regarding the severity of limitation and the factors that contribute to it is vital. In addition to noninvasive exercise testing that quantifies the cardiorespiratory responses, measurement of symptom intensity has proved invaluable in this context (33).

References

1. Agostoni, E., and W.O. Fenn. Abdominal and thoracic pressures at different lung volumes. *J. Appl. Physiol.* 15: 1087-1092, 1960.
2. Aniansson, A., G. Grimby, M. Hedberg, and M. Krotkiewski. Muscle morphology, enzyme activity and muscle strength in elderly men and women. *Clin. Physiol.* 1: 73-86, 1981.
3. Armstrong, B.W., J.N. Workman, H.H. Holcombe, and W.R. Roemmich. Clinicophysiologic evaluation of physical working capacity in persons with pulmonary disease. *Am. Rev. Respir. Dis.* 93: 90-99, 1966.
4. Bazzy, A.R., J.B. Korten, and G.G. Haddad. Increase in electromyogram low-frequency power in nonfatigued contracting skeletal muscle. *J. Appl. Physiol.* 61: 1012-1017, 1986.
5. Bellemare, F., and A. Grassino. Effect of pressure and timing of contraction on human diaphragm fatigue. *J. Appl. Physiol.* 53: 1190-1195, 1982.
6. Belman, M.J., and C. Mittman. Ventilatory muscle training improves exercise capacity in chronic obstructive lung disease patients. *Am. Rev. Respir. Dis.* 121: 273-280, 1980.
7. Belman, M.J. Ventilatory muscle training. In: Sieck, G.C., S.C. Ganderia, and W.E. Cameron, eds. *Respiratory muscles and their neuromuscular control.* (Proceedings of an IUPS Satellite Symposium, Los Angeles, California, July 1986.) New York: Alan R. Liss, 1987, p.363-372.
8. Borg, G.A.V. Psychophysical bases of perceived exertion. *Med. Sci. Sports Exerc.* 14: 377-381, 1982.
9. Bradley, M.E., and R. Crawford. Regulation of breathing during exercise in normal subjects and in chronic lung disease. *Clin. Sci. Molec. Med.* 51: 575-582, 1976.
10. Brown, S.E., R.C. Nagendran, J.W. McHugh, D.W. Stansbury, C.E. Fischer, and R.W. Light. Effects of a large carbohydrate load on walking performance in chronic airflow obstruction. *Am. Rev. Respir. Dis.* 132: 960-962, 1985.
11. Bye, P.T.B., S.A. Esau, R.D. Levy, R.J. Shiner, P.T. Macklem, J.G. Martin, and R.L. Pardy. Ventilatory function during exercise in air and oxygen in patients with chronic airflow limitation. *Am. Rev. Respir. Dis.* 132: 236-240, 1985.
12. Chester, E.H., M.J. Belman, R.C. Behler, G.L. Baum, G. Schey, and P. Buch. Multidisciplinary treatment of chronic pulmonary insufficiency: 3. The effect of physical training on cardiopulmonary performance in patients with chronic obstructive pulmonary disease. *Chest* 72: 695-702, 1977.
13. Clanton, T.L., G.F. Dixon, J. Drake, and J.E. Gadek. Effects of breathing pattern on inspiratory muscle endurance in humans. *J. Appl. Physiol.* 59: 1834-1841, 1985.
14. Daly, J.J., R.S. Duff, E. Jackson, and G.M. Turino. Effect of exercise on arterial lactate, pyruvate and excess lactate in chronic bronchitis. *Br. J. Dis. Chest* 61: 193-197, 1967.
15. De Troyer, A., and J. Yernault. Inspiratory muscle force in normal subjects and patients with interstitial lung disease. *Thorax* 35: 92-100, 1980.
16. Edwards, R.H.T. Human muscle function and fatigue. In: Porter, R., and J. Whelan, eds. *Human muscle fatigue: Physiological mechanisms.* (CIBA Foundation Symposium 82.) London: Pitman Medical, 1981, p. 1-18.
17. El-Manshawi, A., K.J. Killian, E. Summers, and N.L. Jones. Breathlessness during exer-

cise with and without resistive loading. *J. Appl. Physiol.* 61: 896-905, 1986.

18. Gallagher, C.G., and M.K. Younes. Breathing pattern during and following exercise in patients with chronic obstructive lung disease, interstitial lung disease and cardiac disease and in normal subjects. *Am. Rev. Respir. Dis.* 133: 581-586, 1986.

19. Grimby, G., M. Goldman, and J. Mead. Respiratory muscle action inferred from rib cage and abdominal V-P partitioning. *J. Appl. Physiol.* 41: 739-751, 1976.

20. Grimby, G., B. Saltin, and L. Wilhelmsen. Pulmonary flow-volume and pressure-volume relationship during submaximal and maximal exercise in young well-trained men. *Bull. Physiopathol. Respir.* 7: 157-168, 1971.

21. Grimby, G., and J. Stiksa. Flow-volume curves and breathing patterns during exercise in patients with obstructive lung disease. *Scand. J. Clin. Lab. Invest.* 25: 304-313, 1970.

22. Henriksson, J., and J.S. Reitman. Time course of changes in human skeletal muscle succinate dehydrogenase and cytochrome oxidase activities and maximal oxygen uptake with physical activity and inactivity. *Acta Physiol. Scand.* 99: 91-97, 1977.

23. Hughes, R.L., M. Clode, R.H.T. Edwards, T.J. Goodwin, and N.L. Jones. Effect of inspired O_2 on cardiopulmonary and metabolic responses to exercise in man. *J. Appl. Physiol.* 24: 336-347, 1968.

24. Johnson, R.L., H.F. Taylor, and A.C. Degraff. Functional significance of a low pulmonary diffusing capacity for carbon monoxide. *J. Clin. Invest.* 44: 789-800, 1965.

25. Jones, G.L., K.J. Killian, E. Summers, and N.L. Jones. Inspiratory muscle forces and endurance in maximal resistive loading. *J. Appl. Physiol.* 58: 1608-1615, 1985.

26. Jones, N.L. Pulmonary gas exchange during exercise in patients with chronic airflow obstruction. *Clin. Sci.* 31: 39-50, 1966.

27. Jones, N.L., and L.B. Berman. Gas exchange in chronic air-flow obstruction. *Am. Rev. Respir. Dis.* 129: S81-S83, 1984.

28. Jones, N.L., G. Jones, and R.H.T. Edwards. Exercise tolerance in chronic airway obstruction. *Am. Rev. Respir. Dis.* 103: 477-491, 1971.

29. Jones, N.L., K.J. Killian, and D.G. Stubbing. The thorax during exercise. In: Roussos, C., and P.T. Macklem, eds. *The thorax*. New York: Marcel Dekker, 1985, p. 627-661.

30. Jones, N.L., and N. McCartney. Influence of muscle power on aerobic performance and the effects of training. *Acta Med. Scand.* 711: 115-122, 1986.

31. Keens, T.G., T.R.B. Krastins, E.M. Wannamaker, H. Levison, D.M. Crozier, and A.C. Bryan. Ventilatory muscle endurance training in normal subjects and patients with cystic fibrosis. *Am. Rev. Respit. Dis.* 116: 853-860, 1977.

32. Keleman, M.H., K.J. Stewart, R.E. Gillian, C.K. Ewart, S.A. Valenti, J.D. Manley, and M.D. Keleman. Circuit weight training in cardiac patients. *J. Am. Coll. Cardiol.* 1: 38-42, 1986.

33. Killian, K.J. The objective measurement of breathlessness. *Chest* 88: 84S-90S, 1985.

34. Killian, K.J., D.D. Bucens, and E.J.M. Campbell. Effect of breathing patterns on the perceived magnitude of added loads to breathing. *J. Appl. Physiol.* 52: 578-584, 1982.

35. Killian, K.J., and E.J.M. Campbell. Dyspnea and exercise. *Ann. Rev. Physiol.* 45: 465-479, 1983.

36. Killian, K.J., and N.L. Jones. The use of exercise testing and other methods in the investigation of dyspnea. *Clin. Chest Med.* 5: 99-108, 1984.

37. Lane, R., A. Cockroft, L. Adams, and A. Guz. Arterial oxygen saturation and breathlessness in patients with chronic obstructive airways disease. *Clin. Sci.* 72: 693-698, 1987.

38. Leblanc, P., D.M. Bowie, E. Summers, N.L. Jones, and K.J. Killian. Breathlessness and exercise in patients with respiratory disease. *Am. Rev. Respir. Dis.* 133: 21-25, 1986.

39. Leblanc, P., E. Summers, M.D. Inman, N.L. Jones, E.J.M. Campbell, and K.J. Killian. Inspiratory muscles during exercise: A problem of supply and demand. *J. Appl. Physiol.* 64: 2482-2489, 1988.

40. Levine, S., P. Weiser, and J. Gillen. Evaluation of a ventilatory muscle endurance training program in the rehabilitation of patients with chronic obstructive pulmonary disease. *Am. Rev. Respir. Dis.* 133: 400-406, 1986.

41. MacDougall, J.D., G.R. Ward, D.G. Sale, and J.R. Sutton. Biochemical adaptation of human skeletal muscle to heavy resistance training and immobilization. *J. Appl. Physiol: Respir. Environ. Exerc. Physiol.* 43: 700-703, 1977.

42. Mahler, D.A., D.H. Weinberg, C.K. Wells, and A.R. Feinstein. The measurement of dyspnea. *Chest* 85: 751-758, 1984.

43. Matthay, R.A., H.J. Berger, R.A. Davies, J. Loke, D.A. Mahler, A. Gottschaek, and B.L. Zaret. Right and left ventricular exercise

performance in chronic obstructive pulmonary disease: Radionuclide assessment. *Ann. Intern. Med.* 93: 234-239, 1980.

44. Molé, P.A. Exercise metabolism. In: Bove, A.A., and D.T. Lowenthae, eds. *Exercise medicine: Physiologic principles and clinical applications.* Orlando: Academic Press, 1983, p. 43-88.

45. Orenstein, D.M., B.A. Franklin, C.F. Doershuk, H.K. Hellerstein, K.J. Germann, J.G. Horowitz, and R.C. Stein. Exercise conditioning and cardiorespiratory fitness in cystic fibrosis. *Chest* 80: 392-398, 1981.

46. Otis, A.B. The work of breathing. *Physiol. Rev.* 34: 449-458, 1954.

47. Pardy, R.L., and D.E. Leith. Ventilatory muscle training. In: Roussos, C., and P.T. Macklem, eds. *The thorax.* New York: Marcel Dekker, 1985, p. 1353-1372.

48. Pardy, R.L., R.N. Rivington, P.J. Despas, and P.T. Macklem. The effects of inspiratory muscle training on exercise performance in chronic airflow limitation. *Am. Rev. Respir. Dis.* 123: 426-433, 1981.

49. Raimondi, A.C., R.H.T. Edwards, D.M. Denison, D.G. Leaver, R.G. Spencer, and J.A. Siddorn. Exercise tolerance breathing a low density gas mixture, 35% oxygen and air in patients with chronic obstructive bronchitis. *Clin. Sci.* 39: 675-685, 1970.

50. Roussos, C., and P.T. Macklem. The respiratory muscles. *N. Engl. J. Med.* 307: 786-798, 1982.

51. Saltin, B., G. Blomqvist, J.H. Mitchell, R.L. Johnson, K. Wildenthal, and C.B. Chapman. Response to exercise after bed rest and after training: A longitudinal study of adaptive changes in oxygen transport and body composition. *Circulation* 37-38(Suppl. 7): VII-1–VII-78, 1968.

52. Sargeant, A.J., C.T.M. Davies, R.H.T. Edwards, C. Maunder, and A. Young. Functional and structural changes after disuse of human muscle. *Clin. Sci. Molec. Med.* 52: 337-342, 1977.

53. Stubbing, D.G., L.D. Pengelly, J.L.C. Morse, and N.L. Jones. Pulmonary mechanics during exercise in normal males. *J. Appl. Physiol.* 49: 506-510, 1980.

54. Stubbing, D.G., L.D. Pengelly, J.L.C. Morse, and N.L. Jones. Pulmonary mechanics during exercise in subjects with chronic airflow obstruction. *J. Appl. Physiol.* 49: 511-515, 1980.

55. Taylor, R., and N.L. Jones. The reduction by training of CO_2 output during exercise. *Eur. J. Cardiol.* 9: 53-62, 1979.

56. Tobin, M.J., W. Perez, S.M. Guenther, R.F. Lodato, and D.R. Dantzker. Does rib-cage abdominal paradox signify respiratory muscle fatigue? *J. Appl. Physiol.* 63: 851-860, 1987.

57. Weber, K.T., J.R. Wilson, J.S. Janicki, and M.L. Likoff. Exercise testing in the evaluation of the patient with chronic cardiac failure. *Am. Rev. Respir. Dis.* 129(Suppl.): S60-S62, 1984.

58. Wilkie, D.G. Muscle function: A historical view. In: Jones, N.L., N. McCartney, and A.J. McComas, eds. *Human muscle power.* Champaign, IL: Human Kinetics, 1986, p. 3-14.

59. World Health Organization. *International classification of impairment, disabilities and handicaps.* Geneva: Author, 1980.

Chapter 48

Discussion: Exercise and Chronic Airway Obstruction

Brian J. Whipp

The inability to sustain the performance of physical activity for sufficient time to accomplish the imposed task requirements forms the basis for the categorization of work intolerance, or, more properly, power intolerance. This can occur with even modest task demands when the effective operating range of one or more of the physiological systems that support the muscular energy transfer becomes limited.

Chronic airflow obstruction (CAO), such as occurs with bronchial asthma, chronic bronchitis, and pulmonary emphysema, typically leads to a triad of constraining consequences: (a) a reduced range of achievable airflow and, consequently, of ventilation; (b) a ventilatory requirement that is greater than normal because of the influence of the increased physiological dead space fraction of the breath; and (c) the predisposition to shortness of breath, or *dyspnea*, as the system reaches or approaches its airflow and ventilatory limits. With severe airflow limitation, the range of performable physical tasks can therefore be constrained to that of a mild domiciliary routine.

To understand the factors that limit exercise tolerance in such patients, it is necessary to address four interrelated issues:

- To what extent are the requirements met for arterial blood gas and acid base regulation?
- What is the cost of meeting these requirements?
- Are the ventilatory and airflow responses constrained or limited?
- How intensely are the responses perceived as being unpleasant?

Ventilatory Requirements

The ventilatory ($\dot{V}_E$) requirement for regulation of arterial blood CO_2 partial pressure (P_aCO_2) is dependent on three physiological variables: the pulmonary CO_2 exchange rate ($\dot{V}CO_2$), the physiological dead space fraction of the breath (V_D/V_T), and the regulated level of P_aCO_2 itself; that is,

$$\dot{V}_E(BTPS) = \{863 \cdot \dot{V}CO_2 (STPD)\}/\{P_aCO_2 (1 - V_D/V_T)\}$$

where the altitude-independent constant 863 allows for the convention of expressing ventilatory volumes under BTPS conditions, the metabolic exchange under STPD conditions, and the CO_2 level as a partial pressure.

The ventilatory response to the muscular exercise appears to be more closely related to the $\dot{V}CO_2$ response than to the $\dot{V}O_2$ response (14, 37). Consequently, although the respiratory exchange ratio (R, which equals $\dot{V}CO_2/\dot{V}O_2$) at rest and during light exercise in patients with CAO is not significantly different from normal, factors that augment the $\dot{V}CO_2$—such as (a) an increased O_2 (and hence CO_2) cost of breathing (7, 16) or (b) bicarbonate (HCO_3^-) buffering of lactic acid, which may result at low work rates in some patients (18, 36) consequent to the physical deconditioning that commonly occurs with this impairment—can demand a higher ventilation despite the ability to achieve the response being compromised. In fact, dietary-induced increases in R have been shown to reduce exercise tolerance in patients with severe airflow limitation (5). In many patients with CAO, however, blood [lactate] increases and [HCO_3^-] decreases during exercise are small or even nonexistent because of the low degree of stress to the external work-generating muscles and the cardiovascular system (as evidenced by the low maximum heart rate) that results with pulmonary-mechanical limitation to the work. But, although there is evidence that this can be the case with severe CAO, the degree of exercise-induced metabolic acidosis (as assessed by the decrease in the standard bicarbonate [HCO_3^-] STD between rest and the second recovery minute from maximum incremental exercise) has recently been shown (36) to be highly variable between patients with CAO and also to correlate poorly with resting indices of airflow limitation, such as the forced expiratory volume in 1 s (FEV_1) or the maximum voluntary ventilation (MVV): The decrease in $[HCO_3^-]$ STD ranged from 1.0 to 9.5 mEq · 1^{-1} over a range of FEV_1 (% predicted) of 20%–80%, with a correlation coefficient of only 0.06 (36). This finding confirms those previously reported by Kanarek et al. (18). Consequently, there is likely to be a more highly variable potential for trainability in such patients than was previously supposed, particularly with respect to reducing the additional CO_2 load and also the peripheral chemoreceptor stimulation by the metabolic acidemia (38), which may well be potentiated by the characteristic arterial hypoxemia.

The second factor influencing the ventilatory response to exercise is the regulated level of P_aCO_2. A low P_aCO_2 requires a greater increase in alveolar ventilation ($\dot{V}_A$) to clear a given volume of CO_2 (e.g., per liter) from the body, whereas a high P_aCO_2 requires less of a $\dot{V}_A$ response. Patients with CAO, however, have highly variable levels of resting P_aCO_2 and variable patterns of P_aCO_2 change during exercise. Wasserman et al. (35) reported that P_aCO_2 was maintained relatively constant throughout maximal incremental exercise in 11 patients with stable CAO, despite resting P_aCO_2 ranging from 30 to 57 torr; 10 out of 11, however, initially increased P_aCO_2 with the imposition of the lightest work load. In contrast, Jones and Berman (15), however, reported that P_aCO_2 tends to be systematically higher during exercise in patients who fit the bronchitic (i.e., Type B) rather than the emphysematous (i.e., Type A) description and that CO_2 retention is a common consequence in severe CAO.

The resting arterial hypoxemia, which is mainly a consequence of impaired distribution of alveolar ventilation-to-perfusion ($\dot{V}_A/\dot{Q}$) ratios, typically becomes more severe with exercise in Type A CAO patients; the Type B patient tends to experience no further hypoxemia, and in some cases there is even an improvement in arterial oxygenation (15). But, although there is not a good correlation between the degree of arterial O_2 desaturation and the reduction in maximum exercise tolerance between patients, alleviating the hypoxemia by increasing the inspired O_2 fraction has been shown to reduce dyspnea, reduce the level of exercise ventilation (presumably by suppressing the carotid-body afferent neural drive), and consequently to increase

exercise intolerance (13, 35). This is supported by the observation that, although dyspnea was not directly assessed by means of a rating scale, individuals who had previously undergone surgical resection of both carotid bodies could sustain a held breath for appreciably longer than could normal control subjects from either a normoxic or, especially, an hypoxic inspirate (10). Furthermore, there was no hypoxia-induced hyperpnea during exercise in these individuals, unlike the control group (24).

Patients with CAO have impaired pulmonary gas exchange efficiency (15, 35). This is reflected in an increased V_D/V_T and also increased levels of the ideal alveolar-to-arterial PO_2 difference ($P(A-a)O_2$) and the arterial-to-end-tidal PCO_2 difference ($P(a-ET)CO_2$). Consequently, a greater increase in total ventilation ($\dot{V}_E$) is required to effect a given increase in alveolar ventilation. Values of 0.5 or more are not uncommon for V_D/V_T in this condition (15, 35). The ventilatory equivalents for O_2 and CO_2 ($\dot{V}_E/\dot{V}O_2$, $\dot{V}_E/\dot{V}CO_2$) are typically high. And even in those cases in which there is evidence of a lactic acidemia during exercise, there is little or no increase in $\dot{V}_E/\dot{V}O_2$ and $\dot{V}_E/\dot{V}CO_2$ (35) or reduction in P_aCO_2 (15, 35), the normal compensatory hyperventilation being constrained by the limiting pulmonary mechanics.

Cost of Effecting Ventilatory Response

Metabolic energy is expended by the inspiratory muscles mainly (a) to overcome the elastic recoil force of the lung and, at very high thoracic volumes, that of the chest wall (25) and (b) to cause inspiratory flow through the airways or to provide a brake to expiratory flow; that is, other causes of pulmonary impedance, such as tissue viscous flow and inertial influences of accelerating the gas and of the thorax itself, normally represent a small portion of the energy requirements (28). During exhalation, however, lung recoil is an important determinant not only of the airflow that is generated during the breath but also of the maximum attainable airflow (26). Additionally, the metabolic cost of breathing increases when airflow is elevated further by expiratory muscle contraction.

The patient with CAO requires greater-than-normal $\dot{V}O_2$ for breathing (15) because of both the increased resistive work and the inefficient mechanics of respiratory muscle contraction associated with a high functional residual capacity

(FRC). Consequently, a greater respiratory muscle blood flow is required to support the increased respiratory work.

During exercise, the end-expiratory lung volume (EELV) has been shown to increase further in patients with CAO (21), whereas it actually decreases in normal subjects (17, 21, 23) by an amount that continues to be debated; however, the differences may reflect the techniques used to estimate it. Thus, any benefit of thoracic recoil on airflow at the onset of inspiration during exercise that is to be expected in the normal subject (as EELV is less than FRC) will be lost to the patient with CAO in whom EELV increases above FRC. Consequently, the inertial component of the total pulmonary impedance during inspiration needs to be overcome totally by the inspiratory muscles.

Patients with CAO, especially those with reduced lung recoil, can have such a compromised maximum expiratory airflow that the spontaneously generated flow during exercise rapidly encroaches on the constraining envelope of the maximal expiratory flow-volume curve (17, 21). Thus, in addition to increasing EELV (which improves the flow-generating potential but at a cost of less advantageous inspiratory muscle length for force and hence pressure generation), many, but by no means all (4, 32), CAO patients alter their breathing pattern by prolonging the expiratory duration of the breath (T_E) (17, 35). This leads in turn to a reduced inspiratory duration (T_I). The result is that the required inspiratory volume is achieved with both higher peak and higher mean inspiratory flows; that is, V_T/T_I is high and the velocity of shortening of the inspiratory muscles is increased.

Consequently, the greater-than-normal exercise ventilation in patients with CAO is achieved with an even greater respiratory muscle work and increased O_2 (and presumably CO_2) cost of the work. These factors predispose to inspiratory muscle fatigue and the potential for the nutrient flow to the external-work-generating muscles being compromised.

Is the System Limited?

Dyspnea is a common complaint of exercising patients with CAO when the breathing requirements reach or approach the limits of the mechanical performance of the pulmonary system (9, 34). Consequently, the combination of the increased ventilatory demands and the reduced ventilatory capacity predisposes the patient with CAO to pulmonary-mechanical limitation of exercise performance. Maximum exercise $\dot{V}_E$ often reaches values equal to or even in excess of the MVV performed at rest (35). Similarly, the spontaneously achieved expiratory airflow (at a particular lung volume) commonly reaches or in some instance exceeds that obtained during a maximum expiratory flow-volume maneuver (MEVV) (17, 21, 30). The observation that these apparent maxima can be exceeded during spontaneous breathing in some patients reflects: (a) the influence of a small degree of bronchodilation that may occur during the exercise secondary to increased blood concentrations of catecholamines and (b) that maximal expiratory airflow may not be achieved with maximal volitional effort in these patients because of airway compression and even closure at low lung volumes. But, importantly, patients with CAO have been shown not to develop intrathoracic pressures in excess of those required to achieve maximum expiratory flow even when the expiratory flow becomes limited (21). Pressures in excess of this "maximum effective pressure" would lead to airway and alveolar gas compression and consequently to increased expiratory work (power) without an increased airflow. Although the control features of this expiratory pressure optimization remain to be resolved, it does suggest that expiratory muscle fatigue is consequently less likely. It is important to recognize, however, that when the MEVV is not performed in a body plethysmograph, the effects of thoracic gas compression dissociate the actual lung volume from that assessed from the measured expired volume. Furthermore, the MVV or MEVV relationship determined at rest may not reflect the values when the patient experiences pulmonary mechanical limitation during exercise. Cotes (9), for example, cautions the use of the resting MVV as the limiting index of ventilation in those asthmatic patients who develop bronchospasm during exercise. Similarly, the MVV has been reported to be greater when measured during exercise than at rest in normal individuals (33).

Indices such as the FEV_1, which are considered to reflect the MVV (e.g., $FEV_1 \times 40 \cong MVV$), have been shown to be useful as general predictors of the maximum exercise ventilation or power output, but the variability of the reported data is such that three- to fourfold differences in both maximum power output and maximum exercise ventilation (15) have been observed at a particular value of FEV_1.

Although the achievement of expiratory airflow and ventilatory maxima during exercise provides evidence of pulmonary mechanical limitation in patients with CAO, the consequences for inspiratory muscle performance require consideration. As with other skeletal muscles, the respiratory muscles are prone to fatigue when they are required to perform high-intensity respiratory work (6, 30). The duration for which a subject is capable of volitionally sustaining a high level of ventilation (care being taken to avoid hypocapnia) bears (a) an exponential-like or (b) a hyperbolic relationship to the $\dot{V}_E$ of the forms

$$\dot{V}_E = (MVV - MSVC) \cdot e^{-kt}$$

or

$$(\dot{V}_E - MSVC) \cdot t = K_v$$

where MSVC is the ventilatory asymptote (termed the *maximal sustained ventilatory capacity*), k is the rate constant for the decline in the sustainable $\dot{V}_E$ as a function of the tolerable duration (t), and K_v is the curvature constant, which, interestingly, is expressed in units of volume. Normal values for MSVC range from 55% to 80% of MVV, although values of about 90% have been demonstrated in highly fit athletes (for discussion, see ref. 39). The MSVC in patients with CAO bears a proportional relationship to the MVV similar to that reported for normal subjects, but of course the absolute values of both are appreciably lower. This means that when the $\dot{V}_E$ requirements during exercise exceed the MSVC, inspiratory muscle fatigue is likely. This presupposes that the pattern of recruitment and the efficiency of contraction of the respiratory muscles, as well as the level of oxygenation of the blood perfusing them, are similar under the two such diverse conditions (unlikely in the author's judgment). However, inspiratory muscle fatigue, as judged by changes in the electromyographic (EMG) spectrum, has been demonstrated during exercise in patients with CAO (6,12). Furthermore, some authors have reported an improvement in exercise tolerance (despite no systematic changes in indices of maximum airflow) in patients with CAO following a period of specific respiratory muscle training (2, 29). However, this improvement in response to respiratory muscle training is not a consistent finding (13, 22), perhaps in part reflecting differences in the effectiveness of the devices used to induce the training effect. Although there is clear evidence that the ventilatory system can limit maximum exercise performance, it should be noted that system constraint can be present at submaximal work rates. For example, Nery et al. (27) showed that patients with CAO have a longer-than-normal time constant for the

$\dot{V}_E$ response to constant-load exercise and, in many instances, a reduced magnitude of the initial, normally rapid hyperpnea at exercise onset. The slow time constant may reflect the increased pulmonary impedance in this condition (although the $\dot{V}O_2$ time constant was also long, consistent with extreme detraining of these patients), and the reduced initial responses of $\dot{V}O_2$ and $\dot{V}_E$ may reflect impaired pulmonary vascular function.

Perception of the Ventilatory Response

Perhaps the earliest literary use of the term *dyspnea* (breathlessness) was related to exercise when the messenger was addressing King Creon in the opening scene of Sophocles' *Antigone*.[1] And, although a precise and agreed-upon definition of the term remains elusive, its essential elements are given by Scharf et al. (31): "An unpleasant sensation of difficulty of breathing." The topic is a complex one, in part because of the widely differing reported degrees of breathlessness associated with "apparently comparable (pulmonary) mechanical and clinical circumstances" (19), temporal adaptation to the condition, and also possibly different intensities being evoked by different sources of the hyperpneic drive. However, common features of exertional dyspnea in CAO involve increased ventilatory drive and increased respiratory impedance, leading to reduced ventilatory capacity. Tachypnea is also a common finding (34).

The difference between the maximum $\dot{V}_E$ attained during exercise and the resting MVV has been termed *breathing reserve* (35). This was shown to be insignificantly different from zero (ranging between ±10 L · min^{-1}) in patients with stable CAO (35), regardless of whether MVV was directly measured or estimated as the $FEV_1 \times 40$. In a normal control group, the breathing reserve averaged 36 L · min^{-1}. Consequently, the *dyspneic index* (i.e., [$\dot{V}_E \times 100$]/MVV) often approximates 100 in patients with CAO (8, 18, 35); this accounts for the large proportion of these patients who attribute their exercise intolerance exclusively, or in combination with other symptoms, to shortness of breath. For example, Cotes (9) proposed that "breathlessness is inevitable when the ventilation approaches the maximal breathing capacity."

El-Manshawi et al. (11) and Killian and Jones (20) incorporated the relationship between the force

---

[1] I thank Kenneth B. Saunders for bringing this to my attention.

(pressure) generated by the inspiratory muscles during spontaneous breathing (P_{mus}) (as a fraction of the maximum pressure capable of being generated, or P_{max}) to the subject's rating of breathlessness during exercise. They found that subjects who used similar fraction of the maximum inspiratory pressure (P_{mus}/P_{max}) rated a similar degree of dyspnea, as assessed by the Borg scale (3). Similarly, subjects who developed unusually high fractions of P_{max} during spontaneous breathing for a given task (e.g., patients with CAO and those with respiratory muscle weakness) rated an abnormally high level of dyspnea for that task. However, such inferences appear relevant only to reflexly driven breathing, as Adams et al. (1) have demonstrated that volitionally induced changes in ventilation that reproduced the same pattern that was previously induced reflexly by hypercapnia resulted in virtually no perceived dyspnea. On the other hand, the hypercapnia-induced changes were rated high on the visual-analog scale of breathlessness. Therefore, presumably similar P_{mus}/P_{max} and $\dot{V}_E/MVV$ ratios resulted in appreciably different ratings.

In conclusion, patients with CAO are predisposed to pulmonary mechanical limitations to exercise; however, physical detraining as a result of the persistent exertional dyspnea leading to restricted activity levels can also impair exercise tolerance. During exercise these patients are characterized by low values for maximum VO_2, maximum heart rate, and breathing reserve, and little or no respiratory compensation for metabolic acidosis when it develops. High values are typical for V_D/V_T, $P(A-a)O_2$, $P(a-ET)CO_2$, $\dot{V}_E/\dot{V}O_2$, $\dot{V}_E/\dot{V}CO_2$, and heart rate reserve. The combination of increased ventilatory requirement and reduced ventilatory capacity—compounded by arterial hypoxemia and, often, inspiratory muscle fatigue—makes exertional dyspnea the most characteristic cause of the reduced exercise tolerance in these patients.

References

1. Adams, L., R. Lane, S.A. Shea, A. Cockroft, and A. Guz. Breathlessness during different forms of ventilatory stimulation: A study of mechanisms in normal subjects and respiratory patients. *Clin. Sci.* 69: 663-672, 1985.

2. Belman, M.J., and C. Mittman. Ventilatory muscle training improves exercise capacity in chronic obstructive pulmonary disease pa-

tients. *Am. Rev. Respir. Dis.* 121: 273-280, 1980.

3. Borg, G., and B. Noble. Perceived exertion. In: Wilmore, J.H., ed. *Exercise and sports science reviews.* New York: Academic Press, 1974, vol. 2.

4. Bradley, G.W., and R. Crawford. Regulation of breathing during exercise in normal subjects and in chronic lung disease. *Clin. Sci. Molec. Med.* 51: 575-582, 1976.

5. Brown, S.E., R.C. Nagendron, and J.W. McHugh. Effects of a large carbohydrate load on walking performance in chronic air-flow obstruction. *Am. Rev. Respir. Dis.* 132: 960-962, 1985.

6. Bye, P.T.P., G.A. Farkas, and C. Roussos. Respiratory factors limiting exercise. *Annu. Rev. Physiol.* 45: 439-452, 1983.

7. Cherniack, R.M. The oxygen consumption and efficiency of respiratory muscles in health and emphysema. *J. Clin. Invest.* 38: 494-499, 1959.

8. Clark, T.J.H., S. Freedman, E.J.M. Campbell, and R. Winn. The ventilatory capacity of patients with chronic airway obstruction. *Clin. Sci.* 36: 307-316, 1969.

9. Cotes, J.E. *Lung function.* Oxford: Blackwell, 1972.

10. Davidson, J.T., B.J. Whipp, K. Wasserman, S.N. Koyal, and R. Lugliani. Role of the carotid bodies in the sensation of breathlessness during breath-holding. *N. Engl. J. Med.* 290: 819-822, 1974.

11. El-Manshawi, A., K.J. Killian, E. Summers, and N.L. Jones. Breathlessness during exercise with and without resistive loading. *J. Appl. Physiol.* 61: 896-905, 1986.

12. Grassino, A., D. Gross, P.T. Macklem, T. Roussos, and G. Zagelbaum. Inspiratory muscle fatigue as a factor limiting exercise. *Bull. Eur. Physiopathol. Respir.* 15: 105-111, 1979.

13. Hodgkin, J.E. Exercise testing and training. In: Hodgkin, J.E., and T.L. Petty, eds. *Chronic obstructive pulmonary disease.* Philadelphia: W.B. Saunders, 1987, p. 120-164.

14. Jones, N.L. Exercise testing in pulmonary evaluation: Rationale, methods, and the normal respiratory response to exercise. *N. Engl. J. Med.* 293: 541-544, 1975.

15. Jones, N.L., and L.B. Berman. Gas exchange in chronic air-flow obstruction. *Am. Rev. Respir. Dis.* 129(Suppl.): S81-S83, 1984.

16. Jones, N.L., G. Jones, and R.H.T. Edwards. Exercise tolerance in chronic airway obstruction. *Am. Rev. Respir. Dis.* 103: 477-491, 1971.

17. Jones, N.L., K.J. Killian, and D. Stubbing. The thorax in exercise. In: Roussos, C., and P.T. Macklem, eds. *The thorax*. New York: Marcel Dekker, 1985, part B, p. 627-662.

18. Kanarek, D., D. Kaplan, and H. Kazemi. The anaerobic threshold in severe chronic obstructive lung disease. *Bull. Eur. Physiopathol. Respir.* 14: 163-169, 1979.

19. Killian, K.J., and E.J.M. Campbell. Dyspnea. In: Roussos, C., and P.T. Macklem, eds. *The thorax*. New York: Marcel Dekker, 1985, part B, p. 787-828.

20. Killian, K.J., and N.L. Jones. The use of exercise testing and other methods in the investigation of dyspnea. *Clin. Chest Med.* 5: 99-108, 1984.

21. Leaver, D.J., and N.B. Pride. Flow-volume curves and expiratory pressures during exercise in patients with chronic airway obstruction. *Scand. J. Respir. Dis.* 77(Suppl.): 23-27, 1971.

22. Levine, S., P. Weiser, and J. Gillen. Evaluation of a ventilatory muscle endurance training program in the rehabilitation of patients with chronic obstructive pulmonary disease. *Am. Rev. Respir. Dis.* 133: 400-406, 1986.

23. Linnarsson, D. Dynamics of pulmonary gas exchange and heart rate at start and end of exercise. *Acta Physiol. Scand.* 415(Suppl.): 1-68, 1974.

24. Lugliana, R., B.J. Whipp, C. Seard, and K. Wasserman. The effect of bilateral carotid body resection in ventilatory control at rest and during exercise in man. *N. Engl. J. Med.* 285: 1105-1111, 1971.

25. Mead, J. Statics of the respiratory system. In: Fenn, W.O., and H. Rahn, eds. *Handbook of Physiology: Respiration*. Washington, DC: American Physiological Society, 1964, vol. 1, sect. 3, p. 387-410.

26. Mead, J., J.M. Turner, P.T. Macklem, and J.B. Little. Significance of the relationship between lung recoil and maximum respiratory flow. *J. Appl. Physiol.* 22: 95-108, 1967.

27. Nery, L.E., K. Wasserman, J.D. Andrews, D.J. Huntsman, J.E. Hansen, and B.J. Whipp. Ventilatory and gas exchange kinetics during exercise in chronic obstructive pulmonary disease. *J. Appl. Physiol.* 53: 1594-1602, 1982.

28. Otis, A.B. The work of breathing. *Physiol. Rev.* 34: 449-458, 1954.

29. Pardy, R.L., R. Rivington, P.J. Despas, and P.T. Macklem. The effects of inspiratory muscle training on exercise performance in chronic airflow limitation. *Am. Rev. Respir. Dis.* 123: 426-433, 1981.

30. Roussos, C., and J. Moxham. Respiratory muscle fatigue. In: Roussos, C., and P.T. Macklem, eds. *The thorax*. New York: Marcel Dekker, 1985, part B, p. 829-870.

31. Scharf, S., P. Bye, R. Pardy, and P.T. Macklem. Dyspnea, fatigue and second wind. *Am. Rev. Respir. Dis.* 129(Suppl.): S88-S89, 1984.

32. Sergysels, R., S. Degre, P. Garcia-Herreros, R. Willeput, and A. De Coster. Le profil ventilatoire a l'exercise dans les bronchopathies chroniques obstructives. *Bull. Eur. Physiopathol. Respir.* 15: 57-73, 1979.

33. Shephard, R.J. *Alive man! The physiology of physical activity*. Springfield, IL: Charles C Thomas, 1972, p. 105-161.

34. Wasserman, K., and R. Casaburi. Dyspnea: Physiological and pathophysiological mechanisms. *Annu. Rev. Med.* 39: 503-515, 1988.

35. Wasserman, K., J.E. Hansen, D.Y. Sue, and B.J. Whipp. *Principles of exercise testing and interpretation*. Philadelphia: Lea & Febiger, 1986.

36. Wasserman, K., D.Y. Sue, R. Casaburi, and R.B. Moricca. Selective criteria for exercise training in pulmonary rehabilitation. *Eur. Respir. J.* (in press).

37. Wasserman, K., A.L. Van Kessel, and G.G. Burton. Interaction of physiological mechanisms during exercise. *J. Appl. Physiol.* 22: 71-85, 1967.

38. Wasserman, K., B.J. Whipp, S.N. Koyal, and M.G. Cleary. Effect of carotid body resection in ventilatory and acid-base control during exercise. *J. Appl. Physiol.* 39: 354-358, 1975.

39. Whipp, B.J., and R. Pardy. Breathing during exercise. In: Macklem, P., and J. Mead, eds. *Handbook of physiology: Respiration (pulmonary mechanics)*. Washington, DC: American Physiological Society, 1986, p. 605-629.

Chapter 49

Exercise, Immunity, Cancer, and Infection

Leonard H. Calabrese

There is now convincing evidence of a positive correlation between physical activity and reduced overall mortality (34). These data reveal not only an expected protective effect of exercise on cardiovascular mortality (37) but also a less well understood protective effect in the development of certain forms of cancer (20, 22, 34, 39, 45). Given the recognized importance of the immune system in the defense against neoplasia, important questions now exist whether physiological fitness, which clearly is associated with adaptations in a wide variety of physiological systems, may also be associated with adaptation of the human immune response. This chapter attempts to analyze the link between exercise and immunity, its possible relationship to the development of cancer, and its role in the predisposition to infectious disease.

The Human Immune Response

Before one attempts to analyze the relationship between exercise and immunity, the precise role of the immune system in physiological homeostasis must be clarified. The most basic role of the immune system is to provide a system of surveillance for differentiating self from nonself. An examination of the clinical spectrum exhibited in patients with congenitally abnormal immune systems, or with primary immune deficiency diseases, can be revealing. Individuals born with defects of immune responsiveness appear to have two dominating clinical complications: infection and cancer. In addition to these complications, there also appears to be an increased incidence of autoimmune disease, probably resulting from a decreased ability to regulate the overall immune response. The increased incidence of infection observed in immunodeficiency states ranges from life-threatening infections

to very mild disease, depending on the nature and degree of immunodeficiency. In individuals who do not succumb to infective complication, there appears to be a dramatic increase in the incidence of certain forms of cancer, particularly those of the lymphatic system (36). Conversely, it can be reasoned that any modulation of the immune response in a positive or enhancing fashion could theoretically lead to a decreased incidence of cancer and a protective effect against infection. This is particularly relevant in light of numerous studies suggesting that physically active individuals have a decreased incidence of certain forms of cancer (19, 20, 22, 45) as well as the general feeling that exercise and training lead to an increased resistance to infection (3). Whether there is reason to believe that these observations and impressions are in any way related to a beneficial effect of exercise on the immune system is the subject of this chapter.

Several recent reviews have given timely and comprehensive summaries of our current state of knowledge of the human immune system for those who desire an account that is more detailed than in this brief overview (1, 10, 11, 17, 32). For purposes of our understanding, the immune system can be viewed as a compartmentalized system that originates from a pleuripotential stem cell. These primordial cells of immunity develop along alternative pathways either through the thymus, where they ultimately become thymus-derived (T) lymphocytes, or through the bone marrow, where they become bone-marrow derived (B) lymphocytes. Within the physical and hormonal milieu of the thymus, these stem cells undergo dedifferentiation into mature T cells, which can be identified by their ability to form rosettes with sheep red blood cells or, more recently, by one or more cell-surface antigens by monoclonal antibody. These T lymphocytes are primarily responsible for the cell-mediated immune response, which provides protection from a variety of viral, parasitic, mycobacterial, and other intracellular pathogens as well as participating in the delayed hypersensitivity reaction. These T cells are capable of secreting a wide variety of hormones known as *cytokines*, such as interleukin-2 and interferon, which are potent biological response modifiers with anticancer effects. The T cell is also capable of participating in specific cytotoxic reactions, thus possibly giving it a primary role in cancer surveillance; they also play key roles in immunoregulation.

Under the influence of bone marrow, stem cells develop into B cells, the progenitors of plasma cells, which produce antibody. These cells can be identified by immunoglobulin molecules on their surfaces and by a variety of B-cell-specific antigens. Antibody provides defense against the extracellular phase of a variety of infectious agents and serves a role in cytotoxicity when functioning in conjunction with non-T, non-B cells in a system known as *antibody-dependent cellular cytotoxicity* (ADCC). Antibody is also capable of activating the complement system, which has important phlogistic functions as well as potent antiviral and antitumor effects.

An additional line of immune defense is a system of cytotoxic cells known as natural killer (NK) cells. These cells can be of T-cell lineage or of non-T, non-B-cell derivation and are capable of spontaneously (without immunologic memory) killing a wide variety of targets, including tumors and infectious agents. These NK cells, as well as some T cells under the influence of T-cell-derived cytokines, are capable of participating in a form of cellular killing known as *lymphokine-activated killers* (LAK), which recently was shown to be of great importance in anticancer defense (39).

The mononuclear phagocytic system, once thought to provide only a scavenger function for immunologic debris, is now known to be an important part of the afferent limb of immunity. Cells of the monocyte-macrophage lineage serve to process antigen and present it to immunocompetent cells in the context of self-identifying histocompatibility antigens, thus triggering the immune response. These cells not only are capable of antigen presentation but also serve as effectors of phagocytosis and phagocytic killing and under the influence of certain cytokines can become potent members of the anticancer defense.

The complement system is a series of over 20 proteins that is capable of functioning in concert with antibody and other triggering mechanisms to produce inflammation and cellular lysis. It now appears that, in addition to these roles, the complement system in conjunction with immune complexes can be potent regulators of the human immune response.

Although this compartmentalized view of the immune system may appear artificial, it is clinically useful in understanding how external stimuli such as exercise and training influence its various limbs.

Cancer and Immunity

The process by which a cancer or neoplasm develops is not completely understood, but most theories take into account a basic two-step process by which a stem cell produces a genetically altered daughter cell that, during a subsequent division, gives rise to a cancerous cell with additionally altered genetic material. This cancer cell then replicates and eventually forms a tumor.

The signal or cue for this neoplastic process is unknown but can be thought of as resulting from an admixture of stimuli that includes both precancerous and anticancerous influences. These forces have been conveniently viewed as tumor initiators, promoters, or inhibitors. An initiating factor would be one that causes genetic damage directly to the stem cell or intermediate cell and would include such possible agents as chemical carcinogens or ionizing radiation. Promoters of malignancy probably act to enhance tumor growth of stem cells or intermediate cells and would include hormones such as estrogen, which influences the growth of endometrial cells that in certain individuals become cancerous. A number of mechanisms could also theoretically function to inhibit tumor cell growth by neutralizing the effects of initiators or promoters. Such examples of inhibitors include the screening or elimination of ultraviolet irradiation from the skin or the decrease in absorption of carcinogenic chemicals from the gastrointestinal tract.

The immune system, by virtue of its central role in the defense against the nonself, has been viewed by many as an important participant in the defense against cancer. Factors that suppress immunity could function as promoters by decreasing immune elimination of transformed cells or tumor-causing viruses. Alternatively, factors that boost immunity could theoretically inhibit tumor cell growth through enhanced immune surveillance.

A variety of immunologic mechanisms may be central to the defense against cancer. In the past, most theories of immune elimination of tumors have revolved primarily around T-cell-specific killing, which requires not only specificity but also immunologic memory. More recently, the roles of more spontaneously occurring cytotoxic cells, such as NKs and LAKs, have achieved equal if not greater importance in understanding certain tumors' defenses. The ability of the immune system to elaborate lymphokines appears also to be an important tumor defense. Interferons have profound biological effects that interfere with the replication of oncogenic viruses and, along with TNF, inhibit the growth of neoplastic cells. Interleukin-2 promotes the growth of cytotoxic T cells and stimulates the development of highly active LAK cells (11). These LAK cells are notable because they are capable of killing tumor cells both in vitro and in vivo (39).

The theory of immunologic surveillance (5), which states that the immune system serves as a primary defense against newly developing tumor cells by eliminating them before they can develop into cancerous tumors, is supported by many basic scientific and clinical observations. The theory, however, is not without its critics. Frequently cited evidence in favor of immune surveillance includes the increased susceptibility to malignancy in immunosuppressed and aged animals and in humans with primary and acquired forms of immune deficiency, immunosuppression occurring after administration of oncogenic viruses and carcinogens, enhancement of carcinogenesis in animals immunosuppressed by thymectomy, and the inhibition of carcinogenesis by immunostimulation or immune reconstitution.

Critics of immune surveillance cite the fact that if this theory is correct, then an increased incidence of all forms of cancer, not only certain types, would be observed, such as lymphomas and Kaposi's sarcoma. Supporters rebut that it is possible that all forms of tumors would ultimately develop in immunosuppressed hosts, but they die prematurely, and so this possibility is precluded. Another criticism argues that if immune surveillance is important, then tumors would naturally evolve in immunologically privileged areas, such as the anterior chamber of the eye and the brain. Defenders of the theory state that this is unlikely because of the low cell density and turnover in these areas and that lymphomas within the brain indeed are dramatically increased in individuals undergoing renal transplantation and immunosuppression (36).

From these data it is clear that immune function and the factors that lead to adaptation of immune responsiveness must be included in epidemiological analyses of cancer risk and development.

Exercise and Cancer

There is now strong evidence suggesting that exercise is beneficial to health from the prospective of reduced all-cause mortality. The clearest evidence of the protective effects of exercise is reduced cardiovascular disease (37). The suggestion that exercise also reduces mortality from cancer is a more recent one and represents a phenomenon that is decidedly more complex to clarify for a variety of reasons. Cancer, by its very nature, represents an admixture of site-specific diseases, each having highly varying clinical features and courses and probably being influenced by markedly different etiopathogenic factors. Despite these complexities, a growing amount of data suggest that exercise may be a strong influence in the occurrence of at least certain forms of cancer.

Currently, corroborating data from three separate groups support an inverse relationship between cancer of the colon and exercise. The first of these studies (20) examined 2,950 population-based colon cancer cases in males in southern California between 1972 and 1981. Occupational titles were rated as high, moderate, or sedentary to assess physical activity. Men with sedentary jobs had a relative risk of colon cancer 1.6 times that of men with high job intensities. It was interesting to note that this increase occurred in a stepwise manner as activity level decreased. The gradient was unaffected by socioeconomic class, race, or ethnic origin. There was no such relationship between physical activity and the risk of rectal cancer. Anatomically, the largest risk area was the descending colon. Sedentary individuals showed threefold increased risk of cancer of this area, and the relative risk decreased both proximally and distally along the large bowel.

The second study (22) examined the association between physical job activity and colon cancer over a 19-yr follow-up study of 1.1 million Swedish men. Physical activity was gauged by 245 occupational titles obtained from census data and classified according to physical job activity by two individuals with extensive experience in occupational classification who worked independently from each other and had no other link to the investigation. The relative risk of colon cancer in men employed in sedentary occupations was estimated at 1.3, that of men in the high-intensity-work classifications. Anatomically, the highest risk area was the transverse colon, including the flexures (relative risk 1.6), and the lowest risk area was the sigmoid colon (relative risk 1.2). As with the first study there was no increased relative risk for rectal cancer noted. Age, race, and social class were controlled for in this investigation.

The third study (45) examined two populations and came to similar conclusions. The first investigation was a case control study of patients admitted to the Rosewell Park Memorial Institute between 1957 and 1965 composed of 210 white males with cancer of the colon, 276 white males with cancer of the rectum, and 1,431 white males with non-neoplastic digestive disease. Within this group, they compared the amount of lifetime occupational physical activity as judged by lifetime occupational history among the study groups. Findings of this retrospective study appear to corroborate the findings of the other two in that there was an increased risk of colon but not rectal cancer in those with sedentary or light-physical-activity occupations. In a second investigation, they examined the published data of Milham (29) on the occupations and causes of death of 430,000 Washington State males from 1950 to 1979 and 25,000 Washington State females from 1974 to 1979. In this study the risk of cancer of the colon increased consistently with decreased physical activity as determined by job title. Again a strong, consistent association was not found with cancer of the rectum. A similar trend was noted among females, although the number of subjects engaging in strenuous job-related activity was quite small by comparison.

Although these studies demonstrated a strong influence of job-related physical activity on the occurrence of cancer of the colon in men, the recent study by Frisch et al. (19) showed an even more dramatic relationship in women between athleticism in college and the occurrence of cancer of the breast and reproductive organs. They surveyed 5,398 living alumnae, who graduated from 1925 to 1981, by a detailed questionnaire that assessed history of athleticism in college and the development of cancer. The authors stated that this study was suggested by type finding that strenuous exercise delays menarche and that women athletes have a higher incidence of oligomenorrhea and amenorrhea and tend to have lower total body fat than do nonathletes. Accordingly, these variables were examined in detail by their study tool. Following statistical correction for confounding variables such as age, history of pregnancy, family history of cancer, and ingestion of oral contraceptives or other hormones, the prevalence of cancers of the uterus, ovaries, cervix, vagina, and breast was consistently lower for the athletes than for the nonathletes. This study is particularly remarkable because it demonstrated a highly significant statistical correlation between athleticism during college and an event that is considered to have a time course of 20 yr or more.

Clearly, although these studies provide strong data suggesting a link between physical activity and cancer, they are subject to a number of methodological problems that must be kept in mind. Studies relating physical activity as assessed by job title (such as the physical activity data obtained in the Washington State study) must be reviewed with caution because the data were collected from death certificates and may not reflect total lifetime occupational history. It is always possible that workers who are ill in the final phases of their lives may take on more sedentary jobs and thus create a bias toward sedentary occupations in that group. Furthermore, those studies assessing job-related physical activity did not measure avocational physical activity, which could differ in the comparison groups. Also, the association of higher socioeconomic status with sedentary jobs needs to be considered in further studies on this subject. In the study by Frisch et al. (19) it is possible that women who were athletic in college did not continue with this lifestyle or that women who were sedentary in college did take on physically active lifestyles in later life. Additionally, not all studies examining the same question have reached similar conclusions. Paffenbarger et al. (33) did not find similar relationships between cancer of the colon and physical activity in longshoremen, although in their cohort study of college alumni they did find a statistically increased incidence of all cancers in the most sedentary group (34).

Although these studies support a strong link between exercise and cancer, they do not elucidate the mechanism whereby physical activity may protect one from neoplasia, and it is quite possible that markedly different mechanisms influence the predisposition to different types of cancer. Cancer of the colon and rectum, although the leading incident cancer in males and females combined, is not linked to strong risk factors; however, increased dietary fat may be important (31). Exercise could influence the exposure of the bowel to ingested fat by altering bowel habits, thus stimulating peristalsis and reducing transit time. Additionally, although the relationship of this cancer to serum lipids and lipoproteins is far from clear (40), exercise has a profound influence on these variables as well as on percent body fat. Physically active individuals (especially athletes) may eat significantly different diets, and this could impact on certain types of cancer, particularly those of the digestive system. Furthermore, individuals who keep physically active lifestyles, especially athletes such as those in the Frisch study, may take on other attributes, attitudes, and habits that may make them different for nonathletic individuals. These factors deserve further study.

Several other pathogenetic factors need to be considered regarding the association between physical activity and cancer of the reproductive organs in women. In general, cancers of the endometrium and breast are associated with early menarche, later menopause, and greater relative fatness and are opposite to the trend noted in the athletic group, who had significantly later menarche and earlier menopause and who were slightly but significantly leaner (19). These malignancies of reproductive organs are considered hormonally sensitive, and accordingly the athletes may have numerous influences acting on them that cause their hormonal milieus to be significantly different from those of their nonathletic counterparts. Fatness is associated with an increased extraglandular conversion of androgen to estrogen and the metabolism of estrogen to more potent forms that have been observed in association with cancer of the breast (41). Thus, the small but significant difference in leanness may be important.

Aside from these potential etiopathogenetic factors that may influence the occurrence of cancer in physically active individuals, the potential for physical activity to influence the immune response and possibly enhance tumor surveillance is a hypothesis that deserves serious consideration.

Exercise and Immunity

Any critical examination of published studies on exercise and immunity must carefully attempt to analyze a number of variables that potentially could influence results. The relatively few studies published in this area differ markedly in the methodologies used. The differences include the nature, intensity, and duration of exercise; the timing of sample collection for immunologic investigation; the techniques for evaluating immunologic responsiveness; and the use of trained versus untrained subjects. This discussion attempts to weigh these variables whenever possible.

Animal Studies

Animal studies that have examined the influence of exercise stress on immunity have revealed somewhat conflicting results. In a recent study (28) in which healthy mice were trained to run for 10 min twice per day over a prolonged period of time, antibody levels following immunization were compared with those of healthy, sedentary control mice. In this study the antibody titers of the running mice were 2.76 times that of controls. Alternatively, in another study (26) in which male mice were divided into several groups on the basis of different degrees of acute and chronic treadmill exercise splenic T cells were assessed for their responses to the mitogen concanavalin A. The exercised mice had significantly reduced splenic lymphocyte proliferation responses to concanvalin A compared with control animals, and the total number of lymphocytes per spleen was significantly lower in the exercised group. These results suggest that chronic exercise challenge in mice is associated with T-lymphocyte hyporesponsiveness and immunocyte depletion in a secondary lymphoid organ such as the spleen. Clinical interpretations of studies such as these must be made with great caution, as each looks at only one small aspect of immunologic responsiveness. It is interesting to note that a study (27) that examined the effects of exercise on longevity in rats found that those who exercised involuntarily on exercise wheels lived longer than do sedentary controls. Whether immunologic responsiveness is responsible for this phenomenon is not clear.

Human Studies: The Effects of Acute Exercise on Immunity

Polymorphonuclear Leukocyte Distribution and Function

When we consider the hemodynamic changes as well as the biochemical and endocrinologic adaptations to acute exercise, it is not surprising that a number of reports have documented marked alterations in the numbers and distribution of circulating leukocytes with acute physical stress. Most studies (16, 25, 30, 42), but not all of them (38), showed a transient rise in peripheral blood leukocytes that lasted for approximately 15-45 min following acute exercise. The transient nature of this leukocytosis may account for discrepancies in documenting this phenomenon in a number of studies. It appears that in conditioned subjects this postexercise leukocytosis is less pronounced than it is in untrained subjects (6). This phenomenon may be due to a greater rise in cortisone and epinephrine associated with acute physical stress in untrained individuals than that observed in their trained counterparts (38). Studies that examined the physiological function of polymorphonuclear leukocytes following exercise and that included assessments of the hexose monophosphate shunt pathway and the ability to kill bacteria failed to reveal any difference between conditioned and unconditioned subjects in the resting state (23). It does appear that the acute changes in circulating polymorphonuclear leukocyte distribution is a transient phenomenon occurring during and after acute exercise and that it is partially influenced by the conditioning level of the subject. It is doubtful, but not impossible, that such a brief leukocytosis can be responsible for significantly enhanced host defenses.

Lymphocyte Distribution and Function

Lymphocyte trafficking is also temporarily altered during and following acute exercise. A number of studies identified an acute lymphocytosis during and following a variety of forms of acute exercise (6, 38, 42, 49), and this phenomenon again appears to be more pronounced in untrained individuals (42). Robertson et al. (38) felt that the transient lymphocytosis observed in untrained individuals following exercise on a bicycle ergometer regressed coincidentally with a rise in serum cortisol, which has a known lymphopenic effect. Most investigation of lymphocyte subpopulation number and distribution observed that the lymphocytosis following acute exercise is due mainly to a rise in the non-T-cell fraction (2, 24, 25). Earlier studies that utilized nonspecific methodologies inferred from this observation that there was a rise of B cells following acute exercise (24, 25), but recent refinements in subpopulation identification demonstrated clearly that this rise is due primarily to non-T, non-B cells bearing NK phenotypic markers (2). Other studies observed also a transient depletion of T-helper cells with a reciprocal elevation of T-suppressor cells, resulting in a postexercise depression of the helper-to-suppressor ratio (4). The clinical significance of such cell trafficking is difficult to assess, but it could lead to a transient immunologic suppression due to a preponderance of suppressor cells over helper cells. This may not necessarily be so, as it is now known that both the helper cell and the suppressor cell populations can be subdivided into numerous functional subsets that display a variety of counterbalancing immunoregulatory forces. No data are currently available on the relative distribution and number of immunoregulatory T-cell subsets following acute physical exercise.

Lymphocyte function can be assessed by a variety of techniques, depending on the specific function

to be investigated. Humoral immunity can be assessed by the ability of B cells to proliferate to specific T-cell-independent antigens or B-cell mitogens (e.g., Staph aureus Cowan strain I), or by their ability to produce immunoglobulin in culture in response to a variety of stimuli. Cellular immunity can be examined by determining the ability of lymphocytes to respond to specific antigens, alloantigens, or mitogens by secreting cytokines, performing immunoregulatory functions, or proliferating or mediating cytotoxicity.

Studies that examined the effect of exercise on lymphocyte function are limited and appear to indicate clearly that, in addition to the previously described ability to alter the trafficking of lymphocytes, acute exercise also affects their functional capabilities. Studies performed in both trained and untrained subjects revealed varying results in the ability of lymphocytes to proliferate in response to antigen or mitogen immediately following acute physical exercise (6, 30, 38, 42). These data must be interpreted with caution because a postexercise lymphocytosis could alter the results if (a) studies are performed on whole-blood lymphocytes (6) rather than on isolated peripheral blood lymphocytes or (b) the data are expressed as the numbers of proliferating cells in peripheral blood (23) rather than as proliferative ability per cell. When these variables are taken into account, there appears to be a decreased ability of lymphocytes to proliferate to certain mitogens or antigens, at least for a brief period of time.

Cellular cytotoxicity is a complex phenomenon and may be divided into at least three types. The first, T-cell-mediated cytotoxicity, depends on recognition of self-MHC (major histocompatibility complex) gene products and is characterized by demonstrating immunologic memory and specificity. The second type, antibody-dependent cellular cytotoxicity (ADCC), is dependent on antigen recognition by an antibody and the adherence of the antibody to a lymphocyte of non-T, non-B lineage. The third type is mediated by NKs or LAKs, which are not dependent on recognition of MHC gene products, and is mediated by lymphocytes (frequently with large, granular morphologies) of both the T-cell and the non-T, non-B-cell lineages.

Although no studies have examined the effects of exercise on MHC-restricted T-cell-mediated cytoxicity, several studies have investigated both ADCC and NK functions. Hanson and Flaherty (24) and Hedfors et al. (25) both found significant increases in ADCC immediately following acute exercise that was still detected at 24 hr. In a detailed study of

NK function, Brahmi et al. (4) found significantly increased activity immediately following acute exercise that fell below baseline by 2 hr but that returned to normal by 24 hr postexercise. This study demonstrated that postexercise serum had no enhancing effect on this NK-cell activity and that these cells could still be stimulated by interferon, thus suggesting that this lymphokine was not responsible for the observed effect. They further demonstrated that binding of NK cells to their targets was maximal immediately following exercise, suggesting an influx of these types of lymphocytes. This observation is further supported by the study of Berk et al. (2), which demonstrated a significant rise in lymphocytes bearing NK markers immediately following acute exercise.

It thus appears that acute exercise has a transient effect on the ability of lymphocytes to proliferate but a more profound effect on enhancing at least two forms of cellular cytoxicity (i.e., ADCC and NK functions). The clinical significance of these observations is far from clear, but it is conceivable that frequent enhancement of cytotoxic mechanisms during, and then persisting after, acute exercise could be beneficial by enhancing host defenses from infections or neoplasia.

Immunoglobulins and Complement

Only a few studies have examined immunoglobulin concentrations following acute exercise, and none have found significant changes from the preexercise state (23, 24). However, Tomasi et al. (44) found that secretory IgA is depressed in the saliva of nationally ranked Nordic skiers and that this depression is further enhanced by a 50-km race. There was no depression of salivary IgG and no reports of increased respiratory infections in the group. The significance of this observation remains unclear.

Only two studies have examined the effects of exercise on complement components. Hanson and Flaherty (24) found no changes in C3 or C4 in 6 trained runners following an 8-mi race. Dufaux et al. (14) found that intense and prolonged exercise in the form of four 25-km runs per day is followed by elevations of C3 and C4, as well as an elevation of C-reactive protein by the third day that persisted to the end of the race. An additional observation is that these individuals demonstrated increased concentrations of C3 and C4 as well IgG in polyethylene glycol (PEG) precipitates, suggesting the presence of circulating immune complexes in response to severe physical exercise. These observed changes in acute-phase proteins, as well as the development of increased levels of circulating immune complexes, may merely reflect a reparative process in response to tissue injury.

Cytokines

Canon and Kluger (9) demonstrated that human subjects unselected for training elaborate an endogenous pyrogen-like substance immediately after, and for at least 3 hr following, 1 hr of cycling at 60% of maximum aerobic capacity. This substance has been subsequently characterized as a molecule with a 14,000 molecular weight and with the in vitro characteristics of interleukin-1 (IL-1) (8). Furthermore, unstimulated macrophages from 5 of these subjects were found to secrete this IL-1-like substance actively following but not before exercise. Further studies have confirmed the identity of this substance by antibody neutralization. The stimulus for this secretion is unclear but does not appear to be mediated by epinephrine (8).

Viti et al. (46) reported that exercise at 70% maximum oxygen consumption capacity in untrained men results in significant increases in plasma interferon activity that persist for at least 1-2 hr following exercise. This interferon rose only to modest levels (3 IU $\pm$ 1 preexercise to 7 IU $\pm$ 2 postexercise) and was characterized as an acid-labile interferon alpha. Although small in magnitude, this rise in plasma interferon could be clinically significant, as it may reflect a far greater concentration in the lymphoid microenvironment. This form of interferon is atypical because interferon alpha is mainly acid stabile, not acid labile. This form of interferon can be seen in a variety of conditions, including transiently during the course of a variety of viral infections, in sustained levels in connective tissue diseases, and during infection with the human immunodeficiency virus (HIV) (7).

Regarding this clear ability of acute exercise to induce transient release of IL-1 and interferon has a broad range of biological effects, including its presumed primary role in acting as a cofactor during lymphocyte activation. In addition, IL-1 is a potent mediator of the acute-phase response whose effects include the induction of fever; the synthesis of acute-phase proteins; and the release of ACTH, insulin, and neutrophils. Interleukin-1 is cytotoxic for some tumor cells as well and thus theoretically could serve to temporarily enhance resistance to infection and for certain types of neoplasia (12). Alternatively, this response may be only secondary to tissue injury induced by acute exercise and may play only a minor role in other capacities.

The interferon response to exercise is equally difficult to interpret in light of its low level and transient duration. Although interferon alpha acts to increase class 1 MHC molecules on lymphoid surfaces (11) it is also a potent stimulus for NK-cell activity, which has been observed to be increased during and following acute exercise (4, 43). Unfortunately, NK cells obtained following acute exercise are still able to be stimulated by exogenous interferon (4); whereas they would be expected to be interferon refractory if this was the physiological stimulus for their increased postexercise activity. Finally, it should be kept in mind that interferon alpha can act as a potent immunosuppressant (11), so its specific role in immunologic modulation in this setting is unknown.

Human Subjects: The Effects of Training on Immune Responsiveness

Although it is clear from the foregoing discussion that there is some form of immunologic adaptation to exercise, this should not be surprising, considering the cardiovascular, endocrinologic, and biochemical adjustments that occur with acute exercise. An important question that has yet to be answered is whether training can lead to a form of immunologic fitness that potentially affects the host in a beneficial or perhaps deleterious way. In contrast to studies that have examined the effects of acute or brief exercise in human immune responsiveness, confounding variables (e.g., features of lifestyle, diet, and heredity) are likely to be more influential when resting immunologic response in trained individuals is examined, as any observed difference of untrained controls would likely be quite small. The ideal study to address this question would include the serial assessment of a wide variety of immunologic functions that are generally considered to be clinically relevant to host defenses in an untrained cohort undergoing vigorous training with defined physiological end points. Not only the resting immunologic response but also the acute immunologic adaptations that occur in response to exercise at varying degrees of fitness would be assessed. Nutrition, as well as energy balance, would be rigidly controlled. These subjects would be compared to a sedentary control population that would also be studied serially and matched closely for environmental, lifestyle, and demographic features. Finally, this ideal study would examine clinical end points over a long period of time and an attempt to assess the host response to infectious in the development of malig-

nancies. Although this ideal study has yet to be performed (and for many reasons may never be performed), some data examine several of these issues.

Watson et al. (47) performed a detailed immunologic study of 15 sedentary men undergoing a carefully controlled 15-wk training program consisting of 50 min per d of aerobic exercise 5 d per wk. Immunologic studies were performed on several occasions in the resting state in both the pretraining and the posttraining period. A significant training effect was documented by improved maximal oxygen uptake in all subjects. This study documented that training was associated with a significant rise in circulating T lymphocytes from a baseline of 65 + 1.3% (SD to 74 + 1.4% (SD) of circulating lymphocytes. In addition, there was an increase in lymphocyte proliferation to the mitogens phytohemagglutinin and pokeweed that was detected not only by an increase in proliferating cell number but also by an increased proliferation per cell. Alternatively, NK activity dropped significantly with training from a mean lysis of target cells of 38.8 + 3.8% (SD) before to 29.3 + 3.2% (SD) after. No sedentary controls were studied and no clinical assessments performed. Curiously, as previously noted, the relative distribution of NK cells, as well as NK-cell activity, appears to be enhanced immediately following acute exercise (4, 43) and then followed by depression at about 2 hr with a return to baseline by 20 hr postexercise. Furthermore, in the only other study that has examined NK function in detail in both trained and untrained subjects (4), there was a tendency for lower NK function in trained individuals in the resting state. The reasons for these observed discrepancies are presently unknown.

Soppi et al. (42) examined the effect of training on acute immunologic adaptation to exercise by making 17 subjects undergo a 6-wk training period and then performing a variety of immunologic studies before and after exercise on a bicycle ergometer in the pre- and posttraining periods. Although exercise was associated with a transient leukocytosis and a rise in both T-cell and non-T-cell fractions by more than 100% before training, this decreased by 50% after training. The proliferative ability of peripheral blood lymphocytes in the presence of phytohemagglutinin and cocanavalin A remained the same in the trained and the untrained states, although this represented a lower proliferative response per cell. The authors interpreted these data as suggesting that training leads to a decreased ability to mobilize immunocompetent cells, but these fewer cells are capable of responding equally to the greater number mobilized when fitness is low. Finally, a single uncontrolled study of 20 marathon runners (23) assessed complete blood counts, T-cell and non-T-cell numbers, polymorphonuclear leukocyte number, phagocytosis and cytotoxicity, serum immunoglobulins, complement components C3, and C4 and factor B, and the proliferative ability of lymphocytes to phytohemagglutinin and pokeweed mitogens. These were performed in the resting state in 17 subjects and within 1 hr of a 10-mi run in 3 subjects. With the exception of 10 runners with slightly low lymphocyte counts (1,500/mm^3), no subjects were found to have results considered to be clinically abnormal. Although this study suffers from its lack of sedentary controls and statistical analysis, it is in agreement with a similar study performed on 6 trained runners in the resting period (24). Although these studies are limited and not totally in agreement with each other, this can be explained partially by the markedly different immunologic methodologies used over the 6-yr period in which they were conducted. Still, the most carefully controlled studies among these strongly suggest that physical conditioning by means of chronic exercise alters cellular immune functions.

The Clinical Consequences of Immunologic Adaptation to Exercise and Training

The physiological adaptations to exercise and training are heterogeneous, but some of the changes in biological systems that result from training (e.g., cardiovascular, lipoprotein, and body composition) have been clearly demonstrated to be beneficial to the host. If we assume that there is immunologic adaptation to exercise and training, a logical question is whether this resultant change affects the host in a beneficial or a deleterious manner. Teleologically, the immune system is present to provide continuous discrimination of self versus nonself and thus provides both protection from outside invasion from infections or toxins and a system of surveillance and elimination for endogenous tissues undergoing degenerative or neoplastic transformation. The immune system is not an autonomous unit but one that is intimately connected to a host of other biological systems (e.g., cardiovascular, endocrinologic, and neurological). Modulation of the immune system theoretically could be beneficial to the host by enhancing defenses against infection. This could result in less frequent or less severe infections with routine pathogens such as common respiratory and gastrointestinal viruses and the ubiquitous viral agents cytomegalovirus and Epstein-Barr virus. In addition, if the immune system is a critical factor in the surveillance against malignancy (as believed by many), then it may be reasoned that any positive adaptation may result in a lower frequency of cancer. Unfortunately, these types of clinical effects are extremely difficult to prove because the immune systems of most healthy individuals function quite well, providing prompt and effective defense against common pathogens, especially the ubiquitous viral infections mentioned previously. In addition, there is a marked individual variation in the number and intensity of common viral illnesses experienced during the course of a given year. Experimentally, individuals exposed to cold stress demonstrate no enhanced predisposition to infection with cold viruses (13), although no studies have examined predisposition to these infections following physical stress alone. Even more difficult to assess is the impact of immunomodulation of the development of cancer because, as previously stated, the process of neoplastic development may take many decades to occur, and different tumors are highly heterogeneous in their clinical presentations, courses, and predisposing factors. These factors suggest that any study examining the influence of physical training on cancer would take many decades to complete and be difficult to control.

Alternatively, immune adaptation to exercise and training could affect the host in a negative fashion by resulting in an immunologic response that is either deficient or disregulated or both. Again, to prove such an effect may be difficult if the resultant immunologic perturbation is relatively mild. Conceivably, a mild immunodeficiency may result only in the prolongation of a subclinical infection with common pathogens and thus may not be detected by clinical evaluations. Additionally, any suppression of immunologic defense against neoplasia may not be clinically detectable if it is specific for only certain tumors over an extremely prolonged period of time. It is also possible that immunologic adaptation to exercise and training could result in a disregulated immune response that affects the ability of the host to initiate or end a physiological immune response. This could result in heightened immunologic damage in the face of common infections (i.e., immune complex disease) or in the development of spontaneous autoimmune disease. Again, unless the effects are clinically profound, this type of adaptation would be difficult to detect.

Although there are no clear studies that address the question of the clinical effects of immunologic adaptation to exercise or training, there are a number of investigators who have examined limited aspects of this issue. Although popular opinion and the lay literature on exercise maintain that training enhances one's natural resistance to infection (3), there is little evidence of this from existing studies. This paucity may reflect the problem of the limited number of available studies on this subject as well as their experimental designs.

The animal studies previously referred to suggested that chronic exercise stress leads to a variety of immunologic adaptations of both humoral and cellular immunity (26, 28). None of these studies, however, addressed clinical end points with reference to resistance from infection or malignancy. Studies performed in animals with established infection have more often demonstrated a deleterious effect of exercise in the host's ability to clear such infections. Over 30 yr ago it was demonstrated that monkeys infected with poliomyelitis virus and subjected to chilling or marked physical activity close to the end of the incubation period increased sharply the incidence of quadriplegia and death when compared to animals kept at rest or not exposed to cold (48). In a separate study, Gatmaitan et al. (21) demonstrated that in mice with experimental Coxsackie virus B3 myocarditis forced swimming dramatically increased the severity of the infection as well as the viral load within the myocardium These studies may not necessarily be extrapolated to infectious diseases in general because the target organs assessed were physically active tissues and in these cases were themselves infected by the microorganisms. In general, most infectious diseases do not affect skeletal or myocardial muscle and thus may be affected differently by physical stress. Indeed, in a study by Friman et al. (18) that investigated the effects of strenuous, forced exercise on the course and complications and on the myocardial response and performance capacity of rats infected with tularemia, they found that exercise evoked normal training responses even during the generalized infection and no evidence of impaired host responses to the infections as assessed by bacterial counts in blood, liver, and spleen. Limited studies performed in humans have shown that rather strenuous physical exercise in the early convalescent phase of hepatitis may not cause relapse or prolong recovery time (15).

With the exception of several uncontrolled studies that asked trained athletes for subjective impressions of their individual predisposition to infection (23, 44), there is little other data that directly addresses training and predisposition to, or resistance from, infection. In a study of 61 conditioned athletes and 126 unconditioned controls, Douglas and Hanson (12) compared the frequency and severity of specific symptoms of upper-respiratory infection using a validated symptom checklist during a 9-wk period. The athletes were part of the crew team and had more frequent and more severe symptoms than did the control group ($p < 0.05$). The trained athletes saw a doctor and missed class more often than did the untrained controls. They interpreted these data as indicating that a high degree of exercise was associated with selected symptoms of upper-respiratory infection more frequently and with greater severity than it was in the corresponding control group.

This single, controlled observation has some popular support, as evidenced by the opinions of many team physicians who claim that their highly exercising athletes, particularly those at the college level, are often plagued with what they consider to be an unusual frequency and severity of mild infectious disease symptoms. Thus, although the issue is far from settled on the impact of training on host resistance to infection, there does not appear to be any evidence to support a greater resistance to infection at this time.

Finally, could the overall decreased incidence of all forms of cancer observed in physically active individuals (34), the significantly decreased incidence of cancer of the colon in physically active men (20, 22, 45), and the decreased incidence of cancer of the reproductive organs in collegiate women athletes (17) be explained on the basis of enhanced immunosurveillance? Data that support such a hypothesis clearly are lacking at present, and several lines of reasoning seem to suggest that this is not the most plausible explanation:

- Neoplasms that are observed most frequently in immunosuppressed individuals are those of lymphoreticular origin, and it would be suspected that individuals with heightened immunologic surveillance would show a significantly decreased incidence of these tumors when compared to those previously described.
- If heightened immunologic surveillance contributes to a decreased incidence of cancer, there should be observed a decrease in all forms of cancer, not only those of the colon and breast.
- These malignancies least frequently observed in physically active individuals (i.e., colon in

men and reproductive organs in women) are not those frequently associated with immunosuppression.

- Although immunologic adaptation to exercise and training appears to be a real phenomenon, those adaptations thus far described are inconsistent, frequently of small magnitude, and not associated with clear clinical implications.

Alternatively, in light of the general paucity of data published on this subject, there are arguments supporting the role for enhanced immunologic surveillance against malignancy induced by exercise and training:

- Studies performed thus far investigating immunologic adaptation as a function of exercise and training have been limited in number and largely flawed in design and have not utilized the most relative and sophisticated immunologic techniques to assess host defenses against malignancy.
- Observations identifying a significantly decreased incidence of only certain forms of tumors may reflect the fact that immune surveillance is not equally important for all types of cancer.
- The expected decrease in lymphoreticular neoplasms has not been observed in physically active individuals. It is possible that these cancers arise only in immunosuppressed individuals as the result of a complication of immunosuppression (i.e., lack of immunoregulation of lymphocyte proliferation) as opposed to lack of immunosurveillance.
- The protective effect of physical activity on immune surveillance may be at an extremely low threshold of physical activity, as described by Paffenbarger et al. (34), and of extremely small magnitude, limiting its detection in currently published studies.

Thus, in light of the fact that the data thus far reviewed are largely preliminary and controversial, it appears premature to discount totally the role of immunologic adaptation from exercise and training in altering host defenses to infections for malignancies.

Mechanisms

Regardless of the clinical impact of the immunologic adaptations to exercise and training, some consideration should be given to the possible mechanisms involved. First, it is clear that both exercise and training are associated with a variety of physiological events that can at least partially explain the acute immunologic changes observed with exercise. These include the elaboration of epinephrine, ACTH, cortisol, insulin, and the associated hemodynamic changes, all of which are capable of transiently modifying immunologic responsiveness by altering the trafficking and function of immunocytes. Less clear is how training could possibly affect immunologic responsiveness in the resting state. Among the physiological changes that occur with training, one of the more prominent is how the host stores and expends energy. This flow of energy has several key variables, including diet, the metabolism of ingested energy, and the expenditure of this energy. It has been known for decades that animals restricted in energy are resistant to certain forms of tumors, whereas those subjected to overnutrition have a higher incidence of cancer (35). Furthermore, animals mildly restricted in energy experience enhanced longevity associated with an increased immunologic reactivity and a decreased frequency of disease (35). It is conceivable that chronic conditioning leads to similar benefits to the host by maintaining a state of relative leanness and low total body fat. This phenomenon may have strong experimental and practical implications for athletes because diets vary dramatically among different sports in both caloric content and nutritional density and because all the studies that thus far have examined the effects of exercise on immunity have not considered diet as a potential variable. Clearly, future studies must consider not only diet but also energy expenditure and other variables including drugs and emotional stress that are known to impact on immune responsiveness.

References

1. Bach, B.H., and D. Sacks. Current concepts: Immunology, transplantation immunology. *N. Engl. J. Med.* 317: 489-498, 1987.
2. Berk, L.S., B. Nieman, S.A. Tan, S. Nehlson-Cannarella, W.C. Kramer, and M. Owens. Lymphocyte subset changes during acute maximal exercise [Abstract]. *Med. Sci. Sports Exerc.* 18: 706, 1986.
3. Portz, W. Running from infection. *Running World* 19: 78-79, 1984.
4. Brahmi, Z., J.E. Thomas, M. Park, M. Park, and J.R.G. Dowdeswell. The effect of acute

578   Calabrese

exercise on natural killer-cell activity of trained and sedentary human subjects. *J. Clin. Immunol.* 5: 321-328, 1985.

5. Burnet, P.M. The concept of immunologic surveillance. *Prog. Exp. Tumor Res.* 13: 1-12, 1970.

6. Busse, W.W., O.L. Anderson, P.G. Hanson, and J.D. Fots. The effect of exercise in the granulocyte response to isoproterenol in the trained athlete and unconditioned individual. *J. Allergy Clin. Immunol.* 65: 358-364, 1980.

7. Calabrese, L.H., M.R. Proffitt, L. Bocci, K.W. Easly, G. Williams, R. Valenzuela, B. Barna, M.K. Gupta, R.B. Davis, and J.D. Clough. Epidemiologic and laboratory evaluation of homosexual males from an area of low incidence for acquired immunodeficiency syndrome (AIDS). *Cleve. Clin. Q.* 53: 267-275, 1986.

8. Cannon, J.G., W.J. Evans, V.A. Hughes, G.N. Meredith, and C.A. Divarello. Physiologic mechanisms contributing to increased interleukin 1 secretion. *J. Appl. Physiol.* 61: 1869-1874, 1986.

9. Cannon, J.G., and M.O. Kluger. Endogenous pyrogen activity in human plasma after exercise. *Science* 220: 617-618, 1983.

10. Cooper, M.D. Current concepts: B lymphocytes, normal development and function. *N. Engl. J. Med.* 317: 1452-1456, 1987.

11. Dinarello, C.A., and J.W. Mier. Current concepts: Lymphokines. *N. Engl. J. Med.* 317: 440-496, 1987.

12. Douglas, D.J., and P.G. Hanson. Upper respiratory infection in the conditioned athlete [Abstract]. *Med. Sci. Sports.* 10: 55, 1978.

13. Douglas, G.R., K.M. Lindgren, and D.B. Couch. Exposure to cold environment and rhinovirus common cold. *N. Engl. J. Med.* 279: 742-747, 1968.

14. Dufaux, B., K. Höffken, and W. Hollman. Acute phase proteins and immune complexes during several day of severe physical exercise. In: Knuttgen, H.G., ed. *Biochemistry of Exercise.* Champaign, IL: Human Kinetics, 1983: pp. 356-362.

15. Edlund, A. The effect of defined exercise on the early convalescence of viral hepatitis. *Scand. J. Infect. Dis.* 3: 189-196, 1971.

16. Eskola, J., O. Ruuskane, E. Soppi, M.K. Viljaner, M. Järvinen, H. Toivoren, and K. Kouvalainen. Effect of stress on lymphocyte transformation and antibody formation. *Clin. Exp. Immunol.* 32: 339-345, 1978.

17. Frank, M.M. Current concepts: Complement in the pathophysiology of human disease. *N. Engl. J. Med.* 316: 1525-1530, 1987.

18. Friman, G., N.G. Ilbäck, W.R. Beisel, and D.J. Crawford. The effects of strenuous exercise on infection with *Francisella tularensis* in rats. *J. Infect. Dis.* 145: 706-714, 1982.

19. Frisch, R.E., G. Wyshak, N.L. Albright, T.E. Albright, I. Schiff, K.P. Jones, J. Witschi, E. Shiang, E. Koff, and M. Marguglio. Lower prevalence of breast cancer and cancers of the reproductive system among former college athletes compared to non-athletes. *Br. J. Cancer* 52: 885-891, 1985.

20. Garabrant, D.H., J.M. Peters, T.M. Mack, and L. Bernstein. Job activity and colon cancer risk. *Am. J. Epidemiol.* 119: 1005-1014, 1984.

21. Gatmaitan, P.G., J.L. Chuson, and A.M. Lerner. Augmentation of the virulence of murine coxsackie-virus-B3 myocardiopathy by exercise. *J. Exp. Med.* 131: 1121-1136, 1970.

22. Gerhardsson, M., S.E. Norell, H. Kiviranta, N.L. Pedersen, and A. Ahlbom. Sedentary jobs and colon cancer. *Am. J. Epidemiolo.* 123: 775-780, 1986.

23. Gren, R.J., S.S. Kaplan, B.S. Rabin, C.L. Stanitski, and U. Zdziarski. Immune function in the marathon runner. *Ann. Allergy.* 47: 73-75, 1981.

24. Hanson, P.G., and D.K. Flaherty. Immunological responses to training in conditioned runners. *Clin. Sci.* 60: 225-228, 1981.

25. Hedfors, E., G. Holm, and B. Öhnell. Variations of blood lymphocytes during work studied by cell surface markers, DNA synthesis and cytotoxicity. *Clin. Exp. Immunol.* 24: 328-335, 1976.

26. Hoffman-Goetz, L., R. Keier, R. Thorne, and M.E. Housten. Chronic exercise stress depresses splenic T lymphocyte mitogenesis in vitro. *Clin. Exp. Immunol.* 66: 551-557, 1986.

27. Holloszy, J.O., K.K. Smith, and M. Vinins. Effects of voluntary exercise on the longevity of rats. *J. Appl. Physiol.* 58: 826-831, 1985.

28. Liu, Y.G., and S.Y. Wang. The enhancing effect exercise on the production of antibody to Salmonella typhi in mice. *Immunol. Lett.* 14: 117-120, 1987.

29. Milham, S. *Occupational mortality in Washington State, 1950-1979.* (PHHS [NIOSH] Publication No. 83-161). Washington, DC: U.S. Government Printing Office, 1983.

30. Moorthy, A.V., and S.W. Zimmerman. Human leukocyte response to an endurance race. *Eur. J. Appl. Physiol.* 38: 271-276, 1978.

31. Nauss, K.N., L.R. Jacobs, and Newperne, R.M. Dieting, fat and fiber relationship to caloric intake, body growth and colon tumorgenesis. *Am. J. Clin. Nutr.* 45: 243-251, 1987.

32. Nossal, G.J.V. Current concepts: The basic components of the immune system. *N. Engl. J. Med.* 316: 1320-1325, 1987.

33. Paffenbarger, R.S., R.T. Hyde, and A.L. Wing. Physical activity and incidence of cancer in diverse populations: A preliminary report. *Am. J. Clin. Nutr.* 45: 312-317, 1987.

34. Paffenbarger, R.S., R.T. Hyde, A.L. Wing, and C.-c. Hsieh. Physical activity, all-cause mortality of college alumni. *N. Engl. J. Med.* 314: 605-613, 1986.

35. Pariza, M.W., and R.K. Boutwell. Historical perspective: Calories and energy expenditure in carcinogenesis. *Am. J. Clin. Nutr.* 45: 151-156, 1987.

36. Penn, I. The occurrence of malignant tumors in immunosuppressed states. *Prog. Allergy* 37: 259-300, 1986.

37. Protective effect of physical activity on coronary heart disease. *MMWR* 36: 426-429, 1987.

38. Robertson, A.J., K.C.R.B. Ramesar, R.C. Potts, J.H. Gibbs, M.C.K. Browning, R.A. Brown, P.C. Hayes, and J.S. Beck. The effect of strenuous physical exercise on circulating blood lymphocytes and serum cortisol levels. *J. Clin. Lab. Immunol.* 5: 53-57, 1981.

39. Rosenberg, S.A., M.T. Lotze, L.M. Muul, S. Leitman, A.E. Chang, S.E. Ettinghausen, Y.L. Matory, J.M. Skibber, E. Shiloni, J.T. Vetto, C. Seipp, C. Simpson, and C.M. Reichert. Special report: Observation of the systemic administration of autologous lymphokine-activated killer cells and recombinant interleukin-2 to patients with metastatic cancer. *N. Engl. J. Med.* 313: 1485-1492, 1985.

40. Sidney, S., G. Friedman, and R.A. Hiatt. Serum cholesterol and large bowel cancer: A case control study. *Am. J. Epidemiol.* 124: 33-38, 1986.

41. Siiteri, P.K. Adipose tissue as a source of hormones. *Am. J. Clin. Nutr.* 45: 277-282, 1987.

42. Soppi, E., P. Varjo, J. Eskola, and L.A. Laitinen. Effect of strenuous physical stress on circulating lymphocyte number and function before and after training. *J. Clin. Lab. Immunol.* 8: 43-46, 1982.

43. Targan, S., L. Britvan, and F.R. Dorey. Activation of human NKCC by moderate exercise: Increased frequency of NK cells with enhanced capability of effector target lytic interactions. *Clin. Exp. Immunol.* 45: 352-360, 1981.

44. Tomasi, T.B., F.B. Trudeau, D. Czerwinski, and S. Erredge. Immune parameters in athletes before and after strenuous exercise. *J. Clin. Immunol.* 2: 173-178, 1982.

45. Vena, J.E., S. Graham, M. Zielezny, J. Brasure, and M.K. Swanson. Occupational exercise and risk of cancer. *Am. J. Clin. Nutr.* 45: 318-327, 1987.

46. Viti, A., M. Muscettola, L. Paulesu, V. Cocci, and A. Almi. Effect of exercise on plasma interferon levels. *J. Appl. Physiol.* 59: 426-428, 1985.

47. Watson, R.P., S. Moriguchi, J.C. Jackson, L. Werner, J.H. Wilmore, and B.J. Freund. Modification of cellular immune functions in humans by endurance exercise training during β-adrenergic blockade with atenolol on propranolol. *Med. Sci. Sports Exerc.* 18: 95-100, 1986.

48. Weinstein, L. The influence of muscular fatigue, tonsilloadenoidectomy and antigen injections on the clinical course of poliomyelitis. *Boston Med. Q.* 3: 11-16, 1952.

49. Yu, D.T.Y., P.J. Clements, and C.M. Pearson. Effects of corticosteroids on exercise-induced lymphocytosis. *Clin. Exp. Immunol.* 28: 326-331, 1977.

Chapter 50

Discussion: Exercise, Immunity, Cancer, and Infection

Harvey B. Simon

It is indeed a pleasure for me to discuss the review presented by Dr. Leonard Calabrese. His contribution is notable for its elegant and lucid review of the human immune system, for its scholarly summary of the effects of exercise on immunologic mechanisms and cancer risk, and above all for its balanced and sensible conclusions. Let me say at the outset that I agree entirely with those conclusions.

The health consequences of exercise have only recently begun to receive the attention and study they deserve. Yet among the many interactions between exercise and health, the interplay of exercise, immunity, infection, and cancer has received relatively little attention. Although we have much to learn in these important areas, Dr. Calabrese has provided an admirable summary of our current knowledge. Rather than reiterate his review, I restrict my discussion to three areas: First, I offer some brief comments about specific aspects of the interactions between exercise and immunity. Second, I step back and offer some speculations about the big picture, about the likely biological and clinical significance of these phenomena. Finally, I consider the other side of the coin, or how exercise may affect the patient who already has a malignancy or an infection.

Exercise and Immune Function

There is no question that exercise and training can affect immunologic function, at least as measured by a variety of in vitro assays (34, 36). Dr. Calabrese has reviewed many of the pertinent studies in this area, but two additional mechanisms merit consideration.

First, there is a small but growing body of evidence that there are complex interactions between the central nervous system and the immune system. The influence of psychosocial stress on the immune system and on susceptibility to infections, neoplasia, and autoimmune disorders is the subject of ongoing experimental and clinical study. Although much remains to be learned, it appears that a variety of neuroendocrine hormones including corticosteroids, endorphins, interferon, interleukin-1, and catecholamines may mediate bidirectional interactions between the central nervous system and the immune system (19, 32).

Most studies have focused on psychosocial stress or adversive physiological stimuli (such as electric shocks) in studying neuroimmunologic interactions. Although exercise is a very different form of stress, many of these same neuroendocrine transmitters are stimulated by exercise. Interestingly, exercise and psychological stress have been shown to produce a similar rise in blood lymphocyte and monocyte counts, although only the physical stress of exercise causes a significant elevation of plasma catecholamines and of granulocyte counts (23). Additional studies of exercise, neuroendocrine mechanisms, and immunity would be worthwhile.

The second area of interest is the interaction of cytokines, hyperthermia, and host defense against infections and neoplasia. Dr. Calabrese cited two studies (4, 5) that demonstrated that exercise provokes the production and release of interleukin-1 (IL-1). Although these observations are based on small studies, they provide a potentially important link between exercise and host defense mechanisms. Interleukin-1 is an immunostimulator, increasing the activity of both T and B lymphocytes; hence, exercise-induced production of IL-1 might account for the lymphocyte activation reported in other exercise studies and could potentially enhance host defense mechanisms in athletes. In addition, IL-1 mediates the acute-phase response to infection and inflammation; in this capacity, it produces leukocytosis and could therefore be a contributing factor in the leukocytosis of exercise.

Interleukin-1 stimulates hepatic synthesis of acute-phase proteins, including fibrinogen, and is probably responsible for the elevated erythrocyte sedimentation rate observed in many infectious inflammatory states. If IL-1 levels were persistently elevated by exercise, one might expect to find increased erythrocyte sedimentation rates in highly trained athletes. In a small study (observations unpublished) of healthy men engaged in marathon training, I found erythrocyte sedimentation rates normal both at rest and after strenuous running. This indirect observation certainly does not negate the importance of IL-1 in the immunologic response to exercise, but it does underline the need for further studies in this interesting area.

Interleukin-1 and other cytokines, including tumor necrosis factor (TNF) and interferon, are pyrogens, peptide hormones which are carried in the circulation to the anterior hypothalamus, where they act on the thermal control center to produce the vasoconstriction, cessation of sweating, and increased skeletal muscle tone that collectively elevate body temperature (10). Like IL-1, the other cytokines have multiple biological activities; TNF has antitumor activities that can be demonstrated in vivo and in vitro (1). It would be interesting to know whether exercise stimulates host cells to produce and release TNF as it does IL-1 and interferon.

It is possible that cytokines produced during exercise contribute to the elevated body temperature observed during exertion. It is much more likely, however, that the increased metabolic activity of skeletal muscle is the predominant cause of exercise hyperthermia (37). But whatever its genesis, the hyperthermia that accompanies strenuous exertion deserves consideration as a possible defense mechanism in its own right. Elevated temperature per se can enhance recovery from infection of some experimental animals (37), but the effects of pyrexia on clinical host defense in humans remain speculative. Also speculative but warranting mention in the present context is the observation that hyperthermia may play a role in host defense against certain neoplasia (3).

Neuroimmunologic phenomena, cytokine production, and hyperthermia may provide additional links between exercise, immunity, infection, and cancer. But, like the mechanisms reviewed by Dr. Calabrese, the importance of these areas remains conjectural, and further study is required.

Exercise and Host Defense: Clinical Significance

There are many intriguing interactions between exercise and the immune system. In the case of exercise and cancer the available studies are epidemiological, whereas in the case of exercise, immunity, and infection the investigations are based largely on in vitro assays. Although studies have demonstrated the statistical significance of these interactions, the question before us now is a bit different: Are these interactions biologically and clinically significant?

There are no data that suggest an overall relationship between exercise and cancer risk. Nor is this surprising in view of the biological heterogeneity of malignant diseases and the multiple genetic, immunologic, and environmental factors involved in oncogenesis. But, as noted by Dr. Calabrese, there is evidence that exercise decreases the risks of colon cancer (especially in men) and of breast and reproductive cancer in women.

The case for protection against colon cancer is particularly persuasive to me because studies in five different population groups have reached similar conclusions: the three studies reviewed by Dr. Calabrese (16, 17, 39) and an additional study in the European literature (22). All these studies rely on job description for evaluation of energy output; this technique has correlated well with other methods of analysis for the study of exercise and cardiovascular disease, and I believe it is valid here also. We should note, however, that Paffenbarger et al. (27) did not report similar results in their studies of longshoremen and college alumni; more data will be needed to resolve this disparity. At the present I believe that the best evidence suggests that physical activity does protect against colon cancer.

I agree with Dr. Calabrese that the mechanism of such protection is likely to be nonimmunologic. Exercise decreases intestinal transit time (21), and I suspect that this is the mechanism of protection. It is possible also that differences in dietary fiber and fat intake may contribute to the decreased risk of colon cancer in physically active individuals. Obesity appears to increase the risk of colon cancer in men (33) and could contribute to the increased risk observed in sedentary populations. Future studies should investigate these questions and provide more precise evaluations of lifetime vocational and recreational exercise levels in the study subjects.

With regard to cancer of the breast and female reproductive tract, Frisch et al. (14) have presented impressive data suggesting that college athleticism confers substantial protection against the subsequent development of these malignancies. It should be noted that the Washington State study (39), cited by Dr. Calabrese for its data on colon cancer, also shows that women with sedentary jobs are at higher risk for breast cancer than are physically active women. However Paffenbarger et al. (27) studied 4,706 college alumnae but did not find a decreased risk of breast cancer in the physically active women.

The study by Frisch et al. (14) carefully controlled for age, family history of cancer, age at menarche, number of pregnancies, body composition, smoking, and hormone use without finding that any of these variables explain the protective effects of exercise. The study did not control carefully for diet. Although dietary fat intake does not correlate with breast cancer risk (41), alcohol intake does increase risk (31, 42) and should be evaluated in future studies.

On the basis of the available evidence, I think it likely that exercise, particularly if initiated early in the reproductive years, confers protection against breast and reproductive tract cancers in females. The mechanism is probably hormonal and depends on decreased estrogen levels, which result in less end-organ stimulation.

It would be interesting to know whether exercise protects men against hormonally sensitive neoplasia. Two studies (27, 39) include data that suggest that this is not the case with regard to prostate cancer. However, although acute exercise transiently elevates testosterone levels (40), high exercise levels are required to affect gonadotropin secretion (25) and to depress resting testosterone levels (20). Hence, studies of prostate cancer and benign prostatic hypertrophy in very active men seem worthwhile.

While discussing hormonally sensitive neoplasia, we should pause for a moment to issue a reminder to our colleagues in sports medicine. Unfortunately, many athletes still abuse androgenic steroids and are thereby exposed to an increased risk of hepatic neoplasia. Finally, on quite a different clinical note, we should remind outdoor athletes to avoid excessive exposure to the sun and to block ultraviolet radiation with sunscreens to reduce the risk of skin cancer.

In summary, it appears that exercise may exert a clinically significant protective influence, albeit indirectly, on cancers of the colon, breast, and female reproductive tract. But when we turn to exercise, immunity, and infection, the biological significance of the currently available studies is much less clear.

Whereas the studies of exercise and cancer are epidemiological investigations of large numbers of subjects, the studies of exercise and immunity depend on in vitro assays of blood samples from small numbers of subjects. Because of this difference, it is much more difficult to extrapolate from the immunologic studies to clinical medicine.

In most investigations, the immunologic effects of exercise are both modest and transitory. Some studies report findings that contradict other observations; even if we explain such disparities by obvious differences in immunologic methods and exercise protocols, we are left with a very inconclusive picture. I think the reason for this may be in the nature of the immune system itself. One of the great beauties of the intact immune network of humans is that it is self-modulating. Hence, the changes produced by exercise will be met by homeostatic counter-regulation, which restores the status quo.

The in vitro studies cited by Dr. Calabrese support this hypothesis, and several additional papers underline the point. For example, the exercise-induced increase in IL-1 is brief, with peak elevations at 6 hours and a prompt return to baseline levels (6). Similarly, not only is the granulocytosis of exercise brief, but during very prolonged exertion leukocyte counts return to preexercise values even while the exercise itself continues (15). In addition, exercise-induced depressions of salivary 1gA and IgM levels are transient, lasting less than 24 hr (26). Finally, whereas some observers (2) report a decrease in NK-cell activity immediately after exercise, others (38) report a rise in NK-cell activity only to be followed by an equally transient depression that may be caused by an overshoot of homeostatic down-regulatory mechanisms.

Although in vitro studies of the immunology of exercise are very interesting, I suspect that the phenomena they record have statistical significance but not biological significance. As I have already noted, my skepticism is based on the modest magnitude and brief duration of these changes. Of course, this is only supposition on my part, and clinical investigations are needed to resolve the question.

At the present, such studies are sadly lacking. Dr. Calabrese cited a few anecdotes that suggested enhanced "resistance" to infection in athletes, so I feel free to add my own. Despite my professional activities as an infectious disease consultant, I have run for more than 3,800 consecutive days, covering over 43,000 mi, without developing a significant febrile illness. My body might lead me to testify that exercise helps prevent infection, but my mind tells me that this anecdote is not scientifically valid. In fact, the very few objective observations now available suggest opposite conclusions, though they too are methodologically limited.

In an abstract published 10 yr ago, Douglas and Hanson (11) reported that symptoms of upper respiratory tract infection (URI) were more common in members of a college crew team than in their unconditioned classmates. However, fever was equally prevalent in the athletes and the control students. Moreover, although the athletes missed class more often, the controls missed ROTC practice more often, so the functional importance of these observations is uncertain. More recently, Linde (24) studied 44 elite Danish orienteers and age-matched sedentary control subjects over a 1-yr period. The athletes reported more self-diagnosed upper-respiratory infections than did the controls; the difference was statistically significant ($p < .05$). But here too the clinical significance of the data is unclear, as the athletes experienced only 2.5 infections per year and the controls 1.7, and the infections did not differ in severity or duration.

When confronted with such a paucity of data, our usual response is to argue that more studies are needed. Indeed, we cannot draw any firm conclusions about the effects of exercise on immunity and infection without new investigations. However, although I am personally very curious about these interactions, I am not certain that such studies would repay the effort and expense required to do them well, because I suspect that exercise has a relatively minor clinical impact on the risk of developing an infection.

Exercise and the Patient With Cancer or Infection

Thus far I have followed Dr. Calabrese's lead in considering the ways in which exercise may influence the risk of developing cancer or infection. Now I consider the other side of the coin: What are the benefits and risks of exercise in the patient who already has a malignancy or an infection?

To the best of my knowledge, there are no data dealing with the effects of systematic exercise programs on patients with cancer. On the basis of the immunologic and epidemiological factors that Dr. Calabrese and I have discussed, there is little reason to think that exercise per se will help retard the growth of established neoplasia. But there is more to recovery than the control of tumor cells. Depression, fatigue, and diminished function are characteristic responses of many cancer patients, and these symptoms often are much more prominent than one would expect from the extent of the tumor itself. I believe that exercise programs might help alleviate such symptoms in many cancer patients and improve their quality of life in conjunction with critically important medical, surgical, or radiological therapies. Needless to say, exercise programs in these patients must be based on individualized medical evaluation and exercise prescription; sicker patients would also need exercise groups and medical supervision.

We can all cite inspiring examples of amateur and professional athletes who performed splendidly after recovering from cancer. Their examples are an inspiration to cancer patients, and we should learn whether their exercise regimens, when scaled down to individual capacities, could be helpful as well. Exercise programs have produced dramatic psychological, functional, and physiological improvements in cardiac patients, and I believe that exercise in cancer patients deserves systematic study.

Despite the intriguing in vitro immunological data that Dr. Calabrese and I have reviewed, there is little theoretical reason to expect that exercise would assist in recovery from infection, and there are no clinical data to suggest that it does. But there is some important, if incomplete, information about the interactions between exercise and established infections.

Bed rest is part of the traditional regimen that we prescribe for patients with infection. Indeed, in the case of serious, acute infectious processes such advice seems prudent. But in the case of certain subacute or chronic viral infections, prolonged bed rest may produce significant deconditioning and result in weakness and fatigue. All too often fatigue is interpreted by the well-meaning physician as the persistence of an active infection, and the prescription is more rest. The cycle that results can lead to remarkably prolonged debility.

The classic infections in this category are viral hepatitis and infectious mononucleosis. Bed rest is the traditional treatment for hepatitis. More than 30 yr ago, however, Chalmers et al. (7) showed that soldiers with hepatitis who were allowed free activity recovered as quickly as did men who were confined to bed. In 1971 Edlund (13) demonstrated that 6 d of bicycle ergometry did not affect recovery from viral hepatitis, and in 1987 Graubaum et al. (18) showed that 6 wk of training did not alter recovery from acute hepatitis. As a result, it seems quite safe to allow patients with hepatitis to be guided only by symptoms in selecting their own activity levels.

Much the same is true of mononucleosis. In 1964 Dalrymple (8) studied 131 consecutive Harvard students with infectious mononucleosis. Students who were randomized to strict bed rest actually recovered more slowly than did those randomized to unrestricted activity schedules. I allow patients with uncomplicated mononucleosis to remain as active as symptoms permit. In the case of competitive athletes, about 3 wk of rather modest exercise levels should generally precede the resumption of active training. However, because of the risk of splenic rupture, contact sports should not be allowed until splenomegaly has resolved. Finally, although I am not at all sure that so-called chronic mononucleosis exists, I have had some success using graded endurance exercise to reduce fatigue in patients with postinfectious asthenia (the so-called chronic fatigue syndrome).

Exercise appears safe in certain subacute or chronic viral infections, such as mononucleosis and hepatitis. But can exercise have deleterious effects in acute infectious processes? Unfortunately, direct clinical observations are lacking. Popular lore, however, holds that exposure to cold weather decreases resistance to infection; if this were true, winter sports might predispose to respiratory infections. However, a careful study (12) of the results of cold exposure on rhinovirus infection in humans failed to demonstrate any such effects. However, in a very different animal study (29), forced swimming did increase the severity of myocarditis in mice with experimental Coxsackie B-3 virus infections, and the exercise predisposed to cardiomyopathy in surviving animals. These studies were performed with young, vulnerable animals experimentally inoculated with a cardiotropic virus and then forced to swim in heated water. I agree with Dr. Calabrese that this model is very unlike human exercise and infection, but I am a bit more concerned than he is about the risk of myocarditis in humans. Myocarditis is an uncommon cause of sudden death in athletes (35) but is a recognized cause of sudden death during exertion of military recruits (28). These observations should have a sobering effect in athletes who have systemic viral infections.

Can infection adversely effect athletic performance? Here, the widespread anecdotal observations of physicians, coaches, and athletes are supported by experimental (9) and clinical studies (30). Systemic infections do indeed impair physical performance. Clearly, athletes with constitutional symptoms of infection should not be expected to exercise in competition. Even strenuous training should be discouraged because an optimal effort cannot be expected. Moreover, although Linde (24) did not note an increased risk of athletic injury during respiratory infections, I am still concerned that an impairment of strength, endurance, coordination, or concentration during infection could predispose to musculoskeletal injury during exercise.

In practical terms, what can we tell the athlete about exercise in the presence of infection? Mild URIs do not generally require interruptions of exercise schedules; even competitive sports and exposure to cold ambient temperatures may be permitted if the athlete feels well enough to perform. In fact, some athletes who exercise with URIs report symptomatic relief that is probably due to the increased mucus flow associated with exercise. A word of caution may be in order, however, about the use of typical cold remedies, as many of these contain sympathomimetic agents that might cause tachycardia and that could disqualify athletes from high-level competitive events.

In contrast to mild URIs, lower respiratory tract infections may produce bronchospasm, which can be further exaggerated by exercise, especially in cold weather. Thus, it would seem prudent for athletes with these infections to avoid strenuous exertion until recovery has occurred.

Because of the theoretical concern about myocarditis, it also seems prudent to avoid vigorous exertion in the presence of fever, myalgias, and other constitutional symptoms suggestive of systemic infection. Because athletes are notably resistant to such advice, the physician should point out the potential risks of exercise in these circumstance and suggest gentle stretching exercises and strategy sessions as substitutes for intense training until the infection has subsided. And, if the infection-induced layoff is even moderately prolonged, the athlete should be encouraged to resume training at a relatively modest level and to progress only gradually.

It is clear that we have much to learn about the immunologic response to exercise. But even now we know enough to suggest important questions for future biological, clinical, and epidemiological study. And our present knowledge is secure enough to provide a foundation for practical advice to our patients, ranging from individuals with cancer to competitive athletes.

Conclusion

Immunologic Effects of Exercise

A variety of in vitro assays can be used to demonstrate that exercise affects host defense mechanisms including granulocyte counts, lymphocyte counts and functions, cytotoxicity, cytokine production, and secretory immunoglobulin levels. In general, however, these changes are small in magnitude and brief in duration. The biological significance of these phenomena is uncertain.

Exercise and Cancer

Epidemiological studies in five different population groups demonstrated a significantly decreased risk of colon cancer in physically active individuals. Further studies are needed to elucidate the mechanism of this protection; decreased intestinal transit time and lifestyle alterations such as differences in dietary fiber intake are the likely explanations.

A carefully performed epidemiological study demonstrated major reductions in breast and reproductive tract cancer in women who were athletic during their college years. Further studies are needed to confirm this observation, to quantify the intensity and duration of exercise needed to confer protection, and to control for alcohol intake. The mechanism of protection is likely to be decreased estrogenic stimulation, so studies are needed to evaluate this hypothesis as well.

There is little systematic information dealing with the role of exercise in the functional and psychological rehabilitation of cancer patients. There is little reason to expect that exercise training will help induce remissions in these patients, but there is good reason to expect that exercise may improve their quality of life. This question deserves study.

Exercise and Infection

Very little is known about the influence of exercise on the susceptibility to infection. It seems unlikely that exercise training exerts a major effect on the incidence of infection. The few available studies suggest that minor URIs may be slightly more common in athletes. Careful epidemiological investigations are needed to clarify this issue, but it is not likely that the results of such studies will change our understanding of the overall impact of exercise on health.

Bed rest has been prescribed much more often than is necessary in patients with hepatitis and mononucleosis. Such patients may be active to the limits of tolerance, avoiding extreme exertion and contact sports until recovery occurs. Patients with mild URIs need not restrict their exercise schedules. Patients with lower respiratory tract infections and those with fevers and myalgias suggesting systemic infection should probably avoid strenuous exertion until recovery.

References

1. Beutler, B., and A. Cerami. Cachectin: More than a tumor necrosis factor. *N. Engl. J. Med.* 316: 379-386, 1987.
2. Brahmi, Z., J.E. Thomas, M. Park, M. Park, I.R.G. Dowdeswell. The effect of acute exercise on natural killer-cell activity of trained and sedentary human subjects. *J. Clin. Immunol.* 5: 321-328, 1985.
3. Bull, J.M.C. Whole body hyperthermia as an anticancer agent. *CA: A Cancer Journal for Clinicians* 32: 123, 1982.
4. Cannon, J.G., and C. Dinarello. Interleukin-1 activity in human plasma [Abstract]. *Fed. Proc.* 43: 462, 1984.
5. Cannon, J.G., and M.J. Kluger. Endogenous pyrogen activity in human plasma after exercise. *Science* 220: 617-618, 1983.
6. Cannon, J.G., W. Evans, V.A. Hughes, C.N. Meredith, and C.A. Dinarello. Physiological mechanisms contributing to increased interleukin-1 secretion. *J. Appl. Physiol.* 61: 1869-1874, 1986.
7. Chalmers, T.C., R.D. Eckhardt, W.E. Reynolds, J.G. Cigarroa, Jr., N. Deane, R.W. Reifenstein, C.W. Smith, and C.S. Davidson. The treatment of acute infectious hepatitis: Controlled studies of the effects of diet, rest and physical reconditioning on the acute course of the disease and the incidence of relapses and residual abnormalities. *J. Clin. Invest.* 34: 1163, 1955.
8. Dalrymple, W. Infectious mononucleosis. *Postgrad. Med.* 35: 345-349, 1964.
9. Daniels, W.L., J.A. Vogel, D.S. Sharp, J.E. Wright, J.A. Vogel, G. Friman, W.R. Beisel, and J.J. Knapik. Effects of virus infection on physical performance in man. *Milit. Med.* 150: 8-14, 1985.
10. Dinarello, C.A., J.G. Cannon, and S.M. Wolff. New concepts in the pathogenesis of fever. *Rev. Infect. Dis.* 10: 168, 1988.

11. Douglas, D.J., and P.G. Hanson. Upper respiratory infections in the conditioned athlete. [Abstract]. *Med. Sci. Sports* 10: 55, 1978.

12. Douglas, R.G., K.M. Lindgren, and R.B. Couch. Exposure to cold environment and rhinovirus common cold. *N. Engl. J. Med.* 14: 742-747, 1968.

13. Edlund, A. The effect of defined physical exercise in the early convalescence of viral hepatitis. *Scand. J. Infect. Dis.* 3: 189-196, 1971.

14. Frisch, R.E., G. Wyshak, N.L. Albright, T.E. Albright, I. Schiff, K.P. Jones, J. Witschi, E. Shiang, E. Koff, and M. Marguglio. Lower prevalence of breast cancer and cancers of the reproductive system among former college athletes compared to non-athletes. *Br. J. Cancer* 52: 885-891, 1985.

15. Galun, E., R. Burstein, E. Assia, I. Tur-Kaspa, J. Rosenblum, and Y. Epstein. Changes of white blood cell count during prolonged exercise. *Int. J. Sports Med.* 8: 253-255, 1987.

16. Garabrant, D.H., J.M. Peters, T.M. Mack, and L. Bernstein. Job activity and colon cancer risk. *Am. J. Epidemiol.* 119: 1005-1014, 1984.

17. Gerhardsson, M., S.E. Norell, H. Kiviranta, N.L. Pedersen, and A. Ahlbom. Sedentary jobs and colon cancer. *Am. J. Epidemiol.* 123: 775-780, 1986.

18. Graubaum, H.J., C. Metzner, and K. Ziesenhenn. Physical exercise and the course of hepatitis. *Dtsch. Med. Wschr.* 112: 47-49, 1987.

19. Hall, N.R., J.P. McGillis, B.L. Spangelo, and A.L. Goldstein. Evidence that thymosins and other biologic response modifiers can function as neuroactive immunotransmitters. *J. Immunol.* 135: 806, 1985.

20. Hackney, A.C., W.E. Sinning, and B.C. Bruot. Reproductive hormonal profiles of endurance-trained and untrained males. *Med. Sci. Sports Exerc.* 20: 60-66, 1988.

21. Holdstock, D.J., J.J. Misiewicz, T. Smith, and E.N. Rowlands. Propulsion (mass movements) in the human colon and its relationship to meals and somatic activity. *Gut* 11: 91-99, 1970.

22. Husemann, B., M.G. Neubauer, and C. Duhme. Sedentary occupation and rectosigmoidal neoplasms. *Onkologie* 3: 168-171, 1980.

23. Landmann, R.M.A., F.B. Muller, C. Perini, and M. Wesp. Changes of immunoregulatory cells induced by psychological and physical stress: Relationship to plasma catecholamines. *Clin. Exp. Immunol.* 58: 127-135, 1984.

24. Linde, F. Running and upper respiratory tract infections. *Scand. J. Sports Sci.* 9: 21-23, 1987.

25. MacConnie, S.E., A. Barkan, R.M. Lampman, M.A. Schork, and I.Z. Beitins. Decreased hypothalamic gonadotropin-releasing hormone secretion in male marathon runners. *New Engl. J. Med* 315: 411-417, 1986.

26. MacKinnon, L.T., T.W. Chic, A. van As, and T.B. Tomasi. Decreased levels of secretary immunoglobulins following prolonged exercise [Abstract]. *Med. Sci. Sports Exerc.* 86: S40, 1986.

27. Paffenbarger, R.S., R.T. Hyde, and A.L. Wing. Physical activity and incidence of cancer in diverse populations: A preliminary report. *Am. J. Clin. Nutr.* 415: 312-317., 1987.

28. Phillips, M., M. Robinowitz, J.R. Higgins, K.J. Boran, T. Reed, and R. Virmani. Sudden cardiac death in air force recruits. *JAMA* 256: 2696-2700, 1986.

29. Reyes, M.P., K.L. Ho, F. Smith, and A.M. Lerner. A mouse model of dilated-type cardiomyopathy due to coxsackievirus B3. *J. Infect. Dis.* 144: 232-236, 1981.

30. Roberts, J.A. Loss of form in young athletes due to viral infection. *Br. Med. J.* 290: 357-358, 1985.

31. Schatzkin, A., Y. Jones, R.N. Hoover, P.R. Taylor, L.A. Brinton, R.G. Ziegler, E.B. Harvey, C.L. Carter, L.M. Licitra, M.C. Dufour, and D.B. Larson. Alcohol consumption and breast cancer in the epidemiologic follow-up study of the first national health and nutrition examination survey. *New Engl. J. Med.* 316: 1169-1173, 1987.

32. Schindler, B.A. Stress, affective disorders, and immune function. *Med. Clin. N. Amer.* 69: 585-597, 1985.

33. Simopoulos, A.P. Obesity and carcinogenesis: Historical perspective. *Am. J. Clin. Nutr.* 45: 271-276, 1987.

34. Simon, H.B. Exercise and infection. *Phys. Sports Med.* 15: 135-142, 1987.

35. Simon, H.B. Exercise, health and sports medicine. In: Rubenstein, E., and D. Federman, eds. *Scientific American medicine*. New York: Scientific American; 1988.

36. Simon, H.B. The immunology of exercise. *JAMA* 252: 2735-2738, 1984.

37. Simon, H.B., and M.N. Swartz. Pathophysiology of fever and fever of unknown origin. In: Rubenstein, E., and D. Federman, eds. *Scientific American medicine*. New York: Scientific American; 1987.

38. Targan, S., L. Britvan, and F. Dorey. Activation of human NKCC by moderate exercise: Increased frequency of NK cells with enhanced capability of effector-target lytic interactions. *Clin. Exp. Immunol.* 45: 352-360, 1981.

39. Vena, J.E., S. Graham, M. Zielezny, J. Brasure, and M.K. Swanson. Occupational exercise and risk of cancer. *Am. J. Clin. Nutr.* 45: 318-327, 1987.

40. Vogel, R.B., C.A. Books, C. Ketchum, C.W. Zauner, and F.T. Murray. Increase of free and total testosterone during submaximal exercise in normal males. *Med. Sci. Sports Exerc.* 17: 119-124, 1984.

41. Willett, W.C., M.J. Stampfer, G.A. Colditz, B.A. Rosner, C.H. Hennekens, and F.E. Speizer. Dietary fat and the risk of breast cancer. *N. Engl. J. Med.* 316: 22-28, 1987.

42. Willett, W.C., M.J. Stampfer, G.A. Colditz, B.A. Rosner, C.H. Hennekens, and F.E. Speizer. Moderate alcohol consumption and the risk of breast cancer. *N. Engl. J. Med.* 316: 1174-1180, 1987.

Chapter 51

Exercise, Fitness, and Recovery From Surgery, Disease, or Infection

Archie Young

This chapter examines the influence of exercise and of physical fitness on the speed and completeness of recovery from surgery or from acute infection. The evidence is patchy, and the areas discussed should not be taken to be paradigms for all acute ill-health events.

My approach has been guided by two questions:

1. Does a person's fitness before surgery or the onset of acute infection have any effect on the speed of their recovery or on their susceptibility to complications?
2. After surgery or acute infection, does physical training hasten the restoration of well-being and the correction of new impairments?

Before tackling either question, it is necessary to set the scene by reviewing the deconditioning effects of surgery and of acute infection on strength, isometric endurance, general fatigability, and aerobic power.

Illness-Induced Deconditioning

Strength

Strength After Surgery

Even minor surgery (e.g., herniography or breast biopsy) is associated with a 6% reduction in handgrip strength on the first postoperative day (42). This has returned to normal by the following day, but after more significant procedures (e.g., bowel resection or cholecystectomy) a handgrip strength deficit is still present by the eighth postoperative day (42).

An incompletely reported study of 11 patients who had undergone elective surgery and who were ambulant by the second or third postoperative day described approximately 40% reductions in isometric strength at shoulder, hip, and knee (21). These changes were only slight on the second postoperative day, were maximal at 5-10 d, and had disappeared 15-20 d postoperatively. Similar reductions were observed in the total work achieved in repeated isokinetic contractions ($30° \cdot s^{-1}$), but curiously there was no reduction in peak isokinetic strength.

The explanation for the loss of strength after surgery remains obscure. It seems unlikely that is it due merely to bed rest; although 7 d of bed rest may have reduced the isometric strength of the calf muscles of healthy, young men (29), it certainly had no effect on the strength of handgrip, knee flexors or extensors, or vertical or horizontal pushing or pulling movements of the upper limbs (27). Even 6-7 wk of bed rest in a lower-body plaster cast reduced upper-limb strength by only 7%-9% and grip strength not at all (17).

Incomplete voluntary activation of muscle would result in apparent weakness. Patients studied at intervals from 1 hr to 2 wk after arthrotomy and meniscectomy were able to equal their preoperative levels of maximal voluntary activation of the contralateral quadriceps (49, 51). Therefore, it is not possible to assume that the postsurgery weakness observed by Maxwell (42) and Edwards et al. (21) can be explained simply by a reduced ability or willingness to make maximal muscle contractions in the early postoperative days.

If muscle activation is still complete, a loss of strength implies either impaired excitation-contraction coupling or a loss of muscle mass. It is possible that these mechanisms might result from the choice of anesthetic or from the catabolic effect of surgery, respectively.

Strength After Acute Infection

Acute febrile illnesses are often associated with a generalized feeling of weakness and, especially in viral infections, with myalgia. After the febrile phase had passed, 39 patients hospitalized with predominantly viral or mycoplasma infections produced isometric strength measurements about 94% of those recorded 1 mo later and 91% of those recorded after a further 3 mo (27). There were no further increases in strength (with the exception of one muscle group) over the next 8 mo, suggesting that the measurements made 4 mo after the illness may have been a valid indication of the pre-infection strengths of the patients.

For obvious reasons, the only study with premorbid strength measurements involved only a brief illness and a small number of subjects. Seven young men were inoculated with the sand-fly fever virus (16). Isometric strength measurements at the height of the fever (3 or 4 d post-inoculation) averaged 10%-23% less than they were before. Two days later, after the fever had subsided, the mean isometric strength measurements were 1%-19% less than they were before infection, but the differences were no longer statistically significant. Isokinetic knee-extension strength showed losses of 19% (36 • s⁻¹) and 16% (180 • s⁻¹) during the fever and of 16% and 12%, respectively, after the fever; but only the 19% change reached statistical significance. Measurements of the strength of isokinetic elbow flexion at 36 • s⁻¹ and 180 • s⁻¹ were virtually unchanged. The severity of weakness of knee extension correlated with the severity of symptoms rather than with the height of the fever, raising the question of incomplete muscle activation as a result of impaired motivation. The completeness of muscle activation, however, was not measured.

In the same study, biopsies taken from the quadriceps muscles (the muscles with the most clear-cut changes in strength) showed no increase in proteolytic enzymes, no decrease in glycolytic enzymes, and only trivial changes in muscle ultrastructure (31). Circulating levels of creatine kinase (CK), its muscle isoenzyme (CK-MM), and myoglobin (Mgb) were not altered during the illness. This tends to emphasize the mild nature of the infection in this study, as significant elevations of CK have been observed in patients with influenza (25).

Single-fiber electromyography after influenza, echovirus, or mumps infections showed small increases in "jitter" (i.e., small reductions in the safety margin of neuromuscular transmission) but little evidence of impulse blocking (30). This seems unlikely to be an important factor in the weakness experienced after infection by otherwise normal subjects.

Isometric Endurance

Friman (28) also studied the ability of 32 of his 39 patients to sustain an isometric muscle contraction at a force equal to two thirds of their maximal strength at the time. Handgrip endurance did not appear to be affected, but the times for which a two-thirds maximal arm pull and a two-thirds maximal knee extension could be sustained were both 83% of the times achieved 1 yr later. Even 4 mo after the illness, the times were 87% and 93% of those achieved 8 mo later (i.e., not statistically significantly improved). This suggests that the recovery of isometric endurance may be slower than the recovery of strength. Friman suggested that this might be related to impaired glycolytic enzyme activity after he demonstrated lower activities of lactate dehydrogenase and of glyceraldehyde-3-phosphate dehydrogenase after similar infections; the latter enzyme's activity still remained below that of bed-rest controls 4 mo later (4). Theoretically, impairment of isometric endurance could also be explained by a rightward shift of the frequency-force curve (Figure 51.1) increasing the metabolic cost of sustaining a two-thirds maximal contraction. Such a shift could result from impairment of excitation-contraction coupling (60) or from an increased speed of muscle relaxation (55).

Prolonged Fatigue

Postoperative fatigue is an ill-defined complaint of tiredness, lasting sometimes for months, after major surgery (19, 45). The mechanism is completely unknown but could well be similar to whatever it is that impairs isometric muscle endurance after severe infection. A rightward shift of the frequency-force curve seems a potential and readily testable explanation; maximal strength could be fully recovered, whereas submaximal contractions would require an unusually high firing rate of the anterior horn cells, thus contributing to a sensation of exhaustion.

After viral infections, too, a few patients develop a complaint of intermittent, profound fatigue often associated with disordered emotion and thought (36) and that can last for many months or even years (41). This syndrome (or perhaps syndromes)

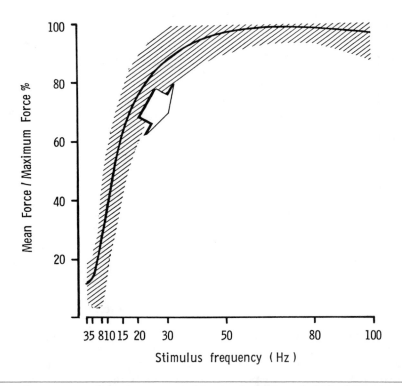

Figure 51.1. Frequency-force curve of the human quadriceps. A rightward shift of the curve will increase the stimulus frequency required to produce a two-thirds maximal contraction.

has many names and may be due to a persistent viral infection (8). Arnold et al. (2) used ^{31}P nuclear magnetic resonance to study energy metabolism in the exercising forearm muscles of a 30-yr-old man with a 4-yr history of a postviral fatigue syndrome since an attack of chicken pox. Muscle pH fell very rapidly with respect not only to time but also the degree of phosphocreatine degradation. It is not yet known whether this is indicative of a specific metabolic lesion or an effect of extreme disuse.

Aerobic Power

Aerobic Power After Surgery and/or Bed Rest

Maximal aerobic power ($\dot{V}O_2$max) and other indices of aerobic fitness may be impaired by reductions in physical activity, in total body hemoglobin, or in circulating blood volume. Any or all of these may occur as a result of surgery. In the most comprehensive study of the effects of surgery on aerobic fitness, Adolfsson (1) made pre- and postoperative measurements on 50 untrained women (aged 20-49) undergoing elective cholecystectomy. One week after surgery their physical working capacities (PWCs) at a heart rate of 170 beats/min (PWC$_{170}$) averaged 8% lower than preoperatively. This defi-

cit had virtually disappeared 1 wk later. Carswell (12) studied patients even earlier, on the fourth day after vagotomy and pyloroplasty, and found a 20% reduction in predicted $\dot{V}O_2$max. Two days later the deficit was only 4% and not statistically significant. In contrast, mean maximal work rates ($\dot{W}_{max}$) were reduced by 13% an average of 10 d after similar procedures (58). Moreover, PWC was still reduced by 12% and 15% in patients whose first postoperative measurements were not made until 1 wk after cholecystectomy or partial gastrectomy, respectively (23).

Taken together (Figure 51.2), these four studies (1, 12, 23, 58) suggest that there may be some doubt about the validity of the first postoperative exercise test, irrespective of when it is performed within the first 2 wk after surgery. However good the preoperative habituation may have been, there may perhaps be an element of rehabituation in the difference between the first and the second postoperative tests. On the other hand, Wood (57) demonstrated a 20%-25% shift in the relationship of blood lactate to work rate 9-12 d after surgery. The individual changes corresponded closely to the respective reductions in $\dot{W}_{max}$, suggesting that the reductions in aerobic fitness were not merely the result of inadequate rehabituation. Other

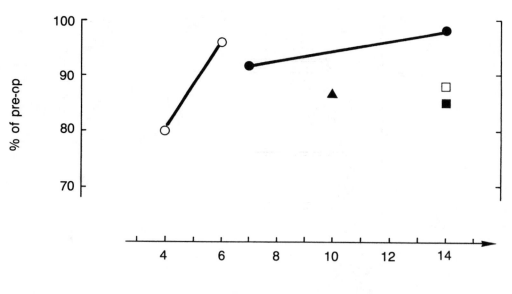

Figure 51.2. Measures of aerobic exercise performance after abdominal surgery: closed circles = PWC_{170} after cholecystectomy (see ref. 1).; open circles = predicted VO_2max after vagotomy and pyloroplasty (see ref. 12); closed triangle = $\dot{W}_{max}$ after major abdominal surgery (see ref. 58); open square = PWC after cholecystectomy (see ref. 23); and closed square = PWC after partial gastrectomy (see ref. 23).

possible mechanisms are discussed in the following sections.

The potential importance of the bed rest itself must be considered. Studies showed that PWC_{170} was reduced by 6% in 22 young men confined to bed for 7 d (26) and $\dot{V}O_2max$ by 15% in 12 middle-aged men confined to bed for 10 d (15). Three weeks of bed rest produced somewhat inconsistent changes, namely, a 9% reduction in $\dot{V}O_2max$ in 8 young men (52) and a 27% reduction in 5 young men (47). On the other hand, other results suggest that the surgery itself may be more important than the duration of bed rest; after meniscectomy, there was a greater increment in the heart rate response to contralateral one-legged pedaling after 4 than after 14 d of bed rest (6).

Mechanism of Loss of Aerobic Power After Surgery. Both atrophy and aerobic deconditioning of muscle by a few days of relative inactivity are possible explanations. The former seems unlikely because the reduction in $\dot{W}_{max}$ after surgery is no less severe when half of the negative nitrogen balance is prevented by amino acid infusion (58). Aerobic deconditioning of muscle also seems less than certain; as young men confined to bed for 17 d showed only a 13% (and nonsignificant) reduction in the citrate synthase activity in biopsies from the

quadriceps and no change in succinic dehydrogenase or cytochrome oxidase activities (53).

Impairment of oxygen delivery to the muscles because of a recumbency-induced reduction in plasma volume (32) is a possibility. It may be particularly relevant after surgery, when there will be both a recumbency-induced diuresis (33) and impaired fluid intake. Despite limited ambulation from the first postoperative day, the patients in the study by Adolfsson (1) showed mean blood volume 1 wk postoperatively that was 6% less than it had been before ($p < 0.05$). Could it be that the normalization of aerobic exercise ability that seems to occur between the first two postoperative exercise tests indicates not habituation but that a single bout of vigorous exercise is sufficient stimulus to restore a normal plasma volume?

Finally, there is the question of the effect of surgical blood loss. Although the apparent operative blood loss was small, Adolfsson's patients had suffered a net 13% fall in total hemoglobin (THb) by 1 wk after surgery. Pre- or postoperative transfusions that eliminated the fall in THb after partial gastrectomy also eliminated the postoperative decrease in PWC (23). Evidence from a venesection experiment, however, suggests that the usual modest blood loss is unlikely to cause significant impairment of aerobic power after the volume loss has been made good. Two to three days after a 10% venesection, mean PWC_{170} was 102% of its prevenesection value despite having been 92% of that value 1 hr after venesection (35).

Aerobic Power After Acute Infection

In children, most of whom had had scarlet fever, there was no suggestion of any deterioration in aerobic fitness when they were exercise tested early after ambulation (9). In contrast, 7 adults who were given sand-fly fever showed significant impairment of their endurance in a previously submaximal walking test (16). The PWC_{170} of 34 adult patients who had suffered more severe infections (including 10 with hepatitis) averaged approximately 14% less than the values obtained 1 mo later (9). In a similar, more recent study the PWC_{150} of 80 postfebrile adults also averaged about 14% less than it did 1 mo later (26). The measurements were repeated after a further 2-1/2 mo of recovery and demonstrated further increases in PWC_{150}, implying that the measurements 1 mo after the event underestimated the true preinfection values (26). These later data suggested that the acute illnesses had reduced PWC_{150} by about 25%.

Only prospective studies of deliberately induced infections can overcome the need to guess the preinfection value of PWC or $\dot{V}O_2max$. Deliberate infection of 12 conscientious objectors with *Plasmodium vivax* malaria produced a 19% reduction in $\dot{V}O_2max$ on the fifth postfebrile day that had resolved 6 wk later (38).

Mechanism of Loss of Aerobic Power After Acute Infection. An explanation for these substantial reductions in aerobic performance may be sought in altered oxygen delivery and utilization at a cellular level, loss of exercising muscle mass, altered cardiovascular control, and/or reduced plasma volume. The citrate synthase activity of biopsies from the quadriceps of 13 patients who had suffered an acute viral infection or mycoplasma pneumonia was some 30% less than in biopsies from normal subjects and 20% less than in biopsies from normal subjects after a week's bed rest (4). Most of the deficit had been recovered about 5 wk later and all of it after a further 11 wk. Changes in cytochrome oxidase activity, however, did not suggest a potential explanation for the postinfection changes in PWC. The reductions in maximal strength observed after infectious illness are too small for mere loss of muscle mass to be an adequate explanation for impaired aerobic exercise performance.

Orthostatic intolerance is a prominent feature after febrile illness (9, 26, 38). The tachycardia, in particular, may explain the post-illness reduction in PWC and in $\dot{W}_{max}$. This may be due in part to a reduced blood volume (due in turn to both recumbency and sweating), but there also seem to be other, unidentified factors operating (37).

The Effects of the Previous Level of Fitness

Previous Fitness and Loss of Aerobic Power

After Bed Rest

There is no evidence to support the notion that the percentage fall in $\dot{V}O_2max$ with bed rest alone is any greater in someone who is well trained than it is in someone who is not (33, 47) (providing the tests are done with the subjects upright).

After Surgery

Bassey and Fentem (7) found that 2 wk of bed rest after meniscectomy increased the heart rate response to cycling at $\dot{V}O_2 = 1.2\ L \cdot min^{-1}$ by an average of 8 beats/min [$\Sigma N = 9$]. Although they interpreted their data as indicating a relatively greater decline in physical condition in those with the best preoperative fitness, they did not allow for the spurious correlation that results from plotting changes against initial values.

In the much larger study by Adolfsson (1), the absolute fall in PWC_{170} after cholecystectomy was greater in women who had undergone 6 wk of preoperative training ($N = 58$). Interpretation of these data is subject to the same difficulty as is that of Bassey and Fentem's data. It is clear, however, that the preoperative training ensured that the lowest postoperative PWC_{170} was essentially unchanged from the pretraining value and was thus about 8% greater than it would have been had there been no preoperative training (Figure 51.3). This was also the conclusion drawn from a similar but incompletely reported study (13).

After Acute Infection

In the 33 female patients in the study by Friman (26), there was a significant positive correlation between the apparent loss of PWC and the presumed preinfection PWC. Once again this may be

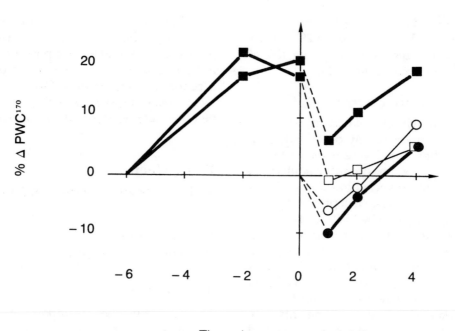

Time since surgery (weeks)

Figure 51.3. Effect of physical training before and/or after surgery on the PWC_{170} of women undergoing elective cholecystectomy. Data are from Adolfsson (1). Postoperative training did not begin until after the first postoperative exercise test. Untrained control groups are indicated by open points and thin lines.

no more than a statistical artifact. That the correlation was less strong in his male patients merely reflects the wider range of body weights in the men (CV = 18%) than in the women (CV = 11%).

Previous Fitness and Recovery From Illness

Irrespective of whether the relative loss of aerobic fitness is greater in those who are well trained, it is appealing to suppose that well-trained patients will benefit from having a postillness PWC greater than it would have been had their illness-associated decline started from a lower, normal level. What evidence is there to support this?

Previous Fitness and Recovery From Surgery

Grimby and Höök argue that preoperative training may be important in "good pre-operative care in order to increase the patient's general condition before he faces the surgical trauma and, possibly, the subsequent inactivity" (34, p. 17). Pugh (43) applied the same logic before subjecting himself to the rigors of a hip arthroplasty, training with crutches so that he could achieve an adequate intensity of exercise.

There is little evidence, however, that this argument has any relevance for young or even middle-aged adults. Adolfsson's patients suffered so few complications after their cholecystectomies that there was no possibility of demonstrating any potential clinical advantage of preoperative training (1). Trained and untrained women had similar lengths of hospital stay and of convalescence after discharge. This possibly reflects surgeons' habits rather than individual need, or it may reflect the considerable reserve capacity between $\dot{V}O_2$max and the rates of oxygen uptake required for most everyday activities. It is only after about age 60 in women and perhaps 70 in men that this safety margin becomes so narrow that a 10%-20% reduction in maximal oxygen uptake becomes potentially limiting for the performance of everyday activities (46, 59).

Figure 51.4 illustrates the consequences of a 15% reduction in the maximal oxygen uptake of a healthy 80-yr-old woman with respect to 40% $\dot{V}O_2$max (the greatest work rate that can be sustained for a full 8-hr day) and 60% $\dot{V}O_2$max (the onset of blood lactate accumulation). Just sitting quietly for 8 hr would become difficult, and dressing and undressing would entail significant lactate accumulation. It seems highly likely that these

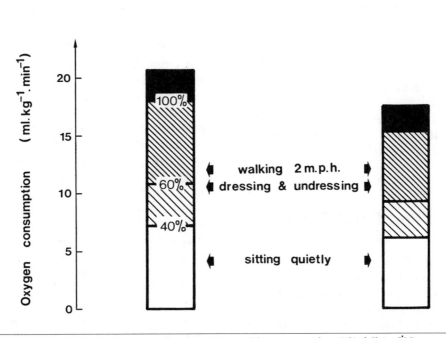

Figure 51.4. Implications for an otherwise healthy 80-yr-old woman of a 15% fall in $\dot{V}O_2$max such as might follow surgery. The top of the solid black part of the column corresponds to the maximal work rate at a metabolic cost greater than $\dot{V}O_2$max.

changes would predispose to a tendency to even greater immobility and its attendant risks of deep-vein thrombosis and pulmonary embolism. Thus, by the age of 80, it seems very possible that the 10%-20% reduction in maximal oxygen uptake that follows surgery might have important clinical consequences.

The 12-min walking distance proved a disappointingly poor predictor of ventilatory complications in patients undergoing lung resection for carcinoma (5). The Canadian Home Fitness Test did not predict circulatory and pulmonary complications in 19 women undergoing abdominal hysterectomy (48). Nevertheless, it was reported as showing a significant negative correlation between "fitness" and length of hospitalization. This claim seems overenthusiastic. First, "fitness" was scored on a 4-point scale, with 9 of the 19 patients in the lowest category (viz., ineligible for testing). Also, the report shows no evidence of any allowance for an age effect in patients aged 18-60. Even if one accepts the validity of the Canadian Home Fitness Test for comparisons of subjects of different ages (which is questionable), the initial exclusion of 9 patients from the performance of the step test is not independent of age.

Neither ischemic changes in an exercise electrocardiogram (ECG) nor an exercise tolerance less than 5 METs was an independent predictor of death, myocardial infarction, or other myocardial damage in a large series of patients undergoing major noncardiac surgery (11). Combining an ischemic exercise ECG and a low exercise tolerance improved predictive specificity (to 82%) but had a sensitivity of only 50% (i.e., half the end-point events were not predicted). Leaving aside the question of whether there is any practical value in a predictive sensitivity of 50%, the findings of this study are of only limited relevance to the question of whether presurgical training has a role in the prevention of postoperative complications. Impaired exercise performance in this study was not so much an indicator of poor aerobic conditioning but rather an indicator of preexisting myocardial or coronary pathology.

Previous Fitness and Recovery From Infection

There is no evidence to refute or support the notion that in humans a good state of aerobic conditioning might enhance recovery from acute infections. Nevertheless, there are some supportive indications from animal studies. Voluntary training in exercise wheels and climbing to the feeding hoppers for 16-18 d produced a small improvement in the survival rate (from 29% to

44%) of mice subsequently infected with *Salmonella typhimurium* (10). A much more severe training program (6 wk of daily swimming to exhaustion) proved beneficial to mice subsequently infected with influenza virus or with *Francisella tularensis* (39). Myocardial catabolism and loss of myocardial cytochrome oxidase activity was less in the trained animals than in controls. Mortality from influenza was also less. These studies support earlier, less well controlled studies of the effect of several bouts of exhaustive exercise before pneumococcal infection (10).

The Effects of Postillness Training

Acute ill health virtually always reduces habitual physical activity. Almost any patient who is admitted to the hospital is put to bed. In addition to the illness, the patient must also contend with the dangers of bed rest (3). Immobilization in bed has several undesirable effects. For example, it allows aerobic deconditioning, muscle atrophy, bone atrophy and demineralization, constipation, skin damage, hyperglycemia, venous thrombosis, and increasing psychological dependence. For these reasons it is well established that the period of bed rest should usually be kept as short as possible. My concern here is whether active physical training confers any additional benefits not gained from conventional early ambulation.

Preventive Exercise During Bed Rest

An hour of exercise per day may attenuate the early loss of interstitial fluid and the later loss of plasma volume that result from bed rest (32). As expected, therefore, 2 hr of training daily during a 3-wk period of bed rest prevented the orthostatic abnormalities that were seen in the controls (52).

Postillness Training and Nitrogen Balance

Exercise is sometimes advocated for patients receiving nutritional supplements in the belief that it may promote nitrogen retention even though it increases not only synthesis but also breakdown of muscle protein. In rats receiving parenteral feeding after laparotomy, treadmill running probably increased muscle turnover of amino acids but did not lessen the negative nitrogen balance or the weight loss (24).

During recovery from polymyositis, there is net retention of nitrogen as muscle tissue is restored. During a detailed study of a single patient, two 4-d periods of physical training were associated with

a more positive nitrogen balance and perhaps also an acceleration in the recovery of strength (22).

Postsurgery Training and Physical Recovery

When meniscectomy was followed by 14 d of bed rest, the relationship of heart rate to $\dot{V}O_2$ during one-legged contralateral ergometry had returned to normal on retesting after 14 d of physiotherapy and returned similarly when the surgery was followed by 4 d of bed rest and then 10 d of ambulation (6). In neither case, however, was a control group retested after a period of less vigorous mobilization. Adolfsson (1) did have adequate controls; both 2 and 4 wk after cholecystectomy the recovery of PWC_{170} was the same in those doing postoperative training as it was in the control group (Figure 51.3). Four weeks after surgery, mean PWC_{170} values were up 5% and 9%, respectively, on the preoperative levels and 17% and 16% on the values 1 wk after the operation.

Neither of these studies (1, 6) indicated any clinical benefit to those who trained after the operation. Where the purpose of surgery is to improve exercise tolerance, however, there is a clear logic to using physical training to ensure that the patient gains the full benefit of surgical intervention, for example, in children with congenital heart disease (40) or in adults after cardiac transplantation (50). In one such study (54), after coronary artery bypass grafting, valve replacement, or both, there was even a strong suggestion that 1 wk of postoperative training resulted in patients being discharged earlier, with greater improvements in walking distance and less restriction of upper-limb range of movement.

Postinfection Training and Physical Recovery

Strenuous physical activity at or shortly after contracting a viral infection can greatly increase the harm caused by the infection. This is best known for Coxsackie myocarditis and myocardiopathy and poliomyelitis paralysis (44). Exhaustive swimming of mice infected with Coxsackie B-3 increased the peak viremia 10-fold, total viremia 75-fold, and myocardial viral content (after 6 d) 1,000-fold. It also prolonged the myocardial and serum interferon peaks and reduced neutralizing antibody levels 16-fold (44). Exhaustive swimming increased mortality among mice infected with influenza virus but not among mice infected with the bacterium *Francisella tularensis* (39), in which it even reduced some of the loss of glycolytic and oxidative enzyme activity in the myocardium.

Very little information is available to guide clinicians in the advice they should give to patients in the later stages of recovery after an acute infection. During convalescence from hepatitis, there is something of a tradition of advising against vigorous activity. There is little or no evidence to justify such advice and some evidence that vigorous exercise does no harm (for relevant data and a review, see ref. 20).

Postillness Training and Psychological Recovery

There are convincing anecdotal and uncontrolled accounts of the benefits of physical activity to promote psychological recovery after surgery or severe illness. The ability to perform physical exercise can improve a patient's self-image and "renews feelings of control over [the] body, promotes self-esteem, and helps dissipate tension and anger" (14, p. 1008). Family and friends change their perceptions of the patient. This is commonly observed with the wives of men performing physical training after myocardial infarction. A small study of teenagers conducted after they underwent surgery for the correction of congenital heart abnormalities suggests that a 1-yr training program helped the mothers be less restrictive of their sons' physical activities and have less anxiety about the possibility of their sons' deaths. It also improved the boys' feelings of adequacy, self-esteem, self-image, and positiveness (18).

Unanswered Questions and Future Directions

Of the many unanswered questions raised in this review, I shall briefly highlight a few that seem both important and potentially answerable.

Loss of Strength After Surgery

The time is ripe for someone to do for the postoperative changes in strength what Adolfsson (1) did for the changes in circulatory and respiratory function. That is, there is a need for a large study of people undergoing a standardized, elective surgical procedure with measurements of muscle strength, cross-sectional area, activation, and frequency-force characteristics. If measurements of muscle fatigability in repeated contractions are included, some light might also be shed on the syndrome of postoperative fatigue. There is considerable scope for further studies into the question of whether exercise can slow the loss of nitrogen that follows major surgery or trauma.

Postoperative Exercise Testing

I should be interested to see the results of a study in which comparable patients had performed their first postoperative exercise tests 2, 4, and 16 d and their second postoperative tests 4, 6, and 18 d after surgery. This would clarify whether there is a need for rehabituation to the exercise test procedure after surgery. Coupled with plasma volume and tilt-table measurements, it would also allow clarification of the role of postoperative hypovolemia and the effectiveness of a single bout of vigorous exercise in correcting postoperative orthostatic intolerance.

Infection Mortality

Preinfection training appears to reduce mortality in mice infected with Salmonella or influenza or that have tularemia. In other situations, there are several beneficial effects of exercise that previously were thought to be due to training but that may be due instead to the most recent single bout of exercise. Examples include changes in lipoprotein profiles, blood pressure, and glucose tolerance. Is the apparent protection against the lethality of some infections an effect of training, or is it an effect of a recent bout of exercise?

Pre- and Postsurgical Training in Old Age

As the population ages and surgical and anesthetic techniques improve, more and more elderly patients are undergoing major surgery. As orthostatic intolerance is more common in old age (56), related postoperative difficulties may well be greater in elderly patients. In addition, as I have already argued, the postoperative loss of PWC may be of much greater practical and clinical significance in older patients. Yet elderly patients and elderly experimental subjects were noticeably absent from the studies that I have reviewed. Modern clinical practice requires that many of these studies be repeated with subjects or patients in their eighth and ninth decades of life.

Conclusion

Both viral infections and surgery may produce a significant loss of strength, a loss greater than that which follows bed rest alone. The explanation is not known.

Maximal aerobic power is reduced by about 8%-20% when first tested during the first 2 wk after surgery. There is some doubt about the interpretation of the first postoperative exercise test, as it is not clear how much rehabituation may be required. The second postoperative test may show little or no deficit. Severe infections are associated with a reduction of $\dot{V}O_2$max by about 15%-25%, which takes more than 1 mo to recover. A reduced plasma volume may explain much of these reductions in $\dot{V}O_2$max. After infections, a reduction in muscle oxidative enzyme activity may also be relevant.

The effect of preoperative training is that the postoperative $\dot{V}O_2$max shows little net change from its pretraining, preoperative value. For most patients this may be of no importance. In elderly patients, however, the safety margins for the performance of some everyday activities may be so narrow that it may be of functional importance to prevent any reduction in $\dot{V}O_2$max.

There is no human evidence that a preexisting good state of aerobic conditioning enhances recovery from acute infections, but there are some supportive indications from animal studies. On the other hand, strenuous exercise shortly after a viral infection is potentially harmful.

The techniques are now available for a detailed, analytical study of postoperative muscle weakness. The effects on plasma volume, orthostatic reactions, and $\dot{V}O_2$max of a single bout of vigorous exercise during the early postoperative period require clarification. There is an urgent need for studies of vigorous pre- and postoperative training for elderly and very elderly surgical patients.

Previous exercise protects mice against the lethality of some infections. Is this an effect of training, or is it an effect of a single bout of exercise? Is there any evidence of a similar effect in humans?

References

1. Adolfsson, G. Circulatory and respiratory function in relation to physical activity in female patients before and after cholecystectomy. *Acta Chir. Scand. Suppl.* 401: 1969.
2. Arnold, D.L., P.J. Bore, G.K. Radda, P. Styles, and D.J. Taylor. Excessive intracellular acidosis of skeletal muscle on exercise in a patient with a postviral exhaustion/fatigue syndrome. A ^{31}P nuclear magnetic resonance study. *Lancet* i: 1367-1369, 1984.
3. Asher, R.A.J. The dangers of going to bed. *Brit. Med. J.* 4: 967-968, 1947.
4. Åström, E., G. Friman, and L. Pilström. Effects of viral and Mycoplasma infections on ultrastructure and enzyme activities in human skeletal muscle. *Acta Pathol. Microbiol. Scand. (A)* 84: 113-122, 1976.
5. Bagg, L.R. The 12-min walking distance; its use in the pre-operative assessment of patients with bronchial carcinoma before lung resection. *Respiration* 46: 342-345, 1984.
6. Bassey, E.J., T. Bennett, A.T. Birmingham, P.H. Fentem, D. Fitton, and R. Goldsmith. Effects of surgical operation and bed rest on cardiovascular responses to exercise in hospital patients. *Cardiovasc. Res.* 7: 588-592, 1973.
7. Bassey, E.J., and P.H. Fentem. Extent of deterioration in physical condition during postoperative bed rest and its reversal by rehabilitation. *Br. Med. J.* 4: 194-196, 1974.
8. Behan, P.O., and W.N.H. Behan. Epidemic myalgic encephalomyelitis. In: Rose, F.C., ed. *Clinical neuroepidemiology*. London: Pitman Medical; 1980: pp. 374-383.
9. Bengtsson, E. Working capacity and exercise electrocardiogram in convalescents after acute infectious diseases without cardiac complications. *Acta Med. Scand.* 154: 359-373, 1956.
10. Cannon, J.G., and M.J. Kluger. Exercise enhances survival rate in mice infected with Salmonella typhimurium (41830). *Proc. Soc. Exp. Biol. Med.* 175: 518-521, 1984.
11. Carliner, N.H., M.L. Fisher, G.D. Plotnick, H. Garbart, A. Rapoport, M.H. Kelemen, G.W. Moran, T. Gadacz, and R.W. Peters. Routine preoperative exercise testing in patients undergoing major noncardiac surgery. *Am. J. Cardiol.* 56: 51-58, 1985.
12. Carswell, S. Changes in aerobic power in patients undergoing elective surgery. *J. Physiol.* 251: 42P-43P, 1975.
13. Carswell, S.H., B.D. Holman, J. Thompson, and W.F. Walker. Acceptable level of aerobic power for patients undergoing elective surgery. *J. Physiol.* 285: 13P, 1978.
14. Cohn, A.H. Chemotherapy from an insider's perspective. *Lancet* i: 1006-1009, 1982.
15. Convertino, V., J. Hung, D. Goldwater, and R.F. DeBusk. Cardiovascular responses to exercise in middle-aged men after 10 days of bedrest. *Circulation* 65: 134-140, 1982.
16. Daniels, W.L., J.A. Vogel, D.S. Sharp, G. Friman, J.E. Wright, W.R. Beisel, and J.J. Knapik. Effects of virus infection on physical performance in man. *Milit. Med.* 150: 8-14, 1985.
17. Deitrik, J.E., G.D. Whedon, and E. Shorr. Effects of immobilization upon various meta-

bolic and physiologic functions of normal men. *Am. J. Med.* 4: 3-36, 1948.

18. Donovan, E.F., R.A. Mathews, P.A. Nixon, R.J. Stephenson, R.J. Robertson, F. Dean, F.J. Fricker, L.B. Beerman, and D.R. Fisher. An exercise program for pediatric patients with congenital heart disease: Psychosocial aspects. *J. Cardiac Rehabil.* 3: 476-480, 1983.

19. Editorial. Postoperative fatigue. *Lancet* i: 84, 1979.

20. Edlund, A. The effect of defined physical exercise in the early convalescence of viral hepatitis. *Scand. J. Infect. Dis.* 3: 189-196, 1971.

21. Edwards, H., E.A. Rose, and T.C. King. Postoperative deterioration in muscular function. *Arch. Surg.* 17: 899-901, 1982.

22. Edwards, R.H.T., C.M. Wiles, J.M. Round, M.J. Jackson, and A. Young. Muscle breakdown and repair in polymyositis: A case study. *Muscle Nerve* 2: 223-228, 1979.

23. Eriksson, F., and S.-O. Liljedahl. Förändringar i arbetskapacitet, blod- och hjärtvolym samt total-Hb efter gall- och ventrikeloperationer. *Nord. Med.* 69: 282, 1963.

24. Freund, H., N. Yoshimura, and J.E. Fischer. Effect of exercise on postoperative nitrogen balance. *J. Appl. Physiol.* 46: 141-145, 1979.

25. Friman, G. Serum creatine phosphokinase in epidemic influenza. *Scand. J. Infect. Dis.* 8: 13-20, 1976.

26. Friman, G. Effects of acute infectious disease on circulatory function. *Acta Med. Scand.* (Suppl. 592): 1976.

27. Friman, G. Effect of acute infectious disease on isometric muscle strength. *Scand. J. Clin. Lab. Invest.* 37: 303-308, 1977.

28. Friman, G. Effect of acute infectious disease on human isometric muscle endurance. *Upsala J. Med. Sci.* 83: 105-108, 1978.

29. Friman, G., and E. Hamrin. Changes of reactive hyperaemia after clinical bed rest for seven days. *Upsala J. Med. Sci.* 81: 79-83, 1976.

30. Friman, G., H.H. Schiller, and M.S. Schwartz. Disturbed neuromuscular transmission in viral infections. *Scand. J. Infect. Dis.* 9: 99-103, 1977.

31. Friman, G., J.E. Wright, N.G. Ilbäck, W.R. Beisel, J.D. White, D.S. Sharp, E.L. Stephen, W.L. Daniels, and J.A. Vogel. Does fever or myalgia indicate reduced physical performance capacity in viral infections? *Acta Med. Scand.* 217: 353-361, 1985.

32. Greenleaf, J.E., E.M. Bernauer, H.L. Young, J.T. Morse, R.W. Staley, L.T. Juhos, and W. Van Beaumont. Fluid and electrolyte shifts during bed rest with isometric and isotonic exercise. *J. Appl. Physiol.* 42: 59-66, 1977.

33. Greenleaf, J.E., and S. Kozlowski. Physiological consequences of reduced physical activity during bed rest. *Exerc. Sport Sci. Rev.* 10: 84-119, 1982.

34. Grimby, G., and O. Höök. Physical training of different patient groups. A review. *Scand. J. Rehabil. Med.* 3: 15-25, 1971.

35. Gullbring, B., A. Holmgren, T. Sjöstrand, and T. Strandell. The effect of blood volume variations on the pulse rate in supine and upright positions and during exercise. *Acta Physiol. Scand.* 50: 62-71, 1960.

36. Hartnell, L. Post-viral fatigue syndrome: A canker in my brain. *Lancet* i: 910, 1987.

37. Hedin, G., and G. Friman. Orthostatic reactions and blood volumes after moderate physical activity during acute febrile infections. *Int. Rehabil. Med.* 4: 107-109, 1982.

38. Henschel, A., H.L. Taylor, and A. Keys. Experimental malaria in man. 1. Physical deterioration and recovery. *J. Clin. Invest.* 29: 52-59, 1950.

39. Ilbäck, N.-G., G. Friman, W.R. Beisel, A.J. Johnson, and R.F. Berendt. Modifying effects of exercise on clinical course and biochemical response of the myocardium in influenza and tularaemia in mice. *Infect. Immunol.* 45: 498-504, 1984.

40. Longmuir, P.E., J.A.P. Turner, R.D. Rowe, and P.M. Olley. Postoperative exercise rehabilitation benefits children with congenital heart disease. *Clin. Invest. Med.* 8: 232-238, 1985.

41. Lyle, W.H., and R.N. Chamberlain. 'Epidemic neuromyasthenia' 1934-1977: Current approaches. *Postgrad. Med. J.* 54: 705-774, 1978.

42. Maxwell, A. Muscle power after surgery. *Lancet* i: 420-421, 1980.

43. Pugh, L.G.C.E. The oxygen intake and energy cost of walking before and after unilateral hip replacement, with some observations on the use of crutches. *J. Bone Joint Surg.* [Br]. 55: 742-745, 1973.

44. Reyes, M.P., and A.M. Lerner. Interferon and neutralizing antibody in sera of exercised mice with coxsackievirus B-3 myocarditis (39204). *Proc. Soc. Exp. Biol. Med.* 151: 333-338, 1976.

45. Rose, E.A., and T.C. King. Understanding postoperative fatigue. *Surg. Gynecol. Obstet.* 147: 97-102, 1978.

46. Saltin, B. Fysisk vedligholdelse hos ældre. I. Aerob arbejdsevne. *Mdskr. Prakt. Lægeg.* 58: 193-216, 1980.

47. Saltin, B., G. Blomqvist, J.H. Mitchell, R.L. Johnson, K. Wildenthal, and C.B. Chapman. Response to exercise after bed rest and after training. *Circulation* 38: Suppl. 7, 1968.

48. Schilling, J.A., and M.T. Molen. Physical fitness and its relationship to postoperative recovery in abdominal hysterectomy patients. *Heart Lung* 13: 639-644, 1984.

49. Shakespeare, D.T., M. Stokes, K.P. Sherman, and A. Young. Reflex inhibition of the quadriceps after meniscectomy: Lack of association with pain. *Clin. Physiol.* 5: 137-144, 1985.

50. Sieurat, P., J.P. Roquebrune, D. Grinneiser, F. Bourlon, J.P. Elbèze, J. Jourdan, and V. Dor. Surveillance et réadaptation des transplantés cardiaques hétérotopiques à la période de convalescence. *Arch. Mal. Coeur* 79: 210-216, 1986.

51. Stokes, M., and A. Young. The contribution of reflex inhibition to arthrogenous muscle weakness. *Clin. Sci.* 67: 7-14, 1984.

52. Sullivan, M.J., P.F. Binkley, D.V. Unverferth, J.-H. Ren, H. Boudoulas, T.M. Bashore, A.J. Merola, and C.V. Leier. Prevention of bedrest-induced physical deconditioning by daily dobutamine infusions. Implications for drug-induced physical conditioning. *J. Clin. Invest.* 76: 1632-1642, 1985.

53. Sullivan, M.J., J. Merola, A.P. Timmerman, D.V. Unverferth, and C.V. Leier. Drug-induced aerobic enzyme activity of human skeletal muscle during bedrest deconditioning. *J. Cardiopulm. Rehabil.* 6: 232-237, 1986.

54. Ungerman-deMent, P., A. Bemis, and A. Siebens. Exercise program for patients after cardiac surgery. *Arch. Phys. Med. Rehabil.* 67: 463-466, 1986.

55. Wiles, C.M., A. Young, D.A. Jones, and R.H.T. Edwards. Muscle relaxation rate, fibre-type composition and energy turnover in hyper- and hypo-thyroid patients. *Clin. Sci.* 57: 375-384, 1979.

56. Wollner, L., and J.M.K. Spalding. The autonomic nervous system. In: Brocklehurst, J.C., ed. *Textbook of geriatric medicine and gerontology* (3rd ed.). Edinburgh: Churchill Livingstone; 1985: pp. 449-473.

57. Wood, C.D. Postoperative exercise capacity following nutritional support with hypotonic glucose. *Surg. Gynecol. Obstet.* 152: 39-42, 1981.

58. Wood, C.D., R. Shreck, R. Tommey, K. Towsley, C.W. Guess, R. Werth, and M. Pollard. Relative value of glucose and amino acids in preserving exercise capacity in the postoperative period. *Am. J. Surg.* 149: 383-386, 1985.

59. Young, A. Exercise physiology in geriatric practice. *Acta Med. Scand. Suppl.* 711: 227-232, 1986.

60. Young, A., and R.H.T. Edwards. Clinical investigations of muscle contractility. *Rheumatol. Rehabil.* 16: 231-235, 1977.

Chapter 52

Discussion: Exercise, Fitness, and Recovery From Surgery, Disease, or Trauma

Neil B. Oldridge

Dr. Young has presented a summary of available data related to exercise and fitness as they affect recovery from surgery and disease and emphasized the paucity of available data. He did not, however, address the third component of this particular topic, that is, trauma or injury. As the objectives of this conference include an examination of exercise and fitness as they relate to health, I have therefore elected to focus on trauma associated with sport. I use the same two questions that guided Dr. Young's approach to this topic:

- Does a person's fitness before a traumatic sport injury have any effect on the susceptibility to injury?
- Does physical conditioning after a traumatic sport injury hasten the restoration of preevent performance?

Participation in exercise and sports is encouraged by various governmental and health agencies, presumably because of their purported associations with health. Unfortunately, participation in competitive and recreational sports will also inevitably result in various types of sport injury. Data on sport injuries in the United States are limited, but there are indications that most drownings, many firearm fatalities, 10% of brain injuries, 7% of spinal cord injuries, and 13% of facial injuries treated in hospitals are related to recreation and sports activities; the greatest risk for sport-related injuries is among persons aged 5-14 yr for most sports and 15-24 yr for sports such as skiing, and males are at greater risk than are females (3). In the United States there are an estimated 3-5 million sport-related injuries per year and some 6,000 deaths resulting from these injuries, and although most sport injuries are not catastrophic, milder,

long-term effects may pose significant public health concerns (3). A recent publication has carefully documented sport injuries in Finland, substantiating that injuries occur in younger persons and males and that most injuries were not severe but may have long-term sequelae (17).

Are there epidemiological, clinical, or experimental data in the sport-injury area that might help us better understand the relationships among exercise, fitness, the prevention of trauma, and rehabilitation after trauma (with or without surgery) in recreational or competitive sports? What rules of evidence should be used when interpreting the available epidemiological and clinical data to answer these questions so that optimal guidelines for the prevention and rehabilitation of sport injuries can be provided?

Sport-injury data are generally available from either anecdotal case studies or case series; these may provide useful clinical information but do not provide incidence of sport injury nor explain the relationships among exercise, fitness, and injury. Case comparison studies, when carefully designed, may provide more useful data on risk factors for specific sport injuries. Retrospective community-based surveys and nonrandomized cohort comparisons with either historical or contemporaneous controls may provide some general incidence data that are, however, not always useful, particularly when the appropriate comparison population-based perspective on which to calculate an injury rate is lacking. Randomized trials and well-designed prospective community surveys are most useful because accurate rates of injuries can be calculated, and interpretations that have high confidence levels about both relationships and treatments can be made. Unfortunately, it is the lack of precisely these kinds of epidemiological studies that is a major obstacle to a better understanding of sport-related injuries. There are no acceptable epidemiological studies on injuries in three of the six most popular aerobic activities (swimming, walking, and calisthenics) and only sparse data on jogging or running (9). This chapter presents available evidence from some of the few appropriately designed studies of injuries in an individual activity, that is, running (7, 14, 15) and in a team sport, that is, soccer (1, 2, 5, 6).

I consider both preventive and rehabilitative aspects of this topic and focus on (a) overuse injury and (b) the impact of immobilization with and without surgery. Overuse is a process rather than an event, and it usually affects the musculoskeletal system and results in the breakdown and fatigue of body structures (generally soft tissue) and then inflammation and swelling; if exercise continues, the process continues and gradually involves both tissue and bone (12).

Prevention: Exercise, Fitness Levels, and Susceptibility to Injury

Does a person's fitness before a sport injury have any effect on their susceptibility to injury? Noakes (13) points out that for an individual who runs regularly "injury becomes not only possible, but inevitable. . . . The factors that make the athlete great . . . training methods, training environment . . . are the same factors responsible for injuries" (p. 326). In a survey of 16,000 recreational runners over a 2-yr span, the investigators identified more than 1,800 overuse injuries, most commonly those of the tibia and fibula, and observed at a local sports medicine clinic that 75% of sport injuries were associated with overuse (12). In an Australian survey (19), most injuries (69%) occurred during competition, 11% during training, and 20% in recreational activities. Further, it is important to accept that, with the boom in exercise and sport, an increase in the number of overuse injuries should be expected.

Among runners, overuse injury has been reported most frequently; acute injuries also occur in runners, either serious injuries (e.g., collisions with motor vehicles), or less serious ones (e.g., being hit by thrown objects or bitten by dogs). However, not all studies of sport injury provide useful incidence data. For example, 550 runners in a race were asked to complete a questionnaire on running habits from which injuries and incidence rates were calculated; 70 questionnaires were not completed (7). The problem is that, although the authors reported a 12.7% (70/550) nonresponse rate to the questionnaire, there were 2,664 runners in the race, which calculates out to a nonresponse rate of 82% (2,184/2,664). Are the data collected and presented in that study representative of the race population?

Powell et al. (15) reported that there are only three epidemiological studies with appropriate definitions of the population at risk from which general running injury rates could be calculated. He stated that although the existing data are so inadequate that firm conclusions about the causes of running injuries are impossible, "a review of three epidemiological studies (one randomized, one retrospective cohort, one cross-sectional survey) shows that the only reasonably well-established cause of running injuries is the number of miles run per week" (p. 100). For example, these authors argue that although the data from one of the studies may appear to suggest that the largest number of injured runners came from the group that ran the fewest miles, this is misleading; the incidence of injuries was in fact greater in those runners who ran the most miles when compared to those running the fewest miles (Table 52.1).

Table 52.1   Injured Runners and Annual Incidence of Injury by Weekly Mileage

Weekly mileage	Injured runners	Total runners	Annual incidence per 100 runners
< 19	168	571	29.4
> 40	52	91	57.1

Note. Data adapted from Powell et al. (15).

An initial interpretation of the available data may be made as follows. If cardiorespiratory fitness improves and the number of miles run during training increases (13) and if the incidence of running injuries correlates directly with the number of miles run (14), then a greater incidence of running injuries could be expected with higher fitness levels. However, although Pollock et al. (14) showed that the number of running injuries was not associated with fitness levels, they clearly made the point that their data must be considered in the "context of running programs of moderate to high intensity" (p. 34). Whether recreational or competitive, the evidence consistently supports the observation that the most important established determinant of overuse injury is the weekly mileage run, whereas fitness has been so infrequently measured before occurrence of the injury that there are no sound supportive data on which to make a valid interpretation.

Overuse injuries have been reported in a number of individual sports other than running. In swimming there is a significant association among so-called breaststroker's knee, an increasing number of years of competitive swimming, and an increased breaststroke training distance (16). As for gymnasts, there is a greater incidence of injury in more skilled gymnasts, presumably largely because of the increased time spent in practice (11). The same holds true for badminton players, in whom there was also a higher incidence of overuse injury per season in elite than in recreational players, although there were more injuries in recreational players per 1,000 hr of match play (8). The latter observation may be associated with lower fitness levels in recreational badminton players compared to elite players, but data to demonstrate this are lacking. The associations between injury incidence and fitness levels among swimmers, gymnasts, and badminton players are not established.

The relationship between fitness and overuse injuries in team sports such as soccer has been reported recently (2). Forty senior male soccer players without injuries requiring absence from matches or training for longer than 4 wk in the previous season were selected as subjects. Using cycle ergometry, maximal oxygen uptake was estimated preseason according to the Astrand-Ryhming nomogram; there were similar numbers of players in the low ($n = 13$), medium ($n = 14$), and high ($n = 14$) $\dot{V}O_2$ groups (Figure 52.1). All new injuries were registered and carefully categorized, including overuse injuries, which were identified as bursitis, tendinitis, and periostitis (2). During a 10-mo period of training and competition, a total of 54 new injuries were registered to 30 subjects; overuse injuries accounted for 26% of the total injuries and occurred significantly less frequently in soccer players with lower $\dot{V}O_2$ (Figure 52.1).

The authors suggest that the lower incidence of overuse injuries in subjects with lower $\dot{V}O_2$ were probably associated with their less intensive training and competition, which placed them at a lower risk of sustaining such injuries than it did those with a higher $\dot{V}O_2$ and more intensive training and competition. This is in contrast to the observation of Pollock et al. (14) that injuries were not related to fitness; however, Pollock et al. specifically excluded beginners (presumably lower $\dot{V}O_2$) from their

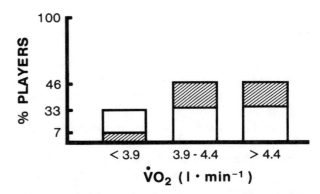

Figure 52.1. Percentage of players with low, medium, and high estimated maximal oxygen consumption (open bars) and percentage of players with overuse injuries in each group (hatched bars). Adapted from Eriksson et al. (2).

study population. It may very well be that there would be a high incidence of injuries in joggers with low $\dot{V}O_2$, particularly if they exercised at relatively high intensities. However, if there is a commonality between injury and weekly mileage in moderate- and high-intensity runners with higher $\dot{V}O_2$ (15) and between injury and intensity of training and competition in soccer players with higher $\dot{V}O_2$ (2) and in other elite athletes (8, 11, 16), then there is congruity in the findings.

In answer to Dr. Young's first question about fitness and susceptibility to injury, the conclusion from the limited and largely indirect information available in runners and soccer players tends to support the observation that a higher incidence of overuse injuries is more likely in individuals who exercise regularly at higher intensities and who therefore presumably have higher levels of fitness. However, because of the lack of well-designed studies, the evidence is patchy, as pointed out by Dr. Young.

Rehabilitation: Exercise, Fitness, and Recovery After Sport Injury

Does physical conditioning after a sport injury hasten the restoration of pre-injury performance? Reports describing rehabilitation regimens after sport injuries frequently provide only a minimal description of the rehabilitation program once immobilization is completed. The importance of appropriate clinical intervention (including rehabilitative and conditioning exercise) in reducing disability, increasing the rate of recovery, or decreasing the incidence of recurrence after a sport injury has been largely the result of the observation of situations for which appropriate intervention has not been prescribed.

Immobilization of a limb or a joint after an acute sport injury with or without surgery results in muscle atrophy, the exact mechanism of which is not yet clear, although there is a loss of both metabolic and contractile proteins. Experimental data are available on the effect of immobilization on the strength characteristics of normal muscle (10) and on the effect of immobilization and different exercise regimens following an acute knee-ligament lesion with and without surgery (5, 6). Reviews of the literature on exercise rehabilitation after knee surgery (4, 18) suggest (a) that patients recover muscular strength more rapidly with active exercise rehabilitation, (b) that $\dot{V}O_2$ recover more rapidly with strength plus one-legged cycling training than with strength training only, (c) that full recovery of range of motion after immobilization of the knee takes as much as four times as long with cylinder casting than with movable cast bracing, and (d) that the movable cast brace results in less reduction in muscle fiber area and no reduction in aerobic energy potential enzyme activity. These data provide evidence that muscle function recovers more rapidly with the early resumption of active motion and the implementation of appropriate exercise rehabilitation and conditioning than it does with no active intervention or inappropriate intervention.

The relationships among immobilization of the normal triceps brachii, atrophy, and strength training were examined in a carefully controlled randomized trial by MacDougall et al. (10). Immobilization of the elbow for 5-6 wk either preceded or followed strength training (high resistance, slow speed); half the subjects were randomized to each group. There were slightly greater decreases in fast-twitch-fiber area (33%) than in slow-twitch-fiber area (25%) and a 41% reduction in slow isokinetic strength of the elbow. The authors reported no beneficial effect of pretraining normal muscle on its susceptibility to immobilization-induced muscle fiber atrophy.

In a carefully controlled study of 84 male soccer players (5), immobilization with and without surgery following an acute lesion of the medial collateral ligament of the knee was prospectively evaluated. The major effect of immobilization was a decrease in both static and dynamic muscle strength and was most apparent in the patients with surgery (5). There was no assessment of fitness levels before the injury, so that issue cannot be discussed with reference to data in this study.

Percutaneous electrical stimulation during immobilization has been reported to prevent muscle fiber atrophy (1, 20); however, this was not demonstrated in this study of soccer players (5). Rehabilitation following a traumatic lesion to one knee has also been investigated in soccer players (6). Following a mean of 33 d of immobilization, the rehabilitation regimen called for treatment three times per week for 4 wk using the following protocols in 107 healthy soccer players with traumatic knee ligament lesions: progressive-resistive exercise, one-legged cycle ergometer exercise training with the injured leg only, and maximum isometric or isokinetic exercise at two different angular velocities. Recovery of all muscle performance variables apparently was unrelated to training method, however, dynamic endurance exercise performance was most improved in the trained leg in those undergoing exercise cycle training (6).

It appears that the essential aspect of resistive training after immobilization is the restoration of muscle volume that is accompanied by a restoration of strength (1, 6). It is important to concentrate efforts on specific functional exercise that emphasizes the neurogenic component of rehabilitation training, as this leads not only to a further increase in muscle mass and strength but also to improved motor relearning and coordination. In addition to dynamic and isometric exercise, isokinetic training is apparently useful, as it provides maximal resistance throughout the midrange of motion of the joint, thus reducing the likelihood of injury that often occurs with eccentric exercise (4, 18).

Unfortunately, much of the clinical evidence for the importance of therapeutic exercise after sport injury is based on the observation of cases in which there has been a failure to initiate and follow through with appropriate rehabilitation strategies or on case series reports of a single treatment technique rather than experimental studies with controls or more than one intervention. Again, on the basis of limited experimental data, the answer to Dr. Young's second question appears to be that physical conditioning after an injury does hasten the rate of recovery to pre-injury performance but that the scientific evidence is patchy although the clinical evidence may be more consistent.

Conclusion

There are more unanswered than answered questions in the areas of exercise, fitness, and health and the prevention and rehabilitation of sport injuries. Future inquiries in the prevention of sport-related injury should attempt to do the following:

- Develop a more comprehensive and sensitive approach to injury definition to permit both intrasport and intersport comparisons.
- Identify prospectively the risk factors associated with sport injury.
- Identify prospectively the long-term sequelae of overuse and acute injuries: What are the long-term effects of injuries in young athletes in different types of sports? With the advent and subsequent popularity of Master's sport competition, what is the effect of aging on the likelihood of injury?
- Determine the differences in injury rates for the same sport played at recreational and elite competitive levels.

These issues are dealt with best in terms of well-designed, large prospective studies and community surveys. Once incidences and patterns of injury have been established, risk factor associations determined, and risks and benefits described, appropriate preventive interventions can be implemented to reduce the potential risk of injury.

In terms of rehabilitation or conditioning exercise and recovery from trauma or injury, future inquiries should attempt to do the following:

- Compare the different effects of different types of rehabilitation and conditioning exercise.
- Determine the optimum time for the initiation of, the duration of, and the dose-response relationships for, rehabilitation and conditioning exercise.
- Define the clinical importance of the specificity of rehabilitation and conditioning exercise.

When possible, these studies should be carried out using experimental methodologies, preferably in a prospective fashion in which different strategies can be compared; clinicians can then decide which strategy is likely to be most effective for which patient.

If exercise and sports are to be advocated as beneficial, it is our responsibility to provide data documenting not only benefit but also risk. Only when the public is provided with data related to both the benefits and the risks of exercise can informed decisions be made about exercise, fitness, and health. As Dr. Young pointed out for surgery and disease, the scientific data on both the prevention and the rehabilitation of injuries associated with sport and exercise are patchy. In addition, as

Dr. Young has done, I reiterate that I too have focused on specific areas and that the paucity of good data on sport injury does not necessarily apply to other areas of exercise, fitness, and health.

References

1. Erikkson, E., and T. Haggmark. A comparison of isometric training and electrical muscle stimulation in the recovery after knee ligament surgery. *Am. J. Sports Med.* 7: 169-171, 1979.
2. Eriksson, L.I., L. Jorfeldt, and J. Ekstrand. Overuse and distortion soccer injuries related to the player's estimated maximal aerobic capacity. *Int. J. Sports Med.* 7: 214-216, 1986.
3. Gerberich, S.G. Sports injuries: Implications for prevention. *Public Health Rep.* 100: 570-571, 1985.
4. Grimby, G. Progressive resistance exercise for injury rehabilitation. *Sports Med.* 2: 309-315, 1985.
5. Halkjaer-Kristensen, J., and T. Ingemann-Hansen. Wasting of the human quadriceps muscle after knee ligament injuries. *Scand. J. Rehabil. Med.* (Suppl. 13): 29-37, 1985.
6. Ingemann-Hansen, T., and J. Halkjaer-Kristensen. Physical training of the hypertrophic quadriceps muscle in man. *Scand. J. Rehabil. Med.* (Suppl. 13): 38-44, 1985.
7. Jacobs, S.J., and B.L. Berson. Injuries to runners: A study of entrants to a 10,000 meter race. *Am. J. Sports Med.* 14: 151-155, 1986.
8. Jorgensen, U., and S. Winge. Epidemiology of badminton players. *Int. J. Sports Med.* 8: 379-382, 1987.
9. Koplan, J.P., D.S. Siscovick, and G.M. Goldbaum. The risks of exercise: A public health view of injuries and hazards. *Public Health Rep.* 100: 189-195, 1985.
10. MacDougall, J.D., G.C.B. Elder, et al. Effects of strength training and immobilization on human muscle fibers. *Eur. J. Appl. Physiol.* 43: 25-34, 1980.
11. McAuley, E.G. Hudaser, K. Shields, et al. Injuries in women's gymnastics. *Am. J. Sports Med.* 15: 558-565, 1987.
12. McKeag, D.B. The concept of overuse: The primary care aspects of overuse syndromes in sports. *Prim. Care* 11: 43-59, 1984.
13. Noakes, T. *Lore of running.* Cape Town, South Africa: Oxford University Press; 1986, p. 326.

14. Pollock, M.L., L.B. Gettman, C.A. Milesis, et al. Effects of frequency and duration of training on attrition and incidence of injury. *Med. Sci. Sports* 8: 31-36, 1977.

15. Powell, K.E., H.W. Kohl, C.J. Casperson, et al. An epidemiological perspective on the causes of running injuries. *Phys. Sportsmed.* 14: 100-114, 1986.

16. Rovere, G.D., and A.W. Nichols. Frequency, associated factors, and treatment of breast-stroker's knee in competitive swimmers. *Am. J. Sports Med.* 13: 99-104, 1985.

17. Sandelin, J., S. Santavirta, R. Lattila, et al. Sports injuries in a large urban population: occurrence and epidemiological aspects. *Int. J. Sports Med.* 8: 61-66, 1988.

18. Sherman, W.M., D.R. Pearson, M.J. Plyley, et al. Isokinetic rehabilitation after surgery. *Am. J. Sports Med.* 10: 155-161, 1982.

19. Smithers, M., and P.T. Meyers. Injuries in sport: A prospective casualty study. *Med. J. Aust.* 142: 457-461, 1985.

20. Wigerstad-Lossing, I., G. Grimby, T. Jonssen, et al. Effects of electrical muscle stimulation combined with voluntary contractions after knee ligament surgery. *Med. Sci. Sports Exerc.* 20: 93-98, 1988.

Chapter 53

Exercise, Fitness, and Mental Health

David R. Brown

Epidemiological investigations have consistently provided support for the relationship between physical activity and physical health (109). For example, in most of these studies it has been observed that physical activity related to occupational status or that regular exercise associated with leisure-time pursuits is inversely related to cardiovascular disease and coronary heart disease (CHD) mortality rates. Indeed, much of the research in exercise science has attended to the relationship between physical activity and the chronic diseases such as CHD that threaten contemporary society. However, a person's health status is multidimensional and includes a mental as well as a physical component. Therefore, it seems important to review research on the relationship among physical activity, physical fitness, and mental health, and this is the intent of this chapter.

Making a distinction between mental and physical health is somewhat artificial. More likely, mental and physical health will covary as a function of exercise and physical or physiological fitness, and this belief is consistent with current holistic health perspectives emphasizing mind-body unity. For example, it is often assumed that the lower cardiovascular morbidity and mortality rates associated with higher levels of activity are due to changes in physical or physiological parameters. However, it is also known that psychological states or traits are related to coronary heart disease (74), as is the level of involvement in activity (105). Therefore, viewing mental and physical health separately rather than as intricately related is simply a convenient means for narrowing the focus of this chapter.

To a large extent, the existing situation in the mental health field is analogous to what is occurring in the physical health field. There are currently millions of people who are disabled and suffering to some degree from mental health problems, and, as with the cardiovascular diseases, these problems are reaching pandemic proportions in many countries. In the United States alone, the cost of mental health care in 1980 was estimated at between $19.4 and $24.1 billion (106).

It has been estimated that 127 million people worldwide and 8-20 million Americans presently suffer from an affective or depressive disorder and that "this is but the tip of the iceberg; only an estimated 25% of those with diagnosable depression ever seek treatment" (107). In the United States,

> As many as 25 percent of the population are estimated to suffer from mild to moderate depression, anxiety, and other indicators of emotional disorder at any given time. The extent and composition of this group varies over time. Although most of these problems do not constitute mental disorders as conventionally diagnosed, many of these persons suffer intensely and seek assistance. By and large, such individuals cope with these stresses with the aid of family, friends or professionals outside the mental health system. (84, p. 8)

The finding that many people suffer from mental health problems and that they attempt to cope and get by on a daily basis with little or no professional mental health intervention is significant. Most of these individuals will be functioning at less than optimal levels personally, socially, and vocationally. For some, such impaired performance may ultimately lead to suicide, which ranked as the eighth-leading cause of mortality in the United States in 1983 (79). It therefore seems critical that efforts continue to be made to identify cost-effective interventions that can be delivered to people in their natural environments and that have the potential to prevent or lessen the severity of mental health problems in the population at large.

In this regard, exercise holds considerable promise. As with physical activity and cardiovascular disease, epidemiological research is encouraging, as there is evidence of a positive relationship between level of activity and mental health. Stephens (105), for example, has completed extensive secondary analyses of four large data bases obtained as a result of surveys conducted in Canada and the United States. The goal of these analyses was to examine the relationship between physical activity and mental health as it exists in household populations in both countries.

> The inescapable conclusion of this study is that the level of physical activity is positively associated with good mental health in the household populations of the United States and Canada, when mental health is defined as positive mood, general well-being, and relatively infrequent symptoms of anxiety and depression. . . . The robustness of this conclusion derives from the varied sources of evidence: four population samples in two countries over a 10-year period, four different methods of operationalizing physical activity, and six different mental health scales. (105, p. 41-42)

This conclusion is encouraging, as physical activity may indeed possess the potential to maintain or promote positive mental health. In other words, involvement in physical activity may prevent the onset of mental health problems (primary prevention) or may ameliorate mental health problems before they escalate to levels of clinical significance (secondary prevention) and require more extensive treatment (tertiary prevention). These forms of prevention were first introduced in the mental health field by Caplan (11) and more recently were applied directly to the prevention of sedentary lifestyles by Kirschenbaum (47). The nature of Stephens's findings, however, do not provide an answer to the question whether involvement in physical activity promotes mental health or whether mental health promotes involvement in physical activity. It remains unknown whether activity enhances psychological well-being or whether happy, relaxed, and nondepressed individuals have the vigor and energy to be active.

Whether improved or maintained mental health is a result of exercise may ultimately depend on one's definition of mental health. For example, respondents in some studies have reported improvements in affect or mood state after they exercise. However, the influence of activity and physical fitness on many other psychological variables is less clear and still unsupported by experimental data (26, 32).

An Operational Definition of Mental Health

To define *mental health* is extremely challenging. The term is used broadly in the exercise literature to encompass such diverse factors as behavior (work, sleep, social behavior), cognition (intelligence, academic performance), personality (self-concept), affect (anxiety, well-being), and perception (32). In addition, one review has focused on the relationship between physical activity and mental illness or disorders that may have a mental component. These disorders include sleep disorders, eating disorders, problems related to alcohol and substance abuse, psychoses, and affective disturbances (26). It is recognized that mental health is related to all these factors or constructs, and there is indeed a fine line between the point where health ends and illness begins. However, from a conceptual and theoretical standpoint it would be advantageous for researchers in exercise science to make distinctions between mental health and mental illness. In the literature on exercise and mental illness, exercise is clearly used as a treatment or as an adjunct to treatment to ameliorate mental problems or decrease mental illness. In the literature on exercise and mental health, by contrast, exercise is used as a health promotion or illness prevention strategy to maintain or enhance mental health and psychological well-being. At minimum, making such a conceptual distinction will help ensure that researchers have clearly articulated the research questions being asked and that at the outset of an investigation they have in mind a clearly defined population of subjects. These are basic methodological considerations, but it is extremely important to identify precisely the psychological characteristics of the subjects used in psychological research in which exercise is employed as an experimental manipulation. This is necessary because individuals who score in the normal range on a psychological inventory and those significantly elevated on the same inventory before exercise may exhibit quite different postexercise responses.

Mental health as used in this chapter implies that the subjects in a research study are from a nonclinical, noninstitutionalized population. In other words, the subjects should not be experiencing any significant degree of psychopathology at the outset of an investigation. This decision is consistent with the intent of the Organizing Committee of this conference to focus as much as possible on the normative population at large. However, research using subjects who are mild or moderately elevated on psychological measures at the commencement of a study and who are at risk for developing more serious mental problems of clinical magnitude is included here. Indeed, such individuals may constitute a large percentage of that one quarter of the general population who at any one time may be suffering from anxiety, depression, or emotional stress (84); for these individuals, exercise may be important in terms of secondary prevention. For this reason, anxiety, depression, and reactivity to stressors are targeted as the key mental health concerns of this chapter.

Methodological Issues

A number of earlier reviews have focused on issues related to exercise and mental health or mental illness (18, 26, 32, 37, 41, 53, 63, 65, 66, 70, 92, 96, 97, 113). In addition, a textbook has been published as a result of a National Institutes of Mental Health workshop conducted in 1984 (72), the purpose of which was to review and analyze the empirical support for using exercise to promote mental health and treat mental illness.

Among the proposed psychological benefits of exercise are improved academic performance, confidence, emotional stability, intellectual functioning, mood, perception, self-control, sexual satisfaction, and work efficiency (41). Although exercise holds promise for maintaining or enhancing mental health (e.g., improving mood state), there are presently few data available to support many of the claims made about other psychological and cognitive benefits of exercise.

As most prior reviews have pointed out, the exercise and mental health literature consists primarily of descriptive, correlational, and cross-sectional studies, and many contain serious methodological problems. Very few well-designed, true experimental investigations possessing good external and internal validity have been conducted. In addition, there is a need to do longitudinal research because many of the psychological benefits that potentially may be derived from exercise may occur or diminish over a period of time.

Methodological problems that are common in much of the research on the relationship between exercise and mental health include (a) the use of inadequate sample sizes, (b) the failure of investigators to assign subjects randomly to experimental conditions, (c) the absence of placebo or control conditions, and (d) the failure to utilize double- or total blind designs. The use of proper sampling procedures and designs employing placebo and control groups will minimize the influence of behavioral artifacts on the outcomes of a study. Such artifacts as demand characteristics, response distortion, the Hawthorne effect, and the Rosenthal effect are especially problematic in exercise research in which psychological responses serve as the dependent variables (67).

The results of many exercise studies are weakened by the fact that subjects are allowed to self-select among the activities or conditions associated with the study. In addition, the responses of subjects may differ based on their expectancies about or beliefs in the efficacy of different experimental conditions. As with problems related to behavioral artifacts, randomization of subjects and a well-designed, properly controlled study possessing placebo and control groups will help safeguard against self-selection and expectancy effects.

One additional methodological problem commonly not controlled for in psychological investigations involving exercise is the assessment of initial differences between subjects on fitness or psychological measures. When relevant to the research question, subjects from fit or unfit and clinical or nonclinical populations need to be identified and their levels of physiological and psychological fitness assessed from the outset of an investigation. This will enhance the external validity of a study.

The foregoing highlighted some of the major methodological limitations of this research area. The remainder of this chapter reviews studies that are relevant to the relationship among exercise, physical fitness, and mental health in the general population. It is not the purpose of this chapter to present a comprehensive narrative review of all the literature related to exercise and mental health. Rather, an attempt is made to identify promising trends in research, consistent long-term research efforts, and unique research endeavors.

Stress and Anxiety

Entire volumes have been devoted to theoretical and conceptual issues related to the constructs of stress or anxiety. Efforts to operationalize these terms have been biological (93), cognitive (54), and psychobiological (102). Conceptual models of stress and anxiety (55, 103) have been expanded to include intervening variables, such as coping behaviors that mediate emotional reactions (e.g., anxiety). These conceptual models have become quite complex. However, these conceptualizations can be simplified to a more basic stimulus-organism-response (S-O-R) model, in which stress is viewed as a process involving the interaction between a person and his or her environment (103, p. 13):

$$\text{Stressor} \rightarrow \begin{array}{c} \text{Perception} \\ \text{of threat} \end{array} \rightarrow \begin{array}{c} \text{Emotional} \\ \text{reaction} \end{array}$$
$$\text{(Stimulus)} \quad \text{(Organism)} \quad \text{(Response)}$$

In the S-O-R model, exercise may be viewed as a stressor that, if perceived as a threat, can lead to emotional distress. This may be how some individuals perceive the pain or discomfort that is sometimes associated with exercise. Other individuals, especially those who have adapted to exercise through training, may perceive exercise as positive stress instead of distress. It is known, for example, that trained or fit individuals have increased cardiovascular efficiency (e.g., reduced blood pressure, reduced heart rate, and increased stroke volume) during physical exertion and recovery from exertion. It therefore may have seemed logical for investigators to hypothesize about whether fit individuals would also respond more efficiently than would unfit individuals to a psychosocial or cognitive stressor (e.g., a timed mental arithmetic test). These types of investigations, in which the response to stressors by fit and unfit subjects is evaluated, make up one area of exercise research related to the construct of stress.

A second major area of research has focused on anxiety, a stress-related emotion. Several studies representative of this area evaluated the efficacy of using acute vigorous physical activity as a means for reducing a person's level of tension or anxiety. These investigations typically involve assessment of an individual's level of physiological arousal, or emotional response (i.e., state anxiety) for a period of time after involvement in a single bout of activity. According to Spielberger (102, 103), state anxiety is a transitory emotional state that fluctuates in response to specific situations or events (e.g., involvement in exercise, taking an examination, or giving a speech). Trait anxiety, an enduring stable personality characteristic, is predicted not to change significantly in response to properly prescribed acute exercise.

Exercise, Physical Fitness, and Reactivity to Stressors

There is currently a great deal of interest in the relationship between fitness and the psychophysio-logical responses of fit and unfit individuals to a variety of stressors. This interest has resulted in a number of investigations in which fitness has been defined as *aerobic* fitness and the stressors are exercise, or laboratory psychosocial stressors. This is not meant to imply that exercise is not a psychosocial stressor. In fact, from a holistic health perspective, all stressors may most appropriately be labeled biopsychosocial stressors, as cognition, physiology, and environment interact in determining a person's interpretation of and response to a stimulus. Evidence has been presented, however, which suggests that it may be theoretically meaningful to distinguish between stressors that elicit active (e.g., a reaction time task) versus passive (e.g., the cold pressor test) coping strategies (57). Nevertheless, it may eventually prove sufficient merely to report findings based on how trained and untrained subjects react to a specific stressor regardless of whether the task is categorized as active, passive, psychosocial, or physical. Perhaps reactivity to stressors within, as well as between, categories will differ. Even if reactivity to an entire class of stressors is ultimately determined to be the same, greater attention needs to be paid to task specificity during efforts to replicate research in this area. Also, several dependent variables have been evaluated in the research on stress reactivity. These include measures of cardiovascular (13, 14, 39, 40, 42, 88, 94, 98, 99, 115), biochemical (13, 42, 98, 101), physiological (e.g., skin temperature) (10, 13, 39, 42, 45, 88, 115), and psychological (40, 42, 88, 98, 99, 101, 115) responses obtained before, during, and after the presentation of different stressors. The fact that researchers have employed a variety of stressors and different dependent measures in their investigations has resulted in findings that are difficult to compare and in a general lack of replication of results across studies. Although some investigators have found significant differences in reactivity to stressors favoring the fit, others have not.

Furthermore, there is a paucity of training investigations of a true experimental nature in which subjects were equated on fitness from the outset of a study; randomly assigned to experimental, placebo, or control conditions; and assessed on the measures of reactivity to the same stressors before and after training and improved fitness effects were documented. However, there are exceptions to this criticism (45, 88, 99). For example, Sinyor et al. (99) randomly assigned 38 male subjects to aerobic training, anaerobic training, or control treatment conditions for 10 wk. The investigators evaluated reactivity to three stressors—a mental arithmetic task, a mental quiz, and the Stroop Color-Word Interference Task—before and after the 10-wk treatment period. Dependent variables, which included heart rate response and measures of subjective arousal, were obtained at different intervals before, during, and after presentation of the stressors.

Sinyor et al. reported that the aerobic training condition led to a significant improvement in the subjects' estimated maximal oxygen uptake ($\dot{V}O_2$max) values and to a significant decrease in their resting heart rates. These differences were not found for the subjects who participated in the anaerobic and the control conditions. In addition, all three groups of subjects showed increased heart rates and subjective arousal responses to the stressors and decreased heart rates and subjective arousal responses following presentation of the stressors. However, none of the three groups differed from one another in reactivity as a function of the treatment conditions.

This study is notable from the standpoint that it was a training study and experimental in nature. Most investigators have employed correlational or cross-sectional designs in attempts to evaluate the influence of aerobic fitness on reactivity to stressors. Groups of subjects are usually established at the outset of a study, theoretically at least, according to high and low aerobic fitness levels. Unfortunately, however, aerobic fitness is seldom assessed in most of the studies representative of this area of research. Direct measures of $\dot{V}O_2$max have been rarely used (13, 101) as a criterion for classifying subjects or evaluating improvements in aerobic fitness. This is true of the studies conducted by Sinyor et al. (99) and of other investigations of an experimental nature (45, 88). This is surprising in light of the fact that aerobic capacity is often of central importance to the questions being asked in this area of research. Normally, the independent variable or measure of aerobic fitness has been some estimate of $\dot{V}O_2$max. In other words, subjects are categorized on the basis of the relationship between submaximal heart rates and direct measures of $\dot{V}O_2$max. In some cases, heart rate values have been used for grouping subjects and subsequently evaluated as a dependent variable. This has led to some confusion about how to analyze and interpret results from investigations in which heart rate values have been used as both dependent and independent measures. Although low resting heart rates may be indicative of a training adaptation resulting from involvement in chronic physical activity, the best indicator of aerobic fitness is cardiorespiratory endurance and the

best measure of physical fitness is a direct measure of $\dot{V}O_2$max. Therefore, it is recommended that whenever the relationship between aerobic fitness and stress reactivity is being evaluated, an investigator assess maximal aerobic power directly, in favor of using predicted $\dot{V}O_2$max measures.

In addition, it is well known that fit individuals often possess lower resting heart rates than do unfit individuals. This means that there may be significant heart rate differences between fit and unfit groups of subjects at the outset of an investigation. It may also mean that during an encounter with a stressor, the increased heart rate response of a fit individual could be greater than that of an unfit individual. This is because a stressor may elevate the heart rates of both the fit and the unfit subjects to comparable levels and because the resting heart rate of the fit individual was lower than that of the unfit individual before the stressor was presented. Some investigators have tried to control for these differences by using a covariance statistical procedure. However, these differences are a very real physiological phenomenon, and the fact is that fit individuals may actually show higher reactivity to stressors (48, 51, 52), not lower reactivity. Training adaptations such as hypertrophy of the adrenal glands might lead to increased reactivity to novel stressors. On the other hand, exercise training has been shown to result in a reduced plasma norepinephrine response to a familiar stressor in stress-sensitive rats (16), and a high level of fitness in men was also associated with an attenuated plasma norepinephrine response to a well-learned familiar stressor (101). Clearly, whether a stressor is novel or well practiced should be specified and controlled for in research exploring the effect of exercise training on reactivity.

The methodological problems that currently permeate the research on aerobic fitness and stress reactivity do not allow for a conclusion to be made supporting the use of chronic exercise to enhance aerobic fitness if the ultimate goal is to modify in a positive manner an individual's reactivity to stressors. Obviously, one exception to this point is in regard to the stressor exercise. It is known that training leading to improvements in cardiorespiratory fitness, as documented by increases in measures of $\dot{V}O_2$max, also leads to alterations in reactivity that are exercise specific. These training adaptations mean that an individual can function more efficiently during exercise as a result of habituating to the exercise stimulus.

The point being made is that no currently available empirical evidence allows one to conclude that aerobic training and improved fitness cause different response patterns to stressors (other than physical activity) that favor the fit when compared to the less fit individual. However, Crews and Landers (17) indicated that available data suggest an association between aerobic fitness and reactivity to stressors. Crews and Landers (17) conducted a meta-analytic review of this area of research and concluded that "aerobically fit subjects had a reduced psychosocial stress response compared to either control group or baseline values" (p. S114). It should be clearly understood, however, that this conclusion is based on a foundation of research possessing serious methodological problems. For example, the statistical manipulations possible in a meta-analysis cannot alter the fact that aerobic fitness has not been evaluated directly in most of the studies included in the review by Crews and Landers. Nor can their meta-analysis rectify other methodological weaknesses in this research. The use of experimental designs, training studies, direct measures of $\dot{V}O_2max$, and replication of findings across studies are required in future research if a definite link between exercise, physical fitness, and reactivity to stressors is to be established.

Animal Studies

The use of an animal model possesses potential for identifying centrally or peripherally mediated mechanisms that elucidate the relationship between exercise and issues related to mental health. For example, neurotransmitter differences have been found between sedentary rats and rats exposed to a chronic exercise stimulus (6). An increase in opiate receptor occupancy has also been reported in rat brains following exercise (81). Therefore, a centrally mediated monamine or endorphin hypothesis may ultimately explain differences between active and inactive people (71). An animal model has also been employed to investigate the relationship between exercise and reactivity to stressors (15, 16).

Cox et al. (15) reported findings from a study in which rats were exposed to a swimming stressor and a predictable tail-shock stressor on different occasions. One group of rats was exposed to the stressors after 5-7 wk of training using swimming as the mode of activity, and a second group of rats was exposed to the same stressors but were not trained. Trained rats showed significantly lower heart rates, lactate values, epinephrine, and corticosterone responses to a swimming stressor (a familiar stressor) than did the nontrained rats, in which swimming was novel. Systolic and diastolic blood pressures were elevated during the swimming stress, but the blood pressure response between the trained and the untrained animals did not differ significantly. The exposure to tail shock, a novel stressor for both the trained and the nontrained rats, resulted in predictable elevations in the dependent measures. However, the trained and the nontrained rats did not differ on any of the measures during shock stress. Therefore, the findings of Cox et al. (15) may mean that any advantages afforded the trained rats were due to habituation to the exercise stimulus rather than to any inherent ability to reduce reactivity to stressors in general. The problem of habituation has also been reported in research with humans (45). These studies (15, 45) point to the need to control for habituation.

Employing a behavioral approach, Weber and Lee (112) and Tharp and Carson (108) found that rats exposed to a chronic swimming (112) and running (108) exercise stimulus were better able to cope with the open field test (a novel stressor) than were less active rats (112) or rats trained using a lighter exercise stimulus of wading and walking (108). Both studies addressed questions regarding the influence of exercise on coping ability.

Reactivity to Stressors
Versus Coping With Stressors

The complex relationship among training, physical fitness, reactivity to stressors, and coping ability has not often been addressed in human research conducted to date. Most research has focused on the relationship between fitness level and subsequent reactivity to stressors. This focus does not address the issue of whether the alterations in reactivity that may accompany improved levels of fitness actually affect the behavioral ability of the organism to better cope with a stressor. The ability or inability to cope with stressors has been identified by Spielberger (102, p. 42-44) as being an important component of the stress process and one that affects the organism's perception and labeling of a stimulus as a stressor. A finding that reactivity to stressors is altered in favor of the fit individual will indeed be important because most individuals encounter numerous stressors each day. Nevertheless, such a finding says nothing about an enhanced ability to cope with stressors, and ultimately this may turn out to be the most critical issue in terms of the relationship between stress and mental or physical health.

Related to this discussion is the fact that the investigations that have dealt with the effects of fitness on reactivity to stressors may also lack ecological validity. Crews and Landers (17) stated that "all of the studies in the present review have used acute, short-term stressors. In some real life settings (i.e., air traffic controllers), individuals may experience more long-term, chronic levels of high stress" (p. 119). There remains the question of whether the results from these laboratory studies will have relevance to the field setting (5) or to the many individuals in the general population who face chronic stress on a sustained basis.

Also, it is not uncommon for individuals to encounter stressors on a daily basis that require isometric (static) or isotonic (dynamic) muscle contraction to perform work successfully. This often occurs as a natural course of employment, for example, in the lifting, pulling, and pushing required of the professional mover, firefighter, or nurse. Perhaps the anaerobic type of chronic activity in the form of strength training will lead to fitness gains that will alter reactivity to some stressors better than will the fitness gains resulting from participation in chronic aerobic activity. Two studies (88, 99) evaluated the influence of strength training on reactivity to stressors, and the outcomes were not positive. Weight training did not significantly alter measures of stress reactivity in either investigation. However, the stressors employed in both investigations did not require the use of muscle strength or endurance. The use of stressors that were more specific to weight-training adaptations may have led to different outcomes in these investigations. However, the research question would be different, being related more to issues of task specificity and habituation than to aerobic fitness per se.

In summary, the theoretical assumption is that the increased cardiovascular endurance or the physiological adaptations that occur with chronic aerobic physical activity (or both) will mediate and attenuate an individual's reactivity across a wide variety of stressors in addition to exercise. Although the theory has intuitive appeal, the research evidence in support of the theory is not particularly strong, has not been replicated, and is based largely on cross-sectional investigations in which $\dot{V}O_2$max has been predicted. Also, the possibility exists that fit individuals may exhibit higher, not lower, reactivity to stressors. In addition, a causal mechanism responsible for the hypothesized differential response patterns in fit and unfit individuals has not been identified, nor

has the relationship between changes in reactivity and the subsequent ability to cope behaviorally with a stressor been elucidated.

Exercise and Reductions in Anxiety and Tension

A second area of study is identified in this chapter as a subarea of the literature on exercise and stress. The focus of researchers in this area has been on anxiety (a stress-related emotion) or its physiological concomitants. There has been increasing interest in using exercise as a means of promoting relaxation. This interest has led to a number of investigations being conducted to document reductions in tension and anxiety that may occur in response to an exercise stimulus.

With few exceptions, studies in this area have not reported the aerobic fitness levels of subjects who participated in the research, nor have training effects been documented. One possible reason is that the reported reductions in anxiety were in response to an acute rather than a chronic exercise stimulus and aerobic fitness per se was not related to the central research question being asked in the investigations. Nevertheless, as hypothesized in the literature on aerobic fitness and stress reactivity, fit individuals may respond differently to an acute stressor when compared to unfit individuals. This would certainly be true in regard to many biochemical and physiological measures obtained during and after the stressor exercise. From a biobehavioral perspective, therefore, it makes theoretical sense to document subjects' fitness levels before a study of acute exercise.

In studies by Farrell et al. (28, 29) the psychophysiological responses of experienced men and women runners were measured during attempts to evaluate the endorphin hypothesis, which could account for some of the psychological effects that result from exercise. Runners possessing high $\dot{V}O_2$max values experienced reductions in tension (29) and mood state (28) following a race (29) and submaximal treadmill exercise (28). The reduction in tension observed in the runners following race conditions may be attributable to a postcompetition response rather than to exercise per se, and the improvements in mood following treadmill running were not significantly different from preexercise levels. The nonsignificant findings obtained in the treadmill study appear to be attributable to the small number of subjects ($n = 6$) involved in the study. Nevertheless, these preliminary findings, which suggest that highly fit athletes may experience improvements in mood following acute vigorous exercise, are similar to findings that have been noted consistently in research using nonathletic populations (68).

Acute Studies

The acute effects of exercise have been documented psychometrically using the *"How do you feel right now?"* state anxiety scale from the Spielberger State-Trait Anxiety Inventory (104) (see also refs. 7, 68, 77, 85, 86) and physiologically using blood pressure measures (38, 85, 86). In addition, the effect of acute exercise on muscle tension has been evaluated electromyographically (19, 20, 24, 25, 95). Morgan (76) and Sime (95) both reported that low-intensity, short-duration physical activity had no significant effect on altering state anxiety. In contrast to these findings, low-intensity, short-duration exercise has resulted in reduced muscle electrical activity (20, 95). Thus, the somatic "tranquilizer effect" associated with exercise, reported by deVries (21) and deVries and Adams (22) to be as potent as the effect obtained from using the tranquilizer drug meprobamate, may have to reach a threshold before it is perceived by an individual as reduced anxiety. These studies suggest that the exercise-anxiety relationship may be affected by exercise intensity, and subsequent research has confirmed the importance of a dose-response function. Although the exercise intensity threshold necessary to promote anxiety reduction has not been specifically determined, it is known that involvement in acute, vigorous exercise of a moderate intensity can lead to such reductions. More important, the research evidence that does exist suggests that the American College of Sports Medicine (1) guidelines for exercise levels that promote increased cardiorespiratory functioning and enhanced body composition may also be sufficient for promoting positive mental health. In other words, an exercise stimulus that requires 15-30 min of aerobic-type activity performed within the target heart rate range of 60%-90% of maximum heart rate reserve appears sufficient to promote an anxiolytic effect due to exercise.

Furthermore, in regard to the potential mental health benefits that are associated with exercise, it is encouraging to note that the tension-reducing effect attributed to involvement in acute exercise is not specific to clinical populations (21, 77, 86). A single bout of vigorous aerobic exercise, for example, has led to reports of reduced anxiety or tension in both normal and clinically anxious individuals (68). It appears that individuals with high, moderate, and low levels of anxiety feel better after exercise, although it has been reported by deVries (20) that the subjects who derived the greatest benefits from exercise were those having the highest levels of muscle electrical activity before exercise. Nevertheless, findings from studies that are correlational, cross-sectional, and quasi-experimental are consistent and encouraging. The findings suggest that one psychological benefit that may occur as a result of properly prescribed chronic physical activity is a reduction in day-to-day tension or anxiety. The anxiety reduction associated with a single bout of exercise is temporary, lasting from 2 to 5 hr (38, 86). Thus, individuals may escape the daily pressure of their job, home, or school environments by taking time out to engage in vigorous physical activity. However, within 2 to 5 hr after returning to the environment from which they escaped, the psychological benefits, in terms of reduced anxiety, are lost. Therefore, exercise may be an important strategy that can help an individual get through the challenges, pressures, and stressors encountered during the day. However, acute exercise will need to be maintained on a chronic basis for the individual to continue reexperiencing the anxiety-reduction effect.

Findings indicating that acute exercise is associated with reductions in anxiety and tension lead to a question about how effective exercise actually is in promoting feelings of relaxation when compared to other strategies. These strategies may include relaxation, meditation, hypnosis, or biofeedback. This question was addressed in part by Bahrke and Morgan (2), who randomly assigned 75 adult male regular exercisers to exercise, meditation, and control conditions. The subjects in the exercise group (*n* = 25) walked on a treadmill at 70% of maximal heart rate, the meditation group (*n* = 25) practiced Benson's relaxation procedure, and the control group (*n* = 25) rested in a reclining chair. All experimental conditions lasted 20 min and state anxiety was assessed before and following each condition. Findings from this investigation indicated that exercise, meditation, and quiet rest all result in significant and comparable reductions in state anxiety. These findings suggest that exercise or meditation per se may not cause reductions in state anxiety and that rest, which is often employed as a control condition, may in fact be considered another form of treatment in research employing psychophysiological measures. Reductions in psychometric measures of anxiety (86), a biochemical measure of anxiety (i.e., epinephrine) (64), and cardiovascular (i.e., blood pressure) (38, 86) and neurophysiological (i.e., EMG) measures (23) have been documented after a rest condition to be equivalent to the decreases that occurred with other tension-reduction strategies, such as biofeedback (23), meditation (64), and exercise (38, 86).

Research by Raglin and Morgan (86) compared the effects of exercise and quiet rest on the state anxiety and blood pressure response of adult male normotensive (*n* = 15) and pharmacologically controlled hypertensive (*n* = 15) subjects. The subjects participated in the quiet-rest or exercise condition on separate days using a counterbalanced design. The research design employed in this investigation also allowed for evaluation of the degree to which treatment effects persisted over the course of a 3-hr period. The findings from this study are generally consistent with previous research in that reductions in state anxiety and blood pressure occurred after the exercise and rest conditions. However, the pattern of response differed over time. In the experiment using normotensive subjects, for example, quiet rest led to a faster and smaller reduction in systolic blood pressure compared to the reductions that occurred postexercise. The quiet rest effect was more transient, however, lasting for only a few minutes following termination of the rest condition. In comparison, the blood pressure reduction that occurred after exercise remained lower during the 1-, 2-, and 3-hr postassessments. Raglin and Morgan (86) concluded that the *quantitative* reductions in blood pressure and state anxiety associated with rest and exercise were comparable but that there may be *qualitative* differences between the two strategies. If this is true, an important question is whether the qualitative differences between strategies reflect inherent differences that are stable across populations (e.g., fit, unfit; high anxious, low anxious; normotensives, hypertensives; males, females).

A biopsychosocial model of behavioral medicine proposed by Schwartz (90) may relate to the findings of Raglin and Morgan. Schwartz predicted that medical treatment effects or outcomes are determined in part by the person, by the person's social or environmental milieu, and by the treatment prescribed. This interactionist approach to medical care may have implications for future research in terms of exercise and mental health, especially in light of findings establishing a relationship between physical fitness and personality characteristics (12, 43, 44, 100, 114) as well as

between exercise and somatic anxiety and between meditation and cognitive anxiety (91). Schwartz et al. (91) reported that exercisers and meditators did not differ with regard to a total or global score of anxiety. However, when anxiety was fractionated into somatic and cognitive subfactors, exercisers scored higher on cognitive and lower on somatic anxiety than did meditators, and meditators scored higher on somatic and lower on cognitive anxiety. It cannot be ascertained from their research design whether subjects gravitated towards involvement in meditation or exercise because of differences in personality or merely whether involvement in meditation and exercise led to the differences observed by Schwartz et al. Nevertheless, it seems reasonable to hypothesize that diverse individuals possessing different preferences, unique state and trait personality characteristics, different physical capabilities, or all these may respond in a qualitatively different manner to active and passive strategies to reduce anxiety or tension.

Although research suggests that vigorous exercise is associated with reductions in tension for most people, the research to date has usually focused on subjects who are physically capable of participating in a wide variety of activities, according to the frequency, duration, and intensity of exercise selected by the subjects or investigator. For many such persons, physical activity does indeed seem to serve as an anxiety- or tension-reducing strategy. However, Brown et al. (7) conducted a study using 5 male and 5 female subjects enrolled in an adaptive physical education class. All the subjects indicated that they were frustrated with their physical limitations, which impaired their ability to exercise at self-imposed desired levels of duration and intensity. The research question posed was whether these subjects were frustrated during exercise by their limitations to the degree that anxiety reduction was impaired. A quasi-experimental, counterbalanced design was employed in which all subjects participated in quiet-rest and exercise conditions. Blood pressure and psychometric measures of state anxiety were assessed before and after each condition. Blood pressure significantly increased during exercise and significantly decreased during rest. Yet the results of the study indicated that both rest and exercise possess the potential to reduce anxiety in individuals who are physically limited to some degree. It was concluded that physically impaired individuals may receive many of the same psychological benefits that are derived by nonimpaired persons.

Chronic Studies

Unlike the relationship between anxiety and acute exercise, the relationship between anxiety reduction and chronic exercise has not been as consistently replicated. deVries (20) found that a group of adult male subjects participating in a 4-wk faculty fitness program experienced a significant reduction in electrical muscle activity following involvement in chronic exercise when compared to a control group. The trained group also had significantly higher estimated $\dot{V}O_2$max values after training, whereas the control group showed no changes on measures of estimated $\dot{V}O_2$max pre- to post- training. Goldwater and Collis (36) found that a 6-wk training program that led to increased cardiovascular fitness was associated with a decrease in a psychometric assessment of anxiety and an increase in a psychological measure of general well-being in a group of young male adults. The fitness measure obtained in this study, however, was based on a step test, so it is unknown whether aerobic fitness was actually associated with the psychological changes that were found. In addition, a true control condition was not used in the study, and the findings could be due to demand characteristics or the Hawthorne effect. Blumenthal et al. (4) and Berger and Owen (3) also provided psychometric evidence that involvement in chronic exercise can lead to enhanced mood state, including decreased anxiety, in nonclinical, healthy middle-aged (4) and college-aged (3) groups of men and women. These investigators caution, however, that selection bias may account for the findings obtained in their studies. Folkins (31) found that chronic exercise led to increased aerobic fitness and decreased anxiety in a group of psychologically normal middle-aged males at high risk for cardiac heart disease. Furthermore, decreases in anxiety did not occur in a control group used in this study. Unfortunately, fitness measures were not reported for the control group, and this limits the importance of finding a relationship between improved aerobic fitness and reductions in anxiety. The psychological findings that were reported in this study could also merely reflect the influence of the Hawthorne effect. Perhaps doing something (i.e., exercise) with the subjects was better than doing nothing. Chronic activity, which led to increases in fitness, did not lead to reductions in anxiety in research with normals in two other studies (33, 62). However, Folkins et al. (33) did find an inverse relationship between estimates of aerobic fitness and anxiety in a group of women who were significantly elevated on anxiety, compared to normative

data, before training. This relationship was not found for men who were elevated on anxiety at the outset of a program of chronic exercise. In addition, McPherson et al. (62) found reductions in anxiety for cardiac rehabilitation patients involved in an exercise program who were elevated on psychological measures at the outset of training.

The methodological problems that characterize the chronic studies do not allow for a conclusion to be made that training that results in improved aerobic fitness is associated with reductions in anxiety or tension. The random assignment of subjects to aerobic exercise, placebo, and control conditions and the documentation of fitness by obtaining $\dot{V}O_2$max values before and after each condition would lead to a clearer understanding of whether a reduction in anxiety is one outcome of training. In addition, greater attention needs to be given to the measure or the directional set used by an investigator to assess anxiety in exercise research. Tests need to be selected on the basis of the research questions being asked. Theoretically, state anxiety would change in response to acute exercise, whereas involvement in chronic exercise may potentially alter trait anxiety. Also, the effects of exercise on somatic anxiety and cognitive anxiety may be quite different (91). In short, there still exists the need to conduct a training study of a true experimental nature employing measures consistent with a theoretical rationale.

An Additional Concern

Although much is being written about using exercise to promote relaxation, the idea has not met with universal acceptance. Pitts (82) and Pitts and McClure (83) suggested that increased levels of lactic acid, an exercise metabolite, may be sufficient to trigger panic attacks in anxiety neurotics or symptoms of anxiety in normals. They base their proposal on research which found that intravenous injections of dl-sodium lactate in anxiety neurotics can provoke an anxiety attack soon after infusion begins (83). Thus, infusion of dl-sodium lactate has shown diagnostic potential for identifying individuals prone to panic attacks (30, 46).

Grosz and Farmer (35), deVries (21), and Morgan (68) refuted the hypothesis of Pitts and McClure. Grosz and Farmer (35) found that lactate infusion and high-intensity anaerobic exercise resulted in completely different acid-base adaptations and concluded that the metabolic changes and shifts in pH that occur during exercise would not be expected to cause anxiety attacks. Although vigorous exercise (especially at the higher intensity levels) can temporarily increase state anxiety during and immediately following activity, these increases have not reached clinical magnitudes or induced panic attacks in highly anxious individuals (21, 68). Because the endogenous production of lactic acid results in physiological responses different than those that occur during lactate infusion, the decreases in lactic acid production associated with chronic training adaptation alternatively will probably not afford a protective mechanism leading to the reduction or elimination of anxiety symptoms, as proposed by Ledwidge (56).

In summary, considerable data have been amassed showing that an association does exist between acute exercise and reduced levels of anxiety and tension. However, the research in this area, which has been primarily correlational, cross-sectional, and quasi-experimental, has not resulted in the identification of underlying mechanisms responsible for the decreases in tension and anxiety that occur postexercise. The research also lacks the methodological controls and designs necessary to conclude that exercise indeed causes such reductions. In addition, the influence of training and improved fitness on the psychological response following acute exercise remains unclear. However, available evidence suggests that both high and low aerobically fit individuals experience enhanced mood after a single bout of vigorous exercise. There remains the need for researchers to conduct methodologically sound studies evaluating the influence of chronic exercise on anxiety and tension. The data that are presently available do not allow for a definitive statement to be made about the relationship among chronic exercise, physical fitness, and anxiety.

Exercise and Depression

The point has been made that most researchers who have focused on questions related to exercise and mental health used correlational or cross-sectional designs to evaluate their hypotheses. This remains true for many researchers who have focused specifically on the relationship between exercise and depression. Nevertheless, research findings consistently suggest that chronic exercise is associated with decreased depression (3, 4, 8, 31, 33, 34, 49, 61, 75, 80), and some studies have documented fitness gains in conjunction with reductions in depression (31, 33, 34, 61). However, only two studies (31, 34) reported fitness gains in

terms of direct measures of $\dot{V}O_2$max. Unfortunately, $\dot{V}O_2$max measures were apparently not obtained for nonexercising subjects in these studies. The failure to obtain $\dot{V}O_2$max values on all subjects attenuates the evidence in support of a hypothesis that improvements in aerobic capacity are responsible for the lowered levels of depression observed in subjects following chronic exercise.

Studies Using Clinical Populations

The efficacy of using exercise as a treatment for depression was established in 1979 by Greist et al. (34), and this research has subsequently been replicated and expanded (49). Greist et al. (34) and Klein et al. (49) found that exercise is just as effective as are time-limited and time-unlimited psychotherapy (34), meditation-relaxation, and group psychotherapy (49) in treating some forms of depression. Results from other clinical studies provide support for using chronic exercise to treat depression (27, 60). Exercise has also been used effectively as an adjunct to psychotherapy and safely with patients who were simultaneously receiving tricyclic antidepressant medication (60). Preliminary evidence by Martinsen et al. (60) suggests that exercise does not potentiate or interact with the effects of tricyclic antidepressants in an additive or synergistic manner, which would contraindicate the combined use of exercise and the tricyclics. This is an important finding, as the effects of both exercise and tricyclic antidepressants are thought to alter brain monoamine levels (71, 87). Additional clinical trials and experimental investigations need to be conducted to replicate the findings of Martinsen et al. (60). The safest course of action, however, would be to require close monitoring of individuals who are exercising while receiving psychotropic medications and to aim toward titrating the exercise-medication dosage when necessary.

Studies Using Nonclinical Populations

Folkins et al. (33), Morgan et al. (75) and Naughton et al. (80) reported findings that training did not lead to lower levels of depressed affect in subjects who scored within the normal range on measures of depression before training. Using a semantic differential scale to assess depressed affect, McPherson et al. (62) also found limited improvement for normal male subjects after training. These findings differ from those of Berger and Owen (3), Blumenthal et al. (4), and Folkins (31), who reported reductions in depression for normal subjects following training programs. The equivocal findings from these studies may be due to differences in the psychometric measures employed, differences in methodology (e.g., selection bias or failure to randomize subjects to experimental, placebo, and control conditions), or to some behavioral artifact (e.g., Rosenthal effect, demand characteristics, or response distortion). In those studies with normals that have reported changes in depression following chronic exercise, explanations other than exercise can be given to explain the findings.

These findings, obtained from investigations using normal subjects, are in contrast to findings from studies using a nonclinical population of subjects who nevertheless exhibit depressive mood state. In 1985, Simons et al. (97) published a review of the research in which exercise has been used as a nonpharmacological treatment of depression. One criticism Simons et al. made of the research was that many studies used subjects who did not have depressive disorders. Instead, subjects were experiencing sadness or a depressed mood or scored in the normal range on a measure of depression. The review by Simons et al. (97), however, ultimately suggests that results from several of these studies could be generalizable to clinical populations. In other words, the findings obtained from research using subjects with depressed moods are similar to the findings in investigations where subjects were suffering from depressive disorders. In both instances, reductions in depression have been documented following chronic exercise.

Chronic Exercise: Prevention Versus Treatment of Depression

The fact that exercise has been used to reduce levels of depressed affect and to treat depressed patients successfully gives little insight into whether exercise maintains positive mental health or whether exercise prevents mental health problems. The distinction between treatment and prevention seems to be especially relevant to the focus of this chapter, which is primarily on health rather than illness issues.

As noted previously, it appears that individuals from the general population who are not depressed at the outset of involvement in a program of chronic exercise will benefit little from training. In other words, people who score within the population average or normal range on a test of depression at the outset of a training program will usually

score within the normal range on the test at the end of the program. However, there it is no empirical evidence available indicating that individuals who exercise and who are fit are provided with a protective factor against depression. Perhaps the maintenance of mental health may ultimately prove to be an important outcome of training or of maintaining a high level of fitness. At present it is probably safest to assume that both the unfit and the fit individual are equally prone to experience depressive episodes, especially those of a secondary or reactive nature. Reactive depression is the type of depression that could occur in response to a life-threatening illness or the loss of a loved one.

Presently, in regard to depression and the population at large, it seems that the greatest potential for chronic exercise lies in its use as an early intervention strategy. Experimental data do suggest that individuals who are mildly or moderately depressed and who may be at risk for experiencing greater or more severe forms of clinical depression have benefited from involvement in aerobic types of chronic exercise.

A study by McCann and Holmes (61) illustrates the potential usefulness of employing exercise as an early intervention strategy. They randomly assigned 43 depressed (scores greater than 11 on the Beck Depression Inventory) undergraduate women to aerobic exercise ($n = 15$), progressive muscle relaxation ($n = 14$), and no-treatment control ($n = 14$) conditions. The fitness levels of) the subjects were estimated using the 12-min-run test before and after a 10-wk treatment period. The Beck Depression Inventory was administered to the subjects at the pretreatment, midtreatment, and posttreatment periods.

The subjects in the aerobic exercise group improved performance on the 12-min-run test and experienced reductions in depression that were greater than those of subjects in either the relaxation or the control groups. Subjects in the relaxation and control groups did not differ on these variables as a function of treatment.

As McCann and Holmes point out, the mechanism causing the reductions in depression that were associated with the aerobic exercise is unknown. Because measures of $\dot{V}O_2$max were not obtained, the reductions in depressions cannot be attributed to changes in aerobic capacity. Nevertheless, the results from this investigation indicate that involvement in chronic exercise can lead to reductions in depression in subjects representative of the general population, in this case mildly to moderately depressed college women.

One additional outcome from the McCann and Holmes research that deserves mentioned was their finding that a significant reduction in depression occurred from the point at which measures of depression were obtained (i.e., during subject selection and screening) to pretreatment measures. This finding suggests that decreases in depression resulted that were independent of treatment effects. This phenomenon is known as *spontaneous remission*, and it reinforces the need for researchers to utilize a control group whenever it is possible and safe to do so. Research in which exercise is used to promote psychological well-being in normals is an example of when a control group should be enlisted. In patient populations, however, the severity of symptoms may be so serious that even a so-called wait-list control, in which treatment is temporarily withheld, may not be considered. In these cases, comparisons of different treatment strategies (e.g., 34, 49) will be the best alternatives to a control group.

In summary, the research has shown that a depressed individual who initiates and maintains a program of chronic exercise may eventually experience a reduction in his or her level of depression as one benefit from training. The reason why this reduction occurs is unknown, and there are insufficient data to claim that decreases in depression are due to changes in aerobic fitness. Almost all studies in this area have employed predicted rather than actual measures of aerobic fitness. Future studies are required to ascertain the reasons behind the positive findings that are being consistently observed in this area of research.

The Causation Issue

Many investigators and reviewers (41, 71, 85, 96, 97) have provided hypotheses that may account for the causal factors that mediate the relationship between exercise and mental health. These hypotheses have been both biological and behavioral.

Behavioral explanations for why acute or chronic exercise may enhance the psychological well-being of an individual include proposals that exercise provides: (a) a personal sense of control or mastery over one dimension of a person's life (41, 97); (b) a means for distracting an individual from the stressors of daily living (41, 71, 73, 85); and (c) an opportunity for receiving extrinsic or intrinsic reinforcement (e.g., awards or the opportunity to socialize) (41). Several of these explanations may also be associated with improved self-esteem or

self-concept, which alone could promote mental health. For example, Tucker (111) provided evidence documenting a relationship between measures of fitness, personality, and self-esteem in a group of male high school students as well as a relationship between the muscular strength and self-concept of male college students (110).

The primary physiological mechanisms that have been suggested as potential mediators of the relationship between exercise and mental health include: (a) hormonal or metabolic adaptations that occur with improved cardiorespiratory efficiency and endurance (41, 97); (b) alterations in the catecholamine or indolamine neurotransmitter substances (i.e., the monoamine hypothesis) (41, 71, 73, 85, 96, 97); (c) increases in levels of endogenous opiates (i.e., the endorphin hypothesis) (41, 71, 73, 85, 96, 97); and (d) an increased core body temperature, resulting in a tranquilizer effect as evidenced by reduced muscle tension, alterations in the brain neurotransmitters, or both (9, 26, 41, 73, 85, 96).

Overtraining and Exercise Abuse

The research reviewed up to this point has dealt with issues important to the relationshiip between exercise and mental health. However, there are also reports of exercise being associated with negative (58, 59, 69, 73, 78) rather than positive psychological changes in an individual. These negative psychological consequences normally occur in response to a training stimulus that is more frequent, longer in duration, and more intense than is required to promote health and physical fitness. In other words, a person will usually be training more than 3-5 d per wk, longer than 15-30 min per exercise session, more intensely than his or her target heart rate or $\dot{V}O_2$max range, or all these (1). It is common for athletes to endure intense training regimens. Yet it is also not unheard of for overfat, sedentary individuals from the general population to become active and eventually to transform into lean, highly competitive individuals who also overtrain (69). A small proportion of these individuals may ultimately become obsessed with exercise and physical fitness (58, 69). They may train to the point that exercise has a deleterious effect on their interpersonal relationships and vocational functioning or to the point of physical self-destruction (69). It has been reported that when these individuals cannot exercise they experience withdrawal symptoms, and these symptoms may include elevated levels of anxiety and depression (69). Elevated anxiety and depression have also been associated with neurotic breakdowns in middle-aged male "fitness fanatics" (59) who experience injury or illness that threatens to deprive them of exercise (58, 59).

Risks from overtraining may also lead to a condition known in sports medicine as staleness. In competitive athletes (78), staleness is characterized by numerous markers that include a decrease in performance and an increase in mood disturbance (e.g., fatigue, depression, and anxiety). Staleness is most commonly observed in endurance athletes who are involved in rigorous training regimens and high-level competition. Nevertheless, recreational exercisers from the general population who become involved in overtraining should be sensitive not only to the physical risks, such as injury, but also to the psychological risks involved. Although appropriate and properly prescribed exercise has the potential to decrease depression, overtraining possesses the potential to produce depression in some individuals.

Conclusion

The study of exercise, physical fitness, and mental health is currently being given high priority in North America. The research interest in the relationship has been fueled in part by reports from the lay population that many individuals feel better after they exercise and from epidemiological data documenting a relationship between physical activity and enhanced psychological well-being. In addition, reports that up to one fourth of the general population at any given time may be functioning at less than optimal levels as a result of stress and the stress-related emotions such as anxiety and depression (84) should intensify the degree of interest and research in exercise and mental health. It is for these reasons that the focus of this review has been on the reductions in depressed affect, anxiety-tension states, and changes in stress reactivity that are purported to result from involvement in exercise.

Several studies in this area used clinical populations in an effort to establish the efficacy of exercise as a potential treatment for individuals suffering from one of the affective disorders. Other investigations utilized subjects who scored within the normal range or who were mild or moderately elevated on some psychological measure. It is important to recognize, however, that in most of the studies focusing on the relationship among

exercise, physical fitness, and mental health subjects were recruited from the general population and not from institutionalized populations. The subjects are usually nonpatients or represent an outpatient clinical population. Therefore, results from most of the research on exercise and mental health are generalizable to segments of the population at large.

The focus of this review was not primarily on investigations in which the research question was directly related to whether exercise was effective as a treatment or adjunct to a treatment. In terms of tertiary prevention, the strongest empirical evidence exists for using chronic exercise as a treatment for depression (27, 34, 49, 60). This chapter addressed whether evidence is available to support the use of exercise as a primary or secondary preventive intervention. Thus, two questions were considered: (a) Can involvement in exercise actually prevent the onset of mental health problems (i.e., primary prevention)? (b) Can individuals who are experiencing a mild or moderate degree of mood or emotional disturbance initiate an exercise program to prevent precursors of mental illness from worsening to clinical proportions (i.e., secondary prevention) and thus requiring tertiary preventive intervention? The use of exercise as a primary, secondary, or tertiary intervention reduces to an issue of timing and of at what point on the continuum of mental health and mental illness a person becomes involved in exercise.

Although preliminary correlational evidence exists (50, 89), there are no experimental data available indicating that people who become involved in acute or chronic exercise are able to prevent the onset of mental health problems. Perhaps the temporary reductions in anxiety or tension associated with acute exercise, when performed on a chronic basis, will prove to be an effective stress management strategy by preventing stress-related emotions from elevating to unhealthy or incapacitating levels. The research designs and lack of longitudinal studies presently do not provide insight into such a possibility. In addition, findings from the research on exercise and mental health in which normal healthy individuals have been used as subjects are not very compelling. Methodological problems associated with much of this research do not allow for a definitive statement to be made that chronic exercise or aerobic fitness is helpful for either maintaining the psychological well-being of normals or reducing psychophysiological arousal during or following encounters with stressors. Alternative explanations, other than training or fitness adaptations, can be given to account for the lowered levels of depression and other enhanced mood states that have been observed in normals following exercise. Furthermore, the few experimental training studies that have been conducted have not clearly established any uniform advantages, or patterns of stress reactivity, that benefit the aerobically fit compared to the unfit. There is also no evidence to indicate that the proposed changes in stress reactivity that may occur in the trained individual are linked either to better-developed adaptive coping behaviors or to a greater ability to withstand mental health problems brought on by exposure to chronic stress.

For the present, it is probably safest to assume that highly active, fit individuals may at some point in their lifetimes be prone to the same reactive mood disorders and mental health problems as are less active, unfit individuals. If and when such problems do occur, there is evidence available to support the view that involvement in exercise may help resolve or lessen the severity of affective disorders. Again, however, it would be premature to claim that such improvements in mental health are a result of enhanced aerobic fitness, as researchers who have studied the relationship between exercise and depression have rarely measured directly the aerobic capacities of the subjects used in these investigations.

In regard to the general population, two findings seem to be consistent. One is that acute vigorous activity that is sufficient to promote increased cardiorespiratory fitness when done on a chronic basis is associated with reductions in state anxiety (68) and muscle tension (21) in normal individuals. In fact, muscle electrical activity was reduced after involvement in low-intensity acute activity (21) and as a result of a chronic activity regimen (20). A second consistent finding is that individuals who are mild or moderately anxious or depressed experience positive mood changes associated with exercise. Involvement in acute vigorous activity resulted in reductions in anxiety (68), whereas chronic activity led to lower levels of depression (97). However, the causal mechanisms mediating these relationships have not been identified.

From a psychological perspective, it can therefore be concluded that exercise does hold promise for both secondary and tertiary preventive efforts, but support does not exist for using exercise as a primary preventive intervention. It is extremely encouraging that exercise possesses the potential to help that one quarter of the population estimated to be experiencing elevated mood states or emotional conflict at any given time. However, it is somewhat discouraging that there is only weak empirical support for recommending exercise and fitness as a means of maintaining or enhancing mental health in individuals possessing normal personality characteristics.

It is hoped that better-designed experimental training studies will result in improved documentation and a greater understanding of the relationship among exercise, physical fitness, and mental health in the population at large. Ultimately, new scales may need to be developed to measure some of the shifts in psychological mood states or sense of well-being that people report after exercise and that to date have remained somewhat elusive and difficult to quantify in normal individuals. Alternatively, there is a need to pursue research questions in which the effects of exercise on a greater number of psychological states or traits are explored. For example, a theoretical rationale can be provided for examining the effects of exercise on anger or hostility, which are behavioral characteristics that have been implicated in the pathogenesis of coronary heart disease (74). The empirical evidence gives reason for optimism. As research methodology improves, as measurement and scaling issues become refined, and as new theoretical avenues are pursued, a more positive picture may emerge during the years ahead. It is hoped that, in time, the use of exercise will be established clearly and unequivocally not only as an effective means for promoting physical fitness but also as a way to maintain and enhance mental health.

For the present it can be concluded that, depending on how mental health is defined, there does seem to be a relationship between exercise and mental health. This relationship has been documented in epidemiological, cross-sectional, correlational, quasi-experimental studies and, on very rare occasions, in research using a true experimental design. However, there is still much to be learned about this relationship:

- The causal mechanism or mechanisms of the relationship remain unknown.
- Direct measures of maximal oxygen uptake are almost never reported in the literature on exercise and mental health, in spite of the fact that aerobic fitness is central to many of the research questions being asked. The influence of physical fitness levels on the relationship between exercise and mental health is unclear.
- The optimal dosage in terms of the frequency, intensity, and duration of exercise needed to promote mental health is unknown.
- The effects of different types of activity on psychological well-being have not been well

documented. To date, most studies have focused on some form of aerobic as opposed to anaerobic activity.

- Finally, the influence of age, gender, race, economic, and occupational status, physical or mental impairments, and personality characteristics as factors that potentially mediate or affect the relationship among exercise, physical fitness, and mental health have generally been ignored.

Nevertheless, the psychological data presently available are sufficiently encouraging to warrant a recommendation to the general public that a program of safe and well-monitored aerobic exercise be initiated. There is reason to believe that many people may derive both physical and mental health benefits from involvement in properly prescribed exercise.

References

1. American College of Sports Medicine. *Guidelines for graded exercise testing and exercise prescription*. Philadelphia: Lea & Febiger, 1980.
2. Bahrke, M.S., and W.P. Morgan. Anxiety reduction following exercise and meditation. *Cog. Ther. Res.* 2: 323-333, 1978.
3. Berger, B.G., and D.R. Owen. Mood alteration with swimming—swimmers really do ''feel better.'' *Psychosom. Med.* 45: 425-433, 1983.
4. Blumenthal, J.A., R.S. Williams, T.L. Needles, and A.G. Wallace. Psychological changes accompany aerobic exercise in healthy middle-aged adults. *Psychosom. Med.* 44: 529-536, 1982.
5. Brooke, S.T., and B.C. Long. Efficiency of coping with a real-life stressor: A multimodal comparison of aerobic fitness. *Psychophysiology* 24: 173-180, 1987.
6. Brown, B.S., T. Payne, C. Kim, G. Moore, P. Krebs, and W. Martin. Chronic response of rat brain norepinephrine and serotonin levels to endurance training. *J. Appl. Physiol.* 40: 19-23, 1979.
7. Brown, D.R., W.P. Morgan, and J.S. Raglin. *Effects of exercise and rest on blood pressure and mood state of physically impaired college students.* Paper presented at the Pan American Sports Medicine Congress, XII, Bloomington, IN, August, 1987.
8. Brown, R.A., D.E. Ramirez, and J.M. Taub. The prescription of exercise for depression. *Phys. Sporstmed.* 6: 34-45, 1978.
9. Bulbulian, R., and B.L. Dorabos. Motor neuron excitability: The Hoffmann reflex following exercise of low and high intensity. *Med. Sci. Sports Exerc.* 18: 697-702, 1986.
10. Cantor, J.R., D. Zillman, and K.D. Day. Relationship between cardiorespiratory fitness and physiological responses to films. *Percept. Mot. Skills* 46: 1123-1130, 1978.
11. Caplan, G. *Principles of preventive psychiatry.* New York: Basic Books, 1984.
12. Chodzko-Zajko, W.J., and A.H. Ismail. MMPI interscale relationships in middle-aged male Ss before and after an 8-month fitness program. *J. Clin. Psychol.* 40: 163-169, 1984.
13. Claytor, R.P., R.H. Cox, E.T. Howley, K.A. Lawler, and J.E. Lawler. Aerobic power and cardiovascular response to stress. *J. Appl. Physiol.* 65: 1416-1423, 1988.
14. Cox, J.P., J.F. Evans, and J.L. Jamieson. Aerobic power and tonic heart rate responses to psychosocial stressors. *Pers. Soc. Psychol. Bull.* 5: 160-163, 1979.
15. Cox, R.H., J.W. Hubbard, J.E. Lawler, B.J. Sanders, and V.P. Mitchell. Cardiovascular and sympathoadrenal responses to stress in swim-trained rats. *J. Appl. Physiol.* 58: 1207-1214, 1985.
16. Cox, R.H., J.W. Hubbard, J.E. Lawler, B.J. Sanders, and V.P. Mitchell. Exercise training attentuates stress-induced hypertension in the rat. *Hypertension* 7: 747-751, 1985.
17. Crews, D.J., and D.M. Landers. A meta-analytic review of aerobic fitness and reactivity to psychosocial stressors. *Med. Sci. Sports Exerc.* 19 (Suppl.): 114-120, 1987.
18. Cureton, T.K. Improvement of psychological states by means of exercise-fitness programs. *J. Assoc. Phys. Mental Rehabil.* 17: 14-25, 1963.
19. deVries, H.A. Effects of exercise upon residual neuromuscular tension. *Bull. Am. Assoc. Electromyogr. Electrodiagnosis* 12: 12, 1965.
20. deVries, H.A. Immediate and long-term effects of exercise upon resting muscle action potential. *J. Sports Med.* 8: 1-11, 1968.
21. deVries, H.A. Tranquilizer effect of exercise: A critical review. *Phys. Sportsmed.* 9: 47-55, 1981.
22. deVries, H.A., and G.M. Adams. Electromyographic comparison of single doses of exercise and meprobamate as to effect on

muscular relaxation. *Am. J. Phys. Med.* 51: 130-141, 1972.

23. deVries, H.A., R.K. Burke, T. Hopper, and J.H. Sloan. Efficacy of EMG biofeedback in relaxation training. *Am. J. Phys. Med.* 56: 75-81, 1977.

24. deVries, H.A., R.A. Wiswell, R. Bulbulian, and T. Moritani. Tranquilizer effect of exercise. *Am. J. Phys. Med.* 60: 57-66, 1981.

25. deVries, H.A., C.P. Simard, R.A. Wiswell, E. Heckathorne, and V. Carabetta. Fusimotor system involvement in the tranquilizer effect of exercise. *Am. J. Phys. Med.* 61: 111-122, 1982.

26. Dishman, R.K. Mental health. In: Seefeldt, V., ed. *Physical activity and well-being.* Reston, VA: American Alliance for Health, Physical Education, Recreation and Dance, 1986, Chapt. 11, p. 304-341.

27. Doyne, E.J., D.L. Chambless, and L.E. Beutler. Aerobic exercise as a treatment for depression in women. *Behav. Ther.* 14: 434-440, 1983.

28. Farrell, P.A., W.K. Gates, M.G. Maksod, and W.P. Morgan. Increases in plasma beta-endorphin/beta-lipotropin immunoreactivity after treadmill running in humans. *J. Appl. Physiol.* 52: 1245-1249, 1982.

29. Farrell, P.A., W.K. Gates, W.P. Morgan, and C.B. Pert. Plasma leucine enkephalin-like radioreceptor activity and tension-anxiety before and after competitive running. In: Knuttgen, H.G., J.A. Vogel, and J. Poortmans, eds. *Biochemistry of exercise.* Champaign, IL: Human Kinetics, 1983, 637-644.

30. Fink, M., M.A. Taylor, and J. Volanka. Anxiety precipitated by lactate. *N. Engl. J. Med.* 281: 1429, 1969.

31. Folkins, C.H. Effects of physical training on mood. *J. Clin. Psychol.* 32: 385-388, 1976.

32. Folkins, C.H, and W.E. Sime. Physical fitness training and mental health. *Am. Psychol.* 36: 373-389, 1981.

33. Folkins, C.H., S. Lynch, and M.M. Gardner. Psychological fitness as a function of physical fitness. *Arch. Phys. Med. Rehabil.* 53: 503-508, 1972.

34. Griest, J.H., M.H. Klein, R.R. Eischens, J. Faris, A.S. Gurman, and W.P. Morgan. Running as a treatment for depression. *Comp. Psychiatry* 53: 20-41, 1979.

35. Grosz, H.J., and B.B. Farmer. Blood lactate in the development of anxiety symptoms: A critical study of Pitts and McClure's hypothesis and experimental study. *Arch. Gen. Psychiatry* 21: 611-619, 1969.

36. Goldwater, B.C., and M.L. Collis. Psychologic effects of cardiovascular conditioning: A controlled experiment. *Psychosom. Med.* 46: 174-181, 1985.

37. Hammett, V.B.O. Psychological changes with physical fitness training. *Can. Med. Assoc. J.* 96: 764-767, 1967.

38. Hannum, S.M., and F.W. Kasch. Acute post exercise blood pressure response of hypertensive and normotensive men. *Scand. J. Sports Sci.* 3: 1, 11-15, 1981.

39. Hollander, B.J., and P. Seraganian. Aerobic fitness and psychophysiological reactivity. *Can. J. Behav. Sci.* 16: 257-261, 1984.

40. Holmes, D.S., and D.L. Roth. Association of aerobic fitness with pulse rate and subjective responses to psychological stress. *Psychophysiology* 22: 525-529, 1985.

41. Hughes, J.R. Psychological effects of habitual exercise: A critical review. *Prev. Med.* 13: 66-78, 1984.

42. Hull, E.M., S.H. Young, and M.G. Ziegler. Aerobic fitness affects cardiovascular and catecholamine responses to stressors. *Psychophysiology* 21: 353-360, 1984.

43. Ismail, A.H., and R.J. Young. The effect of chronic exercise on the personality of middle-aged men by univariate and multivariate approaches. *J. Hum. Ergol.* 2: 45-54, 1973.

44. Ismail, A.H., and R.J. Young. Effect of chronic exercise on the multivariate relationships between selected biochemical and personality variables. *J. Multivar. Behav. Res.* 12: 49-67, 1977.

45. Keller, S., and P. Seraganian. Physical fitness level and autonomic reactivity in psychosocial stress. *J. Psychosom. Res.* 28: 279-287, 1984.

46. Kelly, D., N. Mitchell-Heggs, and D. Sherman. Anxiety and the effects of sodium lactate assessed clinically and psychologically. *Br. J. Psychiatry* 111: 129-141, 1971.

47. Kirschenbaum, D.S. Toward the prevention of sedentary lifestyles. In: Morgan, W.P., and S.E. Goldston, eds. *Exercise and mental health.* Washington, DC: Hemisphere Publishing, 1987, part 2, Chapt. 3, pp. 23-24.

48. Kjoer, M., and H. Galbo. Effect of physical training on the capacity to secrete epinephrine. *J. Appl. Physiol.* 64: 11-16, 1988.

49. Klein, M.H., J.H. Griest, A.S. Gurman, R.A. Neimeyer, D.P. Lesser, N.J. Bushnell, and R.E. Smith. A comparative outcome study of group psychotherapy vs. exercise treatments for depression. *Int. J. Mental Health* 13: 148-176, 1985.

50. Kobasa, S.C., S.R. Maddi, and M.C. Puccetti. Personality and exercise as buffers in the stress-illness relationship. *J. Behav. Med.* 5: 391-404, 1982.

51. Kvetnansky, R. Recent progress in catecholamines under stress. In: Usdin, E.R., R. Kvetnansky, and I.J. Kapin, eds. *Catecholamines and stress: Recent advances*. New York: Elsevier, 1980.

52. Lawler, J.E., R.H. Cox, and J.W. Hubbard. An animal model of environmentally produced hypertension. *Adv. Behav. Med.* 2: 51-97, 1986.

53. Layman, E.M. Contributions of exercise and sports to mental health and social adjustment. In: Johnson, W.R., ed. *Science and medicine of exercise and sports*. New York: Harper, 1960, 560-599.

54. Lazarus, R.S. *Psychological stress and the coping process*. New York: McGraw-Hill, 1966.

55. Lazarus, R.S., and J.R. Averill. Emotion and cognition: With special reference to anxiety. In: Spielberger, C.D., ed. *Anxiety: Current trends in theory and research*. New York: Academic Press, 1972, part IV, Chapt. 7, p. 241-283.

56. Ledwidge, B. Run for your mind: Aerobic exercise as a means of alleviating anxiety and depression. *Can. J. Behav. Sci.* 12: 126-140, 1980.

57. Light, K.C. Cardiovascular responses to effortful active coping: Implications for the role of stress in hypertension development. *Psychophysiology* 18: 216-225, 1982.

58. Little, J.C. The athlete's addiction in runners. *Acta Psychiatr. Scand.* 45: 187-197, 1969.

59. Little, J.C. Neurotic illness in fitness fanatics. *Psychiatr. Ann.* 9: 49-56, 1979.

60. Martinsen, E.W., A Medhus, and L. Sandvik. Effects of aerobic exercise on depression: A controlled study. *Br. Med. J.* 291: 109, 1985.

61. McCann, I.L., and D.S. Holmes. Influence of aerobic exercise on depression. *J. Pers. Soc. Psychol.* 46: 1142-1147, 1984.

62. McPherson, B.D., A. Paivio, M. Yuhasz, P. Rechnitzer, H. Pickard, and N. Lefcoe. Psychological effects of an exercise program for post-infarct and normal adult men. *J. Sports Med. Phys. Fit.* 8: 95-102, 1965.

63. Mellion, M.B. Exercise therapy for anxiety and depression. *Postgrad. Med.* 77: 59-66, 1985.

64. Michaels, R.R., M.J. Huber, and D.S. McCann. Evaluation of transcendental meditation as a method of reducing stress. *Science* 192: 1242-1244, 1976.

65. Mobily, K. Using physical activity and recreation to cope with stress and anxiety: A review. *Am. Corr. J.* 36: 77-81, 1982.

66. Morgan, W.P. Physical fitness and emotional health: A review. *Am. Corr. Ther. J.* 23: 124-127, 1969.

67. Morgan, W.P. Basic considerations. In: Morgan, W.P., ed. *Ergogenic aids and muscular performance*. New York: Academic Press, 1972.

68. Morgan, W.P. Anxiety reduction following acute physical activity. *Psychiatr. Ann.* 9: 36-45, 1979.

69. Morgan, W.P. Negative addiction in runners. *Phys. Sportsmed.* 7: 57-70, 1979.

70. Morgan, W.P. Psychological effects of exercise. *Behav. Med. Update* 4: 25-30, 1982.

71. Morgan, W.P. Affective beneficence of vigorous physical activity. *Med. Sci. Sports Exerc.* 17: 94-100, 1985.

72. Morgan, W.P., and S.E. Goldston, eds. *Exercise and mental health*. Washington, DC: Hemisphere Publishing, 1987.

73. Morgan, W.P., and P.J. O'Connor. Exercise and mental health. In: Dishman, R.K., ed. *Exercise adherence: Its impact on public health*. Champaign, IL: Human Kinetics, 1987, Chapt. 4, pp. 91-121.

74. Morgan, W.P., and J.S. Raglin. Psychologic aspects of heart disease. In: Pollock, M.L., and D.H. Schmidt, eds. *Heart disease and rehabilitation*. New York: John Wiley & Sons, 1985, Chapt. 8.

75. Morgan, W.P., J.A. Roberts, F.R. Brand, and A.D. Feinerman. Psychological effect of chronic physical activity. *Med. Sci. Sports* 2: 213-217, 1970.

76. Morgan, W.P., J.A. Roberts, and A.D. Feinerman. Psychologic effect of acute physical activity. *Arch. Phys. Med. Rehabil.* 52: 422-426, 1971.

77. Morgan, W.P., D.H. Horstman, A. Cymerman, and J. Stokes. Use of exercise as a relaxation technique. *Prim. Cardiol.* 6: 48-57, 1980.

78. Morgan, W.P., D.R. Brown, J.S. Raglin, P.J. O'Connor, and K.A. Ellickson. Psychological monitoring of overtraining and staleness. *Br. J. Sports Med.* 21: 107-114, 1987.

79. National Center for Health Statistics. *Monthly vital statistics report* 32: 8-9, 1984.

80. Naughton, J., J.G. Bruhn, and M.T. Lategola. Effects of physical training on physiologic and behavioral characteristics of cardiac patients. *Arch. Phys. Med.* 49: 131-137, 1968.

81. Pert, C.B., and D.L. Bowie. Behavioral manipulation of rats causes alterations in opiate receptor occupancy. In: Usdin, E., W.E. Bunney, and N.S. Kline, eds. *Endorphins in mental health*. New York: Oxford University Press, 1979, 93-104.

82. Pitts, F.N., Jr. Biochemical factors in anxiety neurosis. *Behav. Sci.* 16: 82-91, 1969a.

83. Pitts, F.N., Jr., and J.N. McClure, Jr. Lactate metabolism in anxiety neurosis. *N. Engl. J. Med.* 277: 1329-1336, 1967.

84. President's Commission on Mental Health. *Report to the President* (Stock No. 040-000-00390-8). Washington, DC: U.S. Government Printing Office, 1978.

85. Raglin, J.S., and W.P. Morgan. Influence of vigorous exercise on mood state. *Behav. Ther.* 8: 179-183, 1985.

86. Raglin, J.S., and W.P. Morgan. Influence of exercise and quiet rest on state anxiety and blood pressure. *Med. Sci. Sports Exerc.* 19: 456-463, 1987.

87. Ransford, C.P. A role for amines in the antidepressant effect of exercise: A review. *Med. Sci. Sports Exerc.* 14: 1-10, 1982.

88. Roskies, E., P. Seraganian, R. Oseasohn, J.A. Hanley, R. Collu, N. Martin, and C. Smilga. The Montreal Type A intervention project: Major findings. *Health Psychol.* 5: 45-69, 1986.

89. Roth, D.L., and D.S. Holmes. Influence of physical fitness in determining the impact of stressful life events on physical and psychological health. *Psychosom. Med.* 47: 164-173, 1985.

90. Schwartz, G.E. Testing the biopsychosocial model: The ultimate challenge facing behavioral medicine? *J. Consult. Clin. Psychol.* 50: 1040-1053, 1982.

91. Schwartz, G.E., R.J. Davidson, and D.J. Goleman. Patterning of cognitive and somatic processes in the self-regulation of anxiety: Effects of meditation versus exercise. *Psychosom. Med.* 40: 321-328, 1978.

92. Scott, M.G. The contributions of physical activity to psychological development. *Res. Q.* 31: 307-320, 1960.

93. Selye, H. *The stress of life*. New York: McGraw-Hill, 1956.

94. Shulhan, D., H. Scher, and J. Furedy. Phasic cardiac reactivity to psychological stress as a function of aerobic fitness level. *Psychophysiology* 23: 562-566, 1986.

95. Sime, W.E. A comparison of exercise and meditation in reducing physiological response to stress [Abstact]. *Med. Sci. Sports Exerc.* 9: 55, 1977.

96. Sime, W.E. Psychological benefits of exercise training in the healthy individual. In: Matarazzo, J.D., S.M. Weiss, J.A. Herd, N.E. Miller, and S.M. Weiss, eds. *Behavioral health: A handbook of health enhancement and disease prevention*. New York: John Wiley & Sons, 1984, 488-508.

97. Simons, A., C.R. McGowan, L.H. Epstein, D.J. Kuper, and R.J. Robertson. Exercise as a treatment for depression: An update. *Clin. Psychol. Rev.* 5: 553-568, 1985.

98. Sinyor, D., S.G. Schwartz, F. Peronnet, G. Brisson, and P. Seraganian. Aerobic fitness level and reactivity to psychosocial stress: Physiological, biochemical, and subjective measures. *Psychosom. Med.* 45: 205-217, 1983.

99. Sinyor, D., M. Golden, Y. Steinert, and P. Seraganian. Experimental manipulation of aerobic fitness and the response to psychosocial stress: Heart rate and self-report measures. *Psychosom. Med.* 48: 324-337, 1986.

100. Sothmann, M.S., and A.H. Ismail. Relationships between urinary catecholamine metabolites, particularly MHPG, and selected personality and physical fitness characteristics in normal subjects. *Psychosom. Med.* 46: 523-533, 1984.

101. Sothmann, M., T. Horn, B. Hart, and A.B. Gustafson. Comparison of discrete cardiovascular fitness groups on plasma catecholamine and selected behavioral responses to psychological stress. *Psychophysiology* 24: 47-54, 1987.

102. Spielberger, C. *Understanding stress and anxiety*. New York: Harper and Row, 1979.

103. Spielberger, C.D. Stress, emotions, and health. In: Morgan, W.P., and S.E. Goldston, eds. *Exercise and mental health*. Washington, DC: Hemisphere Publishing, 1987, part II, Chapt. 2, pp. 11-16,.

104. Spielberger, C.D., R.L. Gorsuch, and R.E. Lushene. *Manual for the State-Trait Anxiety Inventory (STAI)*. Palo Alto, CA: Consulting Psychologists Press, 1970, p. 1-24.

105. Stephens, T. Physical activity and mental health in the United States and Canada:

Evidence from four population surveys. *Prev. Med.* 17: 35-47, 1988.

106. Taube, C.A., and S.A. Barrett (Eds.). *Mental health, United States 1985.* Rockville, MD: U.S. Department of Health and Human Services (NIMH), 1986.

107. Teuting, P., and S.H. Koslow. *Special report on depression research.* Rockville, MD: National Institutes of Mental Health, Science Reports Branch, 1981.

108. Tharp, G.D., and W.H. Carson. Emotionality changes in rats following chronic exercise. *Med. Sci. Sports* 7: 123-126, 1975.

109. Thomas, G.S. Physical activity and health: Epidemiologic and clinical evidence and policy implications. *Prev. Med.* 8: 89-103, 1979.

110. Tucker, L.A. Muscular strength and health. *J. Pers. Psychol.* 45: 1355-1360, 1983.

111. Tucker, L.A. Mental health and physical fitness. *J. Hum. Movement Studies* 13: 267-273, 1987.

112. Weber, J.C., and R.A. Lee. Effects of differing prepuberty exercise programs on the emotionality of male albino rats. *Res. Q.* 39: 748-751, 1968.

113. Weinstein, W.S., and A.W. Meyers. Running as treatment for depression: Is it worth it? *J. Sport Psychol.* 5: 288-301, 1983.

114. Young, R.J., and A.H. Ismail. Personality differences of adult men before and after a physical fitness program. *Res. Q.* 47: 513-519, 1976.

115. Zimmerman, J.D., and M. Fulton. Aerobic fitness and emotional arousal: A critical attempt at replication. *Psychol. Rep.* 48: 911-918, 1981.

Chapter 54

Discussion: Exercise, Fitness, and Mental Health

Wesley E. Sime

A secondary analysis of four large-scale epidemiological surveys conducted in both the United States and Canada has documented a direct relationship between positive mental health and level of physical activity (10). Unfortunately, these studies used cross-sectional, correlational data collected on subjects who were self-selected into physically active versus physically inactive status. The results are also inconclusive because retrospectively it is impossible to know whether the participants exercise to enhance their sense of well-being or whether they are able to exercise only because they already have a sense of well-being. This "which-came-first" type of question is particularly salient in research on exercise habits because the acute, raw sensation of the physical experience of exertion and work for many individuals is predominantly unpleasant. Dyspnea, diffuse muscle and joint pain, and the feeling of fatigue are common symptoms among individuals who do not have very strong compelling motives for exercise (42). Some individuals attempt to deny the initial discomfort of exercise by deriving a sort of masochistic pleasure out of prolonged, moderately intense exertion. Others may be distracted from observing the uncomfortable symptoms because of their external attentional focus (21). Thus, it appears that another possible interpretation of the epidemiological data linking exercise habits to positive mental health is that only those individuals who are already quite mentally strong and healthy and those who have a compelling motivation for exercise will, in effect, have the fortitude to tolerate the acute discomfort of exercise. This motivation may be the desire to achieve the delayed gratification of the post-exercise feeling of calmness and the possible benefits of coronary risk reduction.

Great care must be taken not to promote the benefits of a particular exercise experience to the general population when in fact there may be negative consequences for certain subpopulations. Injury, soreness, obsession, impatience, strain on relationships, and neglect of work are negative outcomes that occur in 7%-20% of individuals who run marathons (48). Regardless, the feeling-good effect following exercise for some individuals is certainly to be encouraged in spite of the inherently uncomfortable nature of the acute experience. For some individuals, exercise can be compared to beating one's head against a wall (i.e., it feels so good when you quit).

The Operational Definition of Mental Health

The operational definition of *mental health*, which includes the intricate relationship between physical and mental functioning as well as the continuum between health and illness, has been well documented (10). The fine line between normal versus abnormal and clinical versus nonclinical must be addressed in greater detail. For example, one recent study documented the prevalence of clinical depression to be 4%-6% in three large U.S. cities (35). The diagnostic criteria included major depressive episodes, manic episodes, and dysthymia. By contrast, nonclinical depression includes less serious symptoms, such as insomnia, tearfulness, sense of failure, indecision, disinterest, and fatigue. Two instruments used to quantify and to diagnose level of depression according to these criteria are the Beck Depression Inventory (8) and the Zung Self-Rating Depression Scale (52).

It should also be noted that life-stress circumstances are also closely related to prevalence of depressive symptoms as well as to anxiety disorders

627

(16). Specifically, several large-scale community studies have shown that stressful life events are moderately correlated to symptoms of demoralization, a common indicator of depression (27). For example, individuals who have recently lost a relative or close friend frequently experience a particular form of distress called *bereavement* (7). All the symptoms commonly seen in a chronically depressed patient are also observed among the bereaved for at least 1 mo after loss (13). Surprisingly, the somatic symptoms (e.g., appetite and weight loss) dissipate after 1 yr, but the psychological symptoms (e.g., death wishes and hopelessness) may persist or even increase in severity over time. Other stressful life changes such as divorce can have a similar influence on the levels of depression, thus confounding the interpretation of epidemiological data on the effects of exercise.

Exercise, Fitness, and Reactivity to Stressors

There is a substantial body of literature describing the relationship between aerobic exercise habit patterns (or fitness levels) and reduced cardiovascular reactivity to psychological stressors (10, 28, 46).

The underlying concern regarding this relationship is based on the related evidence suggesting that cardiovascular reactivity may be a causal factor in the development of coronary heart disease (29). The stability of cardiovascular reactivity is of concern before attributing great significance to the clinical relevance of reactivity. The temporal stability of heart rate, blood pressure, and pre-ejection period in response to a cold pressor test and shock avoidance was examined by test-retest over a 2-1/2-yr period (3). The results showed that heart rate and systolic pressure were very stable over that period but diastolic pressure and pre-ejection period were not (perhaps because of differences in technical methods used in the two tests). It appears that the stability of the measure is sufficient to warrant objective evaluation of the extent to which exercise habit patterns of sufficient intensity and duration are effective in reducing cardiovascular reactivity.

The other remarkable behavior that is known to affect reactivity is the Type A behavior pattern (14). Because Type A causes an increase in reactivity, it is desirable to reduce its prevalence while increasing exercise behavior. Although there are numerous studies showing the effect of interventions to reduce Type A, there is also some evidence

to show that increased physical fitness is associated with a reduction in the Type A behavior pattern (31). Therein lies the potential for one treatment intervention exercise to affect two separate but related coronary risk factors (cardiovascular reactivity and the Type A behavior pattern).

In examining the mechanisms that relate exercise to reactivity, it should be noted that measures of maximal oxygen uptake have not generally been used in most of the previous research (10). One recent exception shows oxygen consumption (as well as heart rate and blood pressure) recorded during graded exercise testing and two psychological stress challenges in both high-fitness and low-fitness subjects (50). The results showed that during both the exercise challenge and the psychological challenge, the high-fitness subjects had similar $\dot{V}O_2$ values; however, they had lower heart rate values than did the low-fitness subjects. Plotting this data as a function of $\dot{V}O_2$, it was determined that the high-fitness groups displayed significantly less additional heart rate during both physical and psychological challenge than did the low-fitness group. Recent animal research demonstrated a significant influence of voluntary exercise on stress-induced hypertension (47). Borderline hypertensive rats that were allowed free access to a running wheel during periods of signaled shock over a 6-wk period showed significantly more attenuation in the stress effect on blood pressure (by 56%) and in heart rate (by 100%) than did the exercise-restricted rats.

There is some controversy whether training that leads to improved fitness in muscle strength or endurance may possibly alter reactivity to some psychological stressor more than does improved cardiorespiratory fitness resulting from chronic aerobic activity (10). One recent study compared the relative effects of 12 wk of aerobic exercise training with strength training in 27 male subjects (44). Some of these individuals were borderline hypertensives. The results showed the aerobic exercise training resulted in a significant reduction in hypertension by down-regulating the absolute magnitude of cardiovascular activity in response to psychological stress. There were no positive benefits from the strength-training intervention in this regard.

Exercise in the Reduction of Anxiety and Tension

There are numerous psychogenic risk factors associated with high levels of striate muscle tension (9).

In particular, a significant volume of research has demonstrated that unnecessarily high levels of skeletal muscle tension are related to adverse psychophysiological problems, such as chronic muscle contraction headache. The personal distress and the documented medical expenses resulting from muscle contraction headache have been significantly high, thus justifying aggressive clinical treatment thereof (9). However, patients that have undergone behavior treatment (biofeedback) to reduce muscle tension levels show significantly reduced headache symptoms as well as reduced medical expenses. Furthermore, it has been demonstrated that even modest levels of anticipatory tension will also cause significant performance reduction (37). High levels of muscle tension preceding a simple motor task disrupted hand steadiness and impaired grip strength.

Low-intensity exercise has been shown to be clearly associated with significant reductions in EMG measures of muscle tension as well as in the Hoffmann reflex, which is an indicator of overall skeletal muscle body tension (15). However, until recently, evidence showed that moderate to high levels of exercise did not decrease these measures of muscle tension. Subsequently, further utilization of the Hoffmann reflex has documented additional benefits of high-intensity aerobic work (11). Subjects participated in a control trial and two 20-min treadmill exercise trials at low (40% $\dot{V}O_2$max) and high (75% $\dot{V}O_2$max) intensities. Low-intensity exercise resulted in a 13% reduction in motorneuron excitability and high-intensity exercise a 21% reduction. The authors hypothesized from this data that one of the possible causes for reduction in overall muscle electrical activity was an increase in body temperature, which was coincidental with the level of the exercise intensity.

A long series of research studies have shown that anxiety and tension levels are significantly reduced by exercise (10). By contrast, a comparable time-out (or rest) condition is equally as effective as is exercise in reducing levels of anxiety, blood pressure, and EMG (38). Further study on the comparative effects of exercise and relaxation has focused on the effect of exercise on muscle tension levels independently and in concert with biofeedback muscle relaxation training (6). The results showed that following a bout of 30 min of bicycle pedaling at a progressively increasing submaximal work load heart rate of 120, 135, and 150 beats/min, the subjects had a significantly higher level of muscle tension for at least 1 hr following the exercise. However, at 90 min following the termination of exercise, the level of muscle tension significantly

decreased below baseline levels. Furthermore, in this study the subjects were randomly assigned to a follow-up phase (nine sessions over a 3-wk period), which included an hour of exercise followed by biofeedback training for the experimental group and a single period of biofeedback training without exercise for the control group. The results showed the biofeedback training produced a significant reduction in muscle tension levels, comparable to the exercise training, but that the combination of exercise and biofeedback was no more effective in reducing muscle tension than was biofeedback training alone.

Exercise and Sleep

The influence of aerobic fitness training on the quality and quantity of sleep has been postulated as a factor in positive mental health. It was demonstrated that exercise deprivation among persons accustomed to exercise is associated with impaired sleep patterns as well as increased anxiety and sexual tension (4). Sleep lab testing with EEG measures on these subjects revealed a reduction in the level of Stage 4 sleep; however, after 1 mo the sleep pattern was normal again. Cross-sectional data on active versus sedentary individuals indicate that runners have a higher proportion of nonrapid eye movement and a lower proportion of rapid eye movement (REM) sleep (51). Reduction in REM sleep occurs with antidepressant medication and electroconvulsive shock therapy as well as exercise (40). The reduction in REM sleep due to exercise and the other treatments causes amnergic synaptic transmissions to be enhanced. Therein lies one physiological mechanism to account for the effect of exercise on mental health. In addition, aerobically fit athletes tend to sleep longer and have elevated slow-wave sleep patterns when compared to matched sedentary control subjects (36).

Exercise and Depression

It has been estimated that the financial cost of depression in the United States is approximately $16.5 billion per year. Of this amount, $3 billion is expended annually for treatment (psychotherapy and pharmacotherapy) and the remainder in the form of sick leave and lower productivity on the job (23). The estimated incidence of depression alone is approximately 10%-25%, and recent data suggest that the prevalence rates are increasing steadily (34). Surprisingly, only about 20% of those who meet the diagnostic criteria for depression are actually seen by trained mental health professionals (psychiatrists or psychotherapists) for treatment. The remainder are seen by a primary care physician, who is not specifically trained to deal with such mental health issues. Furthermore, the physician in these cases is likely to misdiagnose the clinically depressed patient in more than half of all cases. Given the relatively high risk of suicide among individuals with affective, depressive disorders (10%-15%), the concern regarding the proper diagnosis and most effective treatment is very important (49).

Ironically, many of the cases of clinical depression go untreated not only because of failure to diagnose but also because the individual feels stigmatized by the label and the mental health treatment process (34). Therefore, the rationale for prevention-oriented strategies (primary or secondary), including such innovative interventions as exercise, is likely to be very well received by some patients.

Extensive review of the literature shows a large number of studies (mostly correlational) indicating that chronic exercise is associated with decreased depression (10, 22). These effects are more consistent among studies on clinically depressed individuals than on nonclinical populations with less pronounced symptoms of depression at the outset. Clearly, exercise is effective with clinical populations, but the mechanisms and the most effective interventions to achieve an antidepressive effect of exercise are not well established. Not surprisingly, the mechanisms to account for the antidepressant effect of psychotherapy and pharmacotherapy are also not well understood (5).

Recent studies have put forth more evidence supporting exercise benefits for depression. A multiple baseline design using bicycle exercise and placebo with clinically depressed women showed significantly greater symptom reduction for the exercise therapy subjects after 6 wk of treatment, and these effects were maintained at a 3-mo follow-up (18). A follow-up study using aerobic exercise, weight-lifting, and wait-list control groups revealed that both exercise treatments produced significant symptom reduction among clinically depressed women, but the changes were not related to changes in fitness level (19). A similar study that used subjects as their own controls in a multiple baseline design showed that aerobic exercise was more effective in reducing clinical symptoms of depression than was placebo stretching exercise (45). These effects were maintained at a 6-mo follow-up.

Clinical studies on the effects of exercise on mental health are often criticized for lack of comparison to psychotherapy. Another series of studies shed light on this issue. The separate and combined effects of running and cognitive therapy on moderately depressed men and women were examined in two consecutive studies (24, 25). Exercise training was found to be as effective as cognitive therapy, but no additional benefits were observed for a combination of the two. The effects were maintained at 2- and 4-mo follow-ups, but there was no relationship between symptom reduction and change in fitness level. The accumulation of evidence from these respective studies overwhelmingly supports the effects of exercise therapy in the treatment of clinical depression but sheds no light on the mechanism underlying these changes.

The Causal Mechanisms Relating Exercise to Positive Mental Health

There are numerous theories regarding the probable causes of depression. These include (a) life events so overwhelming that adaptive skills fail, (b) heightened neuronal excitability and arousal in the diencephalon, (c) impaired monoamnergic transmission, (d) derangement of neurochemical substrates of reinforcement, (e) the production of faulty neurotransmitters, and (f) decreases in post-synaptic receptor sensitivity (2). There is also a significant association between increasing age and depression (12). However, this relationship is confounded by the influence of fitness differences between subjects of differing ages. Further discussion on the factors related to exercise follows.

Research on middle-aged sedentary and active males demonstrated that depression is significantly related to beta-endorphin levels (32, 41) and enkephalin levels (43). It has been clearly documented that moderate, extended exercise is associated with increased levels of endorphin and plasma beta endorphin (39). It was also demonstrated that the intensity of exercise is proportionally related to responses to beta endorphin, corticotropin, and catecholamine levels (17, 30, 33). Other related studies seeking to replicate these results on beta endorphins found no significant relationship between exercise intensity and endorphin level or between psychological state and endorphin level (26). Exercise at low, moderate, and high intensities was directly proportional to epinephrine and enkephalins responses, but these biochemical variables were not significantly related to the psychological measures of tension (20). By contrast, beta-endorphin levels are positively associated with the mild stress of scuba diving (1). Apparently, the acute experience of being submersed in water in a neutral state of buoyance elicits feelings of well-being or euphoria similar to those reported by many after a strenuous bout of exercise.

Conclusion

The relationship among exercise, fitness, and mental health is based primarily on the subjective effect of feeling good that lasts for 2-6 hr post-exercise in normal subjects and on the reduction in clinical symptoms of anxiety, tension, and depression among patients. Studies to document the mechanisms underlying these effects in both normals and patients have as yet been inconclusive. It is important to remember, however, that the lack of knowledge regarding the mechanisms does not belie the significance of the benefits of exercise training or exercise therapy. A great number of pharmacological treatments are used regularly in the absence of a known mechanism and with a risk of harm in prolonged use far greater than that present in most forms of exercise training and carefully controlled exercise therapy.

The research on cardiovascular reactivity and exercise holds some significant potential because it is linked to coronary risk and to protection from sudden cardiac death. However, the evidence is as yet inconclusive, and the results will not affect mental health per se.

References

1. Adams, M.L., N.W. Eastman, R.P. Tobin, D.L. Morris, and W.L. Dewey. Increased plasma beta-endorphin immunoreactivity in scuba divers after submersion. *Med. Sci. Sports Exerc.* 19(2): 87-90, 1987.

2. Akisal, H.S. A biobehavioral approach to depression. In: Depue, R.A., ed. *The psychobiology of the depressive disorders: Implications for the effects of stress.* New York: Academic Press, 1979, 409-438.

3. Allen, M.T., A. Sherwood, P. Obrist, M. Crowell, and L. Grange. Stability of cardiovascular reactivity to laboratory stressors: A 2-1/2 year follow-up. *J. Psychosom. Res.* 31(5): 639-645, 1987.

4. Baekeland, F. Exercise deprivation: Sleep and psychological reactions. *Arch. Gen. Psychiatry* 22: 365-369, 1970.

5. Baldessarini, R.J. *Biomedical aspects of depression and its treatment.* Washington, DC: American Psychiatric Press, 1983.

6. Balog, L.F. The effects of exercise on muscle tension and subsequent muscle relaxation training. *Res. Q. Exp. Sports* 54(2): 119-125, 1983.

7. Barrera, M. Distinctions between social support concepts, measures and models. *Am. J. Community Psychol.* 14: 413-445, 1986.

8. Beck, A.T. *Depression: Causes and treatment.* Philadelphia: University of Pennsylvania Press, 1972.

9. Blanchard, E.B., J. Jacard, F. Audrasick, P. Guarnieri, and S.E. Jurish. Reduction in headache patients' medical expenses associated with biofeedback and relaxation training. *Bio S-Reg* 10(1): 63-68, 1985.

10. Brown, D.R. Exercise fitness and mental health. In: Bouchard, C., ed. *Exercise fitness and health.* Champaign, IL: Human Kinetics, 1990.

11. Bulbulian, R., and D.L. Daragos. Motor neuron excitability: The Hoffmann reflex following exercise of low and high intensity. *Med. Sci. Sports Exerc.* 18(6): 697-702, 1986.

12. Chodzko-Zajko, W.J., and D.L. Corrigan. The influence of physiological fitness on the relationship between chronological age and depression [Abstract]. *Med. Sci. Sports Exerc.* 19(2): S-67, 1987.

13. Clayton, P.J., and H.S. Darvish. Course of depressive symptoms following the stress of bereavement. In: Barett, J.D., ed. *Stress and mental disorder.* New York: Raven Press, 1979.

14. Contrada, R.J., and D.S. Krantz. Stress reactivity and type A behavior: Current status and future direction. *Ann. Behav. Med.* 10(2): 64-70, 1988.

15. deVries, H.A., C.P. Simard, R.A. Wiswell, E. Heckathorne, and V. Carabetta. Fusimotor system involvement in the tranquilizer effect of exercise. *Am. J. Physical Med.* 61: 111-122, 1982.

16. Dohrenwend, B.S., and B.T. Dohrenwend. Life, stress and illness: Formulation of the issues. In: Dohrenwend, B.S., and B.T. Dohrenwend, eds. *Stressful life events and their*

contacts. New York: Neal Watson Academic Publications, 1981, 1-27.

17. Donevan, R.H., and G.M. Andrew. Plasma beta-endorphin immunoreactivity during graded cycle ergometry. *Med. Sci. Sports Exerc.* 19(3): 229-233, 1987.

18. Doyne, E.J., D.L. Chambles, and L.E. Beutler. Aerobic exercise as a treatment for depression in women. *Behav. Ther.* 14: 434-440, 1983.

19. Doyne, E.J., D.J. Ossip-Klein, E.D. Bowman, K.M. Osborn, I.B. McDugall-Wilson, and R.A. Neimeyer. Running versus weight lifting in the treatment of depression. *J. Consult. Clin. Psychol.* 55: 748-754, 1987.

20. Farrell, P.A., A.B. Gustafson, W.P. Morgan, and C.B. Pert. Enkephalins, catecholamines, and psychological mood alterations: Effects of prolonged exercise. *Med. Sci. Sports Exerc.* 19(4): 347-353, 1987.

21. Fillingim, R.B., and M.A. Fine. The effects of internal versus external information processing on symptom perception in an exercise setting. *Health Psychol.* 5(2): 115-123, 1986.

22. Folkins, C.H., and W.E. Sime. Physical fitness training and mental health. *Am. Psychol.* 36: 373-389, 1981.

23. Frank, R.G., M.S. Camplet, and A. Stoudemire. The social cost of depression. In: A. Stoudemire (Chair), *Perspectives in prevention of depression*. Symposium conducted at the meeting of the American Psychiatric Association, Dallas, May, 1985.

24. Fremont, J., and L.W. Craighead. *Aerobic exercise and cognitive therapy for mild/moderate depression*. Paper presented at the meeting of the Association for Advancement of Behavior Therapy, Philadelphia, 1984.

25. Fremont, J., and L.W. Craighead. Aerobic exercise and cognitive therapy in treatment of dysphoric moods. *Cog. Ther. Res.* 11: 241-251, 1987.

26. Goldfarb, A.H., B.D. Hatfield, G.A. Sforzo, and M.G. Flynn. Serum-endorphin levels during a graded exercise test to exhaustion. *Med. Sci. Sports Exerc.* 19(2): 78-82, 1987.

27. Hirschfeld, R.M.A., and L.K. Cross. Epidemiology of affective disorders. *Arch. Gen. Psychiatry* 39: 35-46, 1982.

28. Keller, S., and P. Seraganian. Physical fitness level and autonomic reactivity to psychosocial stress. *J. Psychosom. Res.* 28(4): 279-287, 1984.

29. Krantz, D.S., and S.B. Marrvick. Acute psychophysiologic reactivity and risk of cardiovascular disease: A review and methodological critique. *Psychol. Bull.* 96: 435-464, 1984.

30. Langenfield, M.P., L.S. Hart, and P.C. Kao. Plasma beta-endorphin responses to one-hour bicycling and running at 60% $\dot{V}O_2$max. *Med. Sci. Sports Exerc.* 19(2): 83-86, 1987.

31. Levenkron, J.C., and L.G. Moore. The type A behavior pattern: Issues for intervention research. *Ann. Behav. Med.* 10(2): 78-83, 1988.

32. Lobstein, D.D., and A.H. Ismail. Basal plasma beta-endorphin and depression scores may be decreased concomitantly by regular training [Abstract]. *Med. Sci. Sports Exerc.* 19(2): 209, 1985.

33. McMurray, R.G., W.A. Forsythe, M.H. Mar, and C.J. Hardy. Exercise intensity-related responses of beta-endorphin and catecholamines. *Med. Sci. Sports Exerc.* 19(6): 570-574, 1987.

34. Munoz, R.F. Depression prevention research: Conceptual and practical considerations. In: Munoz, R.F., ed. *Depression prevention: Research directions*. Washington, DC: Hemisphere Publishing, 1987, 1-30.

35. Myers, J.K., M.M. Weissman, G.L. Tischler, C.E. Holtzer, P.J. Leaf, H. Orvaschel, J.C. Anthony, J.H. Boyd, J.D. Burke, M. Kramer, and R. Stoltzman. Six-month prevalence of psychiatric disorders in three communities. *Arch. Gen. Psychiatry* 41: 959-967, 1980-1982.

36. Paxton, S.J., J. Trinder, and I. Montgomery. Does aerobic fitness affect sleep? *Psychophysiology* 20(3): 320-324, 1983.

37. Pinel, J.P.J., and T.D. Schultz. The effect of antecedent muscle tension levels on motor behavior. *Med. Sci. Sports Exerc.* 10(3): 177-182, 1978.

38. Raglin, J.S., and W.P. Morgan. Influence of exercise and quiet rest on state anxiety and blood pressure. *Med. Sci. Sports Exerc.* 19: 456-463, 1987.

39. Rahkila, P., E. Hakala, K. Salminen, and P. Laatikainen. Response of plasma endorphins to running exercises in male and female endurance athletes. *Med. Sci. Sports Exerc.* 19(5): 451-455, 1987.

40. Ransford, C.R. A role for amines in the antidepressant effect of exercise: A review. *Med. Sci. Sports Exerc.* 14(1): 1-10, 1982.

41. Rasmussen, C.L., and D.D. Lobstein. Beta-endorphin and components of psychological depression are powerful discriminators between joggers and sedentary middle-aged

men [Abstract]. *Med. Sci. Sports Exerc.* 19(2): S-67, 1987.

42. Roth, D.T. Some motivational aspects of exercise. *J. Sports Med.* 14: 40-47, 1974.

43. Sarrell, P.A., A.B. Gustafson, W.P. Morgan, and C.B. Pert. Enkephalins, catecholamines, and psychological mood alterations: Effects of prolonged exercise. *Med. Sci. Sports Exerc.* 19(4): 347-353, 1987.

44. Sherwood, A., K.C. Light, and J.A. Blumenthal. Effects of aerobic exercise training in hemodynamic responses to psychosocial stress in type A men. *Psychosom. Med.* (in press).

45. Sime, W.E., and M. Sanstead. Running therapy in the treatment of depression: Implications for prevention. In: Munoz, R.F., ed. *Depression prevention.* Washington, DC: Hemisphere Publishing, 1987, 12-138.

46. Sinyor, D., S.G. Schwartz, F. Peronnet, G. Brisson, and P. Seraganian. Aerobic fitness level and reactivity to psychosocial stress: Physiological, biochemical, and subjective measures. *Psychosom. Med.* 45(3): 205-217, 1983.

47. Squire, J.N., N.P. Myers, and R. Freed. Cardiovascular responses to exercise and stress in the borderline hypertensive rate. *Med. Sci. Sports Exerc.* 19(1): 11-16, 1987.

48. Summers, J., V. Machin, and G. Sargent. Psychosocial factors related to marathon running. *J. Sports Psychol.* 5(3): 314-331, 1983.

49. Teuting, P., S.H. Koslow, and R.M.A. Hirschfeld. *Special report on depression research* (DHHS Publication No. ADM 81-1085). Washington, DC: U.S. Government Printing Office, 1981.

50. Turner, J.R., D. Carroll, M. Costello, and J. Sims. The effects of aerobic fitness on additional heart rates during activity psychological challenge. *Psychophysiology* (in press).

51. Walker, J.M., T.C. Floyd, G. Fine, C. Cavnes, R. Lualhati, and I. Fineberg. Effects of exercise on sleep. *J. Appl. Physiol.* 44(6): 945-951, 1978.

52. Zunk, W.W.K. A self-rating depression scale. *J. Arch. Gen. Psychiatry* 12: 63-70, 1965.

PART V
Physical Activity and Fitness in Growth, Reproductive Health, and Aging

Chapter 55

Growth, Exercise, Fitness, and Later Outcomes

Robert M. Malina

It is often assumed that regular physical activity during childhood and youth has long-term beneficial effects on growth and maturation and on the health of the individual into adulthood. However, the task of relating regular physical activity and physical fitness to growth and maturation and to health outcomes in adulthood is complex. Physical activity is only one of many factors capable of influencing the developing individual, and it is often difficult to partition effects attributed to physical activity from those associated with normal growth and maturation. Further, growing and maturing individuals are not miniature adults and do not necessarily respond to environmental conditions in a manner similar to that of adults.

Health outcomes in adulthood are influenced by many factors. However, the literature that deals with adult health and physical activity focuses primarily on the status of the cardiovascular system and the risk factors for cardiovascular disease. Because many risk factors for cardiovascular disease are evident in a significant percentage of children and youth, a central question is, Does regular physical activity during childhood and adolescence reduce the risk of atherosclerosis and coronary heart disease in adulthood? The role of childhood physical activity as a factor related to other health outcomes is less often considered and information thus limited.

The objectives of this presentation are fourfold. First, age-, sex-, and maturity-associated variations in several indicators of growth, fitness, physical activity, and cardiovascular health status are briefly considered. Second, the tracking of these indicators during childhood and adolescence is evaluated. Third, effects for regular physical activity during growth on the indicators are discussed. Finally, implications for later health outcomes and needed research are briefly indicated.

Definitions

Growth and Maturation

The terms *growth* and *maturation* occasionally have different meanings to professionals working with children and youth. Growth refers to measurable changes in size, physique, and body composition. Aerobic power, muscular strength, endurance, and power are largely related to body size and show growth patterns that are generally similar to those for stature and weight. Maturity implies a time component that marks the rate of progress toward the mature state. Rate of maturation varies among the systems of the body. Skeletal age, age at appearance of secondary sex characteristics, and age at peak height velocity (PHV) are the most commonly used indicators of biological maturity during childhood and adolescence.

Physical, Physiological, and Motor Fitness

Physical fitness has been operationally defined as including cardiovascular endurance, muscular strength and endurance, flexibility, and body composition (specifically fatness), whereas physiological fitness extends the concept to specific biological systems and tissues that are related to cardiovascular health status (i.e., blood lipids and lipoproteins, blood pressure, and glucose metabolism). Given the role of motor skills as channels of physical activity in children, these skills must be included in any assessment of physical fitness. Components of motor skill include agility, balance, coordination, power, and speed.

Physical Activity

The measurement of habitual physical activity during childhood is a difficult task and needs further attention. Data for relatively large samples of children and youth are derived from questionnaires, interviews, and occasionally diaries, whereas pedometers and heart rate integrators are used less often (51). However, criteria for classifying children as active or inactive vary among studies.

Age-, Sex-, and Maturity-Associated Variation

Somatic Growth

Stature and weight are the two most commonly used measurements of growth. Both follow similar curves of rapid growth during infancy and early childhood, reasonably steady growth during middle childhood, and rapid growth during the adolescent spurt. Growth in stature gradually slows and then eventually ceases, whereas body weight continues to increase into the mid-20s. There is, however, considerable maturity-associated variation in stature and weight. Within a given chronological age-group, those advanced in biological maturity status are on average taller and heavier than those who are delayed. Maturity-associated differences are most pronounced during mid-adolescence. Late maturers generally catch up in stature in late adolescence, whereas body weight differences between children of contrasting maturity status tend to persist.

The adolescent growth spurt in stature occurs on average about 2 yr earlier in girls than in boys, but there is much individual variability. The magnitude of the spurt is greater in boys. Peak weight gain during the adolescent spurt occurs most often after PHV (10, 55).

Body Composition

Body composition is viewed most often in the context of the two-component model, i.e., body weight = fat-free mass (FFM) + fat mass (FM), although changes in adipose, muscle, and skeletal tissues are also important. Body composition and specifically fatness have implications for health status given the association between excessive fatness and complications of several chronic diseases.

Fat-free mass has a growth pattern like that of stature and weight. Sex differences are minor before the adolescent spurt. Major changes occur during adolescence, and sex differences become clearly established. By late adolescence or young adulthood, females have on average only about two thirds of the FFM that males have. Fat mass increases during childhood in both sexes and continues to increase through adolescence in females. However, male adolescence is characterized by stable levels of, or a slight decrease in, FM. Relative fatness of males declines during adolescence because of the marked increase in FFM, especially muscle mass; hence, FM contributes relatively less to body weight at this time. Within a given chronological age-group, children advanced in biological maturity status generally have larger FFMs and FMs than do those who are delayed. This reflects the overall size differences between children of contrasting maturity status (55).

A significant proportion of the changes in body composition during adolescence occur near the time of maximum growth. However, data relating changes in body composition to the timing of the adolescent spurt are limited. Peak growth of FFM occurs close to or just after PHV in boys (65), but corresponding longitudinal data for girls are not available. Measurements of tissue widths on standardized radiographs of the arm and calf indicate growth spurts in bone and muscle that, respectively, occur close to and just after PHV. Subcutaneous fat shows a different pattern. Both sexes lose fat tissue on the arm during the interval of PHV, whereas only males lose subcutaneous fat on the calf at this time (82).

Fat Distribution

An aspect of body composition that has relevance for adult health status is fat distribution, which refers to regional variation in the relative distribution of fat tissue in the body. Evidence currently indicates significant associations among fat distribution, adipose tissue metabolism, abnormalities in lipid and carbohydrate metabolism, and several chronic diseases in adults (13).

The distribution of subcutaneous fat is commonly viewed in terms of the ratio of skinfold thicknesses measured on the trunk to those measured on the extremities. The ratio of the sum of three trunk skinfolds (subscapular, suprailiac, and abdominal) to the sum of three extremity skinfolds (triceps, biceps, and medial calf) indicates, on average, stability in the relative distribution of trunk and extremity subcutaneous fat during childhood. The ratio is similar in boys and girls. Subsequently, sex differences in subcutaneous fat distribution occur. Females, on average, appear to accumulate proportionally more subcutaneous fat on the trunk during early adolescence but then to gain fat on the trunk and extremities at a similar pace. Males, on the other hand, accumulate relatively more fat on the trunk during adolescence, which is accentuated by a reduction in subcutaneous fat on the extremities at this time (54). Among males, however, changes in specific trunk and extremity skinfolds appear to vary relative to the timing of PHV (11).

Presently, there is no effective means of distinguishing between subcutaneous and internal fat in large samples of children. Assuming that the ratio of the sum of skinfolds taken at representative trunk and extremity sites (e.g., the six skinfolds mentioned previously) to FM provides an estimate of the contribution of subcutaneous fat to FM, FM increases at a faster rate than does subcutaneous fat during childhood in both sexes. This trend continues through adolescence in girls, but the relationship between subcutaneous fat and FM is altered during male adolescence. Relative to FM, males have proportionally more subcutaneous fat on the trunk and less on the extremities (54).

Maturity status is related to subcutaneous fat distribution in boys but not in girls. Boys advanced in maturity status tend to have relatively more subcutaneous fat on the trunk than on the extremities compared to boys who are delayed. Early- and late-maturing girls differ only in overall fatness (the former being fatter) and not in the distribution of subcutaneous fat (22, 54).

Physical and Motor Fitness

Absolute aerobic power ($\dot{V}O_2$max, L $\cdot$ min^{-1}) increases from childhood through adolescence in boys but reaches a plateau at about 13-14 yr of age in girls. Before 10-12 yr of age, average $\dot{V}O_2$max of girls reaches about 85%-90% of mean values for boys, but after the adolescent spurt and sexual maturation average $\dot{V}O_2$max of girls reaches only about 70% of mean values for boys (43, 55). There is an adolescent spurt in $\dot{V}O_2$max that occurs close to or just after PHV in both sexes, but peak velocity is greater in boys than in girls (56).

The dependence of aerobic power on body size during growth is indicated in the growth curve of relative $\dot{V}O_2$max (ml $\cdot$ kg^{-1} $\cdot$ min^{-1}). It is rather stable from childhood through adolescence in cross-sectional samples of boys (43), but trends in several longitudinal samples suggest a decline in relative $\dot{V}O_2$max through adolescence (56). On the other hand, relative $\dot{V}O_2$max declines systematically with age from 11 through 17 yr in cross-sectional and longitudinal samples of girls (43, 56). Sex differences in relative $\dot{V}O_2$max are on average slightly less than those for absolute $\dot{V}O_2$max during late childhood and adolescence, about 90%-95%

and 80% of mean values of boys, respectively (55). The decline in relative $\dot{V}O_2$max during adolescence reflects the combined contributions of differential growth rates of aerobic power and body weight, changes in body composition, and perhaps reduced levels of habitual physical activity. When youngsters are categorized as early and late maturing, the former have greater absolute aerobic power, which reflects their larger body size, whereas the latter have greater relative aerobic power, which reflects their smaller body mass (41).

A variety of measures of muscular strength and endurance, agility, balance, coordination, power, and speed show growth curves similar to those of aerobic power. Performance increases on average from middle childhood through adolescence in males but improves until only about 14 yr of age in girls and then remains rather stable or improves only slightly. Mean performances are generally better in boys, except for balance tasks during childhood. The time between 5 and 8 yr of age appears to be a transitional period in the development of motor skills. Basic movement patterns are reaching mature form at this time, but there is much individual variability (34, 55). Application of basic movement patterns to specific test situations also has a significant learning component.

Although longitudinal data are not extensive, several indicators of physical and motor fitness show well-defined adolescent spurts in boys. Tests of strength and power show spurts that tend to follow PHV, whereas tests of speed appear to reach a peak before PHV (10, 11). Corresponding data for girls generally show no clear changes in performance relative to PHV or age at menarche (10).

Strength and motor performance tend to be positively related to biological maturity status in both sexes during childhood, but during adolescence they are positively related only in boys. The maturity relationship reflects the role of body size in strength and motor performance in children and male adolescents and the role of changing body composition and relative fatness in female adolescents.

Flexibility is joint specific, but flexibility of the lower back, hip, and upper thigh as measured by the sit-and-reach task is included in fitness test batteries. Mean scores on this task have a unique growth pattern that is related to the timing of the adolescent spurt and sexual maturity. Females are more flexible than males at all ages. Sit-and-reach scores are stable or decline slightly during childhood in girls, increase during adolescence, and then reach a plateau at about 14-15 yr of age. In contrast, sit-and-reach scores decline from about

7-8 yr through midadolescence in boys and then increase in late adolescence (55). If there is a growth spurt in lower-back and hip flexibility, it probably occurs somewhat before PHV in boys, but the data are not sufficiently definitive (11).

Habitual Physical Activity

Large-scale surveys of habitual physical activity are based primarily on standardized interviews and questionnaires in children 10 yr of age and older. The information ordinarily is converted to an activity score that indicates the overall time spent in physical activities. The intensity of the activities is also occasionally differentiated. Although specific comparisons among studies of habitual physical activity in children and youth are complicated by sampling and seasonal variation, differences in methodology, and probably cultural variation, evidence from national cross-sectional surveys in the United States (71) and Canada (16) and from local longitudinal studies in Europe (26, 39, 40) indicates generally greater activity levels in males than in females and some tendency toward a decrease in level of physical activity during adolescence, especially in late adolescence and more so in males than in females. The adolescent decline in habitual physical activity occurs after the growth spurt and is probably related to the social demands of adolescence, changing interests, and perhaps the transition from school to work or college.

Indicators of Cardiovascular Health

Blood pressure, serum lipids and lipoproteins, and, to a lesser extent, glucose metabolism and insulin sensitivity are used as indicators of cardiovascular health status during childhood and adolescence. Systolic blood pressure increases from about 5 yr of age until adolescence, when boys develop slightly higher values than do girls. Diastolic blood pressure, on the other hand, shows a small increase with age from childhood through adolescence. Sex differences in blood pressure are negligible except for systolic pressure in adolescence. Changes in blood pressure are related primarily to body weight, but both skeletal maturation and subcutaneous fatness are associated with elevated systolic pressure during childhood and adolescence, particularly when weight is deleted as an independent variable. In contrast, sexual maturation is not apparently related to blood pressure during adolescence (19, 33, 47, 76).

After a rapid rise during the first 3 yr of life, mean values of total serum cholesterol (TC) and LDL and HDL cholesterol are rather stable during childhood and then decline circumpuberally. The pubertal decline in HDL-C is more marked in males than in females. Total serum and LDL cholesterol subsequently rise, whereas HDL-C is rather stable and/or then may decline into late adolescence (5, 81). These trends suggest that males, in contrast to females, are progressing toward an atherogenic cholesterol profile after the growth spurt and sexual maturation.

Sex differences in serum lipids are small during childhood, but the rather marked decline in HDL during male adolescence results in higher TC in females at this time. Adolescent variation may be more apparent when lipids are expressed by stage of sexual maturation (7) or skeletal age (76). This probably reflects the more homogeneous grouping of children when an indicator of biological maturity rather than chronological age is used. However, lipid and lipoprotein levels do not differ between children advanced and delayed in biological maturation within a chronological age-group and do not differ when children are grouped relative to age at PHV or age at menarche (76).

Fasting serum triglycerides (TG) are also rather stable during childhood and rise to young adult values during puberty (5, 81). Median TG levels are similar in girls and boys in childhood but rise more so in males during adolescence.

Fasting plasma glucose increases on average gradually with age in both sexes until about 11-13 yr, when it declines more so in girls than in boys. Fasting plasma insulin also increases with age through childhood. It increases through adolescence in girls but declines after about 13-14 yr of age in boys (6). Mean glucose values are higher in boys, whereas mean insulin values tend to be higher in girls. Fasting insulin levels, however, are more variable than are glucose levels.

Generally similar age-associated trends are indicated by glucose tolerance tests, but sample sizes are much smaller. The area under the glucose curve declines from childhood (5-10 yr) into adolescence (11-15 yr) and then increases into young adulthood (16-29 yr). On the other hand, the area under the insulin curve increases from childhood through adolescence into adulthood. On average, mean areas under the glucose curve are greater in males, whereas mean areas under the insulin curve are greater in females, especially in adolescence and young adulthood (64). Thus, adolescent and young adult females apparently produce more insulin in response to a glucose challenge than do males of the same age.

The trends suggest that changes in glucose metabolism and insulin occur during puberty. However, the studies do not control for biological maturity status. Data for prepubertal (no overt development of secondary sex characteristics) and pubertal children derived with the insulin clamp technique suggest a significant change in insulin sensitivity with sexual maturation. Prepubertal children have significantly higher insulin-stimulated glucose metabolism than do pubertal children (1, 14). At two different glucose loads, pubertal children have a 2-3 times greater insulin response than do prepubertal children (14). Puberty is thus associated with a decline in insulin sensitivity or with insulin resistance. Adolescents compensate for the reduction in insulin sensitivity with an increase in insulin secretion at this time. Factors underlying pubertal insulin resistance are apparently several, including changes in body mass and increases in adrenal androgen and growth hormone secretion (14).

Although the preceding considers several indicators of cardiovascular health status in isolation, they are in fact related. Serum TC and TG are related to body weight during childhood and adolescence, especially in individuals at the higher percentiles (5). Impaired glucose tolerance and hyperinsulinemia are also associated with obesity. Fasting plasma glucose and insulin levels are positively related to indices of obesity, serum TG, and VLDL cholesterol and inversely related to HDL (6). Children with high levels of LDL tend to have higher glucose levels and to be fatter, whereas those with high levels of VLDL tend to have high insulin levels following a glucose load (67). Thus, extreme values of fatness, serum lipids and lipoproteins, serum TG, glucose tolerance, and insulin metabolism tend to cluster within individuals.

Tracking of Indicators During Growth

The concept of tracking has been used in growth studies for some time (15, 68), although its use in epidemiological research appears rather recent (18, 70). It is used in the context of prediction and stability. The former refers to the ability to predict subsequent status from earlier measurements, as in predicting adult stature; the latter refers to the maintenance of relative rank or position within a group over time. Tracking, of course, requires longitudinal data. Such data are most often utilized to note relationships between measurements made at one stage of growth with later outcomes in growth or in adulthood and do not imply causal sequences. In general, the closer the time span between measurements, the higher the correlation and thus the greater the stability. As the time span between observations increases, interage correlations generally decline. With few exceptions, interage correlations for indicators of growth, fitness, and cardiovascular status are generally moderate to low and thus have limited predictive utility.

Somatic Growth

Tracking for biological characteristics such as size and fatness is rather poor during infancy and early childhood. Some characteristics begin to track well by 3 yr of age (e.g., stature), whereas others begin to track reasonably well during middle childhood. Correlations between stature at 2 or 3 yr of age and adult stature reach about 0.8 and stay at this level during childhood. There is a slight decline during adolescence due to individual variation in the onset and magnitude of the adolescent spurt. Correlations for body weight during growth and young adult weight are slightly lower (0.6-0.8) than are those for stature (83).

Body Composition

Longitudinal data for FFM and FM are limited, but data for subcutaneous fat are reasonably extensive. Correlations between FFM at 11 and 15 yr and at 11 and 18 yr of age in boys are moderately high (0.7 and 0.6) and those for FM are lower (0.5 and 0.2, respectively) (65). The same trend is generally apparent for several skinfolds in this longitudinal sample, and abdominal and suprailiac skinfolds track slightly better across adolescence than do subscapular and extremity skinfolds.

Interage correlations and analyses of contingency tables for radiographic and skinfold measurements of subcutaneous fat from seven longitudinal studies in the United States and Australia were reported by Roche et al. (69). Before 6 yr of age, the tendency to retain quartile rank is not consistent, but subsequently the tendency to retain quartile rank is significant. Children in the fourth (fattest) quartile after 6 yr of age have a moderate or high risk of remaining in the fourth quartile at subsequent examinations. Using 16 yr as the upper age limit in the longitudinal studies, correlations between subcutaneous fatness during childhood and at 16 yr of age increase gradually before 6 yr of age, are generally stable until puberty, decline during pubescence, and then increase to 16 yr. There is, however, considerable variation among different sites and specific skinfolds. The pectoral (anterior chest), midaxillary, subscapular, and medial calf skinfolds tend to have the highest correlations with values at 16 yr. Interestingly, three of the four are on the trunk. Skinfold measurements at ages beyond 16 yr were also available in several studies. In general, interage correlations decline as individuals progress into young adulthood, and the decline is greater as the interval between measurements increases.

Information on the tracking of fat distribution is limited. In a principal component analysis of fat distribution among adolescent boys, interage correlations between 13 and 18 yr are higher, though moderate, for the total subcutaneous fat component (0.6) than for the trunk-limb component (0.1) (9). These results, though based on four skinfolds (i.e., subscapular, suprailiac, triceps, and calf), suggest that boys with high or low levels of subcutaneous fat at 13 yr of age tend to remain so through adolescence. On the other hand, the low interage correlation for the trunk-limb component suggests that fat distribution changes significantly in individual boys at this time.

Physical and Motor Fitness

Correlations for absolute and relative aerobic power measured at 11 and 18 yr approximate only 0.3 in boys (80). This suggests that $\dot{V}O_2$max does not track well during adolescence. Similar data are not available for girls. Stability of static strength and muscular endurance varies among tasks. Correlations taken at intervals of 5-6 yr during childhood (7 and 12 yr) and adolescence (12 and 17 yr) or over 10 yr (7 and 17 yr) range from low to moderately high (0.0-0.8) (33, 68). Stability of strength measurements of the lower extremity tends to be slightly better than those of the upper extremity. This may be related to the weight-bearing and locomotor functions of the former. Composite strength scores tend to be somewhat more stable than the specific strength measurements that constitute the composite (17). Data for flexibility are limited, but interage correlations between 5 and 10 and between 8 and 14 yr of age are low to moderate, or 0.3 and 0.5, respectively (34). Stability of motor fitness is generally more

variable than the stability of strength and flexibility. Interage correlations for motor fitness items tend to be lower and to vary among specific tasks (34, 68).

Habitual Physical Activity

Information on the tracking of habitual physical activity during growth is not available. Related data on attitudes and involvement in physical activity offer some insights. Attitudes toward physical activity are not stable in upper elementary grades (about 10-12 yr) (77), whereas relationships between attitudes and involvement in physical activity are generally consistent across this span (78). On the other hand, attitudes toward, and involvement in, physical activity are rather stable in high school students followed from about 16 to 18 yr of age. Involvement is generally more stable than attitude. Although attitudes and involvement in physical activity are seemingly stable in late adolescence, the relationship between the two is rather low. The strength of attitudes toward physical activity accounts for only about 20% of the variation in degree of involvement (75). Among junior high school students (approximately 13-15 yr), attitudes toward physical activity, prior experience in physical activity, and current activity habits contribute significantly to the intention to exercise but account for less than half the variance (31). Given the many factors that are actually or potentially related to habitual physical activity, it would be surprising if habitual physical activity is stable during childhood and adolescence.

Indicators of Cardiovascular Health

Tracking of blood pressure is generally moderate to low. Correlations for systolic and diastolic blood pressures taken 6 yr apart during childhood and adolescence are only 0.3 and 0.2, respectively, in the Muscatine Study (18), whereas those for measurements taken 5 yr apart range from 0.4 to 0.6 for systolic and from 0.3 to 0.4 for diastolic blood pressure in the Bogalusa Heart Study (92). Interage correlations for blood pressures measured in adolescence (12-15 yr) and 6 yr later in late adolescence or young adulthood are the same as the correlations across 5 yr at younger ages, ranging from 0.4 to 0.5 for systolic pressure and from 0.3 to 0.4 for diastolic pressure (92). Studies of blood pressure taken during childhood and adolescence and then 13-17 yr later indicate similar interage correlations for systolic pressure (0.3 and 0.4) and a somewhat lower correlation for diastolic pressure (0.2) (35, 44). Although tracking is low to moderate for the general population of children and youth, it is stronger in hypertensive cases; that is, children with elevated blood pressure tend to remain in the higher blood pressure categories over several years.

Correlations between initial and final levels of serum lipids and lipoproteins over periods of 5-6 yr during childhood and adolescence approximate 0.6-0.7 for serum TC, 0.2-0.4 for serum TG, 0.3-0.5 for HDL-C, and 0.6-0.8 for LDL (5). Tracking for serum lipids and lipoproteins is also better at the higher percentiles. More than 40% of children at or above the 90th percentile for TC and LDL-C remain at these high levels 5 or 6 yr after the initial observations. Constancy of ranking for high levels of serum TG and low levels of HDL-C is somewhat lower after 5 or 6 yr, about 20%. The data also indicate a tendency for serum lipids of older children to remain in the upper deciles compared to younger children (5). These trends thus suggest that a significant proportion of children who exhibit an atherogenic profile retain or maintain this profile during childhood and adolescence.

A follow-up of a subsample in the Bogalusa Heart Study over 6 yr from adolescence into young adulthood indicates significant tracking of serum lipids and TG (91). Correlations for small subsamples within specific age categories range from 0.3-0.8 for serum TC, 0.4-0.8 for LDL, 0.3-0.5 for HDL and 0.3-0.7 for serum TG, with one exception: 10- to 11-yr-old girls at the initial observation (0.04). The data for the late adolescent and young adult follow-up are more dramatic when viewed in terms of clinical abnormalities (91) and autopsy results (61). The prevalence of high systolic and diastolic blood pressures in adolescence (10-15 yr) was negligible but 6 yr later was 7%. Although the prevalence of clinically high or low lipid values in adolescence was low, high levels of serum TG and LDL and low levels of HDL were much higher in late adolescence/young adulthood (91). Further, among 35 individuals who died (89% between 15 and 24 yr), antemortem lipid and lipoprotein levels were related to early atherosclerotic lesions of the aorta and coronary arteries. For example, the extent of fatty-streak involvement of the aorta was positively related to antemortem levels of serum TC and LDL (0.7) and negatively related to the HDL ratio (−0.3), whereas fatty-streak development in the coronary arteries was positively related to antemortem levels of VLDL (0.4) (61).

The Role of Regular Physical Activity

Physical activity is often viewed as having a favorable influence on growth, maturation, body composition, and physical and physiological fitness. Inferences about the role of physical activity, however, are based largely on short-term experimental studies. Longitudinal studies that span childhood and adolescence and that control for physical activity are not available. Comparisons of active and inactive individuals or of athletes and nonathletes provide important information. It must be emphasized however, that elite, young athletes are a reasonably select group and differ from the general population in many parameters of growth, maturation, and fitness (49, 52, 53). This qualification also applies to inferences about training based on studies of adult athletes.

Stature

Regular physical activity has no apparent effect on statural growth. Although an increase in stature with activity has been suggested, the observed changes are small and are based on studies that did not control for subject selection and maturity status (2, 48, 49).

Biological Maturation

Age at PHV is not affected by regular physical activity. Boys classified as physically active and inactive for the years before and during the growth spurt do not differ in ages at PHV (42, 56). Similarly, skeletal maturation is not accelerated or delayed by regular training for sport during childhood and adolescence (52, 53). Longitudinal data on the effect of regular physical activity on sexual maturation of boys and girls are limited, and the available cross-sectional data do not indicate a significant effect on sexual maturation (53). Much of the discussion of physical activity and sexual maturation compares the later mean ages at menarche of athletes with those of the general population and infers that intensive training delays menarche (50). However, the data are associational and retrospective, are based on small samples, and do not control for other factors that influence menarche.

Body Weight and Composition

Regular physical activity is an important factor in the regulation of body weight. Activity is associated with a decrease in fatness and occasionally with an increase in FFM (48, 49, 65). However, it is difficult to partition training effects from expected age-associated increases in FFM during growth. Changes in fatness depend on continued activity (or caloric restriction) for their maintenance.

There is generally more concern for the management and correction of excessive fatness in children and youth than for its prevention. Given the importance of regular physical activity in the regulation of fatness (as well as the association among fatness, serum lipids and TG, blood pressure, and poor physical fitness), the potential of regular physical activity initiated during childhood in a preventive role is emphasized. For example, a daily excess of energy intake over expenditure of only 50 kcal can lead to an excess weight gain, most likely fat, of about 2 kg in 1 yr. The imbalance can, of course, be offset with an energy expenditure in excess of intake by 50 kcal per day.

Bone Tissue

Experimental studies of growing animals of several species indicate greater skeletal mineralization and density and increased bone mass with regular training. Corresponding data for children are not extensive, but studies of adult athletes indicate similar results (2, 48, 49). Regular physical activity is also indicated as a significant factor in reducing age-associated bone loss in adulthood (3). In contrast to these positive effects, evidence is accumulating that excessive training associated with altered menstrual function contributes to bone loss in some athletes and increases susceptibility to stress fractures (23, 90). Thus, there may be a threshold for some adolescent and young adult females. Regular physical activity has a beneficial effect on the integrity of skeletal tissue up to a point; when activity is excessive and disturbs menstrual function, it may have a negative influence.

Muscle Tissue

The effects of regular physical activity on muscle tissue are specific to the type of training program. Resistance training is associated with increased strength in females, often without muscular hypertrophy. High resistance programs are associated with hypertrophy. On the other hand, endurance training is associated with increased activity of succinatedehydrogenase (SDH) and phosphofructokinase (PFK) and an increase in the relative area consisting of Type I fibers. The direction of responses to training in growing individuals is similar to those observed in adults, but the magnitude of the responses varies. However, responses to short term training programs are generally not permanent and depend on regular activity for their maintenance (2, 49).

Adipose Tissue

Information on the effects of regular physical activity on adipose tissue cellularity and metabolism of children is lacking. Evidence for adults indicates that the decrease in fatness associated with training is attributable solely to a reduction in adipocyte size (2, 48, 49). Training in adults is also associated with increased ability to mobilize and oxidize fat (21). Because regular training is associated with a decease in fatness in both children and adults, it may be reasonable to assume similar metabolic responses of adipocytes to training in developing individuals.

Aerobic Power

Improvement in aerobic power with endurance activity programs are a function of initial level of $\dot{V}O_2$max and intensity and duration of the training program. Thus, one might expect greater improvement in unfit children with an intensive, long term program. However, most studies of aerobic power have been short term, and many have focused on specialized samples of young athletes, usually runners and swimmers. The evidence suggests a small or limited gain in aerobic power in preadolescent children. It is not certain whether these results are the consequence of low trainability of young children or inadequacies of the training programs. For example, if young children are habitually more active than are adolescents or adults, a more intense and longer program may be required to improve aerobic power significantly. On the other hand, most activities of young children proceed at submaximal work rates, and maximal aerobic power may be an inappropriate indicator. It may be more appropriate to consider changes in submaximal work efficiency (2, 55).

Among adolescents, responses of maximal aerobic power to training improve, but results are not entirely consistent among studies. Results are confounded in part by individual variation in the timing of the growth spurt so that it is difficult to separate training-associated increases in aerobic power from those associated with growth (2, 55). Longitudinal data indicate that boys classified as inactive have lower absolute and relative maximal aerobic power than do highly active boys and those with average levels of activity during childhood and adolescence. The inactive boys also have an adolescent spurt in $\dot{V}O_2$max that is less than that observed in the normally and highly active boys. Although active boys have a higher absolute $\dot{V}O_2$max than do boys with average activity levels before the adolescent spurt, the two groups do not differ during the spurt. However, active boys have greater relative maximal aerobic power before, during, and after the growth spurt (56).

Muscular Strength and Endurance

Although responses are specific to the type of training program, gains in muscular strength and endurance are associated with short-term training programs, but data are more available for boys than for girls (38, 62, 66, 93). Increases in strength are not necessarily accompanied by muscular hypertrophy, which emphasizes neuromuscular responses to the training stimulus. The evidence suggests greater relative strength and endurance increments in young children than in adolescents, but persistence of gains after the cessation of training is not ordinarily considered. As with aerobic power, the short term nature of training programs and the lack of longitudinal data over several years make it difficult to partition training-related changes from those that accompany normal growth and maturation, especially during adolescence, as strength shows a clear growth spurt that occurs, on average, after that for stature (10).

Motor Fitness

The evidence is reasonably clear that regular instruction and practice of motor skills in physical education programs result in improved levels of speed, power, agility, and so on (87). Results, of course, vary among studies, but they all emphasize the importance of physical education programs in the development of motor fitness. It is not possible in the currently available data to evaluate the persistence of gains in motor fitness, to evaluate whether children who are not exposed to physical education catch up in motor fitness, or to partition growth- and maturity-associated improvements from those associated with the physical education programs.

Blood Pressure

Most of the research on the effects of regular physical activity on blood pressure has been done with adults and quite often without satisfactory results. Given the difficulties in deriving consistent blood pressure measurements in children, it is difficult to assess the effects of regular training on blood pressure. Correlations between blood pressure and various measures of fitness ($\dot{V}O_2$max and PWC 150) tend to be low (57), and training studies in children are inconclusive. Some evidence, for example, indicates no change in blood pressure after an 8-wk progressive aerobic program in adolescent males 11-17 yr of age (46), a decline in diastolic pressure in seventh-grade children (about 12-13 yr) after a 12-wk program (27), and a decline in both diastolic and systolic pressures after 6 mo of exercise training in hypertensive male and female adolescents (32). However, because elevated blood pressure is often associated with obesity and because regular physical activity can bring about a reduction in fatness, activity may have positive effects on blood pressure in children and adolescents secondary to its primary effect on fatness.

Lipids and Lipoproteins

Compared to the literature for adults, there are relatively few studies of the effects of regular physical activity on serum lipids and lipoproteins in children and adolescents. The studies are of two types. The first compares lipid profiles of children with different levels of habitual physical activity, and the second compares the effects of specific training programs on lipid levels.

Levels of TC, HDL, and TG are not related to the physical activity habits of 3-yr-old children, but among 12-yr-old children higher levels of HDL and the HDL-to-TC ratio are significantly related (0.2-0.3) to grade in physical education and active membership in school sport clubs (86). Several indicators of habitual physical activity (e.g., number of sports or physical activities engaged in and number of athletic teams) are not related to serum lipids and lipoproteins among 7- to 11-yr-old black children, whereas they are significantly but moderately related to HDL (0.4) and to the LDL-to-HDL and TC-to-HDL ratios (-0.3 to -0.4) in 12- to 15-yr-old black adolescents (25).

Among preadolescent boys 8-11 yr old, those classified as higher active (greater exposure to activities classified as moderate to very highly intense) have significantly lower serum TG and a higher HDL-to-TC ratio than do lower-active boys (84). Small samples of well-trained 11- to 13-yr-old boys and girls (regularly participating in track and field) have significantly higher HDL than do nontrained children. The former also have lower TG and a higher HDL-to-TC ratio, but the differences are significant only among girls (85). Fourteen-year-old boys and girls enrolled in a sports school (ten 45-min periods per week of basketball and light athletics) have significantly higher HDL and lower serum TG than do those enrolled in a standard school (two 45-min periods per week of gymnastics and team games) (63). The former also have slightly lower TC and LDL, but the differences between school programs are not significant. Trained 14- to 16-yr-old boys (regular participation in sports activities for more than 8 hr/wk for at least 1 yr) have significantly higher HDL, lower serum TG, and a higher HDL-to-TC ratio than do normally active and inactive (reluctant to participate in school sports) boys, but the groups do not differ in TC and LDL. On the other hand, trained, normally active and inactive 14- to 16-yr-old girls do not differ in serum lipid and lipoprotein levels (89).

The evidence suggests higher levels of HDL, lower levels of serum TG, and a higher HDL-to-TC ratio in active children, although criteria for estimating degree of habitual physical activity vary, samples are generally small, and some of the active samples are young athletes. Active children also tend to have a higher TC, which is primarily a function of an elevated HDL fraction. The data also suggest an age effect, in that the relationship between habitual physical activity and serum lipids and lipoproteins is generally stronger in adolescents than in children.

Correlations between serum TC and TG and various measures of fitness ($\dot{V}O_2$max and step test) are generally low, especially when fatness is controlled for (57). Nevertheless, it may be of interest that many of the correlations with $\dot{V}O_2$max are negative. Correlations between fitness and HDL in children and youth are more variable. For example, there is no relationship between HDL and $\dot{V}O_2$max in 5- to 12-yr-old children after controlling for age, gender, fatness, and serum TG (72). At the extremes of the HDL distribution, however, children with low HDL have a significantly lower $\dot{V}O_2$max (12%) than do children with high HDL. On the other hand, HDL is significantly related to predicted $\dot{V}O_2$max in combined samples of 12-yr-old Anglo- and Mexican-American children (boys = 0.18, girls = 0.29), but the relationship is reduced to zero when the predicted $\dot{V}O_2$max is

adjusted for the body mass index (73). In other studies, HDL is moderately but significantly (0.4-0.5) related to ergometric exercise tolerance (total work/body weight) in trained and untrained 11- to 13-yr-old boys and girls (85) and 14- to 16-yr-old boys (89), but not in 14- to 16-yr-old girls (89).

Studies of the effects of specific training programs on serum lipids and lipoproteins yield mixed results that probably reflect variation in the intensity and duration of the programs. Several examples are summarized here. A 6-wk program of 40 min of exercise 5 d per week resulted in significant increases in HDL and the HDL-to-TC ratio in 8- to 10-yr-old girls but no change in TC (29), whereas a 12-wk program of 25 min of activity 4 d per week resulted in no significant changes in serum TC and TG in 7- to 9-yr-old boys and girls (30). It is of interest that a Type IV hyperlipidemic child in the trained group was reclassified as normolipidemic after the training program, whereas a Type IV child in the control group retained his status.

Two groups of 8- to 9-yr-old boys undergoing 10 wk of either low (40% $\dot{V}O_2$max) or high (75% $\dot{V}O_2$max) intensity training (walking, jogging, and running) both experienced a decrease in levels of HDL compared to controls, whereas only boys in the high intensity program had a significant decrease in TC. The two training groups also did not differ from each other and the controls in serum TG, LDL, and the HDL-to-TC ratio (74). Adult men also participated in training programs similar to those of the 8- to 9-yr-old boys. Changes in serum lipids and lipoproteins with training did not differ between the prepubescent boys and men.

Among seventh-grade children (about 12-13 yr), a 12-wk program of 30 min of vigorous physical activity 5 d per week resulted in a significant decrease in serum TC and an increase in HDL and the HDL-to-TC ratio (27). It is of interest that groups that received diet education in addition to the exercise program and those that received only diet education experienced a significant decrease only in serum TC.

A 4-wk program of moderate exercise had no effect on lipid levels of black children and adolescents 7-15 yr of age (45), whereas an 8-wk progressive aerobic program had no effect on serum lipids and lipoproteins of 11- to 17-yr-old white boys compared to controls (46). Similarly, 10 wk of moderate (13 METs) and heavy (16 METs) training had no influence on serum lipids and lipoproteins of late adolescent males (mean age 18.1 yr) (37).

Thus, experimental training studies have generally failed to show consistently any significant changes in serum lipids and lipoproteins in normal children and adolescents. These results are in contrast to studies which suggest that habitually more active children have a more favorable lipid profile (higher HDL, higher HDL-to-TC ratio, and lower serum TG) than do normally active and inactive children and adolescents. It is possible that aerobic power and fatness respond more rapidly to training of relatively low intensity than do serum lipids and lipoproteins. On the other hand, longer and more intense training programs may be necessary to alter fractions of HDL and LDL.

Studies of adults indicate that changes in lipid levels with training can be attributed to a reduction in body weight, that is, a negative energy balance (24). Because growth is associated with a positive energy balance as specific tissues and, in turn, body mass increase, the increase in body mass may influence the response of lipids to the training stimulus in developing individuals.

Blood Glucose and Insulin

Evidence on the relationships among physical activity, blood glucose, and insulin is limited for children and youth. Physical activity is negatively related with the product of 1-hr plasma glucose × insulin level during a glucose tolerance test in children (88), whereas habitual physical activity is not significantly related to glucose tolerance in 16- to 24-yr-old males (59). However, the least active subjects tended to have higher glucose scores (glucose concentration adjusted for age, gender, and length of time since the last meal) than did subjects classified as intermediate in activity or most active. Because fatness is related to glucose scores, subjects were classified into tertiles of fatness. Within the leanest tertile, least-active young-adult males had considerably higher glucose scores than did more active males, although there was no association between habitual physical activity and glucose scores in young adult males of average and above-average fatness (59). In contrast, correlations between heart rate response to a step test and blood glucose levels in children and adolescents 10-19 yr of age, although low (0.1-0.2), suggest that poor fitness is associated with diminished glucose tolerance (58). The correlations change negligibly when fatness is statistically controlled.

Trained athletes typically show normal or better glucose tolerance and diminished plasma insulin, which suggests enhanced peripheral sensitivity to insulin (36). These observations presumably reflect the effects of regular training (in addition to selection among athletes). Responses of previously sedentary adults to aerobic training indicate similar results. For example, after 6 wk of aerobic training, sedentary males (mean age 25 yr) show a significant increase in insulin sensitivity that is accompanied by an increase in the concentration of insulin receptors (79). Moreover, the changes in glucose uptake are significantly related to changes in maximal aerobic power with training (0.8). Corresponding data for children are not available.

Implications for Health Outcomes

The role of physical activity and physical fitness during childhood and youth as a favorable influence on the health status of adults or as a preventive factor in diseases of adulthood is not yet established. Nevertheless, the maintenance of a physically active lifestyle and a good level of fitness, as well as the development of positive attitudes toward physical activity, are viewed by many as major components of preventive medicine that should begin in childhood.

Changes in physical, motor, and physiological fitness are influenced by the processes of growth and maturation (among other factors), and it is often difficult to partition the effects of regular physical activity on fitness from changes associated with growth and maturation. The stability of measurements of fatness, aerobic power, strength, flexibility, motor fitness, blood pressure, and serum lipids and lipoproteins is significant but generally low to moderate during childhood and adolescence. Tracking is somewhat better from adolescence into young adulthood for fat and blood pressure and lipids, and better at the extremes of the distributions. Data for aerobic power, strength, flexibility, and motor fitness are less extensive for individuals followed from adolescence into adulthood, and the extremes of the distributions ordinarily have not been considered. The low to moderate stability of these indicators of physical and physiological fitness thus suggests reasonable opportunity for change during childhood and adolescence. Correlations, of course, are influenced by many factors, including measurement variability, normal variation in growth and maturation, and a tendency for the indicators under consideration to cluster and perhaps reinforce one another.

Although regular physical activity has beneficial effects on body composition and specific tissues and on physical fitness, the persistence of training effects is not ordinarily considered. Quite often, gains associated with activity programs revert to pretraining levels when the exercise is stopped; thus, the need for continued activity to maintain the beneficial changes is emphasized. However, just how much activity is necessary to induce and maintain favorable changes in the growing child and adolescent is not certain.

Information on the effects of regular physical activity on risk factors for cardiovascular disease is generally equivocal. Nevertheless, habitually more active children and youth tend to be leaner and to have more favorable lipid and lipoprotein profiles. Data for glucose metabolism are not adequate at present.

A related issue is the potential role for regular physical activity as a factor that can alter what appears to be normal age- and maturity-associated variation in several risk factors. For example, can systematic training during adolescence offset the maturity-associated decline in HDL or insulin sensitivity?

The relationship among aerobic power and blood pressure, lipids and lipoproteins, and glucose metabolism in children and youth tends to be low, whereas effects of experimental activity programs on these parameters of cardiovascular health yield mixed results. Fatness is a confounding variable, and it may be that the positive effects of regular physical activity on fatness secondarily favorably influence blood pressure, lipids and lipoproteins, and glucose metabolism.

Although regular physical activity during childhood and adolescence has the potential to influence favorably a number of parameters related to cardiovascular health, other factors need to be considered, including genotype, normal variation in growth and maturation, fat distribution, and components of lifestyle (especially diet and smoking). Racial and ethnic variations are additional factors. Available evidence indicates variation between black and white children in blood pressure and lipid and carbohydrate metabolism and in the tracking and clustering of various indicators of cardiovascular health (6, 8, 28, 60, 67, 88). Data for Mexican-American children are not as extensive (4). Thus, if physical activity is to be an important agent in the prevention of cardiovascular disease, it is only one component of a multifactorial complex.

Habitual physical activity and fitness are related; more active individuals presumably are more fit. However, physical inactivity is indicated as a risk factor for cardiovascular disease, but a low $\dot{V}O_2max$ may not be so indicated. Hence, which is more important: a satisfactory level of fitness, or a lifestyle with a pattern of regular physical activity? Should more time and effort be devoted to the assessment and encouragement of physical activity in children and youth rather than to fitness per se?

Considerations of the antecedents of adult health and disease in childhood and adolescence focus primarily on risk factors for cardiovascular disease. Other diseases are not generally considered. However, weight regulation and reduction are important aspects of lifestyle and can modify several chronic diseases of adults (e.g, adult onset diabetes, osteoarthritis, and cholelithiasis), whereas regular activity is important in the prevention of osteoporosis (12). Many facets of adult lifestyle are developed during childhood and youth, and the persistence of habits of regular physical activity into adulthood can be a significant factor, as can education about diet and the effects of smoking.

Concerns for antecedents of adult health in childhood generally do not consider motor fitness, which is related in part to strength and flexibility. Motor skill is necessary for physical activity, and the more skilled may be more likely to participate in a greater variety and quantity of physical activities on a regular basis. The need to develop and maintain motor proficiency in childhood and the need to maintain motor proficiency into adulthood are important considerations. An important corollary of motor proficiency is in injury and accident prevention. Poor motor skills may contribute to injuries and accidents in recreational activities and at the workplace.

Finally, most of this discussion has focused on childhood and adolescence. There is a gap in the data for the important transitional years from adolescence into adulthood. This is, of course, a period of transition from high school to career or vocation, and changes in lifestyle associated with the transition may influence many of the parameters considered. For example, smoking, alcohol consumption, and oral contraceptive use are independently related to serum lipids and lipoproteins and blood pressure in late adolescents and young adults 17-24 yr of age (20). Time spent in physical activities also declines at these ages, but some evidence from Sweden suggests a modest increase in physical activity between 20 and 25 yr (26). Thus, lifestyle changes during the transition period between adolescence and adulthood merit closer consideration.

References

1. Amiel, S.A., R.S. Sherwin, D.C. Simonson, A.A. Lauritano, and W.V. Tamborlane. Impaired insulin action in puberty. *N. Engl. J. Med.* 315: 215-219, 1986.

2. Bailey, D.A., R.M. Malina, and R.L. Mirwald. Physical activity and growth of the child. In: Falkner, F., and J.M. Tanner, eds. *Human growth: vol. 2. Postnatal growth, neurobiology.* New York: Plenum Press, 1986: pp. 147-170.

3. Bailey, D.A., A.D. Martin, C.S. Houston, and J.L. Howie. Physical activity, nutrition, bone density and osteoporosis. *Aust. J. Sci. Med. Sport* 18: 3-8, 1986.

4. Baranowski, T., Y.I. Tsong, J. Henske, J.K. Dunn, and P. Hooks. Ethnic variation in blood pressure among preadolescent children. *Pediatr. Res.* 23: 270-274, 1988.

5. Berenson, G.S., and F.H. Epstein. Conference on blood lipids in children: Optimal levels for early prevention of coronary artery disease. *Prev. Med.* 12: 741-797, 1983.

6. Berenson, G.S., B. Radhakrishnamurthy, S.R. Srinivasan, A.W. Voors, T.A. Foster, E.R. Dalferes, and L.S. Webber. Plasma glucose and insulin levels in relation to cardiovascular risk factors in children from a biracial population—The Bogalusa Heart Study. *J. Chron. Dis.* 34: 379-391, 1981.

7. Berenson, G.S., S.R. Srinivasan, J.L. Cresanta, T.A. Foster, and L.S. Webber. Dynamic changes of serum lipoproteins in children during adolescence and sexual maturation. *Am. J. Epidemiol.* 113: 157-170, 1981.

8. Berenson, G.S., A.W. Voors, L.S. Webber, E.R. Dalferes, and D.W. Harsha. Racial differences of parameters associated with blood pressure levels in children—The Bogalusa Heart Study. *Metabolism* 28: 1218-1228, 1979.

9. Beunen, G., A. Claessens, M. Ostyn, R. Renson, J. Simons, J. Lefevre, and D. Van Gerven. *Stability of subcutaneous fat patterning in adolescent boys.* Paper presented at the 5th Congress of the European Anthropological Association, Lisbon, October 1986.

10. Beunen, G., and R.M. Malina. Growth and physical performance relative to the timing of the adolescent spurt. *Exerc. Sport Sci. Rev.* 16: 503-540, 1988.

11. Beunen, G.P., R.M. Malina, M.A. Van't Hof, J. Simons, M. Ostyn, R. Renson, and D. Van Gerven. *Adolescent growth and motor performance: A longitudinal study of Belgian boys.* Champaign, IL: Human Kinetics, 1988.

12. Bierman, E.L., and W.R. Hazzard. Middle age: Strategies for the prevention or attenuation of the chronic diseases of aging. In: Andres, R., E.L. Bierman, and W.R. Hazzard, eds. *Principles of geriatric medicine.* New York: McGraw-Hill, 1985, pp. 862-866.

13. Bjorntorp, P. Fat patterning and disease: A review. In: Norgan, N.G., ed. *Human body composition and fat distribution* (Euro-Nut Report No. 8). Wageningen: Stichting Nederlands Instituut voor de Voeding, 1986, pp. 201-209.

14. Bloch, C.A., P. Clemons, and M.A. Sperling. Puberty decreases insulin sensitivity. *J. Pediatr.* 110: 481-487, 1987.

15. Bloom, B.S. *Stability and change in human characteristics.* New York: John Wiley & Sons, 1964.

16. Canada Fitness Survey. *Canadian youth and physical activity.* Ottawa: Canada Fitness Survey, 1983.

17. Carron, A.V., and D.A. Bailey. Strength development in boys from 10 through 16 years. *Monogr. Soc. Res. Child Dev.* 39(Serial No. 157), 1974.

18. Clarke, W.R., H.G. Schrott, P.E. Leaverton, W.E. Connor, and R.M. Lauer. Tracking of blood lipids and blood pressure in school age children: The Muscatine Study. *Circulation* 58: 626-634, 1978.

19. Cornoni-Huntley, J., W.R. Harlan, and P.E. Leaverton. Blood pressure in adolescence: The United States Health Examination Survey. *Hypertension* 1: 566-571, 1979.

20. Croft, J.B., D.S. Freedman, J.L. Cresanta, S.R. Srinivasan, G.L. Burke, S.M. Hunter, L.S. Webber, C.G. Smoak, and G.S. Berenson. Adverse influences of alcohol, tobacco, and oral contraceptive use on cardiovascular risk factors during transition to adulthood. *Am. J. Epidemiol.* 126: 202-213, 1987.

21. Després, J.-P., C. Bouchard, R. Savard, A. Tremblay, M. Marcotte, and G. Theriault. The effect of a 20-week endurance training program on adipose tissue morphology and lipolysis in men and women. *Metabolism* 33: 235-239, 1984.

22. Deutsch, M.I., W.H. Mueller, and R.M. Malina. Androgyny in fat patterning is associated with obesity in adolescents and young adults. *Ann. Hum. Biol.* 12: 275-286, 1985.

23. Drinkwater, B.L., K. Nilson, C.H. Chestnut, W.J. Bremner, S. Shainholtz, and M.B. Southworth. Bone mineral of amenorrheic and eumenorrheic athletes. *N. Engl. J. Med.* 311: 277-281, 1984.

24. Dufaux, B., G. Assmann, and W. Hollmann. Plasma lipoproteins and physical activity: A review. *Int. J. Sports Med.* 3: 123-136, 1982.

25. Durant, R.H., C.W. Linder, J.W. Harkess, and R.G. Gray. The relationship between physical activity and serum lipids and lipoproteins in black children and adolescents. *J. Adolesc. Health Care* 4: 55-60, 1983.

26. Engstrom, L.M. Physical activity of children and youth. *Acta Paediatr. Scand.* (Suppl. 283): 101-105, 1979.

27. Fisher, A.G., and M. Brown. The effects of diet and exercise on selected coronary risk factors in children [Abstract]. *Med. Sci. Sports Exerc.* 14: 171, 1982.

28. Freedman, D.S., S.R. Srinivasan, A.W. Voors, L.S. Webber, and G.S. Berenson. High density lipoprotein and coronary artery disease risk factors in children with different lipoprotein profiles: Bogalusa Heart Study. *J. Chron. Dis.* 38: 327-338, 1985.

29. Gilliam, T.B., and M.B. Burke. Effects of exercise on serum lipids and lipoproteins in girls, ages 8 to 10 years. *Artery* 4: 203-213, 1978.

30. Gilliam, T.B., and P.S. Freedson. Effects of a 12-week school physical fitness program on peak $\dot{V}O_2$, body composition and blood lipids in 7 to 9 year old children. *Int. J. Sports Med.* 1: 73-78, 1980.

31. Godin, G., and R.J. Shephard. Psychosocial factors influencing intentions to exercise of young students from grades 7 to 9. *Res. Q. Exerc. Sport* 57: 41-52, 1986.

32. Hagberg, J.M., D. Goldring, A.A. Ehsani, G.W. Heath, A. Hernandez, K. Schechtman, and J.O. Holloszy. Effect of exercise training on the blood pressure and hemodynamic features of hypertensive adolescents. *Am. J. Cardiol.* 52: 763-768, 1983.

33. Harlan, W.R., J. Cornoni-Huntley, and P.E. Leaverton. Blood pressure in childhood: The National Health Examination Survey. *Hypertension* 1: 559-565, 1979.

34. Haubenstricker, J., and V. Seefeldt. Acquisition of motor skills during childhood. In: Seefeldt, V., ed. *Physical activity and well-being*. Reston, VA: American Alliance for Health, Physical Education, Recreation and Dance, 1986, pp. 41-102.

35. Higgins, M.W., J.B. Keller, H.L. Metzner, F.E. Moore, and L.D. Ostrander. Studies of blood pressure in Tecumseh, Michigan—II. Antecedents in childhood of high blood pressure in young adults. *Hypertension* 2(Suppl.1): 117-123, 1980.

36. Holm, G., and P. Björntorp. Metabolic effects of physical training. *Acta Paediatr. Scand.* (Suppl. 283): 9-14, 1979.

37. Hunt, J.F., and J.R. White. Effects of ten weeks of vigorous daily exercise on serum lipids and lipoproteins in teenage males [Abstract]. *Med. Sci. Sports Exerc.* 12: 93, 1980.

38. Ikai, M. The effects of training on muscular endurance. In: Kato, K., ed. *Proceedings of the International Congress of Sports Sciences*. Tokyo: University of Tokyo Press, 1966, pp. 145-158.

39. Ilmarinen, J., and J. Rutenfranz. Longitudinal studies of the changes in habitual physical activity of schoolchildren and working adolescents. In: Berg, K., and B.O. Eriksson, eds. *Children and exercise IX*. Baltimore: University Park Press, 1980, pp. 149-159.

40. Kemper, H.C.G. (Ed.). *Growth, health and fitness of teenagers*. Basel: Karger, 1985.

41. Kemper, H.C.G., R. Verschuur, and J.W. Ritmeester. Maximal aerobic power in early and late maturing teenagers. In: Rutenfranz, J., R. Mocellin, and F. Klimt, eds. *Children and exercise XII*. Champaign, IL: Human Kinetics, 1986, pp. 213-225.

42. Kobayashi, K., K. Kitamura, M. Miura, H. Sodeyama, Y. Murasse, M. Miyashita, and H. Matsui. Aerobic power as related to body growth and training in Japanese boys: A longitudinal study. *J. Appl. Physiol.* 44: 666-672, 1978.

43. Krahenbuhl, G.S., J.S. Skinner, and W.M. Kohrt. Developmental aspects of aerobic power in children. *Exerc. Sport Sci. Rev.* 13: 503-538, 1985.

44. Kuller, L.H., M. Crook, M.J. Almes, K. Detre, G. Reese, and G. Rutan. Dormont High School (Pittsburgh, Pennsylvania) Blood Pressure Study. *Hypertension* 2(Suppl. 1): 109-116, 1980.

45. Linder, C.W., R.H. Durant, R.G. Gray, and J.W. Harkess. The effects of exercise on serum lipid levels in children [Abstract]. *Clin. Res.* 27: 797, 1979.

46. Linder, C.W., R.H. Durant, and O.M. Mahoney. The effect of physical conditioning

on serum lipids and lipoproteins in white male adolescents. *Med. Sci. Sports Exerc.* 15: 232-236, 1983.

47. Londe, S., A. Johanson, N.S. Kronemer, and D. Goldring. Blood pressure and puberty. *J. Pediatr.* 87: 896-900, 1975.

48. Malina, R.M. The effects of exercise on specific tissues, dimensions and functions during growth. *Stud. Phys. Anthropol.* 5: 21-52, 1979.

49. Malina, R.M. Human growth, maturation and regular physical activity. *Acta Med. Auxol.* 15: 5-23, 1983.

50. Malina, R.M. Menarche in athletes: A synthesis and hypothesis. *Ann. Hum. Biol.* 10: 1-24, 1983.

51. Malina, R.M. Energy expenditure and physical activity during childhood and youth. In: Demirjian, A., ed. *Human growth: A multidisciplinary review.* London: Taylor and Francis, 1986, pp. 215-225.

52. Malina, R.M. Competitive youth sports and biological maturation. In: Brown, E.W., and C.F. Branta, eds. *Competitive sports for children and youth: An overview of research and issues.* Champaign, IL: Human Kinetics, 1988, pp. 227-245.

53. Malina, R.M. Biological maturity status of young athletes. In: Malina, R.M., ed. *Young athletes: Biological, psychological and educational perspectives.* Champaign, IL: Human Kinetics, 1988, pp. 121-140.

54. Malina, R.M., and C. Bouchard. Subcutaneous fat distribution during growth. In: Bouchard, C., and F.E. Johnston, eds. *Fat distribution during growth and later health outcomes.* New York: Alan A. Liss, 1988, pp. 63-84.

55. Malina, R.M., and C. Bouchard. *Growth and physical activity.* Champaign, IL: Human Kinetics, in press.

56. Mirwald, R.L., and D.A. Bailey. *Maximal aerobic power.* London, Ontario: Sport Dynamics, 1986.

57. Montoye, H.J. Risk indicators for cardiovascular disease in relation to physical activity in youth. In: Binkhorst, R.A., H.C.G. Kemper, and W.H.M. Saris, eds. *Children and exercise XI.* Champaign, IL: Human Kinetics, 1985, pp. 3-25.

58. Montoye, H.J., W. Block, J.B. Keller, and P.W. Willis. Glucose tolerance and physical fitness: An epidemiological study in an entire community. *Eur. J. Appl. Physiol.* 37: 237-242, 1977.

59. Montoye, H.J., W. Block, H. Metzner, and J.B. Keller. Habitual physical activity and glucose tolerance: Males age 16-64 in a total community. *Diabetes* 26: 172-176, 1977.

60. Morrison, J.A., I. deGroot, K.A. Kelly, M.J. Mellies, P. Khoury, D. Lewis, A. Lewis, M. Fiorelli, H.A. Tyroler, G. Heiss, and C.J. Glueck. Black-White differences in plasma lipoproteins in Cincinnati schoolchildren (one-to-one pair matched by total plasma cholesterol, sex, and age). *Metabolism* 28: 241-245.

61. Newman, W.P., D.S. Freedman, A.W. Voors, P.D. Gard, S.R. Srinivasan, J.L. Cresanta, G.D. Williamson, L.S. Webber, and G.S. Berenson. Relation of serum lipoprotein levels and systolic blood pressure to early atherosclerosis: The Bogalusa Heart Study. *N. Engl. J. Med.* 314: 138-144, 1986.

62. Nielsen, B., K. Nielsen, M. Behrendt Hansen, and E. Asmussen. Training of "functional muscular strength" in girls 7-19 years old. In: Berg, K., and B.O. Eriksson, eds. *Children and exercise IX.* Baltimore: University Park Press, 1980, pp. 69-78.

63. Nizankowska-Blaz, T., and T. Abramowicz. Effects of intensive physical training on serum lipids and lipoproteins. *Acta Paediatr. Scand.* 72: 357-359, 1983.

64. Orchard, T.J., D.J. Becker, L.H. Kuller, D.K. Wagener, R.E. LaPorte, and A.L. Drash. Age and sex variations in glucose tolerance and insulin responses: Parallels with cardiovascular risk. *J. Chron. Dis.* 35: 123-132, 1982.

65. Parizkova, J. *Body fat and physical fitness.* The Hague: Martinus Nijhoff, 1977.

66. Pfeiffer, R.D., and R.S. Francis. Effects of strength training on muscle development in prepubescent, pubescent, and postpubescent males. *Phys. Sportsmed.* 14: 134-143, 1986 (Sept.).

67. Radhakrishnamurthy, B., S.R. Srinivasan, L.S. Webber, E.R. Dalferes, and G.S. Berenson. Relationship of carbohydrate intolerance to serum lipoprotein profiles in childhood: The Bogalusa Heart Study. *Metabolism* 34: 850-860, 1985.

68. Rarick, G.L. Stability and change in motor abilities. In: Rarick G.L., ed. *Physical activity: Human growth and development.* New York: Academic Press, 1973, pp. 201-224.

69. Roche, A.F., R.M. Siervogel, W.C. Chumlea, R.B. Reed, I. Valadian, D. Eichorn, and R.W. McCammon. *Serial changes in subcutaneous*

thicknesses of children and adults. Basel: Karger, 1982.

70. Rosner, B., C.H. Hennekens, E.H. Kass, and W.E. Miall. Age-specific correlation analysis of longitudinal blood pressure data. *Am. J. Epidemiol*. 106: 306-313, 1977.

71. Ross, J.G., C.O. Dotson, G.G. Gilbert, and S.J. Katz. The National Children and Youth Fitness Study: After physical education . . . physical activity outside of school physical education programs. *J. Phys. Educ. Dance* 56: 77-81, 1985 (Jan).

72. Sady, S.P., K. Berg, D. Beal, J.L. Smith, M.P. Savage, W.H. Thompson, and J. Nutter. Physical fitness and serum high-density lipoprotein cholesterol in young children. *Hum. Biol*. 56: 771-781, 1984.

73. Sallis, J.F., T.L. Patterson, M.J. Buono, and P.R. Nader. Relation of cardiovascular fitness and physical activity to cardiovascular disease risk factors in children and adults. *Am. J. Epidemiol*. 127: 933-941.

74. Savage, M.P., M.M. Petratis, W.H. Thomson, K. Berg, J.L. Smith, and S.P. Sady. Exercise training effects on serum lipids of prepubescent boys and adult men. *Med. Sci. Sports Exerc*. 18: 197-204, 1986.

75. Schutz, R.W., and F.L. Smoll. The (in)stability of attitudes toward physical activity during childhood and adolescence. In: McPherson, B.D., ed. *Sport and aging*. Champaign, IL: Human Kinetics, 1986, pp. 187-197.

76. Siervogel, R.M., R.N. Baumgartner, A.F. Roche, W.C. Chumlea, and C.J. Glueck. Maturity and its relationship to plasma lipid and lipoprotein levels in adolescents: The Fels Longitudinal Study. *Am. J. Hum. Biol*. 1: 217-226, 1989.

77. Smoll, F.L., and R.W. Schutz. Children's attitudes towards physical activity: A longitudinal analysis. *J. Sport Psychol*. 2: 144-154, 1980.

78. Smoll, F.L., R.W. Schutz, and J.K. Keeney. Relationships among children's attitudes, involvement, and proficiency in physical activities. *Res. Q*. 47: 797-803, 1976.

79. Soman, V.R., V.A. Koivisto, D. Deibert, P. Felig, and R.A. DeFronzo. Increased insulin sensitivity and insulin binding to monocytes after physical training. *N. Engl. J. Med*. 301: 1200-1204, 1979.

80. Sprynarova, S., and J. Parizkova. La stabilite de differences interindividuelles des parametres morphologiques et cardiorespiratoires chez les garcons. In: Lavallee, H., and R.J. Shephard, eds. *Frontiers of activity and child health*. Quebec: Pelican, 1977, pp. 131-138.

81. Tamir, I., G. Heiss, C.J. Glueck, B. Christensen, P. Kwiterovich, and B.M. Rifkind. Lipid and lipoprotein distributions in white children ages 6-19 yr. The Lipid Research Clinics Program Prevalence Study. *J. Chron. Dis*. 34: 27-39, 1981.

82. Tanner, J.M., P.C.R. Hughes, and R.H. Whitehouse. Radiographically determined widths of bone, muscle and fat in the upper arm and calf from ages 3-18 years. *Ann. Hum. Biol*. 8: 495-517, 1981.

83. Tanne, J.M., and R.H. Whitehouse. *Atlas of children's growth: Normal variation and growth disorders*. New York: Academic Press, 1982.

84. Thorland, W.G., and T.B. Gilliam. Comparison of serum lipids between habitually high and low active pre-adolescent males. *Med. Sci. Sports Exerc*. 13: 316-321, 1981.

85. Valimaki, I., M-L. Hursti, L. Pihlakoski, and J. Viikari. Exercise performance and serum lipids in relation to physical activity in schoolchildren. *Int. J. Sports Med*. 1: 132-136, 1980.

86. Viikari, J., I. Valimaki, R. Telama, H. Siren-Tiusanen, H.K. Akerblom, M. Dahl, P.-L. Lahde, E. Pesonen, M. Pietikainen, P. Suoninen, and M. Uhari. Atherosclerosis precursors in Finnish children: Physical activity and plasma lipids in 3- and 12-year-old children. In: Ilmarinen, J., and I. Valimaki, eds. *Children and sport*. Berlin: Springer, 1984, pp. 231-240.

87. Vogel, P.G. Effects of physical education programs on children. In: Seefeldt, V., ed. *Physical activity and well-being*. Reston, VA: American Alliance for Health, Physical Education, Recreation and Dance, 1986, pp. 455-509.

88. Voors, A.W., D.W. Harsha, L.S. Webber, B. Radhakrishnamurthy, S.R. Srinivasan, and G.S. Berenson. Clustering of anthropometric parameters, glucose tolerance, and serum lipids in children with high and low β and pre-β-lipoproteins. *Arteriosclerosis* 2: 346-355, 1982.

89. Wanne, O., J. Viikari, and I. Valimaki. Physical performance and serum lipids in 14-16-year-old trained, normally active, and inactive children. In: Ilmarinen, J., and I. Valimaki, eds. *Children and sport*. Berlin: Springer, 1984, pp. 241-246.

90. Warren, M.P., J. Brooks-Gunn, L.H. Hamilton, L.F. Warren, and W.G. Hamilton. Scoliosis and fractures in young ballet dancers. *N. Engl. J. Med*. 314: 1348-1353, 1986.

91. Webber, L.S., J.L. Cresanta, J.B. Croft, S.R. Srinivasan, and G.S. Berenson. Transitions of cardiovascular risk from adolescence to young adulthood—The Bogalusa Heart Study: II. Alterations in anthropometric, blood pressure and serum lipoprotein variables. *J. Chron. Dis.* 39: 91-103, 1986.

92. Webber, L.S., J.L. Cresanta, A.W. Voors, and G.S. Berenson. Tracking of cardiovascular disease risk factor variables in school-age children. *J. Chron. Dis.* 36: 647-660, 1983.

93. Weltman, A., C. Janney, C.B. Rians, K. Strand, B. Berg, S. Tippitt, J. Wise, B.R. Cahill, and F.I. Katch. The effects of hydraulic resistance strength training in pre-pubertal males. *Med. Sci. Sports Exerc.* 18: 629-638, 1986.

Chapter 56

Discussion: Growth, Exercise, Fitness, and Later Outcomes

Oded Bar-Or

I concur with the approach and recommendations made by R.M. Malina in his comprehensive review. My comments are intended to focus on four additional points: (a) methodological constraints in the assessment of habitual physical activity in children, (b) short- and long-term effects of exercise on the child with a disease, (c) the role of the school in large-scale multidisciplinary interventions, and (d) the implementation of scientific knowledge by society.

Methodological Constraints in the Assessment of Children's Habitual Activity

Because most of the methods used for the assessment of habitual activity in children have been borrowed from studies on adults, their validity for children is questionable. Pedometers, for example, are fairly valid for adults (13) because a predominant part of adult leisure-time activities includes walking and jogging. In contrast, many of the activities of young children include jumping, climbing, and other, upper-limb, exercises that may not be detected by the pedometer. Likewise, most actometers and accelerometers register motion in one plane only. Although these are useful for adults (19, 22), their validity for young children is extremely low. A study by Klesges et al. (19) is a case in point. Although in adults the rank correlation between measurement taken by a single-plane accelerometer and direct observations for 1 hr was 0.81, it was only 0.20 in 20- to 68-mo-old children. After an observation of 7-11 hr, the correlation in the preschoolers was still only 0.54 (18). One solution that needs further assessment is to use several monitors simultaneously, hung on several sites and in different axes.

With the increasing miniaturization and sophistication of electronic devices, the continuous monitoring of heart rate (HR) to assess metabolic level has been gaining attention. However, the validity of such a measurement for children is not yet clear (24). The assumption has been that the metabolic level (reflected by O_2 uptake or $\dot{V}O_2$) is linear with HR and can be predicted from it. This assumption, although correct in general, is too simplistic. The two main, often-quoted intervening factors are the emotional state of the child and the climate, both of which affect changes in HR with little or no change in $\dot{V}O_2$. Although one could correct the observed HR on the basis of climatic conditions that prevail during the experiment (e.g., using the so-called effective temperature as a heat stress index), the relevant correction equations are not yet available for children. More subtle is the correction of HR for the emotional state of the child. This is another issue to consider (5) because in some children the HR-on-$\dot{V}O_2$ regression line is not constant and may vary as a function of exercise intensity.

Some tables are available that have assigned caloric equivalents to various activities. Many of these tables were constructed for adults of supposedly ideal weights and ignore the body mass of the individual in question. It should be realized also that, even when corrected for body mass, the $\dot{V}O_2$ of walking or running children is higher than that of adolescents or adults (2, 21). Thus, adult-based equations that predict the $\dot{V}O_2$ from walking and running speeds and slopes underestimate the actual metabolic cost when used with children.

Although recall questionnaires and self-recording of activities have been found fairly valid with adults (see, e.g., ref. 22), their validity for children needs further study. An inherent limitation of questionnaires is the need to collect information from the parents (and other adults), who may not know the specific activities of their children. As for self-recording logs, it is not known which time intervals are optimal for children, that is, those yielding most information while causing minimal interference in the child's spontaneity. Also unknown is the maximal time period which children of different mental ages can recall in response to a questionnaire. An important observation on the usefulness of self-kept records in children and adolescents is seen in the study by Bouchard et al. (6), who instructed 10- to 18-yr-old girls and boys to record periodically their activities, breaking down the information into 15-min periods. Although the test-retest reliability of this method was high ($r = 0.91$), the authors did not check for validity or assess the degree of interference in spontaneous activity that such detailed recording may have induced.

No doubt, much more research is still needed in this area. The optimal method should probably combine an objective, instrument-based observation with some subjective input by subjects, parents, or both. Quite possibly, the optimal method may be different for different pediatric subgroups.

Health Sequelae of Training in the Child With a Disease

As stated in Malina's review, there is little evidence that increased physical activity can improve children's health or reduce their risk for future diseases such as coronary artery disease. This relates to the general child population, but does it also hold true for children who suffer from a disease or an illness? Table 56.1 summarizes those pediatric diseases for which beneficial effects of enhanced physical activity have been shown or suggested. As yet, randomly allocated, controlled interventions are not available on the long-term effects of training in any of the pediatric diseases. The available information summarized in the table is thus based on short-term studies with small numbers of subjects and with designs that often will not pass epidemiological scrutiny (for a review, see ref. 3).

In spite of this criticism, one should realize that, for some pediatric patients (e.g, those with cystic fibrosis or progressive muscular dystrophy), *later outcomes* refers to adolescence and early adulthood

because the life expectancy of such patients is extremely short.

Table 56.1 Pediatric Diseases in Which Enhanced Physical Activity Has Been Suggested to Be Beneficial to Health

Disease	Possible benefits	Reference
Anorexia nervosa	Behavior modification	Author's data
Asthma	Reduced intensity and frequency of exercise-induced broncho-constriction	16
Cerebral palsy	Prevention of contractures; enhanced ambulation	9, 26, 4
Cystic fibrosis	Higher respiratory muscle endurance; enhanced clearance of bronchial mucus	17, 29
Diabetes mellitus	Better diabetic control	20
Hypertension	Reduction of blood pressure at rest	14, 15
Mental retardation	Increasing environmental stimuli; socialization	1, 7
Muscular dystrophy and atrophy	Strengthening of residual muscle; prolongation of ambulation status; prevention of contractures; weight control	10, 12, 25
Obesity	Weight control; enhanced socialization and self-esteem; improved lipid profile	23, 28

Note. From *Pediatric Sports Medicine for the Practitioner* by O. Bar-Or, 1983, New York: Springer. Adapted by permission.

The School as an Optimal Environment for a Multidisciplinary Approach

For any beneficial long-term effects that they may impart to society, enhanced physical activity and fitness should be promoted in as large a segment of the child population as possible. It is unlikely that such widespread enhancement will be achieved through sports clubs, recreation centers, or individual home programs. On the other hand, the school has much potential as an environment in which exercise and fitness can be promoted for itself or as part of a more comprehensive health education program. Although much research is still needed regarding methodology, feasibility, short- and long-term efficacy, and cost-effectiveness of large-scale school-based programs, some information has already been generated.

Table 56.2 Characteristics That Make the School Environment Suitable for Obesity Prevention and Management Programs

Pooling of multidisciplinary expertise (nurses, counselors, physical educators, and health educators)

Pooling of facilities (gymnasiums, sports fields, and classrooms)

Large critical mass of target population (the obese or children at risk)

Almost year-round daily contact with target population

Streamlined lines of communication with parents

No clinical stigma

A case in point is school-based programs for the prevention and management of obesity. Some of the advantages of the school environment for such programs are listed in Table 56.2. In most societies, the school is the only site where children can meet with a multidisciplinary team of educators and therapists on a daily basis and almost year-round. Because personnel and facilities are already available in many schools, the cost of running prevention and intervention programs can be kept low. Schools also have a built-in infrastructure for communication with parents. In a recent review (27), results were assessed of 13 published programs that had been held in the United States and Canada. It is difficult to reach a general clear-cut conclusion about the efficacy of these programs because they differ in subject selection, presence of appropriate controls, intervention (e.g., duration and whether the intervention should be exercise alone or a multidisciplinary endeavor), and criteria for success. It seems, however, that most of these programs did induce either weight loss or reduc-

tion in percent body fat. Those programs that were successful in inducing reduction of body adiposity had the following common denominators:

- A multidisciplinary intervention that included enhanced activity, nutrition education, and behavior modification
- Exercise classes three to five times per week that promoted and provided incentives for after-school activities
- A team approach that combined input from the nurse, guidance counselor, lunchroom supervisor, and physical education teacher
- Coordinated parental involvement to support new behaviors

An example of such interventions is the studies by Brownell and Kaye (8) and Foster et al. (11). A key question, not yet resolved, is whether such school-based interventions induce long-term weight control once the structured program has been completed.

Strategy for Implementation of Information

Definitive studies on the later outcomes of activity and fitness in childhood must be longitudinal and span long periods of life. Logistically, such designs are almost impossible to perform. They are further complicated by an unknown tracking pattern that takes place over years, as summarized in Malina's review. It is unlikely, therefore, that clear-cut evidence will be available in the foreseeable future for the benefits of optimal activity and fitness in children to their health as adults. Two strategic options are thus available to society: (a) seek the definitive evidence and, only when such evidence is achieved, promote youth exercise for health; or (b) assume that activity, fitness, and positive attitudes toward them are important to future health and, as such, should be promoted even in the absence of clear-cut evidence in their favor.

This author believes that society should not and cannot afford to wait for the definitive evidence. It should instead adopt the latter approach by promoting activity and fitness in youth while supporting research on specific health-related issues. This is analogous to society's commitment to curb smoking long before definitive evidence had been provided about its detrimental effects on health.

References

1. American Academy of Pediatrics. Joint Committee on Physical Fitness, Recreation and Sports Medicine. Activities of children who are mentally retarded. *Pediatrics* 54: 376-377, 1974.
2. Åstrand, P.-O. *Experimental studies of physical working capacity in relation to sex and age.* Copenhagen: Munksgaard, 1952.
3. Bar-Or, O. Physical conditioning in children with cardiorespiratory disease. *Exerc. Sport Sci. Rev.* 13: 305-334, 1985.
4. Berg, K. Effect of physical training of school children with cerebral palsy. *Acta Paediatr. Scand. Supp.* 204: 27-33, 1970.
5. Berg, K., and J. Bjure. Methods for evaluation of the energy expenditure of children with cerebral palsy. *Acta Paediatr. Scand. Suppl.* 214: 15-26, 1970.
6. Bouchard, C., A. Tremblay, C. Leblanc, G. Lortie, R. Savard, and G. Theriault. A method to assess energy expenditure in children and adults. *Am. J. Clin. Nutr.* 37: 461-467, 1983.
7. Brown, B.J. The effect of an isometric strength program on the intellectual and social development of trainable retarded males. *Am. Corr. Ther. J.* 31: 44-48, 1977.
8. Brownell, K.D., and F.S. Kaye. A school-based behavior, nutrition education, and physical activity program for obese children. *Am. J. Clin. Nutr.* 35: 277-283, 1982.
9. Dresen, M.H.W., G. de Groot, J.R. Mesa Menor, and L.N. Bouman. Aerobic energy expenditure of handicapped children after training. *Arch. Phys. Ther. Rehabil.* 66: 302-306, 1985.
10. Florence, J.M., and J.M. Hagberg. Effect of training on the exercise responses of neuromuscular disease patients. *Med. Sci. Sports Exerc.* 16: 460-465, 1984.
11. Foster, G.D., T.A. Wadden, and K.D. Brownell. Peer-led program for the treatment and prevention of obesity in the schools. *J. Consult. Clin. Psychol.* 53: 538-540, 1985.
12. Fowler, W.M., and M. Taylor. Rehabilitation management of muscular dystrophy and related disorders: I. The role of exercise. *Arch. Phys. Med. Rehabil.* 63: 319-321, 1982.
13. Gayle, R., H.J. Montoye, and J. Philpot. Accuracy of pedometers for measuring distance walked. *Res. Q.* 48: 632-636, 1977.
14. Hagberg, J.M., A.A. Ehsani, D. Goldring, A. Hernandez, D.R. Sinacore, and J.O. Holloszy. Effect of weight training on blood pressure and hemodynamics in hypertensive adolescents. *J. Pediatr.* 104: 147-151, 1984.
15. Hagberg, J.M., D. Goldring, A.A. Ehsani, G.W. Heath, A. Hernandez, K. Schechtman, and J.O. Holloszy. Effect of exercise training on blood pressure and hemodynamic features of hypertensive adolescents. *Am. J. Cardiol.* 52: 763-768, 1983.
16. Henriksen, J.M., and T.T. Nielsen. Effect of physical training on exercise-induced bronchoconstriction. *Acta Paediatr. Scand.* 72: 31-36, 1983.
17. Keens, T.G. Exercise training programs for pediatric patients with chronic lung disease. *Pediatr. Clin. North Am.* 26: 517-523, 1979.
18. Klesges, L.M., and R.C. Klesges. The assessment of children's physical activity: A comparison of methods. *Med. Sci. Sports Exerc.* 19: 511-517, 1987.
19. Klesges, R.C., L.M. Klesges, A.M. Swenson, and A.M. Pheley. The validation of two motion sensors in the prediction of child and adult physical activity levels. *Am. J. Epidemiol.* 122: 400-410, 1985.
20. Ludvigsson, J. Physical exercise in relation to metabolic control in juvenile diabetes. *Acta Paediatr. Scand. Suppl.* 283: 45-49, 1980.
21. MacDougall, J.D., P.D. Roche, O. Bar-Or, and J.R. Moroz. Maximal aerobic capacity of Canadian school children: Prediction based on age-related oxygen cost of running. *Int. J. Sports. Med.* 4: 194-198, 1983.
22. Montoye, H.J., and H.L. Taylor. Measurement of physical activity in population studies: A review. *Hum. Biol.* 56: 195-216, 1984.
23. Moody, D.L., J.H. Wilmore, R.N. Girandola, and J.P. Royce. The effects of a jogging program on the body composition of normal and obese high school girls. *Med. Sci. Sports* 4: 210-213, 1972.
24. Saris, W.H.M. Habitual physical activity in children: Methodology and findings in health and disease. *Med. Sci. Sports Exerc.* 18: 253-263, 1986.
25. Scott, O.M., S.A. Hyde, C. Goddard, et al. Effects of exercise in Duchenne muscular dystrophy. *Physiotherapy* 67: 174-176, 1981.
26. Spira, R., and O. Bar-Or. *An investigation of the ambulation problems associated with severe motor paralysis in adolescents: Influence of physi-*

cal conditioning and adapted sport activities (Final Report, Project No. 19-P-58065-F-01). Tel-Aviv: U.S. Department of Health, Education and Welfare, 1975.

27. Ward, S.D., and O. Bar-Or. Role of the physician and the physical education teacher in the treatment of obesity at school. *Pediatrician* 13: 44-51, 1986.

28. Widhalm, K., E. Maxa, and H. Zyman. Effect of diet and exercise upon the cholesterol and triglyceride content of plasma lipoproteins in overweight children. *Eur. J. Pediatr.* 127: 121-126, 1978.

29. Zach, M., B. Purrer, and B. Oberwaldner. Effect of swimming on forced expiration and sputum clearance in cystic fibrosis. *Lancet* ii: 1201-1203, 1981.

Chapter 57

Reproduction: Exercise-Related Adaptations and the Health of Women and Men

Jerilynn C. Prior

This chapter reviews the effects of exercise on reproduction and the implications of reproductive change on health. Reproduction, although important for the preservation of the species, also has basic connections with culture, gender, and sexuality. The value we attach to exercise is tied to its history as part of our culture. Organized sport and competitive athletic events are and historically have been important in most cultures. Because of the interrelation of culture and physiology, a review of reproduction in relation to exercise, fitness, and health should first identify and evaluate the cultural biases that may influence research.

As scientists, athletes, and citizens, we share (to a greater or lesser degree) two presuppositions that affect our concept of health and our way of approaching research:

- Exercise and sport are valued differently depending on the gender of the athlete.
- Altered reproduction means *disease*.

Because I believe that the "facts" are altered by these presuppositions, a short explanation of each is important.

The first presupposition, that exercise has different importance depending on the gender of the athlete, today requires little explanation. The pervasiveness of this belief, despite the major gains in women's sport participation in the last decade, is evident in a written reply from a member of the committee organizing this conference: "You raised the problem of the lack of a woman's perspective in the program. I must say that this was not a concern of the organizing committee, not any more than the representation of francophone or anglophone, or of any other special interest groups were determinant in the selection of speakers" (personal communication, March 13, 1987).

The assumption behind this response could be either that the male perspective is the only pertinent perspective or that gender does not matter in relation to fitness, exercise, and health. However, society still reinforces the value of physical activity for men and only tolerates sports for women. Exercise, for men, is supposedly good, making them stronger, more competitive, and more manly. For women, the turn-of-the-century medical view that "sport wasted vital force, strained female bodies and fostered traits unbecoming to 'true womanhood' " (25) still persists.

The second presupposition is that reproductive change is a serious risk to health and must be evaluated (by complex technology) and treated (by pharmacology) like other significant illnesses are evaluated and treated. "Those experiencing such difficulties (e.g., menstrual irregularity, amenorrhea, or menarcheal delay) should continue exercising while *undergoing thorough evaluation and treatment*" [italics added](49).

If the assumption is that exercise *causes* "athletic amenorrhea" and that amenorrhea is a disease, then exercise must be bad for women. However, if the reproductive system of both males and females is seen as having the capacity to adapt to conditioning exercise, we can begin to build a new paradigm (24) within reproductive physiology. An adaptation model (47) suggests that external factors such as exercise, food deprivation, and stress modulate reproduction. The adaptive changes are temporary, reversible, and therefore not dysfunctional or harmful (39). The adaptation concept fits available data from prospective exercise studies and also resolves the intense dissonance that occurs when a researcher wishes to promote exercise yet desires to document reproductive changes accurately. Table 57.1 contrasts the disease and

Table 57.1   Therapeutic Approach to the Anovulatory Menstruating Athlete

Present or potential problem	Therapeutic options	Rationale
Unexpected asymptomatic menses with or without oligoamenorrhea or metorrhagia)[a]	Medroxyprogesterone 10 mg (2 tabs), days 16-25	Estrogen-primed endometrium will shed after progesterone withdrawal.
Heavy bleeding[a]	Medroxyprogesterone 10-20 mg for 10 d	Medroxyprogesterone will allow complete endometrial shedding.
Midcycle spotting	Medroxyprogesterone 10 mg/d taken at first spotting for 10 d	Prevent estrogen withdrawal bleeding after midcycle estrogen surge.
Infertility	1. Decrease exercise intensity by 10%. 2. Gain 1-2 kg weight. 3. Monitor basal temperature for 3 mo. 4. If above don't allow ovulation or short luteal phase appears, use progesterone suppositories 25 mg bid, days 16-25.	If the hypothalamic system is modulated by exercise, this will allow return to ovulation.
Risk for osteoporosis[a,b]	Increase calcium intake to 1.5 gr/d— 4-6 dairy products and/or supplements (2-5 "Tums"). Medroxyprogesterone 10 mg, days 16-25 cyclically	Decrease negative calcium balance associated with lower gonadal steroids. Has positive effect on bone, mechanism not yet known.
Androgen excess with hirsutism, acne[a,c]	Spironolactone 100-200 mg/d; medroxyprogesterone 10 mg, days 16-25	Antiandrogen medication. Medroxy-progesterone will potentiate anti-androgen effect and prevent heavy bleeding.
Risk of endometrial and/or breast cancer[b]	Medroxyprogesterone 10 mg, days 16-25	Inhibits estrogen's stimulating effect on endometrial and breast tissue.

Note. From "Gonadal Steroids in Athletic Women—Contraception, Complications, and Performance" by J.C. Prior and Y. Vigna, 1985, *Sports Medicine*, **2**(4), p. 293. Reprinted by permission.

[a]Oral contraceptives could be used but will suppress the desired recovery of the hypothalamic-pituitary axis.

[b]If present in women with lower estradiol levels but levels high enough to cause menstrual bleeding.

[c]A rare temporary transition phase from anovulatory to ovulatory cycles.

adaptation models as they relate to reproduction in exercising women.

To promote fitness and foster health we need to acknowledge that exercise is as good for women as it is for men and that reproductive changes are not disease processes but rather adaptive and reversible responses. In addition, we must be clear that overtraining is not healthy in any exercise or sport. It is a reasonable hypothesis to state that most of the reproductive changes blamed on exercise may be the endocrinological consequences of overtraining.

This chapter reviews prospective exercise-training data documenting reproductive changes in men and women. Exercise is viewed as one of several factors (besides weight or fat loss, physical illness, and psychological stress) that can suppress reproductive function at the hypothalamic

level. This chapter reviews implications of these reproductive changes for health, when and how (or if) to treat these changes, and areas needing further study.

The Adaptation Model

Adaptation, as originally described by Selye (47), can occur when a conditioning exercise program is gradual, is not accompanied by a significant negative energy balance, and is without psychological stress. Multiple physiological signals associated with training (e.g., changes in core temperature, increased energy output, central release of endorphins, and corticotrophin-releasing hormone, decreases in insulin, etc.) appear to be centrally integrated.

Precisely which hypothalamic changes guide the subsequent hormonal, reproductive, and behavioral changes is unknown. Alterations in insulin-receptor sensitivity consequent to changes in insulin levels could integrate essential energy balance changes into a neuroendocrinological signal. Another possible sensor could respond to core temperature changes during exercise. It is now clear that hypothalamic signals are translated into changes in pulse frequency and intensity of luteinizing hormone (LH). Hypothalamic-pituitary reproductive changes occurring with conditioning exercise have been reviewed recently (43).

Energy Balance, Nutrition, Weight Loss, and Adaptation

Changes in energy balance are inevitable during a training program. Conditioning exercise requires fuel for working muscles, generates heat, and can decrease basal metabolic rate. In addition, decreases in body fat stores, the most common change during exercise training, tends to suppress reproduction reversibly (16, 51). Numerous cross-sectional studies have attempted to prove that amenorrheic athletes have a lower percent body fat than do menstruating athletes. Hypothalamic amenorrhea has been documented in runners with normal body composition (26) and normal reproductive function has been demonstrated in high-performance athletes who are lean (12% fat with regular ovulation) (44).

No study has shown that negative caloric balance alone accounts for reproductive change during exercise training. A woman channel swimmer with normal (for a sedentary person) percent body fat documented by ultrasound developed anovulation during intense training (17). Percent body fat did not decrease, and fat stores were not different from controls in 5 swimmers who had hormonal changes and oligomenorrhea associated with exercise intensification (46).

Problems with the sensitivity of fat-store measurements (10), difficulties with studies of energy balance, and failure to quantify metabolic rate change over time have hampered efforts to understand the synergistic effect of energy balance and exercise training on the reproductive system. A controlled study of an equal caloric deficit induced first by exercise and then by diet in 6 athletic men showed that exercise-related deficits produced less weight loss and relative nitrogen sparing (28). Until more is understood about energy balance, lean muscle mass and metabolic rate change during exercise and the inter-relationships between nutrition and neurotransmitters, the causes of reproductive change will remain obscure.

Exercise-Related Endocrinological Conditioning

Endocrinological conditioning, in a direct parallel with musculoskeletal or cardiovascular conditioning changes, allows a return of normal reproductive function even when exercise is gradually increased (31). One element suggesting that this is an adaptive process is reversibility (32, 34). Figure 57.1 illustrates the development and resolution of anovulatory cycles of normal length during one woman's training for her first marathon. There was a slight but insignificant increase in weight as her training progressed. Figure 57.2 documents infertility associated with a short luteal phase reversing to pregnancy 6 wk following cessation of training. Adaptability of cycle changes was further documented in a runner's first (but not her second) marathon training sequence (Figure 57.3).

Overtraining

Early studies suggest and recent data confirm that if the exercise program is too intense or rapidly progressive for that individual's physiological state, age, heredity, or other unknown factors, the neuroreproductive equivalent of overtraining occurs. The physiology of this state is unknown but probably represents an excess of hypothalamic output of the primal stress hormones: endorphins and corticotrophin-releasing hormone. Anorexia, insomnia, and decreased exercise performance have been documented in overtrained men (4). In women it is likely that the neuroendocrinologic changes of overtraining may cause amenorrhea (no menses for 6 mo or more). It is at the point of overtraining, or of training and competing despite injury (23), that exercise may result in illness rather than optimum health. Overtraining changes are reversible (5) but require rest from sport in addition to caloric and psychological nurturing.

Male Reproduction During Exercise Training

Very few anecdotal or cross-sectional reports, and only two prospective (unpublished) studies, have

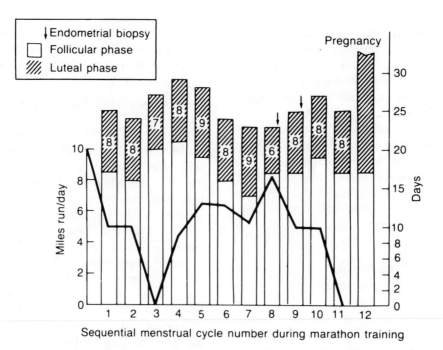

Figure 57.1. Fourteen consecutive menstrual cycles in a woman training for her first marathon. The entire bar represents cycle length and the cross-hatched area luteal length in days. During the course of training, luteal length decreased from normal (≥ 10 d) to short to anovulatory cycles (unshaded bars), before returning to normal after the marathon. Daily mileage is shown the line graph at the bottom. From "Reversible Luteal Phase Changes and Infertility Associated with Marathon Training" by J.C. Prior, B. Ho Yuen, P. Clement, L. Bowie, and J. Thomas, 1982, *The Lancet*, i, pp. 269-270. Reprinted by permission.

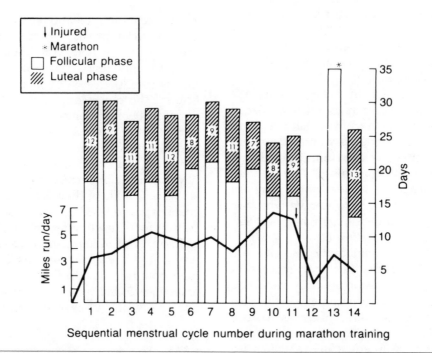

Figure 57.2. Twelve consecutive menstrual cycles from a marathoner who wanted to become pregnant. Cycle length is shown as total bar height and the luteal phase as the cross-hatched area. The line graph at the bottom records daily mileage per cycle. All cycles had short luteal phase lengths (< 10 d). In Cycle 11, she stopped running and became pregnant approximately 6 wk later (Cycle 12). From "Reversible Luteal Phase Changes and Infertility Associated With Marathon Training" by J.C. Prior, B. Ho Yuen, P. Clement, L. Bowie, and J. Thomas, 1982, *The Lancet*, i, pp. 269-270. Reprinted by permission.

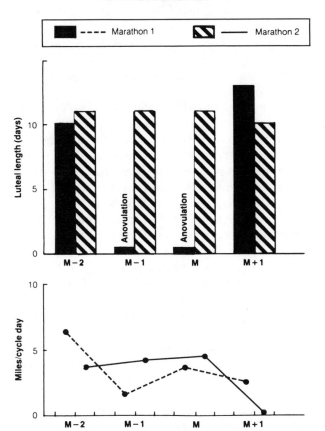

Luteal phase lengths in marathoner

Figure 57.3. Sequential luteal phases in two marathon-training sessions separated by 1 yr. Cycle M is the cycle in which the marathons were run. The luteal phase was normal in M-2 (two cycles before the marathon) the first year, and then anovulatory cycles occurred in the M-1 and M cycles. In the second marathon sequence, the luteal length remained normal. From "The Short Luteal Phase: A Cycle in Transition" by J.C. Prior and Y. Vigna, 1985, *Contemporary Obstetrics/Gynaecology*, **25**, pp. 166-167. Reprinted with permission from CONTEMPORARY OB/GYN, Medical Economics Company.

examined reproductive change in men during a conditioning exercise program. (The ratio of reports on men versus women is approximately 1:100.) Acute hormonal changes are summarized by Wall and Cumming (50), who documented anticipatory and early exercise rises in testosterone, especially free testosterone. Dessypns (15) noted decreased testosterone levels with prolonged exercise. Testosterone increases preceded exercise and could not be explained by an increase in LH.

MacConnie et al. (27) speculated that during acute exercise hormonal increases caused long-

term or steady-state reproductive effects. This seems unlikely because most athletes do not train at a sufficient intensity to provoke increases in gonadal steroids, prolactin, and cortisol that might cause long-term suppression of reproduction.

Cross-sectional studies usually but not always document lower baseline testosterone levels in long-distance runners than in controls. In a study of 31 runners versus 18 controls, testosterone, free testosterone, and prolactin levels were significantly lower in the runners (52). Cross-sectional data suggest that decreased semen volume, semen quality, and fertility may occur in some athletes (2).

Prospective, longitudinal controlled studies of men that begin before the start of a training program and continue as exercise intensifies are rare. Fifteen sedentary men who ran an average of 56 km per week after 6 mo of training had decreases in total testosterone (562 ± 43 to 438 ± 30; $p < 0.01$), free testosterone, and body weight (53). Preliminary prospective data in 5 men taken at the beginning, at 6 wk, and at 6 mo of gradually increasing exercise showed no change in serum testosterone from initial values to 6 mo (618.6-605.4 ng/dl). However, sperm counts tended to decrease (from 228 to 158 million) (Prior et al., personal communication, 1985).

Prospective data provide the most appropriate information about the etiology of reproductive change occurring during training. These data suggest that important changes occur within the hypothalamus. Wheeler et al. (53), in the training study described previously, were the first to document prospectively that there was a decrease in LH pulse frequency during 6 hr of exercise training of from 4.2 ± 0.5 to 3.6 ± 0.5 ($p < 0.05$). These data strongly support the hypothesis that the primary reproductive change takes place in the hypothalamus through decreases in LH pulse frequency. Unfortunately, available data do not clarify the interrelationship of exercise and nutrition as producers of neurotransmitter change as weight and body fat data are not cited.

Reproductive Changes During Exercise Training in Women

The physiological equation we are trying to solve, with exercise on one side and changes in reproduction on the other, has too many person-specific variables (e.g., age, heredity, reproductive state and past experience, nutritional state, and current and previous psychological experience) for cross-sectional studies to provide meaningful data.

Very few studies document specific information about exercise. Exercise data generally include only distance data and disregard duration, intensity, and temporal pattern estimates (e.g., daily short bouts and alternating long and short sessions); and the mix of aerobic, anaerobic, and weight-training components, which are also important. Longer-duration aerobic exercise is more likely to affect reproduction than is weight training.

Acute Exercise-Related Hormone Changes

Acute exercise-related hormone changes in women were first documented by Jurkovski et al. (22) and have been reviewed by Bonen (5). Estradiol and progesterone increased during the luteal phase but were usually unchanged during exercise in the follicular phase. Cumming and Rebar (11) documented early increases in testosterone not associated with LH increases. These changes are similar to those in men and include increases in testosterone and prolactin (sometimes cortisol) and generally no change in LH and FSH.

No prospective studies have documented acute exercise-related gonadal steroid changes with increasing training. Cumming and Rebar (11) reported cross-sectional studies of amenorrheic trained and normally cycling trained and untrained women (data were presented as smoothed curves without variance information). The LH pulse frequency (but not amplitude or the area under the curve) appeared to decrease 6 hr after a 60-min 60% $\dot{V}O_2$max exercise session in 6 menstruating runners (13). Beta-endorphin and met-enkephalin levels tended to decrease with increasing training (20). It is likely that the temporary slowing of LH pulsatility—rather than acute exercise-related increases in estradiol, testosterone, prolactin, and cortisol levels—may contribute to the long-term reproductive changes in women.

Menstrual Cycle Symptom-Related Training Changes

An improved sense of well-being and mood are described by men and women following exercise (29). To document prospectively changes occurring in mood and body symptoms related to exercise and the menstrual cycle, a daily recording form must be used (40). The daily symptom diary (DSD) form has been developed to monitor mood and symptom changes and is kept in parallel with records of exercise distance, duration, and intensity. As a way to quantify a person's percentage of maximal energy output per day, a mathematical equation representing training impulses, or "Trimps," is used (3) that employs exercise time, average exercise heart rate, and basal and maximal heart rates.

Phase characteristics of the menstrual cycle can be monitored by oral basal temperature (BBT) records, which reflect the hypothalamic thermal response to endogenous progesterone. Daily temperatures can be plotted by computer and the data quantified using least mean squares analysis. This analysis finds the day of maximal temperature difference between the follicular and the luteal phase mean temperatures. The LH peak day correlates with the day of maximal temperature difference (onset of the luteal phase) by computer-analyzed BBT data ($r = .880$, $p < 0.001$) (44a).

After 3 mo of conditioning exercise in sedentary ovulatory women, decreased luteal phase breast and fluid symptoms were prospectively documented as the earliest menstrual cycle changes to result from exercise (37). After 6 mo of training either in sedentary women or in runners who intensified exercise before a marathon, decreases in depression, overall luteal phase symptoms, and anxiety were documented (40).

These positive changes are not simply a placebo effect of exercise. In the studies cited previously, women were blind to the hypothesis that premenstrual symptoms would improve and were not troubled by the premenstrual syndrome (PMS). The first changes were not in mood but in breast tenderness and bloating symptoms. Decreased premenstrual symptoms are not due to exercise per se, but to *intensification* of exercise. Controls for the studies did not increase their exercise and had normal moliminal symptoms (e.g., breast, appetite, fluid, and mood symptoms associated with ovulatory menstrual cycles) that did not change significantly over time.

Moliminal symptoms may paradoxically increase in athletes in two situations: (a) a sudden decrease in training related to injury, especially if associated with weight gain; and (b) ovulation for the first time after a prolonged duration of anovulation with either regular or irregular menstruation. Severe PMS may be present in the first one or two luteal phases in a previously anovulatory woman. In figurative terms, it is as though a central "choke" were supplying excess hormones to achieve ovulation. The increased hormonal stimulation is no longer necessary after ovulatory cycles become well established, and PMS becomes normal molimina.

Exercise-Related Menstrual Changes in Cycles of Normal Length

Methodology

Several problems impede the documentation of exercise-related menstrual cycle changes:

- the lack of prospective menstrual cycle data for normals matched for age, gynecologic age, and nutritional balance,
- the lack of noninvasive methodology for documenting menstrual cycle phase characteristics; and,
- the lack of statistical tools for describing and quantifying changing responses to stimuli over time (time series analysis).

We now have prospective menstrual cycle data for sedentary and active (but not training) women across a year to allow the first good comparison with marathon-training women. All 66 women, aged 22-42, had two consecutive ovulatory cycles documented by BBT monitoring before entry into the study. The three groups consisted of 23 sedentary women, 22 women running constant mileage of more than 15 to less than 50 mi per cycle, and 21 women training for a marathon and running more than 50 mi per cycle (44).

To our surprise, the marathon-training women did not experience more short luteal phase or anovulatory cycles than did the sedentary women (44). Average cycle length (28.3 d) and luteal length (10.3 d) were not different among the three groups. Far more women experience intermittent short luteal phases or anovulation, without regard for exercise category, than has been recognized previously. These changes occurred in midreproductive life in women who had normal menstrual cycle and luteal lengths before beginning the study. Only 13 of 66 women had consistently normal cycles across the year (44).

Least mean squares analysis of BBT data, validated against the hormonal "gold standard" of the LH peak, will now permit quantitative longitudinal assessment of the menstrual cycle. The etiology of luteal phase changes will be better understood if studies use BBT data obtained in conjunction with daily records of symptoms, exercise, and intermittent documentation of nutritional balance.

Statistical routines to deal with longitudinal, adaptive, and multifactorial modeling are still inadequate. Forward selection of stepwise regression will aid in assessing the relationships between some changes over time. However, quantification and modeling of adaptive changes are still needed.

Prospective Menstrual Cycle Changes During Exercise Training

The earliest prospective exercise data were obtained in 1939 in rats started abruptly on a treadmill program of 60 min per day who developed anestrus (47). Decreased gonadotropin-releasing hormone pulsatility, manifested as decreased LH pulse frequency and LH quantity, may be the mechanism responsible for exercise-related menstrual cycle alterations. In a cross-sectional study of regularly cycling sedentary and running women (who were not documented to be ovulatory), slower LH pulse frequencies were observed in the runners (12). Figure 57.4 shows the 6-hr LH pulse patterns of the two groups.

Luteal phase shortening has been repeatedly documented during increased training (32, 33, 48). Changes in luteal function (7) and altered folliculogenesis (45) also occur as the intensity of training increases. Although the cycle interval may be lengthened beyond 36 d (oligomenorrhea), maintenance of a normal cycle interval (21-36 d) is more common.

Development of anovulation has been reported more rarely (7, 32, 33). Anovulation may occur (a) with an estrogen and an LH surge without subsequent egg release, (b) with an estrogen but no LH surge, and (c) with no midcycle increase in either estrogen or LH (see Figure 57.5). Although molimina is normally less in exercising women, breast enlargement and other mild symptoms indicate the occurrence of ovulatory cycles in the observant woman. However, if women respond negatively to the question: Can you tell, by the way you feel, that your period is coming? more than 90% of the time they will be anovulatory (41). Data also suggest that the occurrence of dysmenorrhea or menstrual cramps cannot be used to either diagnose or exclude anovulation (41).

Reversibility is characteristic of the menstrual cycle changes related to exercise. Amenorrhea in teenage gymnasts reverses with injury-induced rest (51). Short luteal phases will lengthen with one cycle of decreased exercise or with stabilization of training (32, 34). Although anovulation may reverse to a normal luteal phase in one cycle (32),

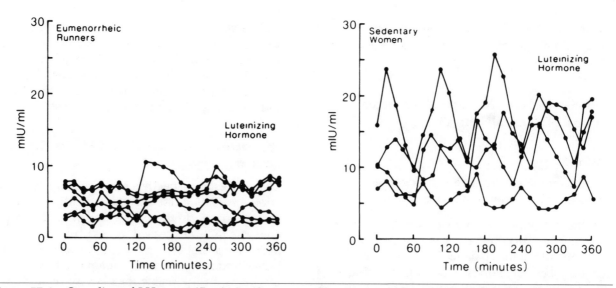

Figure 57.4. Sampling of LH every 15 min in 12 women. Six runners with regular menstrual cycles are shown in the left panel and 4 matched sedentary women with regular cycles in the right panel. Pulse analysis showed decreases in pulse frequency, pulse amplitude, and area under the LH curve in runners compared with sedentary women. From "Defects in Pulsatile LH Release in Normally Menstruating Runners" by D.C. Cumming, M.M. Vickovic, S.R. Wall, and M.R. Fluker, 1985, *Journal of Clinical Endocrinology and Metabolism*, **60**, pp. 810-812. Reprinted by permission.

a 6- to 8-wk lag is more characteristic for return of normal luteal length. Bullen et al. (7) reported that within 6 mo of decreasing exercise training, basal temperature and menstrual cycle interval changes returned to normal.

Exercise-Related Changes in Menstrual Cycle Interval

Menstrual interval is often not prospectively documented during exercise studies. It was not mentioned by Ronkainen et al. (45), was indicated to be unchanged by Carli et al. (8), and was described only as increased and decreased by Boyden et al. (6). Bullen et al. (7) documented delayed menses (oligomenorrhea) in 1 of 9 women in a weight-maintenance group and in 12 of 16 women in a weight-loss group.

Oligomenorrhea (cycle interval > 36 and ≤ 180 d) has been noted in sports such as gymnastics (51) and swimming (46), in which a high percentage of participants are teenagers. As with Bullen's subjects (mean age 22, within 10 yr of menarche), added stressors, such as residence at a summer camp and weight loss, appear to compound the risk.

Amenorrhea (cycle interval ≥ 180 d) may develop in the young woman who is within 12 yr of menarche, who has never ovulated up to the time she starts training, or both, especially if she has associated weight loss. The development of amenorrhea during exercise training has never

been documented in prospective, well-controlled studies of previously ovulatory women who have no added stressors such as weight loss or psychological tension. The frequently used term *athletic amenorrhea* is a misnomer. Age and percent body fat, but not training load or exercise performance, were different for amenorrheic women (19%) who qualified for the U.S. Olympic marathon trials and those who were regularly cycling (65%) (19).

Reproduction and the Overtraining Syndrome

Overtraining is a symptom complex that includes sleep disturbance, depression, anorexia, and decreasing sport performance despite intense training. I feel that amenorrhea is the characteristic reproductive manifestation of overtraining in women. Overtraining is associated with chronically increased cortisol levels (4). Treatment of overtraining must be multifactorial and should include decreases in training, increases in food, and management of associated emotional stress (see the following section).

Evaluation and Therapy of Exercise-Related Reproductive Change

The assessment of reproductive change depends on the assumptions made about the etiology of the

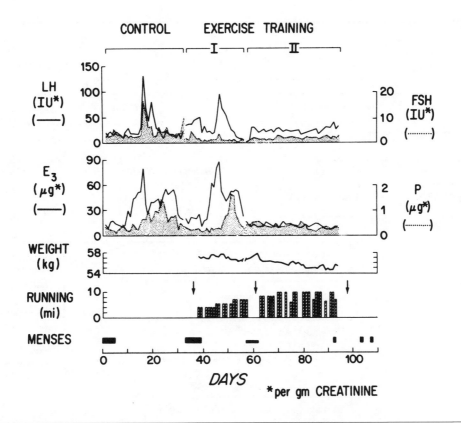

Figure 57.5. Three sequential cycles in a woman who began as sedentary (control cycle) and was running nearly 10 mi/d by Cycle 2. Urinary hormone concentrations show probable luteal phase shortening in Cycle 1 and loss of estradiol and LH surges in Cycle 2. From "Induction of Menstrual Cycle Disorders by Strenuous Exercise" by B.A. Bullen, et al., *New England Journal of Medicine*, **312**, pp. 1349-1353. Reprinted by permission.

changes. A physician who believes in the adaptation model will obtain a detailed history of reproduction, exercise training, weight changes, and present emotional and social environments. Training intensity, weekly weights, and reproductive symptoms and signs will need to be monitored (for women, DSD and BBT).

A physical examination must include measurements of height and weight and some assessment of fat stores (e.g., skinfold measurements) using a formula validated for an athletic population (21). The athlete can be counseled to restore weight (if there is excess loss) and to stabilize training.

A 3- to 6-mo period of monitoring, during which time training and weight are modified, usually allows the return of entirely normal function. Expensive, invasive testing is usually not needed.

The general scheme for investigation of an active woman is shown in Figure 57.6. If changes persist after exercise stabilization, there are usually chronic emotional or nutritional problems. It is important to detect and to counsel appropriately the athlete with compulsive tendencies and the

person with an eating disorder associated with intense exercise (38).

Treatment for potential problems that might develop in an athlete with secondary amenorrhea and in the cycling but anovulatory athlete is shown in Tables 57.2 and 57.3 (36). The principles of therapy rely on the concept that the underlying process is adaptive (38) (Table 57.1). The more information the athlete obtains about her own situation, the more likely her reproductive changes will reverse or mature toward normal. Usually, little pharmacological interference is necessary.

If, however, anovulation or amenorrhea is chronic, cyclic progesterone is an important therapy. Progesterone can prevent or reverse bone loss (42), can prevent endometrial hyperplasia, and may stimulate cyclic function. Recent work showed an 8% 12 mo increase in bone density in sedentary amenorrheic women given 10 mg medroxy-progesterone (Provera) per day for 10 d/mo (42). Chronically short luteal phase cycles may also require treatment, as the average annual luteal length and yearly trabecular bone loss in

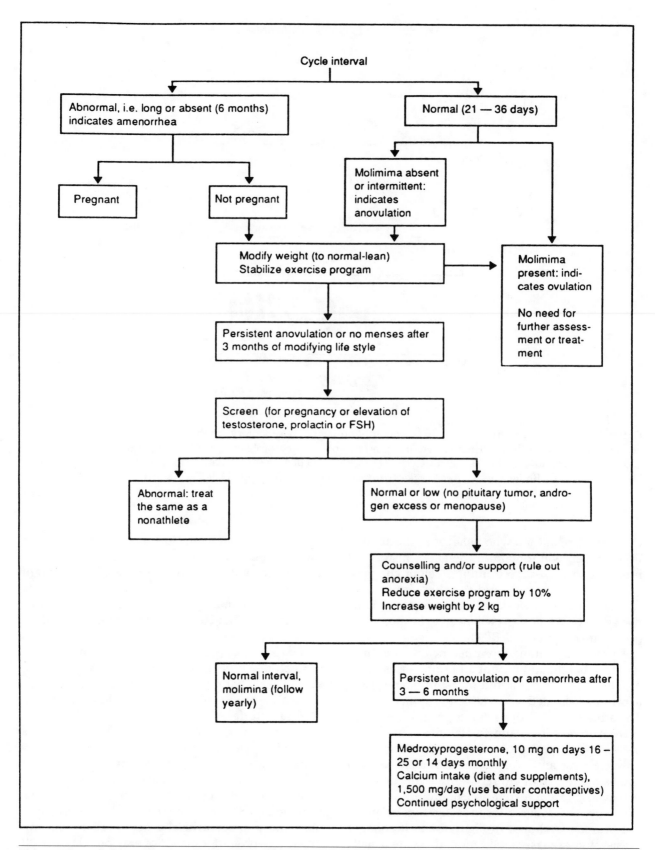

Figure 57.6. A therapeutic approach to establish normal, ovulatory menstrual cycles in active women. Note that, except to exclude pregnancy, no hormonal testing is required until after at least 3 mo of monitoring. From ''Exercise and Reproduction in Women'' by J.C. Prior, 1987, *Medicine North America* (special sports issue), pp. 16-23. Reprinted by permission.

Table 57.2 Therapeutic Approach to the Athlete With Secondary Amenorrhea

Present or potential problem	Therapeutic options	Rationale
Absent menstrual flow[a]	Evaluation to rule out disease	May remove worry-related block
	Explanation and reassurance	
	Medroxyprogesterone 10 mg, days 16-25 monthly whether or not withdrawal bleeding occurs	May stimulate cyclic hypothalamic function.
Vaginal dryness and atrophy[a]	Conjugated estrogen vaginal cream 1/2 applicator (1 g) 1 night/wk	Topical estrogen with little systemic absorption
Risk for osteoporosis[a]	Increase oral calcium to 1.5-2 g/d—4-8 dairy servings and/or supplements ("Tums," 200 mg calcium per tablet)	Decrease negative calcium balance associated with low gonadal steroids.
	Medroxyprogesterone 10 mg/d for 10 d/mo	Positive action on trabecular bone
	Cyclic estrogen and progesterone: i.e., conjugated estrogens 0.3 mg/d, days 1-21 each month	Balanced hormonal replacement
	Medroxyprogesterone 10 mg/d days 16-25	
Infertility	1. Decrease exercise intensity by 10%.	These exercise and diet modifications will allow normal hypothalamic reproductive function to return.
	2. Gain 1-2 kg weight.	
	3. Monitor basal temperature for 3 mo.	
	4. After 3 mo if ovulation has not occurred, give progesterone vaginal suppositories 25 mg bid, days 16-25 of cycle or 10 d/mo.	
	5. Further decreases in exercise, additional weight gain, and stress reduction may be necessary.	
	6. Additional therapy may require ovulation induction measures. However, these methods may not work initially.	

Note. From "Gonadal Steroids in Athletic Women—Contraception, Complications, and Performance" by J.C. Prior and Y. Vigna, 1985, *Sports Medicine,* **2**(4), p. 292. Reprinted by permission.

[a]Oral contraceptives are not desirable because they suppress cyclic hypothalamic-pituitary function.

Table 57.3 The Disease Model Versus the Adaptation Model

Variable	Disease model	Adaptation model
Cause	A single agent or presumed etiology	An integrated interaction of personal and environmental factors
Time course	Continuous or worsening	Labile and reversible
Disability	A present detriment in function/pain/discomfort	A present positive effect; rare discomfort/concern
Prognosis	Risk for chronic disease, harm/discomfort	Excellent, no permanent impairment
Therapy	a. Specific (external) agent	a. Modulation of attitude/environment/lifestyle
	b. Effective	b. Do nothing to interfere with adaptation
	c. Without major side-effects	c. Cause no harm
Therapeutic relationship (patient: physician)	Passive: authoritarian	Active: consultative, supportive

Note. From "Reproductive Changes With Exercise: When and How to Evaluate, Who and Why to Treat," by J.C. Prior, 1988, in J. Puhl, C.H. Brown, and R.O. Voy (Eds.), *Sport Science Perspectives for Women* (pp. 131-150), Champaign, IL: Human Kinetics. Reprinted by permission.

premenopausal women correlated significantly ($r = .47$, $p < 0.001$) (44).

Few, if any, guidelines are available for the evaluation and treatment of men with exercise-related reproductive change. However, it may be assumed that exercise stabilization and some restoration of lost weight would be as appropriate for men as it is for women.

Health Implications of Exercise-Related Reproductive Changes

Few epidemiological studies have addressed the question of exercise-related reproductive change and effects on health and aging. The following discussion deals with some possible exercise-related effects on health and reproduction.

An early, documented positive effect of exercise training for women's health is a decrease in premenstrual symptoms (37, 40). Frisch et al. (18) recently reported decreased reproductive system malignancies in athletic versus sedentary women. Theoretically, the teenage athlete, no matter what her cycle type, is exposed to lower levels of estrogen. Information is needed on the development of hip and spinal fracture in athletic women with menstrual cycle change (because low weight and low levels of progesterone and estrogen are risk factors for fracture).

It can be postulated that the lean, athletic woman has been exposed to lower peak levels of estrogen. If the rapidity or decline from that peak level influences the development of vasomotor instability associated with menopause, then the active woman may have a less symptomatic menopausal transition.

Bone loss may be one health risk related to lower weight and decreased reproductive hormones in the athletic person. The loss is likely to be predominantly trabecular bone because cortical bone loss can be prevented by weight-bearing exercise (1). Dual-photon measurements show significant increases in lumbar bone density (both cortical and trabecular bone) during moderate exercise training (14). Cortical bone, which is present in the trabecular-bone-dominant areas such as the hip and spine, may increase to offset trabecular bone loss.

Increases in HDL cholesterol related to exercise training may compensate for potential decreases that may occur because of lower estrogen levels. Chronic but slight decreases in testosterone in ath-

letic men may also be associated with increases in HDL cholesterol. This positive lipid change, along with coronary artery dilatation, lower blood pressure, lower steady-state catecholamine levels, and decreased body fat, could decrease the athlete's risk of ischemic heart disease.

Areas of Importance in Further Research

One of the key questions that needs to be answered is how changes in nutrition and energy balance during exercise training relate to changes in reproduction. A longitudinal, prospective study is needed on sedentary individuals followed during a gradually increasing training program. Evaluation of energy expenditure during a given work load, weeklong metabolic balance studies, and hormonal documentation at three monthly intervals over a year of increasing training are a necessity. Information must be collected about exercise pattern, reproductive system change, core temperature, diet, and serum levels of triiodothyronine (T3), endorphins, insulin, and growth hormone. In addition, the study should monitor body fat, bone mass, and muscle mass measurements validated for an athletic population. It would also be useful to document whether changes occur in the metabolic pathways for estradiol and adrenal androgens. Only when we have gathered such data will we begin to understand the complex interrelationships among exercise training, energy balance, and reproductive change.

Longitudinal observations of bone mass and the menstrual cycle are needed to see whether differential changes in bone mass occur during short luteal phase and anovulatory cycles in an active versus a sedentary population. Two recent cross-sectional studies suggest the predicted maximal oxygen uptake correlates significantly with dual-photon lumbar bone density ($r = 0.54$) (30) and with calcium in the trunk and thighs by neutron activation ($r = 0.52$) (9). Although progesterone deficiency appears related to bone loss (44), the actual loss or the fracture risk may differ in sedentary versus active populations.

A double-blind, placebo-controlled therapy study is under way in my laboratory to test the reproductive and bone responses of athletic women to various therapies. A randomized two-by-two design will use cyclic Provera (10 mg/d for 10 d/mo) and calcium (1,000 mg/d) as therapeutic agents.

In summary, both men and women experience reversible reproductive changes during exercise training. It is probable that some central hypothalamic signal related to exercise intensity and energy balance decreases the pulse frequency of gonadotropin-releasing hormone and, subsequently, LH. The long-term health implications of these changes are unclear. However, there may be resulting decreases in reproductive cancers, increases in total bone mass (though perhaps trabecular bone loss), and preservation of favorable lipid profiles despite lower estrogen levels in women and because of lower testosterone levels in men. Data are beginning to accumulate that show these changes to be adaptive and that point toward appropriate plans for evaluation and therapy.

References

1. Aloia, J., S.M. Cohn, J.A. Ostuni, R. Cane, and K. Ellis. Prevention of involutional bone loss by exercise. *Am. J. Med.* 89: 356-358, 1978.

2. Ayers, J.W.T., Y. Komesu, T. Romani, and R. Ansbacher. Anthropomorphic, hormonal, and psychologic correlates of semen quality in endurance-trained male athletes. *Fertil. Steril.* 43: 917-921, 1985.

3. Banister, E.W., and C.L. Hamilton. Variations in iron status with fatigue modeled from training in female distance runners. *Eur. J. Appl. Physiol.* 54: 16-23, 1985.

4. Barron, J.L., T.D. Noakes, W. Levy, C. Smith, and R.P. Millar. Hypothalamic dysfunction in overtrained athletes. *J. Clin. Endocrinol. Metab.* 60: 803-806, 1985.

5. Bonen, A. Endocrine alterations with exercise training. In: Puhl, J., and H. Brown, eds. *The menstrual cycle and physical activity.* Champaign, IL: Human Kinetics; 1985: 81-100.

6. Boyden, T.W., R.W. Parmenter, P. Stanforth, T. Rotkis, and J. Wilmore. Sex steroids and endurance running in women. *Fertil. Steril.* 39: 629-632, 1983.

7. Bullen, B.A., G.S. Skrinar, I.Z. Beitins, G. VonMering, B.A. Turnbull, and J.W. McArthur. Induction of Menstrual cycle disorders by strenuous exercise. *N. Engl. J. Med.* 312: 1349-1353, 1985.

8. Carli, G., G. Martelli, A. Viti, L. Baldi, M. Bonifazi, and C. Lupo di Prisco. The effect of swimming training on hormone levels in girls. *J. Sports Med.* 23: 45-94, 1983.

9. Chow, R.K., J.E. Harrison, C.F. Brown, and V. Hajek. Physical fitness effect on bone mass in postmenopausal women. *Arch. Phys. Med. Rehabil.* 67: 231-234, 1986.

10. Cumming, D.C., and R.W. Rebar. Lack of consistency in the indirect methods of estimating percent body fat. *Fertil. Steril.* 41(5): 739-742, 1984.

11. Cumming, D., and R. Rebar. Hormonal changes with acute exercise and with training in women. *Semin. Reprod. Endocrinol.* 3: 55-63, 1985.

12. Cumming, D.C., M.M. Vickovic, S.R. Wall, and M.R. Fluker. Defects in pulsatile LH release in normally menstruating runners. *J. Clin. Endocrinol. Metab.* 60: 810-812, 1985.

13. Cumming, D.C., M.M. Vickovic, S.R. Wall, M.R. Fluker, and A.N. Belcastro. The effect of acute exercise on pulsatile release of luteinizing hormone in women runners. *Am. J. Obstet. Gynecol.* 153: 482-485, 1985.

14. Dalsky, G.P., S.J. Birge, K.S. Kleinheider, and A.A. Ehsani. The effect of endurance training on lumbar bone mass in postmenopausal women [Abstract No. 96]. *Med. Sci. Sport Exerc.* 18: 520, 1986.

15. Dessypns, A. Plasma cortisol, testosterone, androsteindione and LH during a noncompetitive marathon run. *J. Steroid Biochem.* 7: 33-37, 1976.

16. Frisch, R.E., and J.W. McArthur. Menstrual cycles: Fatness as a determinant of minimum weight for height necessary for the maintenance or onset of puberty. *Science* 185: 949-950, 1974.

17. Frisch, R.E., G.M. Hall, T.T. Aoki, J. Birnholz, R. Jacob, L. Landsberg, H. Munro, K. Parker-Jones, D. Tulchinslky, and J. Young. Metabolic, endocrine and reproductive changes of a woman channel swimmer. *Metabolism* 33: 1106-1111, 1984.

18. Frisch, R.E., G. Wyshak, N.L. Albright, T.E. Albright, I. Schiff, K.P. Jones, J. Witschi, E. Shiang, E. Koff, and M. Marguglio. Lower prevalence of breast cancer and cancers of the reproductive system among former college athletes compared to non-athletes. *Br. J. Cancer* 52: 885-891, 1985.

19. Glass, A.R., J.A. Yahiro, P.A. Deuster, R.A. Vigersky, S.B. Kyle, and E.B. Schoomaker. Amenorrhea in Olympic marathon runners. *Fertil. Steril.* 48: 740-745, 1987.

20. Howlett, T.A., S. Tomlin, L. Ngahfoong, L.H. Rees, B.A. Bullen, G.S. Skrinar, and J.W. McArthur. Release of B endorphin and net-enkephalin during exercise in normal women's response to training. *Br. Med. J.* 288: 1950-1952, 1984.

21. Jackson, A.S., M.C. Pollock, and A. Ward. Generalized equations for predicting body density of women. *Med. Sci. Sport Exerc.* 12: 175-182, 1980.

22. Jurkowski, J.E., N.L. Jones, C. Walker, and J. Sutton. Ovarian hormonal responses to exercise. *J. Appl. Sport Sci.* 44: 109-114, 1978.

23. Kirby, S. (1987). *Injury and ill health: The unwritten story about Canada's female Olympic athletes.* Canadian Research Association for the Advancement of Women Conference [Abstract]. Winnipeg, October, 1987.

24. Kuhn, T. The structure of scientific resolutions. 2nd ed. Chicago: University of Chicago Press, 1970.

25. Lenskyj, H. *Out of bounds—Women, sport and sexuality.* Toronto: Women's Press, 1986.

26. McArthur, J.W., B.A. Bullen, I.Z. Beitins, M. Pagano, T.M. Badger, and A. Klibanski. Hypothalamic amenorrhea in runners of normal body composition. *Endocr. Res. Comm.* 7: 13-25, 1980.

27. MacConnie, S.E., A. Barkan, R.M. Lampman, M.A. Schork, and I.Z. Beitins. Decreased hypothalamic gonadotropin-releasing hormone secretion in the male marathon runners. *N. Engl. J. Med.* 315: 411-417, 1986.

28. McMurray, R.G., V. Ben-Ezra, W.A. Forsythe, and A.T. Smith. Responses of endurance-training subjects to caloric deficits induced by diet or exercise. *Med. Sci. Sport Exerc.* 17(4): 574-579, 1985.

29. Murtrie, N. The psychological effects of exercise for women. In: Macloed, D., R. Maughan, M. Nimmo, T. Reilly, and C. Williams, eds. *Exercise—Benefits, limits and adaptations,* London: E. & F.N. Spon; 1987: 270-286.

30. Pocock, N.A., J.A. Eisman, M.G. Yeates, P.N. Sambrook, and S. Eberl. Physical fitness as a major determinant of femoral neck and lumbar spine bone mineral density. *J. Clin. Invest.* 78: 618-621, 1986.

31. Prior, J.C. Endocrine 'conditioning' with endurance training: A preliminary review. *Can. J. Appl. Sports Sci.* 7: 149-157, 1982.

32. Prior, J.C., B. Ho Yuen, P. Clement, L. Bowie, and J. Thomas. Reversible luteal phase changes and infertility associated with marathon training. *Lancet* i: 269-270, 1982.

33. Prior, J.C., K. Cameron, B. Ho Yuen, and J. Thomas. Menstrual cycle changes with marathon training: Anovulation and short luteal phase. *Can. J. Appl. Sport Sci.* 7: 173-177, 1982.

34. Prior, J.C., S. Pride, Y. Vigna, and B. Ho Yuen. Marathon training and reversible luteal phase shortening: A controlled prospective study. *Med. Sci. Sport Exerc.* 15: 174, 1983.

35. Prior, J.C., and Y. Vigna. The short luteal phase: A cycle in transition. *Contemp. Obstet. Gynecol.* 25: 166-167, 1985.

36. Prior, J.C., and Y. Vigna. Gonadal steroids in athletic women: Concerns about contraception, performance and complications. *Sports Med.* 2: 287-295, 1985.

37. Prior, J.C., Y. Vigna, and N. Alojado. Conditioning exercise diseases premenstrual symptoms—a prospective controlled three month trial. *Eur. J. Appl. Physiol.* 59: 349-355, 1986.

38. Prior, J.C. Reproductive changes with exercise: When and how to evaluate, who and why to treat. In: Puhl, J., and H. Brown, eds. *Women and sports sciences.* Champaign, IL: Human Kinetics; 1987.

39. Prior, J.C. Exercise and reproduction in women. [Special sports issue]. *Med. N. Am.* (Fall): 16-23, 1987.

40. Prior, J.C., Y. Vigna, N. Alojado, D. Sciarretta, and M. Schulzer. Conditioning exercise decreases premenstrual symptoms: A prospective, controlled six month trial. *Fertil. Steril.* 47: 402-408, 1987.

41. Prior, J.C., and Y. Vigna. Absence of molimina: The clinical or self-diagnosis of anovulation. Society for Menstrual Cycle Research [Abstract], Ann Arbor, MI, June 1987: 88.

42. Prior, J.C., Y. Vigna, and A. Burgess. Medroxyprogesterone increases trabecular bone density in women with menstrual disorders. Endocrine Society abstracts, 69th Annual Meeting, #560.

43. Prior, J.C. Physical exercise and neuroendocrine control of reproduction. *Baillieres Clin. Endocrinol. Metab.* 1: 299-317, 1988.

44. Prior, J.C., Y. Vigna, A. Burgess, and N. Cunningham. Marathon training in the absence of luteal phase change is not a risk factor for trabecular bone loss. *J. Bone Miner. Res.* 3: S85, 1988.

44a. Prior, J.C., Vigna, Y.M., Schultzer, M., Bonen, A., Lau, W., A new quantitative computerized basal temperature method: Validation against the mid-cycle LH peak in a double blind study. Presented at Society for Menstrual Cycle Research, Salt Lake City, June, 1989.

45. Ronkainen, J., A. Pakarenen, P. Kirkenen, and A. Pauppla. Physical exercise-induced changes and season-associated differences in pituitary-ovarian function of runners and joggers. *J. Clin. Endocrinol. Metab.* 60: 416-422, 1985.

46. Russell, J.B., D.E. Mitchell, P.I. Musey, and D.C. Collins. The role of beta-endorphin and catecholestrogens on the hypothalamic-pituitary axis in female athletes. *Fertil. Steril.* 42: 690-695, 1984.

47. Selye, H. The effect of adaptation to various damaging agents on the female sex organs in the rat. *Endocrinology* 25: 615-624, 1939.

48. Shangold, M., R. Freeman, G. Thysen, and M. Gatz. The relationship between long-distance running, plasma progesterone and luteal phase length. *Fertil. Steril.* 32: 130-133, 1979.

49. Shangold, M.M. Menstrual disturbances in the athlete. *Prim. Care* 11: 109-114, 1984.

50. Wall, S.R., and D.C. Cumming. Effects of physical activity on reproductive function and development in males. *Semin. Reprod. Endocrinol.* 3: 65-80, 1985.

51. Warren, M. The effects of exercise on pubertal progression and reproductive function in girls. *J. Clin. Endocrinol. Metab.* 51: 1150-1157, 1980.

52. Wheeler, G.D., S.R. Wall, A.N. Belcastro, and D.C. Cumming. Reduced serum testosterone and prolactin in male distance runners. *JAMA* 252: 514-516, 1984.

53. Wheeler, G.D., S. Williamson, M. Singh, W.D. Pierce, W.F. Epling, A.N. Belcastro, and D.C. Cumming. Decreased serum total and free testosterone and LH pulse frequency with endurance training in men. Paper presented at the 69th Annual Meeting of the Endocrine Society, Indianapolis, 1987.

Chapter 58

Discussion: Reproduction: Exercise-Related Adaptations and the Health of Women and Men

David C. Cumming

Research into exercise-associated reproductive dysfunction in women has been criticized by reason of possible harm to women's exercise programs because it focuses on the negative aspects of women's sports. To promote fitness and foster health, we need to consider that exercise is beneficial for both men and women. It is unfortunate that there is concern that women's athletics programs may suffer from the results of research into reproductive changes with exercise, but that concern should not close our minds. As a result of such investigation, many of the initial fears about the prevalence of athletic amenorrhea and the roll of exercise have been dismissed. It is clear from the many studies that have been performed over the last 2 decades that strenuous exercise, particularly endurance training, can influence hypothalamic-pituitary-gonadal (HPG) axis function in both men and women. In most circumstances, the changes appear physiological and subclinical, whereas reproductive dysfunction occurs in only a small percentage of athletes. Nevertheless, the risk-benefit ratio of exercise-induced changes in the reproductive system, both clinical and subclinical, is not well defined in women and not at all defined in men.

The purpose of this chapter is to review the physiological responses of the HPG axis to exercise and to examine how those changes interact with other factors to produce reproductive dysfunction. In addition, a brief review of the effects of exercise and training during pregnancy is presented.

Subclinical Change in the HPG Axis Associated With Exercise in Women and Men

The changes in reproductive function associated with exercise have been well documented in men and women in good cross-sectional and prospective studies. Collectively, studies from several institutions (Table 58.1) have shown that strenuous training induces decreased pulsatile LH release at rest (with a further decrease in LH pulse frequency following acute exercise in women), that serum gonadotropin responses to GnRH are blunted, and that sex steroids are generally lowered (1, 5, 6, 10, 13, 14, 48, 53, 54). The neuroendocrinologic background of these changes has resisted definition.

Dr. Prior's prospective studies have suggested that inadequate luteal phase and anovulation are found in a majority of women undergoing increased training (37). The findings generally correspond with hormonal investigations. Dr. Prior makes a strong case for the use of symptothermal methods as a convenient and accurate method of prospective research. In clinical situations, the use of basal body temperature graphing has been found wanting, as up to 75% of patients displaying monophasic basal body temperature graphs were proven ovulatory on progesterone measurement, endometrial biopsy, or both (4, 30, 34, 36). The accuracy of absent cyclical molimina as an index of anovulation must also be questioned.

Table 58.1   Subclinical Changes in HPG Function in Men and Women With Training

	Type of study	Reference
Changes in men		
Decreased circulating testosterone	Cross-sectional	53
Decreased circulating testosterone	Longitudinal	48
Decreased circulating testosterone	Cross-sectional	1
Decreased circulating testosterone	Prospective	54
Decreased LH and FSH response to GnRH	Cross-sectional	29
Decreased LH pulse frequency	Cross-sectional	29
Decreased LH pulse frequency	Prospective	54
Changes in women		
Decreased late follicular estradiol levels	Prospective	5
Decreased luteal progesterone levels	Cross-sectional	19
Decreased LH and FSH response to GnRH	Prospective	6
Decreased LH pulse frequency	Cross-sectional	13
Further decrease in LH pulse frequency following acute exercise	Correlated samples	14

From an analysis of 1,400 patients attending an infertility clinic, we found 10 patients with regular menses (25- to 35-day intervals) and absent cyclical molimina (author's unpublished data). Eight of the 10 patients were ovulatory by criteria of mid-luteal serum progesterone measurement and late-luteal endometrial biopsy. Hormonal measurement, however inconvenient, remains the cornerstone of an accurate assessment of change. Large-scale prospective studies using the most accurate technology would clarify the questions raised by Dr. Prior's comparisons among groups of runners and nonrunners.

Overt Reproductive Dysfunction in Women Athletes

In some women, at an individual threshold based on factors to be discussed here, subclinical reproductive change becomes overt reproductive dysfunction with oligomenorrhea or amenorrhea occurring. Corresponding clinically apparent changes may occur in some men. Abnormally low levels of gonadal steroids and impaired spermatogenesis have been described in runners with high exercise loads, decreased body fat, and high stress scores (1).

Menarche is delayed in competitive athletes and ballet dancers when compared with nonexercising control groups or the population mean (22, 24, 31,

32, 33, 51). Although a variety of explanations unrelated to exercise were offered for the delay in menarche (11), Frisch et al. (22) suggested that physical activity itself is responsible for the delay because it is proportional to the number of years spent in training. In a longitudinal study of teenage ballet dancers in a professional ballet school, advancement of pubertal stages, onset of menstruation, and resumption of menstruation occurred at times of rest during vacations or following injuries (51). The findings of this study cannot explain the mechanisms involved because factors other than activity (e.g., small changes in body composition, changes in relative energy expenditure, and reduced physical stress) are also occurring.

In the first significant study of secondary amenorrhea in women runners, Feicht et al. (20) sent a questionnaire to 400 collegiate athletes and received 128 replies from women not taking birth control pills. Women runners who had experienced three periods or less in the previous year were defined as having secondary amenorrhea. The frequency of amenorrhea, as defined, varied from 6% to 43% depending on weekly mileage. Speroff and Redwine (46) found 46 of 872 (5.3%) respondents to be amenorrheic. Only 18.6% of respondents were running more than 20 mi per week and there did not appear to be an increase with increasing mileage. Dale et al. (15) found the frequency of oligomenorrhea in runners, joggers, and nonexercising controls to be 34%, 23%, and 4%, respectively. Similarly, Shangold and Levine

(45) found 16% and 2% of women during marathon training to be oligomenorrheic and amenorrheic, respectively, and Lutter and Cushman (28) found 19.3% to be irregular and 3.4% to be amenorrheic in a similar group. The point prevalence of amenorrhea in nonathletic women of similar age has been estimated at approximately 2% in studies based on representative samples (11). No similar estimates are available for the frequency of oligomenorrhea. Estimates of point prevalence of amenorrhea in the studies of women runners have relied on responses to questionnaire surveys. These may give a somewhat biased view because it may be assumed that runners with problems may respond to the survey with greater frequency than do normally menstruating runners. On the basis of these cross-sectional studies, Shangold and Levine (45) suggested that there is not in fact a significant increase in exercise-associated amenorrhea.

Runners with secondary amenorrhea generally have a hypothalamic amenorrhea with low normal or low serum gonadotropin and estradiol levels (Table 58.2). Others have reported similar results. The findings suggest that women with exercise-associated amenorrhea or oligomenorrhea have a symptomatic exaggeration of the subclinical changes. The question of why menstrual irregularity should occur in runners has received considerably more attention in recent years. Amenorrheic runners may have significant advantages in speed compared with their normally menstruating peers (42, 45), but it is not essential to develop oligomenorrhea to be involved in exercise at the highest levels (16). Other factors are summarized in Table 58.3 and are discussed in more detail.

Physical Stress of Training and Competition

Acute exercise is physically stressful, producing alterations in cardiac, pulmonary, and metabolic function at several sites including hepatic, pancreatic, and muscle metabolism. As discussed previously, cross-sectional studies to determine whether increasing training load increases frequency of oligomenorrhea have produced conflicting data and varied interpretations (11). The question of exercise intensity (e.g., speed of running) has received scant attention.

Prospective training studies have supported the contention that most women who have regular menses when they initiate training continue to do so with increased training volume (37). None of

Table 58.2 Findings on Investigation of 25 Runners With Runners' Amenorrhea

Hormone levels	n
Serum gonadotropin levels	
Low normal LH and FSH	16
Hypogonadotropic	8
High LH-FSH ratio	1
Serum estradiol levels	
Low normal	17
Subnormal	8

Table 58.3 Pathophysiological Factors of Exercise-Induced Changes in Reproductive Function

The physical stress of training or competing
The emotional stress of training or competing
Abnormalities of nutrition and energy drain
Altered lean-to-fat ratio
Loss of weight
Predisposition
Acute hormonal changes with exertion
Chronic hormonal effects of training

18 normally menstruating runners who added 50 mi per week to their training volume became amenorrheic despite clear effects on the reproductive system (5, 6). Women in Prior's studies retained cycles, although there were some very clear effects of training on BBT and perimenstrual symptomatology (37, 38). In contrast, 5 of 13 regularly menstruating swimmers became oligomenorrheic when weekly training volume was increased from 60 to 100 km per week (40, 41). An effect of training intensity, volume, or both in the genesis of the reproductive dysfunction seems to be a commonsense finding, but the evidence is far from conclusive.

Overtraining has become accepted as a clinically recognizable syndrome following the excellent study by Barron et al. (3), which summarized the clinical features of overtraining and documented elevated basal serum cortisol levels and a subnormal cortisol response to exogenous ACTH. The study did not examine the reproductive status of runners. Most of the women who complain of oligomenorrhea or amenorrhea present as healthy young women without specific complaint other than their change in menses. There is no evidence linking reproductive dysfunction with the over-training syndrome.

Emotional Stress of Training and Competing

Early authors suggested that trying to fit exercise or competition into a busy schedule was bound to cause psychological stress. When women runners were asked to evaluate subjectively to the degree of stress associated with training, amenorrheic runners reported significantly more stress than did their normally menstruating counterparts (42). Time of menarche was normal in young musicians seeking a professional career, but was delayed by approximately 3 yr in ballet dancers (51). Assuming that the goal-oriented lifestyle provided a similar degree of stress for each group, the author suggested that the delay in menarche was not entirely related to stress. Studies of psychological changes in women runners have not produced any characteristic findings and have been reviewed in detail (11). There is scant evidence that the menstrual irregularity associated with physical activity has as its primary origin either psychological or psychiatric problems. Even when differences in psychological well-being have been shown between normally menstruating and amenorrheic runners, these differences have statistical rather than clinical significance.

Nutrition, Body Composition, and Physical Activity

Physical activity tends to be anorexigenic; studies have reported inappropriately low increases in caloric intake when energy expenditure is increased. Absolute decrease in caloric intake in circumstances in which nutrition is not in doubt may have a direct influence on gonadotropin secretion (17, 26) and some evidence has supported the concept of a specific nutritional cocktail that can stimulate gonadotropin secretion (47). Cross-sectional studies have attempted to address the question of specific dietary deficiencies being responsible for symptomatic reproductive change but have provided conflicting evidence of various macronutrient deficiencies in amenorrheic athletes (7, 16, 27, 42, 43). In general, there are problems with the methodology for assessing nutritional status, as the accuracy of diet diaries and the data banks used to assess them is open to question.

Low body fat is not a prerequisite for, nor is it invariably accompanied by, symptomatic reproductive change in runners. Nevertheless, thin athletes and those with a history of a large weight loss following the initiation of running are more likely to be symptomatic (42). A prospective study has also indicated that a controlled caloric intake in association with strenuous exercise leads to a greater number and degree of hormonal and cycle reproductive changes than does a diet designed to maintain body weight (8). The various methods of assessing body fat can produce conclusions that are method specific in the same population (12). Despite the methodological problems—that is, despite the difficulties in clarifying the mechanism(s) of action through which body composition, nutrition, and exercise are linked to symptomatic and asymptomatic reproductive changes—the link is clear and worthy of further investigation.

Predisposition to Menstrual Irregularity

Women with reproductive dysfunction associated with exercise tend to be younger than those reporting regular menstrual cycles (15, 28, 42, 44, 49). Exercise at a young age may influence both the timing of menarche and subsequent menstrual function while continuing exercise (21). Women with regular cycles or a pregnancy before beginning exercise have less tendency to develop irregularity (28, 42, 44). The consistent findings suggest a predisposition to menstrual irregularity in some women. It is unclear how this might be investigated further.

Risk-Benefit Ratio

Warren et al. (52) investigated the relationship between delay in menarche and secondary amenorrhea and the occurrence of scoliosis or fractures in a population of professional ballet dancers. There is a clear association of primary and secondary amenorrhea, abnormal eating attitudes, and scoliosis or fractures. Dr. Prior has raised questions about bone loss even in women who continue to menstruate. In contrast, a large retrospective study has suggested that, if activity-associated fractures are excluded, former college athletes are no more likely to fracture than are controls (55). Other benefits were suggested, such as reductions in the prevalence of hormone-dependent tumors and diabetes mellitus (21, 23). It would appear from the series of studies from Harvard that there may indeed be benefits from exercise at college and that some of our fears can be laid to rest. Unfortunately, these kinds of retrospective studies cannot differentiate among some very pertinent questions, such as the effects of prolonged amenorrhea.

Management of Exercise-Associated Reproductive Dysfunction in Women

Delay in puberty, secondary amenorrhea, and oligomenorrhea should be evaluated. Potentially significant symptoms should not be ignored merely because they occur in women athletes. The patients are individuals with anxieties, stresses, questions, and problems that may include lethal disease, and they must be dealt with as individuals to resolve the questions that relate to them (Table 58.4). Shangold's suggestion that women with symptomatic change "should continue exercise while undergoing thorough evaluation and *where appropriate* treatment" (p. 110, emphasis added) is reasonable to define the significance of a symptom (44).

Table 58.4 Management of Exercise-Associated Amenorrhea

Full medical history including lifestyle information and physical examination

Exclude significant disease (or manage specific disorders if found)

Evaluate and manage individual needs and problems

1. Consequences of amenorrhea
   Risk of osteoporosis?
   Dyspareunia?
   Risk of endometrial carcinoma?
2. Reproductive needs
   Contraception?
   Ovulation induction?

Despite the early research it appears that amenorrhea is only slightly more frequent in women who exercise. Minimal investigation (measurement of LH, FSH, prolactin, estradiol, and thyroid screen including TSH) should be performed to locate the focus of the change. If this is not clearly central in nature, the question of a significant incidental disease process is clearly paramount. Exclusion of a central structural lesion using coned pituitary X rays will provide reassurance that the problem is functional. Earlier assessment of the relative contributions of predisposition, dietary deficiencies, body composition,

stress, and exercise will permit an assessment of nonpharmacological interventions.

Pharmacological interventions may be required if there are specific problems or reproductive needs. The question of bone loss in amenorrheic athletes has become foremost in the concerns related to amenorrheic athletes. Most centers do not have access to methodology that is sufficiently accurate to pick up the loss of bone (10). The question of the need to provide support for the skeleton needs to be addressed in the light of findings that risk of subsequent fractures is not increased in former college athletes. The problem of management of minimal bone losses is likely to be as controversial in athletes as it is in perimenopausal and postmenopausal women. Estrogen replacement has been the drug of choice, although, as was shown a decade ago, progestational agents (norethindrone and medroxyprogesterone) were effective in preventing bone loss (10).

The question of needing to reduce the risk of endometrial cancer is also debatable because again, as Frisch has shown, the risk is reduced in former college athletes. Perhaps it is appropriate at this time to start investigating women with exercise-associated reproductive function with endometrial biopsies to see whether changes occur in the endometrium. Dyspareunia can be solved by estrogen cream or lubricants. It may seem illogical to discuss contraception in amenorrheic women, but clearly in these women ovulation can occur without warning and may result in pregnancy. The management of the runner for whom adequate contraception is essential is not different from that of other amenorrheic women.

In runners seeking pregnancy, the primary management approach involves a change in lifestyle that returns to the physiological norms of body composition and diet, as well as a reduction in exercise load. I and others have had difficulty in inducing ovulation in runners who continue to maintain low body fat and high exercise loads even with the complex technology of GnRH pumps available. There are no data that I am aware of that support the use of cyclic progesterone to induce the return of normal menses, and it is not recommended.

Clinically Apparent Reproductive Changes in Men

In contrast to the cyclic nature of the endocrine control of reproduction in women, the endocrine control of the male reproductive system is steady state with a typical endocrine servomechanism. Symptomatic changes in testicular androgenesis and spermatogenesis are slower and less clearly definable. There is some evidence that males with a high level of physical activity do have some impairment of fertility (2). In an artificial insemination program, donors with a high physical activity profile and low semen volume had significantly lower pregnancy rates than did those with normal activity and low semen volume. When semen volume was normal, there was no reduction in fertility. We have anecdotal evidence from several subjects that semenanalysis may be maintained normal despite a very high weekly training mileage.

Anecdotal data has also suggested that libido may be impaired in some runners during periods of intense endurance training (53). Reduced testosterone levels may play a role in this, but chronic fatigue could also be a significant factor. The only large-scale study of sexuality in runners was published in *The Runner* (18). Although the scientific validity of the findings may be questioned, it is surprising that almost one quarter of the male respondents to the questionnaire would be prepared to give up sex before running, and almost half admitted that they sometimes felt too tired from running to engage in sex. The positive replies to this question increased with increasing mileage.

So little is known of short- or long-term problems with exercise-induced symptomatic reproductive change in men that it is impossible at present to provide advice on the management of the situation other than to review with the athlete the possibility of decreasing the exercise load. It is generally thought that puberty is not influenced by physical activity in men (50), but perhaps it is time to take a closer look at some specific questions. I have been made aware of teenage wrestlers whose growth potential appears to be reduced by "making weight." Such anecdotal information provides only questions that must be answered.

Exercise and Pregnancy

Because more women are involved in physical activity during their reproductive years, it may be anticipated that they would wish to continue their usual exercise regimens during their pregnancies. Speroff and Redwine (46) found that 7.3% of respondents to their questionnaire were running while pregnant. Pregnancy is associated with specific adaptations in the mother because the fetus is dependent on her for nutrition, respiration, and excretion. Possible maternal hazards include the physiological and anatomical difficulties of exercising in late pregnancy, the problems of joint laxity, postural change, and the increased tendency to minor accidents that occurs during pregnancy. From a fetal point of view, the questions essentially concern short- and long-term supply of oxygen and their essential nutrients, although the possibility of major injury through direct trauma to the uterus and exercise-induced increases in temperature are of at least theoretical importance.

Hard physical work has been associated with poorer pregnancy outcome, but the need for manual labor may be associated with inadequate nutrition and suboptimal health care. Extrapolation of these data and the findings from various animal experiments where stressful, forced exercise was employed is difficult to justify. The belief that exercise, including antenatal exercise, is beneficial to pregnancy by shortening labor and improving neonatal outcome is not generally confirmed in prospective studies. Small, prospective studies, with one recent exception (25), have not shown any significant benefit for exercising women who were accustomed to physical exercise during pregnancy compared with those who were not. Retrospective studies have not shown any convincing evidence of significant benefit or, equally important, of significant harm from chronic repeated exercise during pregnancy. There is some evidence that heavy exercise loads throughout pregnancy may adversely affect neonatal outcome with spontaneous premature rupture of the membranes and premature delivery being associated (11). Prospective studies have tended to suggest that babies are smaller than average when the mother exercised throughout pregnancy. Some studies have reported a higher frequency of obstetric complications and operative deliveries in runners, whereas others have reported no significant problems in women who exercised extensively during their pregnancies.

Measurement of fetal well-being during acute exercise has been indirect, relying on fetal heart rate measurements of short-term responses; but varying patient types, exercise load, and monitoring systems have made comparison of the studies difficult. Studies have suggested that fetal heart rate patterns may change with exercise with an intraexercise bradycardia being most commonly seen (11). Fetal breathing movements responded to maternal exercise more readily than did fetal heart rate, and it was suggested that this may provide a more sensitive test of fetal well-being. Because of the technical difficulties of obtaining adequate recordings, studies of breathing movements and fetal heart variability, both of which are sensitive to fetal difficulties, have not provided good indications of fetal well-being during exercise. Fetal activity has been reported to be reduced following exercise (9). It may be assumed that acute effects on the fetus result from a decreased oxygen supply through a redistribution of blood supply. Although the venerable study by Morris et al. (35) supports the concept that this may happen in humans, most data result from animal experiments in which forced exercise was used.

Many questions remain to be answered about exercise in pregnancy. Does exercise during pregnancy have any demonstrable benefit in terms of labor and delivery, pregnancy outcome, or recovery? What types of exercise are safe? Is there a point beyond which the exercise becomes unsafe for mother or fetus? Do some medical problems contraindicate exercise in pregnancy? There is clearly conflict in studies that deal with the effect of exercise. In general, the well-being of the mother and fetus are not harmed by physical activity that is kept within reasonable bounds. Unfortunately, these bounds are not well defined. Recommendations about exercise tend to be common sense and have little hard fact to back them up (11).

Conclusion

Early studies focus on the abnormalities of reproduction that occur in women athletes. The suggestion of an abnormally high frequency of amenorrhea has not been supported by cross-sectional and prospective studies, although physical activity is associated with some interesting changes in the neuroendocrinologic control of the gonads in both men and women.

Exercise-associated reproductive changes can be induced by training and can provide some of the most interesting insights on how neuroendocrinologic systems work with data that have been among the most fascinating in the last decade. Patients with overt reproductive dysfunction who fall outside the bounds of normality need to be investigated and managed. Management of most patients does not involve the use of medications but rather a reduction of exercise load and the correction of abnormalities of diet and body composition. Present research into, for example, bone loss is picking up subclinical decreases in bone by a methodology that generally is not available for

clinical use and that and that may be clinically irrelevant in the long term.

We do not have a full picture of the significance of reproductive dysfunction and the subclinical changes associated with exercise. The challenge of investigating exercise-associated reproductive dysfunction is still with us. We need to understand mechanisms and long-term significance much better. We need to understand exercise in pregnancy much better. We need to be unafraid that findings will be used for political purposes. Nothing has been discovered in any of the research that should stop women or men from exercising. We suggested several years ago (39) that exercise-associated reproductive dysfunction was reversible, and nothing has contradicted that.

References

1. Ayers, J.W.T., Y. Komesu, T. Romain, and R.A. Ansbacher. Anthropometric, hormonal and psychologic correlates of semen quality in endurance trained male athletes. *Fertil. Steril.* 43: 917-921, 1985.
2. Baker, E.R., R. Leuker, and P.G. Stumpf. Relationship of exercise to semen parameters and fertility success of artificial insemination donors. *Fertil. Steril.* 41: 107S, 1984.
3. Barron, J.L., T.D. Noakes, W. Levy, C. Smith, and R.P. Millar. Hypothalamic dysfunction in overtrained athletes. *J. Clin. Endocrinol. Metab.* 60: 803-806, 1985.
4. Bauman, J.E. Basal body temperature unreliable method of ovulation detection. *Fertil. Steril.* 36: 729-732, 1981.
5. Boyden, T.W., R.W. Pamenter, P. Stanforth, T.C. Rotkis, and J.H. Wilmore. Sex steroids and endurance running in women. *Fertil. Steril.* 39: 629-632, 1983.
6. Boyden, T.W., R.W. Pamenter, P. Stanforth, T.C. Rotkis, and J.H. Wilmore. Impaired gonadotropin responses to gonadotropin releasing hormone stimulation in endurance trained women. *Fertil. Steril.* 41: 359-363, 1984.
7. Brooks, S.M., C.F. Sanborn, B.H. Albrecht, and W.W. Wagner. Diet in athletic amenorrhea [Letter]. *Lancet* i: 559-560, 1984.
8. Bullen, B.A., G.S. Skrinar, I.Z. Beitins, G. von Mering, B.A. Turnbull, and J.W. McArthur. Induction of menstrual disorders by strenuous exercise in untrained women. *N. Engl. J. Med.* 312: 1349-1353, 1985.

9. Clapp, J.F. Fetal heart rate response to running in middle and late pregnancy. *Am. J. Obstet. Gynecol.* 153: 251-252, 1985.

10. Cumming, D.C. Osteoporosis: Investigation and management of women at risk. *SOGC Bull.* 10: 17-29, 1988.

11. Cumming, D.C. The reproductive effects of exercise. *Curr. Probl. Obstet. Gynecol.* 10: 231-285, 1987.

12. Cumming, D.C., and R.W. Rebar. Lack of consistency in the indirect methods of estimating percent body fat. *Fertil. Steril.* 41: 739-742, 1984.

13. Cumming, D.C., M.M. Vickovic, S.R. Wall, and M.R. Fluker. Defects in pulsatile LH release in normally menstruating runners. *J. Clin. Endocrinol. Metab.* 60: 810-812, 1985.

14. Cumming, D.C., M.M. Vickovic, S.R. Wall, M.R. Fluker, and A.N. Belcastro. The effect of acute exercise on pulsatile release of luteinizing hormone in women runners. *Am. J. Obstet. Gynecol.* 153: 482-485, 1985.

15. Dale, E., D.H. Gerlach, and A.L. Wilhite. Menstrual dysfunction in distance runners. *Obstet. Gynecol.* 54: 47-53, 1979.

16. Deuster, P.A., S.B. Kylem, P.B. Moser, R.A. Vigersky, A. Singh, and E.B. Schoomaker. Nutritional intakes and status of highly trained amenorrheic and eumenorrheic women runners. *Fertil. Steril.* 46: 636-643, 1986.

17. Dubey, A.K., J.L. Cameron, R.A. Steiner, and T.M. Plant. Inhibition of gonadotropin secretion in castrated male Rhesus monkeys (Macaca mulatta) induced by dietary restriction: Analogy with the prepubertal hiatus of gonadotropin release. *Endocrinology* 118: 518-525, 1986.

18. Editorial. Special survey: Running and sex. *The Runner,* May 1982, p. 26-35.

19. Ellison, P.T., and C. Lager. Exercise-induced menstrual disorders. *N. Engl. J. Med.* 313: 825-826, 1985.

20. Feicht, C.B., T.S. Johnson, B.J. Martin, K.E. Sparkes, and W.W. Wagner, Jr. Secondary amenorrhea in athletes [Letter]. *Lancet* ii: 1145-1146, 1978.

21. Frisch, R.E., G. Wyshak, N.L. Albright, T.E. Albright, I. Schiff, K.P. Jones, J. Witischi, E. Shiang, E. Koff, and M. Marguglio. Lower prevalence of breast cancer and cancers of the reproductive system among former college athletes compared to non-athletes. *Br. J. Cancer* 52: 885-891, 1985.

22. Frisch, R.E., A.V. Gotz-Welbergen, J.W. McArthur, T.E. Albright, J. Witischi, B. Bullen, J. Birnholtz, R.B. Reed, and H. Hermann. Delayed menarche and amenorrhea of college athletes in relation to age of onset of training. *JAMA* 246: 1559-1563, 1981.

23. Frisch, R.E., G. Wyshak, T.E. Albright, N.L. Albright, and I. Schiff. Lower prevalence of diabetes in female former college athletes compared with nonathletes. *Diabetes* 35: 1101-1105, 1986.

24. Frisch, R.E., G. Wyshak, and L. Vincent. Delayed menarche and amenorrhea in ballet dancers. *N. Engl. J. Med.* 303: 17-19, 1980.

25. Hall, D.C., and D.A. Kauffman. Effects of aerobic and strength conditioning on pregnancy outcomes. *Am. J. Obstet. Gynecol.* 157: 1199-1203, 1987.

26. Klibanski, A., I.Z. Beitins, T. Badger, R. Little, and J.W. McArthur. Reproductive function during fasting in men. *J. Clin. Endocrinol. Metab.* 53: 258-263, 1981.

27. Lloyd, T., J.R. Buchanan, S. Bitzer, C.J. Waldman, C. Myers, and B.G. Ford. Interrelationships of diet, athletic activity, menstrual status and bone density among collegiate women. *Am. J. Clin. Nutr.* 46: 681-684, 1987.

28. Lutter, J.M., and S. Cushman. Menstrual patterns in female runners. *Phys. Sportsmed.* 10(9): 60-72, 1982.

29. MacConnie, S.E., A. Barkan, R.M. Lampman, M.A. Schork, and I.Z. Beitins. Decreased hypothalamic gonadotropin releasing hormone secretion in male marathon runners. *N. Engl. J. Med* 315: 411-417, 1986.

30. Magyar, D.M., S.P. Boyers, J.R. Marshall, and G.E. Abraham. Regular menstrual cycles and premenstrual molimina as indicators of ovulation. *Obstet. Gynecol.* 53: 411-414, 1979.

31. Malina, R.M., C. Bouchard, R.F. Shoup, A. Demirjian, and G. Lariviere. Age at menarche, family size and birth order in athletes at the Olympic Games, 1976. *Med. Sci. Sports Exerc.* 11: 354-358, 1979.

32. Malina, R.M., W.W. Spirduso, C. Tate, and A.M. Baylor. Age at menarche and selected menstrual characteristics in athletes at different competitive levels and in different sports. *Med. Sci. Sports Exerc.* 10: 218f-222, 1978.

33. Malina, R.M., A.B. Harper, H.H. Avent, and D.E. Campbell. Age at menarche in athletes and non-athletes. *Med. Sci. Sports* 5: 11-13, 1973.

34. Moghissi, K.S. Accuracy of basal body temperature for ovulation detection. *Fertil. Steril.* 34: 89-98, 1980.

35. Morris, N., S.B. Osborn, and H.P. Wright. Effective uterine blood flow during exercise in normal and pre-eclamptic pregnancies. *Lancet* ii: 481-484, 1956.

36. Orrell, K.G.S., W. Wrixon, and A.C. Irwin. The prediction of ovulation. *Nova Scotia Med. Bull.* 59: 119-124, 1980.

37. Prior, J.C. Menstrual cycle changes with training: Anovulation and short luteal phase. *Can. J. Appl. Sports Sci.* 7: 173-177, 1982.

38. Prior, J.C., Y. Vigna, N. Alojado, D. Sciaretta, and M. Schulzer. Conditioning exercise decreases premenstrual symptoms: A prospective controlled six month trial. *Fertil. Steril.* 47: 402-408, 1987.

39. Rebar, R.W., and D.C. Cumming. Reproductive function in women athletes. *JAMA* 246: 1590, 1981.

40. Russell, J.B., D. Mitchell, P.I. Musey, and D.C. Collins. The relationship of exercise to anovulatory cycles in female athlete: Hormonal and physical characteristics. *Obstet. Gynecol.* 63: 452-456, 1984.

41. Russell, J.B., D. Mitchell, P.I. Musey, and D.C. Collins. The role of β-endorphin and catecholestrogens on the hypothalamic-pituitary axis in female athletes. *Fertil. Steril.* 42: 690-695, 1984.

42. Schwartz, B., D.C. Cumming, E. Riordan, M. Selye, S.S.C. Yen, and R.W. Rebar. Exercise associated amenorrhea: A distinct entity? *Am. J. Obstet. Gynecol.* 1141: 662-670, 1981.

43. Schweiger, U., F. Herman, R. Laessle, W. Riedel, M. Schweiger, and K.-M. Pirke. Caloric intake, stress and menstrual function in athletes. *Fertil. Steril.* 49: 447-450, 1988.

44. Shangold, M.M. Menstrual disturbances in the athlete. *Prim. Care* 11: 109-114, 1984.

45. Shangold, M.M., and H.S. Levine. The effect of marathon training on menstrual function. *Amer. J. Obstet. Gynecol.* 143: 862-869, 1982.

46. Speroff, L., and D.B. Redwine. Exercise and menstrual function. *Phys. Sportsmed.* 8(5): 42-52, 1979.

47. Steiner, R.A. Nutritional and metabolic factors in the regulation of reproductive hormone secretion in the primate. *Proc. Nutr. Soc.* 46: 159-175, 1987.

48. Strauss, R.H., R.R. Lanese, and W.B. Malarkey. Weight loss in amateur wrestlers and its effect on testosterone levels. *JAMA* 254: 3337-3338, 1985.

49. Wakat, D.K., K.A. Sweeney, and A.D. Rogol. Reproductive system function in women cross country runners. *Med. Sci. Sports Exerc.* 14: 263-269, 1982.

50. Wall, S.R., and D.C. Cumming. Effects of physical activity on reproductive function and development in males. *Semin. Reprod. Endocrinol.* 3: 65-80, 1985.

51. Warren, M.P. The effects of exercise on pubertal progression and reproductive function in girls. *J. Clin. Endocrinol. Metab.* 51: 1150-1157, 1980.

52. Warren, M.P., J. Brooks-Gunn, L.H. Homlek, W.G. Hamilton, and L.F. Warren. Scoliosis and fractures in young ballet dancers: Relation to delayed menarche and secondary amenorrhea. *N. Engl. J. Med.* 314: 1348-1353, 1986.

53. Wheeler, G.D., S.R. Wall, A.N. Belcastro, and D.C. Cumming. Reduced serum testosterone and prolactin levels in male distance runners. *JAMA* 252: 514-516, 1984.

54. Wheeler, G.D., S. Williamson, M. Singh, W.D. Pierce, W.F. Epling, A.N. Belcastro, and D.C. Cumming. *Decreased serum total and free testosterone and LH pulse frequency with endurance training in men.* Endocrine Society Meeting, Indianapolis, June 1987 [Abstract].

55. Wyshak, G., R.E. Frisch, T.E. Albright, N.L. Albright, and I. Schiff. Bone fractures among former college athletes compared with nonathletes in the menopausal and postmenopausal years. *Obstet. Gynecol.* 69: 121-126, 1987.

Chapter 59

Exercise, Fitness, and Aging

Elsworth R. Buskirk

The relationship of physical activity to health status is one of major interest, particularly as it applies to the elderly. Some data on the prevalence of physical activity in the United States have been available since the 1960s, but they are relatively incomplete in regard to our elderly citizens (48). Information about regular exercise among the elderly was reported from the first National Health and Nutrition Examination Survey (30). Related exercise data were obtained in Canada during a 1976 survey (42). Although the collection of data on activity patterns continues, there are problems in assessing the true levels of physical activity among the elderly. Thus, our descriptions of physical activity in populations remain suspect, and the relationship among physical activity, health outcomes, and chronic disease are only beginning to be understood, with the possible exception of coronary heart disease and atherosclerosis.

Health status, physical fitness, exercise patterns, and the effectiveness of exercise prescription all are inextricably interrelated. Thus, the definition of a physically active population remains variable, and inferences from studies of physical activity versus health status remain tenuous. An improved understanding of the essential features of an appropriate physical activity regimen plus more definitive assessments of regular exercise and health status should be sought. Important steps in this direction have recently surfaced and include the recent review by Powell et al. (35) and the concerted efforts of Paffenbarger and his colleagues as well as investigations by many of those participating in this conference.

More information is also needed about the performance capabilities among the elderly, particularly strength and power. We have paid only moderate attention to these variables, whereas cardiovascular and oxygen delivery have been relatively well studied.

Initiation of Habitual Exercise and Subsequent Adherence to a Regimen

Although some attention has been given the question of subject or patient compliance with regular exercise regimens (11), less attention has been paid to the postprogram maintenance of the exercise habit (3, 19, 25, 26, 33, 45).

It has been our experience that adherence to a regularly scheduled exercise program by formerly relatively sedentary men is approximately 40%-50% participation in scheduled sessions at 18 mo. Others have found somewhat better adherence or compliance under special circumstances, particularly in those involved in rehabilitation from a myocardial infarction (33). In 1978 to 1981 we had the opportunity to evaluate exercise participation among those who had taken part in an earlier collaborative study of physical activity and cardiovascular disease at Pennsylvania State University (27, 47). The group of men randomly assigned to a supervised physical activity program in 1967 was restudied approximately 13 yr later. About 28% of these men engaged in some form of regular exercise (e.g., jogging), but their average time commitment was quite low, about 30 min per week during the year before the follow-up measurement (Tables 59.1 and 59.2).

Only 2 of the original 58 exercisers who were studied maintained an exercise regimen that approximated the original program amount. One subject at follow-up exceeded the amount of exercise in the original program. A plot of the jogging or running time for the exercise group revealed a year-by-year decline so that by 13 yr of follow-up the former exercise group and the control group participated in regular exercise to approximately the same extent, or about 40 min per week of what

Table 59.1 Mean Jogging or Running Hours per Week Immediately Before Exercise Program and During Follow-Up

Study group	n	Preprogram, 1967 Mean	± SE_M	Follow-up, 1979 Mean	± SE_M	Student's t test on difference (p)
N	89	0.02	0.01	0.19	0.07	.0145
W	51	0.04	0.04	0.08	0.05	.5656
ME	47	0.01	0.01	0.16	0.09	.1012
E	58	0.00	0.00	0.31	0.08	.0002
C	46	0.01	0.01	0.30	0.14	.0402
VA	22	0.00	0.00	1.10	0.39	.0102
All subjects	313[a]	.01	.01	.27	.05	.0001
One-way ANOVA: F		0.58		5.88		
p		.7209		.0001		
Duncan's Multiple Range Test[b]		$\underline{W\ ME\ N\ C\ E}$ VA				

Note. SE_M = standard error of the mean; N = normals; W = withdrawals; ME = medical exclusions; E = exercise group; C = control group; VA = volitionally active. From "A 13-year Follow-up of a Coronary Heart Disease Risk Factor Screening and Exercise Program for 40- to 59-year Old Men: Exercise Habit Maintenance and Physiologic Status" by P.C. MacKeen, J.L. Rosenberger, J.S. Slater, W.C. Nicholas, and E.R. Buskirk, 1985, *Journal of Cardiopulmonary Rehabilitation*, **5**, pp. 510-523. Reprinted by permission.

[a]Unless otherwise indicated, total sample size in the tables that follows ranges from 310 to 315 (data incomplete for some variables).

[b]Groups connected by <u>bar</u> are not significantly different.

Table 59.2 Leisure-Time Physical Activity in Follow-Up

Study group	Aerobic activity (hr · wk^{-1})[a] Mean ± SE_M		Heavy AMI[b] (kcal · d^{-1}) Mean ± SE_M		Total leisure activity (kcal · d^{-1}) Mean ± SE_M	
N	0.62	0.18	62	8	336	22
W	0.25	0.10	77	13	325	32
ME	0.53	0.15	63	10	339	33
E	0.70	0.17	68	8	430	38
C	0.70	0.20	68	14	381	41
VA	4.53	0.79	331	37	755	80
All subjects	0.85	0.11	86	6	388	16
One-way ANOVA: F	25.34		36.87		11.13	
p	.0001		.0001		.0001	
Duncan's Multiple Range Test[c]	$\underline{W\ ME\ N\ E\ C}$ VA		$\underline{N\ ME\ C\ E\ W}$ VA		$\underline{W\ N\ ME\ C\ E}$ VA	

Note. Data derived from the Minnesota Leisure Time Physical Activity Interview. SE_M = standard error of the mean; N = normals; W = withdrawals; ME = medical exclusions; E = exercise group; C = control group; VA = volitionally active (as classified in 1966-1968 study). From "A 13-year Follow-up of a Coronary Heart Disease Risk Factor Screening and Exercise Program for 40- to 59-year Old Men: Exercise Habit Maintenance and Physiologic Status" by P.C. MacKeen, J.L. Rosenberger, J.S. Slater, W.C. Nicholas, and E.R. Buskirk, 1985, *Journal of Cardiopulmonary Rehabilitation*, **5**, pp. 510-523. Reprinted by permission.

[a]Includes activities with an aerobic component and assigned an intensity code of 5.5 or greater (Minnesota Leisure Time Physical Activity Interview), with the exception of cycling, which was included although its intensity code is 4.

[b]AMI = activity metabolic index, following the convention of Taylor et al. (46) as adapted from Buskirk et al. (8). Heavy AMI includes activities with an intensity code of 6 or greater.

[c]Groups connected by <u>bar</u> are not significantly different.

might be regarded as regular aerobic exercise (Table 59.1). The equality suggested a clear case of regression toward the mean. In contrast, a group of volitionally active men remained so and participated in about 4.5 hr per week of aerobic exercise. When risk factor profiles for coronary heart disease were compared at follow-up, there were no major differences between those in the exercise and those in control groups. A comparable study on women that involved only an 18-mo follow-up revealed comparable results, that is, a gradual but marked reduction in regular exercise (25) (Table 59.3).

Ilmarinen and Fardy (19) found much better retention of the exercise habit in a 3-yr follow-up of middle-aged Finnish men who were at a somewhat higher risk than were the men studied at Penn State. Twenty-eight percent of the subjects actually increased the amount of their regular exercise, 28% maintained about the same amount, and 43% decreased the amount compared to program quantities. Similarly, Oldridge (33) reported that 56% still exercised regularly 6 mo after completing a 6-mo exercise program. Bengtsson (3) reported that 43% of his subjects exercised regularly 1 yr following a 3-mo program, and Synder et al. (45) reported that 81% still exercised 9 mo or more following a 4- to 6-wk exercise program. Because these three studies involved myocardial infarction patients, these patients may have had greater motivation to continue regular exercise. Nevertheless, with the exception of the especially high participation at follow-up by the patients studied by Synder et al. (and this at about 9 mo), even the best studies imply a significant reduction in regular exercise once a supervised program of regular exercise is stopped.

Several factors may be responsible for the lack of adherence to a regular exercise program, but the subject's age appears to be an important factor, as does length of the follow-up period. The degree of specificity with which regular physical activity can be assessed by questionnaire or interview may play a role as well. In this regard, it should be noted that among the men studied at Penn State the maximal aerobic power ($\dot{V}O_2max$) results were consistent with the intergroup differences in regular physical activity (Table 59.4). There were no significant differences in $\dot{V}O_2max$ at follow-up when expressed in $L \cdot min^{-1}$ and only a modest difference favoring the exercise group when expressed as $ml \cdot kg^{-1} \cdot min^{-1}$. Because maximal heart rates were almost identical and maximal exercise intensities (METs) achieved, we concluded that there was an equivalent propensity to exercise to exhaustion.

Somewhat at variance with the picture of recidivism that has been painted are the exercise participation data obtained by Kasch et al. (21), who have been able to follow regular exercisers for a period of 20 yr. Although these men engage in different activities, they continue to do so three or more times per week and expend in excess of 2,000 kcal per week in following their exercise regimens. Our data for the volitionally active men generally yielded comparable information over the 13-yr period. Two important questions are How physically active are we? and What motivates some people to continue regular exercise while others decide against doing so? Some reasons for slacking off from the exercise habit are given in Table 59.5.

Although it was suggested in the previous section that the exercise habit is not easy to instill in most adults, there is limited evidence indicating

Table 59.3 Jogging Activity: Intention at Conditioning Program

	Program termination versus adherence at follow-up		
	Women with normal % body fat ($n = 10$)	Obese ($n = 18$)	All follow-up women ($n = 28$)
Intending to jog			
Number	8	14	22
Percentage of group	80	78	79
Actually jogging at follow-up			
Number	4	6	10
Percentage of group	40	33	36
Women not carrying out an intention to jog			
Number	4	8	12
Percentage of intending	50	57	54

Note. From "Body Composition, Physical Work Capacity and Physical Activity Habits at 18-month Follow-up of Middle-aged Women Participating in an Exercise Intervention Program" by P.C. MacKeen, B.A. Franklin, W.C. Nicholas, and E.R. Buskirk, 1983, *International Journal of Obesity, 7*, pp. 61-71. Reprinted by permission.

Table 59.4   Maximal Oxygen Uptake (ml · kg^{-1} · min^{-1}) Achieved in 1967-1968 and at Follow-Up (1978-1981)

Study group	n	Best test, 1967-1968 Mean ± SE_M		Follow-up, 1979-1981 Mean ± SE_M		Student's t test (p)
E	51	37.71	0.68	31.67	0.95	.0001
C	38	32.22	0.69	28.39	0.99	.0001
VA	21	41.88	0.96	36.45	1.65	.0006
All subjects	110	36.61	0.55	31.45	0.69	.0001
One-way ANOVA: F		32.76		9.76		
p		.0001		.0001		
Duncan's Multiple Range Test[a]		C̲ ̲E̲ VA		C̲ ̲E̲ VA		

Note. SE_M = standard error of the mean; E = exercise group; C = control group; VA = volitionally active (as classified in 1966-1968 study). From "A 13-year Follow-up of a Coronary Heart Disease Risk Factor Screening and Exercise Program for 40- to 59-year Old Men: Exercise Habit Maintenance and Physiologic Status" by P.C. MacKeen, J.L. Rosenberger, J.S. Slater, W.C. Nicholas, and E.R. Buskirk, 1985, *Journal of Cardiopulmonary Rehabilitation,* **5**, pp. 510-523. Reprinted by permission.

[a]Groups connected by <u>bar</u> are not significantly different.

Table 59.5   Reasons Given for Decreased Adherence to Activities of the Conditioning Program Following Its Termination, and Frequency of Mention

Stated reason	% of N[a]	% of O[b]	% of all subjects
1. Inability to find or make time, job demands, young children and family demands, pressure of university coursework or research, sick relative to care for, and move to new house	90 (9)	61 (11)	71 (20)
2. Poor self-discipline or motivation, no car for transportation to an exercise program, no parking proximal to exercise facilities, no exercise facilities near home, and hiatus between program termination and availability of other supervised exercise	44 (4)	44 (8)	43 (12)
3. Loss of social support afforded by the conditioning program group	20 (2)	33 (6)	28 (8)
4. Another leisure-exercise mode with aerobic component pursued	0	17 (3)	11 (3)
5. Less energy	20 (2)	0	7 (2)
6. Disappointment with lack of weight loss during program	0	6 (1)	4 (1)
7. High physical activity demand in occupation (but not at aerobic training intensity)	10 (1)	0	4 (1)
8. Significant weight gain following program	10 (1)	0	4 (1)
9. Dislike of jogging	10 (1)	0	4 (1)
10. Three rather than four or five sessions per week preferred	10 (1)	0	4 (1)

Note. Data are percentages of women citing reasons; the number of women citing reasons is given in parentheses. Many participants cited multiple reasons, and all are included. From "Body Composition, Physical Work Capacity and Physical Activity Habits at 18-month Follow-up of Middle-aged Women Participating in an Exercise Intervention Program" by P.C. MacKeen, B.A. Franklin, W.C. Nicholas, and E.R. Buskirk, 1983, *International Journal of Obesity,* **7**, pp. 61-71. Reprinted by permission.

[a]N = Women with normal percent body fat.

[b]O = Obese women.

an increase in regular participation in physical activity in the United States in recent years (4, 44). Still, present data are inadequate to quantify this suggested upward trend with precision. But what is some of the evidence? On the basis of a U.S. Public Health Service survey, Stephens et al. (44) reported that less than 20% of adults in the United States engage in an amount of exercise (frequency, intensity, and duration) sufficient to enhance their cardiovascular status. They found that about 40% of those surveyed were sedentary and that although another 40% did participate in some exercise, they did so infrequently. Blair et al. (4) found that among those presenting themselves in 1973 for evaluation and exercise prescription at the Cooper Clinic in Dallas, Texas, about 13% of the men and 11% of the women engaged in regular exercise. Those presenting themselves in 1985 indicated much greater participation in regular exercise, that is, 78% of the men and 60% of the women. The implication was that the population of those who seek evaluation and exercise prescription, at least in Texas, had changed during the 12-yr interval and that many more were physically active in 1985 compared to 1973. Similarly, Powell and Paffenbarger (34) reported an increased participation in vigorous sports activity among Harvard alumni over the period 1962-1977. Only 22% of those surveyed participated in vigorous sports activity in 1962. In 1977, 82% among those aged 45-49 yr did so, with 62% among those aged 60-64 showing reduced activity.

The additional point should be made that participation in vigorous sports tends to decrease with age despite organizational efforts to promote such events as competition for master's athletes. On review of the limited data, one has the overall impression of increased regular physical activity among today's citizens compared to 10-20 yr ago. Despite this impression, convincing longitudinal comparisons of regular physical activity of people as they age are rare, and the available data on adherence and compliance to a supervised exercise program and the results of follow-up studies run counter to the perceived national trend. The opportunity and necessity to obtain good longitudinal population statistics about regular exercise is clear, as is the need for better cross-sectional information.

Measurement of Physical Activity in Surveys

Physical activity implies participation in body movement, a complex behavior that can take many forms and for which there are a variety of types of assessments. Unfortunately, there are no standard measurement procedures short of the utilization of ergometers. The methods of assessment of regular physical activity have utilized a variety of techniques, including questionnaires and interviews, time motion studies, accelerometers, cumulative heart rate meters, pulmonary ventilation or oxygen uptake monitors, doubly labeled water turnover, and so on. For obvious reasons of practicality in surveys, most attention has been focused on the questionnaire interview approach. Wilson et al. (49) reviewed assessment methods and found most to be heterogeneous and insufficiently validated. Use of a person's history of physical activity and recall of physical activity for specific periods of time constitute the retrospective method. Here, acquisition of historical information is obtained by a self-administered questionnaire, and recall information is usually obtained by interview. An advantage of these procedures is that large groups can be surveyed at a reasonable cost but with some sacrifice in objectivity. Memory bias plays an important role and induces reasonably large variances with respect to precise designation of type, frequency, and duration of physical activity. Nevertheless, several investigators have attempted to refine the historical techniques.

A continuing effort to obtain reliable information has been under way for some time at the University of Minnesota (16, 47). These efforts have focused on leisure-time physical activity, as have our own (8). The University of Minnesota investigators reported high reliability with Spearman rank correlation coefficients between test and retest of 0.79-0.88 for total activity, ranging from 0.69 to 0.86 among the light-, moderate-, and heavy-intensity subcategories. In employing such techniques and using intertechnique comparisons, Salonen and Lakka (36) found three distinct dimensions for physical activity: activity at work, leisure-time exercise, and very strenuous sports activity. These three accounted for about 63% of the total variance in physical activity. However, one would like to do better.

Because of the problems in assessing regular physical activity, Powell et al. (35) set up several criteria for including studies in their review of exercise in the prevention of coronary heart disease. These included a clear operational definition of physical activity, a valid and reliable measurement instrument, a specific assignment identified with an individual, a clear description of the exercise dose, a description of the individual's past activity, and identification of the fact that the data were collected systematically so that summarization could take place. The selective process that Powell et al. (35) took in screening studies for well-documented physical activity participation provides a useful model for other researchers who are engaged in attempts to relate regular participation in physical activity to health status or incidence of chronic disease.

A complete history of activities documented with respect to type, frequency, intensity, and duration can serve several purposes. If a physical activity index is calculated, such as the activity metabolic index (AMI) (8), subpopulations or groups can be described and compared. If the index is translatable into standardized units such as METs or kcal $\cdot$ kg^{-1} $\cdot$ d^{-1}, dose-response effects or relationships can be examined, categories established, and estimates made of the prevalence of beneficial exercise. Estimates of benefit versus risk can also be obtained and effective comparisons made with similarly treated data in the literature.

Performance of Common Activities and Perception of Fitness in Relation to Age

The National Health Interview Survey has been conducted in approximately 42,000 households, and in 1984 a special supplement on aging was designed to collect information about physical limitations plus health-related and pertinent social information. Despite the fact that estimates of the prevalence of disability were based on "Yes" or "No" responses, useful approximations of the prevalence of disability were obtained because of the large sample (31). The report revealed that a greater percentage of women than of men had difficulty performing work-associated activities. Examples are provided in Tables 59.6 and 59.7. Although the gender-associated difference was minimal with respect to walking, it was quite marked with respect to lifting or carrying loads. Difficulty in performing the activities increased with age, as did the percentage of those unable to perform the respective tasks. People who were still employed were much less likely to have difficulty with a task than were those who were retired. Those who had retired because of ill health were the most likely to have difficulty with an activity. Essentially the same conclusions were drawn in relation to home-management activities that included the performance of heavy housework (32).

Although the elderly tend to underestimate their ability to exercise, they also tend to be satisfied

Table 59.6 Percentage of People 55-74 Years of Age Who Have Worked Since Age 45 With Difficulty or Inability to Walk 1/4 Mile

Sample	Age (yr)			
	55-59	60-64	65-69	70-74
Men				
Difficulty	12.3	17.0	20.1	23.3
Unable	5.0	7.9	9.4	8.7
Women				
Difficulty	12.6	15.8	19.9	26.6
Unable	5.8	8.0	7.9	10.2

Note. Data adapted from National Center for Health Statistics (31).

Table 59.7 Percentage of People 55-74 Years of Age Who Have Worked Since Age 45 With Difficulty or Inability to Lift or Carry 25 Pounds

Sample	Age (yr)			
	55-59	60-64	65-69	70-74
Men				
Difficulty	11.6	15.4	16.8	23.1
Unable	3.5	3.8	5.6	7.5
Women				
Difficulty	22.9	31.0	33.8	40.8
Unable	9.1	8.7	9.3	10.7

Note. Data adapted from National Center for Health Statistics (31).

with their physical fitness. Thus, McAvoy (27) found that among those 65 and older a perceived barrier to regular exercise was their concept of their physical ability. The physical fitness of those elderly city dwellers observed by Sidney and Shephard (40) was average or below, yet they perceived themselves as engaging in sufficient physical activity. It seems, therefore, that perception and reality among the elderly with respect to physical activity can be quite different and that the differences presumably are as great for activities involving strength and flexibility as for those involving respiratory-cardiovascular fitness. It seems important to improve the elderly's perceptions of physical activity through education that uses behavioral modification techniques and simple testing to effect a change in lifestyle that involves regular exercise.

Aspects of Skeletal Muscle Related to Regular Exercise

Attempts to counter the trend for becoming physically less active with age are only partially successful for most people, with an exception possibly for those who remain motivated as habitual exercisers. Although considerable attention has been paid to the changes in cardiovascular fitness with age, much less emphasis has been placed on what occurs in skeletal muscle. It is well known that maximal static and dynamic strength and maximal speed and power are reduced with diminished activity, particularly among the elderly. These reductions have been reviewed by several authors (2, 7, 17, 18, 29, 39, 41). The lack of willingness by many elderly people to engage in activities requiring strength and power may well be related to a somewhat erroneous perception of weakness. The emphasis here is on a brief, partial summarization of representative cross-sectional and longitudinal appraisals of muscular strength, endurance, and power in relation to aging and on the structural and functional changes that occur in skeletal muscle.

Strength represents the force developed by contracting muscles, and power represents the application of force per unit time. Both strength and speed are conceptually involved with power. Changes within skeletal muscle are associated with the age-related decline in strength and therefore in power. Nevertheless, the decline in power is enhanced because speed is reduced through lessened nerve-conduction velocity and synaptic transmission. An associated diminution in the speed of contraction of Type II fibers may occur, as may an increased threshold for muscle excitability.

The dramatic decrease in power is illustrated vividly by the performances in age-group competition in events such as the shot put, the discus throw, and the vertical and long jumps. Nor does training prevent a substantial decline, although the master's athlete seldom trains at the intensity that a younger counterpart does.

An experiment by Bosco and Komi (6) tested the ability of male subjects aged 4-73 yr to perform vertical jumps from a force platform following an initial squat (Table 59.8). Interpretation of the results indicated that the contractile force, power, and elastic properties increased up to the third decade and then decreased progressively thereafter. Several investigators have observed a profound decline in both knee-flexion and knee-extension capabilities. The investigation of Murray et al. (personal communication, 1984) serves as a good example (Table 59.9). Davies et al. (12) assessed the ability to develop power during cycling

Table 59.8 Force and Power Developed During Squatting Jump in Male Age Groups

Age group (yr)	n	Body weight (kg)	Average force (N)	Average power (W) (kg BW^{-1})
4-6	10	18 ± 2	114 ± 40	16 ± 4
13-17	19	56 ± 9	402 ± 92	22 ± 3
18-28	35	80 ± 10	618 ± 137	23 ± 4
29-40	16	79 ± 7	508 ± 153	17 ± 4
41-49	18	77 ± 12	435 ± 96	14 ± 3
54-65	4	76 ± 12	320 ± 23	19 ± 4
71-73	11	74 ± 8	315 ± 118	7 ± 3

Note. Data expressed as mean ± SE_M. Adapted from Bosco and Komi (6).

Table 59.9 Isometric Knee Flexor and Extensor Muscle Strength (kg/cm)

Age group (yr)	n	Flexor strength in 3 knee-joint positions			Extensor strength in 3 knee-joint positions		
		30°a,b	45°a,b	60°a,b,c	30°a	45°a,b,c	60°a,b,c
20-35	24	719 ± 37	792 ± 38	792 ± 36	1188 ± 58	1728 ± 83	1797 ± 69
42-61	24	682 ± 38	721 ± 40	676 ± 39	1056 ± 58	1444 ± 69	1402 ± 69
70-86	24	502 ± 33	510 ± 32	505 ± 31	903 ± 45	1110 ± 68	1124 ± 56

Note. Data expressed as mean ± SE_M and adapted from Murray et al. (personal communication, 1984).

[a]Youngest different from oldest ($p < .01$).

[b]Middle-aged different from oldest ($p < .01$).

[c]Youngest different from middle-aged ($p < .01$).

and vertical jumping in older (60 yr) and younger (22 yr) men. Significant decrements in contractile force and power were observed with age. Electrical stimulation experiments indicated that maximal plantar flexion force in the older men was 50%-60% of that in the younger men and that the muscles of older men contracted and relaxed less rapidly. The electrical stimulation experiments suggest that changes within skeletal muscle are relatively more important than is a change in the ability to recruit fibers.

There is some support for the concept that the force per cross-sectional area of functional contractile tissue remains relatively constant (23, 37). Thus, any loss of contractile tissue or gain in noncontractile material would decrease force per unit area of a limb and thereby apparent strength.

Experiments in which total body nitrogen and ^{40}K (10) were assessed indicated a loss of body cell mass with age and a greater loss of muscle mass than of nonmuscle lean tissue. Borkan et al. (5) found not only less lean tissue among the elderly but also greater fat content within and between muscles. Muscle biopsy investigations have found not only intramuscular fat and more connective tissue but also more lipofuscin granules as well as fiber atrophy in the elderly (38). Steen (43) has reviewed such studies and concluded that by age 70 there has been a 40% loss, compared to early adulthood, in skeletal muscle in contrast to losses of 20% or less in the mass of other tissues. Total body water tended to decrease in proportion to body cell mass.

It has been demonstrated repeatedly that regular resistance exercise can increase strength in the elderly (18, 28), perhaps through recruitment of more motor units but also because of some hypertrophy. Most of us are aware of examples of the preservation of strength into later life. Dummer et al. (14) provide an interesting example of two women who were master's swimmers. The women

(ages 70 and 71 yr) demonstrated superior strength and flexibility for their ages and, importantly, felt free to complete all strength tests at maximal levels and through a full range of motion because of confidence in their abilities.

Thus, a strong argument can be made for large interindividual differences with respect to functional differences in strength and power with age. The variance is largely dependent on the extent of participation in regular exercise. Nevertheless, a decline in muscular performance eventually is inevitable with advanced age.

Reductions in muscle tissue oxidative capacity (15), oxygen delivery (20), and contractile tissue suggest impaired muscular endurance, at least at relatively high intensities of strength. At low to moderate intensities of contraction, muscular endurance declines little with age until senescence intervenes (1).

To summarize, advanced age has significant deleterious effects on skeletal muscle that in turn reduce strength and power. Some of the changes in skeletal muscle with age are listed in Table 59.10. Muscle mass reduction with aging involves losses of muscle fibrils and muscle fibers (24) that may involve past injury and loss of motoneurons (Table 59.11). Injured muscle fibers may be lost because

Table 59.10 Changes in Skeletal Muscle With Age

Decreases	Increases
Muscle fiber size	Collagen cross-linking
Muscle fiber number	Ratio of Type I to
Myofibrillar ATPase activity	Type II fibers
ATP: creatine phosphate	Membrane excitability
Glycogen; glycolytic enzymes	threshold
Oxidative enzymes	Connective tissue
Mitochondrial protein	
Impulse conduction velocity	

Table 59.11 Estimates of Characteristics Determined From Cross Sections of Whole Vastus Lateralis Muscle

n	Age group (yr)	Age range (yr)	Muscle area (A) (mm²/48)[a]	Fiber density (D) (M/mm²)	Total fiber (A · D · 10³)	Type I fibers (%)
9	20	15-22	76 ± 10	179 ± 43	648 ± 164	50 ± 5
9	30	26-37	75 ± 9	168 ± 20	599 ± 85	50 ± 4
8	50	49-56	69 ± 11	175 ± 38	579 ± 173	52 ± 15
9	70	70-75	56 ± 7	142 ± 19	380 ± 70	52 ± 6
8	80	80-83	43 ± 9	158 ± 32	323 ± 79	55 ± 11

Note. Data expressed as mean ± SE_M. Adapted from Lexell et al. (24).

[a]48 areas counted.

of degeneration and a depressed regenerative capacity.

In rats, Daw et al. (13) have estimated that only about 25% of the observed skeletal muscle atrophy with aging can be accounted for by the loss in muscle fibers. Inactivity, through lack of fiber recruitment, can produce hypotrophy of existing fibers, and both Type I and Type II fibers are probably equally susceptible. The observation that there is selective loss of Type II fibers (22) may be associated with the limitations of needle biopsy samples obtained on a cross-sectional basis (9, 17). Muscle mass reduction also occurs from atrophy of existing fibers as well as from a reduction in fiber number (24). Regular exercise can modify the magnitude of functional decrement through the attenuation of fiber atrophy and perhaps the preservation of motoneuronal integrity. Nevertheless, some fiber loss is inevitably due to a centrally oriented loss of motoneurons and a lessened capacity for muscle fiber regeneration.

Conclusion

This chapter explored some aspects of regular physical activity as they relate to elderly people. It examined problems associated with the initiation and retention of, and adherence to, the exercise habit and has assessed the relative lack of information about our status as a physically active population. The difficulties with appraisal of physical activity in large surveys the decrease in ability to perform common activities, a less-than-accurate perception of fitness, and the modified aspects of skeletal muscle that appear related to the decrease in strength and power among the elderly all contribute to our relatively incomplete knowledge of exercise and aging. Little was said about the effects of disability or disease, both of which are important modifiers of function. Nevertheless, even among relatively healthy people, the problems identified are well worthy of pursuit, particularly on a longitudinal basis. Cross-sectional data have provided useful insights, but longitudinal appraisals are certainly needed. More attention should also be paid to the modifying effects that are possible through regular participation in well-planned exercise regimens. It is apparent that morphological and functional changes can be attenuated by regular activity and thus that capabilities can be retained, possibly well into advanced age. Simultaneous modifications in lifestyle that involve good nutrition, no smoking, no social drug use, moderation in use of alcohol, and so on may well supplement the effects of regular exercise. Also needed are basic studies of how mechanisms related to the neuro-motor-muscular system are modified by aging and affected by exercise. Activation and receptor physiology, together with cellular and subcellular metabolic interactions, deserve attention. Opportunities for significant research abound.

Acknowledgments

My thanks are expressed to Steven Segal, who conceptually contributed to the content of this manuscript and participated in the process of proofreading and to Becky Nilson, who typed and assembled the manuscript in its final form.

References

1. Aniansson, A., G. Grimby, N. Hedberg, A. Rungren, and L. Sperling. Muscle function in old age. *Scand. J. Rehabil. Med.* 6(Suppl.): 43-49, 1978.
2. Asmussen, E., and K. Heebøll-Nielsen. Isometric muscle strength of adult men and women. In: Asmussen, E., A. Fredsted, and E. Ryge, eds. *Communications from the Testing and Observations Institute of the Danish National Association for Infantile Paralysis.* Copenhagen, 1961, no. 11.
3. Bengtsson, K. Rehabilitation after myocardial infarction. *Scand. J. Rehabil. Med.* 15: 1-9, 1983.
4. Blair, S.N., R.T. Mulder, and H.W. Kohl. Reaction to "Secular trends in adult physical activity: Exercise boom or bust?" *Res. Q. Exer. Sport* 58: 106-110, 1987.
5. Borkan, G.A., D.E. Hults, A.F. Gerzof, A.H. Robbins, and C.K. Silbert. Age changes in body composition revealed by computer tomography. *J. Gerontol.* 38: 673-677, 1983.
6. Bosco, C., and P.V. Komi. Influence of aging on the mechanical behavior of leg extensor muscles. *Eur. J. Appl. Physiol.* 43: 209-219, 1980.
7. Buskirk, E.R. Health maintenance and longevity: Exercise. In: *Handbook of the Biology of Aging* (2nd ed.). Finch, C.E. and E.L. Schneider, eds. New York: Van Nostrand Reinhold, 1985: 894-931.
8. Buskirk, E.R., D. Harris, J. Mendez, and J. Skinner. Comparison of two assessments of physical activity and a survey method for caloric intake. *Am. J. Clin. Nutr.* 24: 1119-1125, 1971.

9. Buskirk, E.R., and S.S. Segal. The aging motor system: Skeletal muscle weakness. In: Spirduso, W.W., and H.M. Eckert, eds. *Physical Activity and Aging*. Champaign, IL: Human Kinetics, 1988: 19-36.

10. Cohn, S.H., D. Vartsky, S. Yasumura, A. Sawitsky, I. Zanzi, A. Vaswani, and K.J. Ellis. Compartmental body composition based on total-body nitrogen, potassium, and calcium. *Am. J. Physiol.* 239: E524-E530, 1980.

11. Compliance with Exercise. Part I: *J. Cardiac Rehab.* 4: 119-155; Part II: *J. Cardiac Rehab.* 4: 166-208, 1984.

12. Davies, C.T.M., J. White, and K. Young. Electrically evoked and voluntary maximal isometric tension in relation to dynamic muscle performance in elderly male subjects, aged 69 years. *Eur. J. Appl. Physiol.* 51: 37-43, 1983.

13. Daw, C.K., J.W. Starnes, and T.P. White. Muscle atrophy and hypoplasia with aging: Impact of training and food restriction. *J. Appl. Physiol.* 64: 2428-2432, 1988.

14. Dummer, G.M., P. Vaccaro, and D.H. Clarke. Muscular strength and flexibility of two female masters swimmers in the eighth decade of life. *J. Orthoped. Sports Phys. Therap.* 6: 235-237, 1985.

15. Farrar, R.P., T.P. Martin, and C.M. Arides. The interaction of aging and endurance exercise upon the mitochondrial function of skeletal muscle. *J. Gerontol.* 36: 642-647, 1981.

16. Folsom, A.R., D.R. Jacobs, C.J. Casperson, O. Gomez-Marin, and J. Knudsen. Test-retest reliability of the Minnesota leisure time physical activity questionnaire. *J. Chron. Dis.* 39: 505-511, 1986.

17. Green, H. Characteristics of aging human skeletal muscle. In: Sutton, J.R. and R.M. Brock, eds. *Sports medicine for the mature athlete*. Indianapolis: Benchmark Press, 1986, 17-26.

18. Hettinger, T. *Physiology of strength*. Springfield, IL: Charles C Thomas, 1961.

19. Ilmarinen, J., and P.S. Fardy. Physical activity intervention for males with high risk of coronary heart disease: A three-year follow-up. *Prev. Med.* 6: 416-425, 1977.

20. Irion, G.L., U.S. Vasthare, and R.F. Tuma. Age-related changes in skeletal muscle blood flow in the rat. *J. Gerontol.* 42: 660-665, 1987.

21. Kasch, F.W., J.P. Wallace, S.P. VanCamp, and L. Verity. A longitudinal study of cardiovascular stability in active men aged 45 to 65 years. *Phys. Sportsmed.* 16: 117-124, 1988.

22. Larsson, L. Morphological and functional characteristics of the aging skeletal muscle in man. *Acta Physiol. Scand. Suppl.* 457: 1-36, 1978.

23. Larsson, L., G. Grimby, and J. Karlsson. Muscle strength and speed of movement in relation to age and muscle morphology. *J. Appl. Physiol.* 46: 451-456, 1979.

24. Lexell, J., C.C. Taylor, and M. Sjöstrom. What is the cause of the aging atrophy? *J. Neurol. Sci.* 84: 275-294, 1988.

25. MacKeen, P.C., B.A. Franklin, W.C. Nicholas, and E.R. Buskirk. Body composition, physical work capacity and physical activity habits at 18-month follow-up of middle-aged women participating in an exercise intervention program. *Int. J. Obes.* 7: 61-71, 1983.

26. MacKeen, P.C., J.L. Rosenberger, J.S. Slater, W.C. Nicholas, E.R. Buskirk. A 13-year follow-up of a coronary heart disease risk factor screening and exercise program for 40-to 59-year old men: Exercise habit maintenance and physiologic status. *J. Cardiopulm. Rehabil.* 5: 510-523, 1985.

27. McAvoy, L.H. *Recreation preferences of the elderly persons in Minnesota*. Unpublished doctoral dissertation, University of Minnesota, Minneapolis, 1976.

28. Moritani, T., and H.A. deVries. Neural factors versus hypertrophy in the time course of muscle strength gain in young and old men. *J. Gerontol.* 36: 294-297, 1981.

29. Muir-Gray, J.A. Exercise and aging. In: MacLeod, D., R. Maughan, M. Nimmo, T. Reilly, and C. Williams, eds. *Exercise: Benefits, limits and adaptations*. New York: E. and F.N. Spon; 1987: 33-48.

30. National Center for Health Statistics. Plan and operation of the second National Health and Nutrition Examination Survey, 1976-1980. *Vital and Health Statistics* (Series 1, No. 15). Hyattsville, MD: Public Health Service, July 1981.

31. National Center for Health Statistics. M.G. Kovar and A.Z. LaCroix. Aging in the eighties: Ability to perform work-related activities. Data from the Supplement on Aging to the National Health Interview Survey, United States, 1984. *Advance Data from Vital and Health Statistics. No. 136.* (DHHS Pub. No. [PHS] 87-1250). Hyattsville, MD: Public Health Service, May 8, 1987.

32. National Center for Health Statistics. D. Dawson, G. Hendershot, and J. Fulton. Aging in the eighties, Functional limitations

of individuals age 65 years and over. *Advance Data from Vital and Health Statistics. No. 133.* (DHHS Pub. No. [PHS] 87-1250). Hyattsville, MD: Public Health Service, June 10, 1987.

33. Oldridge, N. Compliance and dropout in cardiac exercise rehabilitation. *J. Cardiac Rehabil.* 4: 166-177, 1984.

34. Powell, K.E., and R.S. Paffenbarger, Jr. Workshop on epidemiological public health aspects of physical activity and exercise: A summary. *Public Health Rep.* 100: 118-125, 1985.

son, and J.S. Kendrick. Physical activity and the incidence of coronary heart disease. *Ann. Rev. Public Health* 8: 253-287, 1987.

36. Salonen, J.R., and T. Lakka. Assessment of physical activity in population studies—Validity and consistency of the methods in the Kuopio ischemic heart disease risk factor study. *Scand. J. Sports Sci.* 9: 89-95, 1987.

37. Segal, S.S., J.A. Faulkner, and T.P. White. Architecture, composition and contractile properties of rat soleus muscle grafts. *Am. J. Physiol.* 250: C474-C479, 1986.

38. Shafiq, S.A., S.G. Lewis, L.C. Dimino, and H.S. Schutta. Electron microscopic study of skeletal muscle in elderly subjects. In: Kaldor, G., and W.J.D. Battista, eds. *Aging.* New York: Raven Press; 1978: vol. 6.

39. Shock, N.W. Systems integration. In: Finch, C., and L. Hayflick, eds. *Handbook of the biology of aging.* New York: Van Nostrand Reinhold; 1977: 639-665.

40. Sidney, K.H., and R.J. Shephard. Activity patterns of elderly men and women. *J. Gerontol.* 32: 25-32, 1977.

41. Skinner, J.S., C.M. Tipton, and A.C. Vailas. Exercise, physical training and the aging process. In: A. Viiduk, ed. *Lectures in Gerontology.* New York: Academic Press; 1982: vol. 1B, 407-439.

42. Statistics Canada. *Culture statistics/recreation activities 1976.* Ottawa: Minister of Supply and Services, 1980.

43. Steen, B. Body composition in aging. *Nutr. Rev.* 46: 45-51, 1988.

44. Stephens, T., D.R. Jacobs Jr., and C.C. White. A descriptive epidemiology of leisure time physical activity. *Public Health Rep.* 100: 147-158, 1985.

45. Synder, G., B. Franklin, M. Foss, and M. Rubenfire. Characteristics of compliers and non-compliers to cardiac exercise therapy programs [Abstract]. *Med. Sci. Sports Exerc.* 14: 179, 1982.

46. Taylor, H.L., E.R. Buskirk, and R.D. Remington. Exercise in controlled trials of the prevention of coronary heart disease. *Fed. Proc.* 32: 1623-1627, 1971.

47. Taylor, H.L., D.R. Jacobs Jr., B. Schucker, J. Knudson, A.S. Leon, and G. DeBacker. A questionnaire for the assessment of leisure time physical activity. *J. Chronic Dis.* 31: 741-755, 1978.

48. The Gallup Poll. Six of ten adults exercise regularly. *The Los Angeles Times Syndicate,* May 1984.

49. Wilson, P.W.F., R.S. Paffenbarger, J.N. Morris, and R.J. Havlik. Assessment methods for physical activity and physical fitness in population studies: Report of a NHLBI workshop. *Am. Heart J.* 111: 1177-1192, 1986.

Chapter 60

Discussion: Exercise, Fitness, and Aging

D.A. Cunningham
D.H. Paterson

The age-related changes observed in many physiological capacities have often been described as a linear decline. The minimal capacity of the system under study remains by the eighth or the ninth decades of life. There is evidence, however, that this relationship of linear decline with age may not be accurate. There are two possible problems with this description of aging and its relationship with many functional capacities. First, the variability among the elderly is considerable, such that many of the elderly can function as well as can many younger persons. Second, the linear relationship of physiological capacities with age, as determined primarily from cross-sectional data, may not represent the actual rate of decline, and a curvilinear relationship with an accelerated rate of decline in the older groups has been observed for several age-related changes.

Extremes of variability in function of 70- and 80-yr-old men and women are witnessed among master's athletes, who are capable of exceptional physical performances such as the reported times for the completion of a marathon. Active elderly men have established times of less than 4 hr (Figure 60.1) for this very long and demanding race. On the other extreme, many elderly in this age-group are not able to carry out normal daily activities and are dependent on others for such basic requirements as washing and cooking meals. The reasons for such large discrepancies are varied and may be related to disease processes. However, in the absence of clinical symptoms, interindividual differences among the elderly remain high.

Recent studies of elderly muscular and cardiorespiratory systems have shed light on physiological and functional losses with age. Changes in limb muscle mass with aging are dramatic. Comparisons of muscle morphology between the young and the elderly and between arm and leg muscle dramatically illustrate such changes. The

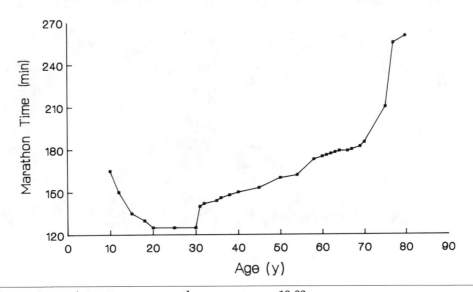

Figure 60.1. Approximate times to run a marathon across ages 10-80 yr.

loss of muscle tissue in the elderly is clearly seen with computerized tomographic imaging (CT scans). Comparisons of CT scans of elderly arms or legs with those of younger subjects illustrate these changes (unpublished observations) (Figure 60.2). Elderly arms have a larger component of skin plus subcutaneous tissue, whereas there is little difference in the amount of these tissues in the legs. Infiltration of both arm and leg muscle by fat and other nonmuscle tissues is greater in the elderly and is particularly pronounced in the "older" plantar flexor muscles. These changes in muscle have also been detailed in a study by Lexell et al. (12), who studied muscle mass in the vastus lateralis in 43 autopsies from healthy sudden-death victims. The age-associated changes in muscle area and total number of fibers described a curvilinear relationship. The point of most rapid decline in muscle mass appeared to be late in the sixth decade of life. This loss was caused by a loss of fibers, with no predominant effect on any fiber type and, to a lesser extent, in fiber size (mostly Type II fibers).

A functional correlate of the decrement in muscle mass change has been shown to occur in measurements of muscle strengths (17, 20) and measurements of normal walking performances (10). Changes in both muscle strength (plantar flexor muscles) and normal speed of walking were described by a curvilinear relationship with age. The similarity of these observations strongly suggests a causal relationship; that is, the loss of muscle mass and strength may determine the choice of walking speed. The similarity of these changes is illustrated in Figure 60.3, in which the curvilinear relationship has been adapted from other studies (10, 12, 20).

The age-related changes in plantar flexor muscle isokinetic strength have been measured on the Cybex. The study involved cross-sectional determination of force of contraction at several movement speeds (3). This study demonstrated that at slow movements (30°/s) there was no significant difference between the young and the elderly subjects. However, at faster movements (180°/s), the

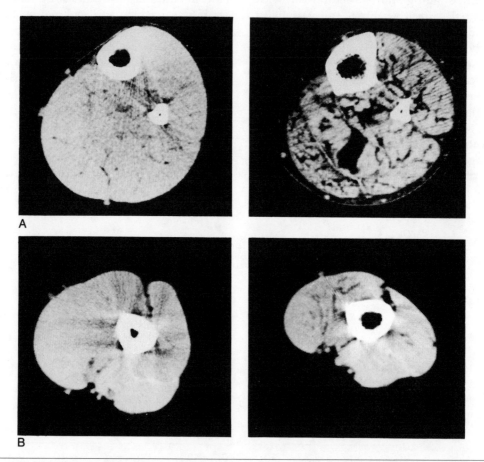

Figure 60.2. A) computed tomography cross section of right leg at level of maximum girth from an elderly man (83 yr) on the right and a young man (27 yr) on the left; B) computed tomography cross section of right arm from an elderly man (83 yr) on the right and a young man (27 yr) on the left.

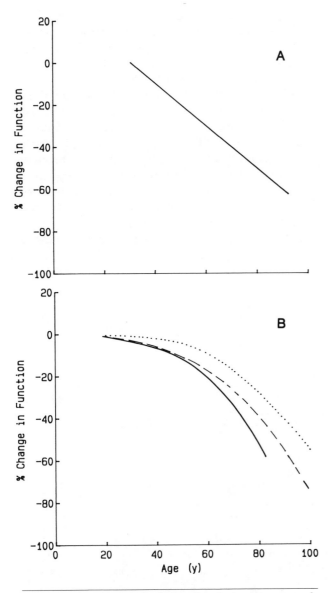

in muscle mass (CT scans). It is interesting that self-selected walking speeds have also been found to be increased following a period of exercise training (2).

The changes in cardiorespiratory fitness, measured as maximum oxygen uptake ($\dot{V}O_2$max), with aging have been reviewed in several reports (1, 11, 14). Regular exercise in the seventh decade of life has resulted in measured changes in $\dot{V}O_2$max and in submaximal work capacity (4, 18). The normal gain in $\dot{V}O_2$max is approximately 10%-15% over 1 yr of exercise training; however, increases as high as 40% have been observed. The change in $\dot{V}O_2$max is dependent on two factors (19): (a) the initial $\dot{V}O_2$max; that is, the lower the $\dot{V}O_2$max at the start of the exercise program, the greater the gain (Figure 60.4); and (b) the intensity of the exercise-training program.

Figure 60.3. A) usual relationship between age and percent change in function as found in cross-sectional data; B) age-related change in percent of functional loss. Adapted from Himann et al. 10 (———), Vandervoort and McComas 20 (........), and Lexell et al. 12 (———).

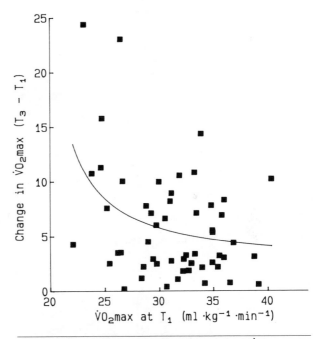

Figure 60.4. Relationship between initial $\dot{V}O_2$max and change in $\dot{V}O_2$max following a 1-yr exercise-training program. The curve is a rectangular hyperbola $Y = (2.224\ X/(-18.437 + X)$. Adapted from Cunningham et al. (2, 4).

elderly subjects had significantly lower force generation than had the young active or the sedentary subjects. The elderly appear to have greater inability to generate force at high speeds than if the action is slow. Recently, strength training of the elderly has been shown to increase knee extensor and flexor strength (6); thus, losses in functional capacity of muscle appear to be reversible. Although further study is needed, it appears that these changes were accompanied by an increase

The rate of adaptation to exercise training of elderly men (66 yr) has been studied and was found to be similar to that of younger subjects. The 4-wk training program consisted of walking or jogging that was held constant at 70% of the initial $\dot{V}O_2$max. The change in aerobic capacity was determined with weekly measurements of $\dot{V}O_2$max (Figure

60.5). The $\dot{V}O_2$max increased 7.5% over the 4 wk of training. This change was fit by an exponential curve ($r = 0.75$). The one-half time for the rate of adaptation of $\dot{V}O_2$max was 8.3 training sessions over 13.8 d (8). This rate of adaptation is very similar to that found in a study on younger men (9) in which the one-half time value was 10.3 training sessions (over 10.3 d) after a similar 4 wk of training at a constant stimulus.

A few studies have reported results of exercise training programs over extended periods of time (> 1 yr). MacKeen et al. (13) reported a 13-yr study of exercise training of middle-aged men identified for coronary heart disease risk factors. They found that the group that maintained a regular program

of exercise training over this time reduced the loss of fitness with time. Those who stopped exercise after the first year of training had values for $\dot{V}O_2$max that regressed toward pretraining levels. In a similar study of 63- to 68-yr-old men, three groups of subjects were formed following an initial 1-yr training period (4). The groups were (a) those men in the training group who chose to continue to exercise for an additional 4 yr (still active), (b) those who stopped (were active), and (c) a random sample of the control group (control) (14). Those who stopped soon returned to control values for $\dot{V}O_2$max, whereas the still active group maintained a significantly greater level of fitness over the 5 yr (Figure 60.6). Figure 60.7 illustrates the age-related

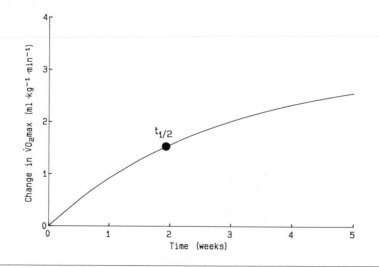

Figure 60.5. Rate of adaptation to exercise training in the elderly. Weekly $\dot{V}O_2$max measures during 4 wk of training were fit with an exponential association to determine one-half time of adaptation (13.8 d). Adapted from Govindasamy et al. (9).

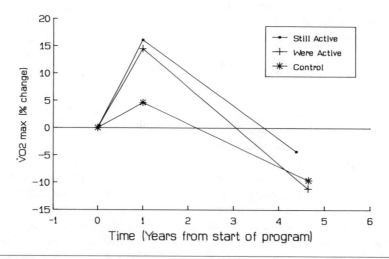

Figure 60.6. Relationship between the time from the start of the exercise program for the three groups and the percent change in $\dot{V}O_2$max.

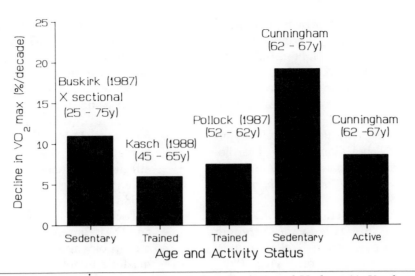

Figure 60.7. The yearly decline in $\dot{V}O_2$max for four studies (Buskirk and Hodgson 1, Kasch et al. 11, Pollock et al. 15, and Cunningham from Paterson et al. 14).

decline in $\dot{V}O_2$max in several studies and the influence of long-term exercise training. Although further longitudinal data are needed, there is some evidence that the age-related decline of $\dot{V}O_2$max in the elderly is amenable to retardation.

It is of considerable interest that exercise training in the elderly resulted in marked and significant increases in $\dot{V}O_2$max that averaged about 15% over 1 yr. Of perhaps greater importance is the observation that if the same men are tested on a submaximal work task, their time to fatigue may increase as much as 150% (16). This has considerable implications that are important with regard to the ability of the elderly to maintain independent lifestyles. In conclusion, the following appear to be good working hypotheses:

- Variability in physiological function among the elderly is much greater than it is in younger persons.
- The critical age when accelerated decline in function begins is the seventh decade of life (on average).
- The loss in body strength is related to the loss in muscle tissue and is more critical in faster movements.
- Exercise training in elderly will attenuate the normal age-related decline in $\dot{V}O_2$max.
- Exercise training will increase submaximal performance to a greater degree than the change in $\dot{V}O_2$max.
- The degree of change in $\dot{V}O_2$max with training is dependent on initial $\dot{V}O_2$max and, to a lesser degree, the intensity of training.

- The rate of adaptation to training in the elderly is similar to that in the young.

The mechanisms of age-related decline in cardiorespiratory function in the elderly have to date not been delineated. Studies of heart function have suggested an altered responsiveness to preload (5), reduced responsiveness to catecholamine stimulation (7), and a heightened after-load (5). Future studies in ventilatory control, gas exchange dynamics, and blood flow distribution in the elderly in response to exercise stressors will yield valuable information regarding the mechanisms governing functional losses with aging and the reversibility of these losses with physical activity.

Acknowledgments

The authors wish to thank E. Nowicki and Dr. S. Higgs for their help in the preparation of this manuscript. Grant support was from NSERC (A2787).

References

1. Buskirk, E.R., and J.L. Hodgson. Age and aerobic power: The rate of change in men and women. *Fed. Proc.* 46: 1824-1829, 1987.
2. Cunningham, D.A., P.A. Rechnitzer, and A.P. Donner. Exercise training and the speed of self-selected walking pace in men at retirement. *Can. J. Aging* 5: 19-26, 1986.

3. Cunningham, D.A., D. Morrison, C.L. Rice, and C. Cooke. Aging and isokinetic plantar flexion. *Eur. J. Appl. Physiol.* 56: 24-29, 1987.

4. Cunningham, D.A., P.A. Rechnitzer, J.H. Howard, and A.P. Donner. Exercise training of men at retirement: A clinical trial. *J. Gerontol.* 42: 17-23, 1987.

5. Cunningham, D.A., R.J. Petrella, D.H. Paterson, and P.M. Nichol. Comparison of cardiovascular response to passive tilt in young and elderly men. *Can. J. Physiol. Pharm.* 66: 1425-1432, 1988.

6. Frontera, W.R., C.N. Merideth, K.P. O'Reilly, H.G. Kruttgen, and H.J. Evans. Strength conditioning in older men: Skeletal hypertrophy and improved function. *J. Appl. Physiol.* 64: 1038-1044, 1988.

7. Gerstenblith, G., D.G. Renlund, and E.G. Lakatta. Cardiovascular response to exercise in younger and older men. *Fed. Proc.* 46: 1834-1839, 1987.

8. Govindasamy, D., D.H. Paterson, M. Poulin, and D.A. Cunningham. Time course of cardiorespiratory adaptation in elderly men. *Can. J. Sport Sci.* 13: 75P, 1988.

9. Hickson, R.C., J.M. Hagberg, A.A. Ehsani, and J.D. Holloszy. Time course of the adaptive responses of aerobic power and heart rate to training. *Med. Sci. Sports Exerc.* 13: 17-20, 1981.

10. Himann, J.E., D.A. Cunningham, P.A. Rechnitzer, and D.H. Paterson. Age-related changes in speed of walking. *Med. Sci. Sports Exerc.* 20: 161-166, 1988.

11. Kasch, F.W., J.P. Wallace, S.P. VanCamp, and L. Verity. A longitudinal study of cardiovascular stability in active men aged 45 to 65 years. *Phys. Sports Med.* 16: 117-124, 1988.

12. Lexell, J., C.C. Taylor, and M. Sjöstrom. What is the cause of the aging atrophy? *J. Neurol. Sci.* 84: 275-294, 1988.

13. MacKeen, P.C., J.L. Rosenberger, J.S. Slater, W.C. Nicholas, and E.R. Buskirk. A 13-year follow-up of a coronary heart disease risk factor screening and exercise program for 40-59 year old men: Exercise habit maintenance and physiologic status. *J. Cardiopulm. Rehabil.* 5: 510-523, 1985.

14. Paterson, D.H., D.A. Cunningham, J.E. Himann, and P.A. Rechnitzer. Long term effects of exercise training on $\dot{V}O_2$max in older men. *Can. J. Sport Sci.* 13: 124P-125P, 1988.

15. Pollock, M.L., C. Foster, D. Knapp, J.L. Rod, and D.H. Schmidt. Effect of age and training on aerobic capacity and body composition of master athletes. *J. Appl. Physiol.* 62: 725-731, 1987.

16. Poulin, M., D.H. Paterson, D. Govindasamy, and D.A. Cunningham. Endurance training of elderly men: Responses to submaximal exercise. *Can. J. Sport Sci.* 13: 132-133P, 1988.

17. Rice, C.L., D.A. Cunningham, D.H. Paterson, and M.S. Lefcoe. Morphological investigation of elderly and young limbs using computed tomography. *Can. J. Sport Sci.* 13: 138P, 1988.

18. Seals, D.R., J.M. Hagberg, B.F. Hurley, A.A. Ehsani, and J.O. Holloszy. Endurance training in older men and women: I. Cardiovascular responses to exercise. *J. Appl. Physiol.* 57: 1024-1029, 1984.

19. Thomas, S.L., D.A. Cunningham, P.A. Rechnitzer, A.P. Donner, and J.H. Howard. Determinants of the training response in elderly men. *Med. Sci. Sports Exerc.* 17: 667-672, 1985.

20. Vandervoort, A.A., and A.J. McComas. Contractile changes in opposing muscles of the human ankle joint with aging. *J. Appl. Physiol.* 61: 361-367, 1986.

PART VI
The Risks of Exercising

Chapter 61

Risks of Exercising:
Sudden Cardiac Death and Injuries

David S. Siscovick

The role of exercise and fitness in the promotion of health has long been a source of controversy (19). On the one hand, there is mounting epidemiological evidence that vigorous exercise reduces the occurrence of several major noncommunicable diseases (24). On the other hand, clinical observations raise concerns about the potential risks of exercising (12, 27). The balance between the benefits and risks of exercise has been difficult to assess, in part because few epidemiological studies have examined the risks of exercising.

The purpose of this chapter is to consider the epidemiological evidence related to two risks of exercising: sudden cardiac death and musculoskeletal injuries. For each condition, we estimate the magnitude of the risk related to exercise, determine whether the risk is modified by the presence of other factors, and examine the extent to which the specific risks detract from the benefits of exercising. In addition, we discuss briefly the implications of these observations for public health and clinical recommendations regarding exercise in apparently healthy individuals.

Sudden Cardiac Death During Exercise

The occurrence of myocardial ischemia, cardiac arrythmias, and sudden cardiac death during exercise raise concerns about the cardiac hazards of exercising. Several studies suggest that among adults approximately 5% of sudden deaths occur during strenuous physical activity (21, 25). If events during moderate physical activity also are considered, approximately 15% of sudden cardiac deaths occur during activity. Given the overall mortality rate from sudden cardiac death in the setting of arteriosclerotic heart disease, the prevention of exercise-related sudden death remains a challenge.

Absolute Risk During Exercise

Several studies have estimated the magnitude of the risk of sudden death during exercise among adults. The incidence of death during jogging among apparently healthy joggers in the state of Rhode Island was 1 case per 15,240 exercisers per year (26). We observed a similar rate of cardiac arrest during exercise in a study of vigorous leisure-time activity in Seattle, Washington (25). Somewhat higher rates were reported among joggers at the Aerobics Center in Dallas, Texas (5), and marathon runners in South Africa (17). It is likely that differences in the absolute rates estimated from these studies reflect differences in the study population, the nature of the exercise, the time at risk from exercise, or all these.

Vouri (29) estimated the incidence of sudden cardiac death during jogging or running and cross-country skiing in the total Finnish male population, 20-69 yr of age. Incidence rates were lowest among younger men and were similar for middle-aged and older men. These data suggest that sudden death during exercise is a rare occurrence. To determine whether the risk is increased during exercise, it is necessary to determine whether the incidence during exercise is increased compared to the incidence at other times.

Transient Increase in Risk During Exercise

The risk of sudden death is transiently increased during exercise. Thompson (26) reported that the risk of sudden death during jogging in Rhode Island was increased 7-fold compared to that during more sedentary activities. Vouri (29) reported that the risk of sudden death during prolonged cross-country skiing in Finland was increased 4.5-fold. In Seattle we observed a similar overall estimate of the increase in risk during vigorous exercise compared to the risk at other times (25). These observations suggest that the occurrence of sudden death during exercise is not a random event. Vigorous exercise can occasionally precipitate sudden death.

Factors That Modify Risk During Exercise

Several studies have examined the influence of other factors (e.g., intensity, habitual activity level, age, gender, and prior morbidity) on the risk of sudden cardiac death during exercise. Vouri (29) demonstrated that the magnitude of the increase in risk during activity, compared to the risk at other times, was greater for strenuous than for nonstrenuous exercise; there was a 9-fold increase in risk during strenuous exercise but only a 3.2-fold increase during nonstrenuous exercise.

We demonstrated in Seattle that the magnitude of the transient increase in risk of primary cardiac arrest during vigorous leisure-time physical activity was influenced by the level of habitual physical activity (25). With increasing levels of habitual high-intensity activity, there was a reduction in the transient increase in risk during activity. Among apparently health men with low levels of habitual activity, the risk was increased 56-fold (95% confidence limits for estimate of relative risk, 23-131). However, among men who were habitually active, the risk was increased only 5-fold (95% confidence limits for estimates of relative risk, 2-14).

Several studies have observed that the relative risk of sudden cardiac death during exercise, compared to the risk at other times, was highest among younger men (25, 26). However, we demonstrated that the increased relative risk among men under age 45 primarily reflects a lower risk of primary cardiac arrest at other times (25). Among apparently healthy men under age 45, 6 of 12 cases of primary cardiac arrest occurred during vigorous exercise. When differences in the amount of time spent in exercise are considered, the incidence of primary cardiac arrest is similar for younger and older men.

The risk of sudden cardiac death during activity appears to be lower in women than in men. Vouri (29) noted that sudden cardiac death during activity was 14 times less frequent among women than among men in Finland despite the fact that the proportion of women and the frequency of participation in recreational activity were similar to those of men.

The presence of clinical cardiac disease also modifies the absolute risk of cardiac arrest during activity (7, 25). The incidence of cardiac arrest during exercise is higher for patients with prior clinical cardiac disease than for apparently healthy persons (28). However, the magnitude of the transient increase in risk during activity, compared to the risk at other times, is similar to that observed among apparently healthy persons. For persons with prior clinical cardiac disease, there is a six-fold increase in risk during strenuous exercise. Of note, 85% of patients who suffer cardiac arrest in the setting of supervised cardiac rehabilitation are successfully resuscitated (28).

Risk factors for coronary heart disease, such as hypercholesterolemia, hypertension, cigarette smoking, obesity, and alcohol consumption, may also influence the risk of sudden cardiac death during activity. Because these factors are related to the risk of coronary heart disease, it has been assumed that their presence increases the risk of exercise-related acute cardiac events. Although clinical coronary heart disease has been shown to increase the risk of exercise-related sudden cardiac death, whether these factors increase risk has not been investigated.

Other forms of comorbidity may also influence the risk of sudden cardiac death during exercise. A recent report from the U.S. armed forces suggested that the presence of sickle-cell trait (hemoglobin AS) increased the risk of exertion-related deaths among a large cohort of young-adult black male recruits (10). Among black males with sickle-cell trait, the cumulative incidence of sudden death during exertion during a 6-wk basic training period was 1 death per 3,200 recruits.

Balance of Cardiac Risks and Benefits

Few studies have examined the cardiac risks and benefits of exercise in the same population. In Seattle we examined both the risk of primary cardiac arrest during vigorous exercise and the potential benefit of habitual exercise in the same population (25). We determined the extent to which the transient increase in risk of primary cardiac arrest during exercise detracts from the benefits of habitual vigorous exercise.

The overall incidence of primary cardiac arrest reflects the weighted average of the risk during and not during exercise, where the weights are the amount of time spent in and out of vigorous activity. Among men who engaged in habitual vigorous exercise, the transient increase in risk during activity was outweighed by a decrease in risk at other times, so that the overall risk for vigorous exercisers was lower than that for more sedentary men (25). Men who did not engage in vigorous exercise were not at risk for cardiac arrest during exercise. However, these sedentary men had the highest overall rates of primary cardiac arrest.

After simultaneous adjustment for hypertension history and current cigarette smoking, the estimate of the overall relative risk for primary cardiac arrest for men who engaged in vigorous exercise for more than 20 min per week, compared to more sedentary men, was 0.40 (95% confidence limits, 0.23-0.67) (25). In short, among habitually vigorous men, the overall risk of primary cardiac arrest (both during and not during vigorous exercise) was only 40% that of sedentary men. These data suggest that although the risk of primary cardiac arrest is transiently increased during vigorous exercise, habitual vigorous exercise is associated with an overall reduced risk of primary cardiac arrest.

The net effect of exercise training in cardiac rehabilitation programs was reviewed by May et al. (15). Although pooled results from six studies suggest a possible 19% lower total mortality in patients who engage in exercise, none of the studies individually were large enough to show statistically significant reductions in total mortality. On the other hand, there was no evidence that the cardiac hazards of exercise outweigh the cardiac benefits in supervised cardiac rehabilitation programs.

Exercise-Related Musculoskeletal Injuries

Although sudden death during exercise is a rare event, clinicians have long recognized that musculoskeletal injuries are one of the more common risks of exercising. Injuries result from physical trauma to bone, soft tissue, or both. The occurrence of macrotrauma during collision or impact sports causes a variety of musculoskeletal injuries. On the other hand, microtrauma from repetitive overloading in a cumulative manner over time results in overuse syndromes. For persons who engage in regular recreational exercise such as jogging, swimming, aerobic dance, and racket sports, overuse syndromes are of particular concern. With increased participation in regular exercise, the size of the population at risk for overuse injuries has grown. For these reasons, there is a need to estimate the risks of exercise-related musculoskeletal injuries and the factors that influence these risks. However, few epidemiological studies have examined the incidence of exercise-related injuries for the aerobic activities that most people choose to improve fitness (11).

We limit our review to studies of the relation between exercise and musculoskeletal injuries in adults. We recognize that musculoskeletal injuries represent only a subset of all exercise-related injuries; because they are common and have the potential to affect functional ability adversely over both the short and the long term, we consider them the most important type of exercise-related injury. For similar reasons, we restrict our review to the risk of injuries related to the most popular forms of aerobic exercise in the United States and Canada; each of these activities has the potential to enhance an individual's cardiorespiratory capacity when properly performed on a regular basis. Finally we consider only epidemiological studies that were designed to determine risk or the factors that influence risk. Recently, Walter et al. (30) reviewed the methodologies for examining the etiology of sport injuries. This review emphasized the limitations of case series and the need for comparison groups to make valid inferences regarding risk and risk factors for injuries.

Running- or Jogging-Related Injuries

The risk of musculoskeletal injuries related to running or jogging were examined in several retrospective cohort studies (1, 8, 10, 14). In each case, the study population was a cohort of individuals who had attended a health and fitness club or participated in a road race. The occurrence of musculoskeletal injuries related to running was assessed retrospectively by self-report. Blair et al. (1) estimated that 24% of the participants in the Aerobics Center in Dallas experienced an injury during the prior year that was severe enough to cause them to stop running for at least 7 d. Koplan et al. (10) reported that 35% of participants in the Peachtree Road Race in Atlanta, Georgia, experienced a musculoskeletal injury attributed to running that was severe enough to require a decrease in weekly mileage run in the year following the race. In addition, 13% of men and 17% of women runners were injured and sought medical attention during this 1-yr period. Jacobs and Berson (8) reported that 47% of entrants in a 10-km race indicated a running-related injury during the 2 yr before the race. Approximately 15% of the runners had sought medical attention for their running-related injuries, and a similar proportion experienced pain that prevented running. Maughan (14) found that 58% of runners preparing for a marathon incurred an injury in preparation for the race. Of those injured, approximately 75% interrupted their formal training as a result of the injury. However, the length of the training period and whether medical attention was sought were not specified in this report. Given the select nature of these study populations, it is possible that these rates either underestimate or overestimate the risk of injuries. Furthermore, without a nonrunning comparison group, it is not possible to determine whether running increases the risk of musculoskeletal injury.

Running Increases Risk of Injuries

Blair et al. (1) conducted a retrospective cohort study of running and self-reported, physician-diagnosed orthopedic injuries among patients seen at the Cooper Clinic for health maintenance examinations, physical fitness assessments, and lifestyle counseling. The incidence of orthopedic injuries was higher among runners at each site examined; only the difference in rates of knee injury was statistically significant at conventional levels.

Factors That Modify Risk of Running

Factors that might influence the risk of running-related musculoskeletal injuries have been examined in several studies. Blair et al. (1) hypothesized that several factors (i.e., gender, age, obesity, weekly miles run, time per mile during training, time and place of running, and stretching habits) might be associated with the risk of running-related injuries. Of these, only distance run per week was positively related to the risk of injuries; this association remained statistically significant ($p = .03$) after controlling for age, stretching, and time per mile. Koplan et al. (10) also found that the risk of injury increased with increasing mileage, a finding that was similar for men and women, for all types of injuries, and for those with and without a medical consultation for the injury. Of note, age, obesity, speed of running, and years of running did not contribute independently to the risk of running-related injury. Similarly, Jacobs and Berson (8) observed that running-related injuries were positively associated with running more miles per week, running more days per week, and running more races over the last year. In this study, injured runners also were less likely to participate regularly in other sports. In contrast to Koplan et al., Jacobs and Berson reported that running at a faster pace also increased the risk of injury.

However, Jacobs and Berson did not consider these different factors simultaneously, so it is not possible to determine whether each was independently related to the risk of injury.

Aerobic Dance-Related Injuries

Recently, Garrick et al. (4) prospectively examined the risk of musculoskeletal injuries among participants in aerobic dance and rhythmic calisthenics performed to music. Students from six aerobic dance facilities were followed for up to 16 wk with weekly phone contacts to assess their activity levels and the occurrence of musculoskeletal injuries. Forty-four percent of students reported at least one musculoskeletal complaint during follow-up. However, 75% of participants experienced no disability, such as a reduction or cessation of dance activities. In addition, 2.5% of students experienced injuries that required medical care.

Factors That Modify Risk of Aerobic Dance

Several factors that might influence the risk of musculoskeletal injury among participants in aerobic dance were considered in the study by Garrick et al. (4). Injury rates were higher among persons with prior orthopedic problems, those with a minimal weekly commitment to aerobic dance (once per week), and those who did not engage in other types of exercise. The type of flooring or the brand of shoe was not related to injury rates. Whether these negative findings reflect the limited range or a lack of effect related to these forms of passive protection remains unclear. This observational study did not examine injury rates among sedentary persons who were beginning an aerobic dance program. For this reason, and given the select nature of the study population, it remains unclear whether the rates of injury observed are generalizable to those persons who are beginning aerobic dance.

Other Exercise-Related Musculoskeletal Injuries

Even fewer epidemiological studies examine the risk of musculoskeletal injuries related to other popular forms of regular aerobic exercise (e.g., swimming, racket sports, cycling, and walking). For example, the prevalence of injuries to the shoulder and knee among competitive swimmers has been previously estimated (20, 22). The limitations of prevalence rates of exercise-related musculoskeletal injuries have been discussed elsewhere

(30). We are unaware of studies that have examined the risks of musculoskeletal injury related to noncompetitive swimming and the factors that might influence these risks. On the other hand, the incidence of injuries to British Club badminton players has been estimated at .09 per male and .14 per female per year (6); most of these injuries were leg strains, sprains, blisters, and cramps. Although the prevalence of tennis elbow has been reported (2), the incidence of tennis elbow or factors that influence the risk have not been investigated. Finally, there are no epidemiological studies of nontraumatic musculoskeletal injuries related to regular walking or cycling for exercise.

Discussion

This review suggests that exercising to promote fitness and health has risks. Epidemiological studies have estimated the incidence of sudden death during exercise, identified several factors that might alter this risk, and put into perspective the risks and benefits of vigorous exercise that relate to sudden cardiac death. On the other hand, there are limited data regarding both the risks of musculoskeletal injuries related to running or jogging and aerobic dance and the factors that might influence these risks. The incidence of exercise-related injuries for persons who engage in regular walking, swimming, cycling, and most racket sports are not currently available.

Limitations of Available Evidence

Several limitations of the evidence regarding the risk of exercise-related sudden cardiac death need to be considered. First, the definition of *exercise-related events* differs in different studies. Should an acute cardiac event that occurs several hours after exercise be considered exercise related? Or should only those events that occur during or immediately after exercise, such as within 1 hr, be considered exercise related? Second, few studies have been large enough to consider factors that might confound or modify the transient increase in risk during exercise. In addition, detailed information regarding prior activity levels or other risk factors is frequently not available. For these reasons, few studies have tried to identify predictors of exercise-related sudden cardiac death using multivariable techniques. Finally, the risk of nonfatal myocardial infarction may also be increased transiently during exercise; however, both clinically silent myocardial

infarction and stuttering chest pain syndromes, such as unstable angina pectoris, limit estimates of exercise-related nonfatal myocardial infarction.

The limitations of available evidence regarding the risks of exercise-related musculoskeletal injuries are summarized elsewhere (30). Several prospective studies currently in progress have attempted to address some of the methodological limitations of available data. These studies involve active surveillance of both activity levels and the occurrence of injuries. However, whether the findings of studies of current exercisers will be generalizable to less select populations that are beginning regular exercise remains unclear.

Application of Knowledge

The application of available knowledge related to the risks of exercise presents additional challenges. For example, efforts to minimize the cardiac hazards of exercise have focused on (a) the identification of susceptible individuals based on a preexercise examination and (b) the identification of groups of individuals at risk based on the presence of potential risk factors for exertion-related sudden cardiac death. In adults, sudden cardiac death during exercise most commonly occurs in the setting of coronary heart disease. For this reason, screening of apparently healthy middle-aged men with coronary heart disease risk factors with exercise electrocardiography has frequently been used to assess the safety of strenuous exercise. Recommendations regarding preexercise evaluation covering the spectrum of cardiovascular diseases have recently been published (13, 16). Given the large number of persons involved in recreational exercise, the small absolute risk of cardiovascular complications during exercise, the high costs of adequate screening (including the need for trained personnel), and the large number of false positive and negative findings in an apparently healthy population, screening programs to detect cardiac disease among sedentary persons who plan to enter vigorous exercise programs may not be feasible (3). For these reasons, preparticipation screening of middle-aged and older subjects remains a major area of controversy. Unfortunately, there are few empirical data that specifically address the utility of preexercise evaluation in reducing the risk of exercise-related sudden cardiac death.

Another approach to minimize the cardiac hazards of exercising is to inform exercisers of symptoms of possible coronary heart disease and of other factors that might contribute to the occurrence of exercise-related sudden cardiac death.

Personal habits (cigarette smoking or alcohol consumption before exercise), factors related to exercise itself (not warming up, competition, intensity of effort, and not cooling down), or factors related to the environment (extremes of temperature or humidity) increase cardiac work load and electrical instability of the myocardium and may increase the risk of cardiac events during exercise. Although epidemiological studies have not demonstrated that these factors increase the risk of sudden death during exercise, this may reflect only a lack of evidence rather than evidence of a lack of effect. Given the rate of sudden cardiac death during exercise, it is unlikely that epidemiological studies will have adequate power to explore fully the potential interactions between these factors and exercise. Nevertheless, there is concern that when these factors occur (especially in combination) in the setting of vigorous exercise, they may increase the risk of sudden death during exercise among apparently healthy individuals with clinically inapparent coronary heart disease.

Exercise-related musculoskeletal injuries appear relatively common, although only a minority of such injuries result in impairment of functional ability. On the basis of available epidemiological data, it appears that the risk of exercise-related musculoskeletal injuries to the lower extremities increases with increasing mileage run per week. In addition, the risk of musculoskeletal injury related to aerobic dance is increased among those persons with prior orthopedic injuries and a minimal weekly commitment to aerobic dance and among those who do not engage in other types of sports. However, additional epidemiological studies of exercise-related musculoskeletal injuries are needed to define better the potential risks of exercising and to suggest targets for preventive interventions that might reduce the risk of exercise-related injuries.

Conclusion

The need to consider both the benefits and risks of physical activity and exercise when making clinical and public health recommendations was noted in the summary of a workshop (sponsored by the Centers for Disease Control) on epidemiological and public health aspects of physical activity and exercise. The workshop was held in September 1984, several months after Jim Fixx collapsed and died during exercise. In the summary, Powell and Paffenbarger (18) noted that

a recurrent theme of discussion was that the benefits and risks cannot be considered in isolation. It may be necessary to study them separately, but the overall effect of physical activity on the health of the population requires that both be known, both be studied with equal care, and that both be considered dispassionately. The potential overall beneficial impact of physical activity on health will be poorly served if activity patterns are recommended indiscriminately for all groups without regard for the sub-group specific benefits and risks.

References

1. Blair, S.N., H.W. Kohl, and N.N. Goodyear. Rates and risks for running and exercise injuries: Studies in three populations. *Res. Q. Exerc. Sport.* 58: 221-228, 1987.
2. Carroll, R. Tennis elbow: Incidence in local league players. *Br. J. Sports Med.* 15: 250-256, 1981.
3. Epstein, S.E., and B.J. Maron. Sudden death and the competitive athlete: Perspectives on preparticipation screening studies. *J. Am. Coll. Cardiol.* 7: 220-230, 1986.
4. Garrick, J.G., D.M. Gillian, and P. Whiteside. The epidemiology of aerobic dance injuries. *Am. J. Sports Med.* 14: 67-72, 1986.
5. Gibbons, L.W., K.H. Cooper, B.M. Meyer, and R.C. Ellison. The acute cardiac risk of strenuous exercise. *JAMA* 244: 1799-1801, 1980.
6. Hensley, C.D. A survey of badminton injuries. *Br. J. Sports Med.* 13: 156-160, 1979.
7. Hossack, K.F., and R. Hartwig. Cardiac arrest associated with supervised cardiac rehabilitation. *J. Cardiac Rehabil.* 2: 402-406, 1982.
8. Jacobs, S.J., and B.L. Berson. Injuries to runners: A study of entrants to a 10,000 meter race. *Am. J. Sports Med.* 14: 151-155, 1986.
9. Kark, J.A., D.M. Posey, H.R. Schumacher, and C.J. Ruehle. Sickle-cell trait as a risk factor for sudden death in physical training. *N. Engl. J. Med.* 317: 781-787, 1987.
10. Koplan, J.P., K.E. Powell, R.K. Sikes, R.W. Shirley, and C.C. Campbell. An epidemiologic study of the benefits and risks of running. *JAMA* 248: 3118-3121, 1982.
11. Koplan, J.P., D.S. Siscovick, and G.M. Goldbaum. The risks of exercise: A public view of injuries and hazards. *Public Health Rep.* 100: 189-195, 1985.

12. Kraus, J.F., and C. Conroy. Mortality and morbidity from injuries in sports and recreation. *Annu. Rev. Public Health* 5: 163-192, 1984.

13. Maron, B.J., and S.E., Epstein (Eds.). Symposium on the athlete heart. *J. Am. Coll. Cardiol.* 7: 189-243, 1986.

14. Maughan, R.J., and J.D.B. Miller. Incidence of training-related injuries among marathon runners. *Br. J. Sports Med.* 17: 162-165, 1983.

15. May, G.S., K.A. Eberlein, and C.D. Furberg. Secondary prevention after myocardial infarction: A review of long term trials. *Prog. Cardiovasc. Dis.* 24: 331-352, 1982.

16. Mitchell, J.H., B.J. Mason, and S.E. Epstein (Eds.). 16th Bethesda conference: Cardiovascular abnormalities in the athlete: Recommendations regarding eligibility for competition. *J. Am. Coll. Cardiol.* 6: 1189-1232, 1985.

17. Noakes, T.D., L.H. Opie, and A.G. Rose. Marathon running and immunity to coronary heart disease: Fact versus fiction. *Clin. Sports Med.* 3: 527-543, 1984.

18. Powell, K.E., and R.S. Paffenbarger. Workshop on epidemiologic and public health aspects of physical activity and exercise: A summary. *Public Health Rep.* 100: 118-126, 1985.

19. Rennie, D., and N.K. Hollenberg. Cardiomythology and marathons. *N. Engl. J. Med.* 301: 103-104, 1979.

20. Richardson, A.B., F.W. Jobe, and H.R. Collins. The shoulder in competitive swimming. *Am. J. Sports Med.* 8: 159-163, 1980.

21. Romo, M. Factors related to sudden death in acute ischemic heart disease. *Acta Med. Scand. Suppl.* 547, 1973.

22. Rovere, G.D., and A.W. Nichols. Frequency, associated factors, and treatment of breast stroker's knee in competitive swimmers. *Am. J. Sports Med.* 13: 99-104, 1985.

23. Shepherd, R.J. Exercise in coronary heart disease. *Sports Med.* 3: 26-49, 1986.

24. Siscovick, D.S., R.E. LaPorte, and J.M. Newman. The disease-specific benefits and risks of physical activity and exercise. *Public Health Rep.* 100: 180-188, 1985.

25. Siscovick, D.S., N.S. Weiss, R.H. Fletcher, and T. Lasky. The incidence of primary cardiac arrest during vigorous exercise. *N. Engl. J. Med.* 311: 874-877, 1984.

26. Thompson, P.D., E.J. Funk, R.A. Carleton, and W.Q. Sturner. Incidence of death during jogging in Rhode Island from 1975 to 1980. *JAMA* 247: 2535-2538, 1982.

27. Thompson, P.O., W.P. Stern, P. Williams, K. Duncan, W.L. Haskell, and P.D. Wood. Death during jogging or running: A study of 18 cases. *JAMA* 242: 1265-1267, 1979.

28. VanCamp, S.P., and R.A. Peterson. Cardiovascular complications of outpatient cardiac rehabilitation programs. *JAMA* 256: 1160-1163, 1986.

29. Vouri, I. The cardiovascular risks of physical activity. *Acta Med. Scand. Suppl.* 711: 205-214, 1984.

30. Walter, S.D., J.R. Sutton, J.M. McIntosh, and C. Connolly. The etiology of sport injuries: A review of methodologies. *Sports Med.* 2: 47-58, 1985.

Chapter 62

Discussion: Risks of Exercising: Sudden Cardiac Death and Injuries

Stephen D. Walter

It matters not how a man dies, but how he lives. The act of dying is not of importance, it lasts so short a time.
—Samuel Johnson, 1769

From this remark it might seem as if Johnson interpreted deaths from all causes as having been sudden. It also suggests that we should concentrate our research efforts on risks (e.g., injuries) among the living and put relatively little weight on mortality outcomes. Siscovick has taken a wider perspective on both mortality and morbidity outcomes than did Johnson, perhaps suggesting the contemporary desire for a more balanced and integrated evaluation of all the relevant risks and benefits.

The association of physical activity with health has been under investigation for over 30 yr, at least since Morris's studies of London transport workers and British civil servants (2, 4, 5). Whereas most of the older studies concentrated on activity levels defined by occupational group, a more recent trend has been to study recreational exercise patterns. Participation in many forms of recreational activity has increased substantially over the past few years to the point where the potential impact on population morbidity and mortality patterns is considerable. It is therefore extremely important to establish a more accurate epidemiological picture of the risks and benefits of various kinds of exercise at various frequencies and intensities. In so doing, we may offer rational advice to individuals wishing to improve their health by exercising and at the same time assess the societal benefits from the development and encouragement of exercise programs.

Risks and Benefits of Exercise

The choice of appropriate study protocols for this purpose presents considerable methodological challenges. Problems arise from the diverse nature of the potential risks and benefits of exercise. Siscovick has confined his attention to benefits in the form of reduced risk from sudden cardiac death and risks in the form of increased musculoskeletal injury rates. But it is clear that as yet we have only an incomplete picture of all the risks and benefits. For example, most recreational studies to date have been on runners, but we know much less about injury rates for many other popular sports, such as swimming, hiking, or skiing.

On the benefits side we know little about the psychosocial benefits of exercise, although regular exercisers cite health-related reasons most commonly as the rationale for their participation. Canadian national survey data (10) have suggested that the most common reasons for exercising were "for good health," "good for me in general," "to lose weight," and "for release of tension"; each of these has a strong health connotation. Other effects that were not considered by Siscovick but that have been studied by others include premature degenerative joint disorders in long-term runners (6), thermal illness (11), functional capacity changes (3), and reduced usage of medical services (3). A methodological challenge is how all these positive and negative effects of exercise may be quantified and compared.

Choice of Participants for Epidemiological Studies of Exercise and Health

The movement away from occupational to recreationally based definitions of activity levels has presented new problems in the selection of appropriate populations to study. Many recent projects

715

have sampled from entrants in mass-participation events such as road races. Although this is a convenient way to identify and study large numbers of athletes, the generalizability of such studies is perhaps questionable. By choosing people who are sufficiently fit to participate in these events, we may induce a "healthy athlete bias" analogous to the familiar "healthy worker effect" in occupational epidemiology. Individuals who are already injured may be discouraged from or unable to enter sporting events; in contrast, the "survivors" who remain sufficiently free of injury to enter the event may be healthier on average. Furthermore, even once sampling is completed there may be different probabilities of athletes continuing to be enrolled in a cohort study, according to the intensity of exercise and the likelihood of injury. Preliminary data have suggested that runners who are younger, who are running less miles per week, and who have not experienced an injury are more likely to drop out and be lost to follow-up. Differential dropout rates of this kind may limit study generalizability.

An equally important concern is that the subset of habitual exercisers who enter organized events may not be representative of all exercisers. Selection bias is obviously a problem if one samples from elite, highly competitive events. It is probably less so if we study athletes in community events and fun runs, but there will still be a certain number of athletes in the general population who never enter even casual, noncompetitive events and so cannot be involved in studies using this sampling strategy.

Choice of Study Design

Despite this possible lack of generalizability, the prospective use of athlete cohorts defined by participation in specific events offers some considerable methodological and practical advantages (14). In particular, the risk profile of each athlete can be established before the occurrence of an injury or cardiac event, thereby reducing the likelihood of reporting bias in the physical activity level of each subject.

The alternative case-control design has been used by several authors. In this approach the activity level must be estimated for cases (e.g., cardiac deaths) and controls (e.g., randomly selected members of the community) for a certain time period before the case event; this usually requires memory recall (14). If the cases are cardiac deaths, the data on prior exercise levels must be obtained from a proxy, such as the spouse; to avoid bias, proxies must also be used to obtain the control exposure information. Reliance on memory in this way may impair both precision and bias. Imprecision will occur because it is difficult to recall exercise status accurately from several years previous. Bias may occur because the case respondents have a different motivation to recall and report accurately than do the controls.

The problem of recall bias is particularly acute for outcomes such as cardiac events that occur *during* exercise. A related problem (and one that has not been extensively investigated) is the possibility of diagnostic reporting bias for exercise-related deaths. Intensive publicity typically follows a death during exercise; an example is the death of James Fixx, a noted exponent of exercise (12). It is possible that whereas cardiac deaths during exercise are almost certain to be reported as "sudden," cardiac deaths occurring at other times may sometimes be misattributed to other causes. If so, we would overestimate the risk elevation for cardiac deaths during exercise itself.

Indices of Risk

Various indices have been proposed to express the risk of health events. First, there is the *number of exercise sessions corresponding to one event*. For example, Vuori (13) calculated that there was 1 death per 2.6 million exercise sessions for men aged 40-49 yr. Second, if we know the duration of exercise, the *risk per hour* during exercise can be calculated (9, 13). For example, Siscovick et al. (9) estimated the risk of cardiac arrest per 10 million man-hours during exercise and, by complementarity, not during exercise. A third index, the *relative risk per hour* during versus not during exercise can then be derived. The final indices are the *overall risk* of exercisers and their *risks relative to nonexercisers*.

Each of these indices gives a slightly different message. The first index conveys information about the risk per session (which turns out to be numerically very low for most people), but it does not say anything about background risk so is difficult to put into perspective. The second and third indices based on risk per hour suggest to an athlete what the risk elevation might be during the exercise period itself, rather than the background risk. For persons whose relative risk is substantially above 1 and whose absolute risk during exercise is sufficiently high, we may contemplate preventive measures such as the provision of first aid and resuscitation services, information about the risks of various forms of exercise, and so on.

The final two indices are probably the most important because they convey the overall benefit of exercise to an individual. For example, if the risk of a cardiac death during a limited period of exercise turns out to be low, then it can be tolerated to achieve the overall risk reduction. In this context, the transient risk elevation during exercise is almost irrelevant.

The risk-per-hour indices rely critically on the accurate estimation of the duration of the exercise session. Even if this can be accurately timed, we may also elect to include an additional period to allow biological recovery, for example, until heart rate and blood pressure had returned to normal values. This approach would recognize that certain body systems remain under stress even after the actual period of exercise exertion.

Further interpretation of the risk-per-session, the risk-per-hour, and the overall indices can be achieved by reexpressing them in the more familiar scale of an *annual rate*. For example, Vuori (13) estimated the average exercise session for 40- to 49-yr-old men to be 30 min long. Combining this with his estimated 1 death per 2.6 million exercise sessions, we may calculate the equivalent annual death rate as $(60/30) \times 24 \times 365 \times 1,000/2.6 \times 10^6$, or 6.74 per 1,000 persons. This rate may then be compared to usual vital statistics.

A further type of index can be calculated if a detailed dose-response relationship between exposure and risk is available, for example, the *risk per mile* of running. Preliminary data have shown that the risk per mile may be lower for higher-mileage runners. This is consistent with Siscovick's evidence that the risk of musculoskeletal injury is higher for persons who have relatively little commitment to the sport.

Measurement of Recreational Exercise Levels

Another problem in population-based studies of recreation concerns the accurate measurement of exposure and outcome. It is relatively easy to ask runners about the frequency, intensity, and duration of their exercise, and indeed they do report these variables reliably. However, it is almost impossible to validate this information. In our own studies we have established reasonable levels of internal reliability of runner-reported mileage by comparing their responses on the average number of miles run per day, the number of days run per week, and the total weekly mileage, each of which is obtained in different parts of the questionnaire. Similarly, to assess respondent reliability in reporting their general level of sedentary, walking, and standing activities during the day, we have examined the internal consistency of responses to these three components. However, much more work is needed in this area.

Ascertainment of Injuries

For the case of musculoskeletal injuries, there are several other measurement problems that concern the health outcome itself. Depending on the study circumstances, it may be necessary to use athlete self-reports of injury, the clinical accuracy of which is open to doubt. We have found that there is good agreement between the athlete self-reports and clinical findings when the classification is restricted to the body site but that more detailed diagnosis by the athlete is unreliable.

A related issue is in distinguishing new and recurrent injuries. Musculoskeletal problems frequently recur over period of years, but it is often difficult to say whether a particular episode is a new or an old problem. Only about half these injuries may be treated clinically (15), so there is a tradeoff between obtaining clinically validated data on only a selected subset of injuries and obtaining unvalidated information on a higher percentage of injuries.

A further limitation of many previous studies is that they have been restricted to participants in one sport. In fact, exercisers typically participate in several other sports. For example, we have found that 95% of runners have at least one other regular activity (15). Because at least some morbidity among runners is actually caused by these other types of exercise, we are faced with difficult problems in attributing appropriate numbers of cases to each type and in deciding which forms of exercise are safe.

Generalizability of Observational Studies of Exercise

As Siscovick discussed, one of the difficulties in interpreting much epidemiological evidence on exercise is its observational nature, as randomized experiments are rare. So, for example, we must be concerned about the possibility of selection bias; perhaps participants in exercise programs were actually fitter to begin with. Some indirect evidence against this hypothesis is provided in a review by Powell et al. (8), who found that cohort studies that had used medical screening to exclude preclinical disease before beginning follow-up of study participants showed approximately the same risk reduction for cardiac events with exercise as did studies that did not use medical prescreening. Also, the beneficial effect of exercise persists over time, making it less likely that the groups of inactive persons contain many cases of preclinical disease at baseline. In other words, inactivity appears not to be a consequence of preclinical disease.

Nevertheless, there are risks in extrapolating the results of observational studies to predict the effects of intervention. Further studies are needed on the effects of changes in exercise level, some of which occur naturally. For example, in a long-term cohort study in Finland there was a relatively low correlation between the activity level of adult men in 1964 compared to their activity level 20 yr later (7). The men initially classified as having high physical activity had reduced overall mortality for approximately 10 yr when compared to men with low physical activity. However, by the end of the 20-yr follow-up period, the overall survival curves of these two groups had converged once again. On the other hand, the survival curves for coronary heart disease in particular were relatively close for the first few years of follow-up and then gradually diverged. Twenty years after enrollment into the study, the main mortality benefit for the exercisers was in coronary heart disease and was a sustained and late effect despite the low correlation of initial and final activity levels. In terms of overall mortality, these data suggest that exercise may not extend the maximum life span but rather postpones some early deaths. More studies of this kind are needed to provide information on the pattern of risk over the lifespan, especially as major changes in exercise patterns occur.

It is difficult to predict from available data what might be the impact of gradual or sudden *increases* in activity levels. Existing studies do suggest some important qualitative differences in the risks for habitual low or high exercisers. As Siscovick has demonstrated, persons with little (but nonzero) activity experience very high levels of risk of cardiac arrest during their limited activity, but their overall reduction in cardiac mortality may be quite small. Also, the risk of musculoskeletal injury appears to be higher among persons with relatively little commitment, especially if the "dose" of activity exposure is taken into account.

Implications for Exercise Prescriptions

The available data present a paradox for how exercise programs might be recommended for persons with no current activity. These people are at high risk for cardiovascular events; but if they begin exercise at a modest initial level, Siscovick's data suggest that their risks during exercise itself are substantially elevated and that the overall benefit may be relatively small. Persons initiating exercise may also raise their risk of musculoskeletal injuries, although it should be recognized that there is substantial musculoskeletal morbidity even in sedentary populations (1).

An encouraging feature of the evidence to date is that age appears to be a relatively unimportant factor for musculoskeletal injuries. Cross-sectionally derived injury rates appear approximately equal for men and women of all ages. But once again the implications for interventions are less clear. We should not necessarily conclude the initiation of exercise will produce the same risks and benefits for people of all ages. Drawing an analogy from cancer etiology, it may be that the age at which exercise is initiated and its cumulative duration may be equally important.

Conclusion

In summary, it appears that there are still gaps in our knowledge of the determinants of risks and benefits in general populations. Powell et al. (8) have indicated that studies with stronger methodology have generally been more likely to show a beneficial effect of exercise on cardiac-related deaths than have weaker studies. Attention to methodological rigor will become more important as we attempt to answer some of the more outstanding etiological questions: How quickly do health benefits accrue to persons initiating exercise programs? What is the optimal frequency and intensity of exercise to maximize these benefits? For how many years does the exercise need to be sustained to maintain the benefit?

Even when epidemiological data can answer these questions, we will still face policy issues of how to combine the evidence on risks and benefits of qualitatively different types. For example, how do we balance higher levels of musculoskeletal injury with lower levels of cardiac death? How are the psychological benefits of exercise to be taken into account? And how are the costs of the exercise itself to be factored into the calculation?

The techniques of cost-benefit and cost-effectiveness analysis appear most suited to weigh the various advantages and disadvantages. Costs should include the personal and social costs of the exercise activity itself, the health care costs of treating resultant morbidity, and the indirect costs such as lost productivity at work. Benefits should include reductions in future health care costs and gains in quality-adjusted life years. Another relevant quantity is the individual's willingness to pay the costs to receive the health benefits. Also, it is of interest to consider the personal utility of various states of health; for some persons, increased musculo-skeletal morbidity may be acceptable to reduce cardiac mortality, but for others a low- or non-exercising state may be preferred. Each of these areas presents significant problems of definition and measurement but all are essential ingredients to a meaningful, integrated approach to the problem.

Finally, we must not consider the health effects of exercise in isolation from other risk factors. For example, initiation of exercise by an individual will likely be correlated with other lifestyle changes, such as cessation of smoking or dietary changes. These additional factors must be taken into account when the effects of exercise are assessed.

Many challenges remain in elucidating these etiologic and policy questions. Sound epidemiological methods will be an important component in addressing them. Private decision making and public policy on exercise will depend on an integrated assessment of all the health risks and benefits and their associated costs, and of implications for personal utility. Cost-benefit and cost-utility methods will be useful in this regard.

Acknowledgments

I am grateful to my colleague Prof. Roberta Labelle for helpful discussions concerning the health economics aspects of exercise. Partial support of this work was through a National Health Scientist Award to Dr. Walter from the National Health research and Development Program.

References

1. Blair, S.N., H.W. Kohl, and N.N. Goodyear. Rates and risks for running and exercise in-juries: Studies in three populations. *Res. Q. Exerc. Sport* 58: 221-228, 1987.

2. Heady, J.A., J.N. Morris, A. Kagan, and P. Raffle. Coronary heart disease in London busmen: A progress report with special reference to physique. *Br. J. Prev. Soc. Med.* 15: 143-153, 1961.

3. Lane, N.E., D.A. Bloch, P.D. Wood, and J.F. Fries. Aging, long distance running, and the development of musculoskeletal disability. *Am. J. Med.* 82: 772-780, 1987.

4. Morris, J.N., J.A. Heady, P. Raffle, C.G. Roberts, and J.W. Parks. Coronary heart disease and physical activity of work. *Lancet* ii: 1053-1057, 1111-1120, 1953.

5. Morris, J.N., A. Kagan, D. Pattison, C. Gardner, and M.J. Raffle. Incidence and prediction of ischemic heart disease in London busmen. *Lancet* ii: 553-559, 1966.

6. Panush, R.S., C. Schmidt, J.R. Caldwell, N.L. Edwards, S. Longley, R. Yonker, E. Webster, J. Nauman, J. Stork, and H. Pettersson. Is running associated with degenerative joint disease? *JAMA* 255(9): 1152-1154, 1986.

7. Pekkanen, J., A. Nissinen, B. Marti, and J. Tuomilehto. Reduction of premature mortality by high physical activity: A 20-year follow-up of middle-aged Finnish men. *Lancet* i: 1473-1477, 1987.

8. Powell, K.E., P.D. Thompson, C.J. Caspersen, and J.S. Kendrick. Physical activity and the incidence of coronary heart disease. *Annu. Rev. Public Health* 8: 253-287, 1987.

9. Siscovick, D.S., N.S. Weiss, R.H. Fletcher, and T. Lasky. The incidence of primary cardiac arrest during vigorous exercise. *N. Engl. J. Med.* 311: 874-877, 1984.

10. Statistics Canada. *Recreational activities*. (Publication No. 87-501). Ottawa, Govt. of Canada: 1978.

11. Sutton J.R., and O. Bar-Or. Thermal illness in fun running. *Am. Heart J.* 100: 778-781, 1980.

12. Guru of jogging promoted value of physical fitness. *Toronto Globe and Mail*, July 23, 1984.

13. Vuori, I. The cardiovascular risks of physical activity. *Acta Med. Scand. Suppl.* 711: 205-214, 1984.

14. Walter, S.D., J.R. Sutton, J.M. McIntosh, and C. Connolly. The etiology of sport injuries: A review of methodologies. *Sports Med.* 2: 47-58, 1985.

15. Walter, S.D., L.E. Hart, J.R. Sutton, J.M. McIntosh, and M. Gauld. Training habits and

injury experience in distance runners: Age and sex-related factors. *Phys. Sports Med.* 16: 101-113, 1988